jtraill@mtsinai.on.ca

LVEDP	left ventricular end-diastolic pressure
LVEDV	left ventricular end-diastolic volume
m^2	meters squared
μm	micrometers
MABP	mean arterial blood pressure
MalvP	mean alveolar pressure
MAP	mean arterial pressure
MAS	meconium aspiration syndrome
mcg	micrograms
MDI	meter dose inhaler
mEq/L	milliequivalents/liter
MEP	maximum expiratory pressure
MetHb	methemoglobin
mg	milligram
mg%	milligram percent
mg/dl	milligrams per deciliter
MI-E	mechanical insufflation-exsufflation
MIF	maximum inspiratory force
min	minute
MIP	maximum inspiratory pressure
mL	millimeter(s)
MLT	minimum leak technique
mm	millimeters
mm Hg	millimeters of mercury
mmol	millimole
MMV	mandatory minute ventilation
Mo	month
MOV	minimum occluding volume
ms	millisecond
MVV	maximum voluntary ventilation
NaBr	sodium bromide
NaCl	sodium chloride
NEEP	negative end-expiratory pressure
NICU	neonatal intensive care unit
NIF	negative inspiratory force (also see MIP and MIF)
NIH	National Institutes of Health
NIPPV	noninvasive positive pressure ventilation
nM	nanomole
nM/L	nanomole/liter
nm	nanometers
NO	nitric oxide
N_2O	nitrous oxide
NPO	nothing by mouth
NP	nasopharyngeal
NPV	negative pressure ventilation
O_2	oxygen
O_2Hb	oxygenated hemoglobin
OH^-	hydroxide ions
OHDC	oxyhemoglobin dissociation curve
P	pressure
ΔP	change in pressure
P_{50}	PO_2 at which 50% saturation of hemoglobin occurs
P_{100}	Pressure on inspiration measured at 100 milliseconds
P_A	alveolar pressure
P_a	arterial pressure
PA	pulmonary artery
$P(A\text{-}a)O_2$	alveolar-to-arterial partial pressure of oxygen
P_ACO_2	partial pressure of carbon dioxide in the alveoli
P_aCO_2	partial pressure of carbon dioxide in the arteries
Palv	alveolar pressure
P_AO_2	partial pressure of oxygen in the alveoli
P_aO_2	partial pressure of oxygen in the arteries
PaO_2/F_IO_2	ratio of arterial PO_2 to F_IO_2
PaO_2/P_AO_2	ratio of arterial PO_2 to alveolar PO_2
PAP	pulmonary artery pressure
$\overline{PAP}$	mean pulmonary artery pressure
$P(a\text{-}et)CO_2$	Arterial-to-end [illegible] ide also, a-et PCO_2
PAGE	perfluorocarbon associated gas exchange
PAug	pressure augmentation
PAV	proportional assist ventilation
P_{aw}	airway pressure
$\bar{P}aw$	mean airway pressure
P_{awo}	airway opening pressure
PB	barometric pressure
P_{bs}	pressure at the body's surface
PCEF	peak cough expiratory flow
PCIRV	pressure control inverse ratio ventilation
PCO_2	partial pressure of carbon dioxide
PCV	pressure control ventilation
PCWP	pulmonary capillary wedge pressure
$PCWP_{tm}$	transmural pulmonary capillary wedge pressure
PDA	patent ductus arteriosus
PEA	pulseless electrical activity
$P_{\bar{E}}CO_2$	partial pressure of mixed expired carbon dioxide
PEEP	positive end expiratory pressure
$PEEP_E$	extrinsic PEEP (set-PEEP)
$PEEP_I$	intrinsic PEEP (auto-PEEP)
$PEEP_{total}$	total PEEP (the sum of intrinsic and extrinsic PEEP)
PEFR	peak expiratory flow rate
P_{es}	esophageal pressure
$P_{ET}CO_2$	partial pressure of end-tidal carbon dioxide; also $PetCO_2$
P_{FLEX}	pressure at the inflection point of a pressure/volume curve
P_{GA}	gastric pressure
P_{high}	high pressure during APRV
PHY	permissive hypercapnia
PIE	pulmonary interstitial edema
PIF	pulmonary interstitial fibrosis
P_{Imax}	maximum inspiratory pressure; also MIP, MIF, NIF
P_{inside}	inside pressure
$P_{intrapleural}$	intrapleural pressure; also P_{pl}
P_IO_2	partial pressure of inspired oxygen
PIP	peak inspiratory pressure; also P_{peak}
P_L	transpulmonary pressure
P_{low}	low pressure during APRV
PLV	partial liquid ventilation
P_M	mouth pressure
P*mus*	muscle pressure
PO_2	partial pressure of oxygen
$P_{outside}$	pressure outside
P_{Peak}	peak inspiratory pressure; also PIP
PPHS	persistent pulmonary hypertension in the newborn
P_{pl}	intrapleural pressure
$P_{plateau}$	plateau pressure
ppm	parts per million
PPST	premature pressure-support termination
PPV	positive pressure ventilation
PRA	plasma renin activity
PRVC	pressure regulated volume control
PS	pressure support
Pset	set pressure
PSmax	maximum pressure support
PSV	pressure support ventilation
psi	pounds per square inch
psig	pounds per square inch gauge
P_{TA}	transairway pressure
$PtcCO_2$	transcutaneous PCO_2
$PtcO_2$	transcutaneous PO_2
P_{TM}	transmural pressure
P_{TR}	transrespiratory pressure
P_{TT}	transthoracic pressure; also P_w
PV	pressure ventilation

PVCs premature ventilation contractions
$P_{\bar{v}}O_2$ partial pressure of oxygen in mixed venous blood
PVR pulmonary vascular resistance
PVS partial ventilatory support
P_w transthoracic pressure; also P_{TT}
Q2H every two hours
$\dot{Q}_T$ cardiac output
$\dot{Q}_S/\dot{Q}_T$ shunt
R respiratory exchange ratio
RAM random access memory
RAP right atrial pressure
Raw airway resistance
RCP respiratory care practitioner
RDS respiratory distress syndrome
Re Reynold's number
R_E expiratory resistance
REE resting energy expenditure
R_I inspiratory resistance
ROM read only memory
RQ respiratory quotient
RT respiratory therapist
RV right ventricle
RVP right ventricular pressure
RVEDP right ventricular end-diastolic pressure
RVEDV right ventricular end-diastolic volume
SA sinoatrial
SaO_2 arterial oxygen saturation
S.I. system internationale (international system)
SIMV synchronized intermittent mandatory ventilation
Sine sinusoidal
sp. species
sPEEP spontaneous PEEP
SpO_2 oxygen saturation measured by pulse oximeter
STPD standard temperature, pressure saturated; zero degrees Celsius, 760 mm Hg, dry
SV stroke volume
SVC slow vital capacity
$S_{\bar{v}}O_2$ mixed venous oxygen saturation
SVN small volume nebulizer
SVR systemic vascular resistance
T temperature
TCT total cycle time
T_E expiratory time
TGI tracheal gas insufflation
T_I inspiratory time
TID three times a day
T_I/TCT duty cycle
T_{high} time for high pressure delivery in APRV
T_{low} time for low pressure delivery in APRV
TLV total liquid ventilation
torr measurement of pressure equivalent to mm Hg
TPTV time-triggered, pressure-limited, time-cycled ventilation
U unit
UN urinary nitrogen
V volume
$\dot{V}$ flow
$\dot{V}_A$ alveolar ventilation per minute
VA venoarterial
VAI ventilator-assisted individuals
VAPS volume assured pressure support
VC vital capacity
V_C volume lost to tubing compressibility
VCIRV volume controlled inverse ration ventilation
$\dot{V}CO_2$ carbon dioxide production per minute
V_D volume of dead space
$\dot{V}_D$ dead space ventilation per minute
V_{Dalv} alveolar dead space
V_{Danat} anatomical dead space
V_{Dmech} mechanical dead space
$\dot{V}_E$ minute ventilation
VEDV ventricular end-diastolic volume
$\dot{V}O_2$ oxygen consumption per minute
VS volume support
V_T tidal volume
V_D/V_T dead space-to-tidal volume ratio
vol% volume per 100 mL of blood
$\dot{V}/\dot{Q}$ ventilation/perfusion ratio
VV volume ventilation; also venovenous
W work
WOB work of breathing
WOBi imposed work of breathing
yr year

MOSBY'S RESPIRATORY CARE EQUIPMENT

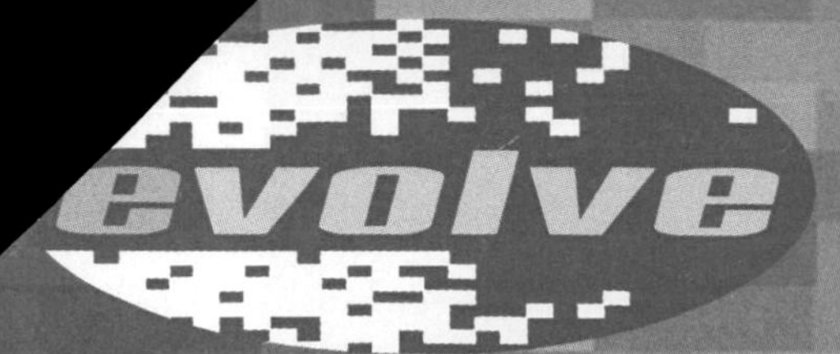

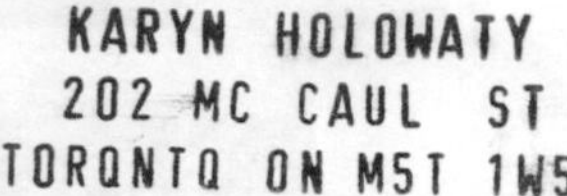

The Latest Evolution in Learning.

Evolve provides online access to free learning resources and activities designed specifically for the textbook you are using in your class. The resources will provide you with information that enhances the material covered in the book and much more.

Visit the Web address listed below to start your learning evolution today!

LOGIN: http://evolve.elsevier.com/Cairo

Evolve Online Courseware for *Mosby's Respiratory Care Equipment,* 7th edition, offers the following features:

- **Weblinks**
  Links to places of interest on the web specific to respiratory care.
- **Content Updates**
  Find out the latest information on equipment, including the newest models, and other issues in the field of respiratory care.
- **Additional Content**
  Find information about older, but not obsolete, ventilators and other equipment.
- **Frequently Asked Questions**
  Additional materials to enhance the textbook content.
- **Links to Related Products**
  See what else Elsevier Science has to offer in a specific field of interest.

Think outside the book...evolve.

Seventh Edition

MOSBY'S RESPIRATORY CARE EQUIPMENT

J.M. CAIRO, PHD, RRT
Professor of Cardiopulmonary Science and Physiology
Department Head, Cardiopulmonary Science
Assistant Dean for Educational Technology
School of Allied Health Professions
Louisiana State University Health Sciences Center
New Orleans, Louisiana

SUSAN P. PILBEAM, MS, RRT, FAARC
Respiratory Education Consultant
Staff Therapist, Flagler Hospital
St. Augustine, Florida

with 721 illustrations

Mosby

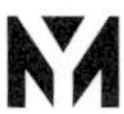

An Affiliate of Elsevier

11830 Westline Industrial Drive
St. Louis, Missouri 63146

Mosby's Respiratory Care Equipment ISBN 0-323-02215-4

Copyright © 2004, Mosby, Inc. All rights reserved.

No part of this publication may be reproduced or transmitted in any form or by any means, electronic or mechanical, including photocopying, recording, or any information storage and retrieval system, without permission in writing from the publisher. Permissions may be sought directly from Elsevier's Health Sciences Rights Department in Philadelphia, PA, USA: phone: (+1) 215 238 7869, fax: (+1) 215 238 2239, e-mail: healthpermissions@elsevier.com. You may also complete your request on-line via the Elsevier Science homepage (http://www.elsevier.com), by selecting "Customer Support" and then "Obtaining Permissions."

NOTICE

Respiratory Therapy is an ever-changing field. Standard safety precautions must be followed, but as new research and clinical experience broaden our knowledge, changes in treatment and drug therapy may become necessary or appropriate. Readers are advised to check the most current product information provided by the manufacturer of each drug to be administered to verify the recommended dose, the method and duration of administration, and contraindications. It is the responsibility of the licensed health care provider, relying on experience and knowledge of the patient, to determine dosages and the best treatment for each individual patient. Neither the publisher nor the author assumes any liability for any injury and/or damage to persons or property arising from this publication.

Previous editions copyrighted 1999, 1995, 1992, 1989, 1986, 1983.

Library of Congress Cataloging in Publication Data
Cairo, Jimmy M.
Mosby's respiratory care equipment.—7th ed./J.M. Cairo, Susan P. Pilbeam.
p.; cm.
Includes bibliographical references and index.
ISBN 0-323-02215-4
1. Respiratory therapy—Equipment and supplies. 2. Respiratory intensive care—Equipment and supplies. I. Title: Respiratory care equipment. II. Pilbeam, Susan P., 1945- III. Title.
[DNLM: 1. Respiratory Therapy—instrumentation. WF 26 C136m 2004]
RC735.I5R4728 2004
615.8'36'028—dc21 2003051369

Managing Editor: Mindy Copeland
Publishing Services Manager: Deborah L. Vogel
Design Manager: Kathi Gosche

Printed in United States of America

Last digit is the print number: 9 8 7 6 5 4 3 2 1

To Rhonda, the love of my life,
And to Robert C. Allen, MD, PhD, mentor, colleague, friend.
"La simplicité est la vérité; la symétrie est la beauté."
JMC

To my husband, Bob Wazgar, for his love and his faith in me.
"Do not conform any longer to the pattern of this world, but be transformed by the renewing of your mind."
SPP

Contributors

Charles G. Durbin, Jr., MD, FAARC
Professor of Anesthesiology and Surgery
Medical Director of Respiratory Care
University of Virginia Health System
Charlottesville, Virginia

Kevin Lord, MHS, RRT
Instructor
Department of Cardiopulmonary Science
School of Allied Health Professions
Louisiana State University
New Orleans, Louisiana

Kenneth F. Watson, MS, RRT
Respiratory Care Research Coordinator
Respiratory Care Department
Children's Hospital
Boston, Massachusetts

Dennis R. Wissing, PhD, RRT
Associate Professor and Program Coordinator
Department of Cardiopulmonary Science
School of Allied Health Professions
Louisiana State University
Shreveport, Louisiana

Reviewers

Ken Drechny, RRT, RCP
Clinical Technical Supervisor
University of Chicago–Mitchell Hospital
Chicago, Illinois

Jim Fink, MS, RRT
Administrative Director, Respiratory Sciences
Edward Hines Jr. Veteran's Administration Hospital
Hines, Illinois

Theresa Gramlich, MS, RRT
Assistant Professor
Department of Respiratory Care
University of Arkansas for Medical Sciences
Education Coordinator
Veteran's Administration Medical Center
Little Rock, Arkansas

Robert Hirnle, MS, RRT
Program Director
Highline Community College
Des Moines, Washington

Chris Kallus, MEd, RRT
Program Director
Respiratory Care Program
The Victoria College
Victoria, Texas

Sindee Kalminson Karpel, MPA, RRT
Adjunct Professor and Clinical Associate
Respiratory Therapy Technology Program
Edison Community College
Fort Myers, Florida

Joe Koss, MS, RRT
Director of Clinical Education
Respiratory Therapy Program
Indiana University
Indianapolis, Indiana

S. Gregory Marshall, PhD
Associate Professor
Department of Respiratory Care
Southwest Texas State University
San Marco, Texas

Timothy Op't Holt, EdD, RRT
Associate Professor
Cardiorespiratory Care Program
University of South Alabama
Mobile, Alabama

Fran Piedalue, RRT
Clinical Coordinator of Respiratory Care
University Hospital
University of Colorado
Denver, Colorado

Joe Ross, MS, RRT
Program Director
Respiratory Care Program
Baltimore City Community College
Baltimore, Maryland

James R. Sills, MEd, CPFT, RRT
Director, Respiratory Care Programs
Rock Valley College
Rockford, Illinois

William V. Wojciechowski, MS, RRT
Chairman and Associate Professor
Department of Cardiorespiratory Care
University of South Alabama
Mobile, Alabama

Foreword

As I sit down to work on this foreword to the 7th edition of JM Cairo and Sue Pilbeam's *Mosby's Respiratory Care Equipment*, I am at a great disadvantage! In one fell swoop, I have managed to misplace my file that contained the first draft of my comments, my favorite writing instrument (cost, $1.75), and my "writing" glasses (cost, considerably more!). How will the job get done? Where are those tools when I need them? How will I proceed without this *equipment*? Without my *equipment*, indeed, I am at loose ends.

Equipment is what this book is all about. After the more than 35 years that I have worked, taught, and written in the discipline of respiratory care, I have felt an interesting sense of déjà vu recently. While learning about the tools of the trade was still important, the evolution of the respiratory care practitioner from "technician" to "therapist" has been accompanied by a shift from emphasis on equipment to problem-based learning, therapist (patient)-driven protocols, and (believe it or not!) case management.

More mature readers of these pages will remember the old NBRC "oral examinations," which probed the candidate's knowledge of, and familiarity with various kinds of respiratory care equipment. I recall that some examiners would go so far as to alter a simple device such as a medication nebulizer, and would expect the hapless candidate to reassemble it correctly, and THEN discuss its appropriate application! The current Clinical Simulation Examination does its best to accomplish this task. The learning understanding and application of the ever-more-complex equipment has never been more important.

Readers of the 6th edition of *Mosby's Respiratory Care Equipment* will find much in the current edition that is familiar, though presented in an updated and innovative fashion. Learning objectives still appear at the beginning of each chapter, and review questions and references appear at the end. A unique feature for this edition is an online website. This website will provide an updated source of information on innovations in respiratory care equipment, such as selected adult and pediatric ventilators, as well as home care and alternative site ventilating devices. All in all, I counted at least 15 new ventilators since the 6th edition!

Another addition to this version of *Mosby's Respiratory Care Equipment* is a feature called "Clinical Rounds," which replaces the previous Decision Making and Problem Solving questions. This feature provides more clinically related questions and answers to test the reader's comprehension of the material covered in the text. Readers will appreciate an in-depth update on the myriad of new devices. A solid chapter on cardiovascular monitoring, including electrocardiography and hemodynamics, is also included. These topics have become an integral part of Respiratory Therapy curricula.

For my own part, I would like to see this valuable text become required reading for physicians in pulmonary medicine/critical care fellowships. These individuals, who care for the sickest of patients, need to have more than a passing knowledge of the capabilities, as well as the limitations, of devices in use by their respiratory care practitioner colleagues.

One more thing to note is the outstanding clarity and precision of the figures, highlighted summary boxes, and tables that appear throughout the text. In a text devoted to explaining complex operation and application of mechanical devices in a highly readable fashion, great attention to detail has been given by the authors, and it shows.

Finally, this volume does not attempt to be everything to everybody. The clinical indications for, application of, and complications from the devices described are short, but they are accurate. The task undertaken by the authors is to describe the equipment in the respiratory care practitioner's "bag of tricks," and to assure a smooth transition for application of these devices in the care of patients. In this cornucopia of information, ideas, and treatment strategies, the reader will learn the "nuts and bolts" of this honored profession, information that will be useful for the remainder of the practitioner's professional life.

By the way, I still am looking for my "writing" glasses!

George G. Burton, MD, FCCP, FAARC
Clinical Professor Medicine
Wright State University School of Medicine
Dayton, Ohio

Preface

Revising a textbook can be a formidable task. This challenge is particularly evident for authors who are confronted with a dynamic field of study like Respiratory Care. Technological innovations in health care are occurring at a pace that some might characterize as daunting. Indeed, health care practitioners spend a considerable amount of time just trying to stay abreast of the latest advances in new devices and techniques, computer-assisted technologies, pharmacologic agents, and clinical practice guidelines in their respective field.

In the seventh edition of *Mosby's Respiratory Care Equipment*, we have attempted to provide an up-to-date and comprehensive review of the devices and techniques used by respiratory therapists to treat patients with cardiopulmonary dysfunction. As you read through this edition of *Mosby's Respiratory Care Equipment*, you will see that we have tried to present this material in a concise and readable fashion. Comments that we have received from students, educators, and practitioners who read the 6th edition of this text have reinforced our belief that we should write in a style that reflects our experiences as teachers of respiratory care students. We hope that educators who have used our text in their respiratory care curricula will continue to find it useful and recognize that we have maintained this philosophy.

Throughout the text, we use pedagogical aids that we believe will assist the reader in seeing applications for the various devices and concepts in clinical practice. Chapter outline and learning objectives, along with a list of key terms, are included in each chapter. Practical scenarios commonly encountered by respiratory therapists appear in "Clinical Rounds" boxes throughout the text. Summaries of the most current AARC clinical practice guidelines, updated and expanded reference lists including computer and internet resources, and national board style review questions are also included in every chapter. Figures and tables have been updated when necessary and every effort has been made to ensure that readers are provided with high-quality photographs and illustrations that are descriptive and easy to follow. A new feature of this edition of *Mosby's Respiratory Care Equipment* is the addition of a website that is designed to provide readers with continual updates related to respiratory care equipment. The EVOLVE website includes important updates on medical devices, historical vignettes, clinical practice guideline updates, and materials that can be used to enhance educational experiences for students enrolled in respiratory care education programs.

The structure of the text is designed to follow a typical respiratory therapy curriculum. The text begins with a review of those physical principles that the reader will encounter in later chapters. Chapters 2 and 3 provide a detailed discussion of the devices and concepts that are used in medical gas therapy. Chapter 4 describes basic concepts and equipment related to the administration of aerosols and humidity therapy. Particular emphasis has been placed on providing strategies for selecting, applying, and troubleshooting these devices.

Educators who used the sixth edition of *Mosby's Respiratory Care Equipment* will notice that we moved the chapter on infection-control procedures to Chapter 5. Our decision to move this information was based on feedback from readers who felt that this material should be presented during the early phases of respiratory therapy education. As with the previous edition, we have attempted to focus on those infection-control procedures that apply to respiratory care equipment. This information includes recommendations from the Centers for Disease Control and Prevention on methods to reduce the risk of infection to both patients and respiratory care practitioners. Chapter 6 presents a clinically useful approach to airway management. It includes an extensive review of various artificial airways and related ancillary equipment, such as manual resuscitators. The indications, applications, and contraindications (including complications) associated with the use of each device are also included. Lung expansion devices, including incentive spirometers, IPPB apparatus, and chest physiotherapy devices are reviewed in a concise manner in Chapter 7.

Chapter 8 includes detailed descriptions of the devices and techniques that are commonly used by respiratory care practitioners to monitor physiologic function specifically related to pulmonary diagnostic tests. In Chapter 9 we present a summary of the theory of operation and appropriate use of electrocardiography and hemodynamic monitoring. As with Chapter 8, discussions of how physiologic measurements can be used in the care of patients are also included. Chapter 10 contains information related to blood gas analysis. Standard invasive devices and techniques are discussed along with noninvasive devices and techniques, such as pulse oximetry and transcutaneous monitoring.

The chapters on mechanical ventilators have been updated, and in the case of Chapter 11, reorganized. Chapter 11 reviews basic technical operation and physical function of ventilator components and includes coverage of such subjects as fluidics, ventilator graphics, and the basic function of high-frequency ventilators. We have maintained our philosophy of not attempting to cover management of the patient-ventilator system, which is handled in other texts. Chapter 12 reviews multipurpose ventilators that are used primarily for ICU patients. Previous generation ventilators covered in the sixth edition, such as the Bear 3, Adult Star, and Hamilton AMADEUS, will now be available on the EVOLVE site. A new section has been added to this chapter that previews newly released ventilators, such as the Dräger Savina and the Servo^{i}. Chapter 13 provides an update of mechanical ventilators that are specifically used in pediatric and neonatal care, with helpful clinical information about these devices. Chapter 14 contains information related to those ventilators that are routinely used in home care, for noninvasive ventilation and for transport of ventilator dependent patients. From any of the ventilator chapters the reader can select the unit appropriate for their school laboratory or clinical setting and review its operation with the ventilator in front of them, or by using the illustrations of the front panels provided within the text itself.

As we mentioned earlier, providing up-to-date information on current technology is one of the most important challenges of revising a text of this nature. Choosing what ventilators to include in this text is an obvious example. Readers will notice that we did not attempt to include every commercially available ventilator. Actually, it is reasonable to assume that one or more new ventilators will be introduced shortly after this book is published. This does not change the fact that it is essential for clinicians using these devices to stay informed. In an attempt to address this issue and to update practitioners of software changes that are now common to microprocessor-controlled ventilators, we will use our EVOLVE website. Readers are encouraged to check this site regularly for updates on existing and new ventilator technologies. We hope that this approach will enhance the usefulness of this text for students and practitioners.

The final chapter of *Mosby's Respiratory Care Equipment* contains a review of the equipment and procedures used in sleep diagnostics. Recent changes in the Standards for Educational Programs for Respiratory Therapy emphasize the need for this material to be included in any text related to respiratory care. For this reason, we have included a discussion of the physiology of sleep, the pathophysiologic consequences of sleep apnea, and graphic plots of EEG, respiratory flow, chest-wall motion, and oxygen saturation to illustrate these concepts.

As with the previous edition of this text, our intent in writing this book was to provide students, teachers, practicing respiratory therapists, and other members of the health care team with a text that is comprehensive, up-to-date, and easy to read. Every attempt was made to provide clinically applicable information that could help practitioners provide better patient care.

Acknowledgments

There were a number of individuals who generously contributed to this project. We wish to thank Charles Durbin, MD; Dennis Wissing, PhD, RRT; and Kevin Lord, MHS, RRT for their insightful contributions and dedication to purpose in their specialty areas. We offer our profoundest gratitude and respect to Ken Watson, MS, RRT for his extraordinary efforts on this project. His dedication to our profession is evident in the excellent chapter on infant and pediatric ventilators. We are especially grateful to Michael G. Levitzky, PhD, for his review and insightful comments related to electrocardiography and hemodynamic monitoring. We also want to recognize those individuals who graciously offered assistance during this project. They include Andy Pellett, PhD, RCVT; John Zamjahn, MHS, RRT; Espisito McClarty, AS, RRT; Kim Simmons, MHS, RRT; Yvon Dupuis, RRT; Fran Piedalue, RRT; Barbara Gair; and Demitirus Frazier.

We would like to offer a special thanks to all of the manufacturers and distributors represented in this text and for their tremendous cooperation. They include Glen and Helen Philmon, Asepsis Product Consultants, Inc; Rich Sobel, Cardiopulmonary Corporation; Geoffrey F. Lear, Jeff Fisher, Estella Baytan, Drager, Inc; Beth Keiffer, Bruce Bray, David Thompson, Tim Rossman, Hamilton Medical; Greg Martin, Les Sherman, Innovative Medical Concepts, Inc; Cyndy Miller, Janus Angus, Dwayne Sell, Lily Chang, Newport Medical; Angela King, Mark Barch, Barb Rogers, Michelle Reilly, Dan Morell, Randy Reed, David Fowler, Geri Robinson, Pulmonetics; Dave Hyde, Barbara Sullivan, Bud Reeves, Tammy Billings, Puritan Bennett, a division of Tyco Medical; Barry Feldman, Steve Birch, Wayne Johnson, Sandra Binder, Respironics; Michael Schultz, Sechrist; Sara Corocoran, Mike MacGregor, Michael Beebie, Siemens Servo; Christine Reilly, Greg Oliver, Roger Renaud, Rebecca Mabry, Viasys Healthcare, Critical Care Division. We want to also thank all of the clinical specialists we consulted for their support of this endeavor and the profession of Respiratory Care.

We want to express our appreciation to Elsevier Publishing Company for providing an editorial group that can only be described as outstanding. We sincerely appreciate the dedication of Mindy Copeland, Karen Fabiano, and Shelly Dixon to this project. Their suggestions helped us to improve the organization and readability of this text. We offer special thanks to Ann Rogers, whose kind and gentle manner guided us through the final manuscript preparation and made it an enjoyable process.

We wish to thank George G. Burton, MD, for writing the foreword to this edition. Dr. Burton's contributions to the profession of Respiratory Care are well recognized and we are grateful for his willingness to participate in this project.

Finally, we would like the reader to know that our work on this project continues to be a rewarding experience. Our feelings can best be summarized in the words of A.G. Sertillanges, "The reward of a work is to have produced it; the reward of effort is to have grown by it."

Jim Cairo
New Orleans, Louisiana

Sue Pilbeam
St. Augustine, Florida

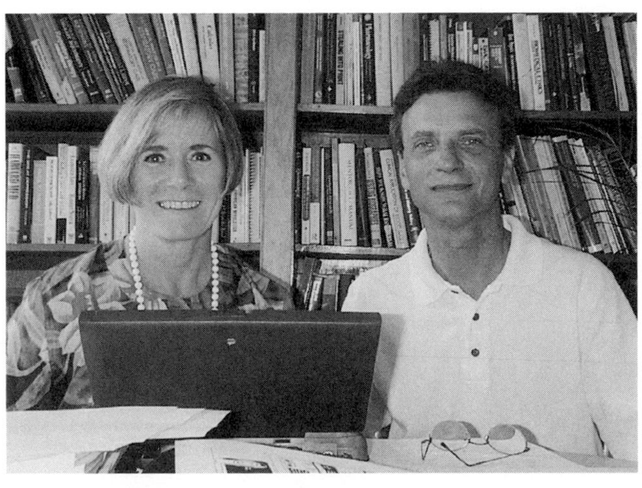

Contents in Brief

Detailed Contents

5

PRINCIPLES OF INFECTION CONTROL, 130

J.M. Cairo

6

AIRWAY MANAGEMENT, 152

Charles G. Durbin, Jr.

7

LUNG EXPANSION DEVICES, 189

J.M. Cairo

8

ASSESSMENT OF PULMONARY FUNCTION, 215

J.M. Cairo

9

CARDIOVASCULAR DIAGNOSTIC TESTING, 254

J.M. Cairo

14

Transport, Home-Care, and Alternative Ventilatory Devices, 727

Kevin Lord
Susan P. Pilbeam

15

Sleep Diagnostics, 790

J.M. Cairo

American Association for Respiratory Care Clinical Practice Guideline Excerpts

Chapter 1

Basic Physics for the Respiratory Therapist

J.M. Cairo

Chapter Outline

Chapter Learning Objectives

Upon completion of this chapter, the reader should be able to:

1. Differentiate between kinetic and potential energy.
2. Compare the physical and chemical properties of the three primary states of matter.
3. Explain why large amounts of energy are required to accomplish the changes associated with solid-liquid and liquid-gas phase transitions.
4. Convert temperature measurements from the Kelvin, Celsius, and Fahrenheit temperature scales.
5. Define pressure and describe two devices that are commonly used to measure it.
6. List various pressure equivalents for 1 atmosphere (atm).
7. Calculate the density and specific gravity of liquids and gases.
8. Explain how changes in pressure, volume, temperature, and mass affect the behavior of an ideal gas.
9. Calculate the partial pressure of oxygen in a room air sample of gas obtained at 1 atm.
10. List the physical variables that influence the flow of a gas through a tube.
11. Explain how the pressure, velocity, and flow of a gas change as it moves from part of a tube with a large radius to another part with a small radius.
12. Describe the Venturi and Coanda effects and how both can be used in the design of respiratory care equipment.
13. State Ohm's law and relate how changes in voltage and resistance affect current flow in a direct-current series circuit.
14. Describe three strategies that can be used to protect patients from electrical hazards.

Key Terms

Absolute Humidity
Acoustics
Adhesive Forces
Ammeter
Amorphous Solids
Ampere
Archimedes's Principle
Atomic Theory
Atoms
Avogadro's Number
Boiling Point
Boltzmann's Universal Gas Constant
Chemical Potential Energy
Cohesive Forces
Compounds
Condensation
Critical Pressure
Critical Temperature
Diffusion
Dipole-Dipole Interactions
Elastic Potential Energy
Electricity and Magnetism
Electromotive Force
Elements
Evaporation
Fahrenheit
Fluids
Freezing Point
Gravitational Potential Energy
Horsepower
Hydrogen Bonding
Hydrometer
Insulators
Joules
Kelvin
Kilowatt
Kinetic Energy
Latent Heat
Macroshock
Mechanics
Melting Point
Microshock
Molecules
Mixtures
Newtons
Ohm
Optics
Potential Energy
Power
Relative Humidity
Resistors
Sublimation
Supercooled Liquids
Système International
Thermistor
Thermodynamics
Thermometers (Electrical and Nonelectrical)
Van der Waals Forces
Vaporization
Vapor Pressure
Vapors
Volt
Voltmeter
Watt
Wheatstone Bridge

Physics is the most fundamental and all-inclusive of all the sciences, and has had a profound effect on all scientific development. In fact, physics is the present-day equivalent of what used to be called natural philosophy, from which most of our modern sciences arose. Students of many fields find themselves studying physics because of the basic role it plays in all phenomena.

Richard P. Feynman
Six Easy Pieces[1]

Physics is the branch of science that deals with the interactions of matter and energy. Classical physics comprises the fields of **mechanics, optics, acoustics, electricity and magnetism,** and **thermodynamics**. The laws of classical physics describe the behavior of matter and energy under ordinary, everyday conditions. Modern physics, which began at the end of the nineteenth century, seeks to explain the interactions of matter and energy under extraordinary conditions, such as in extreme temperatures or when moving near the speed of light. Modern physics is also concerned with the interactions of matter and energy on a very small scale (i.e., nuclear and elementary particle physics). It is noteworthy that, at the subatomic level, the laws of classical physics governing space, time, matter, and energy are no longer valid.

Knowing the principles of classical physics is fundamental to having a clear understanding of how various types of respiratory care equipment operate. Indeed, this chapter began with a quote from Nobel laureate Richard Feynman to underscore the idea that physics is not only part of the foundation of respiratory care but also serves the same function in all of the clinical sciences.

This chapter presents a review of classical physics applicable to respiratory care equipment. It is not intended to present a compendium of physics, but rather focuses its discussion on how these physical principles are commonly encountered in respiratory care equipment. A list of several physics textbooks is included in the reference list at the end of the chapter to facilitate a more detailed study of physics.[2-4]

Energy and Matter

Energy and Work

The concepts of energy and work are closely related. In fact, energy is usually defined as the ability to do work, where work (W) equals the product of a force (F) acting on an object to move it a distance (d), or

$$W = F \times d.$$

Note that this definition is more specific than our everyday description of work. In everyday life, we say that work is anything that requires the exertion of effort. In physics, work is performed only when the effort produces a change in the position of the matter (i.e., the matter moves in the direction of the force). In the **Système International** (SI) of measurements, energy and work are expressed in **joules** (J), where 1 J equals the force of 1 **Newton** (N) acting on a 1-kilogram (kg) object to move it 1 meter (m). **Power** (P), which is a measure of the rate at which work is being performed (P = W/t), is expressed in **watts** (W), with 1 W equivalent to 1 J/second. Because the watt is a relatively small number, we rely more on the **kilowatt** (kW), which equals 1000 watts (e.g., a 2-kW motor can perform work at a rate of 2000 J/second). Another common term used for power is **horsepower** (hp). Approximately, 1 hp equals 746 W of power, or 0.746 kW.

The energy required to perform work can exist in various forms, including mechanical energy, thermal energy, chemical energy, sound energy, nuclear energy, and electrical energy. According to the law of conservation of energy, energy cannot be created or destroyed but can only be transferred. For example, a fossil fuel such as coal, which is a form of chemical energy, can be converted to electrical energy, which, in turn, can provide the power to operate a fan or compressor. Therefore, we can think of work as the transfer of energy by mechanical means. As such, mechanical energy is usually divided into two categories: **kinetic energy** and **potential energy**.

Kinetic and Potential Energy

Kinetic energy is the energy that an object possesses when it is in motion; potential energy is stored energy, or the energy that an object possesses because of its position. The kinetic energy (KE) of an object can be quantified with the formula:

$$KE = 1/2(mv^2),$$

where m is the mass of the object and v is the velocity at which it is traveling. Intuitively, one might guess that the greater the mass, the greater the kinetic energy. It is not necessarily obvious that the kinetic energy of the substance increases to a greater extent with similar increases in the velocity at which the object is traveling. In fact, when looking at the formula, one can see that the kinetic energy increases exponentially when velocity increases. That is, kinetic energy is proportional to the square of the velocity at which the object is moving (e.g., a twofold increase in mass increases the kinetic energy twofold, and a twofold increase in velocity results in a fourfold increase in the kinetic energy).

One can think of potential energy as the energy that an object has by virtue of its position. For example, a weight raised above your head has the potential to exert a force when it falls. The energy that the weight gains as it falls is the result of gravity. (In this example, however, potential energy is more correctly referred to as **gravitational potential energy.**) The amount of potential energy (PE) that an object possesses can be calculated as:

$$PE = mgh,$$

where m is the mass of the object, g is the force of gravity (32 feet/sec^2), and h is the height that the object is raised. Potential energy can also be stored in a compressed spring or a chemical bond. With a spring, energy is required for compression. This elastic PE is then converted into kinetic energy when the spring is allowed to uncoil. Petroleum reserves of coal, oil, and gas, which represent chemical PE stores, can be converted to KE when chemical bonds are broken to provide the power required to operate lights, automobiles, and other devices we use in our daily lives.

States of Matter

Matter is generally defined as anything that has mass and occupies space. The **atomic theory** states that all matter is composed of tiny particles called atoms. Although it can appear in various forms, all matter is made up of only about 100 different types of atoms called elements.[5,6] These elements can combine in fixed proportions to form molecules, which, in turn, can form compounds and mixtures.

All matter can exist in three distinct states: solid, liquid, and gas. The physical properties of each of these states can be explained by the kinetic theory, which states that the atoms and molecules that make up matter are in constant motion. Figure 1-1 is a schematic illustrating the three states of matter. Solids are usually characterized as either crystalline or amorphous. Notice that crystalline solids are highly organized structures whose atoms and molecules are arranged in a lattice. Amorphous solids, such as glass or margarine, have constituent particles that are less rigidly arranged. Amorphous solids are sometimes called supercooled liquids because of this random arrangement.

Of the three states of matter, solids possess the least amount of kinetic energy. Most of their internal energy is PE that is contained in the intermolecular forces holding the individual particles of solids together. In solids, these forces are strong enough to limit the motion of the atoms and molecules to what appear to be vibrations or oscillations about a fixed point. Because of these features, solids are characterized as incompressible substances that can maintain their volume and shape.

Liquids possess attractive forces as do solids, but the cohesive forces in liquids are not as strong. Liquid molecules have greater freedom of movement and possess more kinetic energy than those of solids. It is difficult to illustrate exactly how liquid particles move, but one can envision that these particles can slide past each other, thus giving liquids fluidity, or the ability to flow. Although the intermolecular forces holding liquids together are relatively weak when compared with solids, these forces lend enough cohesiveness to liquid molecules to allow them to maintain their volumes. Liquids are essentially incompressible—that is, a liquid can be made to occupy a smaller volume only if an incredible amount of force is exerted upon it.

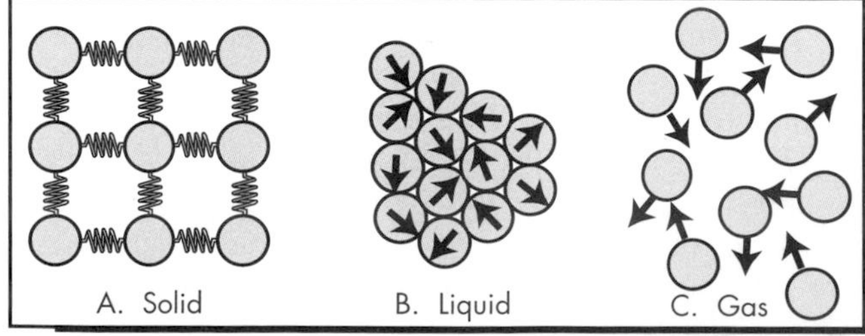

Figure 1-1 Simplified models illustrating the three states of matter: **A,** solid; **B,** liquid; **C,** gas.

Box 1-1 Substances Existing as Gases at Room Temperature and 1 atm

Oxygen
Nitrogen
Helium
Hydrogen
Chlorine
Nitrogen dioxide

Gases have extremely weak—if any—cohesive forces between their constituent particles. Therefore, gases possess the greatest amount of KE of the three states of matter, though their PE is minimal compared with the other two states of matter. The motion of the atoms and molecules that make up gases is random. Gases do not maintain their shapes and volumes but expand to fill the available space. Gases are similar to liquids in that the particles composing them can move freely, thus giving gases the ability to flow. For this reason, gases and liquids are described as fluids.

Box 1-1 lists some of the more common substances that normally exist as gases at room temperature. Most of the gases encountered in everyday life (i.e., nitrogen, oxygen, carbon dioxide, and carbon monoxide) are colorless and odorless; however, a notable exception is nitrogen dioxide (NO_2), which is an atmospheric pollutant that is dark brown and has a pungent odor. The properties of individual medical gases are discussed in Chapter 2.

Change of State

It should be apparent from the discussion so far that the physical state of any substance is determined from the relation of its kinetic energy content and the potential energy stored in its intermolecular bonds. Changes of state involve the interconversion of solids, liquids, and gases, which can be accomplished by altering the relationship between the KE and PE of a substance, such as by changing its temperature (i.e., by adding or removing heat). Consider the example of converting the solid form of water, ice, to liquid and then to steam. Adding heat to ice increases the kinetic activity (i.e., vibration of the water molecules) in ice, thus melting or weakening the intermolecular attractive forces and producing liquid water. (Freezing, which is the opposite of melting, can be accomplished by transferring

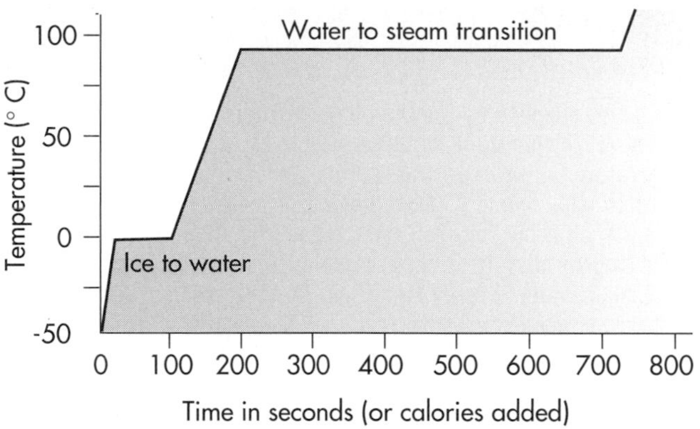

Figure 1-2 Energy-temperature relationship for the conversion of solid ice to liquid water to steam. Energy is added at a rate of 1 cal/sec. (Redrawn from Nave CR, Nave BC: *Physics for the health sciences*, ed 3, Philadelphia, 1985, WB Saunders.)

Table 1-1 Melting and boiling points and latent heats of fusion and vaporization of some common substances

Substance	Melting Point (°C)	Heat of Fusion (cal/g)	Boiling Point (°C)*	Heat of Vaporization (cal/g)
Water	0	80	100	540
Ammonia	-75	108	-33	327
Ethyl alcohol	-114	26	78	204
Nitrogen	-210	6.2	-196	48
Oxygen	-219	3.3	-183	51
Lead	327	5.9	1620	208
Mercury	-39	2.7	357	68

From Scanlan CL, Spearman CB, Sheldon RL: Egan's fundamentals of respiratory care, *ed 6, St Louis, 1995, Mosby.*

**At standard atmospheric pressure of 760 mm Hg.*

the KE of a substance to its surroundings, such as when a substance is exposed to cold temperatures.) Adding more heat causes the liquid water molecules to move more vigorously and escape into the gaseous state, or vaporize **(evaporation).** The temperature at which a solid converts to a liquid is a substance's **melting point.** (Note that the **freezing point** is the same temperature as the melting point, that is, the temperature at which a liquid is changed to a solid state.) The temperature at which a liquid converts to a gaseous state is its **boiling point.**

Figure 1-2 shows the phase changes associated with the conversion of 1 gram (g) of ice to steam.[7] As heat is added, ice begins to change to liquid at a temperature of 0° C. Note that although the addition of heat effects a change in state, the temperature of the water does not change immediately (i.e., there is a plateau in temperature). The temperature will change only after all of the ice is converted to liquid. The amount of heat that must be added to a substance to cause a complete change of state is called the **latent heat** of fusion and is expressed in calories per gram. Therefore, the amount of heat that must be added to effect the change from solid to liquid is called the latent heat of melting. In the case of water, approximately 80 calories (cal)/g of ice must be added to completely liquefy ice when the temperature reaches 0° C. After the ice has been completely liquefied, the temperature will increase 1° C per second if heat continues to be added at a rate of 1 cal/sec. This same type of phenomenon occurs at the substance's boiling point when water is converted to steam. The amount of heat that must be supplied to completely change liquid to steam (i.e., vaporize water) is the latent heat of vaporization. As one can see, a considerably greater amount of heat (540 cal/g) must be added to convert water to steam when compared with the amount of heat that must be added to melt ice into water. More energy is required in the process of vaporization because intermolecular forces must be essentially removed to allow the molecules to break loose and enter into the gaseous state.[8] Table 1-1 lists the melting and boiling points, along with the latent heats of fusion and vaporization for some commonly used substances.

Sublimation

Under certain conditions, solid molecules can completely bypass the liquid state and change to gas. This process, called **sublimation,** occurs when the heat content of a substance increases to a point at which the molecules in the solid state gain enough energy to break loose and enter the gaseous state while remaining below its melting point. The conversion of solid carbon dioxide (i.e., dry ice) to gaseous carbon dioxide is the most common example of this process.

Evaporation and Condensation

The conversion of a liquid to the gaseous state has been discussed in terms of boiling (e.g., the transition from water to steam occurs at a temperature of 100° C). Although it may not be obvious, this phase transition (evaporation) begins at temperatures between 0° C and 100° C. Evaporation occurs when some of the liquid molecules gain enough kinetic energy to break through the surface of the liquid and convert to free gaseous molecules. The rate of evaporation increases with an increase in temperature, an increase in surface area, or a decrease in pressure.

Two forces must be overcome for evaporation to occur: the mass attraction of the molecules for each other (i.e., **dipole-dipole interactions, hydrogen bonding,** and **Van der Waals forces**) and the pressure of the gas above the liquid. We can enhance the process of evaporation by either increasing the kinetic energy of the liquid molecules or reducing the pressure above the liquid. Raising the temperature of a liquid increases the velocity and the force of the molecules hitting each other and moves them farther apart. This increased kinetic activity increases the force that

Box 1-2 Evaporation and Condensation

A fairly common example that can be used to illustrate concepts of evaporation and condensation relates to the water-vapor content, or humidity, of the air surrounding us. This concept is obvious to anyone who has ever spent a hot August day somewhere in the southern part of the United States, such as New Orleans. As stated in the section on evaporation, one of the main factors influencing evaporation is temperature. Increasing the temperature increases water evaporation (in New Orleans, the water is from the lakes and bayous all around the city) by increasing the molecular activity of the water and increasing the capacity of the air to hold water vapor. If the actual amount of water vapor in the air is to be measured, the water-vapor content must be determined. The amount or weight of water that can be contained (to capacity) in the air is called the absolute humidity and is expressed in grams of water vapor per cubic meter (gm/m^3) or milligrams per liter (mg/L). (The absolute humidity can be measured or it can be computed with tables supplied by the United States Weather Bureau.[8]) Note that at a temperature of 37° C (98.6° F), which is a typical temperature in New Orleans during August, air that is 100% saturated will contain 43.80 mg of water per liter of air. In most cases, the air is not fully saturated but is only 90% saturated with water vapor; that is it only contains 0.90 = 43.80 mg/L, or 39.42 mg of water in every liter of air. For this reason, the National Weather Service chooses to report relative humidity, or the ratio of actual water content to its saturated capacity, at a given temperature (in this case, the relative humidity would be 90%).

One might ask how condensation can be included in this example, but consider that nearly every afternoon between 4 and 5 PM it rains in New Orleans. The rain occurs because the air cools (the sun begins to set), and the capacity of the air to hold water decreases. This decreased capacity to hold water vapor causes condensation, and rain results.

these molecules possess as they hit the surface of the liquid, thus allowing the liquid molecules to escape more easily and frequently. **Vapor pressure** is a measure of the force that molecules exert as they hit the surface of the liquid and escape into the gaseous phase.

The concept of vapor pressure can be used to define the boiling point of a liquid in more precise terms, that is, the boiling point is the temperature at which the vapor pressure of a liquid equals the atmospheric pressure. Reducing the pressure above the liquid lowers its boiling point because the forces opposing the escape of molecules from the liquid are decreased. This concept explains why water boils at a lower temperature at high altitudes. It also explains the process of freeze-drying as a means of food preservation. In the latter procedure, a substance is placed in a vacuum, thus reducing the opposition that liquid molecules must overcome to evaporate, therefore boiling off any liquid present.

The opposite of evaporation is condensation, which is simply defined as the conversion of a substance from a gas to a liquid. In evaporation, heat energy is removed from the air surrounding a liquid and transferred to the liquid, thus cooling the air. In contrast, during condensation, heat is removed from the liquid and transferred to the surrounding air, warming it. Box 1-2 contains an example of how evaporation and condensation can affect a person's daily life.

Evaporation and condensation are essential components in respiration. Specifically, effective ventilation requires that there is a balance between the evaporation and condensation of the moisture of respired gases so that airway mucosa are not dried and irritated. Therapeutic procedures, such as administration of dry medical gases or insertion of an endotracheal tube into the patient's airway to provide mechanical ventilatory support, can severely interfere with the patient's ability to maintain this balance. The potential problems associated with bypassing the body's mechanisms for humidifying inspired gases can be minimized by ensuring that all gases delivered to the patient are adequately humidified. Devices, such as humidifiers and hygroscopic condenser filters, or artificial noses, are two examples of devices that can be used to ensure adequate humidification of inspired gases. We will revisit these concepts in our discussion of humidity and aerosol therapy (see Chapter 4).

Critical Temperature and Critical Pressure

When a liquid is placed in a closed container, the force of the molecules trying to escape from the liquid eventually equilibrate with the force or pressure of the liquid molecules that have entered into the gaseous state, and no more liquid molecules will escape. If the temperature of the liquid is raised, however, the velocity its molecules are traveling will increase, whereas the mass attraction between its constituent molecules is reduced. Raising the temperature also increases the capacity of the air above the liquid to hold liquid vapor. Thus the vapor pressure also increases with increases in temperature, necessitating a higher opposing force to equilibrate the molecule's escape from the liquid state. At its boiling point, the force of the molecules in the liquid equals the surrounding pressure, and the molecules may fail to escape. So, in essence, the boiling point is the temperature at which the force exerted by the molecule of the liquid trying to escape equals the forces opposing its escape (i.e., atmospheric pressure and mass attraction). As gas molecules are heated above the boiling point, the force (pressure) required for converting them back to a liquid also increases. Ultimately, a temperature is reached above which gaseous molecules of a substance cannot be converted back to a liquid, no matter what pressure is exerted on them. This temperature is called the **critical temperature.**[7] Therefore, the critical temperature can be thought of as the highest temperature at which a substance can exist in a liquid state. **Critical pressure** is the pressure that must be applied to the substance at its critical temperature to maintain equilibrium between the liquid and gas phases.[8] The term ***critical point*** is used to describe the critical temperature and the critical pressure of a substance. Substances that exist as liquids at

Table 1-2 Critical temperatures and pressures required for maintaining the liquid state of gases at room temperature

	Critical Temperature		*Critical Pressure*		*Approximate Pressure in Commercial Cylinder at Room Temperature*	
Gas	°C	°F	atm	psi	atm	psig
Cyclopropane	125	257	54.2	797	5.4	79
Nitrous oxide	36.5	97.7	71.8	1054	50.6	745
Carbon dioxide	31.1	87.9	73.0	1071	57.0	838

From Scanlan CL, Spearman CB, Sheldon RL: Egan's fundamentals of respiratory care, ed 6, St Louis, 1995, Mosby.

ambient conditions have critical temperatures that are greater than room temperature (i.e., 20° C to 25° C). Substances that normally exist as gases at ambient conditions have critical temperatures that are usually well below room temperature. (Table 1-2 lists critical temperatures and pressures of some commonly encountered substances.)

Two commonly encountered substances can be used to demonstrate the principles of critical temperature and critical pressure. For example, water boils at 100° C and has a critical temperature of 374° C. At temperatures below 100° C, water exists as a liquid. As its temperature is raised above 100° C, water converts to a gas, steam. Between 100° C and 374° C, steam can be converted back into liquid by applying progressively greater amounts of pressure to it. In fact, to maintain equilibrium between the liquid and gaseous states of water at 374° C, 218 atm of pressure must be applied. Furthermore, above 374° C, water can only exist as a gas—no matter how much pressure is applied. Oxygen has a boiling point of –183° C and a critical temperature of about –119° C. At temperatures below –183° C, oxygen can exist as a liquid. After its temperature is raised above –183° C, liquid oxygen becomes a gas. At temperatures between –183° C and –119° C, the gaseous oxygen can be converted back to a liquid by compression. As with water, greater amounts of pressure must be applied to cause this conversion until the critical temperature of –119° C is reached. At oxygen's critical temperature, a pressure of 49.7 atm must be applied to maintain equilibrium between the gaseous and liquid phases of oxygen. After the temperature is raised above the critical temperature, oxygen cannot be converted to a liquid no matter how much pressure is applied to it.

Application of the concepts of critical temperature and critical pressure can be seen in medical gas therapy. As discussed in Chapters 2 and 3, medical gases can be supplied in cylinders and bulk storage systems. Substances such as N_2O and carbon dioxide have critical temperatures above room temperature and thus can exist as vapors (i.e., as a mixture of liquid and gas when placed in a compressed-gas cylinder [gases and vapors will be discussed in the next section of this chapter]). Air, oxygen, and helium, on the other hand, have critical temperatures well below room temperature and exist as gases when placed under pressure in a compressed-gas cylinder. Liquid air and oxygen, which must be kept at very low temperatures (i.e., below their boiling points), are stored in specially insulated containers. When needed, the liquid oxygen or air is allowed to exceed its critical temperature and convert to gas.[8]

Gases Versus Vapors

A gas is a state of matter that is above its critical temperature. Free molecules of the same substance below its critical temperature are a vapor. Simply stated, a vapor is the gaseous form of any substance that can exist as a liquid or a solid at ordinary pressures and temperatures. For example, under conditions of 1 atm and a room temperature of 25° C, oxygen exists in the gaseous state because it is above its critical temperature (–119° C) and is therefore classified as a true gas. Water, on the other hand, is below its critical temperature (374° C) and is considered a vapor. Water vapor can be converted back to liquid or ice if sufficient pressure is applied.

Two commonly used vapors are carbon dioxide and N_2O. Both of these substances can be converted to liquid at room temperature if enough pressure is applied. In fact, both gases are supplied to hospitals in pressurized cylinders in which most of the vapor is converted to liquid. As will be discussed in Chapter 2 (Manufacture, Storage, and Transport of Medical Gases), the amount of carbon dioxide or N_2O remaining in cylinders containing substances below their critical temperature (liquids) must be determined by weighing the cylinders instead of reading the pressure level within the cylinder. Gases such as oxygen, nitrogen, and helium are examples of substances that are usually supplied in compressed-gas cylinders above their critical temperatures. In these cases, the pressure gauge gives an accurate estimate of the amount of gas remaining in the cylinder.

Physical Properties of Matter

Temperature

As already stated, temperature is a measure of the average kinetic energy of the molecules of an object,[9] but it is also a measure of the relative warmth or coolness of a substance. Recall that adding heat to a substance changes its physical properties. This phenomenon of changing physical

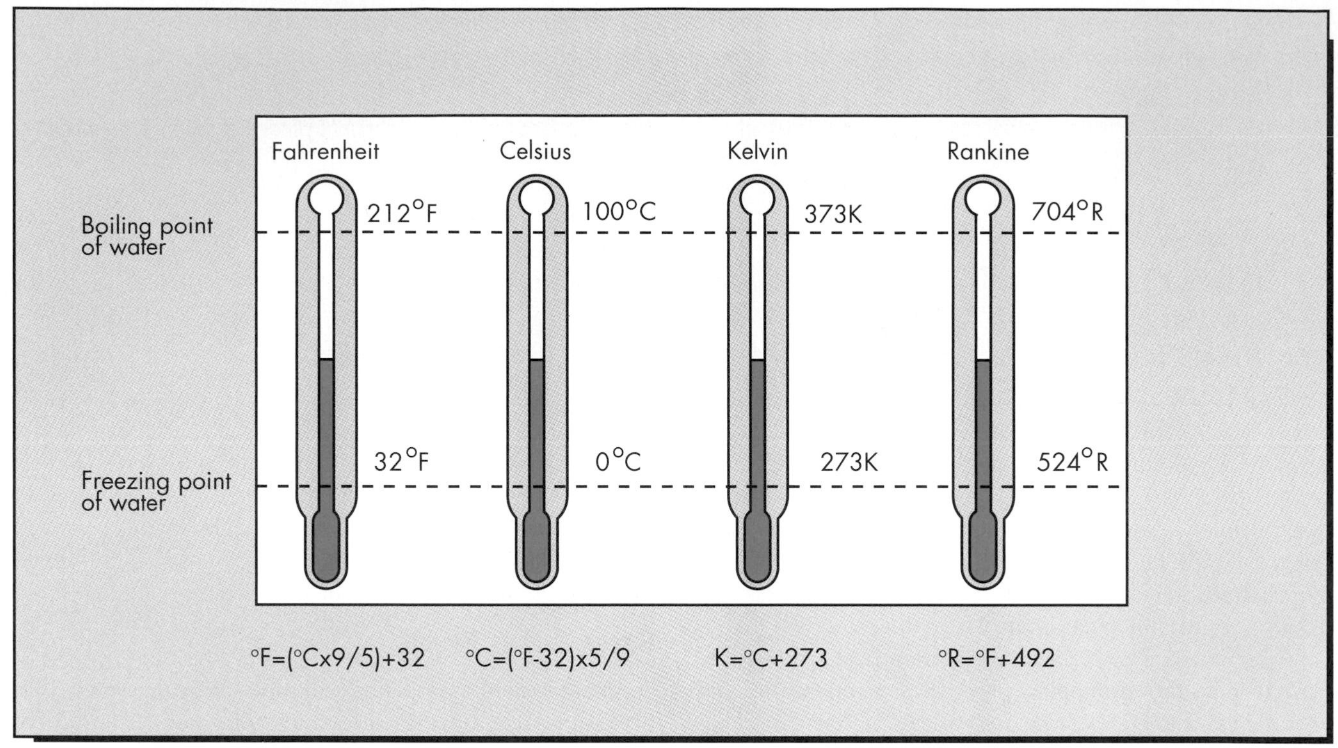

Figure 1-3 Temperature scales.

properties can be used in temperature measurements and in designing temperature scales.[10]

Thermometers are devices used to measure temperature. They are made with materials that undergo physical changes as their temperature changes. Thermometers are generally classified as nonelectrical and electrical thermometers.[10] The most commonly used nonelectrical devices are mercury and alcohol thermometers. Resistance thermometers, thermistors, and thermocouples are examples of electrical thermometers.

The mercury thermometer is probably the best-known example of a nonelectrical thermometer. This device is the product of Gabriel Daniel Fahrenheit's work on temperature measurement during the early part of the eighteenth century. Fahrenheit (1686-1736) used mercury because he found that it expands and contracts as its temperature changes. He constructed the first thermometer and ultimately the first mercury temperature scale (i.e., the Fahrenheit temperature scale).

Electrical thermometers operate on the principle that the electrical resistance of metal increases linearly with increases in temperature.[10] A typical resistance thermometer consists of a platinum wire resistor, a battery, and an ammeter for measuring current flow. Because the amount of current flowing through the platinum wire is directly related to the resistance of the wire, the ammeter can detect temperature changes by measuring the changes in current flow that occur when the resistor's temperature is changed.*

**Actually, the electrical circuit consists of multiple resistors arranged in a configuration called a Wheatstone bridge. We will limit our discussion of electrical circuits at this point because we will discuss the principles of electricity later in this chapter.*

Another common example of an electrical thermometer is the **thermistor.** It is typically a metal oxide bead, whose resistance changes as its temperature rises and falls. An ammeter connected to an electrical circuit measures temperature in a manner similar to that described for the resistance thermometer. Thermistors are incorporated into a number of medical devices, including mechanical ventilators, spirometers, capnographs, and metabolic monitors. Thermistors are also an integral part of the balloon-flotation catheters that are used with thermodilution cardiac output monitors. All of these devices will be discussed in more detail in Chapters 8 and 9 when monitoring physiologic function is considered.

Temperature Scales

A temperature scale is constructed by choosing two reference temperatures and dividing the difference between these points into a certain number of degrees. The size of the degree depends on the particular temperature scale being used. The most common reference temperatures are the melting point of ice and the boiling point of water because recognizable changes take place and thus can be given a value against which other temperatures can be measured.

Three temperature scales are routinely used in science and medicine: the absolute (**Kelvin**) scale, the **Celsius** scale, and the **Fahrenheit** scale. A fourth temperature scale, the **Rankine** scale is used in the engineering sciences.[7] Figure 1-3 shows the scalar relationships between the Kelvin, Celsius, and Fahrenheit, and Rankine scales.

The SI units for temperature are based on the Kelvin scale, with the zero point equal to 0 K or absolute zero, and the boiling point equal to 100 K. Theoretically, absolute zero is the temperature at which all molecular motion stops. Notice that the Kelvin scale is described as a centigrade scale because there are 100 divisions between the freezing and boiling points of water.

The metric or centimeter-gram-second (cgs) system is based on the Celsius scale, which can also be characterized as a centigrade scale. In the Celsius scale, the freezing point for water is designated as 0° C, whereas the boiling point of water equals 100° C. It is important to recognize that although the Celsius and Kelvin scales are both considered centigrade scales, the same temperature will have different values on each. Notice in Figure 1-3 that a temperature of 0 K (i.e., absolute zero or the temperature at which all of the kinetic activity of a substance stops) corresponds to a temperature of −273° C, and that the zero point on the Celsius scale (0° C; i.e., the freezing point of water) therefore corresponds to a temperature of 273 K on the Kelvin scale. Similarly, the boiling point of water on the Celsius scale (100° C) corresponds to a temperature of 373 K.

Box 1-3 Temperature Scales

Conversions Between the Kelvin and Celsius Scales

K = ° C + 273

° C = K - 273

Example 1

37° C equals how many Kelvin?

K = 37° C + 273

= 310 K

(Note that Kelvin is not preceded by the symbol for degrees)

Example 2

373 K equals how many degrees Celsius?

° C = 373 K - 273

= 100° C

Conversions Between the Celsius and Fahrenheit Scales

° C = 5/9 (° F - 32)

° F = (9/5 × ° C) + 32

Example 1

98.6° F equals how many degrees Celsius?

° C = 5/9 (98.6° F - 32)

= 5/9 (66.6)

= 37° C

Example 2

25° C equals how many degrees Fahrenheit?

° F = (9/5 × 25) + 32

= 45 + 32

= 77° F

The Fahrenheit scale, which is used in British or the foot-pound-second (fps) system, sets the freezing point of water at 32° F and the boiling point of water at 212° F. The Fahrenheit scale has 180 divisions between the freezing and the boiling points of water, and therefore cannot be considered a centigrade scale.

Box 1-3 contains formulae for converting temperatures between the various scales. As will be seen later in this chapter, the Kelvin scale is used when the gas and other physical laws are described; and although there is increased emphasis on using the Celsius scale in the scientific literature and clinical medicine, clinicians in the United States continue to use the Fahrenheit scale for recording patient temperatures.

Pressure

When gas molecules collide with solid or liquid surfaces, they exert a pressure. Pressure (P) is usually defined as the force that a gas exerts over a given area (P = Force/Area). Pressure measurements are reported in a variety of units, including pounds per square inch (psi, or lb/in^2), millimeters of mercury (mm Hg), torr, centimeters of water (cm H_2O), and kilopascals (kPa).[11] Box 1-4 contains formulae for converting pressure units.

Atmospheric pressure is the pressure that atmospheric gases exert on objects within the Earth's atmosphere. It exists because the gases that make up the atmosphere are attracted to the Earth's surface by gravity, thus forming a column of air around the Earth. Atmospheric pressure is highest near the Earth's surface; at sea level, atmospheric pressure equals 760 mm Hg. As you move away from the surface of the Earth, the atmospheric pressure decreases because of a reduction in the force of gravity pulling air molecules toward the Earth. For example, the atmospheric pressure in

Box 1-4 Pressure Conversions

Pressure can be measured in a variety of units, including:

- Centimeters of water (cm H_2O)
- Millimeters of mercury (mm Hg), or torr
- Pounds per square inch (lb/in^2, or psi)
- Atmospheres (atm)
- Kilopascals (kPa)

The following formulae enable conversions between these units:

- cm H_2O × 0.7355 = mm Hg (torr)
- mm Hg (torr) ÷ 0.7355 = cm H_2O
- cm H_2O × 0.098 = kPa
- kPa ÷ 0.098 = cm H_2O
- mm Hg × 0.1333 = kPa
- kPa ÷ 0.1333 = mm Hg
- mm Hg ÷ 760 = atm
- atm × 14.7 = lb/in^2 (psi)

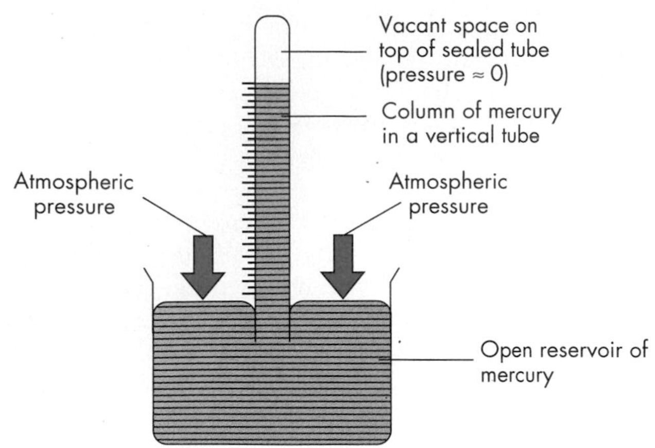

Figure 1-4 A mercury barometer. (From Eubanks DH, Bone RC: *Comprehensive respiratory care*, ed 2, St Louis, 1990, Mosby.)

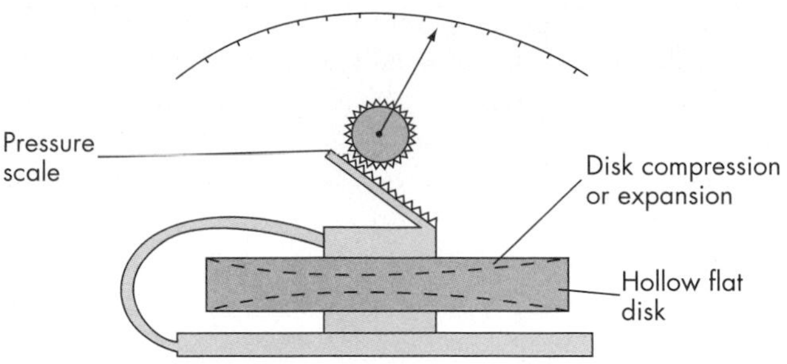

Figure 1-5 An aneroid barometer. (From Eubanks DH, Bone RC: *Comprehensive respiratory care*, ed 2, St Louis, 1990, Mosby.)

Chicago, which is located at sea level, averages around 760 mm Hg. The atmospheric pressure in Denver, which is located 1 mile above sea level, averages about 630 mm Hg.

Atmospheric pressure can be measured with a barometer similar to the one shown in Figure 1-4. The mercury barometer, which was invented by Evangelista Torricelli (c. 1608-1647), is the most commonly used device for measuring atmospheric pressure. (Torricelli was the first person to recognize the existence of atmospheric pressure; the pressure measurement *torr* is named in his honor.) The mercury barometer uses the weight of a column of mercury to equilibrate with the force of the gas molecules hitting the surface of a mercury reservoir. A column is completely filled with mercury and erected with its open end below the surface of a mercury reservoir. The mercury in the column tries to return to the reservoir as a result of gravity. The force, which gas molecules exert as they hit the surface of the reservoir, counteracts the force of gravity and pushes the mercury upward in the tube. The atmospheric pressure equals the height of the mercury column.

The aneroid barometer (Figure 1-5) measures atmospheric pressure by equilibrating the atmospheric gas pressure with a mechanical force, or the expansion force of an evacuated metal container. As atmospheric pressure increases, the pressure on the surface of the metal container tends to compress it. The change in the container's dimensions is recorded by a gearing mechanism, which changes the location of an indicator on the recording dial. Likewise, a decrease in atmospheric pressure surrounding the container allows the metal container to expand toward its normal shape.

Density

Density (d) is the measure of a substance's mass per unit volume under specific conditions of pressure and temperature, or:

$$d = \text{mass/volume.}$$

For measurements taken near the surface of the earth, mass may be replaced by a substance's weight, so that **weight density** (d_w) equals weight divided by its volume, or:

$$d_w = \text{weight/volume.}$$

As one travels away from the surface of the earth, the force of gravity diminishes, and thus the relationship between mass and weight changes (i.e., as the force of gravity decreases, so does weight, even though mass stays the same).

For solids and liquids, density can be expressed in grams per liter (g/L) or in grams per cubic centimeter (g/cm^3). The density of gases is also expressed in grams per liter. Because of the influence of pressure and temperature on the density of gases, density is calculated under standard temperature and pressure conditions. Note that standard temperature and pressure (STPD) is defined as 0° C, 760 mm Hg, and dry. The density of gases will be discussed in more detail with the discussion of Avogadro's law later in this chapter.

Buoyancy

When an object is immersed in a fluid, it appears to weigh less than it does in air. This effect, **buoyancy,** can be explained by **Archimedes's principle.**[7-9] Archimedes's principle states that when an object is submerged in a fluid, it will be buoyed up by a force equal to the weight of the fluid that is displaced by the object. The weight of the displaced liquid can be calculated as the product of the volume (V) of displaced liquid and the weight density (d_w) of the liquid:

$$F_{buoyancy} = Vd_w.$$

Consider what happens when an object is submerged in water. Water has a weight density of 1 gm/cm^3. If the weight density of the object being submerged is less than the weight density of water, the object will float. If the weight density of the submerged object is greater than that of water, the object will sink. Figure 1-6 illustrates a practical example of this concept. In this case, the weight density of a block of Styrofoam is considerably less than a block of lead. It should be apparent from this example that the Styrofoam has a weight density less than water, and floats, whereas block of lead has a weight density greater than water, and sinks.

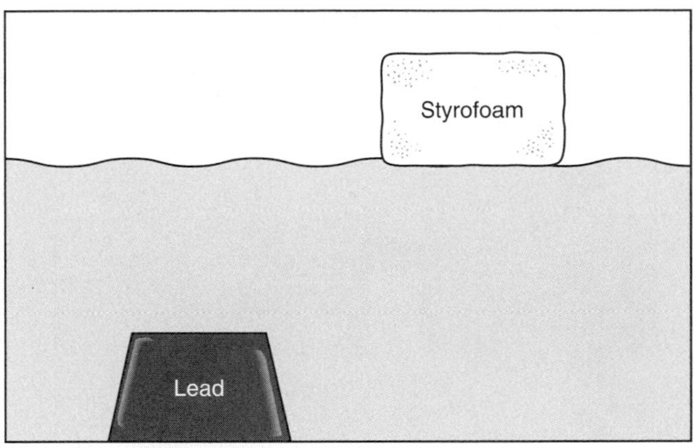

Figure 1-6 A practical example of buoyancy. Notice that a block of Styrofoam floats because its weight density is less than that of water, whereas the block of lead sinks because its weight density is greater than the weight density of water.

The measurement of the specific gravity of a liquid or a gas represents another practical application of Archimedes's principle. Specific gravity is a comparison of a substance's weight density relative to a standard. For liquids, water is used as the standard, and gases are compared with oxygen or hydrogen.[6] The device shown in Figure 1-7, a hydrometer, is used clinically to measure the weight density or specific gravity of liquids, such as urine. The density of a liquid is measured by the level at which the hydrometer floats in the liquid. Thus if the liquid is very dense, the hydrometer floats near the surface because only a small volume of liquid needs to be displaced to equal the weight of the hydrometer. Conversely, as the density of the liquid decreases, the hydrometer sinks to the bottom of the beaker containing the liquid. Notice in Figure 1-7 that the specific gravity can be read from the tube. Thus a reading of 1.025 indicates that the liquid weighs 1.025 times more than water.[8]

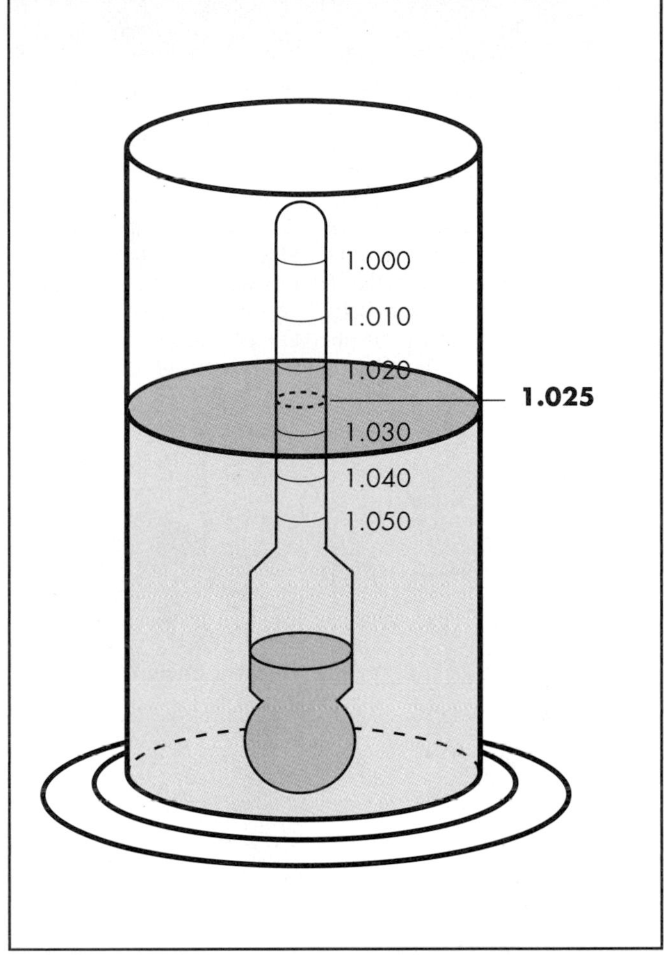

Figure 1-7 A hydrometer for measuring specific gravity. (Modified from Nave CR, Nave BC: *Physics for the health sciences*, ed 3, Philadelphia, 1985, WB Saunders.)

Viscosity

Viscosity can be defined as the force opposing deformation of a fluid. The viscosity of a fluid is dependent on its density and on the cohesive forces between its constituent molecules (i.e., as the cohesive forces of a fluid increase, so does its viscosity).

Viscosity is manifest differently in liquids and gases.[9] The viscosity of a liquid is primarily determined by the cohesive forces between its molecules, whereas the viscosity of a gas is determined by the number of collisions of the gas molecules. For example, raising the temperature of a liquid such as cooking oil weakens the cohesive forces between its molecules and decreases its viscosity. As the oil is heated and its temperature increases, it flows more freely than at a lower temperature (e.g., room temperature). Conversely, increasing the temperature of a gas increases its kinetic energy (i.e., the frequency of collisions of its constituent molecules). The greater number of collisions results in a higher internal friction, and thus an increase in viscosity.

Viscosity is an important factor to consider when describing laminar or streamlined flow. How viscosity influences fluid mechanics, specifically as it relates to Poiseuille's law, will be discussed later in this chapter.

Surface Tension

Before the phenomenon of surface tension is described, the difference between **adhesive** and **cohesive** forces should be discussed. Adhesive forces are attractive forces between two different kinds of molecules. Cohesive forces, on the other hand, are attractive forces between like kinds of molecules. The difference between these two forces can be envisioned by taking two dishes and filling one with water and the other with mercury. If a paper towel is gently submerged into each liquid, the results will be different. When the towel is placed in the water dish, it absorbs the water. This is because the attractive, adhesive forces between the molecules of the towel and the water are greater than the attractive forces of the water molecules for each other. When the towel is submerged in the mercury dish, it does not absorb the mercury because the attractive, cohesive forces between the mercury molecules are greater than the

Box 1-5 Adhesive and Cohesive Forces

The properties of adhesion and cohesion can be demonstrated by placing liquid in a small-diameter glass tube like those shown below. Notice that at the top of the column of liquid, the liquid forms a curved surface, or meniscus. In Tube *A*, which contains water, the meniscus is concave; but in Tube *B*, which contains mercury, the meniscus is convex. In Tube *A*, the meniscus is turned up because the attractive, adhesive forces between the water and the glass cause the water to adhere to the wall of the tube. In Tube *B*, the meniscus is turned down because the cohesive forces within the mercury are stronger than the adhesive forces between the mercury and the glass.

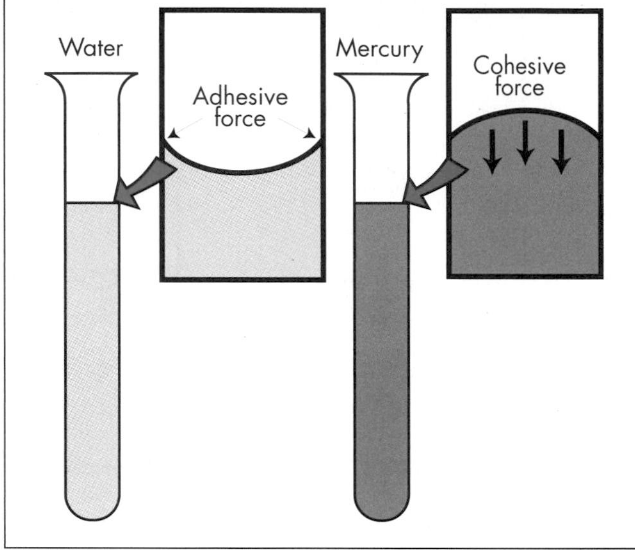

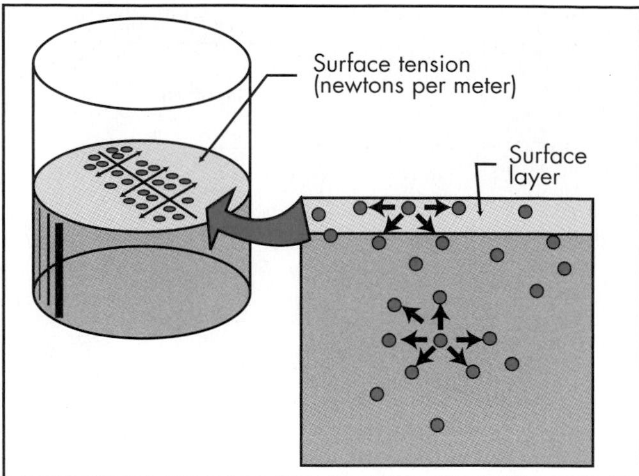

Figure 1-8 The molecular basis for surface tension. See text for explanation.

Table 1-3 Examples of surface tension

Substance	°C	Surface Tension (dynes/cm)
Water	20	73
Water	37	70
Tissue fluid	37	50
Whole blood	37	58
Plasma	37	73
Ethyl alcohol	20	22
Mercury	17	547

From Scanlan CL, Wilkins RL, Stoller JK: Egan's fundamentals of respiratory care, *ed 7, St Louis, 1999, Mosby.*

attractive forces between the molecules of the towel and the mercury. (See Box 1-5 for another application involving adhesive and cohesive forces.)

Surface tension is generated by the cohesive forces between liquid molecules at a gas-liquid interface or at the interface of two immiscible (i.e., unable to mix) liquids like oil and water. Figure 1-8 illustrates the molecular basis of surface tension at a gas-liquid interface. At some depth, the molecules within a liquid are attracted equally from all sides, whereas the molecules near the surface experience unequal attractions.[10] Notice that near the surface of the liquid, some of the forces in the liquid act in a direction that is parallel to the surface, whereas others are drawn toward the center of the liquid mass by this net force. Those forces acting parallel to the surface of the liquid cause the liquid to behave as though a film is present at the gas-liquid interface. The forces drawn toward the center of the liquid tend to reduce its exposed surface to the smallest possible area, which is usually a sphere.

We can measure the surface tension of a liquid by determining the force that must be applied to produce a "tear" in this film.[7] As such, in the SI system of measurements, surface tension is usually expressed in dynes per centimeter (dyn/cm). Table 1-3 lists surface tensions for several liquids that are commonly encountered in respiratory care. Note that the surface tension of a given liquid varies inversely with its temperature. Thus surface tension decreases as the temperature of a liquid increases.

LaPlace's Law

As just stated, surface tension forces cause a liquid to have a tendency to occupy the smallest possible area, which is usually a sphere. The pressure within a liquid sphere should be influenced both by the surface tension forces offered by the liquid and by the size of the sphere. Indeed, Pierre-Simon LaPlace (1749-1827), a French astronomer and mathematician, found that pressure within a sphere is directly related to the surface tension of the liquid and inversely related to the radius of the sphere, or:

$$P = 2(ST/r),$$

where P is the pressure within the sphere, ST is the surface tension of the liquid, and r is the radius of the sphere.

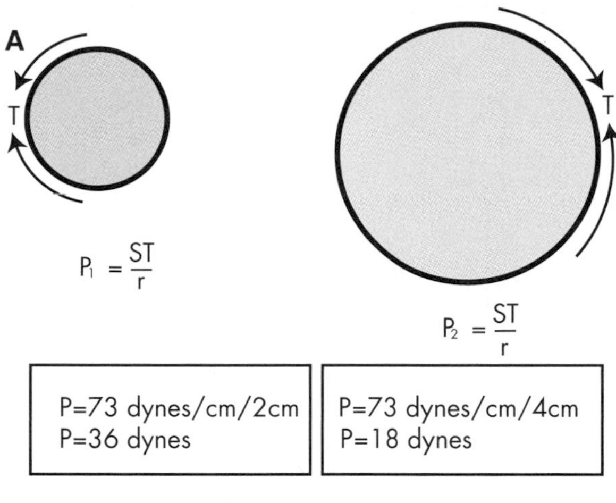

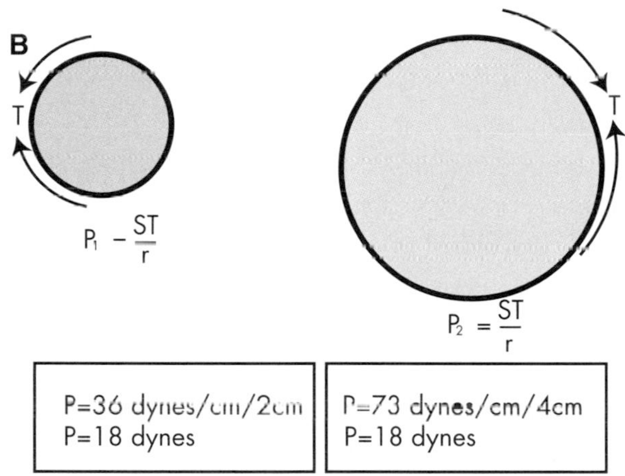

Figure 1-9 LaPlace's law. **A,** water bubble; **B,** soap bubble. See text for discussion.

The examples shown in Figure 1-9 should help to illustrate this principle. In Figure 1-9, A, two droplets of water are shown. One droplet has a radius of 2 cm and the other droplet has a radius of 4 cm. If we assume that the surface tension is equal in both droplets (i.e., the surface tension of water is 73 dyn/cm), then the pressure in the smaller droplet is twice that of the larger droplet.

Now consider what happens when the surface tension of the smaller droplet is reduced by, for example, adding a surface-active agent (i.e., soap) to the water. As shown in Figure 1-9, *B*, the surface tension of the larger water droplet remains at 73 dyn/cm, but half as much reduces the surface tension of the smaller soap bubble (36 dyn/cm). By a simple calculation, one can see that the pressures within both of the spheres are now equal.

Applications of LaPlace's law can be found in the discussion of aerosol therapy in Chapter 4. As will be seen, surface tension explains why liquid particles retain their spherical shape when suspended in an aerosol suspension.

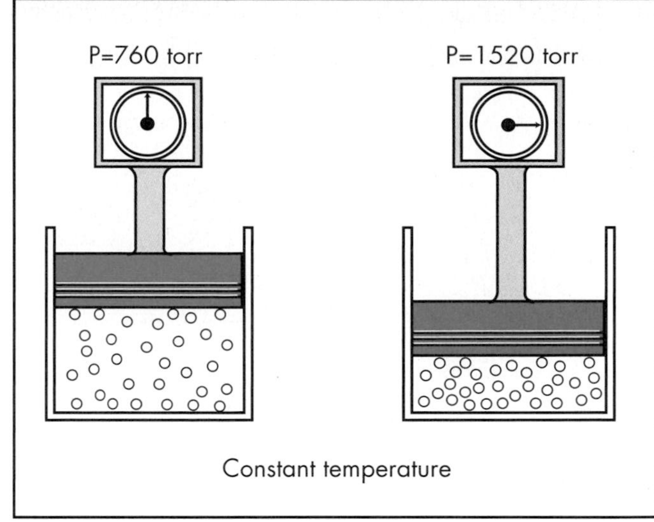

Figure 1-10 Boyle's law. (Redrawn from Levitzky MG, Cairo JM, Hall SM: *Introduction to respiratory care*, Philadelphia, 1990, WB Saunders.)

The Gas Laws

The gas laws presented in this section are important generalizations about the macroscopic behavior of gaseous substances. These laws can be seen as summaries of numerous experiments that were conducted over the course of several centuries. The importance of these laws in the development of physics and chemistry is undeniable, and their relevance to the practice of respiratory care cannot be overstated.

Boyle's Law

Robert Boyle (1627-1691), a British chemist, was the first scientist to systematically investigate the pressure-volume relationships of a gas sample. Using an apparatus like the one shown in Figure 1-10, Boyle found that the volume that a gas occupies when it is maintained at a constant temperature is inversely proportional to the absolute pressure exerted on it, or:

$$V = 1/P, \text{ or } V = k(1/P).$$

Note that the absolute pressure of a gas equals the atmospheric pressure plus the pressure measured with a gauge. For example, the pressure of a gas compressed into a 10-L tank is measured to be 29.4 psi. The absolute pressure of the gas equals the atmospheric pressure (14.7 psi) plus the gauge pressure of 29.4 psi. Thus the absolute pressure of the gas is 44.1 psi.

Boyle's law can be expressed in a more useful form:

$$V_1P_1 = V_2P_2, \text{ or } V_1/V_2 = P_2/P_1,$$

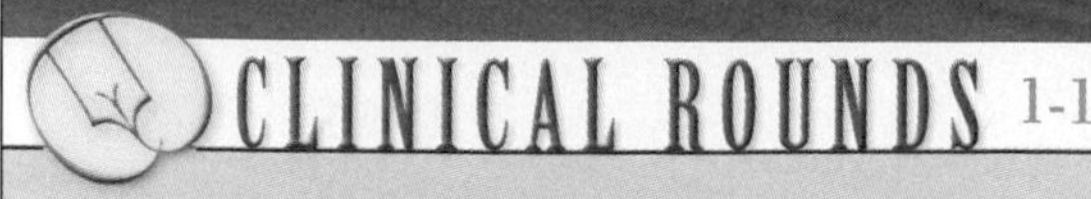

A snorkel diver is preparing to descend a freshwater pond to a depth of 66 ft. At sea level, his lungs contain about 3000 mL of air. As he descends below the surface of the water, what will happen to the gas volume in his lungs as he descends to 33 ft and then to 66 ft below the surface of the pond?

See Appendix A for the answer.

which allows an unknown volume or pressure to be calculated when the other variables are known. For example, one can solve for an unknown volume by rearranging the equation to read:

$$V_2 = V_1P_1/P_2.$$

Applications of Boyle's law can be found in a number of topics included in this text, such as the mechanics of ventilation, medical gas therapy, blood-gas measurements, and pulmonary function testing, which includes spirometry and body plethysmography (See Clinical Rounds 1-1).

Charles's and Gay-Lussac's Laws

Jacques Charles (1746-1823), a French chemist, is recognized as the first scientist to demonstrate experimentally how the volume of a gas varies with changes in temperature. He showed that the volume of a given amount of gas held at a constant pressure increases proportionately with increases in the temperature of the gas[12] (Figure 1-11). The relationship between volume and temperature can be explained by the fact that as the temperature of the gas increases, the kinetic energy of the gas molecules increases. This increased kinetic energy content causes the gas molecules to move more vigorously, so the gas expands. Conversely, as the temperature of the gas decreases, its molecular activity diminishes, so the gas volume contracts.

William Thomson (Lord Kelvin, 1824-1907) realized the significance of these findings and suggested that there should theoretically be a temperature at which all molecular activity ceases and the associated gas volume is zero. This temperature is called *absolute zero* and has been calculated to be –273.15° C. Although the absolute zero of any substance has not been achieved in a laboratory setting, this temperature serves as a starting point for the Kelvin temperature scale. As mentioned earlier, 1° C corresponds to 1 K. Also, notice that temperature is expressed without degrees in the Kelvin scale (e.g., 0 K equals –273.15° C). Using the work of Kelvin, Charles's Law is now stated as: when the pressure of a gas is held constant, the volume of a gas varies directly with its absolute temperature expressed in Kelvin, or:

$$V/T = k, \text{ or } V_1/T_1 = V_2/T_2.$$

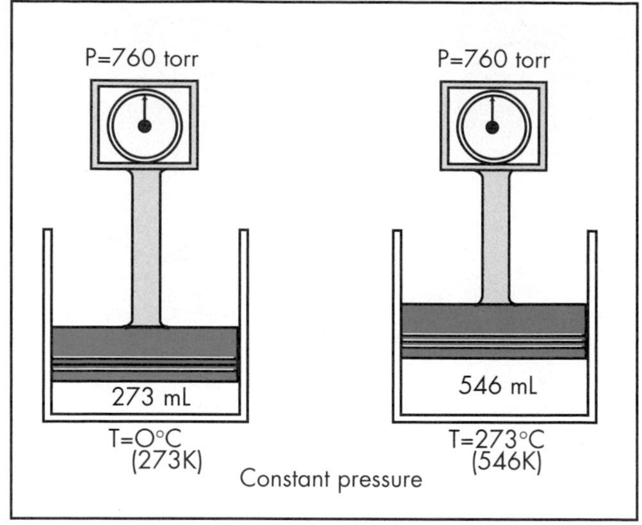

Figure 1-11 Charles's law. (Redrawn from Levitzky MG, Cairo JM, Hall SM: *Introduction to respiratory care*, Philadelphia, 1990, WB Saunders.)

Therefore, doubling the absolute temperature of a gas increases the volume of the gas twofold. Conversely, reducing the temperature of a gas by half decreases the volume of the gas by half.

Joseph Gay-Lussac (1778-1850) extended Charles's work by showing that if the volume of a gas is held constant, the gas pressure rises as the absolute temperature of the gas increases, or:

$$P/T = k, \text{ or } P_1/T_1 = P_2/T_2.$$

Figure 1-12 illustrates Gay-Lussac's law. An example of Gay-Lussac's law that might be encountered in clinical practice can be found in Clinical Rounds 1-2.

Combined Gas Law

In the discussions of the gas laws so far, it was assumed that one or more of the variables in each law were constant. For example, Boyle's law describes the relationship between pressure and volume when temperature is constant. Charles's law specifies the relationship between temperature and volume when pressure is constant; and Gay-Lussac's law describes the relationship between temperature and pressure while volume is constant.

The combined gas law describes the macroscopic behavior of gases when any or all of the variables change simultaneously. As such, the combined gas law states that the absolute pressure of a gas is inversely related to the volume it occupies and directly related to its absolute temperature, or:

$$PV/T = nR,$$

where n is the number of moles of gas (a mole is a quantity of substance with a mass equal to its molecular weight expressed in grams), and R is **Boltzmann's universal gas constant.**[3,7,8]

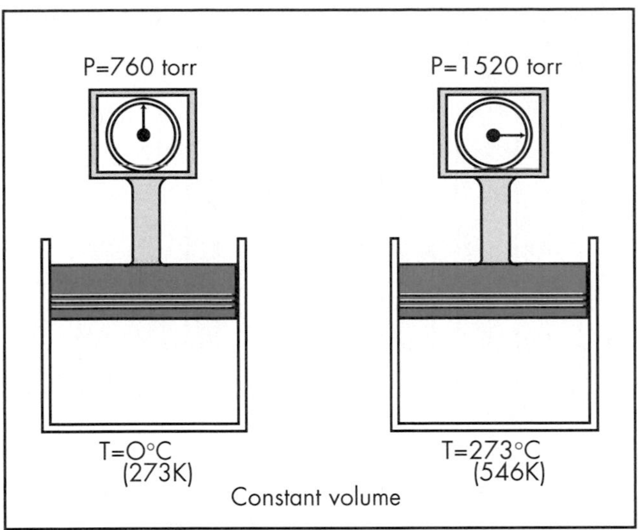

Figure 1-12 Gay-Lussac's law. (Redrawn from Levitzky MG, Cairo JM, Hall SM: *Introduction to respiratory care*, Philadelphia, 1990, WB Saunders.)

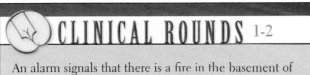

An alarm signals that there is a fire in the basement of the hospital. Although the fire is confined to an area that is approximately 300 ft from the room where the compressed-gas cylinders are stored, you are asked to move the cylinders to a safer location. Why is it necessary to move the cylinders?

See Appendix A for the answer.

A more practical expression of the combined gas law equation that is used throughout this text is:

$$P_1V_1/T_1 = P_2V_2/T_2.$$

In this form of the combined gas law, the gas constant (R) and the number of moles of gas (n) are not included because it is assumed that they will not be affected by changes in pressure, volume, and temperature. See Clinical Rounds 1-3 for an example of a calculation using this form of the combined gas law.

Applications of the combined gas law are found throughout this text. Pressure, volume, and temperature corrections are used extensively in arterial blood-gas measurements (see Chapter 10) and during pulmonary function testing (see Chapters 8 and 9).

Dalton's Law of Partial Pressures

Dalton's law states that the sum of the partial pressures of a gas mixture equals the total pressure of the system. Furthermore, the partial pressure of any gas within a gas mixture is proportional to its percentage of the mixture.[7,8] The partial pressure of a gas in a mixture can be calculated

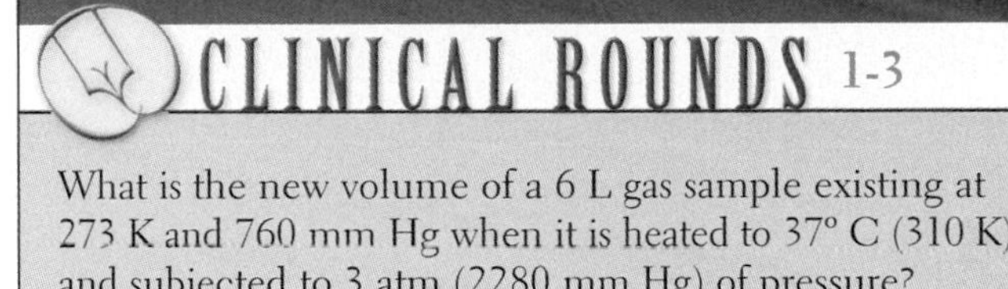

What is the new volume of a 6 L gas sample existing at 273 K and 760 mm Hg when it is heated to 37° C (310 K) and subjected to 3 atm (2280 mm Hg) of pressure?

See Appendix A for the answer.

by multiplying the total pressure of the mixture by the percentage of the mixture that the gas in question occupies. For example, the partial pressure of oxygen in room air when the barometric pressure equals 1 atm (760 mm Hg) can be calculated by multiplying the total barometric pressure by the percentage of oxygen in the room air. (Note that oxygen makes up approximately 21% of the atmosphere, or 0.21.) Thus:

$$PO_2 = (760)\ (0.21)$$
$$PO_2 = 159.6 \text{ mm Hg}$$

Continuing with this example, the total atmospheric pressure equals the sum of the partial pressures for oxygen (21%), nitrogen (78%), carbon dioxide (0.03%), and other trace gases (~0.7%), or:

$$P_B = PO_2 + PN_2 + PCO_2 + P\text{ (trace gases)}$$
$$P_B = (760)\ (0.21) + (760)\ (0.78) + (760)\ (0.0003) + (760)\ (0.07)$$
$$P_B = 760 \text{ mm Hg}$$

It should be noted that water vapor pressure does not follow Dalton's law because such pressure primarily depends on temperature. Because water vapor displaces the partial pressure of other gases, the water vapor pressure (P_{H2O}) must be subtracted from the total pressure of the gas mixture when the partial pressure of a gas saturated with water vapor is calculated. For example, to calculate the partial pressure of oxygen in a sample of gas that is saturated with water vapor at 37° C, the following formula* is applied:

$$PO_2 = (P_B - P_{H2O})\ (F_iO_2)$$
$$PO_2 = (760 \text{ mm Hg} - 47 \text{ mm Hg})\ (0.21)$$
$$PO_2 = 149.73 \text{ mm Hg}$$

Avogadro's Law

This law states that equal volumes of gas at the same pressure and temperature contain the same number of molecules. It is based on the work of Amedeo Avogadro (1776-1856), who determined that 1 gram molecular weight (gmw), or mole, of any gas occupies 22.4 L at a temperature of 0° C (273 K) and a pressure of 1 atm. Subsequently, it was determined that 1 mole of gas at this volume contains 6.02×10^{23} molecules (**Avogadro's number**). For example, 1 mole of oxygen (mw = 32g) occupies a volume of 22.4 L and contains 6.02×10^{23} molecules when measured at 0° C (273 K) and 1 atm.

**Note that the vapor pressure of water at 37° C is 47 mm Hg; Table 1-4 lists the vapor pressures for water at selected temperatures.*

Table 1-4 Water-vapor pressure and content at selected temperatures and 760 mm Hg

°C	Vapor Pressure (mm Hg)
0	4.58
10	9.21
11	9.84
12	10.52
13	11.23
14	11.99
15	12.79
16	13.63
17	14.53
18	15.48
19	16.48
20	17.54
21	18.65
22	19.83
23	21.07
24	22.38
25	23.76
26	25.21
27	26.74
28	28.35
29	30.04
30	31.82
31	33.70
32	35.66
33	37.73
34	39.90
35	42.18
36	44.56
37	47.07
38	49.70
39	52.44
40	55.32

A practical application of Avogadro's law is seen in the calculation of gas densities and specific gravity. The density of a gas per unit volume can be calculated with the following formula:

$$\text{Density (gm/L)} = \text{mw of gas}/22.4 \text{ L}.$$

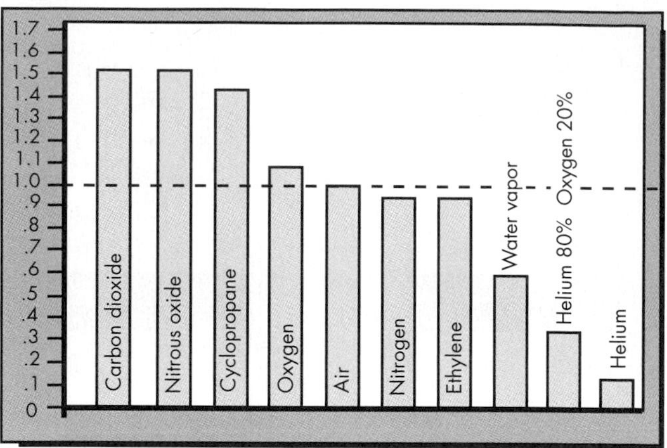

Figure 1-13 Specific gravity for several gases that are used in respiratory care and anesthetics. Comparisons have been made with air at 25° C and 1 atm. (Redrawn from Adriani J: *The chemistry and physics of anesthesia*, ed 3, Springfield, Ill, 1979, Charles C Thomas.)

The specific gravity of a gas is defined as the ratio of the density of a gas relative to the density of a standard gas, such as air, oxygen, or hydrogen. Figure 1-13 shows the specific gravity of several gases used in respiratory care and anesthetics.

Laws of Diffusion

Up to this point, the discussion of gases has focused on the ability of a gas to expand and to be compressed. Another property that must be discussed in any analysis of gas behavior is **diffusion,** which can be defined as the net movement of gas molecules, by virtue of their kinetic properties, from an area of high concentration to an area of low concentration. Graham's law, Henry's law, and Fick's law will be used to describe diffusion and its applications in respiratory care.

Graham's Law

In 1832, Thomas Graham (1805-1869) stated that when two gases are placed under the same temperature and pressure conditions, the rates of diffusion of the two gases are inversely proportional to the square root of their masses, or:

$$r_1/r_2 = \sqrt{M_1/M_2},$$

where r_1 and r_2 represent the diffusion rates of the respective gases, and M_1 and M_2 are the molar masses.

If the mass of a gas is considered directly proportional to its density at a constant temperature and pressure, then:

$$r_1/r_2 = \sqrt{d_1/d_2}$$

where d_1 and d_2 are the densities of the gases in question.

Henry's Law

When a gas is confined in a space adjacent to a liquid, a certain number of gas molecules dissolve in the liquid phase. Joseph Henry found that for a given temperature, the mass of a gas that dissolves (and does not combine chemically) in a specified volume of liquid is directly proportional to the product of the partial pressure of the gas and its solubility coefficient, or:

$$c \alpha P \times S$$

where c is the molar concentration (in mol/L) of the dissolved gas, P is the pressure (in atm) of gas over the liquid, and S is the solubility coefficient (also known as Bunsen's coefficient) for the gas in that particular liquid (in L/atm or L/mm Hg). The solubility of a gas in a liquid is equal to the volume of gas (in liters) that will saturate 1 L of liquid at standard temperature and pressure (0° C and 1 atm). In respiratory care, Henry's law is encountered in discussions of the solubility of gases, such as oxygen, in blood. In the latter case, we express the solubility of a gas in milliliters of gas dissolved in milliliters of blood. For example, it is known that 0.023 mL of oxygen dissolve in every milliliter of blood at a temperature of 38° C and 1 atm of pressure.

Fick's Law of Diffusion

Thus far, the diffusion rate of a gas into another gas and the diffusion rate of a gas into a liquid have been discussed. In respiratory care, the diffusion of gases across semipermeable membranes (e.g., the diffusion of oxygen and carbon dioxide across the alveolar-capillary membrane) is also a concern.[12,13] A semipermeable membrane is not freely permeable to all components of a mixture. Thus the membrane may be impermeable to a substance because of its size or chemical composition (e.g., electrical charge).

Adolph Fick stated that the flow of a gas across a semipermeable membrane per unit time ($\dot{V}$gas) into a membrane fluid phase is directly proportional to the surface area (A) available for diffusion, the partial pressure gradient between the two compartments (ΔP), and the solubility of the gas (S). This flow is inversely proportional to the square root of the molecular weight of the gas (√MW) and the thickness of the membrane (T) (Figure 1-14). Fick's law can be shown as:

$$\dot{V}gas = A \times S \times \Delta P/\sqrt{MW} \times T.$$

Considering that the diffusivity of a gas equals its solubility divided by the square root of its molecular weight, or

$$D = S \div \sqrt{MW},$$

where D is the diffusivity, S is the solubility, and MW is the molecular weight, then Fick's law can be restated as:

$$\dot{V}gas = A \times D \times \Delta P/T.$$

Test your understanding of the laws of diffusion by answering the question in Clinical Rounds 1-4.

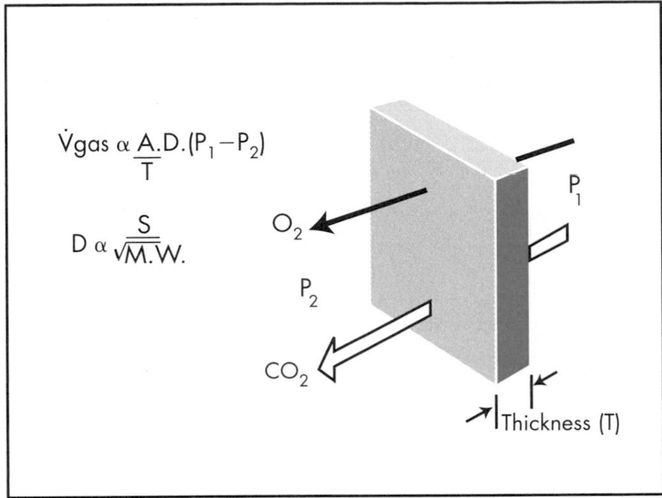

Figure 1-14 Fick's law of diffusion. (Modified from West JB: *Respiratory physiology: the essentials*, ed 3, Baltimore, 1985, Williams & Wilkins.)

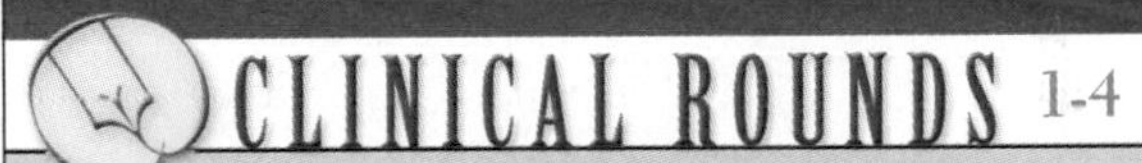

Using Fick's law of diffusion, describe several conditions during which the diffusion of oxygen across the alveolar-capillary membrane is reduced.

See Appendix A for the answer.

Fluid Mechanics

Fluid mechanics is the branch of physics dealing with the properties and behavior of fluids in motion. This field involves fluid dynamics, which is subdivided into hydrodynamics (the study of liquids in motion) and aerodynamics (the study of gases in motion). With diffusion, gas movement was described as being the result of the spontaneous intermingling of the individual gas molecules as a result of random thermal motion. In the section that follows, bulk gas flow, which deals with the transport of whole groups of molecules (i.e., a volume of gas) from one location to another rather than the movement of individual gas molecules, will be discussed.

Patterns of Flow

This text is primarily concerned with the flow of fluids through various types of tubes. Whether this flow involves the movement of liquids or gases, all fluid flow may be characterized as being laminar, turbulent, or transitional in nature. Figure 1-15 shows the three types of flow.

In laminar flow, the fluid flows in discrete cylindrical layers or streamlines.[8] Laminar flow is normally associated with the movement of fluids through tubes with smooth

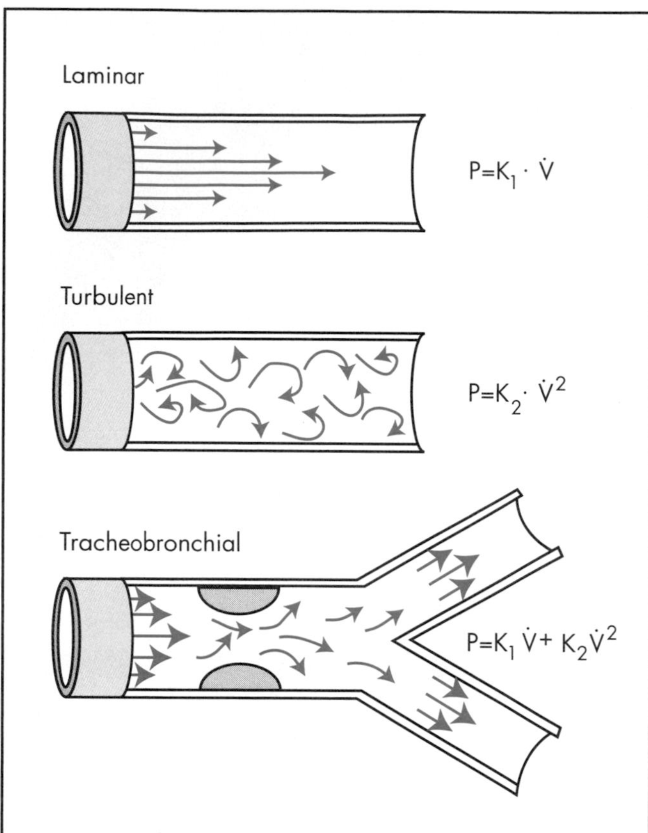

Figure 1-15 Three patterns of flow: laminar, turbulent, and transitional.

surfaces and fixed radii. With laminar flow, the pressure required to produce a given flow is directly related to the viscosity of the fluid and the length of the tube and inversely related to the radius of the tube. These relationships will be discussed in detail in the section on Poiseuille's law.

With turbulent flow, the movement of fluid molecules becomes chaotic and the orderly pattern of concentric layers seen with laminar flow is lost. As will be seen, Poiseuille's law cannot be used to predict the amount of pressure required for a given flow when turbulence is present. When turbulence is present, the pressure required to produce a given flow is influenced less by the viscosity of the fluid and more by its density. Additionally, the driving pressure required to achieve a given flow is proportional to the *square* of the flow. Turbulent flow occurs when there is a sharp increase in the velocity at which the fluid is moving, when the tube's radius varies, and when tubes have rough, uneven surfaces. The likelihood of developing turbulent flow can be predicted by Reynolds's number, which will be discussed shortly.

Transitional flow is simply a mixture of laminar and turbulent flows. In cases when laminar flow predominates, the driving pressure varies linearly with the flow. When turbulent flow dominates, the driving pressure varies with the *square* of the flow. Transitional flow typically occurs at points where tubes divide into one or more branches. Figure 1-15 illustrates the types of flow that can be observed as gas flows into the lungs. Gas flow in the larger airways is turbulent, but laminar flow predominates in the smaller airways. Transitional flow (or tracheobronchial flow, as it appears in Figure 1-15) occurs at points where the airways divide (e.g., where the mainstem bronchi divide into the lobar bronchi).

Poiseuille's Law

When considering the flow of a liquid or gas through a tube, there are two factors that must be considered: the driving pressure forcing the fluid through the tube (i.e., the pressure gradient) and the resistance that the fluid must overcome as it flows through the tube. Jean L.M. Poiseuille (1797-1869), a French physiologist, described the interrelationships between pressure, flow, and resistance for a liquid flowing through an unbranched rigid tube with the formula:

$$\Delta P = \dot{Q} \times R,$$

where ΔP is the pressure gradient from the beginning to the end of the tube ($P_1 - P_2$), $\dot{Q}$ is the flow of the liquid through the tube, and R is the resistance opposing the flow of the liquid. (Note that in discussions of the mechanics of breathing, $\dot{Q}$ is replaced with $\dot{V}$, which is used to symbolize the flow of a gas.) The pressure gradient can be described as the difference in pressure at the entrance of the tube and the exit point, or $P_1 - P_2$. Poiseuille found that the factors determining resistance to flow include the viscosity of the fluid, as well as the length and radius of the tube, or

$$R = (8\eta l)/\pi(r^4)$$

where η is the viscosity of the liquid, l is the length of the tube, and r is the radius of the tube. Incorporating these findings, Poiseuille's law can be rewritten as,

$$\Delta P = \dot{Q} \times [(8\eta l)/(\pi r^4)].$$

Based on these equations, the following can be stated:

1. The more viscous a fluid, the greater the pressure gradient required to cause it to move through a given tube.
2. The resistance offered by a tube is directly proportional to its length; the pressure required to achieve a given flow through a tube must increase in direct proportion to the length of the tube.
3. Because the resistance to flow is inversely proportional to the fourth power of the radius, small changes in the radius of a tube will cause profound decreases in the flow of the fluid through the tube. For example, decreasing the radius by one half increases the resistance sixteenfold.

Applications of Poiseuille's law are found in the discussion related to medical gas therapy, physiologic pressure monitoring, and mechanical ventilation.

Reynolds's Number

As discussed earlier, fluid flow becomes turbulent when there is a sharp increase in the velocity at which the liquid or gas molecules are traveling. Several other factors can also produce turbulent flow, including changes in the density and viscosity of the gas or in the diameter of the tube. These factors can be combined mathematically to determine Reynolds's number:

$$N_R = v \times d \times (2r/\eta),$$

where v is the velocity of flow, r is the radius of the tube, and d and η are the density and viscosity of the gas, respectively. Note that the Reynolds's number does not have units. Turbulent flow predominates when the Reynolds's number exceeds 2000, although turbulent flow may occur at lower Reynolds's numbers when the surface of the tube is rough or irregular.[8,14]

Turbulent flow is produced by an increase in the linear velocity of the gas, the density of the gas, or the radius of the tube; it can also be produced by reductions in the viscosity of the gas. Applications of Reynolds's number will be seen in the discussions of the mechanics of breathing and mechanical ventilation later in this text.

Bernoulli Principle

This principle is the result of work by Daniel Bernoulli (1700-1782), a Swiss mathematician who stated that as the forward velocity of a gas (or liquid) moving through a tube increases, the lateral wall pressure of the tube will decrease.[7,15] This can be demonstrated with an apparatus like that in Figure 1-16, which consists of a fluid flowing through a tube that has a series of manometers attached to its wall. The manometers register the lateral wall pressure as the fluid flows through the tube. Notice that as the fluid flows through a tube of uniform diameter, there is a progressive drop in pressure over the length of the tube. The gradual decrease in pressure can be determined by looking at the first three manometers in Figure 1-16. Notice that as the fluid flows through a constriction in the tube, the pressure in the fourth manometer shows an even greater drop in pressure. If it is assumed that the total flow of liquid is the same before and after the constriction, then the flow of liquid must accelerate as it enters the constriction. Thus it is reasonable to assume then that the drop in fluid pressure is directly related to the increase in fluid speed.

Venturi Principle

This principle, which is related to the work of Bernoulli, was first described by Giovanni Venturi (1746-1822) and can be illustrated with an apparatus like the one in Figure 1-17. Notice that this apparatus is similar to the tube used to explain the Bernoulli principle. The Venturi principle states that the pressure drop that occurs as the fluid flows through a constriction in the tube can be restored to the preconstriction pressure if there is a gradual dilatation in the tube distal to the constriction. Using a gradual dilation of the tube (e.g., with an angle of divergence not exceeding 15 degrees) helps to prevent the generation of turbulent flow.[7,8]

Venturi tubes are used in many devices in respiratory care. Air entrainment masks, aerosol generators, and humidifiers are the most common examples. With these devices, a lateral port located just distal to the constriction is used to entrain the second gas or a liquid into the main gas flow. The increased gas flow is accommodated by a gradual dilation of the tube located downstream of the constriction. Other applications of the Venturi principle are described throughout this text.

Coanda Effect

The Coanda effect, which is also based on the Bernoulli principle, is illustrated in Figure 1-18. As was previously explained, the lateral wall pressure of the tube decreases when the fluid flows through a narrowing of the tube because of the increased forward velocity of the fluid flow. If the wall does not have a side port for entraining another fluid, the low pressure adjacent to the wall draws the stream of fluid against the wall. When a specially contoured tube, such as the one in Figure 1-18, is attached distal to the narrow part of the tube, the flow exiting the narrow part of the tube tends to adhere to the wall of the contoured tube because of two factors: a negative pressure is generated past

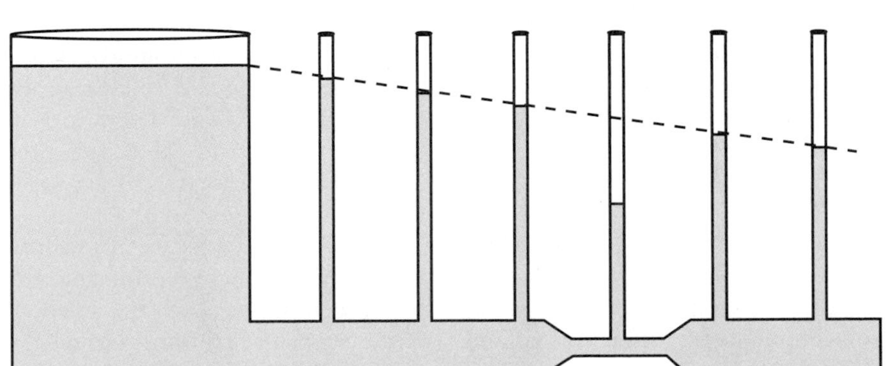

Figure 1-16 The Bernoulli principle. (Redrawn from Nave CR, Nave BC: *Physics for the health sciences*, ed 3, Philadelphia, 1985, WB Saunders.)

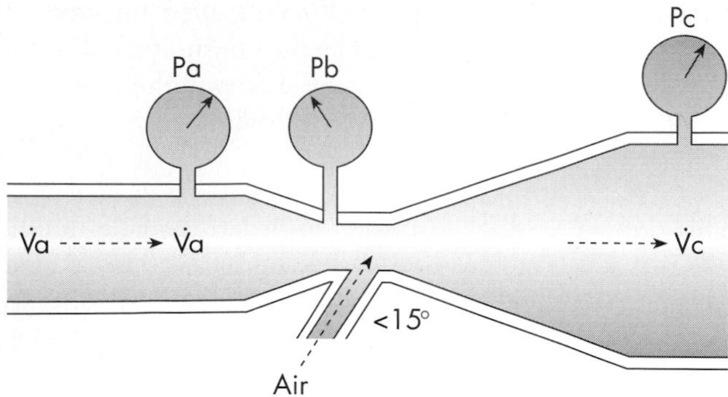

Figure 1-17 The Venturi principle. See text for discussion. (From Scanlan CL, Wilkins BL, Stoller JK: *Egan's fundamentals of respiratory care*, ed 7, St Louis, 1999, Mosby.)

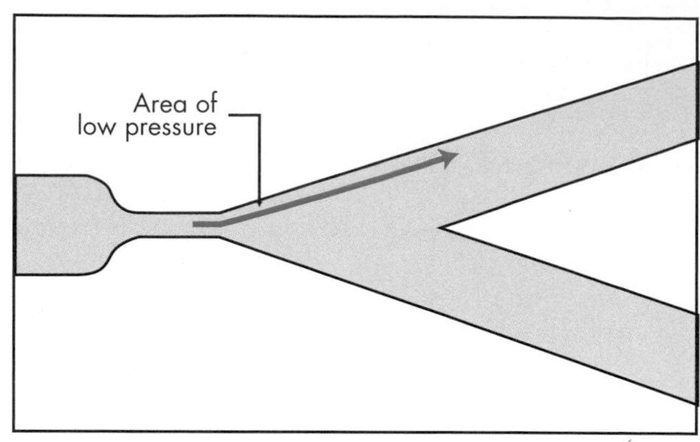

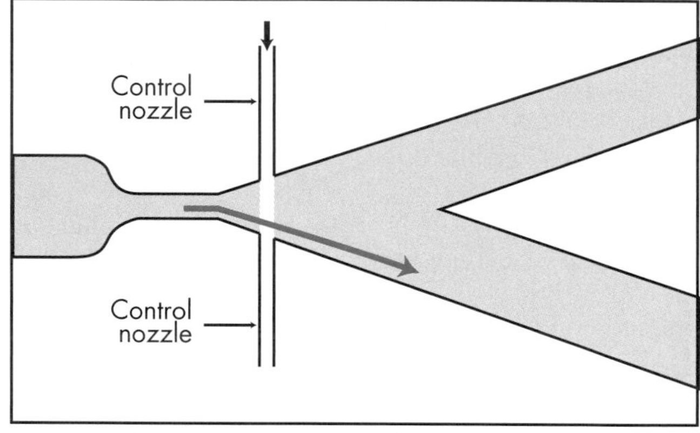

Figure 1-18 The Coanda effect.

the constriction, thus drawing the fluid toward the curved extension; and the ambient pressure opposite the extension pushes the fluid stream against the wall, where it remains locked until interrupted by a counterforce, such as a pulse of air.[8] Using these findings, Coanda was able to demonstrate that with careful placement of the postconstriction extensions, he could deflect a stream of air through a full 180-degree turn by extending the wall contour.[10]

The Coanda effect is the basis for **fluidic** devices that are used in several mechanical ventilators (see Chapter 12). Such devices use gates that are regulated by gas flow from side jets, which operate on the principle that pulses of air are used to redirect the original gas stream. The main advantage of using these fluid logic devices is that they have fewer valves and moving parts that can break (i.e., gas flow is regulated by gas jets, not typical mechanical metal or plastic valves). The primary disadvantage is that these devices consume more gas than more conventional devices because gas flow is used to power the various fluid logic gates. Chapter 11 includes an extensive discussion of fluidic elements used in mechanical ventilators.

Principles of Electricity

Many respiratory care devices are powered by electricity and, in many cases, are also controlled by computers that use solid-state electronic circuitry. Mechanical ventilators, blood-gas analyzers, physiologic transducers and monitors, cathode ray tube displays, strip chart and X-Y recorders are some examples.[8] Because of the importance of these devices in respiratory care, it is essential to have a basic understanding of electronics and electrical safety.

Principles of Electronics

Electricity is produced by the flow of electrons through a conductive path or circuit. This flow, electric current, is influenced by: (1) the force pushing the electrons through a conductive path (i.e., electromotive force or voltage) and (2) the resistance that the electrons must overcome as they flow through the conductive path.

Electric current, which is symbolized as I, can be measured with an **ammeter.** The standard unit of measurement of electric current is the **ampere** (A), where 1 A is equivalent to 6.25×10^{18} electrons passing a point in 1 second. (Note that in electronics, the term *coulomb* is used as a shorthand notation for 6.25×10^{18} electrons. Thus 1 A equals 1 coulomb per second). Amperes can be subdivided into smaller quantities, such as milliamperes (mA, or milliamp) and microamperes (μA or microamp), using scientific notation. For example, 1 mA is 1/1000 of an ampere, and 1 μA is 1/1,000,000 of an ampere. Ammeters typically have scales calibrated in amperes, milliamperes, and microamperes.

As previously stated, voltage is the electrical force (more correctly termed **electromotive force,** or emf) that drives electrons through the conductive path. In most physics textbooks, voltage is also described as the potential difference between two points. Voltage sources include batteries, hydroelectric generators, solar cells, and piezoelectric crystals.

Voltage is measured using a **voltmeter;** and the standard unit of measurement for voltage is the **volt** (V), which can be defined as the electrical potential required for 1 A of electricity to move through 1 **ohm** (Ω) of resistance. As with amperes, volts can be subdivided into smaller units, such as millivolts (mV) and microvolts (μV).

Resistance in electric circuits, as with resistance in fluid circuits, is the opposition to flow. Resistance, which is measured in ohms, is a property of conductors that is influenced by its chemical composition or specific resistance (ρ), as well as by its length and cross-sectional area. Most metals and salt solutions are good conductors (i.e., they offer low resistance to current flow). Rubber, plastic, and glass are poor conductors because they offer high resistance to current flow. Because these materials are such poor conductors, they can be used as protective coverings on conductive wires. As such, these latter materials are often called **insulators.** With regard to physical dimensions, the resistance of a conductor increases as its length increases or its cross-sectional area decreases.

Resistance is not limited to conductors alone. Electronic components called resistors are manufactured to have specific amounts of resistance. **Resistors** serve to limit current and to develop voltages that are less than the source voltage.

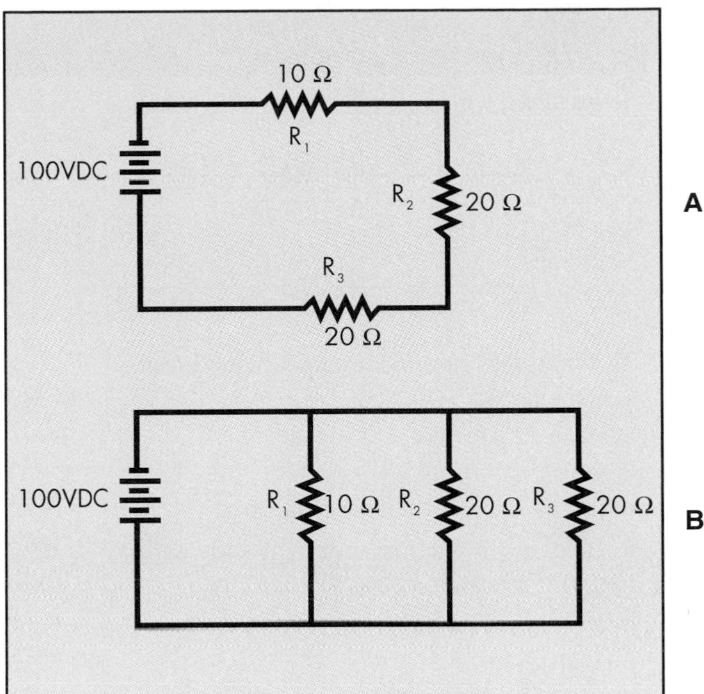

Figure 1-19 Schematic illustrating two types of electric circuits: **A,** direct current (DC) series circuit; **B,** direct current (DC) parallel circuit.

Ohm's Law

The relationships among current, voltage, and resistance can be explained with **Ohm's law:**

$$V = I \times R.$$

According to Ohm's law, voltage and current are directly related, which simply means that if the resistance is constant, increases in voltage cause increases in current flow. Conversely, decreases in source voltage cause a reduction in current flow (assuming resistance is constant). Now consider how changes in resistance affect current flow. If voltage is held constant, increases in resistance will cause a decrease in current flow, whereas decreases in resistance will cause an increase in current flow. Thus current and resistance are inversely related.

It should be apparent from this discussion that any one variable can be solved for if the other two are known. Thus, by rearranging the above equation, the current can be solved for:

$$I = V/R.$$

Similarly, resistance can be solved for with the following rearrangement:

$$R = V/I.$$

It is important to grasp these concepts in order to understand circuit analysis. These principles will now be applied in an analysis of simple electric circuits.

Electrical Circuits

An electrical circuit consists of a voltage source, a load, and a conductive path. An applied voltage causes a current to flow through a conductive path containing one or more loads before returning to the voltage source.

Figure 1-19 shows two types of electric circuits: series circuits and parallel circuits. Notice that in a series circuit, the current flows through one path. The current flows from the voltage source through the conductor and through a series of resistive loads, which are arranged end-to-end (i.e., through R_1 then R_2, etc.), and then back to the voltage source. This is contrasted by the parallel circuit, which may be depicted as two or more series circuits connected to a common voltage source.

There are several principles to remember when analyzing series and parallel circuits. These principles, which are referred to as Kirchhoff's laws, provide the framework for performing circuit analysis.

Kirchhoff's laws governing series circuits may be summarized as follows:

1. A series circuit can have one or more voltage sources. The total source voltage equals the sum of the individual sources if their direction of polarity is the same.
2. In a series circuit, current is the same through all components.
3. The total resistance in a series circuit can be computed by finding the sum of all resistance in the circuit. That is, $R_T = R_1 + R_2 + R_3 \ldots$
4. The sum of voltage drops across resistance in the circuit equals the applied voltage, or $V_T = IR_1 + IR_2 + IR_3 \ldots$

Parallel circuits must adhere to the following guidelines:

1. All branches of parallel circuit have the same applied voltage.
2. Each branch of a parallel circuit may have a different current flow, depending on the resistance of the branch.

Box 1-6 Electrical Circuit Analysis

Series Circuits

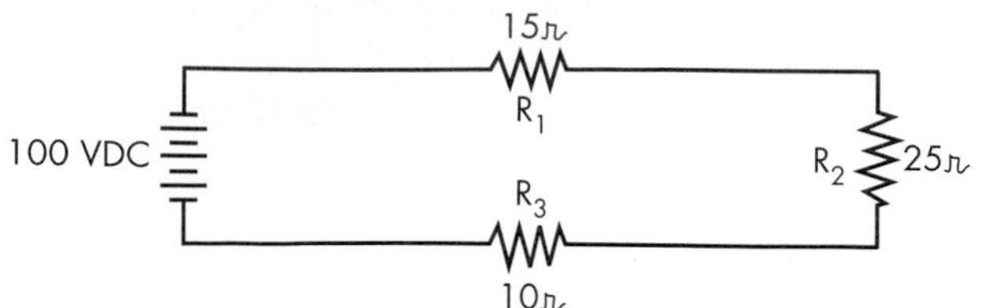

What is the total electrical resistance of this circuit?

$R_T = R_1 + R_2 + R_3$

$R_T = 15\Omega + 25\Omega + 10\Omega$

$R_T = 50\Omega$

What is the total current through the circuit?

$I_T = VT/RT$

$I_T = 100\ V/50\Omega$

$I_T = 2\ A$

Parallel Circuits

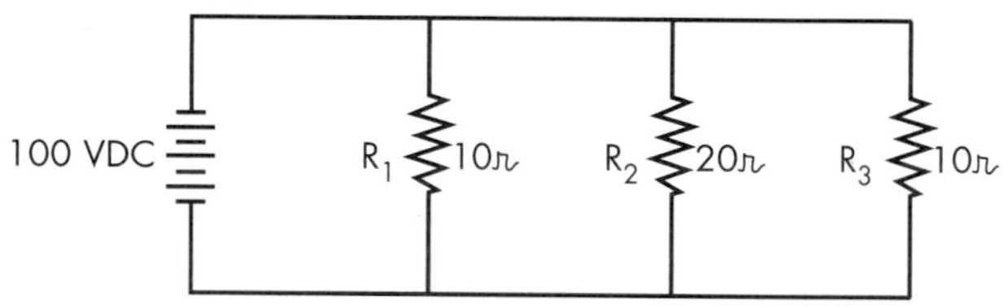

What is the total electrical resistance of this circuit?

$R_T = 1/1/R_1 + 1/R_2 + 1/R_3$

$R_T = 1/(1/10\Omega) + 1/(1/20\Omega) + 1/(1/10\Omega)$

$R_T = 4\ \Omega$

What is the current flow through each branch of the circuit?

$I_1 = 100\ V/10\Omega$

$I_1 = 10\ A$

$I_2 = 100\ V/20\Omega$

$I_2 = 5\ A$

$I_3 = 100\ V/10\Omega$

$I_3 = 10\ A$

What is the total current flow through the circuit?

$I_T = I_1 + I_2 + I_3$

$I_T = 25\ A$

The total current flow can also be calculated in the following manner:

$I_T = V_T/R_T$

$I_T = 100\ V/4\Omega$

$I_T = 25\ A$

3. The total current flowing through a parallel circuit can be computed by finding the sum of the currents flowing through the various branches of the circuit. Thus, $I_T = I_1 + I_2 + I_3 \ldots$
4. The total resistance in a parallel circuit can be computed by finding the sum of the reciprocals for each resistance. That is, $R_T = 1/(1/R_1 + 1/R_2 + 1/R_3 \ldots)$.

Box 1-6 provides several examples of simple circuit analysis.

Electrical Safety

Electrical accidents occur when current from an electrical device interacts with body tissue, impairing physiologic function. It is important to recognize that electrical hazards only exist when the current path through the body is complete. That is, two connections to the body are required for an electrical shock to occur.[8,16] One connection (the "hot" wire) brings the current to the body while the second connection (the neutral wire) completes the circuit by sending the charge to a point of lower potential or ground.

The extent of impairment depends on the amount of current flowing through the body, the duration that the current is applied, and the path that the current takes through the body.[8] Figure 1-20 shows the approximate current ranges and the physiologic effects of a 1-second exposure to various levels of 110 V, 60 Hz alternating currents applied externally to the body.[16]

Two types of electric shock hazards are usually described: **macroshock** and **microshock.** A macroshock occurs when a relatively high current is applied to the body surface. Generally, a current of 1 mA is required to elicit a macroshock. A microshock occurs when a low current (usually less than 1 mA) is allowed to bypass the body surface and flow directly into the body.

Electric current can damage body tissues by causing thermal burns and inadvertently stimulating excitable tissue, such as cardiac muscle. Burns are caused when electric energy dissipates in body tissues, causing the temperature of the tissues to rise. If the temperature gets high enough, it can cause burns. Inadvertent stimulation of excitable tissue can occur when an extraneous electric current of sufficient magnitude causes local voltages that can trigger action potentials. Action potentials triggered in sensory nerves cause a tingling sensation that is associated with electric shock. Action potentials generated in motor nerves and muscles result in muscle contractions, which—if the intensity of the stimulation is high enough—can cause tetanus or sustained contraction of the muscle.

It should be noted that the heart is the organ most susceptible to electrical hazards. Its susceptibility to electrical hazards arises from the fact that when current exceeds a certain value, extra systolic contractions can occur in cardiac muscle. Further increases in current can cause the heart to fibrillate and can ultimately cause sustained myocardial contraction.

Preventing Electrical Hazards

Various strategies should be employed to reduce the likelihood of electrical accidents. These include ensuring the proper grounding of medical equipment, installing ground-fault circuit interrupters, and avoiding contact with transcutaneous conductors.[16]

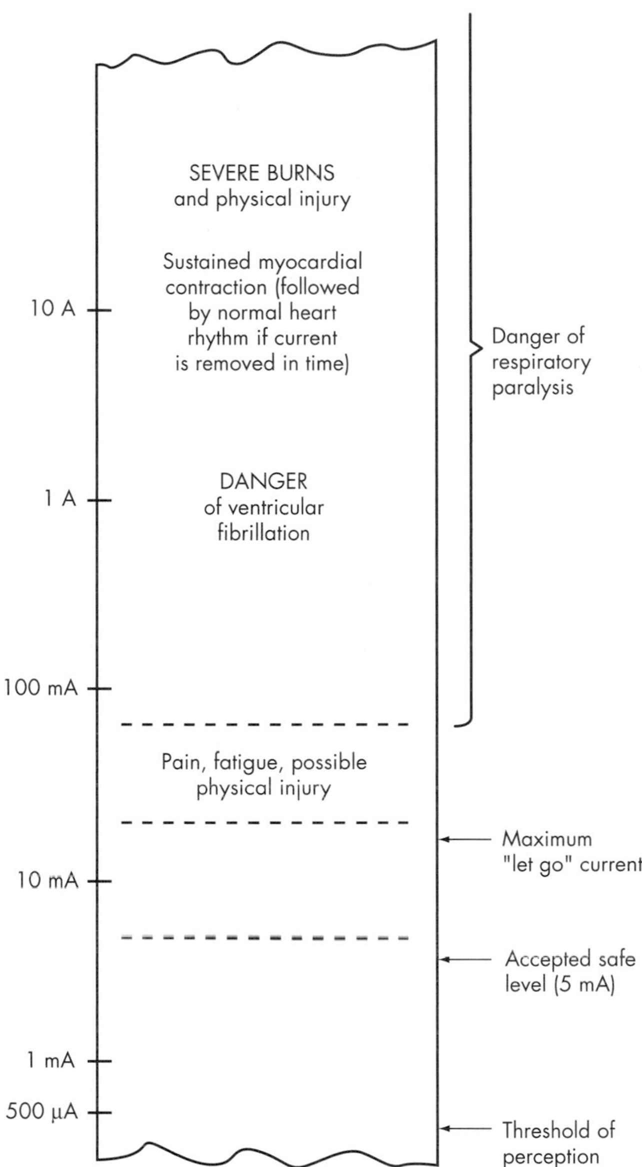

Figure 1-20 Physiologic effects of electrical current associated with a 1-second external contact with a 110 VAC current at 60 Hz. (Redrawn from Cromwell L, Weibell FJ, Pfeiffer EA: *Biomedical instrumentation and measurements,* ed 2, Englewood Cliffs, NJ, 1980, Prentice-Hall.)

Grounding

The principle of this protection method for medical equipment is to provide a low-resistance conductive path that allows the majority of fault current to bypass the patient and return to ground. In cord-connected electrical equipment, this ground connection is established by a third round or U-shaped contact in the plug.

It is important to recognize that grounding is only effective if a good ground connection exists. Worn or broken wires, inadvertent disconnection of ground wires from receptacles, and deliberate removal of ground contacts from plugs interfere with the protection associated with grounding. Because conventional receptacles, line cords, and plugs do not hold up to hospital use, most manufacturers provide hospital-grade receptacles and plugs that must meet Underwriters' Laboratory specifications. Hospital-grade receptacles and plugs can usually be identified by a green dot.[16]

Ground-Fault Circuit Interrupters

Normally, all of the power entering a device through the hot wire returns through the neutral wire. Circuit interrupters monitor the difference between the hot and neutral wires of the power line with a differential transformer and an electrical amplifier. When this difference exceeds a predetermined level (e.g., 5 mA), as occurs when the current bypasses the neutral wire and flows through the patient, the power is interrupted by a circuit breaker. Notice that this interruption occurs rapidly so that the patient does not encounter any harmful effects.

Avoiding Contact with Transcutaneous Conductors

The resistance offered by the skin represents the greatest part of the body's electrical resistance.[16] This resistance can be significantly reduced by permeating the skin with conductive fluid, by cuts and abrasions to the epithelium, or by the introduction of needles through the skin surface. Electrically conductive catheters inserted through a vein or artery can also bypass the natural electrical resistance offered by the skin.

It should be apparent from the discussion so far that these conditions can place patients in compromised states and make them susceptible to microshock hazards. These hazardous effects can be lessened if all electrical devices being used with a microshock-sensitive patient are well-insulated and connected to outlets with a common low-resistance ground.[8] Additionally, devices should be inspected regularly for frayed or bare wires.

Summary

Physics provides a basic framework for any discussion of respiratory care equipment. Under ordinary conditions, all matter behaves according to a group of physical laws, such as the gas laws and the laws of fluid dynamics. Medical application of these laws can be found in a variety of devices, including compressed-gas cylinders, oxygen therapy apparatuses, aerosol generators and humidifiers, mechanical ventilators, and spirometers and medical gas analyzers.

In the following chapters, the operational theories for various devices used in respiratory care will be described. A working knowledge of topics such as matter and energy, temperature and pressure measurements, the gas laws, fluid mechanics, and electricity is necessary to fully appreciate how various respiratory care devices operate.

Review Questions

See Appendix A for answers.

1. Convert the following temperatures:
   a. 37° C = ________ ° F
   b. ________ ° C = 54° F
   c. ________ K = 98.6° F
   d. 25° C = ________ K

2. Perform the following pressure conversions:
   a. ________ kPa = 30 cm H_2O
   b. 760 mm Hg = ________ cm H_2O
   c. ________ cm H_2O = 25 mm Hg
   d. 303.9 kPa = ________ atm

3. Calculate the partial pressures of each of the following gases in room air when the barometric pressure is 750 mm Hg (assume that room air contains 21% oxygen, 78% nitrogen, and 0.03% carbon dioxide):
   a. PO_2 = ________ mm Hg
   b. PN_2 = ________ mm Hg
   c. PCO_2 = ________ mm Hg

4. What is the total pressure of a gas mixture if PO_2 = 90 mm Hg, PCO_2 = 40 mm Hg, PN_2 = 573 mm Hg, and PH_2O = 47 mm Hg?
   a. 573 mm Hg
   b. 713 mm Hg
   c. 750 mm Hg
   d. 760 mm Hg

5. A compressed-gas cylinder at 760 mm Hg and 25° C is moved into a room where the temperature is 38° C. What is the new pressure of the cylinder, assuming that the volume of gas within the cylinder remains constant?

6. A patient's lung capacity is measured to be 5 L at an initial temperature of 25° C and an ambient pressure of 760 mm Hg. What will be the new volume if the temperature increases to 37° C and the pressure to 1520 mm Hg?

7. Calculate the densities of oxygen and carbon dioxide. The molecular weight of oxygen is 32 gmw, and the molecular weight of carbon dioxide is 44 gmw.

8. According to Poiseuille's law, the gas flow through a tube is inversely proportional to the:
   I. length of the tube
   II. driving pressure of the gas through the tube
   III. viscosity of the gas
   IV. radius of the tube
   a. IV only
   b. I and III only
   c. I, II, and III only
   d. II, IV, and V only

9. Which of the following will increase the flow of a gas across a semipermeable membrane according to Fick's law of diffusion?
   I. Increasing the surface area of the membrane
   II. Increasing the partial pressure gradient of the gas across the membrane
   III. Increasing the density of the gas
   IV. Increasing the thickness of the membrane
   a. I and II only
   b. III and IV only
   c. I, II, and III only
   d. II, III, and IV only

10. Which of the following variables will lead to an increase in turbulent airflow?
   I. Increased density of the gas
   II. Decreased linear velocity of the gas flow
   III. Increased radius of the conducting tube
   IV. Decreased viscosity of the gas
   a. I and III only
   b. II and IV only
   c. I, II, and III only
   d. I, III, and IV only

11. What is the total current flowing through a DC circuit containing a 100-V power source and a total resistance of 50Ω?

12. List three strategies that can be used to protect patients from electrical hazards.

13. Calculate the energy cost of operating a 1000-watt air compressor for 24 hours if the electrical energy cost is 10 cents per kilowatt-hour.

14. Macroshock can occur when a person has a 1-second external contact with a 110 VAC current at 60 Hz. What is generally considered the minimum current that the person must contact to experience macroshock?
   a. 100 μA
   b. 1 mA
   c. 10 mA
   d. 1A

15. A respiratory therapist traveling from Chicago, Illinois, to Denver, Colorado, notices that he becomes short of breath while walking to the luggage area of the airport. His wife who is also a respiratory therapist comments that his breathlessness is due to the thinness of the air in Denver. He says that he knew that could explain the breathlessness but also remembered that the air in Denver contains 21% oxygen just like in Chicago. Bemused by his comment, she asks him what is the PO_2 of the air in Denver. Note that the barometric pressure in Denver was recorded as 630 mm Hg.
   a. 147 mm Hg
   b. 132 mm Hg
   c. 122 mm Hg
   d. 90 mm Hg

References

1. Feynman R: *Six easy pieces*, Reading, Mass, 1995, Addison-Wesley.
2. Krauskoff KB, Beiser A: *The physical universe*, ed 9, New York, 2000, McGraw-Hill.
3. Asimov I: *Understanding physics*, New York, 1993, Barnes and Noble.
4. Bevelacqua JJ: Basic health physics, New York, 1999, Wiley-Interscience.
5. Chang R: *Chemistry*, ed 7, New York, 2001, McGraw-Hill.
6. Lide DR, editor: *Handbook of chemistry and physics*, ed 83, Cleveland, 2001, Chemical Rubber Co.
7. Nave CR, Nave BC: *Physics for the health sciences*, ed 3, Philadelphia, 1985, WB Saunders.
8. Scanlan CL: Physical principles in respiratory care. In Scanlan CL, Spearman CB, Sheldon RL, editors: *Egan's fundamentals of respiratory care*, ed 7, St Louis, 1999, Mosby.
9. Wojciechowski WV: *Respiratory care sciences, an integrated approach*, ed 3, Albany, 2001, Delmar.
10. Davis PD, Parbrook GD, Kenny, GNC: *Basic physics and measurement in anaesthesia*, ed 4, Oxford, 1995, Butterworth-Heinemann.
11. Adriani J: *The chemistry and physics of anesthesia*, ed 3, Springfield, Ill, 1979, Charles C Thomas.
12. West JB: *Respiratory physiology: the essentials*, ed 3, Baltimore, 1985, Williams & Wilkins.
13. Guyton AC, Hall, JE: *Textbook of medical physiology*, ed 10, Philadelphia, 2000, WB Saunders.
14. Cromwell L, Weibell FJ, Pfeiffer EA: *Biomedical instrumentation and measurements*, ed 2, Englewood Cliffs, NJ, 1980, Prentice-Hall.
15. Levitzky MG, Cairo JM, Hall SM: *Introduction to respiratory care*, Philadelphia, 1990, WB Saunders.
16. Kacmarek RM, Mack CM, Dimas S: *The essentials of respiratory care*, ed 3, St Louis, 1995, Mosby.

Internet Resources

American Association for Respiratory Care: http://www.aarc.org

American Physical Society: http://www.aps.org

How Things Work—Louis A. Bloomfield: http://howthingswork.virginia.edu

Physics Reference Guide: http://www.physlink.com

The Internet Public Library: http://www.ipl.org

United States Library of Medicine: http://www.nlm.nih.gov

University of Winnipeg Introductory Physics Notes: http://theory.uwinnipeg.ca/physics/

Virtual Physics Laboratory: http://jersey.uoregon.edu/vlab

Chapter 2

Manufacture, Storage, and Transport of Medical Gases

J.M. Cairo

Chapter Outline

Chapter Learning Objectives

Upon completion of this chapter, the reader should be able to:

1. Describe the chemical and physical properties of the medical gases most often encountered in respiratory care.
2. Identify various types of medical gas cylinders (e.g., Types 3, 3A, 3AA, and 3AL).
3. Identify the following cylinder markings: Department of Transportation (DOT) specifications, service pressure, hydrostatic testing dates, manufacturer's identification, ownership mark, serial number, and cylinder size.
4. List the color codes used to identify medical gas cylinders.
5. Discuss *United States Pharmacopeia (USP)* purity standards for medical gases.
6. Compare the operation of direct-acting cylinder valves with diaphragm type of cylinder valves.
7. Explain the American Standards Association (ASA) indexing, the Pin Index Safety System (PISS), and the Diameter Index Safety System (DISS).
8. Identify and correct a problem with cylinder valve assembly.
9. Calculate the gas volume remaining in a compressed-gas cylinder and estimate the duration of gas flow based on the cylinder's gauge pressure.
10. Describe the components of a bulk liquid oxygen system and discuss National Fire Protection Agency (NFPA) recommendations for the storage and use of liquid oxygen in bulk systems.
11. Discuss the operation of a portable liquid oxygen system and describe NFPA recommendations for these systems.
12. Calculate the duration of a portable liquid oxygen supply.
13. Identify three types of medical air compressors and describe the operational theory of each.
14. Summarize NFPA recommendations for medical air supply safety.
15. Compare continuous- and alternating-central–supply systems.
16. Identify a DISS station outlet and a quick-connect station outlet.
17. Compare the operational theory of a membrane oxygenator with that of a molecular sieve oxygenator.

Key Terms

Alternating-Supply Systems
American Standards Association (ASA) Indexing
Check Valves
Continuous-Supply Systems
Cryogenic
Cylinder Volume-Pressure Constants
Diameter Index Safety System (DISS)
Diaphragm Compressors
Diaphragm Valves
Direct-Acting Valves
Fractional Distillation
Frangible (Rupture) Disks
Fusible Plugs
Isolation Valve
Joule-Kelvin (Joule-Thompson) Effect
Liquefaction
Molecular Sieves
Oxygen Concentrators
Physical Separation
Pin Index Safety System (PISS)
Piston Compressors
Pressure Swing Adsorption (PSA)
Quick-Connect Adapters
Rotary Compressors
Semipermeable Membranes
Spring-Loaded Devices
Thorpe-Tube Flowmeter
Volume-Pressure Constant
Wood's Metal

Compressed gases are routinely used in the diagnosis and treatment of patients with cardiopulmonary dysfunction. The appropriate quality, purity, and potency of these medical gases are subject to government regulations. These regulations, along with recommendations proposed by the Compressed Gas Association (CGA) and other private agencies, provide guidelines for the manufacture, storage, and transport of compressed gases. As such, the primary purpose of these guidelines is to protect public safety. Respiratory therapists should be familiar with these regulations, as well as the indications, contraindications, and adverse effects associated with breathing medical gases.

Properties of Medical Gases

Air

At normal atmospheric conditions, air is a colorless, odorless gas mixture that contains varying amounts of water vapor. For practical purposes, we can assume that atmospheric air contains about 78% nitrogen and 21% oxygen by volume. Trace gases, including argon, carbon dioxide, neon, helium, methane, krypton, nitrous oxide, and xenon, make up the remaining 1% of atmospheric air. Table 2-1 shows a typical analysis of dry air at sea level.

Air is a nonflammable gas but it supports combustion. It has a density of 1.2 kg/m^3 at 21.1° C (70° F) and 760 mm Hg.[1] Because air is used as a standard for

Table 2-1 Composition of room air

Component	% by Volume	% by Weight
Nitrogen	78.084	75.5
Oxygen	20.946	23.2
Argon	0.934	1.33
Carbon dioxide	0.0335	0.045
Neon	0.001818	–
Helium	0.000524	–
Methane	0.0002	–
Krypton	0.000114	–
Nitrous oxide	0.00005	–
Xenon	0.0000087	–

From Compressed Gas Association, Inc: Handbook of compressed gases, *ed 3, New York, 1990, Van Nostrand Reinhold.*

measuring the specific gravity of other gases, it is assigned a value of 1 at 21.1° C and 1 atmosphere (atm).[1] At its freezing point, –195.6° C (–320° F), air is a transparent liquid with a pale bluish cast.

Compressed air is prepared synthetically from nitrogen and oxygen and shipped as a gas in cylinders at high pressure. Liquid air can be obtained through a process called **liquefaction** and shipped in bulk in specially designed **cryogenic** containers. For many medical applications, air is filtered and compressed at the point of use. The theory of operation of portable air compressors is described later in this chapter.

Oxygen (O_2)

Oxygen is an elemental gas that is colorless, odorless, and tasteless at normal temperatures and pressures. It makes up 20.9% of the Earth's atmosphere by volume and 23.2% by weight. It constitutes about 50% of the Earth's crust by weight. Oxygen is slightly heavier than air, having a density of 1.326 kg/m^3 at 21.1° C and 760 mm Hg (specific gravity = 1.105).[1] At temperatures less than –183° C (–300° F), oxygen exists as a pale bluish liquid that is slightly heavier than water.

Oxygen is classified as a nonflammable gas, but it readily supports combustion (i.e., the burning of flammable materials is accelerated in the presence of oxygen). Some combustibles, such as oil and grease, burn with nearly explosive violence if ignited in the presence of oxygen.[1] All elements except the inert gases combine with oxygen to form oxides; oxygen is therefore characterized as an oxidizer.

The two methods most commonly used to prepare oxygen are the **fractional distillation** of liquid air and the **physical separation** of atmospheric air. The fractional distillation of liquid air, which relies on the Joule-Kelvin or the Joule-Thompson effect, was introduced by Karl von Linde in 1907.[2] Box 2-1 describes the fractional distillation process; Figure 2-1 illustrates the components of a typical fractional distillation system. The fractional distillation process is used commercially to produce bulk oxygen, which can be stored as a liquid in cryogenic storage tanks or converted into a gas and shipped in metal cylinders.

Box 2-1 Fractional Distillation of Liquid Air

1. Room air is drawn through scrubbers to remove dust and other impurities.
2. Air is cooled to near the freezing point of water (0° C) to remove water vapor.
3. Air is compressed to 200 atm, causing the temperature of the gas mixture to increase.
4. Compressed air is cooled to room temperature by passing nitrogen through coils surrounding the gas mixture.
5. As the temperature drops, the gas mixture expands. The temperature achieved is less than the critical temperature of nearly all gases in air, thus producing a liquid gas mixture.
6. The liquid air is transferred to a distilling column where it is warmed to room temperature. As the air warms, various gases boil off as their individual boiling points are reached.
7. Liquid oxygen is obtained by maintaining the temperature of the gas mixture just below the boiling point of oxygen (–183° C, or –297.3° F at 1 atm).
8. The process is repeated until the liquid oxygen mixture is 99% pure with no toxic impurities.
9. The liquid oxygen is then transferred to cold converters for storage and later transported either in bulk as a liquid or in compressed gas cylinders as a gas.

The physical separation of atmospheric air is accomplished with devices that use **molecular sieves** and **semipermeable membranes** to filter room air. These devices, which are called **oxygen concentrators,** are primarily used to provide enriched oxygen mixtures for oxygen therapy in home-care settings. How oxygen concentrators operate will be discussed in more detail later in this chapter.

Carbon Dioxide (CO_2)

Carbon dioxide is a colorless, odorless gas at normal atmospheric temperatures and pressures. It has a density of 1.833 kg/m^3 at 21.1° C and 1 atm; it is therefore about 1.5 times heavier than air (specific gravity = 1.522).[1] Carbon dioxide is nonflammable and does not support combustion or life.

Carbon dioxide can exist as a solid, liquid, and gas at a temperature of –56.6° C (–69.9° F) and a pressure of 60.4 psig (the triple point of CO_2).[1] At temperatures and pressures below its triple point,* carbon dioxide exists as a

**The triple point is a specific combination of temperature and pressure in which a substance can exist in all three states of matter in a dynamic equilibrium.*

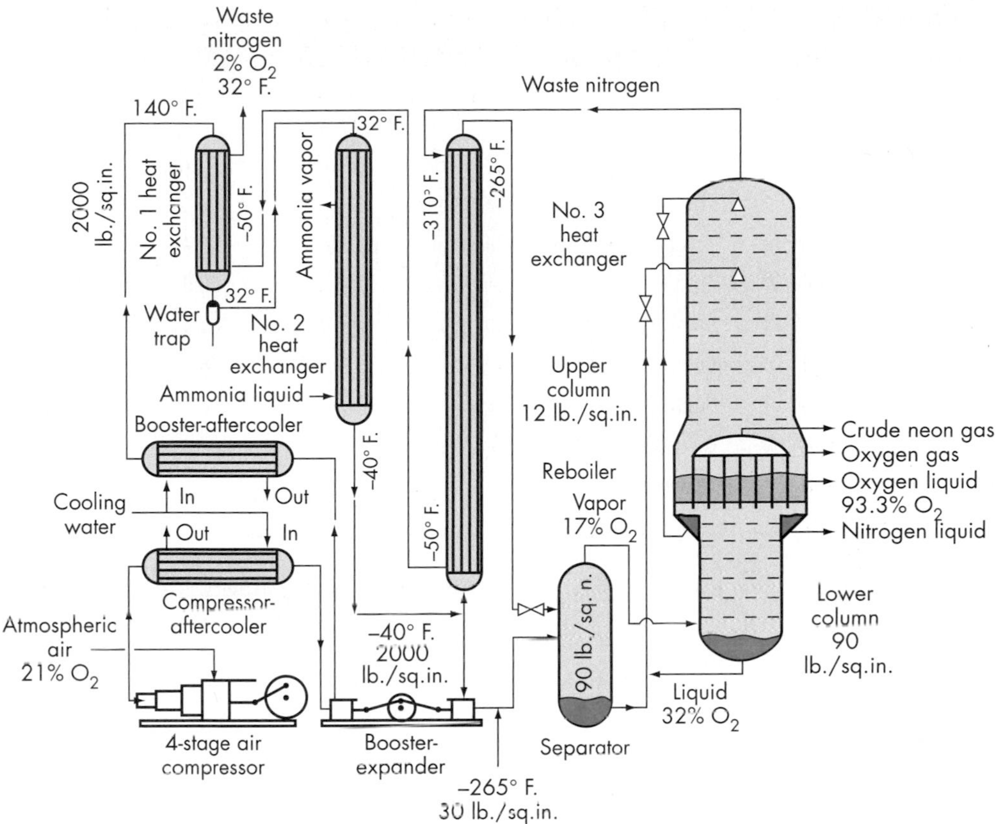

Figure 2-1 Fractional distillation apparatus for producing liquid oxygen. (Courtesy Nellcor Puritan Bennett, Pleasanton, Calif.)

solid ("dry ice") or a gas, depending on the temperature. At temperatures and pressures above its triple point but below its critical temperature (31.1° C or 87.9° F), carbon dioxide can exist as a liquid or as a gas. Thus when carbon dioxide is stored at these temperatures in a pressurized container, such as a metal cylinder, the liquid and gaseous forms of carbon dioxide exist in equilibrium. Above 31.1° C, carbon dioxide cannot exist as a liquid, regardless of the pressure.[1]

Unrefined carbon dioxide can be obtained from the combustion of coal, natural gas, or other carbonaceous fuels.[1] Carbon dioxide can also be obtained as a byproduct in the production of ammonia, lime, and kilns, among other products. Purified carbon dioxide is prepared through the liquefaction and fractional distillation processes.

Solid carbon dioxide is used to refrigerate perishable materials while in transport (e.g., food and laboratory specimens). Liquid carbon dioxide can be used as an expendable refrigerant[1] and is used extensively as a fire-extinguishing agent in portable and stationary fire-extinguishing systems. Gaseous carbon dioxide is used in food processing (e.g., carbonation of beverages), water treatment, and as a growth stimulant for plants.[1]

Carbon dioxide is primarily used for the treatment of singultus (hiccups) and as a stimulant/depressant of the central nervous system (CNS). It is also used as a standard calibration gas for blood-gas analyzers, transcutaneous partial pressure of carbon dioxide (PCO_2) electrodes, and capnographs. Because carbon dioxide cannot support life, it must be combined with oxygen before being administered to patients. Carbon dioxide/oxygen mixtures (carbogen mixtures) are prepared by combining 5% to 10% carbon dioxide with 90% to 95% oxygen. The United States Food and Drug Administration (USFDA) purity standard requires that carbon dioxide used for medical purposes is 99.0% pure.[3]

Helium (He)

Helium is the second lightest element, having a density of 0.165 kg/m^3 at 21.1° C and 1 atm (specific gravity = 0.138).[1] It is an inert gas that has no color, odor, or taste. Helium is only slightly soluble in water and is a good conductor of heat, sound, and electricity.[4]

Helium occurs naturally in the atmosphere in very small quantities (see Table 2-1). It can be prepared commercially from natural gas, which contains as much as 2% helium.[1] Helium can also be obtained by heating uranium ore. Purity standards for the preparation of helium require that commercially available helium be 95% pure. Helium is chemically and physiologically inert and is classified as a nonflammable gas that will not support combustion or life. Breathing 100% helium will lead to severe hypoxemia. Because of its low density, He is combined with oxygen (i.e., heliox is a mixture of 80% helium and 20% oxygen) to deliver oxygen therapy to patients with severe airway obstruction

Table 2-2 Properties of commonly used medical gases

Medical Gas	Chemical Symbol	Molecular Weight	Physical Characteristics: Color	Odor	Taste	Boiling Point	Critical Temperature	Physical State	Combustion Characteristics
Air	Air	28.97	Colorless	Odorless	Tasteless	−194.3	−140.6	Gas/liquid	NF/SC
Oxygen	O_2	31.99	Colorless	Odorless	Tasteless	−182.9	−118.4	Gas/liquid	NF/SC
Carbon dioxide	CO_2	44.01	Colorless	Odorless	Slightly acid	−29.0	+31.0	Liquid/gas	NF
Carbon monoxide	CO	28.01	Colorless	Odorless	Tasteless	−191.5	−140.2	Gas	F
Nitrous oxide	N_2O	44.01	Colorless	Odorless	Tasteless	−88.5	+36.4	Liquid/gas	NF
Nitric oxide	NO	30.01	Colorless	Odorless	Tasteless	−151.8	−92.9	Gas	NF
Helium	He	4.00	Colorless	Odorless	Tasteless	−268.9	−267.0	Gas	NF

NF, *Nonflammable;* SC, *supports combustion;* F, *flammable.*

(i.e., it decreases the work of breathing by decreasing turbulent airflow). It is also used in pulmonary function testing for measuring residual volume and diffusing capacity.

Nitric Oxide (NO)

Nitric oxide is a diatomic molecule that exists as colorless gas at room temperature. It is nonflammable and will support combustion. It has a density of 1.245 kg/m^3 and a specific gravity of 1.04 (21.1° C, 760 mm Hg).[1] Nitric oxide is highly unstable in the atmosphere and can exist in three biologically active forms in tissues: nitrosonium (NO^+), nitroxyl anions (NO^-), and as a free radical ($NO^{\cdot}$).

In the presence of air, nitric oxide combines with oxygen to form brown fumes of nitrogen dioxide (NO_2), which is a strong oxidizing agent. It is not corrosive, and most structural materials are unaffected; in the presence of moisture, however, it can form nitrous and nitric acids, both of which can cause corrosion. Nitric oxide and nitrogen dioxide combined form a potent irritant that can cause chemical pneumonitis and pulmonary edema.[4]

Nitric oxide can be prepared by oxidizing ammonia at high temperatures (500° C) in the presence of a platinum catalyst or by reducing acid solutions of nitrates.[1] Chemiluminescent analysis is used to determine the final concentration of nitric oxide and nitrogen dioxide with a stated accuracy of ±2% (see Chapter 8 for a discussion of chemiluminescent analysis of nitric oxides). Nitric oxide is supplied with nitrogen in compressed-gas aluminum alloy cylinders.[5] Before 1997, nitric oxide was supplied in cylinders with a volume capacity of 152 ft^3 with 660 CGA valve outlets. It is now supplied in smaller cylinders (82 ft^3) with 626 CGA valve outlets.

Although nitric oxide is toxic in high concentrations, experimental results suggest that low doses of it are a powerful pulmonary vasodilator.[5] Very low concentrations (2 to 80 parts per million [ppm]) combined with oxygen have been used successfully to treat persistent pulmonary hypertension of the newborn (PPHN)[6] and adult respiratory distress syndrome.[7]

CLINICAL ROUNDS 2-1

Based on the discussion of compressed gases, name the appropriate gas for each of the following situations:
As a refrigerant.
For reducing the work of breathing in a patient with airway obstruction.
To treat hypoxemia in a patient with chronic obstructive pulmonary disease.
For reducing pulmonary vasoconstriction, such as occurs in PPHN.

See Appendix A for the answer.

Although many investigators have suggested that inhalation of low-dose nitric oxide is relatively safe, special precautions apply. Specifically, the levels of nitrogen dioxide and nitrogen trioxide, as well as the patient's methemoglobin levels, should be monitored throughout the procedure.[5]

Nitrous Oxide (N_2O)

Nitrous oxide is a colorless gas at normal temperatures and atmospheric pressures. It is odorless, tasteless, and nonflammable but will support combustion, and is slightly soluble in water, alcohol, and oils. Nitrous oxide is noncorrosive and may therefore be stored in commercially available cylinders. Because it is an oxidizing agent, it will react with oils, grease, and other combustible materials.

Nitrous oxide is prepared commercially by the thermal decomposition of ammonium nitrate and as a byproduct from adipic acid manufacturing processes.[1] At elevated temperatures (>649° C), it decomposes into nitrogen and oxygen.

The major use of nitrous oxide is as a CNS depressant (i.e., an anesthetic). As such, it is a potent anesthetic when

Box 2-2 Agencies Regulating Manufacture, Storage, and Transport of Medical Gases

Regulating Agencies

Center for Devices and Radiological Health (CDRH)

An agency of the FDA that provides standards for medical devices.

Department of Health and Human Services (HHS)

Department of the federal government that oversees health care delivery in the United States. Formerly known as the Department of Health, Education, and Welfare (HEW).

Department of Transportation

Provides regulations for the manufacture, storage, and transport of compressed gases. Before 1970, this responsibility was vested with the Interstate Commerce Commission (ICC).

Environmental Protection Agency (EPA)

Government agency that establishes standards and administers regulations concerning potential and actual environmental hazards.

Food and Drug Administration (FDA)

An agency of the Department of Health and Human Services (HHS) that sets purity standards for medical gases.

Occupational Safety and Health Administration (OSHA)

An agency of the Department of Labor that oversees safety issues related to the work environment.

Transport Canada (TC)

Canadian government agency that administers regulations concerning manufacture and testing of compressed gas cylinders and their distribution.

Recommending Agencies

American National Standards Institute (ANSI)

Private, nonprofit organization that coordinates the voluntary development of national standards in the United States. Represents US interests in international standards.

American Society of Mechanical Engineers (ASME)

Issues information on design, manufacture, and structural standards for components of central piping systems.

Compressed Gas Association (CGA)

Comprises companies involved in the manufacture, storage, and transport of all compressed gases. Provides standards and safety systems for compressed-gas systems.

International Standards Organization (ISO)

International agency that provides standards for technology.

National Fire Protection Association (NFPA)

Independent agency that provides information on fire protection and safety.

United States Pharmacopoeia/National Formulary (USP/NF)

A not-for-profit private organization founded to develop officially recognized quality standards for drugs, including medical gases.

Z-79 Committee

ANSI committee for establishing standards for anesthetic and ventilatory devices, including anesthetic machines, reservoir bags, tracheal tubes, humidifiers, nebulizers, and other oxygen-related equipment.

administered in high concentrations; in low concentrations, other depressant drugs must be used concomitantly to achieve effective anesthesia. (Nitrous oxide is often called "laughing gas," a term that was coined in 1840.[8]) Note that inhalation of nitrous oxide without provision of a sufficient oxygen supply may cause brain damage or be fatal.

Long-term exposure of health care workers to nitrous oxide has been associated with adverse side effects, including neuropathy and feto-toxic effects (spontaneous abortions).[1] The National Institute of Occupational Safety and Health has recommended limits for exposure to nitrous oxide of health care providers working in surgical suites and dental offices. Systems to trap exhaled nitrous oxide are used to capture any unused gas, preventing inadvertent exposure of health care workers.

Table 2-2 provides a summary of the properties of commonly used medical gases. Clinical Rounds 2-1 provides an exercise for you to test your understanding of the aforementioned discussion of medical gases.

Storage and Transport of Medical Gases

Medical gases can be classified as nonliquefied and liquefied. Nonliquefied gases are stored and transported under high pressure in metal cylinders. Liquefied gases are stored and transported in specially designed bulk liquid storage units. The design of compressed gas cylinders, bulk storage containers, and their valve outlets, as well as their transportation, testing, and periodic examination, are subject to national standards and regulations.[9,10] Box 2-2 contains a list of agencies that provide recommendations and regulations for the manufacture, storage, transport, and use of medical gases.

Cylinders

Metal cylinders have been used for storing compressed gases since 1888.[10] Federal regulations issued by the Department of Transportation (DOT) require that all cylinders used to store and transport compressed gases conform to well-defined specifications.* These specifications, along with recommendations from the NFPA and the CGA, provide industry standards for cylinder design and maintenance and the safe use of compressed gases. Appendix 2-1 contains a summary of NFPA and CGA recommendations for compressed-gas cylinders.

**Before 1970, the Interstate Commerce Commission served as the regulatory agency for the construction, transport, and maintenance of compressed gases, but in 1970 the DOT took over this responsibility.*

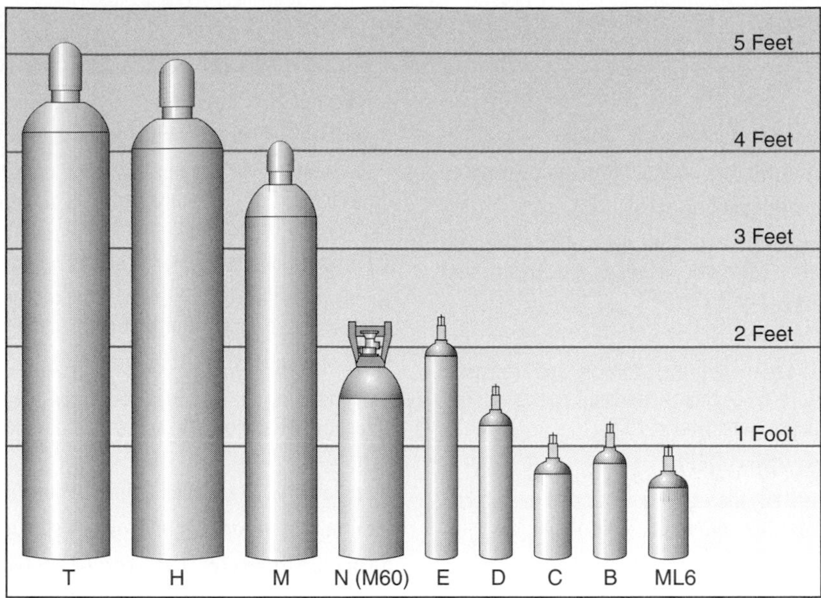

Figure 2-2 Various types of high-pressure cylinders used in medical gas therapy. (From Hess D, MacIntyre N, Adams A, et al: *Respiratory care, principles and practice*, Philadelphia, 2002, WB Saunders.)

Construction and Maintenance of Compressed-Gas Cylinders

Compressed-gas cylinders are constructed of seamless, high-quality steel, chrome-molybdenum, or aluminum that is either stamped into shape using a punch-press die or spun into shape by wrapping heated steel bands around specially designed molds. The bottom of the cylinder is welded closed and the top of the cylinder is threaded and fitted with a valve stem (Figure 2-2).

Type 3AA cylinders are produced from heat-treated, high-strength steel; type 3A cylinders are made of carbon-steel (non-heat–treated). Type 3AL cylinders are constructed of specially prescribed seamless aluminum alloys. Type 3 cylinders, which are made of low-carbon steel, are no longer produced. Note that the steel used in the construction of cylinders must meet the chemical and physical standards set by the DOT. (In Canada, the specifications for the construction of cylinders are set by Transport Canada.[8])

Compressed-gas cylinders should be capable of holding up to 10% more than the maximum filling pressure as marked.[11,12] This added capacity is required because of variations in cylinder pressure that occur with changes in ambient temperature. The Bureau of Explosives requires that all cylinders contain a pressure-relief mechanism to prevent explosion.[13]

Type 3AA and 3A cylinders must be hydrostatically reexamined every 10 years to determine their expansion characteristics. (The asterisk following the reexamination date on the cylinder markings [see Figure 2-4] indicates that the cylinder must be retested every 10 years.[11]) Type 3AL cylinders must be reexamined every 5 years to test their expansion characteristics. Hydrostatic examination involves measuring a cylinder's expansion characteristics when it is filled to a pressure of five-thirds its working pressure. This examination consists of placing a cylinder filled with water in a vessel that is also filled with water. When pressure is applied to the interior of the cylinder, the cylinder expands, displacing water from the jacket surrounding the cylinder. The volume of water displaced when pressure is applied equals the total expansion of the cylinder. The permanent expansion of the cylinder equals the volume of water displaced when the pressure is released. This information is then used to calculate the elastic expansion of the cylinder, which is directly related to the thickness of the cylinder. Increases in the elastic expansion of a cylinder indicate a reduction in the wall thickness. Reductions in wall thickness can occur when the cylinder is physically damaged or is attacked by corrosion.[8]

Filling Medical Cylinders

As you might expect, filling and refilling medical gas cylinder is a potentially dangerous process. The United States Department of Transportation (DOT), United States Food and Drug Administration (FDA), and United States Pharmacopeia/National Formulary (USP/NF) have established a series of guidelines (i.e., good manufacturing practices) that set strict controls over large commercial cylinder filling operations, as well as small home medical equipment dealers refilling relatively small numbers of cylinders.[8] Companies performing cylinder filling and refilling procedures must register with the FDA, which monitors compliance through bi-annual on-site inspections.

Good manufacturing practices are designed to ensure that only properly trained individuals are involved in the refilling process and that the procedure is performed using certified equipment. These guidelines also specify that only safe and clean cylinders can be refilled. Gases used in this process must meet USP/NF standards for purity and each cylinder must have a current intact label that is readable and meets FDA and DOT regulations. In addition, each batch of cylinders must be identified by an assigned lot number that is traceable if recall is necessary.

The process of filling and refilling gas cylinders involves four elements: (1) cylinder pre-fill inspection, (2) cylinder filling, (3) post-fill procedures, and (4) appropriate documentation.[8] Cylinder pre-fill inspection focuses on removal of any residual gas before refilling, visual inspection of each cylinder for any signs of damage, verification that the last hydrostatic testing date does not exceed DOT retest criteria, and ensuring that the cylinder is properly labeled. As mentioned, cylinder refilling must be done with certified equipment. Cylinders are attached to a specially designed manifold (Figure 2-3) that allows for cylinder evacuation before filling of the cylinder from a gas supply source. Gas from the supply source is introduced into the cylinders at a controlled flow that permits a filling rate of no more than 200 psig per minute until the permitted full pressure is attained. (Note that the full pressure is corrected for temperature so that the accurate volume is present at STP conditions.[8]) Once the cylinders are filled, the valves of the cylinders are closed and removed from the manifold. A post-fill procedure is then performed on each cylinder to ensure that the cylinder valve does not leak and that the cylinder contents meet the minimum purity standards set by the USP/NF. Documentation of each of the previous steps and the signature of the individual who filled the cylinders must be recorded in a transfilling log. Company records should also include daily calibration of oxygen analyzers used to test purity of cylinder contents along with evidence that the manifold and gauges are inspected according to an established schedule.

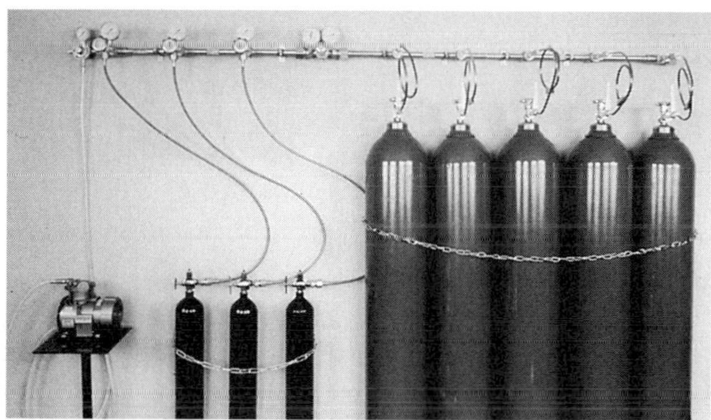

Figure 2-3 Example of a transfilling manifold.

Cylinder Sizes and Capacities

Table 2-3 summarizes the weights and volume capacities for various cylinders and gases that are used in respiratory care. The most commonly used cylinders for medical gas therapy are the "E" and "H" types of cylinders. "D" cylinders are also used for the storage of nitric oxide.

"E" cylinders are frequently used as a source of oxygen in emergency situations (e.g., CPR carts, etc.) and for transporting patients requiring oxygen therapy. These smaller cylinders also store gases used in anesthetics, as well as calibration gases for portable diagnostic equipment (e.g., capnographs and pulse oximeters).

Table 2-3 Physical characteristics of common-sized aluminium and steel cylinders

	Aluminium							*Steel*				
	B or M6	ML6	C or M9	D	E	N or M60	M or MM	D	E	M	H	T
Service pressure (psig)	2216	2015	2015	2015	2015	2216	2216	2015	2015	2015	2265	2400
Height without valve (inches)	11.6	7.7	10.9	16.5	25.6	23	35.75	16.75	25.75	43	51	55
Diameter (inches)	3.2	4.4	4.4	4.4	4.4	7.25	8	4.2	4.2	7	9	9.25
Weight without valve (pounds)	2.2	2.9	3.7	5.3	7.9	21.7	38.6	7.9	11.3	58	117	139
Capacity at Listed Pressure at STPA												
Oxygen (cubic feet	6	6	9	15	24	61.4	122	15	24	110	250	300
Oxygen (L)	170	170	255	425	680	1738	3455	425	680	3113	7075	8490

From Hess D, MacIntyre N, Adams A, et al: Respiratory care: principles and practice, *St Louis, 2002, WB Saunders.*

STPA, *Standard temperature and pressure, atmospheric.*

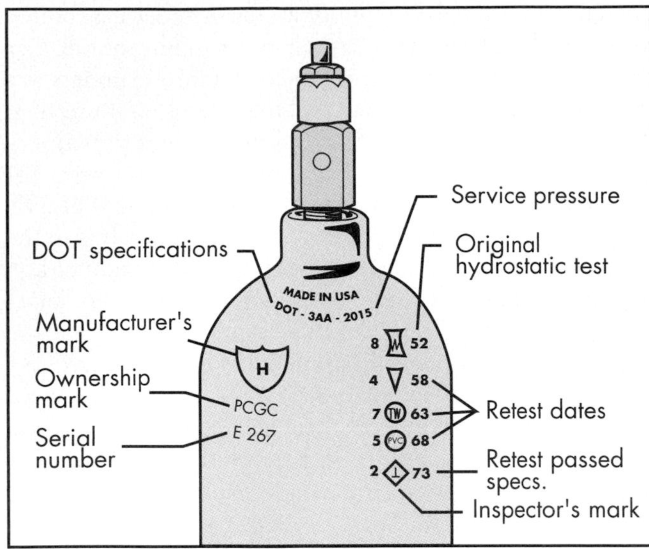

Figure 2-4 Standard markings for compressed gas cylinders. (Modified from Nellcor Puritan Bennett, Pleasanton, Calif.)

"H" type cylinders are used as the primary source of oxygen and other medical gases in smaller hospitals without bulk liquid systems (see the following section). Hospitals and other facilities with bulk liquid oxygen systems use these larger cylinders as a secondary or reserve source of medical gases. Large cylinders are frequently used for home-care patients requiring long-term oxygen therapy. These larger cylinders are also routinely used to store calibration gases that are required in the blood-gas and pulmonary function laboratories.

Cylinder Identification

Cylinders are engraved with information that is primarily designed to identify where the cylinder was manufactured, the type of material used in its construction (i.e., 3AA, 3A, or 3AL), the service pressure of the cylinder, the date of its original hydrostatic test, and its reexamination dates.[1] Additionally, the manufacturer's name, the owner's identification number, and the size of cylinder are usually engraved on the cylinder. Figure 2-4 illustrates the standard markings that appear on compressed-gas cylinders. Note that a "+" following the stamped hydrostatic examination date indicates that the cylinder complied with requirement of the examination. A "+" does not follow the reexamination date on aluminum cylinders.

Medical gas cylinders are color-coded for easy identification. Table 2-4 shows the color codes prescribed by the United States National Formulary.[3] Generally, these colors conform to the international cylinder color-coding system. Two major exceptions in the international system are oxygen cylinders, which are painted white, and compressed-air cylinders, which

Table 2-4 Color codes for medical gases

Gas	Chemical Symbol	Purity*	Color Code
Air	–	99.0	Yellow or black and white†
Carbon dioxide	CO_2	99.0	Gray
Carbon dioxide/oxygen	CO_2/O_2	99.0	Gray and green‡
Cyclopropane	C_3H_6	99.0	Orange
Ethylene	C_2H_4	99.0	Red
Helium	He	99.0	Brown
Helium/oxygen	He/O_2	99.0	Brown and green‡
Nitrogen	N_2	99.0	Black
Nitrous oxide	N_2O	97.0	Light blue
Nitric oxide	NO	99.0	Teal and black
Oxygen	O_2	99.0	Green and white†

**National Formulary Standards.*
†International color code system.
‡Always check labels to determine the percentages of each gas.

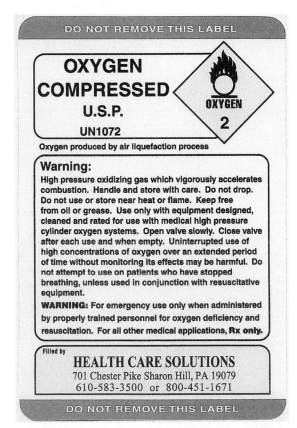

Figure 2-5 Example of compressed gas cylinder labeling. (From Hess D, MacIntyre N, Adams A, et al: *Respiratory care: principles and practice*, Philadelphia, 2002, WB Saunders.)

are painted yellow or black and white. Cylinders containing gas mixtures, such as helium-oxygen and carbon dioxide-oxygen are divided into two categories of color-coding, each based on the percentage of gases contained. For example, cylinders of carbon dioxide-oxygen mixtures that contain more than 7% carbon dioxide are predominantly gray with the shoulder of the tank painted green. Cylinders containing carbon dioxide-oxygen mixtures with less than 7% carbon dioxide are predominantly green with a gray shoulder. Helium-oxygen cylinders containing more than 80% helium are painted brown with a green shoulder. Cylinders of helium-oxygen mixtures containing less than 80% helium (balanced with oxygen) are predominantly green with a brown shoulder.

Color codes are only a guide; printed labels are still the primary way to identify the contents of a gas cylinder. Figure 2-5 is a standard label for an oxygen cylinder. The CGA and the American Standards Association (ASA) specify that all labels should include the name and chemical symbol of the gas in the cylinder. The label should also show the volume of the cylinder (in liters) at a temperature of 21.1° C (70° F).[1] Generally, labels will also include any specific hazards related to use of the gas and precautionary measures and instructions in case of accidental exposure or contact with the contents.

The USFDA requires that compressed gases used for medical purposes meet certain minimum requirements for

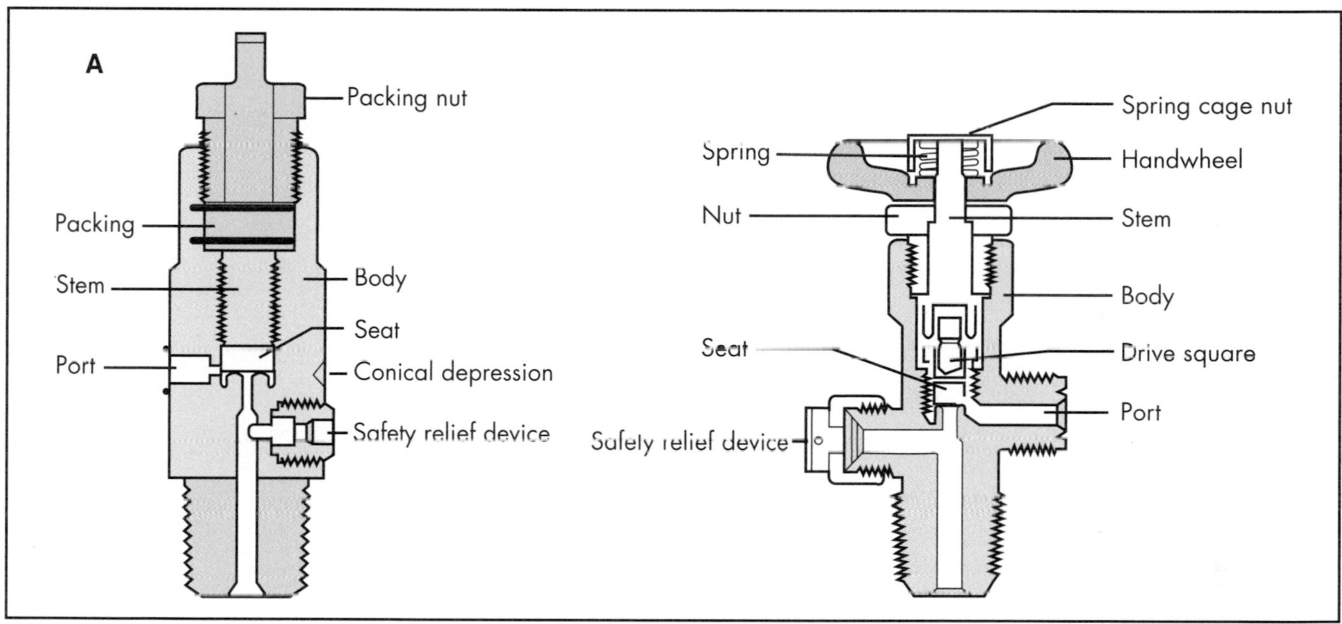

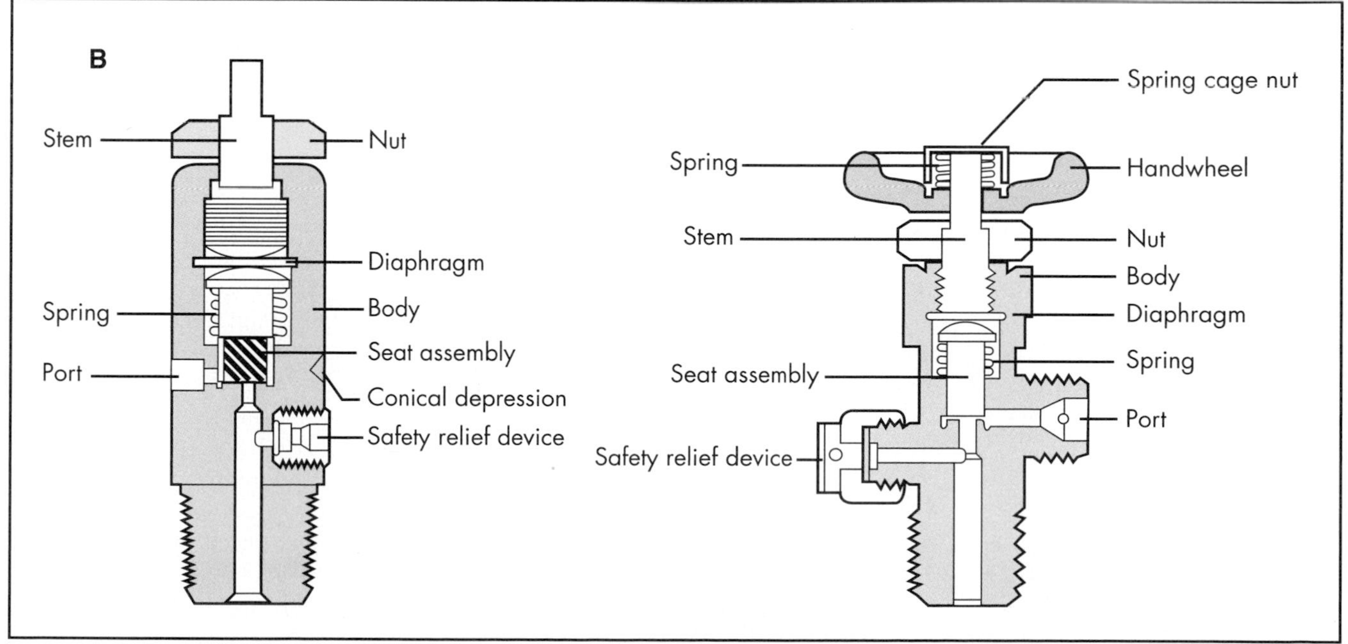

Figure 2-6 Cylinder valves: **A,** direct-acting valve; **B,** diaphragm valve. (Courtesy Nellcor Puritan Bennett, Pleasanton, Calif.)

purity, and the purity of the gas must be indicated on the label identifying the contents of the cylinder. These standards are listed in the NF/USP. (See Table 2-4 for a list of these purity requirements.) The USFDA also requires that the names of the manufacturer, packer, and distributor be included on the label.

Cylinder Valves

Cylinder valves are control devices that seal the contents of a compressed cylinder until it is ready for use. A cylinder valve is composed of the following elements:

1. A chrome-plated, brass body
2. A threaded inlet connector for attachment to the cylinder
3. A stem that opens and closes the cylinder when turned by a handwheel or handle
4. An outlet connection that allows for attachment of regulators and pressure-reducing valves
5. A pressure-relief valve

Figure 2-6 shows the two different types of cylinder valves that are affixed to compressed medical gas cylinders: **direct-acting valves** and **diaphragm valves**. A direct-acting valve (Figure 2-6, *A*) contains two fiber washers and a Teflon packing to prevent gas leakage around the threads. The term direct-acting is derived from the arrangement of movements in the valve wheel. These movements are directly reflected in the valve seat because it is one piece moved by threads. Direct-acting valves can withstand high pressures (i.e., more than 1500 psi).

Diaphragm type of valves (Figure 2-6, *B*) use a threaded stem in place of the packing found on the direct-acting valves. The stem is separated from the valve seat and spring by two diaphragms, one made of steel and one made of copper. When the stem is turned counterclockwise and raised because of the threading, the diaphragm is pushed upward with the stem by the valve seat and spring, causing the valve to open. Turning the stem clockwise resets the diaphragm and closes the valve.

Diaphragm type of valves have several advantages, including: (1) the valve seat does not turn and is therefore resistance to scoring, which could cause leakage; (2) no stem leakage can occur because of the diaphragm; and (3) the stem can be opened with a partial rotation rather than with two turns of the wheel as in direct-acting type of valves. Diaphragm valves are generally preferable when pressures are relatively low (i.e., less than 1500 psi). They are also ideal for situations where no gas leaks can be allowed, such as with flammable anesthetics.

Pressure Relief Valves

Figure 2-7 illustrates three types of pressure-relief mechanisms: **rupture disks, fusible plugs**, and **spring-loaded devices.**[1] A rupture disk (also called a frangible disk) is a thin, metal disk that ruptures or buckles when the pressure inside the cylinder exceeds a certain predetermined limit. A fusible plug is made of a metal alloy that melts when the temperature of the gas in the tank exceeds a predetermined temperature. Fusible plugs operate on the principle that as the pressure in a tank increases, the temperature of the gas increases, causing the plug to melt. After the plug melts, excess pressure is released.* Spring-loaded devices are designed to release excessive cylinder pressure and reseal, preventing further release of gas from the cylinder after the cause of the excessive pressure is removed.[1] With these devices, a metal seal is held in place by an adjustable spring. The amount of pressure required to force the seal

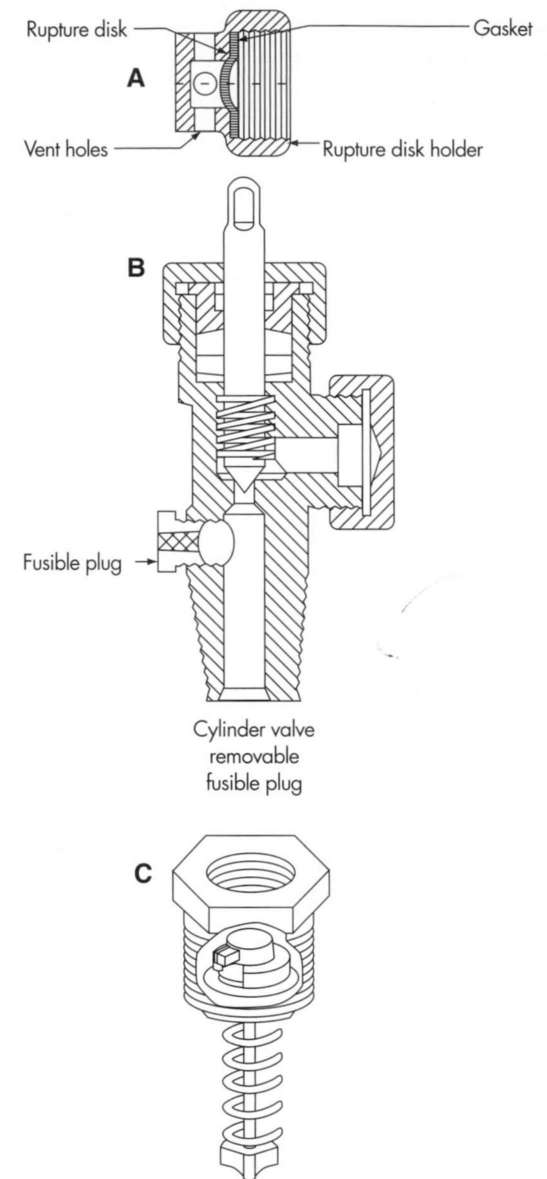

Figure 2-7 Pressure-relief valves: **A,** rupture (frangible) disks; **B,** fusible plug; **C,** spring-loaded device. (Redrawn from Compressed Gas Association: *Handbook of compressed gases*, ed 3, New York, 1990, Van Nostrand Reinhold.)

**A commonly used metal alloy is called Wood's metal; fusible plugs made of this alloy generally have melting temperatures of 208° to 220° F.*

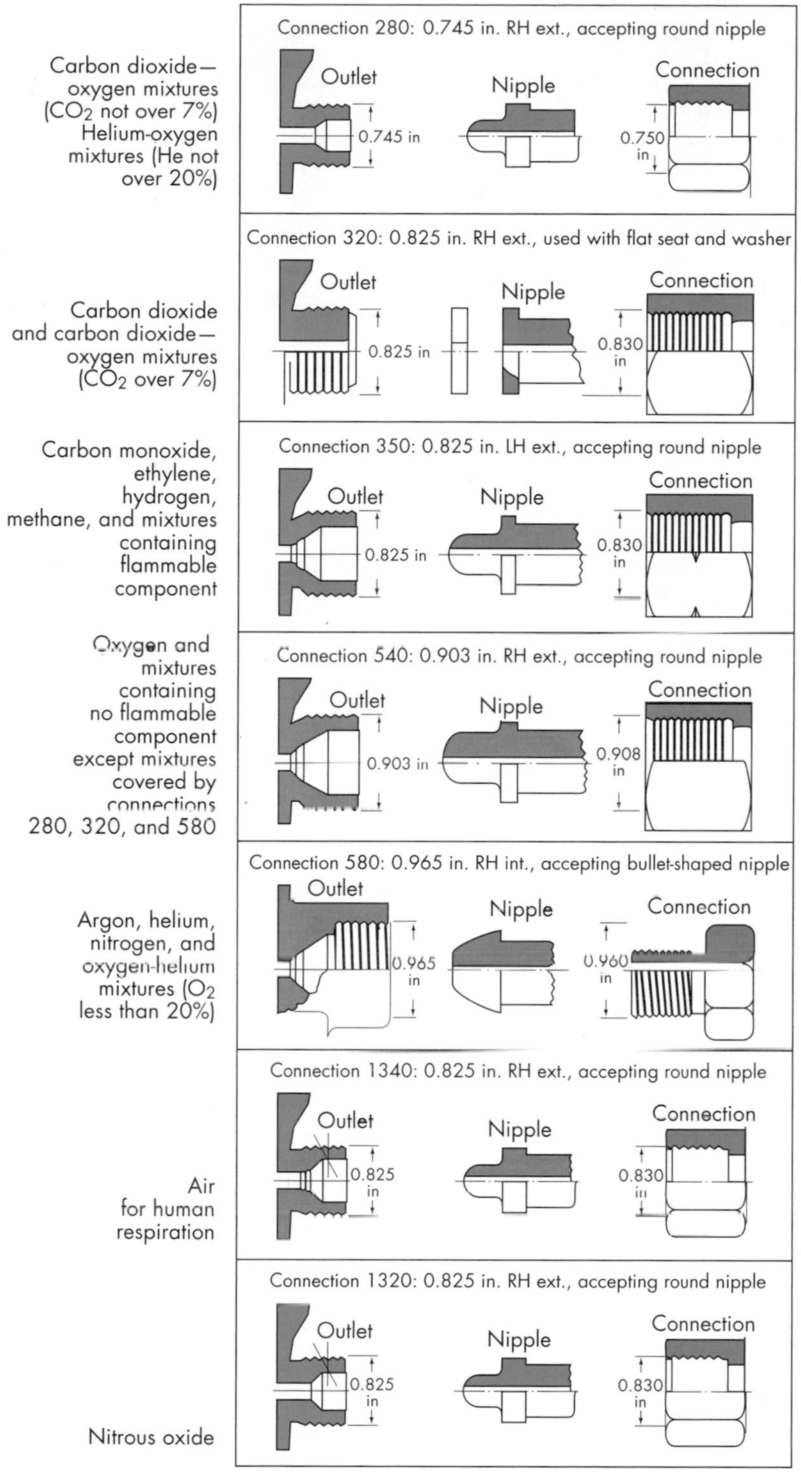

Figure 2-8 American Standard system for large cylinders. (Courtesy Datex-Ohmeda, Madison, Wisc.)

open depends on the tension of the spring holding the metal seal in place. Spring-loaded devices are usually more susceptible to leakage around the metal seal than rupture disks and fusible plugs.[1] Note that spring-loaded devices may also be affected by changes in environmental conditions (i.e., freezing, sticking).

Safety Systems

Outlet connections of cylinder valves are indexed according to standards that were designed by the CGA and adopted by the ASA and the Canadian Standards Association. American Standard connections are noninterchangeable to prevent the interchange of regulating equipment between gases that are not compatible.

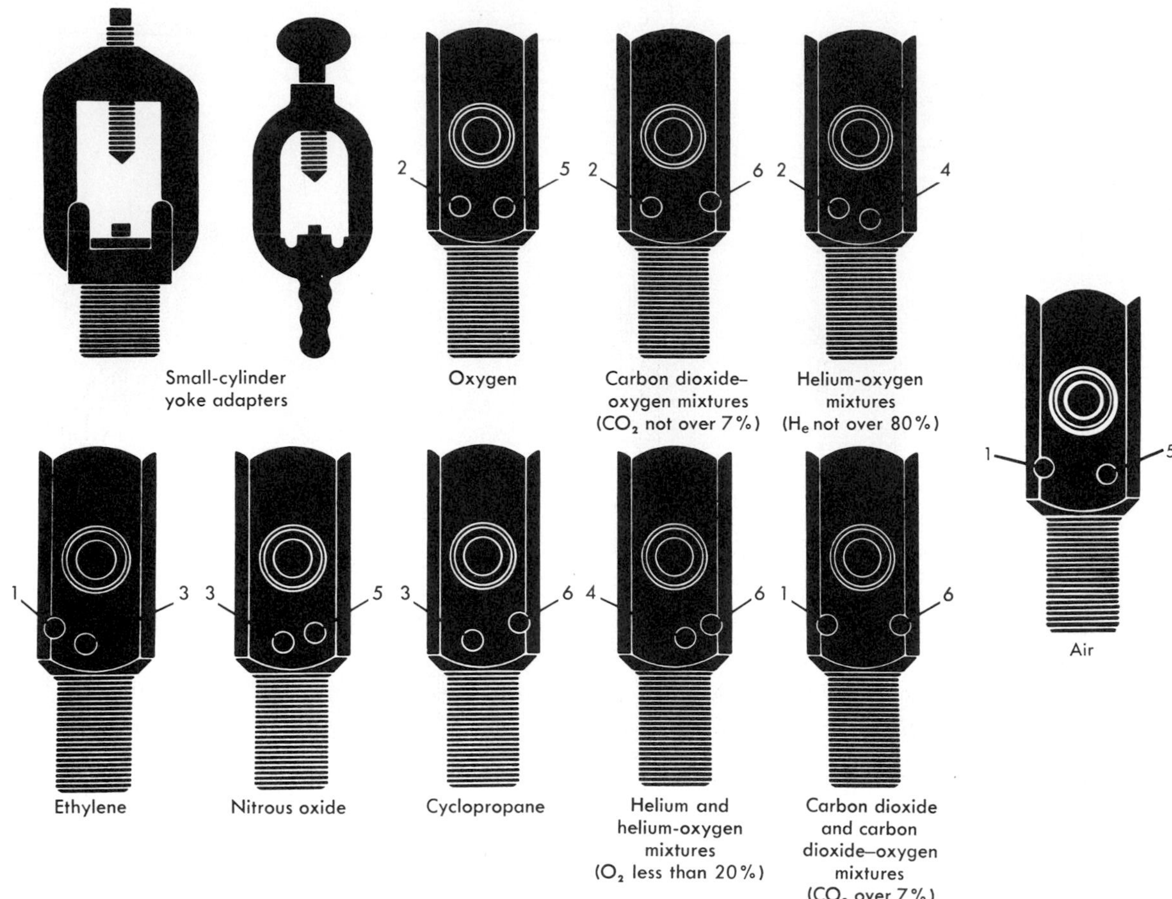

Figure 2-9 PISS system for small cylinders. (Courtesy Datex-Ohmeda, Madison, Wisc.)

American Standard indexing includes separate systems for large and small cylinders. Large cylinder-valve outlets and connections (e.g., for sizes H and K) are indexed by thread type, thread size, right- or left-handed threading, external or internal threading, and nipple-seat design.[12] Figure 2-8 illustrates the American Standard connections for medical gases that are commonly used in respiratory care. Look at the oxygen connection shown in this figure. The diameter of the cylinder's outlet is listed in thousandths of inches (e.g., oxygen connection is 0.903 in). The letters following these numbers indicate the type of threading used (i.e., right-handed [RH] vs. left-handed [LH]). The abbreviations Ext and Int specify whether the threads are external or internal. Note that the connections for oxygen and other life-support gases are right-handed and external. The remaining information indicates if the outlet requires a nipple attachment. Oxygen valves require a rounded nipple.

Small cylinders (e.g., sizes A to E) with post type of valves use a different American Standard indexing called the **Pin Index Safety System (PISS).** In this system, indexing is accomplished by the exact placement of two pins into holes in the post valve. Note that the hole positions are numbered from 1 to 6; each medical gas uses a specified pin sequence. Figure 2-9 shows the different combinations that are used to differentiate the most commonly used medical gases. For example, the pins for an oxygen regulator must be placed in the 2 and 5 positions for it to attach to the oxygen cylinder's post valve. Cylinder regulators will be discussed in Chapter 3.

Setting Up and Troubleshooting of Compressed-Gas Cylinders

Box 2-3 contains the steps that should be followed when setting up a compressed-gas cylinder.[14] The following is a list of simple suggestions that should be kept in mind when handling compressed gas cylinders:

1. Cylinder contents should be clearly labeled. If the contents of a cylinder are questionable, do not use it.
2. Full and empty cylinders should be appropriately labeled and kept separate.
3. Cylinder valves should be fully opened when in use and always closed when the gas contained in the cylinder is not being used. Cylinder valves should be closed if the cylinder is empty.
4. Large cylinders have a protective cap that fits over the valve stem. This cap should be kept on cylinders when moving or storing them. Small cylinders with PISS valve stems do not have protective caps but

Box 2-3 Procedure for Setting up a Compressed-Gas Cylinder

1. Make sure that the cylinder is properly secured.
2. Remove the protective cap or wrap and inspect the cylinder valve to ensure that it is free of dirt, debris, or oil.
3. Alert others nearby that you are about to "crack" the cylinder valve, making a loud noise. Turn the cylinder valve away from anyone present. Then quickly open and close the valve to remove dirt or small debris from the valve outlet.
4. Inspect the inlet of the device to be attached to ensure that it is free of dirt and debris.
5. Securely tighten—but do not force—the device onto the cylinder outlet. Use appropriate wrenches that are free of oil and grease; never use pipe wrenches. Remember to only use cylinder valve connections that conform to ANSI and PISS B57. Low-pressure, threaded connections must comply with DISS or must be noninterchangeable, low-pressure, quick-connecting devices. Never connect fixed or adjustable orifices or metering devices directly to a cylinder without a pressure-reducing valve.
6. Be certain that the regulator or reducing valve is in the closed position, and then slowly open the cylinder valve to pressurize the reducing valve or regulator that is attached. After pressurization has occurred, open the cylinder valve completely and turn it back a quarter- to half-turn to prevent "valve freeze" (i.e., when the valve cannot be turned).

CLINICAL ROUNDS 2-2

A respiratory therapist "cracks" an H cylinder of oxygen and then attaches an oxygen regulator to the cylinder outlet. She slowly opens the valve stem and hears a sudden, loud hissing sound coming from the connection between the cylinder outlet and the regulator. What should she do?

See Appendix A for the answer.

have an outlet seal that must be removed before the appropriate regulator is attached.

5. Regulators and other appliances intended for use with a specific gas should not be used with other gases.
6. Cylinders should be properly secured at all times either in a stand, chained to a wall, or in a cart to prevent them from tipping over.

Most problems encountered with cylinders and regulators involve: (1) gas leakage at the valve stem or in the regulator, and (2) failure to achieve adequate gas flow at the cylinder regulator outlet. Leaks typically occur from large cylinders because of loose connections between the regulator and the cylinder valve. Gas leaks from small cylinders are most often associated with damage to the plastic washer that fits between the valve stem and the regulator. Gas leaks at the regulator outlet can be caused by a loose connection between the regulator and attached equipment. (See Clinical Rounds 2-2.) Failure to achieve a desired gas flow from a cylinder regulator can result from inadequate pressure (e.g., low gauge pressure) or from an obstruction at the regulator outlet.

Table 2-5 Volume-pressure conversion factors

Cylinder Size	Conversion Factor
E	622.0 L/2200 psi = 0.28
G	5269.0 L/2200 psi = 2.41
H to K	6600.0 L/2200 psi = 3.14

Determining the Volume of Gas Remaining in a Cylinder and the Duration of Cylinder Gas Flow

Calculating the gas volume remaining in a cylinder requires knowledge of either the pressure or the weight of the cylinder. (See Table 2-3 for a list of values for commonly used medical gas cylinders.) For nonliquefied gas cylinders (e.g., compressed air, oxygen, helium), the gas volume contained in a cylinder is directly related to the regulator's gauge pressure. Table 2-5 shows these constants, or "tank factors," for the more commonly used medical gas cylinders. The volume of gas remaining in a cylinder can then be calculated by multiplying the cylinder's **volume-pressure constant** by the gauge pressure. Box 2-4 is an example of this calculation. The resultant volume can then be divided by the flow rate of gas being used to determine the duration of gas flow remaining in minutes.

Determining the gas volume remaining in a liquefied gas cylinder (e.g., carbon dioxide and nitrous oxide) is more of a challenge. The gas volume remaining in a liquefied gas cylinder cannot be determined by the method just described because the liquid remains in equilibrium with the gas above it until the liquid is depleted. The volume of liquefied gas remaining is best determined by weighing the cylinder before and after it is filled. Thus the volume of liquid gas remaining in the cylinder is directly related to the weight of the cylinder. After the volume is determined, the duration of gas flow can be calculated by dividing that volume by the flow rate of gas being used.

Liquid Oxygen Systems

Hospitals and larger health care facilities typically rely on bulk liquid supply systems for medical air and oxygen needs. The increased use of bulk liquid supply systems is the result of a couple of factors: (1) gases shipped in bulk are less expensive than gases shipped in cylinders, and (2) liquefied oxygen occupies a fraction of the space required to store

Box 2-4 Estimating the Duration of a Medical Gas Cylinder Supply

The amount of time that it will take a cylinder filled with compressed gas to provide a set flow rate of gas can be calculated with the following formula:

$$\frac{\text{cylinder pressure (psi)} \times \text{cylinder factor*}}{\text{flow rate of gas (L/min)}} = \text{duration of flow in min}$$

Example:

You are asked to transport a patient who is receiving oxygen from a nasal cannula at 4 L/min. The pressure gauge on the cylinder reads 1800 psi. How long will the cylinder provide the appropriate oxygen flow?

$$1800 \text{ psi} \times (0.28) \div 4 \text{ L/min} = 126 \text{ min, or about 2 hours}$$

**The cylinder factor represents the relationship between cylinder volume and gauge pressure. Thus an E cylinder can hold 622 L of gas at a filling pressure of 2200 psi. The volume-pressure cylinder factor for E cylinders equals 622 L/2200 psi, or 0.28 L/psi. Table 2-5 shows the cylinder factors for the several commonly used cylinders.*

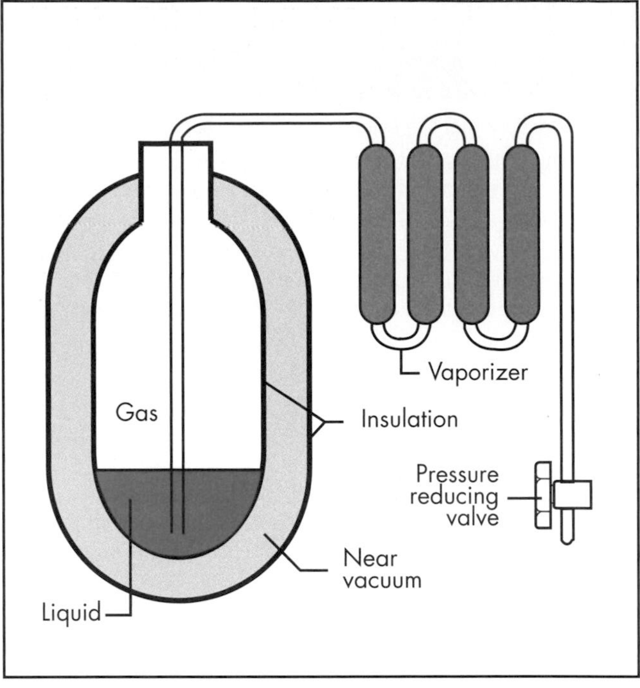

Figure 2-10 Components of a bulk oxygen supply.

gaseous oxygen. Note that gaseous oxygen occupies a volume 860 times that of liquid oxygen.

Construction of bulk gas systems is regulated by the NFPA and the American Society of Mechanical Engineers (ASME). The Bureau of Explosives of the United States Department of the Treasury provides regulations for the design and operation of pressure-release valves.[1,13]

Bulk Liquid Oxygen Systems

The NFPA defines a bulk oxygen system as more than 20,000 ft^3 of oxygen (at atmospheric temperature and pressure), including unconnected reserves, that are on hand at the site.[13] Figure 2-10 illustrates the major components of a bulk oxygen system. It consists of an insulated reservoir, a vaporizer with associated tubing attached to the reservoir, a pressure-reducing valve, and an appropriate pressure-release valve. The reservoir stores a mixture of liquid and gaseous oxygen. The vaporizer acts a heat exchanger where heat is absorbed from the environment and used to warm the liquid oxygen to room temperature, thus forming gaseous oxygen. The pressure-reducing valve serves to reduce the working pressure of the gas to a desired level (usually 50 psi for hospitals and other health care facilities) before it enters the hospital's compressed gas piping system (see Figure 2-20 for a description of piping systems). The pressure-release valve allows some of the gas on top of the liquid to escape if the contents are warmed too much. This release of gas allows the gas within the container to expand, thus lowering the temperature (see Gay-Lussac's law in Chapter 1). This maintains the gas under pressure between its boiling point and its critical temperature so that the majority of the reservoir's contents will be maintained in the liquid state.

As previously stated, bulk reservoir systems must meet specifications provided by the NFPA.[13] Appendix 2-1 contains a summary of the NFPA recommendations and regulations for bulk oxygen systems. Proper installment of these systems is critical to maintain public safety. Figure 2-11 illustrates the minimum distances between bulk oxygen storage facilities and other structures.

Portable Liquid Oxygen Systems

Smaller versions of the bulk oxygen system are available for home-care settings. Figure 2-12 illustrates the Linde PC 500/Walker unit (Union Carbide). Figure 2-13 shows the Linde/Walker portable unit. The main unit contains a liquid reservoir, a vaporizer coil, and a pressure-relief valve. The smaller, portable device, which has a similar design, is filled from the main unit. Most portable systems are designed to provide a working pressure of 20 psi. The Linde unit, however, can provide a working pressure of 90 psi.

Bulk systems used in home care can provide an economical source of oxygen for patients requiring long-term oxygen therapy. These systems generally can provide a reliable source of oxygen for 4 to 6 weeks, depending on the demand. Portable units can provide an 8- to 12-hour supply of oxygen for patients during times of greater mobility. As will be

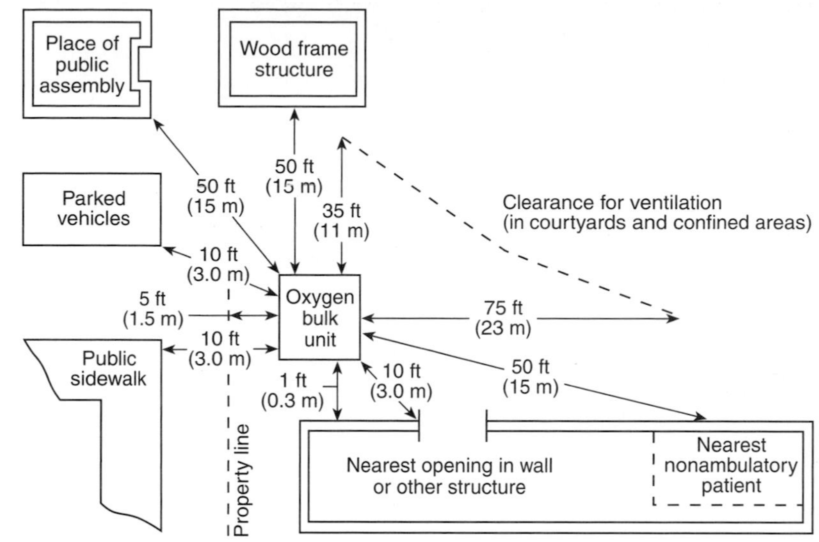

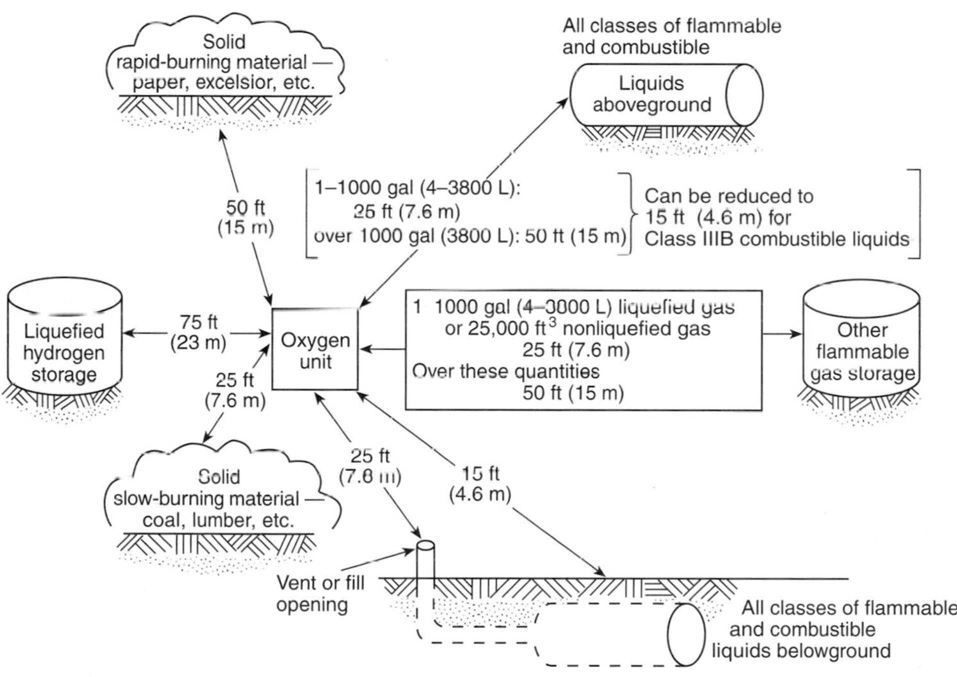

Figure 2-11 Minimum distances for locating structures around a bulk oxygen supply.

discussed in Chapter 3, oxygen-conserving devices can increase the amount of time that these smaller systems can provide oxygen. Box 2-5 shows how to calculate the duration of a liquid oxygen supply. Remember that the amount of time that a supply will last depends on the weight of the liquid remaining in the reservoir—not the pressure, as for cylinders. Because 1 L of liquid oxygen weighs 2.5 lb, the number of liters of liquid oxygen present can be calculated by dividing the weight of the liquid oxygen by 2.5. Considering that oxygen expands to 860 times its liquid

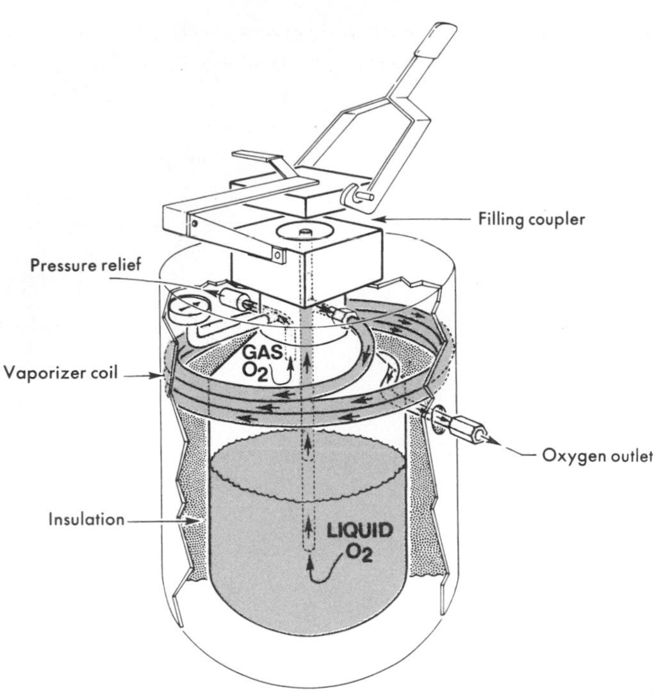

Figure 2-12 Linde PC500/Walker liquid oxygen system. (Modified from Lampton LM: Home and outpatient oxygen therapy. In Brasher RE, Rhodes MI, editors: *Chronic obstructive lung disease*, St Louis, 1978, Mosby.)

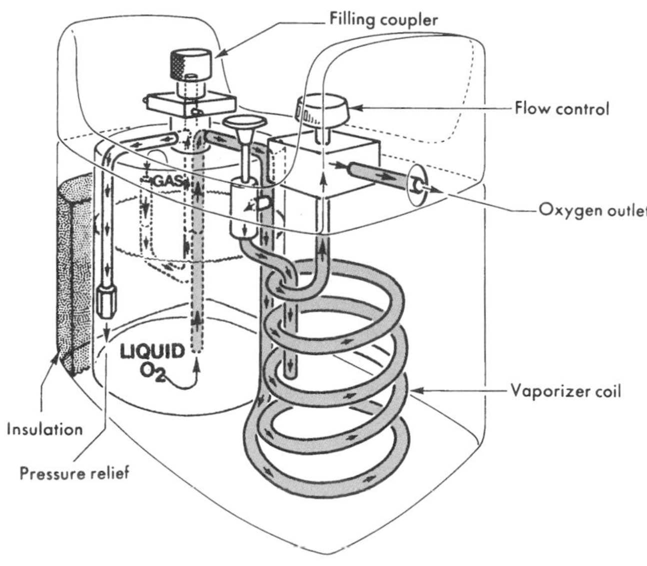

Figure 2-13 Linde/Walker portable liquid oxygen unit. (Modified from Lampton LM: Home and outpatient oxygen therapy. In Brasher RE, Rhodes MI, editors: *Chronic obstructive lung disease*, St Louis, 1978, Mosby.)

volume at 25° C and 1 atm, the total volume of gaseous oxygen available can be calculated by multiplying the number of liters of liquid oxygen by 860. Then the amount of time in minutes that the supply will last can be determined by dividing this volume by the flow rate of the gas being delivered.

Box 2-5 Calculating the Duration of a Liquid Oxygen Supply

1. A liter of liquid oxygen weighs 2.5 lb, so:
   liquid weight ÷ 2.5 = # of liters of liquid oxygen.
2. Gaseous oxygen occupies a volume that is 860 times the volume of liquid oxygen, so:
   liters of liquid × 860 = liters of gas.
3. Duration of supply (minutes) = gas supply remaining (in liters) ÷ flow (liters/minute).

Example:

How long would a liquid oxygen supply weighing 10 lb last if a patient were receiving oxygen through a nasal cannula at 2 L/min?

Amount of gas (liters) = (10 lb ÷ 2.5 lb/L) × 860

Amount of gas = 3440 L

Duration of supply (minutes) = amount of gas ÷ flow (in liters)

Duration of supply = 3440 L ÷ (2 L/min)

Duration of supply = 1720 min,

or about 28 hours and 40 min

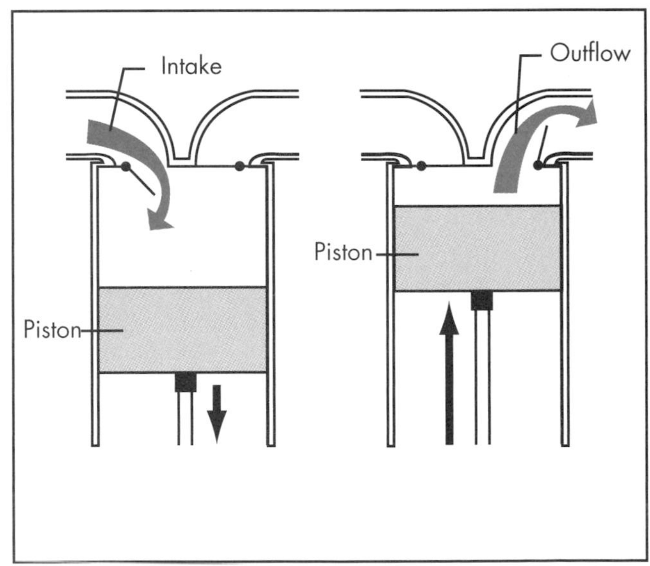

Figure 2-14 Piston air compressor.

It is important to know the operating pressure of the device before attaching flowmeters or restrictors to control gas flow out of the system. Failure to recognize the actual delivery pressure of these devices can result in injury to the patient or damage to the attached equipment. The actual flow delivered can be determined with a **calibrated Thorpe-tube flowmeter** (see Chapter 3 for a discussion of flowmeters). Appendix 2-3 lists the NFPA safety recommendations for portable oxygen systems.

Medical Air Supply

Portable Air Compressors

Compressed air is used to power many respiratory care devices. In many cases, air can be compressed at the point of administration by portable air compressors. Larger portable systems can produce compressed air with a standard working pressure of 50 psi; these units can therefore be used to power devices such as pneumatically powered ventilators. Smaller portable compressors, which are unable to achieve these high working pressures, are used for bedside applications (e.g., powering small-volume nebulizers).

Three types of compressors are currently available: piston, diaphragm, and rotary units. **Piston compressors** use the action of a motor-driven piston to compress atmospheric air. The piston is seated within a cylinder casing and is sealed to it with a carbon or Teflon ring. Figure 2-14 illustrates the operational principle of a typical piston air

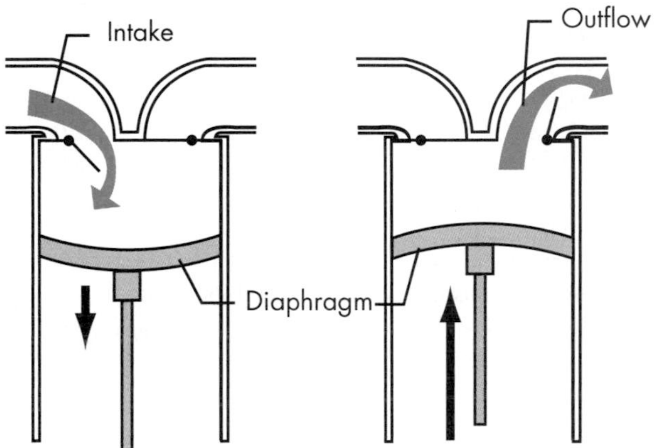

Figure 2-15 Diaphragm compressor.

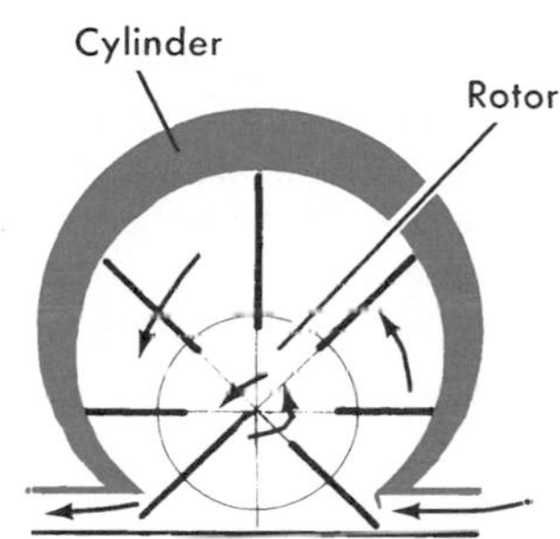

Figure 2-16 Rotary compressor.

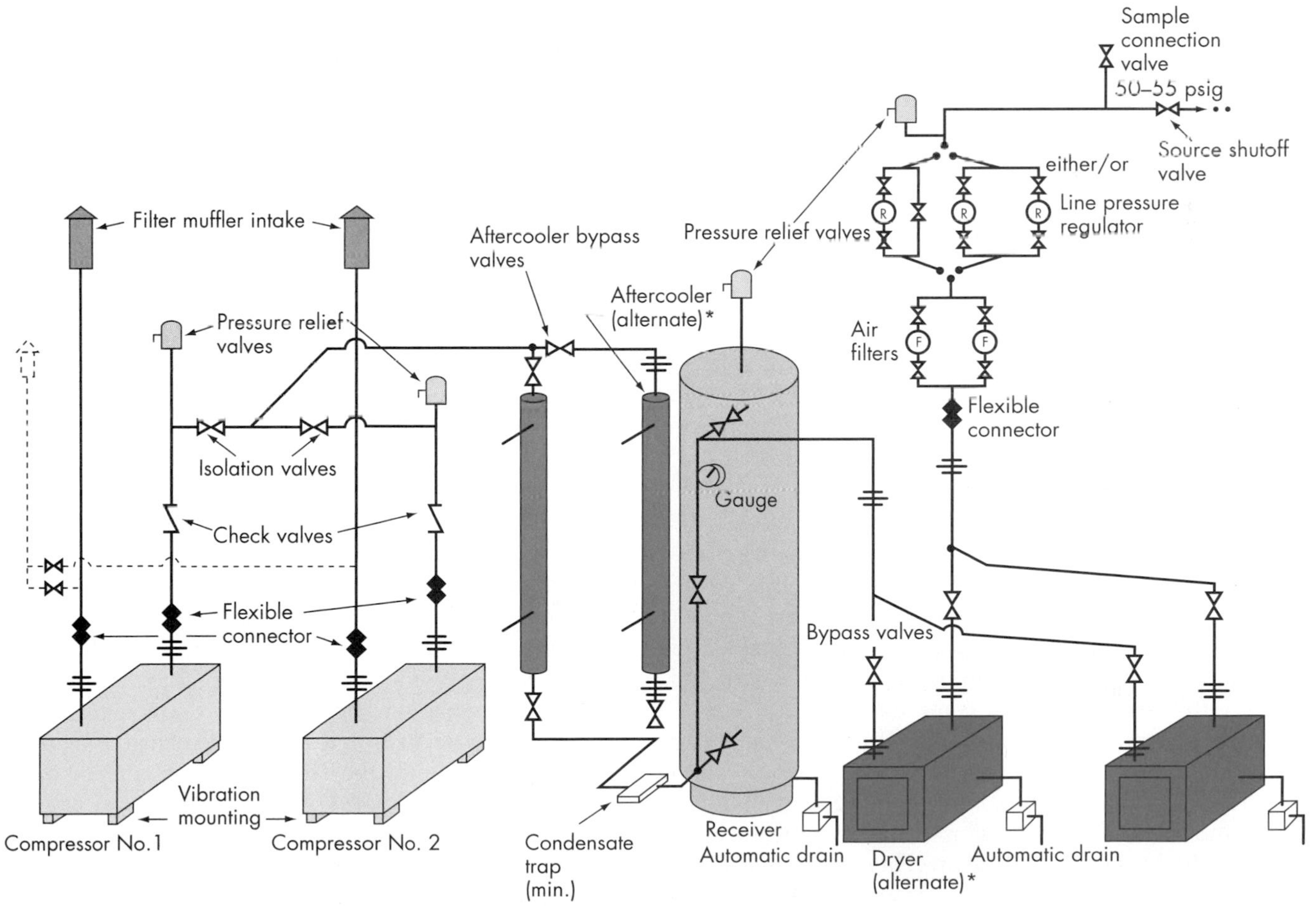

Figure 2-17 Bulk medical air supply. (Modified from *Standard for health care facilities,* [NFPA99], 1996, copyright National Fire Protection Association, Quincy, Mass.)

Box 2-6 NFPA Recommendations for Medical Air Supply

1. The source of medical air must be from the outside atmosphere and should not contain contaminants such as particulate matter, odor, or other gases.
2. The air-intake port must be located outdoors, above roof level, at a minimum distance above the ground, and 10 ft from any door, window, or other intake opening in the building. Intake ports must be turned downward and screened.
3. Air taken into the system must contain no contamination from engine exhaust, fuel storage vents, vacuum system discharges, or other particulate matter because odor of any type can be drawn into the system.
4. A minimum of two oil-free compressors must be duplexed together, with provisions for operating alternately or simultaneously, depending on the demand. Each compressor or duplex must be capable of maintaining the air supply to the system at peak demand.
5. Backflow through compressors that are cycled off must be prevented automatically.
6. Each duplex system should be provided with disconnection switches, motor-starting devices with overload protection, and a means of automatically alternating the compressor(s). Use of the compressors should be divided evenly and automatic means of activating additional compressor(s) should be provided in case the supply source unit becomes incapable of maintaining adequate pressure.
7. Air storage tanks or receivers must have a safety valve, an automatic drain, a pressure gauge, and the capacity to ensure practical on-off operation.
8. The type of medical air compressor and the local atmospheric conditions govern the need for intake filters/mufflers, after-coolers for air dryers, and additional downstream regulators.
9. Antivibration mountings are to be installed (in accordance with manufacturer's recommendations) under the components and flexible couplings that connect the air compressors, receivers, and intake and supply lines.
10. A maintenance program must be established following the manufacturer's recommendations.

From Compressed Gas Association: Handbook of compressed gases, *ed 3, New York, 1990, Van Nostrand Reinhold.*

compressor used to power a mechanical ventilator. As the piston retracts, atmospheric air is drawn in through a one-way intake valve. When the piston protracts, the intake valve closes, and gas leaves through a one-way outflow valve. A small gas reservoir is placed in a coiled tube to allow the hot, compressed gas to cool to room temperature before it is delivered to the output valve. The reservoir also removes some of the humidity from the intake gas. There is usually a water drain near the compressor's output, and it is recommended that a water trap be placed between the output and the device to be attached to the compressor to avoid problems with moisture accumulation. Examples of portable piston compressors include the Bennett MC-1 and MC-2 compressors, the Ohio High Performance Compressor, and the Timemeter PCS-1 units.

Diaphragm compressors (Figure 2-15) use a flexible diaphragm attached to a piston to compress gas. As the piston moves down, the diaphragm is bent outward, and gas is drawn through a one-way valve into the cylinder. Upward movement of the piston forces the gas out of the cylinder through a separate one-way outflow valve. Examples of diaphragm compressors are the Air Shields Diapump and the DeVilbiss small nebulizer compressor.

Rotary compressors use a rotating vane to compress air from an intake valve. As the rotating vane turns, gas is drawn into the cylinder through a one-way valve (Figure 2-16). While the rotor turns, the gas is compressed as the oval-shaped cylinder becomes smaller. The compressed gas is then forced out of the compressor through another one-way outflow valve. Low-pressure, rotary compressors are used in ventilators such as the Bennett MA-1.

Bulk Air Supply Systems

Bulk systems of compressed air for hospitals and other health care facilities can be supplied by a system like the one shown in Figure 2-17. Most bulk air systems use two compressors that can operate together or independently, depending on the demand for compressed air. Each compressor should also be able to deliver 100% of the average peak demand if the other compressor is turned off for maintenance or fails to operate. Box 2-6 summarizes the NFPA recommendations for safely operating medical air-supply systems.

Air compressors used in bulk supply systems are usually piston or rotary compressors. Large piston compressors can typically provide a high-flow output and working pressures of at least 50 psi. A reservoir is incorporated into the design of the compressor unit to accommodate varying peak flow needs. The reservoir receives the compressed air and stores it at a higher pressure than in the piping system. A dryer attached to the outflow of the reservoir removes humidity (from refrigeration) from the air entering the piping system. A reducing valve on the reservoir outflow line reduces the pressure to 50 psi or the desired working pressure. In most cases, a pneumatic sensing unit turns the compressor off when the reservoir pressure reaches a preset high level. This sensing unit also turns the compressor back on when the reservoir pressure falls below 50 psi.

High-pressure rotary units require a liquid sealant to efficiency produce high pressures. These systems typically include a reservoir for storing gas under high pressure, a dryer to remove humidity, and a pressure-relief valve to control the output pressure of the compressed gas. A

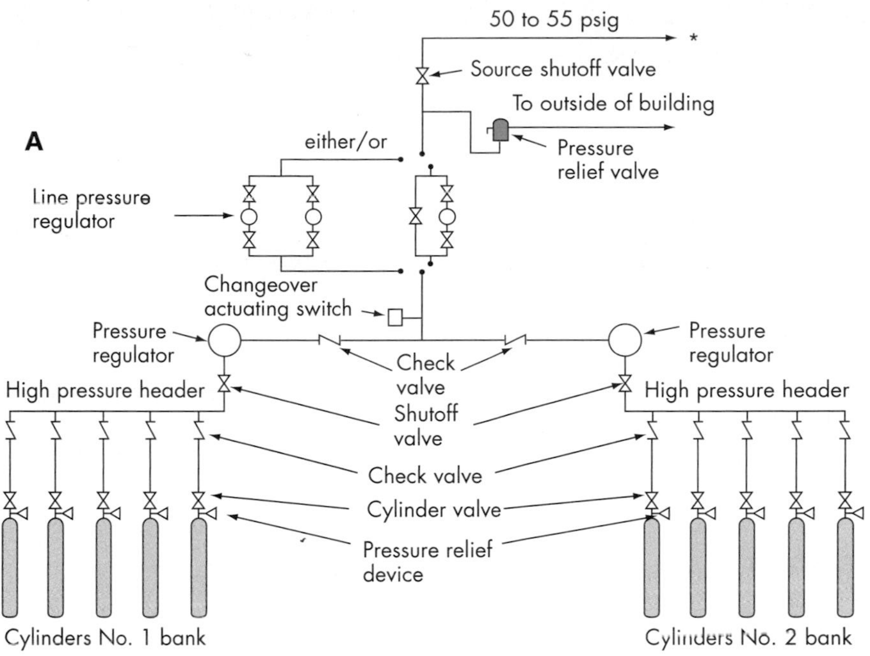

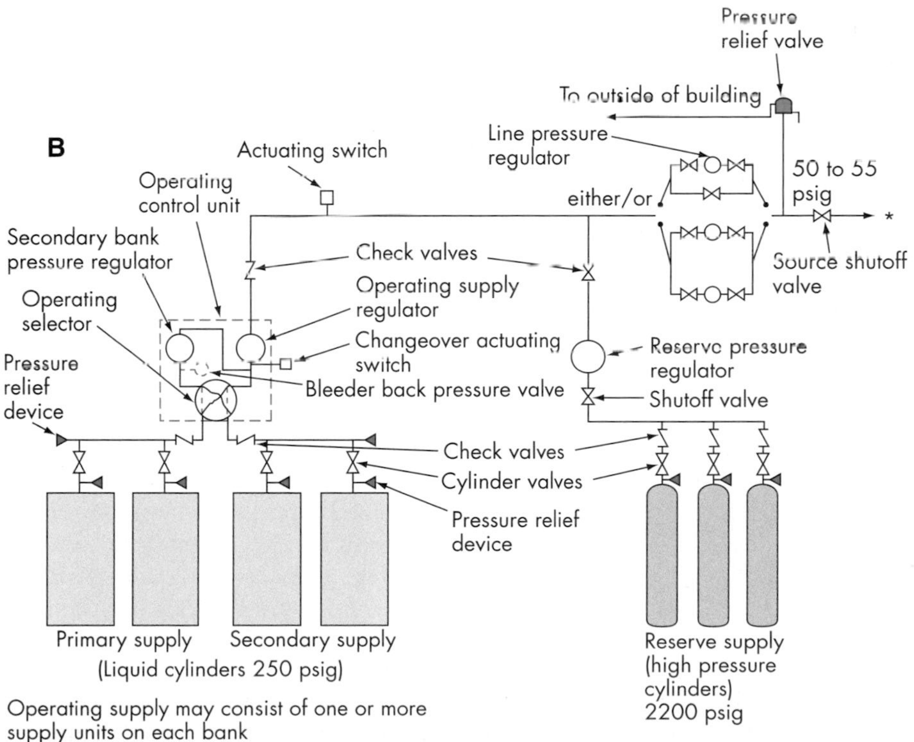

Figure 2-18 Alternating supply systems for medical air or oxygen: **A,** alternating supply without reserve supply; **B,** alternating supply with primary and secondary cylinders. (Modified from Standard for health care facilities, [NFPA99], 1996, copyright National Fire Protection Association, Quincy, Mass.)

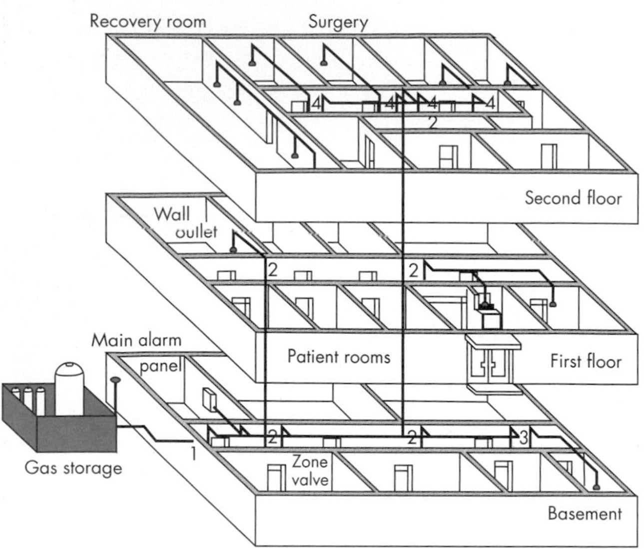

Figure 2-19 Hospital piping system. Zone valves must be placed (1) at the entrance to the hospital, (2) at each riser, (3) at each branch supplying an area, and (4) at each operating room. (Courtesy Nellcor Puritan Bennett, Pleasanton, Calif.)

pneumatic sensing unit such as those used in piston type of compressors is also used to maintain a constant working pressure of 50 psi and avoid unnecessary high pressures.

Central Supply Systems

Hospitals and other health care facilities, such as freestanding clinics, rehabilitation centers, and diagnostic laboratories, typically rely on central-supply systems to provide medical gases to multiple sites within the institution.

Large hospitals usually rely on continuous supply systems. A continuous-supply system contains two sources of gas supply, one of which serves as a reserve source for use only in an emergency.[13] The primary source is usually a large liquid oxygen or air reservoir, whereas the reserve supply is a smaller liquid reservoir or a bank of compressed-gas cylinders. The primary source must be refilled at regular intervals. NFPA regulations require that the reserve supply contain an average day's supply of oxygen. The NFPA also requires that these systems include a pressure regulator, **check valves,** and a pressure-relief valve between each gas supply and main piping system.

Alternating-supply systems usually consist of two banks of cylinders, one designated as the primary source and the other as the secondary source. Each bank of cylinders must contain a minimum of two cylinders or at least an average day's supply of oxygen or air. After the primary source is depleted or unable to meet system demands, the secondary system automatically becomes the primary source of oxygen or air. The empty bank is simply refilled or replaced. As a safety feature, an actuating switch must be connected to the master control panel to indicate when the change to the secondary bank is about to occur.[13] Check valves are installed between each cylinder and the manifold to prevent the loss of gas from the manifold cylinders in the event the pressure-relief devices on an individual cylinder functions or a cylinder lead fails.

Figure 2-18 illustrates an alternating system that contains liquid oxygen cylinders as the primary and secondary oxygen sources, along with a reserve oxygen supply of compressed-gas cylinders. The reserve supply is used only when the primary and secondary sources are unable to supply system demands.[13] Note that the system must contain check valves and pressure-relief devices between the gas source and the main supply line. As with the previously described alternating system, an actuating switch signals when the changeover from the primary to the secondary source occurs.

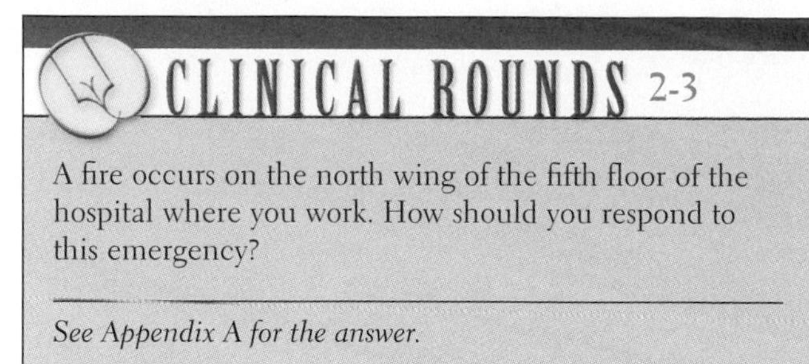

CLINICAL ROUNDS 2-3

A fire occurs on the north wing of the fifth floor of the hospital where you work. How should you respond to this emergency?

See Appendix A for the answer.

Piping Systems

Gases stored in central-supply units are distributed to various sites or zones within a hospital or health care facility via a piping system such as the one shown in Figure 2-19. NFPA regulations govern the construction, installation, and testing of these systems.[13] Pipes used to transport gases must be seamless type K or L (ASTMB-8) copper tubing or standard weight brass pipe. The size of the pipes must be sufficient to maintain proper delivery volumes and to conform to good engineering practices. The gas contents of the pipeline must be labeled at least every 20 ft and at least once in each room or story through which the pipeline travels.

Pressure-regulating devices located between the bulk and the main supply lines must be capable of maintaining a minimum delivery pressure of 50 psi to all station outlets at the maximum delivery-line flow. Pressure-relief valves should be installed downstream from the mainline pressure regulator. A pressure-relief valve should also be installed upstream of any zone valve to prevent excessive pressure in a zone where the shutoff valve is closed. All pressure-relief valves are set 50% higher than the system working pressure (e.g., 75 psi for a 50-psi system pressure).

As previously stated, piping systems in hospitals are organized into zones, which allow for quick isolation of all independent areas if maintenance is required. In case of fire, affected zones can be isolated, thus preventing the problem from spreading to other areas of the hospital (See

Clinical Rounds 2-3). Shutoff valves are located at the point where the mainline enters the hospital, at each riser, and between each zone and the main supply line. Zone shutoff valves for oxygen must be located outside of each critical care unit. Shutoff valves for every oxygen or nitrous oxide line must also be located outside of each surgical suite.

Shutoff valves are generally located in a large box with removable windows large enough to permit manual operation of the valve. They should be installed at a height where they can be operated from the standing position in an emergency. All valves must be labeled as shown in Figure 2-20.

Piping systems must be tested for leaks and to ensure that gas-supply lines have not become crossed. Visual inspection of the system can identify obvious problems, such as worn or loose connections, damaged pipes, pipes soiled with oil, grease, or other oxidizable materials, and crossing of gas supplies (e.g., crossing of compressed air and oxygen supply lines). Crossing of supply lines can be checked by reducing the system pressure to atmospheric and then purging each supply line separately with oil-free dry air or nitrogen. It can also be determined if the gas lines are crossed by analyzing gas samples from the appropriate station outlets. Gases used to purge the supply lines should be passed through a white filter at a flow of 100 L/min to determine if the purge gas is clean and odor-free. The content of gas lines should be tested for purity with the appropriate gas analysis.

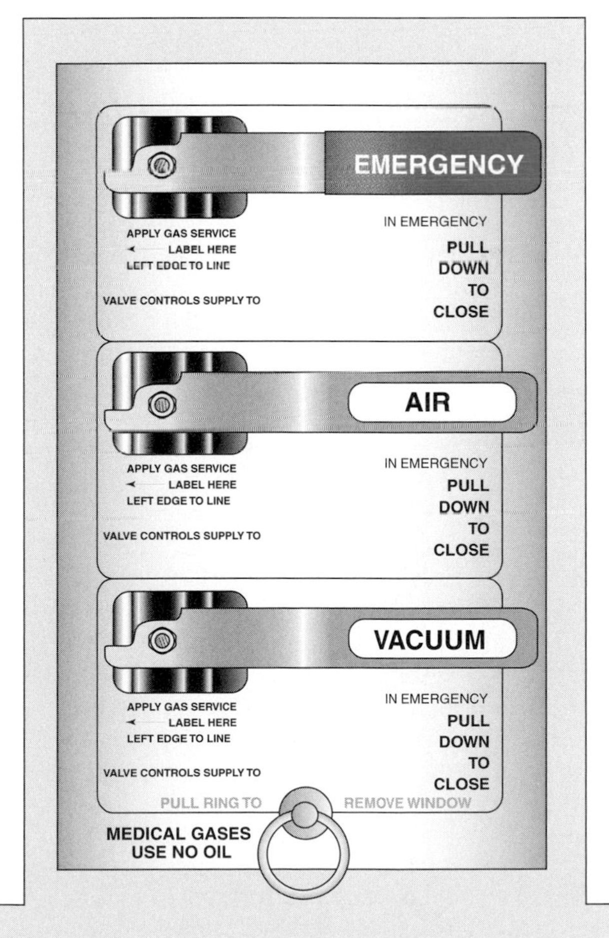

Figure 2-20 Zone shutoff valves for a bulk oxygen supply.

All medical gas supply lines should contain alarm systems that alert hospital personnel of system malfunctions (e.g., loss of system pressure, change from the primary system supply source to the secondary and reserve supplies, and reduction in reserve supply below an average day's amount). Alarm panels should include visual and audible alerting signals and should be placed in locations that allow for continuous surveillance (e.g., in the engineering department of the hospital). Alarm systems should also be located in critical care areas where life-support systems such as mechanical ventilators are used. The Joint Commission on Accreditation of Healthcare Organizations requires that there is a written policy for responding to alarms and that personnel working in areas where alarms are located are instructed on how to respond.[14] Failure to respond appropriately can end in disaster. Response plans should include ensuring that all patient equipment is working properly and that appropriate personnel (i.e., respiratory care services and engineering) are immediately notified.

Station Outlets

Station outlets provide connections for gas-delivery devices, such as flowmeters and mechanical ventilators. These outlets consist of a body mounted to the supply line, an outlet faceplate, and primary and secondary check valves, which are safety valves that open when the delivery device's adapter is inserted into the station outlet and which close automatically when the adapter is disengaged from the outlet. Station outlets must not be supplied directly from a riser unless they are supplied through the manual shutoff valve located in the same story as the outlet. Outlet faceplates must be labeled with the name or symbol of the delivered gas. They may also be color-coded for easy identification.

Station outlets are designed with safety systems that prevent connection of incompatible devices. Two safety systems are currently available: the **Diameter Index Safety System (DISS)** and **quick-connect adapters.** Figure 2-21 shows an outlet that uses DISS. This system, which was designed by the CGA, uses noninterchangeable, threaded fittings to connect gas-powered devices to station outlets. Each outlet must be fitted with a cap on a chain or installed in a recessed box that is equipped with a door to protect the outlet when not in use. Outlets are typically located about 5 ft above the floor or are recessed to prevent physical damage to the valve or control equipment. Delivery lines that serve anesthetic devices must have a backflow of gas into the system, and the check valves must be able to hold a minimum of 2400 psi.[1,13,15]

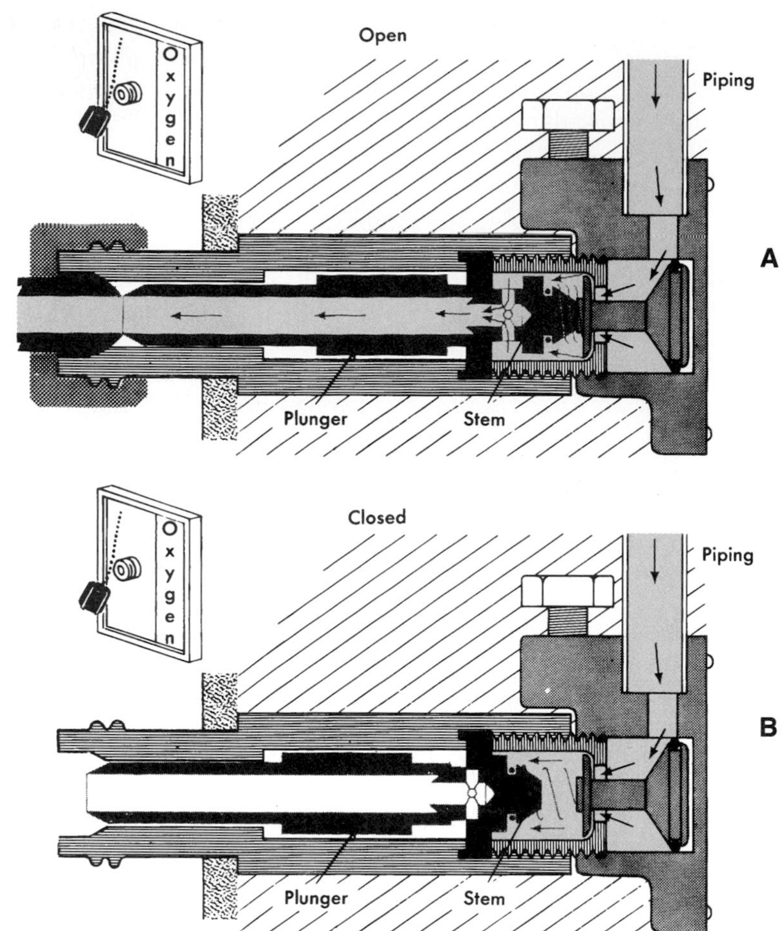

Figure 2-21 Station outlets for a DISS system. (Courtesy Nellcor Puritan Bennett, Pleasanton, Calif.)

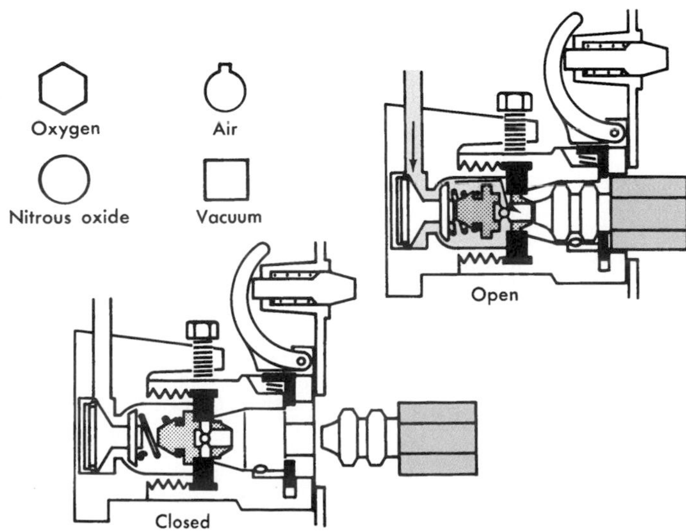

Figure 2-22 Schematic of typical quick-connect type of connection. (Courtesy Nellcor Puritan Bennett, Pleasanton, Calif.)

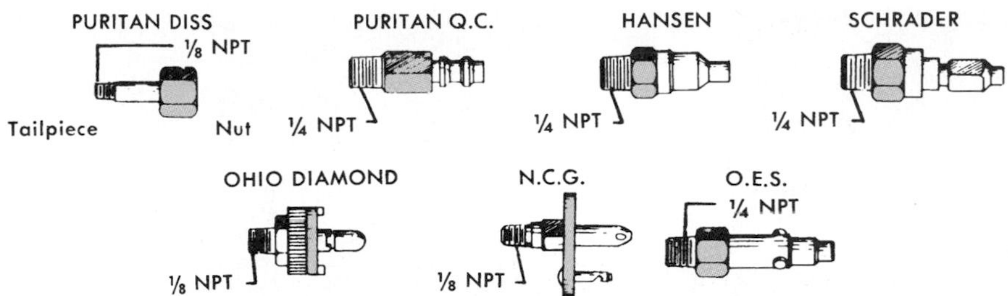

Figure 2-23 Common types of quick-connect adapters. (Courtesy Nellcor Puritan Bennett, Pleasanton, Calif.)

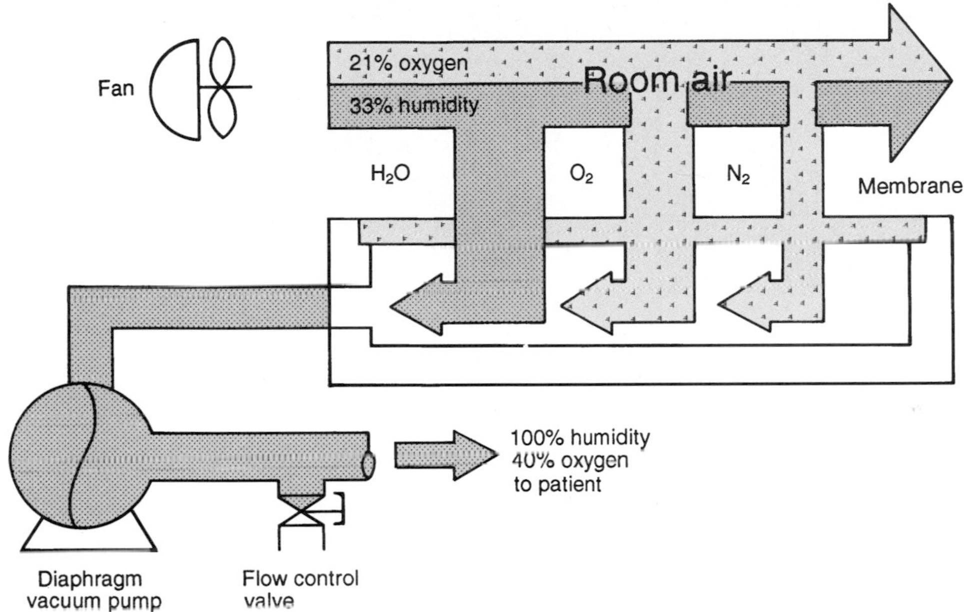

Figure 2-24 Oxygen concentrator that uses semipermeable membrane. (Courtesy Oxygen Enrichment Co, Schenectady, NY.)

Figure 2-22 shows a schematic of a quick-connect type of connection, and Figure 2-23 shows examples of quick-connect adapters. These connections use a plunger that is held forward by a spring to prevent gas from leaving the outlet. Inserting the appropriate adapter pushes the plunger backward, allowing gas to flow into the striker and into the equipment that is attached to the adapter. When the adapter is removed, the spring resets the plunger and closes the outlet.

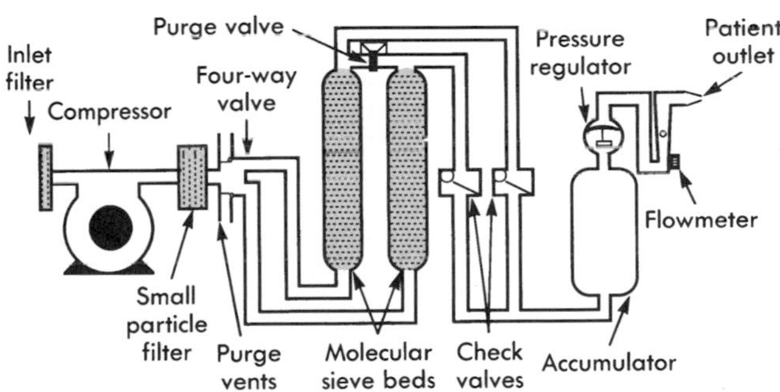

Figure 2-25 Oxygen concentrator that relies on a molecular sieve.

Oxygen Concentrators

Oxygen concentrators are devices that produce enriched oxygen from atmospheric air. They provide an alternative to compressed-gas cylinders, particularly in the delivery of respiratory therapy to home-care patients. Two types of concentrators are currently available: those using semipermeable plastic membranes and those using molecular sieves.

Concentrators using semipermeable membranes to separate oxygen from room air are composed of plastic membranes containing pores that are 1 μm in diameter (1 μm = 1/25,000 in). Atmospheric gases diffuse through the membrane at different rates. The rate at which a gas diffuses depends on its diffusion constant and solubility for the plastic membrane and the pressure gradient for the gas across the membrane. A diaphragm compressor is used to provide a constant vacuum across the membrane.

Oxygen and water vapor diffuse through these membranes faster than nitrogen. Generally, a constant flow of humidified 40% oxygen can be provided for 1 to 10 L/min.[16] Figure 2-24 is a functional diagram of an oxygen concentrator that uses a semipermeable membrane.

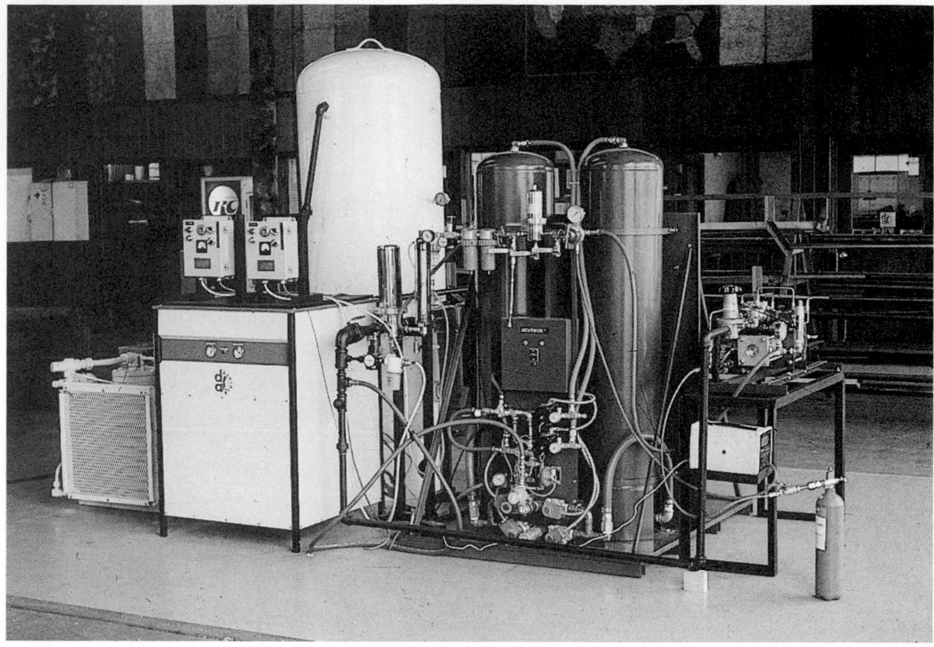

Figure 2-26 Large oxygen concentrator for producing bulk oxygen for a hospital. (Courtesy Dri-Aire, Columbus, Calif.)

Figure 2-25 shows an oxygen concentrator that relies on molecular sieves to produce an enriched oxygen mixture. Such systems use a compressor to pump room air at pressures of 15-25 psig to one of two sets of sieves. Nitrogen is removed by passing room air through sodium-aluminum silicate (zeolite) pellets producing an enriched oxygen mixture. It is important to mention that nitrogen and other gases absorbed by the zeolite pellets must be purged to ensure that the unit functions properly. In the **pressure swing adsorption (PSA) method,** intermittent pressurization of one of the sieve beds occurs while the other bed is purged to remove any absorbed gases and moisture.

The concentration of oxygen leaving the system depends on the flow rate set. For example, at flows less than 6 L/min, the gas contains about 92%-97% oxygen.[8] Note that flowmeters calibrated for low inlet pressures must be used to assure accurate delivery of oxygen to the patient because the outlet pressure from these concentrators is approximately 5 to 10 psig. The DeVilbiss 303 DS/DZ and 515 DS/DZ oxygen concentrators are examples of molecular sieve concentrators.

Figure 2-26 is a picture of a large concentrating system for producing enriched oxygen mixtures in bulk. This system contains a compressor that supplies air to a refrigerated drying system. Gas exits the refrigeration unit and passes through a 0.015-μm filter. Part of the air flows through a molecular sieve bed at 120 psi. The resulting gas that leaves the molecular sieve contains 92% to 95% oxygen. Air and oxygen are reduced to 50 psi and stored in reservoir tanks. These systems are available for smaller hospitals and for recharging oxygen cylinders on site.

Summary

The information contained in this chapter represents some of the basic principles of respiratory care. Respiratory care practitioners are responsible for administering medical gases and therefore must know the standards for the manufacture, storage, and transport of such gases. These standards provide guidelines for safely using medical gases in the diagnosis and treatment of patients with cardiopulmonary dysfunctions.

Compressed-gas cylinders and bulk gas supplies provide the source gas for the operation of many respiratory care devices. Oxygen concentrators have added another dimension to the home treatment of patients with chronic cardiovascular and pulmonary diseases. Respiratory care practitioners should understand the theory of operation of medical gas supply systems and be able to identify malfunctions that can interfere with the proper delivery of medical gases.

Review Questions

See Appendix A for answers.

1. Which of the following is classified as a nonflammable gas that does not support combustion?
   a. Oxygen
   b. Carbon dioxide
   c. Helium
   d. Nitric oxide

2. Medical gas cylinders are color-coded for easy identification. E cylinders of carbon dioxide are painted:
   a. yellow
   b. green
   c. black
   d. gray

3. A respiratory therapist is having trouble attaching a regulator to an E cylinder. One possible cause might be that the:
   a. outlet threads of the cylinder do not match the threads of the regulator
   b. regulator diaphragm is jammed
   c. pin positions of the regulator are not the same as the cylinder
   d. cylinder has not been cracked

4. Bulk liquid oxygen supplies should not be closer than ________ to public sidewalks.
   a. 2 ft
   b. 4 ft
   c. 7 ft
   d. 10 ft

5. Calculate the duration of the liquid oxygen supply if the liquid supply weighs 30 lb and the oxygen demand is 4 L/min.
   a. 10 hours
   b. 23 hours
   c. 35 hours
   d. 43 hours

6. What is the duration of oxygen flow from an H cylinder containing 1200 psi of oxygen when the flow to a nasal cannula is 4 L/min?
   a. 9 hours, 42 minutes
   b. 12 hours, 15 minutes
   c. 15 hours, 42 minutes
   d. 16 hours, 10 minutes

7. Large-piston air compressors employed in bulk supply systems can typically provide working pressures of:
   a. 50 psi
   b. 75 psi
   c. 100 psi
   d. 120 psi

8. Alternating supply systems for medical gases that are used in hospitals should include a reserve supply for oxygen in case the primary system fails. How much reserve oxygen should be available?
   a. An average 8-hour supply
   b. An average day's supply
   c. An average 3-day supply
   d. An average week's supply

9. Oxygen concentrators that use semipermeable membranes can usually provide what percentage of oxygen at flows of 1 to 10 L/min?
   a. 24%
   b. 40%
   c. 60%
   d. 100%

10. The percentage of oxygen delivery provided by molecular sieve O_2 concentrators depends on which of the following factors?
   I. The size of the concentrator
   II. The rate of gas flow
   III. The temperature of the refrigeration unit
   IV. The age of the sieve beds
   a. II only
   b. I and IV only
   c. I, II, and III only
   d. I, II, and IV only

11. The pressure inside a cylinder increases dramatically when the cylinder is exposed to extremely high temperatures. What prevents cylinders with frangible discs from exploding when exposed to extremely high temperatures?
   a. The frangible disc will rupture from the increased pressure, allowing gas to escape from the cylinder
   b. The cylinder stem will blow off when the temperature reaches 200° F
   c. The stem diaphragm will rupture, allowing gas to escape
   d. The frangible disc will melt when the temperature reaches 100° F

12. A respiratory therapist is checking cylinder markings to determine if any of the cylinders need to be tested. The labeling reads as follows:
   9 83+
   6 94+
   This information indicates:
   a. The cylinder is due for retesting
   b. The time between the test dates shown exceeds recommendations
   c. The cylinder is made of aluminum
   d. The owner of the cylinder

13. Before using an H cylinder of oxygen, a respiratory therapist opens it, and gas at high pressure comes out of the cylinder outlet. Which of the following statements is true?
   a. This was an accident and should not be repeated
   b. Allowing gas to escape from the cylinder lets the therapist smell the gas to ensure it is oxygen
   c. This action clears debris from the connector
   d. This action should be performed after a regulator is attached to the cylinder outlet

14. A respiratory therapist is helping design a new hospital wing. Which of the following agencies should be contacted so that the piping system of oxygen and air is correctly installed?
   a. NFPA
   b. USFDA
   c. HHS
   d. DOT

15. A hospital uses a large air compressor system to supply air through its piped gas lines. This gas will be free from pollutants found in the local environment-true or false? Why?

References

1. Compressed Gas Association, Inc: *Handbook of compressed gases,* ed. 4, New York, 1999, Van Nostrand Reinhold.
2. Dorsch JA, Dorsch SE: *Understanding anesthesia equipment: construction, care, and complications,* ed 4, Baltimore, 1999, Williams & Wilkins.
3. Howder C: *Cardiopulmonary pharmacology,* ed 2, Baltimore, 1996, Williams & Wilkins.
4. Scanlan CL, Spearman CB, Sheldon RL: *Egan's fundamentals of respiratory care,* ed 7, St Louis, 1999, Mosby.
5. Rau J: *Respiratory care pharmacology,* ed 6, St Louis, 2001, Mosby.
6. Kinsella JP, et al: Clinical response to prolonged treatment of persistent pulmonary hypertension of the newborn with low doses of inhaled nitric oxide, *J Pediatr* 123(1):103, 1993.
7. Gerlach H, et al: Long term inhalation with evaluated low doses of nitric oxide for improvement of oxygenation in patients with adult respiratory distress syndrome, *Intensive Care Med* 19(8):443, 1993.
8. Hess D, MacIntyre N, Adams A, et al: *Respiratory care: principles and practice,* Philadelphia, 2002, WB Saunders.
9. Schreiber P: *Anesthetic equipment,* New York, 1972, Springer-Verlag.
10. McPherson S: *Respiratory care equipment,* ed 5, St Louis, 1995, Mosby.
11. Code of Federal Regulations: Title 49, Parts 1-199, Washington, DC, 1974, US Government Printing Office.
12. National Fire Protection Association: *Standard for health care facilities,* New York, 2002, ANSI/NFPA 99.
13. Blaze C: *Quick reference to respiratory care equipment assembly and troubleshooting,* St Louis, 1995, Mosby.
14. Klein BR, editor: *Health care facilities handbook,* ed 4, Quincy, Mass, 1993 National Fire Protection Association.
15. Lampton LM: Home and outpatient oxygen therapy. In Harchear RE, Rhodes MI, editors: *Chronic obstructive lung disease: clinical treatment and management,* St Louis, 1978, Mosby.
16. Kacmarek RM: Delivery systems for long-term oxygen therapy, *Respir Care* 45(1):84, 2000.

Internet Resources

American Association for Respiratory Care: http://www.aarc.org

Compressed Gas Association: http://www.cganet.com

GasNet—Global Anesthesiology Server Network: http://gasnet.med.yale.edu

Joint Commission on Health Care Organizations: http://www.jcaho.org

Mallinckrodt: http://www.mallinckrodt.com

National Fire Protection Association: http://www.nfpa.org

Ohmeda Medical: http://www.ohmedamedical.com

US Food and Drug Administration: http://www.fda.gov

Appendix 2-1

NFPA and CGA Recommendations for Cylinders

Storage

1. Storage rooms must be dry, cool, and well-ventilated. Cylinders should not be stored in an area where the temperature exceeds 51.67° C (125° F).
2. No flames should have the potential of coming in contact with the cylinders.
3. The storage facility should be fire-resistant where practical.
4. Cylinders must not be stored near flammable or combustible substances.
5. Those gases supporting combustion must be stored in a separate location from those that are combustible.
6. The storage area must be permanently posted.
7. Cylinders must be grouped by content.
8. Full and empty cylinders must be segregated in the storage areas.
9. Below-ground storage should be avoided.
10. Cylinders should never be stored in the operating room.
11. Large cylinders must be stored upright.
12. Cylinders must be protected from being cut or abraded.
13. Cylinders must be protected from extreme weather to prevent rusting, excessive temperatures, and accumulations of snow and ice.
14. Cylinders should not be exposed to continuous dampness or corrosive substances that could promote rusting of the cylinder and its valve.
15. Cylinders should be protected from tampering.
16. Valves on empty cylinders should be kept closed at all times.
17. Cylinders must be stored with protective caps in place.
18. Cylinders must not be stored in a confined space, such as a closet or the trunk of a car.

Transportation

1. If protective valve caps are supplied, they should be used whenever cylinders are in transport and until they are ready for use.
2. Cylinders must not be dropped, dragged, slid, or allowed to strike each other violently.
3. Cylinders must be transported on an appropriate cart secured by a chain or strap.

Use

1. Before connecting equipment to a cylinder, be certain that connections are free of foreign materials.
2. Turn valve outlet away from personnel, and crack cylinder valve to remove any dust or debris from outlet.
3. Cylinder valve outlet connections must be American Standard or CGA pin indexed, and low-pressure connections must be CGA diameter indexed.
4. Cylinders must be secured at the administration site and not to any movable objects or heat radiators.
5. Outlets and connections must only be tightened with appropriate wrenches and must never be forced on.
6. Equipment designed to use one gas should not be used with another.
7. Never use medical cylinder gases when contamination by backflow of other gases may occur.
8. Regulators should be off when the cylinder is turned on, and the cylinder valve should be opened slowly.
9. Before equipment is disconnected from a cylinder, the cylinder valve should be closed and the pressure released from the device.
10. Cylinder valves should be closed at all times, except when in use.
11. Do not transfill cylinders because this is hazardous.
12. Cylinders may be refilled only if permission is secured from the owner.
13. Cylinders must not be lifted by the cap.
14. Equipment connected to cylinders containing gaseous oxygen should be labeled: OXYGEN—USE NO OIL.
15. Enclosures intended to contain patients must have the minimum text regarding NO SMOKING and the labels must be located (1) in a position to be read by the patients and (2) on two or more opposing sides visible from the exterior. It should be noted that oxygen hoods fall under the classification of oxygen

enclosures and require these labels as well. In addition, another label is required that instructs visitors to get approval from hospital personnel before placing toys into an oxygen enclosure.

16. High-pressure oxygen equipment must not be sterilized with flammable agents (for example, alcohol and ethylene oxide), and the agents used must be oil-free and nondamaging.
17. Polyethylene bags must not be used to wrap sterilized high-pressure oxygen equipment because when flexed, polyethylene releases pure hydrocarbons that are highly flammable.
18. Oxygen equipment exposed to pressures of less than 60 psi may be sterilized with either a nonflammable mixture of ethylene oxide and carbon dioxide or with fluorocarbons.
19. Cylinders must not be handled with oily or greasy hands, gloves, or clothing.
20. Never lubricate valve outlets or connecting equipment. (Oxygen and oil under pressure cause an explosive oxidation reaction.)
21. Do not flame test for leaks. (Usually a soap solution is used.)
22. When in use, open valve fully and then turn it back a quarter- to a half-turn.
23. Replace cap on empty cylinder.
24. Position the cylinder so that the label is clearly visible. The label must not be defaced, altered, or removed.
25. Check label before use; it should always match the color code.
26. No sources of open flames should be permitted in the area of administration. A NO SMOKING sign must be posted at the administration site. It must be legible from a distance of 5 ft and displayed in a conspicuous location.
27. Inform all area occupants of the hazards of smoking and of the regulations.
28. Equipment designated for use with a specific gas must be clearly and permanently labeled accordingly. The name of the manufacturer should be clearly marked on the device. If calibration or accuracy is dependent on gas density, the device must be labeled with the proper supply pressure.
29. Cylinder carts must be of a self-supporting design with appropriate casters and wheels, and those intended for use in surgery where flammable anesthetics are used must be grounded.
30. Cold cylinders must be handled with care to avoid hand injury resulting from tissue freezing caused by rapid gas expansion.
31. Safety-relief mechanisms, uninterchangeable connections, and other safety features must not be removed or altered.
32. Control valves on equipment must be closed both before connection and when not in use.

Repair and Maintenance

1. Use only the service manuals, operator manuals, instructions, procedures, and repair parts that are provided or recommended by the manufacturer.
2. Allow only qualified personnel to maintain the equipment.
3. Designate and set aside an area clean and free of oil and grease for the maintenance of oxygen equipment. Do not use this area for the repair and maintenance of other types of equipment.
4. Follow a scheduled preventive maintenance program.

Appendix 2-2

NFPA Recommendations and Regulations for Bulk Oxygen Systems

1. Containers that are permanently installed should be mounted on noncombustible supports and foundations.
2. Liquid oxygen containers should be constructed from materials that meet the impact test requirements of paragraph UG-48 of the ASME Boiler and Pressure Vessel Codes, Section VII, and must be in accordance with DOT specifications and regulations for 4 L liquid oxygen containers. Containers operating above 15 psi must be designed and tested in accordance with the ASME Boiler and Pressure Vessel Code, Section VII, and the insulation of the liquid oxygen container must be of noncombustible material.
3. All high pressure gaseous oxygen containers must comply with the construction and test requirements of ASME Boiler and Pressure Vessel Code, Section VIII.
4. Bulk oxygen storage containers must be equipped with safety-release devices as required by ASME Code IV and the provisions of ASME S-1.3 or DOT specifications for both the container and safety releases.
5. Isolation casings on liquid oxygen containers shall be equipped with suitable safety-release devices. These devices must be designed or located so that moisture cannot either freeze the unit or interfere in any manner with its proper operation.
6. The vaporizing columns and connecting pipes shall be anchored or sufficiently flexible to provide for expansion and contraction as a result of temperature changes. The column must also have a safety-release device to properly protect it.
7. Any heat supplied to oxygen vaporizers must be done in an indirect fashion, such as with steam, air, water, or water solutions that do not react with oxygen. If liquid heaters are used to provide the primary source of heat, the vaporizers must be electrically grounded.
8. All equipment composing the bulk system must be cleaned to remove oxidizable material before the system is placed into service.
9. All joints and connections in the tubing should be made by welding or using flanged, threaded slip, or compressed fittings; and any gaskets or thread seals must be of suitable substance for oxygen service. Any valves, gauges, or regulators placed into the system must be designed for oxygen service. The piping must conform to ANSI B 31.3; piping that operates below –20° F must be composed of materials meeting ASME Code, Section VIII.
10. Storage containers, piping valves, and regulating equipment must be protected from physical damage and tampering.
11. Any enclosure containing oxygen control or operating equipment must be adequately ventilated.
12. The location shall be permanently posted to indicate "OXYGEN—NO SMOKING—NO OPEN FLAMES" or an equivalent warning.
13. All bulk systems must be regularly inspected by qualified representatives of the oxygen supplier.
14. Weeds and tall grass must be kept a minimum of 15 ft from any bulk oxygen container. The bulk oxygen system must be located so that its distance provides maximum safety for other areas surrounding it. The minimum distances for location of a bulk oxygen system near the following structures (Figure 2-11) are as follows:
    a. 25 ft from any combustible structure.
    b. 25 ft from any structure that consists of fire-resistant exterior walls or buildings of other construction that have sprinklers.
    c. 10 ft from any opening in the adjacent walls of fire-resistant structures.
    d. 25 ft from flammable liquid storage above ground that is less than 1000 gallons in capacity, or 50 ft from these storage areas if the quantity is in excess of 1000 gallons.
    e. 15 ft from an underground flammable liquid storage that is less than 1000 gallons, or 30 ft from one in excess of 1000 gallons capacity. The distance from the oxygen storage containers to connections used for filling and venting of flammable liquid must be at least 25 ft.

f. 25 ft from combustible gas storage above ground that is less than 1000 gallons capacity, or 50 ft from the storage of over 1000 gallons capacity.
g. 15 ft from combustible liquid storage underground and 25 ft from the vent or filling connections.
h. 50 ft from flammable gas storage less than 5000 ft^3; 90 ft from flammable gas in excess of 5000 ft^3 NTP.
i. 25 ft from solid materials that burn slowly (e.g., coal and heavy timber).
j. 75 ft away in one direction and 35 ft away at an approximately 90-degree angle from confining walls unless they are made from a fire-resistant material and are less than 20 ft high. (This is to provide adequate ventilation in the area in case venting occurs.)
k. 50 ft from places of public assembly.
l. 50 ft from nonambulatory patients.
m. 10 ft from public sidewalks.
n. 5 ft from any adjoining property line.
o. Must be accessible by a mobile transport unit that fills the supply system.

15. The permanent installation of a liquid oxygen system must be supervised by personnel familiar with the proper installation and construction as outlined in the NFPA 50.
16. The oxygen supply must have an inlet for the connection of a temporary supply in emergency and maintenance situations. The inlet must be physically protected to prevent tampering or unauthorized use and must be labeled: "EMERGENCY LOW-PRESSURE GASEOUS OXYGEN INLET." The inlet is to be installed downstream from the main supply line shutoff valve and must have the necessary valves to provide the emergency supply of oxygen as well as isolate the pipeline to the normal source of supply. There must be a check valve in the main line between the inlet connection and the main shutoff valve and another check valve between the inlet connection and the emergency supply shutoff valve. The inlet connection must have a pressure-relief valve of adequate size to protect the downstream piping from pressures in excess of 50% above normal pipeline operating pressure.
17. The bulk oxygen system must be mounted on noncombustible supports and foundations.
18. A surface of noncombustible material must extend at least 3 ft beyond the reach of liquid oxygen leaks during system operation or filling. Asphalt or bitumastic paving is prohibited. The slope of the area must be considered in the sizing of the surface.
19. The same type of surface must extend at least the full width of the vehicle that fills the bulk unit and at least 8 ft in the transverse direction.
20. No part of the bulk system should be underneath electrical power lines or within reach of a downed power line.
21. No part of the system can be exposed to flammable gases or to piping containing any class of flammable or combustible liquids.
22. The system must be located so as to be readily accessible to mobile supply equipment at ground level as well as to authorized personnel.
23. Warning and alarm systems are required to monitor the operation and condition of the supply system. Alarms and gauges are to be located for the best possible surveillance, and each alarm and gauge must be appropriately labeled.
24. The master alarm system must monitor the source of supply, the reserve (if any), and the mainline pressure of the gas system. The power source for warning systems must meet the essentials of NFPA 76A.
25. All alarm conditions must be evaluated, and necessary measures taken to establish or ensure the proper function of the supply system.
26. Two master alarm panels, with alarms that cannot be canceled, are to be located in separate locations to ensure continuous observation. One signal must alert the user to a changeover from one operating supply to another, and an additional signal must provide notification that the reserve is supplying the system.
27. If check valves are not installed in the cylinder leads and headers, another alarm signal should be initiated when the reserve reaches a 1-day supply.
28. All piping systems must have both audible and visible signals that cannot be canceled to indicate when the mainline pressure increases or decreases 20% from the normal supply pressure. A pressure gauge must be installed and appropriately labeled adjacent to the switch that generates the pressure alarm conditions.
29. All warning systems must be tested before being placed in service or being added to existing service. Periodic retesting and appropriate recordkeeping are required.

Appendix 2-3

NFPA Safety Recommendations and Regulations for Portable Liquid Oxygen Systems

1. Liquid oxygen units will vent gas when not in use, creating an oxygen-enriched environment. This can be particularly hazardous in the following situations:
   a. When the unit is stored in a closed space.
   b. When the unit is tipped over.
   c. When the oxygen is transferred to another container.
2. Liquid oxygen units should not be located adjacent to heat sources, which can accelerate the venting of oxygen.
3. The unit surface should not be contaminated with oil or grease.
4. Verify the contents of liquid containers when setting up the equipment, changing the containers, or refilling the containers at the home.
5. Connections for containers are to be made with the manufacturer's operating instructions.
6. The patient and family must be familiar with the proper operation of the liquid devices along with all precautions, safeguards, and troubleshooting methods.
7. Transfill one unit from another in compliance with CGA pamphlet P-26, "Transfilling of Low Pressure Liquid Oxygen to be Used for Respiration," and in accordance with the manufacturer's operating instructions.
8. All connections for filling must conform to CGA V-1, and the hose assembly must have a pressure release set no higher than the container's rated pressure.
9. Liquid containers must have a pressure release to limit the container pressure to the rated level, and a device must also be incorporated to limit the amount of oxygen introduced into a container to the manufacturer's specified capacity.
10. Delivery vehicles should be well-vented to prevent the buildup of high oxygen levels, and transfilling should take place with the delivery vehicle doors wide open.
11. "No smoking" signs must be posted, and there can be no sources of ignition within 5 ft.
12. The transfiller must affix the labels required by DOT and FDA regulations, and records must be kept stating the content and purity. Instructions must be on the container, and the color-coding and labeling must meet CGA and NFPA standards.
13. All devices used with liquid oxygen containers must be moisture-free, and pressure releases must be positioned correctly to prevent freezing and the buildup of high pressures.
14. When liquid oxygen is spilled, both the liquid and gas that escape are very cold and will cause frostbite or eye injury. When filling liquid oxygen containers, wear safety goggles with side shields, along with loose-fitting, properly insulated gloves. High-top boots with cuffless pants worn outside of the boots are recommended.
15. Items exposed to liquid oxygen should not be touched because they cannot only cause frostbite, but can stick to the skin. Materials that are pliable at room temperature become brittle at the extreme temperatures of liquid oxygen.
16. If a liquid oxygen spill occurs, the cold liquid and resulting gas condense the moisture in the air, creating a fog. Normally, the fog will extend over an area that is larger than the area of contact danger, except in extremely dry climates.
17. In the event of a spill, measures should be taken to prevent anyone from walking on the surface or wheeling equipment across the area for at least 15 minutes. All sources of ignition must be kept away from the area.
18. Liquid oxygen spilled onto asphalt or oil-soaked concrete constitutes an extreme hazard because an explosive reaction can occur.
19. If liquid oxygen or gas comes in contact with the skin, remove any clothing that may constrict blood flow to the frozen area. Warm the affected area with water at about body temperature until medical personnel arrive. Seek immediate medical attention for eye contact or blistering of the skin.
20. Immediately remove contaminated clothing and air it away from sources of ignition for at least an hour.

Chapter 3

Administering Medical Gases: Regulators, Flowmeters, and Controlling Devices

J.M. Cairo

Chapter Outline

Chapter Learning Objectives

Upon completion of this chapter, the reader should be able to:

1. Compare the design and operation of single-stage and multistage regulators.
2. Identify the components of preset and adjustable regulators.
3. Explain the operational theory of a Thorpe-tube flowmeter, a Bourdon flowmeter, and a flow restrictor.
4. Demonstrate a method for determining if a flowmeter is pressure-compensated.
5. Compare low-flow and high-flow oxygen delivery systems.
6. Name several commonly used low-flow oxygen delivery systems.
7. Discuss the advantages and disadvantages of oxygen-conserving devices.
8. Explain the operational theory of air-entrainment devices.
9. Compare the operation of oxygen blenders with that of oxygen mixers and adders.
10. Describe the physiologic effects of hyperbaric oxygen therapy.
11. List the indications and contraindications of nitric oxide therapy.
12. Describe the appropriate use of mixed-gas (e.g., heliox, carbogen) therapy.

Key Terms

Adjustable, Multiple-Orifice Flow Restrictors
Adjustable Regulators
Back Pressure-Compensated
Boothby-Lovelace-Bulbulian (BLB) Mask
Bourdon Flowmeters
Carbogen
Fixed-Performance Oxygen Delivery System
Fixed-Orifice Flow Restrictors
Fixed-Performance Devices
Flow-Restrictor Multistage Regulators
Flow Restrictors
French
Heliox
Monoplace Hyperbaric Chamber
Multiplace Hyperbaric Chamber
Multistage Regulators
Mustache Cannula
Non—Pressure-Compensated
Oxygen Adder
Oxygen Blender
Pendant Cannula
Pulse-Demand Oxygen Delivery System
Preset Regulators
Pressure-Compensated
Single-Stage Regulators
Thorpe-Tube Flowmeters
Variable-Performance Oxygen Delivery System

Administering medical gases is one of the primary responsibilities of respiratory therapists. This responsibility stems from work that began in several eighteenth-century physiology laboratories and came to fruition in the clinical settings of the middle of the 20th century. Barcroft, Davies and Gilchrist, Barach, Petty, and others made significant contributions to the theory and practice of oxygen therapy by designing apparatuses to deliver oxygen to dyspneic patients.[1,2] Cogent studies performed by these and other scientists demonstrated the value of oxygen therapy and laid the foundation for respiratory care professions.

As the responsibilities of respiratory therapists continue to grow, all practitioners must understand the principles of oxygen therapy, as well as other forms of medical gas therapy, including nitric oxide and hyperbaric oxygen therapy. Therefore, this chapter will review the operational principles of devices commonly used to administer medical gases.

Regulators and Flowmeters

Regulators (or reducing valves) are devices that reduce high-pressure gases from cylinders or bulk storage units to lower working pressures, usually to 50 psi. Flowmeters are devices that control and indicate the gas flow delivered to patients.

Regulators

Regulators are generally classified as **single-stage** or **multistage.** They can be further divided into **preset** and **adjustable regulators.** Preset regulators deliver a specific outlet pressure; adjustable regulators can deliver a range of outlet pressures.

Single-Stage Regulators

Figure 3-1 shows the components of a typical preset single-stage regulator, which consists of a body that is divided in half by a flexible metal diaphragm. The area above the diaphragm is a high-pressure chamber. The lower chamber has a spring attached to the lower surface of the diaphragm and is exposed to ambient pressure. A valve stem attached to the upper half of the diaphragm sits on the high-pressure inlet to the upper chamber. Note that excess pressures in the upper chamber can be released through a pressure-relief valve that opens if the regulator malfunctions and the pressure inside the high-pressure chamber rises to 200 psig.

The gas flow into the high-pressure side of the regulator is dependent upon the effects of two opposing forces: gas pressure above the diaphragm and spring tension below the diaphragm. When the force offered by the high-pressure gas above the diaphragm equals the force offered by spring tension, the diaphragm is straight and the inlet valve is closed. If the force offered by the spring exceeds the force offered by the gas pressure, the spring expands the diaphragm and opens the inlet valve.

For a preset single-stage regulator, the spring tension is calibrated to deliver gas at a preset pressure (usually 50 psig). Adjustable regulators such as the one in Figure 3-2 allow the operator to adjust the spring tension (and thus control the outlet pressure) by using a threaded hand control attached to the spring-diaphragm apparatus. Most adjustable regulators can be set to deliver pressures between 0 and 100 psig.

Multistage Regulators

Multistage regulators are simply two or more single-stage regulators in a series. Figure 3-3 is a schematic of a two-stage regulator. Notice that the tension of the spring in the first stage of the regulator is usually preset by the manufacturer, but the spring tension in the second stage is typically adjustable. Each stage of the regulator contains a pressure-relief valve to release excess pressure if there is a malfunction in either stage. (The number of stages of a regulator can be determined by counting the number of pressure-relief valves on the regulator.)

Multistage regulators operate on the principle that gas pressure is gradually reduced as gas flows from a high-pressure source through a series of stages to the outlet. For example, gas from a compressed cylinder (e.g., 2200 psig) enters the first stage of a two-stage regulator, and the gas pressure is reduced to an intermediate pressure (e.g., 700 psig). This lower pressure gas then enters into the second stage of the regulator, where the gas pressure is further reduced to the desired working pressure (e.g., 50 psig) before the gas reaches the outlet.

Multistage regulators can control gas pressures with more precision than single-stage regulators because the pressure is gradually reduced. Additionally, multistage regulators produce gas flow that is much smoother than that from single-stage regulators. Multistage regulators are more expensive and larger than single-stage regulators, so they are usually reserved for tasks requiring precise gas flow (e.g., for research purposes).

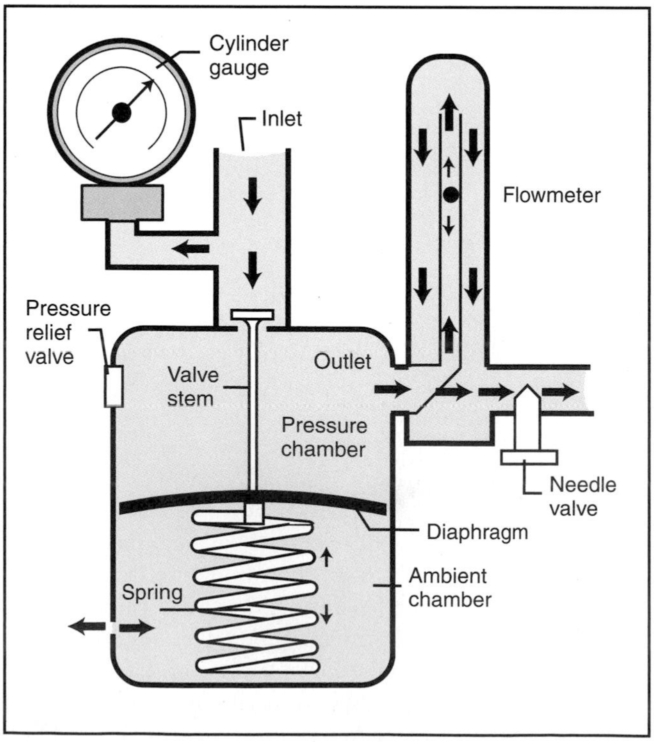

Figure 3-1 Components of a single-stage regulator. (Redrawn from Persing G: *Entry level respiratory care review,* Philadelphia, 1992, WB Saunders.)

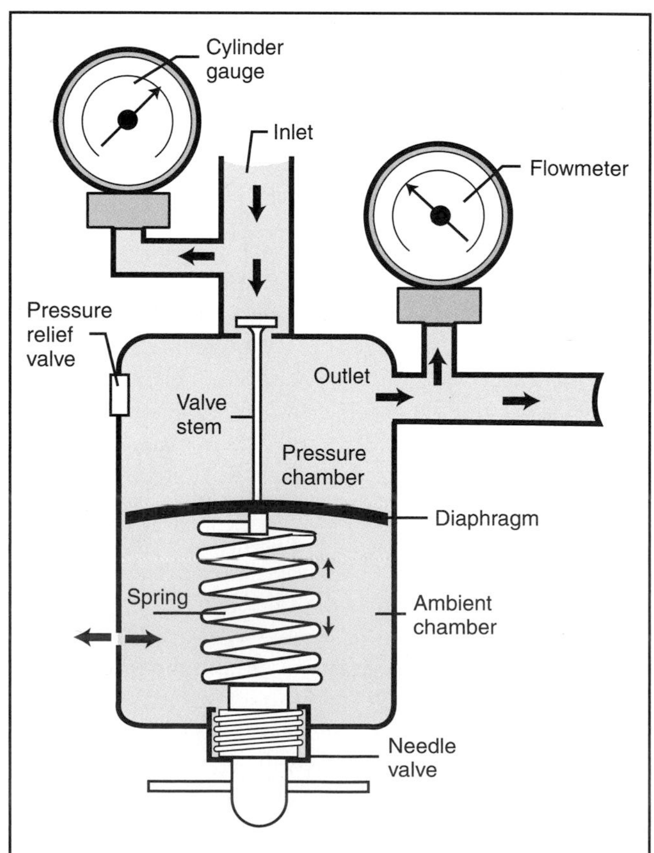

Figure 3-2 Components of an adjustable, single-stage regulator. (Redrawn from Persing G: *Entry level respiratory care review,* Philadelphia, 1992, WB Saunders.)

Flowmeters

As mentioned previously, flowmeters are devices that control and indicate flow. Three types are usually described: **Thorpe-tube flowmeters, Bourdon flowmeters, and flow restrictors.**

Thorpe-Tube Flowmeters

Thorpe tubes are the most common flowmeters used in respiratory care. As Figure 3-4 shows, these devices consist of a tapered, hollow tube engraved with a calibrated scale (usually in L/min), a float, and a needle valve for controlling the flow rate of gas. (Flowmeters used in neonatal and pediatric care may be calibrated in mL/min.) The flow rate of gas delivered is read by locating the float on the calibrated scale. It is important to use the center of the float as the reference point when reading flow rates on the calibrated scale. This is particularly evident when trying to adjust flows of 1 to 3 L/min.

The operational principle for these devices can be explained in the following manner. As gas flows through the unit, it pushes the ball float higher. As the ball float moves

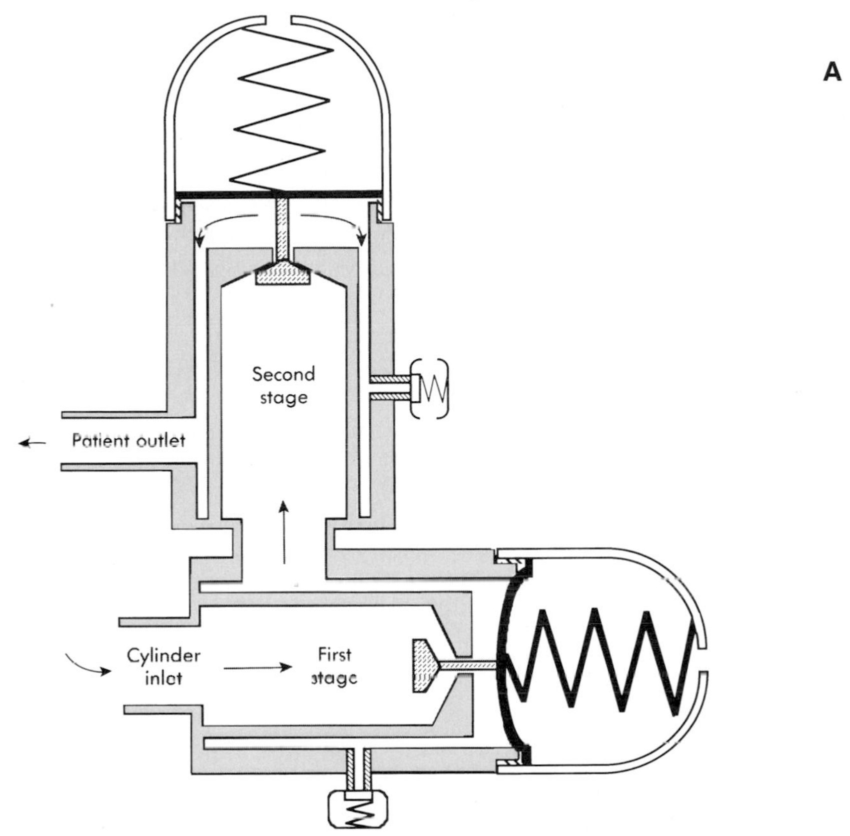

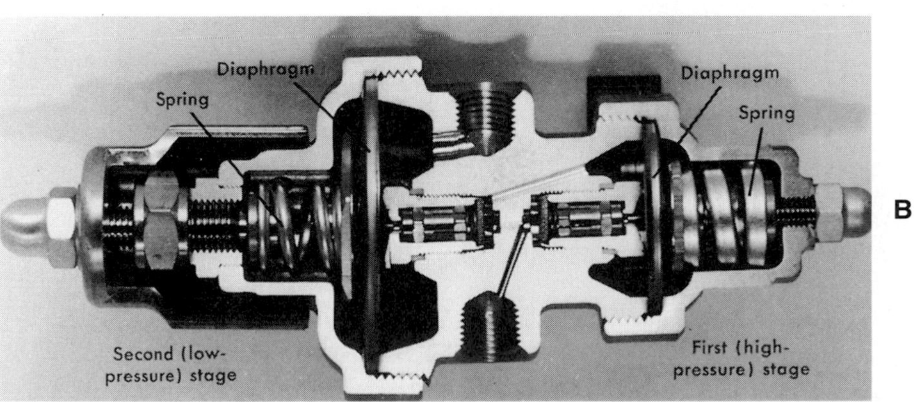

Figure 3-3 **A,** Multistage reducing valve. Double-stage valve is functionally two single-stage reducing valves in tandem. Gas enters the first stage (first reducing valve) and its pressure is lowered. Gas then enters the second stage (second reducing valve), and pressure is lowered to the desired working pressure (usually 50 psig). A three-stage reducing valve would have one more reducing valve in the series. **B,** National double-stage reducing valve. (Courtesy National Welding Equipment Co., Richmond, Calif.)

higher in the tube, more gas is allowed to travel around it as a result of the gradually increasing diameter of the indicator tube. The height that the ball float is raised depends on the force of gravity pulling down on it and the force of the molecules trying to push it up. The ball float will rise until enough molecules can go around it to restore the equilibrium between gravity and the number of molecules hitting the bottom of the ball float.

Back Pressure Compensation

Thorpe-tube flowmeters are usually described as being **pressure-compensated** and **non—pressure-compensated.** On pressure-compensated flowmeters (Figure 3-5), the needle valve controlling gas flow out of the flowmeter is located distal to the Thorpe tube. This arrangement allows the pressure in the indicator tube to be maintained at the source gas pressure (i.e., 50 psig). Pressure-compensated flowmeters provide accurate estimates of flow, regardless of the downstream pressure. (Note that pressure-compensated flowmeters indicate actual flow unless the source gas pressure varies, the flowmeter is set to deliver a higher flow than is actually available from its source gas supply, or the float in the tube is not set in a vertical position.[1]) The following example may help to illustrate how these devices operate. When a restriction or high-resistance device is attached to a pressure-compensated flowmeter, the pressure gradient between the source gas pressure and the outlet pressure is decreased. The float within the Thorpe tube registers the true gas flow out of the flowmeter because back pressure created by a downstream resistance only increases the pressure distal to the needle valve. It should be apparent, however, that if the back pressure exceeds the source gas pressure (e.g., 50 psig), gas flow stops.

In the case of non—pressure-compensated flowmeters (Figure 3-6), the needle valve is located before the indicator tube. Restriction or high-resistance devices attached to the outlet of a non—pressure-compensated Thorpe-tube flowmeter create back pressure, which is transmitted back to the needle valve. Because the needle valve is located proximal to the Thorpe tube, the back pressure causes the float to fall to a level that indicates a flow lower than the actual flow.

Pressure-compensated flowmeters are usually labeled as such on the back of the flowmeter. A flowmeter can also be determined to be pressure-compensated if the following test is performed. With the needle valve closed, the flowmeter is plugged into a high-pressure gas source (i.e., bulk storage wall outlet). If the float in the indicator tube jumps and then falls to zero, the flowmeter is pressure-compensated. This float movement occurs because the source gas must pass through the indicator tube before it reaches the needle valve.[1]

The most common problem associated with Thorpe-tube flowmeters is gas leakage because of faulty valve seats. This problem is usually detected when the flowmeter is turned off completely, but gas can be heard continuing to flow from the flowmeter outlet; the flowmeter should be replaced.

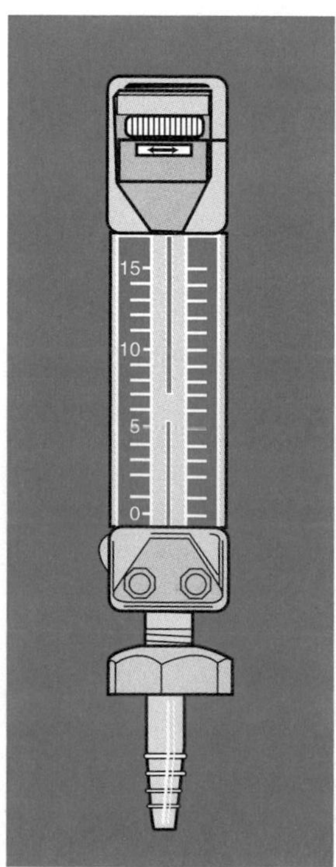

Figure 3-4 Thorpe-tube flowmeter.

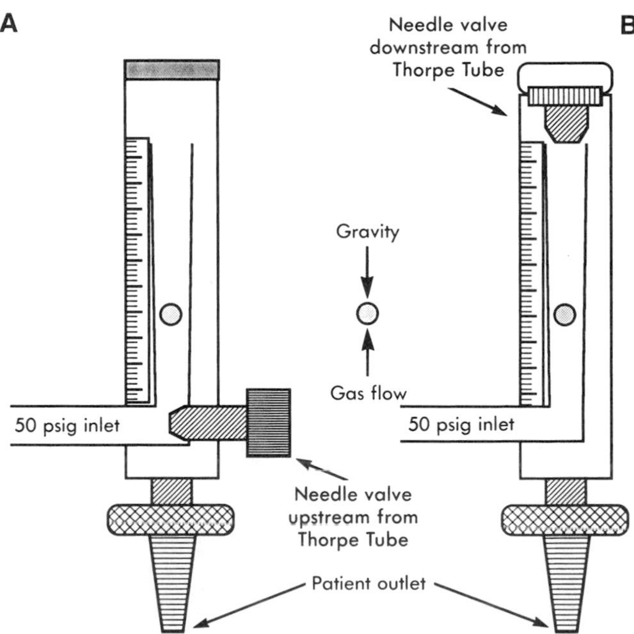

Figure 3-5 **A,** Non-pressure-compensated Thorpe flowmeter. **B,** Pressure compensated Thorpe flowmeter. The two opposing forces are (1) gravity pulling the float downward and (2) the driving pressure of the gas flow pushing the float upward. When these two forces reach a balance (equilibrium), the float remains stationary, "floating" in the gas column. Because the gas column consists of a tapered tube, as the gas flow increases and the float is displaced upward, greater volumes of gas pass by the float and enter the patient outlet. Needle valve placement determines if the device is back-pressure-compensated.

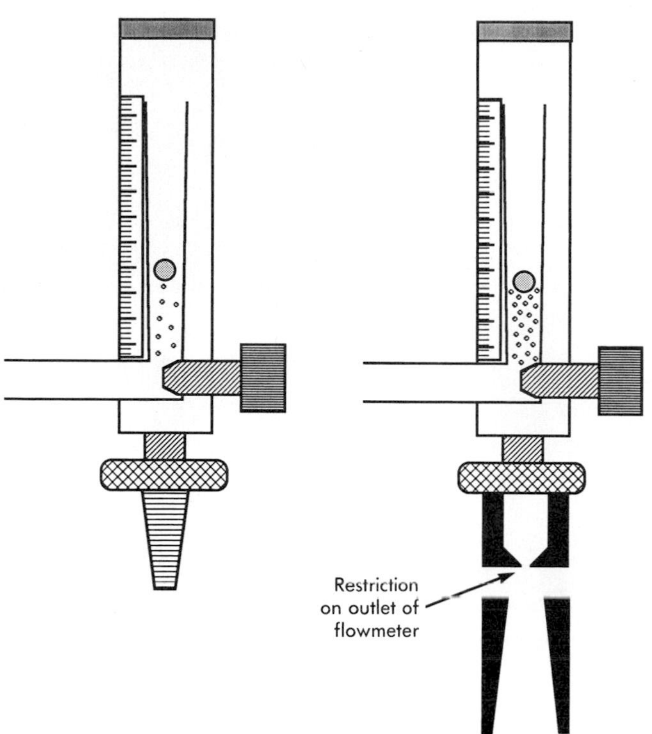

Figure 3-6 Non-pressure-compensated Thorpe-tube flowmeter.

Bourdon Flowmeters

As Figure 3-7 shows, the Bourdon flowmeter is actually a reducing valve that controls the pressure gradient across an outlet with a fixed orifice. The operational principle of this device is simple: as the driving pressure is increased, the flow from the flowmeter outlet increases.

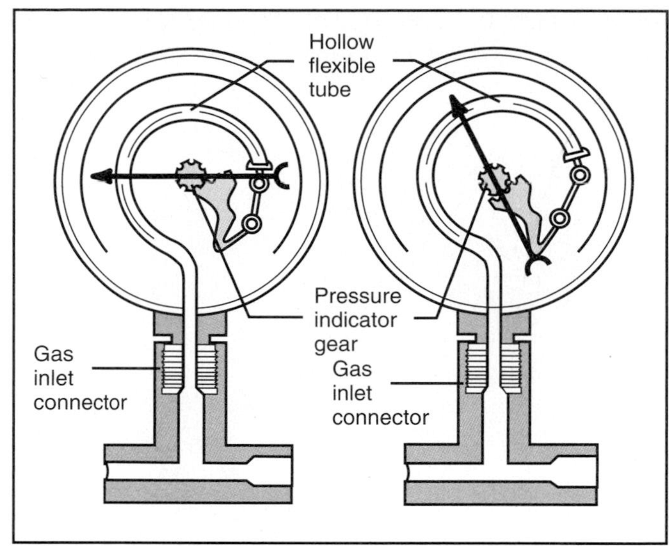

Figure 3-7 Schematic of a Bourdon flowmeter. (Redrawn from Ward JJ: Equipment for mixed gas and oxygen therapy. In Barnes TA, editor: *Core textbook of respiratory care practice*, ed 2, St Louis, 1994, Mosby.)

The flow rate of gas can be measured because the Bourdon flowmeter gauge is calibrated in liters per minute. As long as the pressure distal to or downstream from the orifice remains atmospheric, the indicated flow is accurate. As resistance to flow increases, the indicated flow reading becomes inaccurate (i.e., these devices are not back-pressure—compensated). Figure 3-8 demonstrates how increasing resistance at the gas outlet affects the flow reading. Note that although the outlet becomes totally occluded, the flow reading remains constant. Figure 3-9 is a picture of a commonly used Bourdon flowmeter.

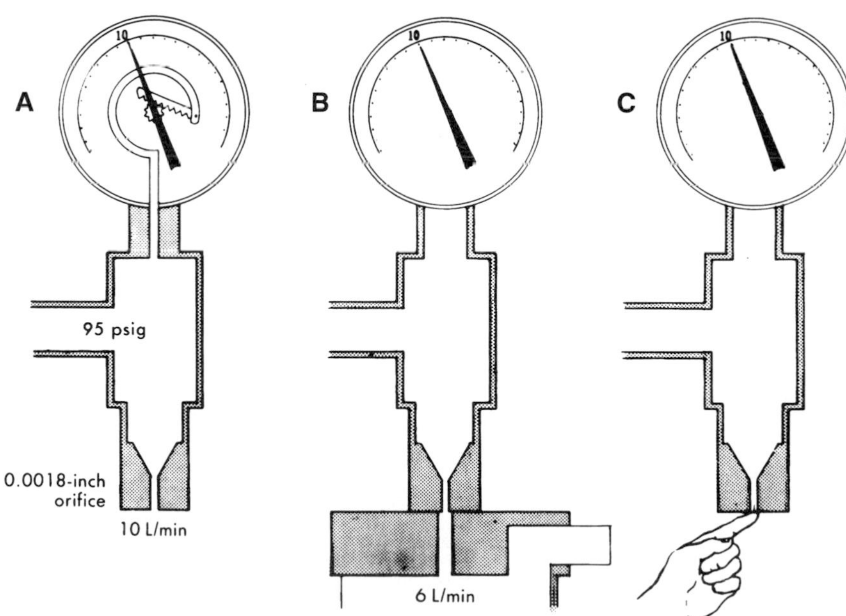

Figure 3-8 Bourdon gauge **(A)** with resistance **(B)** downstream. If resistance is placed on the outlet of the Bourdon regulator, the postrestriction pressure is no longer constant because it will be somewhat higher than atmospheric. Pressure gradient is then decreased; because only prerestriction pressure—not actual pressure gradient—is monitored, the reading will be erroneously high **(C)**. (Courtesy Nellcor Puritan Bennett, Pleasanton, Calif.)

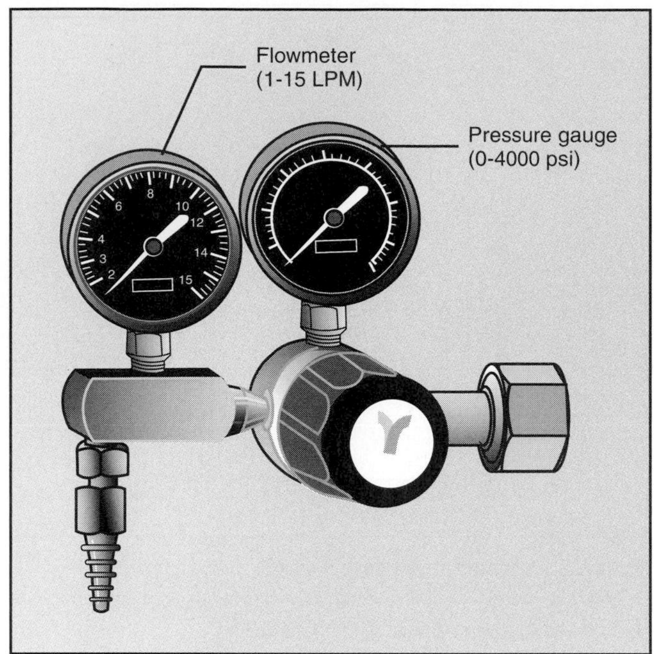

Figure 3-9 Bourdon gauge flowmeter.

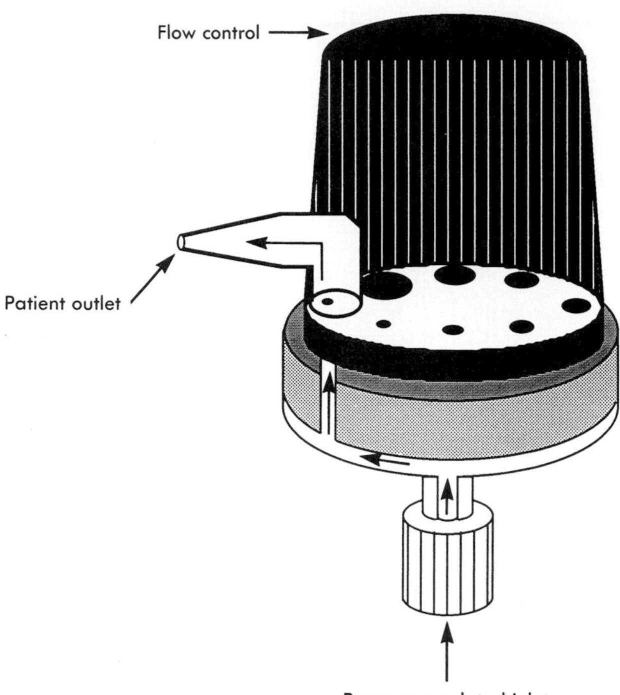

Figure 3-10 Schematic of a variable-orifice flow restrictor. These devices employ a series of calibrated ports to deliver a set flow at a designated pressure. Per NFPA requirements, the delivery pressure is included on the restrictor label.

Flow Restrictors

These devices operate on the same principle as Bourdon flowmeters (i.e., the gas flow through these devices can be increased by raising the driving pressure across a fixed resistance). Like Bourdon flowmeters, flow-rate readings are inaccurate when resistance increases downstream from the gas outlet. There are two types of flow restrictors: **fixed-orifice** and **adjustable, multiple-orifice** types albeit the fixed-orifice devices are no longer manufactured. The adjustable, multiple-orifice type of flow restrictor employs a series of calibrated openings in a disc that can be adjusted to deliver different flows. As with the fixed-orifice type of flow restrictor, the operating pressure is crucial to the accuracy of the device. Figure 3-10 shows an example of a variable-orifice flow restrictor.

It is essential to use the appropriate operating pressure for these devices to function properly. Some are designed for use with hospital gas sources (i.e., 50-psi gas sources), whereas others are designed to work on portable liquid oxygen used in home-care settings (i.e., 20-psi gas source).

Devices for Administering Medical Gases

Oxygen Therapy

The goal of oxygen therapy is to treat or prevent hypoxemia. Many different devices can be used to achieve this goal in spontaneously breathing patients. It is important that respiratory therapists understand how to select and assemble these devices and to ensure that they are working properly. The American Association for Respiratory Care has developed clinical practice guidelines for oxygen administration in acute care facilities and in home- and extended-care facilities.[3-5] These guidelines inform practitioners of indications, contraindications, precautions, and possible complications of oxygen therapy. Each guideline lists the devices that can be used to administer oxygen to spontaneously breathing patients, along with a brief description of criteria that should be used to assess the need for and the outcome of oxygen therapy. These guidelines should be reviewed and used as a resource when treating patients who require oxygen therapy. Clinical Practice Guidelines 3-1 and 3-2 summarize guidelines for oxygen therapy for adults in acute care and extended care facilities. Clinical Practice Guideline 3-3 summarizes the guidelines for oxygen therapy for neonatal and pediatric patients.

Low-Flow versus High-Flow Devices

Oxygen therapy systems are generally classified as **low-flow (variable performance)** and **high-flow (fixed performance)** devices.[4,5] The terms *low-flow* and *variable performance devices* are used because these devices supply oxygen at flow rates that are lower than a patient's inspiratory demands; thus varying amounts of room air must be added to provide part of the inspired volume. Low-flow devices deliver fractional inspired oxygen (F_IO_2) levels that can vary from 0.22 to approximately 0.60, depending on the patient's inspiratory flow, tidal volume, and the oxygen flow used.

Nasal cannulas and catheters (Historical Note 3-1), transtracheal catheters, simple oxygen masks, partial-rebreathing reservoir masks, and nonrebreathing reservoir masks are examples of low-flow oxygen therapy devices.

High-flow or fixed performance devices provide oxygen at flow rates high enough to completely satisfy a patient's inspiratory demands. Such devices supply the inspiratory demands of the patient either by entraining fixed quantities of ambient air or by using high-flow rates and reservoirs. The most important characteristic of high-flow devices is that they can deliver fixed F_IO_2 levels (i.e., from 0.24 to 1.00), regardless of the patient's breathing pattern. Air-entrainment masks, incubators, oxygen tents, and oxygen hoods are high-flow systems. High-volume aerosol devices and humidifiers that are used to provide continuous humidification through face masks and tracheostomy collars incorporate air-entrainment devices and thus can also be considered high-flow oxygen therapy devices.

It is a common misconception that low-flow systems can only deliver low F_IO_2 and that high-flow systems can only deliver high F_IO_2. As will be seen, both low- and high-flow systems can deliver a wide range of F_IO_2. **Do not confuse the terms *low flow* and *high flow* with the terms *low* F_IO_2 and *high* F_IO_2.**

Low-Flow Devices

Nasal Cannulas

Nasal cannulas (Figure 3-11) are used extensively to treat spontaneously breathing, hypoxemic patients in emergency rooms, in general and critical care units, during exercise in cardiopulmonary rehabilitation, and for long-term oxygen therapy in home-care settings.[2,6] The standard nasal cannula is a blind-ended, soft plastic tube that contains two prongs that fit into the patient's external nares. The prongs, which are approximately a half inch long, can be straight or curved. The cannula is held in place either with an elastic band that fits over the ears and around the head or with two small-diameter pieces of tubing that fit over the ears and can be tightened with a bolo tie type of device that fits under the chin. Cannulas are available in infant, child, and adult sizes.

The most common problems with these devices are related to (1) nasopharyngeal-mucosal irritation, (2) twisting of the connective tubing between the patient and the oxygen flowmeter, and (3) skin irritation at pressure points where the tubing holding the cannula in place touches the patient's face and ears. Irritation of the nasal mucosa and the paranasal sinuses occurs most often when high-flow rates of oxygen

Clinical Practice Guidelines 3-1

Oxygen Therapy for Adults in the Acute Care Facility—2002 Revision and Update*

Definition/Description

Oxygen therapy is the administration of oxygen at concentrations greater than ambient air with the intent of treating or preventing the symptoms and manifestations of hypoxia. The procedure addressed is the administration of oxygen therapy in the acute care facility other than with mechanical ventilators and hyperbaric chambers.

Indications

- Documented hypoxemia. Defined as a decreased PaO_2 in the blood below normal range (i.e., PaO_2 <60 torr, or SaO_2 <90% in subjects breathing room air or with a PaO_2 or SaO_2 below desirable range for specific clinical situation
- An acute situation in which hypoxemia is suspected; substantiation of hypoxemia is required within an appropriate period of time following initiation of therapy
- Severe trauma
- Acute myocardial infarction
- Short-term therapy (postanesthesia) or surgical intervention

Precautions and/or Complications

- With a PaO_2 ≥60 torr, ventilatory depression may occur in spontaneously breathing patients with chronically elevated $PaCO_2$.
- With F_IO_2 ≥0.50, absorption atelectasis, oxygen toxicity, and/or depression of ciliary and/or leukocyte function may occur.
- Bacterial contamination associated with certain nebulization and humidification systems is a possible hazard.
- Oxygen administration should be administered with caution to patients suffering from paraquat poisoning and patients receiving bleomycin.
- During laser bronchoscopy, minimal levels of supplemental oxygen should be used to avoid intratracheal ignition.

Limitations

- Oxygen therapy has only limited benefit for the treatment of hypoxia due to anemia and may be of limited benefit with circulatory disturbances.
- Oxygen therapy should not be used in lieu of, but in addition to mechanical ventilation when ventilatory support is indicated.

Monitoring

- Patient monitoring should include clinical assessment along with oxygen tension or saturation measurements. This should be done at the following times: when therapy is initiated; within 12 hours of initiation of therapy for F_IO_2s <0.40; within 8 hours for F_IO_2s ≥0.40; within 72 hours of an acute myocardial infarction; within 2 hours for patients diagnosed with COPD.
- All oxygen delivery systems should be checked at least once per day. More frequent checks with calibrated analyzers are indicated for systems susceptible to variations in F_IO_2.

**For a copy of the complete AARC Clinical Practice Guideline, see* Respir Care *47(6):717-720, 2002.*

Clinical Practice Guidelines 3-2

Oxygen Therapy in the Home or Extended-Care Facility*

Setting

This guideline is confined to oxygen administration in the home or extended care facility.

Indications: Documented Hypoxemia

- In adults, children, and infants older than 28 days: P_aO_2 <55 torr, or SaO_2 <88% in subjects breathing room air.
- P_aO_2 of 56 to 59 torr, or SaO_2 or SpO_2 <89% in association with specific clinical conditions (e.g., cor pulmonale, congestive heart failure, or erythrocythemia with hematocrit >56%).
- Some patients may not qualify for oxygen therapy at rest but will qualify for oxygen during ambulation, sleep, or exercise; oxygen therapy is indicated during these specific activities when the S_aO_2 falls to less than 88%.

Precautions and/or Complications

These are the same as those cited for oxygen therapy in the acute care hospital.

Limitations

These are the same as those cited for oxygen therapy in the acute care hospital.

Monitoring

- Clinical assessment should be performed by the patient and/or the caregiver to determine changes in clinical status (e.g., dyspnea scales or diary cards).
- Baseline oxygen tension and saturation must be measured before oxygen therapy is begun; these measurements should be repeated when clinically indicated or following the course of the disease.
- SpO_2 may be made to determine appropriate oxygen flow for ambulation, exercise, or sleep.
- All oxygen delivery equipment should be checked at least once daily by the patient or caregiver. Checks should include proper equipment function, prescribed flow rates, fractional concentration of delivered oxygen (FDO_2), remaining fluid or compressed gas content, and backup supply. During monthly visits, a respiratory care practitioner should reinforce appropriate practices and performance by the patient and/or caregiver and ensure that the oxygen equipment is maintained in accordance with manufacturer's recommendations.

Frequency

Oxygen should be administered continuously, unless it has been shown to be necessary only in specific situations (e.g., exercise, sleep).

Infection Control

Normally, low-flow oxygen systems without humidifiers do not present a clinically important risk of infection and need not be routinely replaced. High-flow systems that employ heated humidifiers or aerosol generators, especially when applied to patients with artificial airways, should be cleaned and disinfected on a regular basis.

**For a complete copy of this guideline, see* Resp Care 37:918-922, 1992.

Clinical Practice Guidelines 3-3

Selection of an Oxygen Delivery Device for Neonatal and Pediatric Patients—2002 Revision and Update*

Definition/Description

The administration of supplemental oxygen to neonatal and pediatric patients requires the selection of an oxygen delivery system that suits the patient's size, needs, and the therapeutic goals.

Indications

- Documented hypoxemia
- An acute situation in which hypoxemia is suspected or in which suspected regional hypoxia may respond to an increase in PaO_2. Substantiation of PaO_2 is required within an appropriate period of time following initiation of therapy

Contraindications

- No specific contraindications to delivering oxygen exist when indications are judged to be present.
- Nasal cannulas and nasopharyngeal catheters are contraindicated in patients with nasal obstruction (e.g., nasal polyps, choanal atresia).
- Nasopharyngeal catheters are contraindicated in the presence of maxillofacial trauma, in patients in whom a basal skull fracture is present or suspected, or those in whom coagulation problems exist.
- It is the expert opinion of the Clinical Practice Guideline Steering Committee (2002) that nasopharyngeal catheters are not appropriate for oxygen administration in the neonatal population.

Hazards/Precautions/Possible Complications

- The etiology of retinopathy of prematurity, especially the role of oxygen, is controversial. Care should be taken when supplemental oxygen is provided to preterm infants (<37 weeks' gestation). It is suggested that oxygen supplementation should not result in a PaO_2 >80 torr.

Continued

Clinical Practice Guidelines 3-3—cont'd

Selection of an Oxygen Delivery Device for Neonatal and Pediatric Patients—2002 Revision and Update*

- The administration of supplemental oxygen to patients with certain congenital heart lesions (e.g., hypoplastic left-heart, single ventricle) may cause an increase in alveolar oxygen tension and compromise the balance between pulmonary and systemic blood flow.
- The administration of supplemental oxygen to patients suffering from paraquat poisoning or to patients receiving certain chemotherapeutic agents (e.g., bleomycin) may result in pulmonary complications (e.g., oxygen toxicity and pulmonary fibrosis).
- Stimulation of the superior laryngeal nerves may cause alterations in respiratory pattern if the gas flow from the oxygen source is cool and is directed at the face of the infant.
- Inappropriate selection of FDO_2 or oxygen flow may result in hypoxemia or hyperoxemia.
- Skin irritation can result from material used to secure the cannula or from local allergic reaction to polyvinyl chloride. Improper sizing can lead to nasal obstruction or irritation.
- Displacement can lead to loss of oxygen delivery.
- Inadvertent CPAP may be administered depending upon the size of the nasal cannula, the gas flow, and the infant's anatomy.
- Irritation can result if flows are excessive; improper insertion can cause gagging and nasal or pharyngeal trauma; improper sizing can lead to nasal obstruction or irritation.
- Excessive secretions and/or mucosal inflammation can result.
- Skin irritation may result from material used to secure the cannula and/or from local allergic reaction to polyvinyl chloride.
- Excessive flow may cause gastric distention.
- Transtracheal catheters may be associated with an increased risk of infection compared to nasal cannulas and catheters.
- Aspiration of vomitus may be more likely with oxygen masks. Rebreathing of CO_2 may occur if total O_2 flow to the mask is inadequate.
- It is the expert opinion of the Clinical Practice Guideline Steering Committee (2002) that partial rebreathers or non-rebreathers are not appropriate for the neonatal population.

Limitations

Nasal cannulas: Changes in minute ventilation and inspiratory flow affect air entrainment and result in fluctuations in F_IO_2. Prongs are difficult to keep in position, particularly with small infants. The effect of mouth versus nose breathing on F_IO_2 remains controversial. Use may be limited by the presence of excessive mucus drainage, mucosal edema, or a deviated septum. Maximum flow should be limited to 2 L/min in infants and newborns. Care should be taken to keep the cannula tubing and straps away from the neck to prevent airway obstruction in infants. Discrepancies between set and delivered flow can occur in the same flowmeter at different settings and among different flowmeters. Discrepancies in flow and oxygen concentration between set and delivered values can occur in low-flow blenders at flows below the recommended range of the blender.

Nasopharyngeal catheters: Method is in less common use because of the complexity of care. F_IO_2 is difficult to control and measure. Effect of mouth versus nose breathing on F_IO_2 remains controversial. Use may be limited by excessive mucus drainage, mucosal edema, or the presence of a deviated septum. Catheter should be cleared frequently to prevent occlusion of the distal holes. Patients should be observed for evidence of catheter occlusion, and the catheter should be alternated between nares every 8-12 hours and changed daily. Catheter sizes less than 8 Fr are less effective in oxygen delivery. Lower oxygen concentrations are delivered if the catheter is placed in the nose rather than in the pharynx. Low-flow flowmeters (<3 L/min) should be used. Discrepancies between set and delivered flow can occur in the same flowmeter at different settings and among different flowmeters. Discrepancies in flow and oxygen concentration between set and delivered values can occur in low-flow blenders at flows below those recommended by the manufacturer.

Transtracheal catheters: Method is in less common use because of the complexity of care. Requires frequent medical monitoring. Replacement catheters are costly. Increased time needed for candidate evaluation and teaching.

Masks provide variable F_IO_2 depending on inspiratory flow and construction of the mask's reservoir and are not recommended when precise concentrations are required; are confining and may not be well tolerated; interfere with feeding; may not be available in sizes appropriate for all patients; require a minimum flow per manufacturer's instructions to avoid possible rebreathing of CO_2. The maximum F_IO_2 attainable with a simple, non-rebreathing or partial-rebreathing mask in neonates, infants, and children has not been well documented. The performance of air-entrainment masks may be altered by resistance to flow distal to the restricted orifice (resulting in higher FDO_2 and lower total flow delivered). The total flow from air-entrainment masks at settings greater than 0.40 may not equal or exceed the patient's inspiratory flow. Performance is altered if the entrainment ports are blocked.

Hoods: O_2 concentrations may vary within the hood. O_2 concentrations should be measured as near the nose and mouth as possible. Opening any enclosure decreases the O_2 concentration. For infants and children confined to hoods, nasal O_2 may need to be supplied during feeding and nursing care. Flows >7 L/min are required to wash out CO_2. Devices can be confining and isolating. Concentration in a hood can be varied from 0.21 to 1.0. Temperature of the gases in the hood should be maintained to provide a neutral thermal environment. High gas flows may produce harmful noise levels.

Assessment of Need

Need is determined by measurement of inadequate oxygen tensions and saturations by invasive or noninvasive methods and/or the presence of clinical indicators as previously described. Supplemental oxygen flow should be titrated to maintain adequate oxygen saturation as indicated by pulse oximetry SpO_2 or appropriate arterial or venous blood gas values.

Continued

Clinical Practice Guidelines 3-3—cont'd

Selection of an Oxygen Delivery Device for Neonatal and Pediatric Patients—2002 Revision and Update*

Monitoring

Clinical assessment should include but is not limited to cardiac, pulmonary, and neurologic status and apparent work of breathing; noninvasive or invasive measurement of oxygen tensions or saturation in any patient treated with oxygen-within 1 hour of initiation for the neonate.

All oxygen delivery systems should be checked at least once each day. More frequent checks by calibrated analyzer are necessary in systems susceptible to variation in oxygen concentration or applied to patients with artificial airways. Continuous analysis is recommended in hoods. Oxygen should be analyzed as close as possible to the infant's face.

All heated delivery systems should be continuously monitored for temperature.

For a copy of the complete AARC Clinical Practice Guideline, see Resp Care 47(6):707-716, 2002.

HISTORICAL NOTE 3-1
Nasal Catheters

Nasal catheters were introduced by Lane in 1907.[1,6] It is important to recognize that although these devices are still available, they are used infrequently. Nasal catheters consist of a hollow, soft plastic tube that contains a blind distal tip with a series of side holes. They are available in 8 to 10 French (F) for children and 12 to 14 F for adults.

Note that the term ***French*** is a method of sizing catheters according to outside diameters (OD). Each unit in the French scale is approximately 0.33 mm. Thus an 10 F tube has an outside diameter or 3.3 mm, etc.

The catheter can be placed with relative ease and minimal patient discomfort if done properly. First, it should be coated with a water-soluble lubricant, and its patency should be checked (by observing if oxygen flows through it unobstructed). Once the patency has been confirmed, the catheter is inserted into an external naris and advanced along the floor of the nasal cavity until it can be seen at the back of the patient's oropharynx. It should then be positioned just behind the uvula. For blind insertion, the distance that the catheter must be inserted can be estimated by measuring the distance from the tip of the patient's nose to the earlobe, which can then be marked on the catheter with a small piece of surgical tape. The catheter can be held in place by taping it to the nose.

Nasal catheters can deliver F_IO_2s of approximately 0.22 to 0.35 when the oxygen flow is set at 2 to 5 L/min. Higher F_IO_2s can be obtained by increasing the oxygen flow to the patient. Notice that the actual F_IO_2 varies considerably depending on the patient's tidal volume and respiratory rate and whether respiration is occurring primarily through the nose or the mouth.

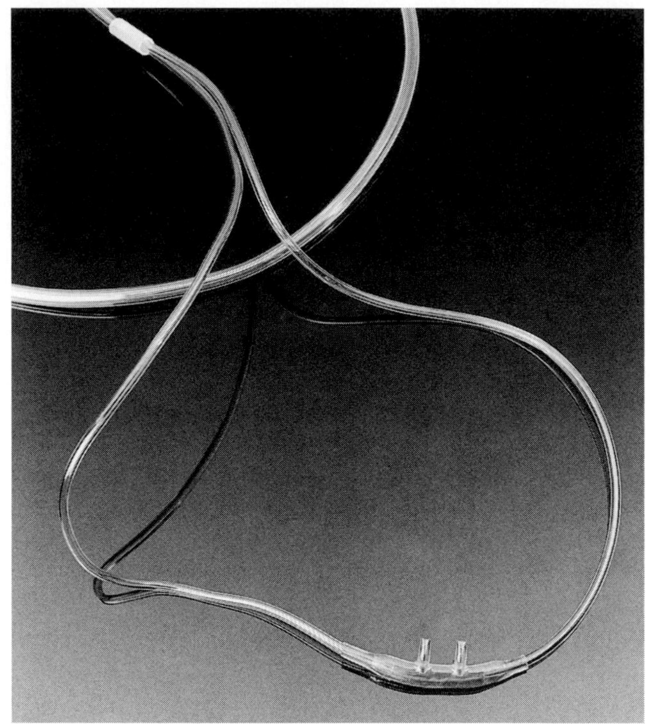

Figure 3-11 Nasal cannula.

are used. The problem appears to be increased with nasal cannulas that use straight instead of curved prongs. With straight prongs, oxygen flow is directed toward the superior aspects of the nasal cavity, thus promoting turbulent flow; with curved prongs, oxygen entering the nose is directed across the nasal turbinate, thus enhancing laminar flow as the gas flows through the nasal cavity. Twisting of connective tubing is an insidious problem that is difficult to prevent. Avoiding excessive lengths of connective tubing, as well as periodically checking for patency appear to be the most reliable means of dealing with this problem. The problems of skin irritation and pressure-point soreness associated with using these devices can be minimized by placing cotton gauze padding between the tubing and the patient's face and ears.

For adult patients, nasal cannulas can theoretically produce F_IO_2 levels of 0.24 to 0.44 with oxygen flow rates of 1 to 6 L/min. Oxygen flows higher than 6 L/min do not produce significantly higher F_IO_2s and are poorly tolerated by patients because they cause nasal bleeding and drying of the nasal mucosa. For neonates, oxygen flows of 0.25 to 2.0 L/min can produce F_IO_2 levels of 0.35 to 0.70.[5-7] Keep in mind that the actual F_IO_2 delivered is influenced by the patient's tidal volume and respiratory rate and whether breathing is predominantly occurring through the nose or the mouth.

Table 3-1 lists the approximate F_IO_2 levels delivered by flow rates of 1 to 6 L/min to an adult patient. Generally, the F_IO_2 increases by about 4% for each liter of flow increase. A problem-solving exercise for calculating the approximate F_IO_2 when using a variable-performance device such as a nasal cannula is provided in Clinical Rounds 3-1. It should be emphasized that this is simply an estimate and that the actual delivered F_IO_2 for any given oxygen flow rate may be significantly different.[2] In a clinical setting, adjusting the flow rate of oxygen delivered to the patient is generally an empirical process (i.e., it is adjusted according to the patient's oxygen needs). This empiric approach should be based on observations of the patient's breathing pattern and level of comfort, as well as pulse oximetry or arterial blood gas data, if available.

Table 3-1 Guidelines for Estimating F_IO_2 with Low-Flow Oxygen Delivery Systems

100% Oxygen Flow Rate (L)	F_IO_2
Nasal cannula or catheter	
1	0.24
2	0.28
3	0.32
4	0.36
5	0.40
6	0.44
Oxygen mask	
5-6	0.40
6-7	0.50
7-8	0.60
Mask with reservoir bag	
6	0.60
7	0.70
8	0.80
9	0.80+
10	0.80+

From Shapiro BA, et al: Clinical application of respiratory care, ed 4, St Louis, 1991, Mosby.
F_IO_2, fractional inspired oxygen.

CLINICAL ROUNDS 3-1

A Simple Method for Estimating Theoretical F_IO_2

A 150-lb, spontaneously breathing patient is receiving oxygen at 6 L/min through a nasal cannula. The patient's tidal volume is 500 mL and respiratory rate is 20 breaths per minute (inspiratory time = 1 second; expiratory time = 2 seconds). Estimate the theoretical F_IO_2.

See Appendix A for the answer.

Oxygen-Conserving Devices

Transtracheal oxygen (TTO) catheters, reservoir cannulas, and pulse-demand oxygen delivery systems are recent developments that have significantly improved the delivery of oxygen therapy, especially with regard to conserving oxygen supplies during long-term oxygen therapy.

Transtracheal Catheters. The concept of TTO therapy was first described by Heimlich in 1982.[8] The guiding principle of such oxygen therapy is that oxygen delivered directly into the trachea should provide the patient with adequate oxygen, while reducing the amount of oxygen used. That is, the direct delivery of oxygen into the trachea reduces dilution with room air on inspiration because the upper airways (the anatomic reservoir) are filled with oxygen. Consequently, lower oxygen flows from the source gas (e.g., 0.25 to 2 L/min) are required to achieve a desired level of oxygenation. Indeed, TTO catheters can produce overall oxygen savings of 54% to 59%.[1]

Catheter placement requires minor surgery. A small, plastic stent is inserted into the patient's trachea between the second and third tracheal rings.[1,9] The stent remains in place for about a week to ensure that a permanent tract is

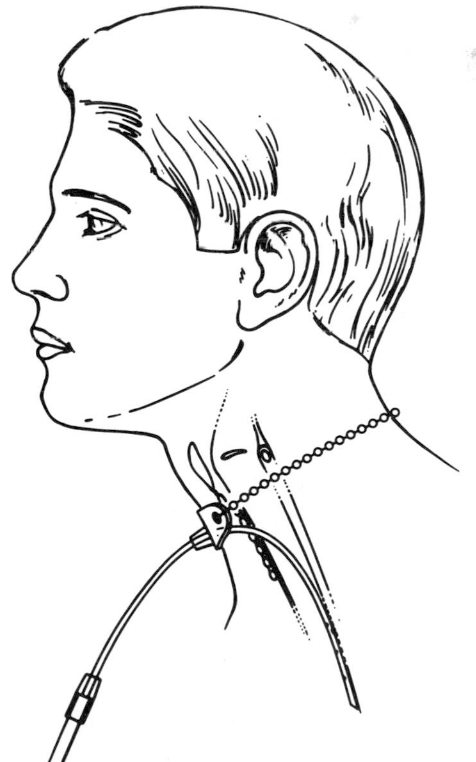

Figure 3-12 Transtracheal catheter. (From Scanlan CL, Wilkins RL, Stoller JK: *Egan's fundamentals of respiratory care*, ed 7, St Louis, 1999, Mosby.)

formed between the trachea and the outer skin. Removal of the stent is accomplished over a guide wire. After the stent is removed, a 9 F Teflon catheter is inserted into the tract over the guide wire. The catheter is held in place with a neck chain to prevent inadvertent dislodgment or removal (Figure 3-12). It is recommended that catheters are replaced at 90 days or earlier before they become cracked, kinked, or occluded by pus or mucus.[1,9,10] Patients must be educated on proper care of these devices to avoid complications. Routine care should include cleaning, lavage, and use of a cleaning rod to remove mucus that can occlude the lumen of the catheter.[9,10]

As previously stated, transtracheal catheters reduce oxygen costs by requiring lower oxygen flows to prevent hypoxemia. Therefore patients can purchase smaller, lighter cylinders or reservoirs for greater convenience. Using special, low-flow regulators or flow restrictors may also lead to greater cost savings.[1,10] Other important advantages of transtracheal catheters include improved patient compliance with oxygen therapy because of cosmetic appearance (these devices are relatively inconspicuous), increased patient mobility, and the avoidance of nasal irritation associated with the use of nasal cannulas. Finally, it should be mentioned that TTO devices use standard oxygen therapy equipment, which is important because if there is a problem with the catheter, emergency equipment (e.g., a conventional nasal cannula) can be easily set up and used by the patient.

The primary disadvantage of using transtracheal catheters is related to complications associated with minor surgery (i.e., hemoptysis, infection, and subcutaneous emphysema).[9,10] Mucous obstruction and occlusion of the distal end of the tube can also present complications, which can be minimized with proper care, including saline instillation and periodic clearing of the catheter lumen with a guide wire or cleaning rod. Clinical Rounds 3-2 illustrates a common example of how TTO can increase patient compliance with oxygen therapy.

Reservoir Cannulas. Figures 3-13 and 3-14 show two commercially available reservoir cannulas: the **mustache cannula** and the **pendant cannula.** The mustache cannula

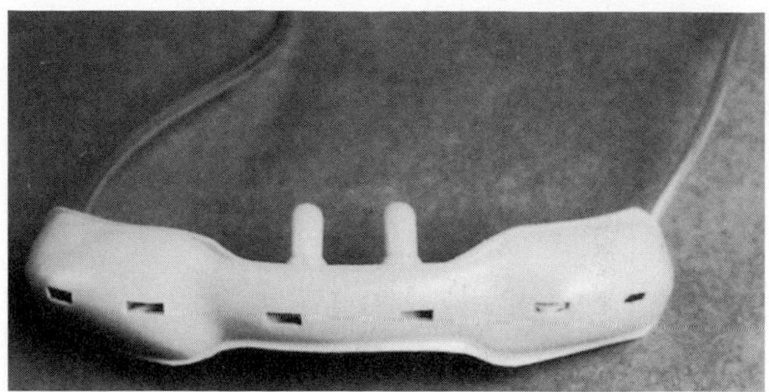

Figure 3-13 Mustache reservoir cannula. (Courtesy Chad Therapeutics, Chatsworth, Calif.)

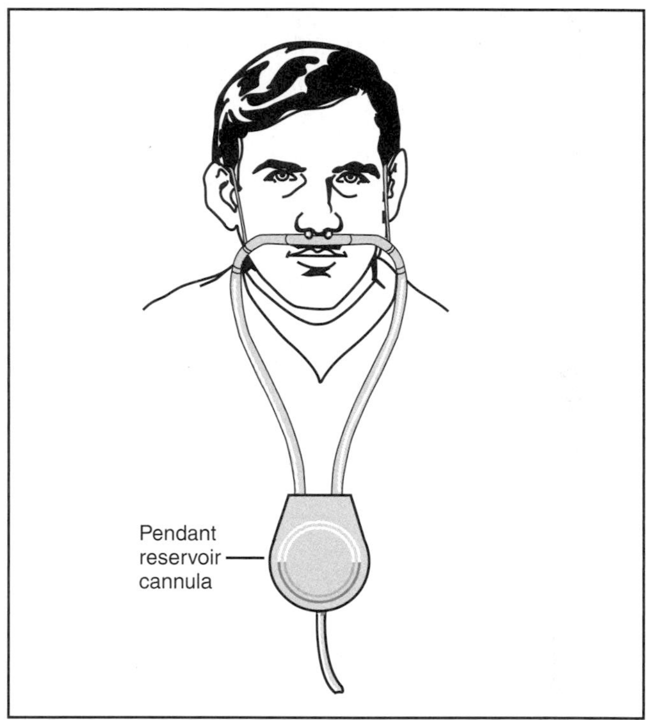

Figure 3-14 Pendant reservoir cannula.

can hold about 20 mL of gas and works in the following manner. During the early part of exhalation, gas derived from the patient's dead space inflates the reservoir. As exhalation continues, oxygen from the source gas (e.g., 100% oxygen from a 50-psi source) flows into the lateral aspects of the cannula, forcing the dead space gas medial and out of the nasal prongs and filling the reservoir with 100% oxygen. On inspiration, the initial part of the inhaled gas entering the patient's airway is drawn from this reservoir. As the reservoir collapses, the device then functions like a conventional nasal cannula. Thus the reservoir adds 20 mL of 100% oxygen as a bolus in addition to the continuous oxygen flow from the supply source. The added bolus of gas therefore reduces the amount of oxygen that must be derived from the continuous-flow source to achieve a desired F_IO_2.

Pendant cannulas operate in a similar manner, except that the reservoir is attached with connective tubing that serves as a conduit to a pendant that hangs below the chin.

CLINICAL ROUNDS 3-2

A home-care patient requiring continuous oxygen therapy is instructed to use a nasal cannula at a flow of 2 L/min. After a short period, the patient is admitted to the hospital with signs of hypoxemia. When asked if he had been using the prescribed oxygen, the patient explains that he used it only intermittently because it was uncomfortable, and furthermore he felt self-conscious about wearing it in public. What would you suggest to help this patient overcome the problems he described?

See Appendix A for the answer.

The added tubing between the reservoir and the pendant increases the amount of gas that can be stored so that these types of devices can hold nearly 40 mL of 100% oxygen. As with mustache cannulas, the main advantage of these devices is their ability to conserve gas flow.

Mustache and pendant cannulas can significantly reduce oxygen supply use compared with continuous-flow nasal cannulas. Studies indicate that mustache and pendant systems may reduce oxygen supply use by 50%,[11] though the cost of reservoir cannulas is higher than that of standard nasal cannulas. Also, many patients feel that mustache type of cannulas are heavier, larger, and more obvious than conventional nasal cannulas. Pendant cannulas, however, can be concealed by the patient's clothing.

Pulse-Demand Oxygen Delivery Systems. As the name implies, these systems deliver oxygen to the patient on demand. That is, they provide oxygen only during inspiration. Electronic, fluidic, and combined electronic-fluidic sensors are used to control gas delivery to the patient. Demand systems can operate with nasal catheters, nasal cannulas, and transtracheal catheters.[11,12] Figure 3-15 is a schematic of a demand system for a nasal cannula.[1] With this type of system, oxygen is delivered to the patient only after a sufficient inspiratory effort is made (i.e., $<^{-}1$ cm H_2O). After it is activated, the demand valve opens, delivering oxygen at a preset flow rate, and closes during exhalation to conserve oxygen. The demand valve connects directly to the oxygen source (50 psig), therefore replacing the flowmeter that is used with continuous-flow cannulas. Note that demand systems can function as pulsed or continuous-flow sources of oxygen. Settings allow the operator to select the equivalent of 1 to 5 L/min of oxygen flow from a conventional flowmeter. Shigeoka and Bonnekat[12] calculated that a patient receives about 17 mL of oxygen at the 1 L/min setting, 35 mL at the 2 L/min setting, 51 mL at the 3 L/min setting, and so on. It should be pointed out that oxygen delivered from these devices is not humidified because the system is delivering small pulses of oxygen. Thus humidification is not necessary because drying of the mucous membranes, as might occur with continuous-flow delivery systems, does not occur with these devices.

A common problem encountered with demand devices involves improper placement of the sensor. This type of problem can interfere with detection of an inspiratory effort, malfunction of the demand (solenoid) valve, and inadequate inspiratory flows. Improper placement of the sensor and malfunction of the demand valve can usually be detected by carefully observing the patient during initial set-up. Determining the adequacy of inspiratory flow requires feedback from the patient, either through verbal comments or oximetric analysis.

Simple Oxygen Mask

Although modern oxygen masks are made of different materials than earlier masks, their overall design has hardly changed since their introduction in the late eighteenth century.[6] Modern oxygen masks, as with the one shown in Figure 3-16, are cone-shaped devices that fit over the patient's nose and mouth and are held in place with an elastic band that fits around the patient's head. During inspiration, the patient draws gases both from oxygen flowing into the mask through small-bore tubing connected to the base of the mask and from room air via ports on the sides of the mask. These ports also serve as exhalation ports. A typical adult oxygen mask has a volume of approximately 100 to 200 mL and may be thought of as an extension of the anatomic reservoir because the patient will inhale its contents during the early part of inspiration. As such,

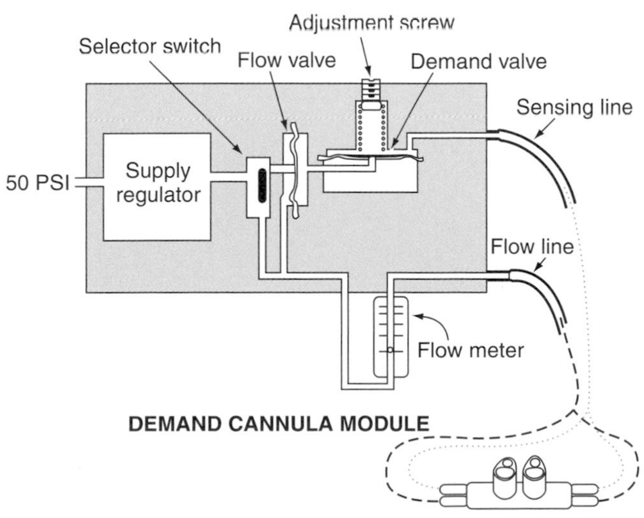

Figure 3-15 Pulse-demand oxygen-delivery system for nasal cannula. (Redrawn from Barnes TA: *Core textbook of respiratory care practice*, ed 2, St Louis, 1994, Mosby.)

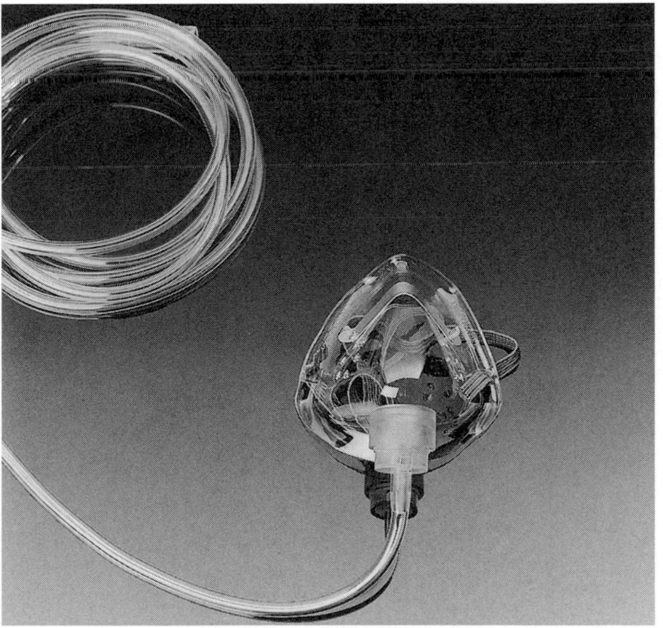

Figure 3-16 Simple oxygen mask.

simple oxygen masks can deliver higher F_IO_2 levels than do nasal cannulas because of a "reservoir effect." Note that the oxygen flow into the mask must be sufficient to wash out exhaled carbon dioxide, which can accumulate in this potential reservoir.

Generally, simple oxygen masks can deliver F_IO_2s of 35% to 50% at oxygen flows of 5 to 10 L/min. The F_IO_2 that is actually delivered to the patient depends on the flow of oxygen to the mask, the size of the mask, and the patient's breathing pattern. See Table 3-1 for a list of approximate F_IO_2 levels for flows of 5 to 8 L/min. Simple oxygen masks are reliable and easy to set up. Disposable plastic masks are available in infant, child, and adult sizes. They are ideal for delivering oxygen during minor surgical procedures and emergency situations.

There are, however, several disadvantages to using oxygen masks. For example, the delivered F_IO_2 can vary significantly, thus limiting the use of these devices for patients who require well-defined inspired oxygen concentrations. Carbon dioxide rebreathing can occur if the oxygen flow to the mask is not sufficient to wash out the patient's exhaled gases. For this reason, it is generally recommended that the minimum flow set on an oxygen mask is 5 L/min. Oxygen masks are confining and may not be well-tolerated by some patients. Furthermore, they must be removed during eating, drinking, and facial and airway care. Patients often complain that these oxygen masks cause skin irritation, especially when they are tightly fitted. Finally, aspiration of vomitus may be more likely when the mask is in place.

Partial-Rebreathing Masks

The partial-rebreathing mask is derived from the **Boothby-Lovelace-Bulbulian (BLB) mask,** which was introduced by Boothby and associates in 1940.[13] As Figure 3-17 shows, the partial-rebreathing mask consists of a facepiece, which is similar to the simple oxygen mask described previously, and a reservoir bag that is attached to the base of the mask. In a typical, adult partial-rebreathing mask, the reservoir bag has a volume capacity of about 300 to 500 mL. Gas flow from the oxygen source is directed into mask and the reservoir via small-bore tubing that connects at the junction of the mask and bag.

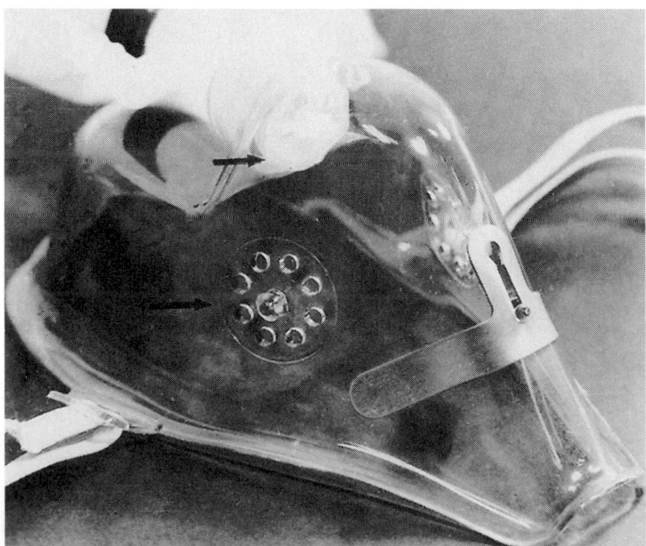

Figure 3-17 Partial-rebreathing mask. (From Gilmore TJ, Shoup CA: *Laboratory exercises in respiratory care*, ed 3, St Louis, 1988, Mosby.)

The operational theory of these devices is fairly straightforward. When the patient inhales, gas is drawn from the bag, the source gas flowing into the mask, and potentially from the room air through the exhalation ports. As the patient exhales, the first third of the exhaled gas fills the reservoir bag, and the last two thirds of the exhaled gas are vented through the exhalation ports. Notice that the volume that fills the reservoir bag is roughly equivalent to the volume of the patient's anatomical dead space volume. Because the volume that fills the reservoir bag represents gas that has not participated in gas exchange, it will have a high partial pressure of oxygen (PO_2) and a low partial pressure of carbon dioxide (PCO_2). Thus the patient inhales this gas mixture during the next breath.

Partial-rebreathing masks can deliver F_IO_2s of 0.40 to 0.60 for oxygen flows of 6 to 8 L/min (see Table 3-1). The actual percentage of oxygen delivered is also influenced by the patient's ventilatory pattern. Note that the minimum flow of oxygen should be sufficient to ensure that the bag does not completely deflate when the patient is inhaling (i.e., the flow should be sufficient to maintain the reservoir bag at least one third to one half full on inspiration).[4,14] Partial-rebreathing masks are available in child and adult sizes.

Nonrebreathing Masks

These masks look very similar to the partial-rebreathing masks except that they contain two valves (Figure 3-18). The first set of valves is a one-way valve (*B*) located between the reservoir bag and the base of the mask. This valve allows gas flow to enter the mask from the reservoir bag when the patient inhales and prevents gas flow from the mask back into the reservoir bag during the patient's exhalation, as

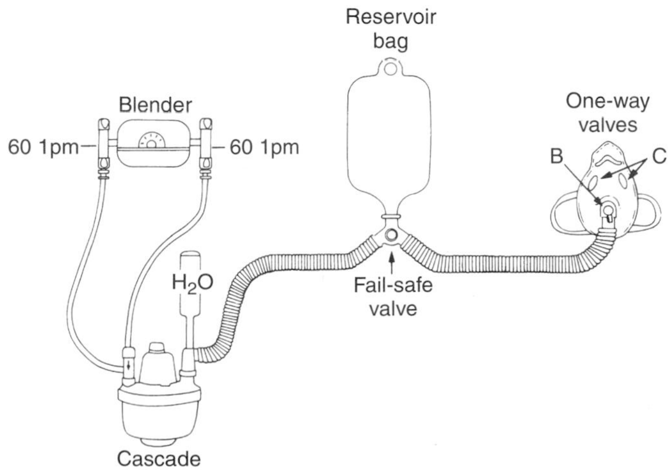

Figure 3-18 Nonrebreathing mask. (From Foust GN, et al: *Chest* 99:1346, 1991.)

occurs with the partial-rebreathing mask. The second set of valves is at the exhalation ports *(C)*. The one-way valves placed there prevent room air from entering the mask during inhalation. They also allow the patient's exhaled gases to exit the mask on exhalation. As with the partial rebreathing mask, the flow of oxygen to the mask should be sufficient to maintain the reservoir bag at least one third to one half full on inspiration.

Nonrebreathing masks can theoretically deliver 100% oxygen, assuming that the mask fits snugly on the patient's face and the only source of gas being inhaled by the patient is derived from the oxygen flowing into the mask-reservoir system. In actual practice, disposable nonrebreathing masks can deliver F_IO_2s of 0.6 to 0.8.[14] The discrepancy between disposable nonrebreathing masks and the original BLB masks is primarily related to the fact that manufacturers usually supply disposable masks with one of the exhalation valves removed. The valve is removed as a precaution in case the oxygen flow to the mask is interrupted or inadequate for the patient's needs (i.e., safety regulations require that the patient can still entrain room air if there is an interruption in source gas flow). Original BLB masks contain a spring-disk safety valve that opens if oxygen flow to the mask is interrupted.

Nonrebreathing masks are effective for administering high F_IO_2s to spontaneously breathing patients for short periods. Prolonged use of these masks can be associated with valve malfunctions (i.e., sticking due to moisture accumulation, or deformity from wear).

High-Flow Oxygen System

Air-Entrainment Masks

Air-entrainment masks are the result of the pioneering work of Barach and associates[15-17] from the 1930s to the 1960s. Figure 3-19 is a schematic of a typical air-entrainment mask. It consists of a plastic mask connected to a jet nozzle, which is encased within a plastic housing that contains air-entrainment ports. Oxygen flowing through the nozzle "drags" in room air through the entrainment ports as a result of viscous, shearing forces between the gas exiting the jet nozzle outlet and the surrounding ambient air.[18] The concentration of oxygen delivered to the patient, therefore, depends on the flow of oxygen exiting the jet nozzle, the size of the jet nozzle outlet, and the size of the entrainment port.

For most commercially available masks, the concentration is varied by changing the size of the nozzle outlet or the entrainment ports. The flow of oxygen to the nozzle is constant and set to a minimum value, usually between 2 and 10 L/min. Note that partial obstruction of oxygen flow downstream of the jet orifice or partial obstruction of the entrainment ports will decrease the amount of room air entrained, thus raising the F_IO_2 of the delivered gas.[19-21]

Figure 3-20 presents a simple method for calculating the air:oxygen entrainment ratio and the total gas flow delivered for a given F_IO_2.[20] Table 3-2 contains a list of the air:oxygen entrainment ratios required to achieve a given F_IO_2, evidencing that the total flow of gas delivered is

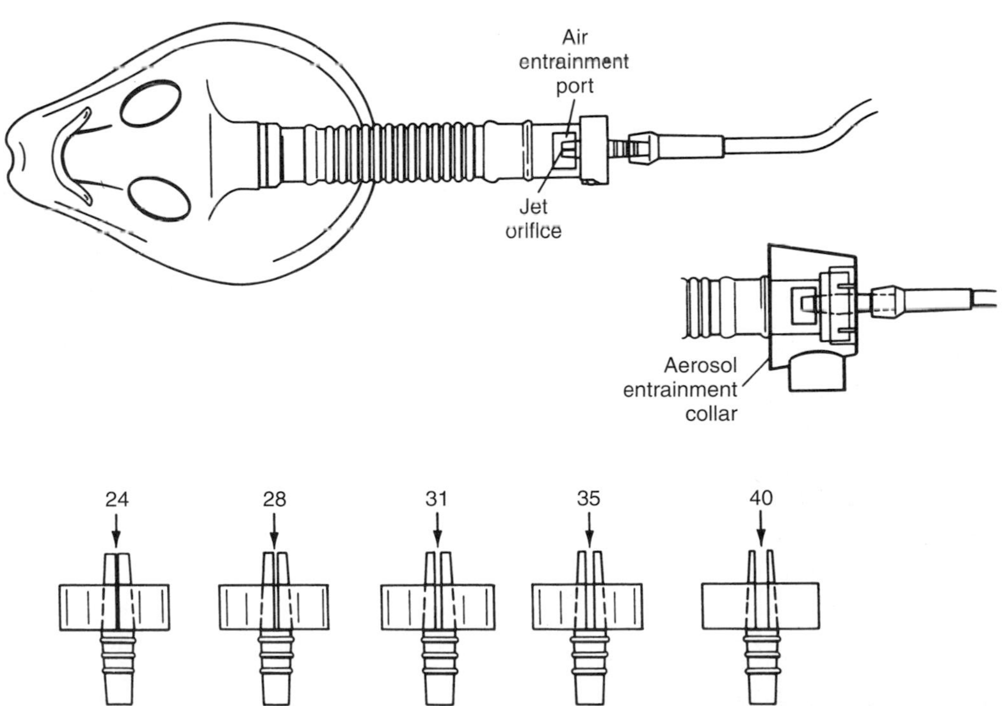

Figure 3-19 Schematic illustrating the components of an air-entrainment mask. Aerosol collar allows high humidity or aerosol entrainment from an air source. (From Kacmarek RM: In-hospital O_2 therapy. In Kacmarek RM, Stoller J, editors: *Current respiratory care,* Toronto, 1988, BC Decker.)

$$O_2 \text{ flow} = \frac{\text{Total flow} \times (F_IO_2 - 0.2)}{0.8}$$

EXAMPLE:
Known: Total flow = 10 L/min
$F_IO_2 = 0.4$

$$O_2 \text{ flow} = \frac{10 \times (0.4 - 0.2)}{0.8}$$

$$O_2 \text{ flow} = \frac{10 \times 0.2}{0.8}$$

$$O_2 \text{ flow} = \frac{2}{0.8}$$

O_2 flow = 2.5 L/min

(Air flow = Total flow – O_2 flow)

$$F_IO_2 \text{ flow} = \frac{O_2 \text{ flow} + (0.2 \times \text{Air flow})}{\text{Total flow}}$$

EXAMPLE:
Known: O_2 flow = 2.5 L/min
Air flow = 7.5 L/min
Total flow = 10 L/min

$$F_IO_2 = \frac{2.5 + (0.2 \times 7.5)}{10}$$

$$F_IO_2 = \frac{2.5 + 1.5}{10}$$

$$F_IO_2 = \frac{4}{10}$$

$F_IO_2 = 0.4$

$$\text{Total flow} = \frac{O_2 \text{ flow} \times 0.8}{F_IO_2 - 0.2}$$

EXAMPLE:
Known: O_2 flow = 2.5 L/min
$F_IO_2 = 0.4$

$$\text{Total flow} = \frac{2.5 \times 0.8}{0.4 - 0.2}$$

$$\text{Total flow} = \frac{2}{0.2}$$

Total flow = 10 L/min

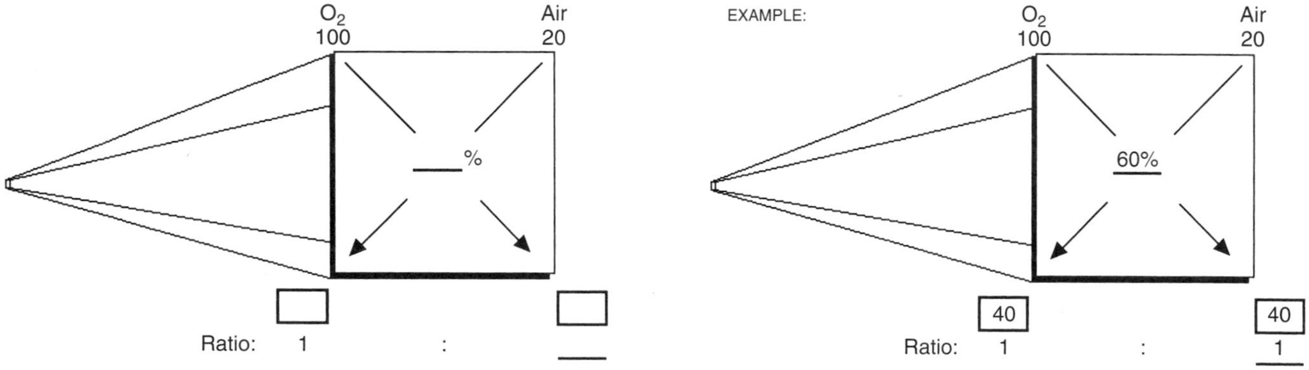

Figure 3-20 Method for calculating air-oxygen entrainment ratios.

Table 3-2 Approximate Entrainment Ratios for Commonly Used Oxygen Concentrations*

Oxygen Percentage	Air:Oxygen Ratio	Total Parts†
100	0:1	1
70	0.6:1	1.6
60	1:1	2
50	1.7:1	2.7
40	3:1	4
35	5:1	6
30	8:1	9
28	10:1	11
24	25:1	26

*Assuming F_IO_2 is 20.9%.
†Total parts × Oxygen flow = Total flow estimate.

greater for low F_IO_2 than it is for high F_IO_2. Air-entrainment masks are able to function much better as fixed-performance devices at low F_IO_2s (<0.4) than at higher F_IO_2s (>0.4).[19,21,22] The discrepancy between the set F_IO_2 and the actual delivered F_IO_2 is exaggerated by abrupt increases in inspiratory flow. Campbell and associates[23] suggest that many commercially available masks produce variable F_IO_2 when patients generate high inspiratory flows because of insufficient mask volume.

Air-entrainment masks are excellent for providing oxygen therapy to hypoxemic chronic obstructive pulmonary disease patients, who typically require fixed F_IO_2 between 0.24 and 0.35.[17] The total flow of gas delivered (oxygen plus air) by such masks for lower F_IO_2 levels is usually sufficient to meet peak inspiratory flow requirements for these patients. Supplemental humidification of the delivered gas is usually not required when the oxygen flow is low (e.g., <4 L/min) because the oxygen flow is a small percentage of the total flow. Increased moisture can be delivered by attaching a compressed, air-driven aerosol to the air-entrainment port via an open, plastic collar. (Such collars work best with masks that have large air-entrainment ports.[20]) Alternatively, high humidity can be delivered with fixed F_IO_2s with large-volume aerosol nebulizers and humidifier units that use air-entrainment devices, which can provide increased levels of moisture at several fixed oxygen percentage settings (e.g., 0.4, 0.6, and 1.0). A number of appliances, including aerosol masks, face tents, T-tubes, and tracheostomy collars, can be used to deliver these moisture-rich gases. Care should be taken not to allow moisture to accumulate in the tubing downstream from the air-entrainment device. Accumulated moisture acts as an obstruction, which can decrease the amount of room air entrained and raise the F_IO_2 delivered to the patient. Notice that the total flow of gas provided by this type of apparatus may not be sufficient to meet patients' high ventilatory demands. Thus the F_IO_2 may vary considerably in these situations because the patient will be forced to entrain room air to meet increased ventilatory needs.[24,25] Large-volume nebulizers and humidifiers will be discussed in more detail in Chapter 4.

Oxygen Hoods

Oxygen hoods were introduced in the 1970s as a means of maintaining a relatively constant F_IO_2 to infants requiring supplemental oxygen. Figure 3-21 shows a typical hood used to deliver oxygen therapy to pediatric patients. It is a clear plastic enclosure that is placed around the patient's head. Fixed oxygen concentrations (from an air-entrainment device or an oxygen/air blender [see the section on oxygen blenders later in this chapter]) can be connected to the hood via an inlet port that is located at the rear of the hood. The flow rate of gas entering the hood is set to ensure that the exhaled carbon dioxide is flushed out (i.e., the flow rate should be approximately 5 to 10 L/min).

The F_IO_2 must be measured intermittently or monitored continuously with an oxygen analyzer. Several studies have shown that in hoods, the oxygen seems to be layered, with the highest concentration near the bottom of the hood. The partial pressure of oxygen in the arteries (PaO_2) should also be measured by arterial blood gas analysis at regular intervals. The noise levels inside these devices can present problems, and every effort should be made to minimize this effect.[26]

Incubators

Incubators, along with oxygen tents, can be classified as environmental delivery systems because they provide large volumes of oxygen-enriched gas to the atmosphere immediately surrounding the patient. The first incubator was designed by Denuce in 1857.[20] Several years later (c. 1880), Tarnier designed an enclosed incubator to provide a warm environment for premature infants.[20] Current incubators (Figure 3-22) allow for variable control of the environmental temperature, humidity, and F_IO_2. The temperature and humidity of the gas within the incubator are controlled by a servo-controlled mechanism connected to a fan that circulates environmental gas over heating coils and a blow-by humidifier. Supplemental oxygen can be provided by connecting a heated humidifier directly to the incubator.

The F_IO_2 is controlled with an air-entrainment apparatus that allows the selection of high and low F_IO_2s. Generally, when the air entrainment port remains open, an F_IO_2 of 0.4 or less is delivered. The port must be occluded to deliver higher F_IO_2 levels. (Opening and closing of the port is accomplished by moving an occluder that is attached to a red metal flag. This feature is incorporated into the design of the system to alert the medical staff that high concentrations of oxygen are being delivered.)

It is important to remember that the actual concentration of oxygen delivered to the patient can vary considerably when the enclosure is opened for nursing-care procedures. Because of the variability in oxygen concentrations that can occur when oxygen is provided through the incubator's oxygen inlet, it may be necessary to deliver oxygen directly to the infant via an oxygen hood placed directly over the infant's head inside the incubator.[9] Regardless of the method used to deliver oxygen to the infant, the actual F_IO_2

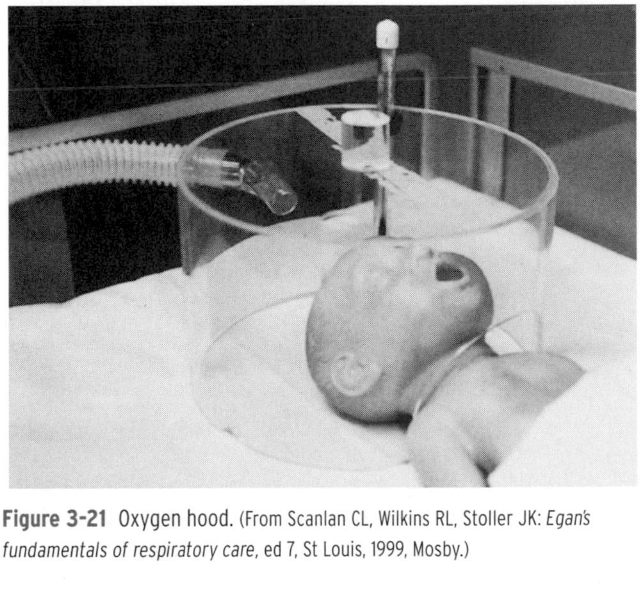

Figure 3-21 Oxygen hood. (From Scanlan CL, Wilkins RL, Stoller JK: *Egan's fundamentals of respiratory care*, ed 7, St Louis, 1999, Mosby.)

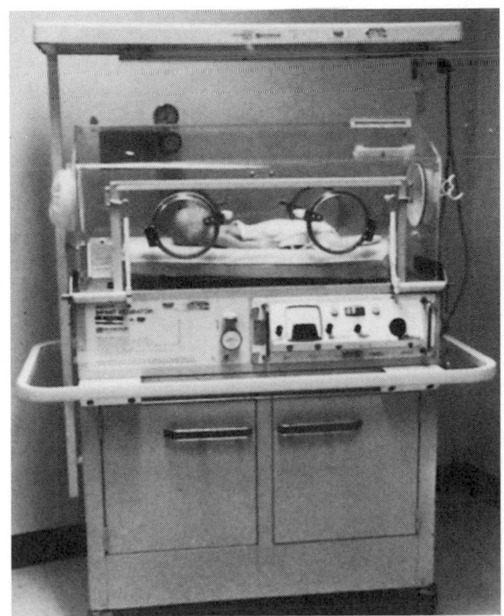

Figure 3-22 Infant incubator. (From Scanlan CL, Wilkins RL, Stoller JK: *Egan's fundamentals of respiratory care*, ed 7, St Louis, 1999, Mosby.)

in the incubator should be intermittently measured or continuously monitored. Additionally, blood gases should be sampled at regular intervals to ensure that the infant is receiving the appropriate oxygen therapy. (The partial pressure of arterial oxygen should be monitored in infants receiving oxygen therapy. High PaO_2 values in these patients are associated with a high incidence of retinopathy and loss of sight.)

Recent studies have demonstrated that noise levels within incubators can be quite high.[26] Although noise may be a difficult problem to control, every effort must be made to minimize noise levels within these devices.

Oxygen Tents

Sir Leonard Hill is credited as being the first clinician to use the oxygen tent,[3] but Alvin Barach improved the operation of these devices by conditioning the air within the tent.[4] (Barach accomplished this early form of air conditioning by adding a fan to circulate the air over a cooling tower containing ice.) During the early 1900s, oxygen tents were often used to provide oxygen to hypoxemic adults and children. Modern oxygen tents are primarily used for pediatric patients requiring enriched oxygen and high humidity levels. Today's oxygen tents can provide environmental control of (1) oxygen concentration, (2) humidity, and (3) temperature (Figure 3-23). The F_IO_2 and the humidity content delivered to the patient are controlled by a high-flow aerosol unit, which is incorporated into the tent. Ultrasonic nebulizers (see Chapter 4) can also be used to increase the humidity inside the tent. Temperature is controlled with refrigeration coils containing Freon. These systems can typically reduce the temperature inside of the tent from 10° to 12° F below room temperature.

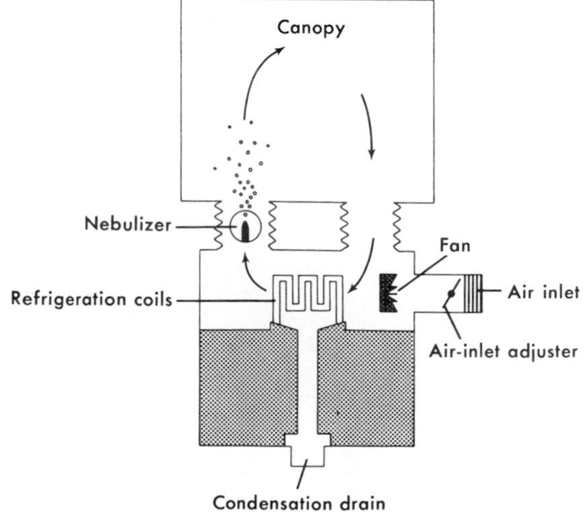

Figure 3-23 Oxygen tent.

Oxygen Proportioners

Oxygen Adders

The simplest example of an oxygen proportioner is an **oxygen adder,** such as the one shown in Figure 3-24. This system consists of two flowmeters: one attached to an oxygen supply and the other attached to an air supply. The outputs of the two flowmeters are directed to humidifiers and then to the patient via any of the delivery systems previously described. The F_IO_2 of the gas delivered to the patient depends on the ratio of air:oxygen flow. The concentration can be calculated using the same principle as for calculating air:oxygen entrainment ratios for air-entrainment masks. For example, if the air and oxygen flowmeters are each set to deliver 15 L/min, then the ratio is 1:1, which corresponds to an F_IO_2 of 0.60. However, if the air flowmeter was set to 15 L/min and the oxygen flowmeter was set to 5 L/min, then the air:oxygen entrainment ratio would be 3:1, corresponding to an F_IO_2 of 0.40 (see Table 3-2).

Oxygen Blenders and Mixers

A more sophisticated device for accomplishing air-oxygen mixing is the **oxygen blender** (or oxygen mixer). Figure 3-25 illustrates a typical oxygen blender and its components. Compressed air and oxygen from a high-pressure source enter into a chamber where the pressures of the two gases are equalized. (An alarm system is incorporated into the design of these devices to alert the practitioner if the pressures of the source gases are not comparable [i.e., >10 psi difference between the air and oxygen pressures].) Unequal source gas pressures can cause the blender to malfunction and deliver unreliable F_IO_2s. This is accomplished by reducing the higher pressure gas to match the lower pressure gas, which is usually 50 psig. The gases are then routed to a precise metering device that controls the amount of each gas reaching the outlet. This metering device can be adjusted with a rotary mixing-control knob on the faceplate. Turning the knob counterclockwise decreases the amount of oxygen reaching the outlet, therefore

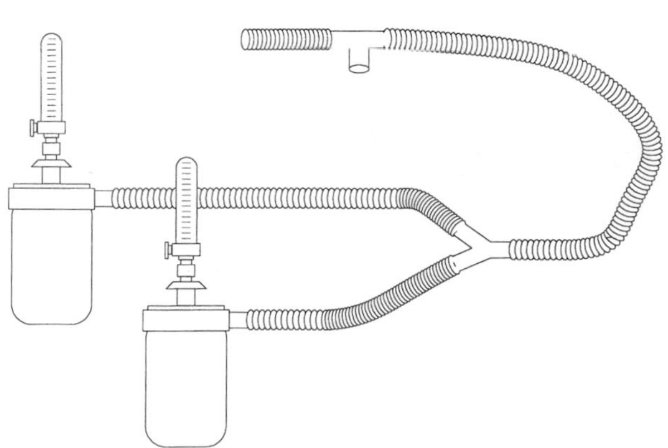

Figure 3-24 Schematic of an oxygen adder. (From Scanlan CL, Wilkins RL, Stoller JK: *Egan's fundamentals of respiratory care*, ed 7, St Louis, 1999, Mosby.)

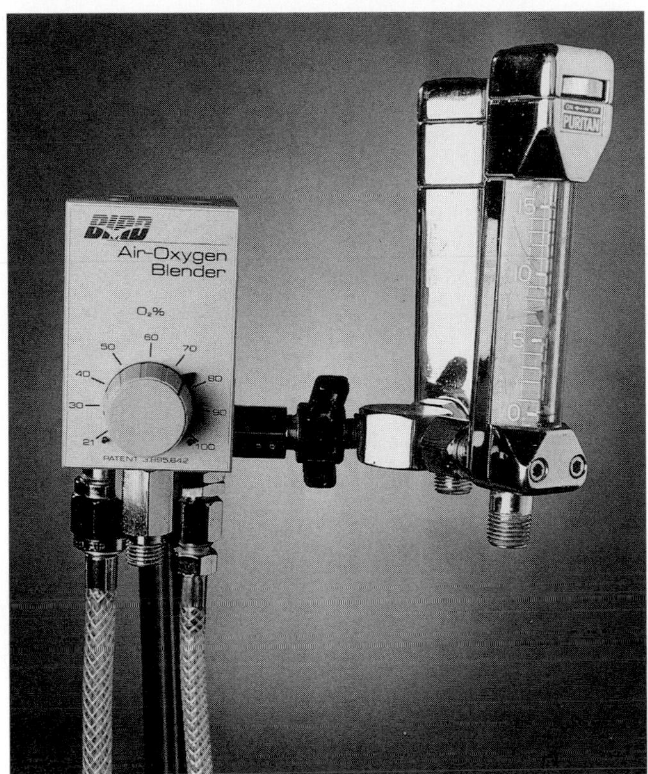

Figure 3-25 Oxygen blender.

Depth in feet	Pressure in ATA	Relative volume	Relative diameter
0	1	100%	100%
33	2	50%	79.3%
66	3	33.3%	69.3%
99	4	25%	63%
132	5	20%	58.5%
165	6	16.6%	55%

Figure 3-26 Pressure-volume relationships during hyperbaric oxygen therapy. (Redrawn from Davis JC, Hunt TK: *Hyperbaric oxygen therapy,* Kensington, Md, 1977, Undersea Medical Society.)

reducing the delivered F_IO_2. Conversely, turning the knob clockwise reduces the amount of air reaching the outlet, thus increasing the F_IO_2.

Oxygen blenders are a reliable means of providing a variety of F_IO_2 levels. Flowmeters can be connected to the blender's outlet, as can ventilators or any other devices that use 50 psig source gas. Because moisture and particulate matter introduced into the blender by the source gases can cause the blender to malfunction, it is important to filter the gas before it enters the blender housing.

Hyperbaric Oxygen Therapy

Hyperbaric oxygen therapy exposes patients to a pressure greater than atmospheric while they breathe 100% oxygen either continuously or intermittently. Historically, hyperbaric therapy has been used most often to treat subjects with decompression sickness and air embolism associated with deep sea diving. More recently, it has been successfully used to treat patients with a variety of disorders, including carbon monoxide poisoning and smoke inhalation, anaerobic infections that are refractory to conventional therapy, thermal injuries, skin grafts, and refractory osteomyelitis. Although hyperbaric oxygen therapy has increased significantly during the past decade, its use is somewhat limited because it is expensive to purchase and maintain hyperbaric units. A brief discussion of the physiologic basis of hyperbaric oxygen therapy and a description of the equipment required follow. For a more detailed analysis of hyperbaric oxygen therapy, consult the references at the end of this chapter.[27-29]

Physiologic Principles

Effects on Respiratory Function

Exposure to elevated barometric pressures during hyperbaric oxygen therapy can directly affect a number of physiologic parameters related to respiration, including lung volume, arterial and alveolar partial pressures for oxygen, the temperature of the gases being breathed, and the work of breathing.

Lung Volumes. The effects on lung volume can be explained by Boyle's law, which states that if the temperature of a gas remains constant, the volume of a gas is inversely related to its pressure. That is, as pressure exerted on the container increases, the gas volume decreases. Thus when a person is exposed to elevated pressures, the gas volume contained in any body cavity tends to be compressed. For example, as the ambient pressure is doubled (1520 mm Hg, or 2 atm), the air volume in the lung is reduced to half of what it would occupy at normal ambient pressures (760 mm Hg, or 1 atm). Figure 3-26 illustrates pressure/volume relationships that are typically encountered during hyperbaric oxygen therapy.

Alveolar and Arterial Partial Pressures of Oxygen. The effect of increased ambient pressure on the partial pressure of alveolar oxygen (P_AO_2) can be explained by Dalton's law, which states that the total pressure of a gas mixture, such as air, equals the sum of the partial pressures of each of the constituent gases in the mixture. Considering that air is 21% oxygen and 79% nitrogen, then ambient air (assuming that the barometric pressure is 760 torr) will have a partial oxygen pressure (PO_2) of about 160 torr (0.21×760 torr) and a partial nitrogen pressure of about 600 torr (0.79 × 760 torr). This same logic can be applied to the alveolar air equation for calculating the P_AO_2 that follows:

$$P_AO_2 = (P_{bar} - PH_2O)\ F_IO_2 - P_aCO_2 \div 0.8$$

Therefore, if the barometric pressure (P_{bar}) equals 760 torr, PH_2O equals 47 torr, $PaCO_2$ equals 40 torr, and the F_IO_2 equals 0.21, then the P_AO_2 would be about 100 torr. Consider if the barometric pressure is doubled to 1520 torr, or 2 atm. If all other variables in the equation remain constant, then the P_AO_2 would equal 333 torr.

Henry's law is used to explain the changes in the PaO_2 that occur with exposure to elevated ambient pressures. It states that the degree to which a gas enters into physical solution in body fluids is directly proportional to the partial pressure of gas to which the fluid is exposed. Remember that Henry's law states that the relative quantities of gas entering a fluid are related to the pressure of gas exerted on the fluid and the solubility of the gas in the fluid in question. Thus oxygen's solubility in plasma is about 0.003 vol % (mL of oxygen/100 mL of whole blood) for every torr of PaO_2. If it is assumed that the ventilation-perfusion relationship for a patient's lungs is normal, then the PaO_2 would be slightly less than 100 torr when the patient is breathing room air at 1 atm. Furthermore, the PaO_2 would be approximately 333 torr for breathing room air when the ambient pressure is increased to 2 atm. Then it can be calculated that as the PaO_2 increases from about 100 torr (at 1 atm) to approximately 333 torr (at 2 atm), the amount of dissolved oxygen increases from 0.3 vol % (100 torr × 0.003 vol %/torr) to 1.0 vol % (333 torr × 0.003 vol %/mm Hg). So, the oxygen-carrying capacity of plasma increases considerably under hyperbaric conditions. It is therefore reasonable to assume that this form of therapy is beneficial to the treatment of patients who have abnormally functioning hemoglobin and thus a reduced ability to carry oxygen attached to hemoglobin, such as occurs with carbon monoxide poisoning.

Gas Temperatures. According to Gay-Lussac's law, if the volume of a gas remains constant, there is a direct relationship between the absolute pressure of a gas and its temperature. It is reasonable to suggest that if the volume of a hyperbaric chamber remains constant, increasing the pressure would raise the temperature inside of the chamber. (Indeed, this problem should limit the usefulness of this form of therapy.) In practice, gas temperature changes encountered during hyperbaric therapy are easily controlled by regulating the rates at which pressures are increased and decreased, the temperature of the air used for compression and decompression, and the flow rate of ventilation used to dissipate heat.[27]

Work of Breathing. As the barometric pressure increases, there is an increase in the density of the gas being breathed. The increase in gas density results in an increased work of breathing, which is not noticeable and can easily be accommodated in normal subjects. In patients with reduced lung reserves, however, this increased work may present problems and require ventilatory support. It is also important to recognize that many ventilators will malfunction when placed in a hyperbaric chamber.[30]

Vascular Function

Several studies have demonstrated that hyperbaric oxygen therapy increases the synthetic ability of tissues by increasing collagen deposition, thus enhancing the growth of new blood vessels in damaged tissues and the revascularization of these tissues.[27] This effect has been used to successfully treat patients with skin grafts.

Immunologic Function

It is well-established that leukocyte function is enhanced during hyperbaric oxygen therapy. This improved function is thought to be related to an increase in the oxygen available for microbicidal metabolism (i.e., H_2O_2, OH^-). Coupled with this enhanced microbicidal activity of leukocytes, oxygen appears to directly inhibit the growth of certain bacteria, particularly those involved in anaerobic infections, such as *Clostridia* sp., which are responsible for gas gangrene.

Equipment

Hyperbaric chambers are generally classified as either monoplace or multiplace units (Figure 3-27). **Monoplace hyperbaric chambers** are specified by the National Fire Protection Association (NFPA) as Class B chambers and are rated for single occupancy.[27] There are several monoplace units available commercially. Although they differ considerably in appearance, they all use the same principle of operation, generally relying on a single gas source for compression and respiration. (Some newer systems provide connections for a separate source gas for respiration.)

A typical chamber is generally about 8 to 10 ft long and 3 ft in diameter. The outer shell of the unit is constructed of steel and clear, double-thick acrylic. Some newer units contain a separate chamber compartment to accommodate attendants working with the patient. Most units are mounted on wheels for portability but are usually treated as stationary systems; therefore, they are placed in a room that is designated for the purposes of hyperbaric therapy.

Multiplace hyperbaric chambers are walk-in units that provide enough space to treat two or more patients simultaneously. They vary in size (2 to 13 occupants), but usually contain a main chamber for treating patients and a smaller chamber allowing attendants to enter and leave without altering the pressure within the main chamber. Multiplace chambers provide two gas sources: one for compression and one for respiration. Hyperbaric oxygenation is achieved by having the patient breathe oxygen by mask or through a specially designed hood while being exposed to elevated barometric pressures in the compressed air chamber. Treatment schedules (i.e., the amount of time that the patient breathes 100% oxygen vs. air) are tailored to the specific needs of the patient. Generally, patients are placed on schedules in which intermittent air breathing periods of 5 minutes or

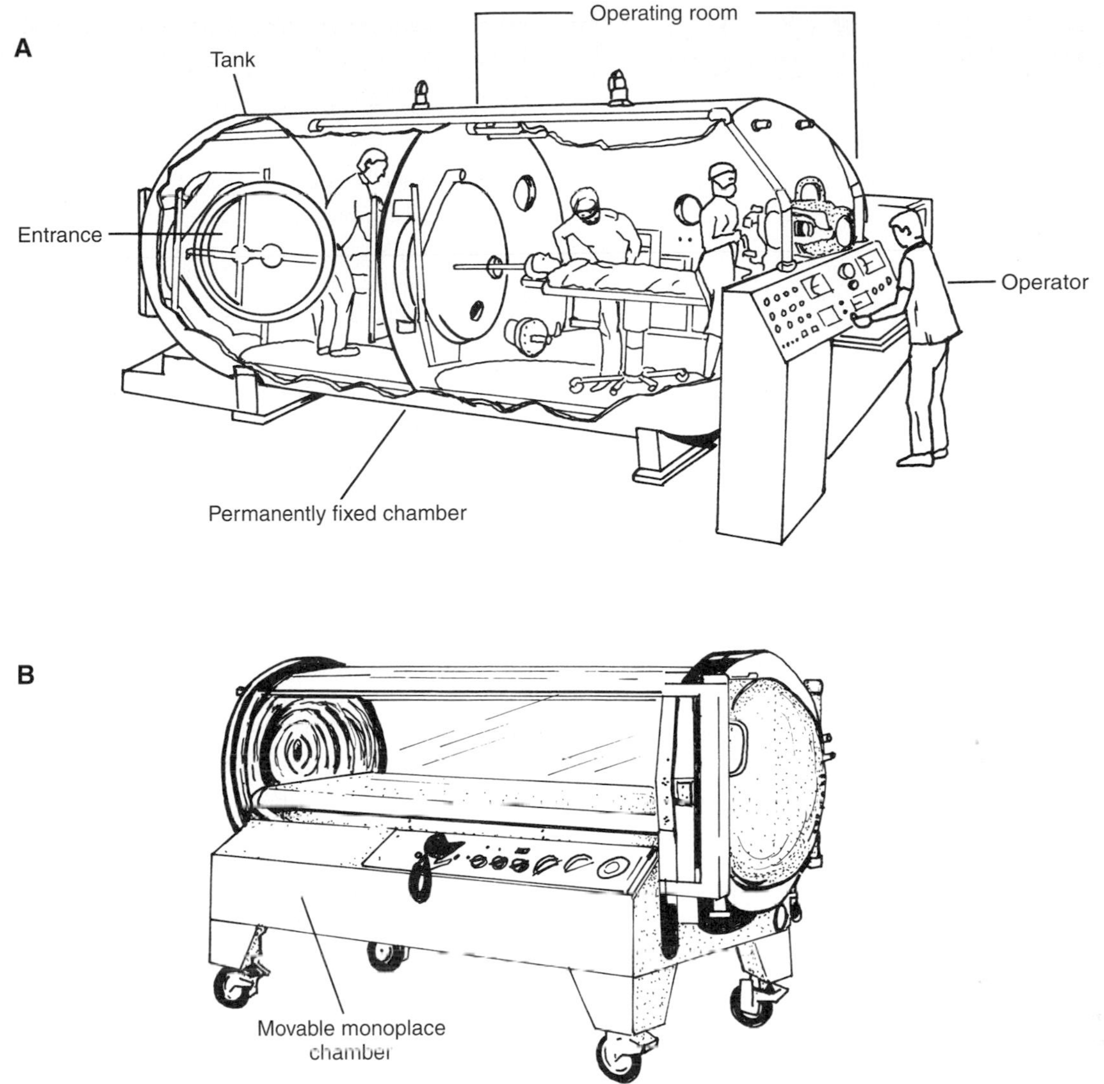

Figure 3-27 Schematics of a multiplace **(A)** and a monoplace **(B)** hyperbaric oxygen chamber. (From Scanlan CL, Wilkins RL, Stoller JK: *Egan's fundamentals of respiratory care*, ed 7, St Louis, 1999, Mosby.)

more are programmed approximately every 20 minutes. This intermittent air breathing is used to prevent oxygen toxicity.

Monitoring Devices

All hyperbaric facilities should have the capability to monitor the oxygenation status of patients undergoing hyperbaric oxygen therapy. Transcutaneous monitoring has proven to be valuable in assessing the overall oxygenation status of a patient undergoing hyperbaric therapy. Selective placement of the probe can also provide information on the localized effects of hyperbaric oxygen therapy on ischemic tissue.

Arterial blood gas monitoring can provide information on the oxygenation status of patients receiving hyperbaric therapy and is also an indication of their ventilatory status. Arterial blood samples can be drawn from patients and removed from the chamber for analysis. Care must be taken to ensure that the sample remains tightly sealed until it is analyzed. Transcutaneous monitoring and arterial blood gas analysis is discussed further in Chapters 8 and 10.

Indications and Contraindications for Hyperbaric Oxygen Therapy

As stated previously, hyperbaric oxygen therapy is most often associated with the treatment of individuals who have experienced decompression sickness and other maladies associated with deep-sea diving. Box 3-1 lists several other conditions that have been successfully treated with this type of oxygen therapy.[31-33] Although the effectiveness of hyperbaric oxygen therapy may vary among patients, patients with any of these conditions should respond to it.

Box 3-2 lists some of the known contraindications for hyperbaric oxygen therapy. The only absolute contraindication is pneumothorax. If pneumothorax occurs during hyperbaric treatment, chest tubes should be immediately inserted; failure to treat pneumothorax can have dire consequences.

Box 3-1 Indications for Hyperbaric Oxygen Therapy

Air embolism
Carbon monoxide poisoning
Cyanide poisoning
Decompression sickness
Gas gangrene
Refractory anaerobic infections
Refractory osteomyelitis
Skin grafts
Thermal burns
Wound healing

Box 3-2 Contraindications for Hyperbaric Oxygen Therapy

High fevers
Hypercapnia (>60 torr)
Obstructive airway disease
Optic neuritis
Pneumothorax
Seizure disorders
Sinusitis
Upper respiratory infections
Viral infections

From Kindall EP: Clinical hyperbaric oxygen therapy. In Bennett P, Elliot D, editors: Physiology and medicine of diving, *ed 4, Philadelphia, 1993, WB Saunders.*

The other conditions listed are relative contraindications. Note that serious problems can arise when patients with obstructive bronchial disease caused by asthma, bronchitis, or emphysema are treated with hyperbaric therapy. Gas trapping can result in barotrauma. Similarly, patients who have upper respiratory infections and nasal congestion are usually unable to clear their ears during compression and decompression and thus are prone to eardrum rupture during treatment.

Nitric Oxide Therapy

As discussed in Chapter 2, nitric oxide has been shown to be a potent pulmonary vasodilator. It has been used successfully to treat persistent pulmonary hypertension of the newborn,[31,34] as an adjunct to the treatment of congenital cardiac defects, to reverse pulmonary vasoconstriction associated with adult respiratory distress syndrome, and possibly to reverse the bronchoconstriction induced by histamine and methacholine.[35-38]

Nitric oxide is supplied as a compressed gas mixture of nitric oxide and nitrogen (minimum purity 99%) in cylinders constructed of aluminum alloy.[39] It is supplied this way because it is a highly reactive molecule that is rapidly oxidized to nitrogen dioxide in the presence of oxygen and to nitric acid in the presence of water. Nitrogen dioxide and nitric acid are toxic if inhaled. In low concentrations, they can cause a chemical pneumonitis; higher concentrations can cause lung injury, such as pulmonary edema, which can ultimately lead to death.[31,40]

The therapeutic dose of nitric oxide is between 2 and 80 parts per million.[39] Figure 3-28 is a commercially available nitric oxide delivery system manufactured by Ohmeda. The Ohmeda I-NOvent delivery system is designed for use with most conventional critical care ventilators and can be adapted for use with both adult and pediatric ventilators. Figure 3-29 illustrates the principle of operation.[39] An injection module that consists of a sensor and a gas injection tube is inserted into the inspiratory circuit at the ventilator outlet. Flow in the ventilator circuit is measured, and nitric oxide is injected proportional to the flow to provide the desired dose. The system includes sensors for monitoring oxygen, nitric oxide, and nitrogen dioxide. Gas is sampled downstream of the injection point near the Y-piece in the inspiratory circuit. The gas concentrations are measured with electrochemical cells that are calibrated at regular intervals by the user.[39] Several alarm systems are available to alert staff members when problems arise, including alarms for high and low nitric oxide, high nitrogen dioxide, and high and low oxygen. Other alarms can be set to notify the user when source gas pressure is lost, the electrochemical cells fail, and calibration is required.[39]

Helium-Oxygen (Heliox) Therapy

Helium-oxygen (**heliox**) mixtures have been used on a limited basis to treat patients with airway obstruction.[41,42] Specifically, heliox has been used to manage asthmatic patients with acute respiratory failure, to administer anesthetic gases to patients with small-diameter endotracheal tubes, to treat postextubation stridor in pediatric trauma patients, as an adjunct in the treatment of pediatric patients with refractory croup, and to provide ventilatory support for patients with severe airway obstruction due to chronic bronchitis and emphysema.[43-47]

As stated in Chapter 2, the benefit of breathing heliox is related to its lower density when compared with pure oxygen or air. Remember that the density of a 80%:20% (helium:oxygen) mixture is 0.43 g/L, and that 100% oxygen has a density of 1.43 g/L. Thus an 80%:20% mixture is 1.8 times less dense than 100% oxygen. The lower density promotes laminar flow and reduces the amount of turbulent flow. This relationship is important to remember when administering heliox because the actual flow rate of gas delivered will be approximately 1.8 times greater than the set flow.

Heliox mixtures are supplied in compressed gas cylinders. Two concentrations are generally available: an 80%:20% (helium:oxygen) mixture and a 70%:30% mixture (density = 0.554 g/L). Heliox is usually administered to

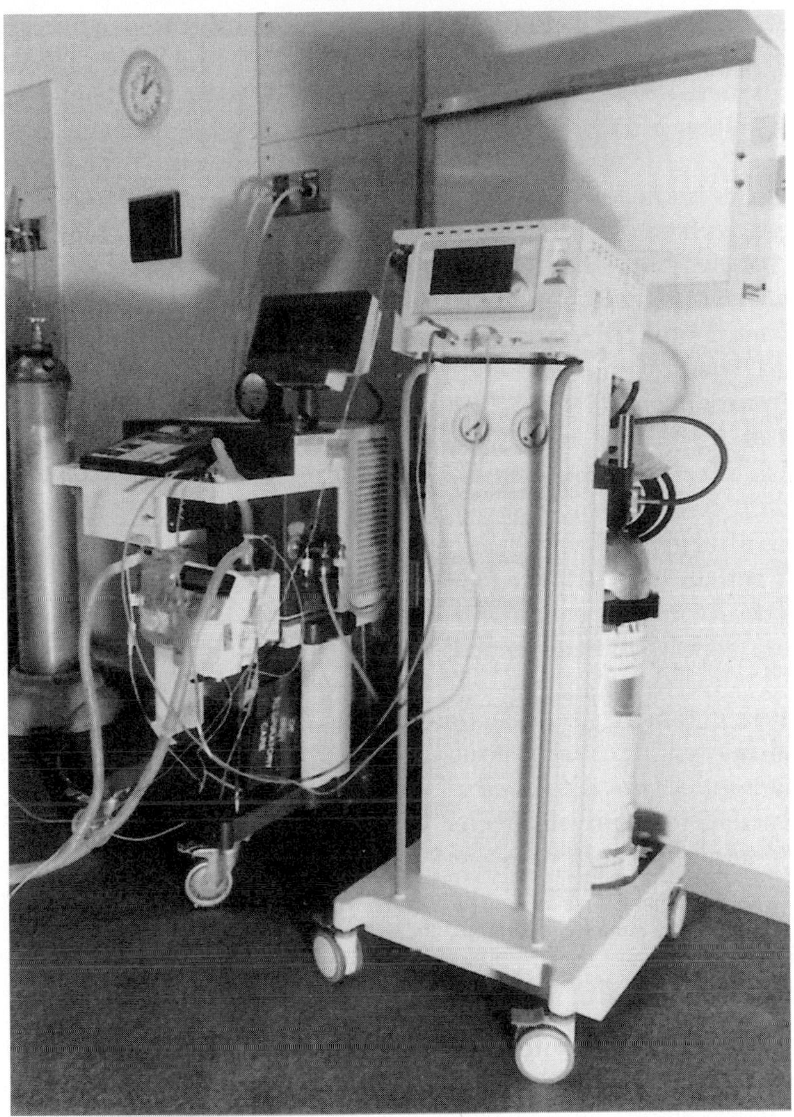

Figure 3-28 Commercially available nitric oxide delivery system. (From Hess D, Ritz R, Branson RD: Delivery systems for inhaled nitric oxide, *Respir Care Clin North Am* 3[3]:371, 1997.)

intubated patients with an intermittent positive pressure device. For nonintubated patients, a well-fitted, nonrebreathing mask attached to a reservoir bag should be used. The flow rate of gas should be high enough to prevent the reservoir bag from collapsing during inspiration. Nasal cannulas are ineffective for delivering heliox because of leakage. Large-volume enclosures, such as hoods, are also unsatisfactory because helium tends to concentrate at the top of these devices.

It is important to monitor the fractional concentration of oxygen delivered to the patient when administering a heliox mixture. In some cases, commercial cylinders containing helium and oxygen may be "unmixed" (i.e., because of the difference in densities between helium and oxygen, a layering effect can occur). If a sufficient amount of oxygen is not mixed with the helium being breathed by the patient, hypoxemia can result.[48] (See Clinical Rounds 3-3 for a problem-solving exercise involving heliox therapy.)

Carbon Dioxide–Oxygen (Carbogen) Therapy

Carbon dioxide–oxygen mixtures (**carbogen**) are used to treat hiccoughs and carbon monoxide poisoning, as a stimulant/depressant of ventilation, and to prevent the complete washout of carbon dioxide during cardiopulmonary bypass. The frequency of this procedure is limited because of the adverse effects associated with breathing elevated concentrations of carbon dioxide. Box 3-3 lists the clinical manifestations of carbon dioxide toxicity.

Carbogen is supplied in compressed-gas cylinders as either 5%:95% (carbon dioxide:oxygen) or as 7%:93% (carbon dioxide:oxygen). It can be administered to patients with a nonrebreathing mask connected to a reservoir bag. The mask should fit snugly on the patient's face, and the flow rate of gas should be high enough to prevent the bag from collapsing when the patient inhales.

To prevent adverse reactions when administering this type of therapy, it is essential to monitor pulse, blood pressure,

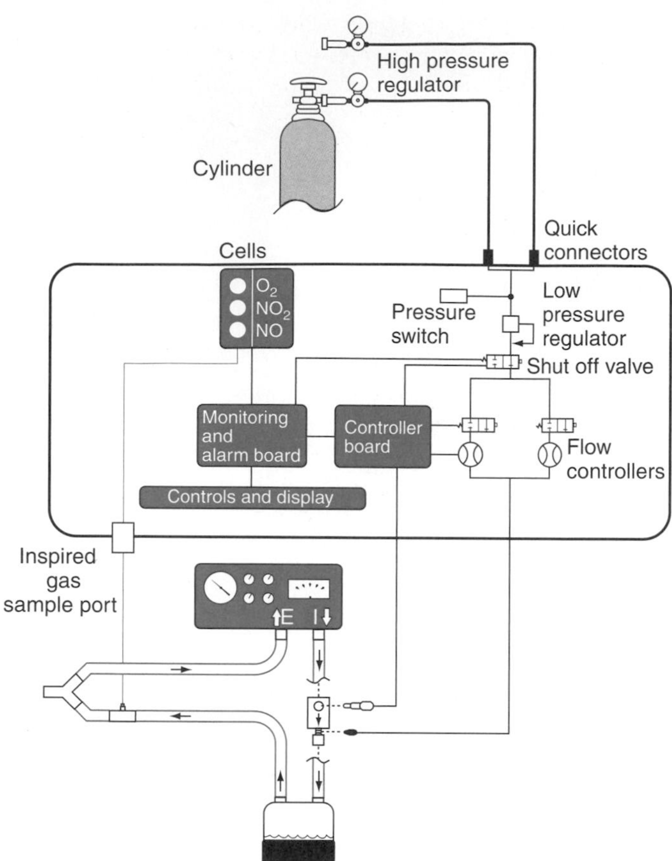

Figure 3-29 Schematic illustrating the principle of operation of the Ohmeda I-NOvent delivery system. (See text for description.) (Redrawn from Hess D, Ritz R, Branson RD: Inhaled nitric oxide I, *Respir Care Clin North Am* 3[3]:398, 1997.)

and respiration as well as the patient's mental status. Pulse, arterial blood pressure, and minute volume normally increase as the patient breathes carbogen, but the rapidity and level of these changes depend on the concentration of the mixture. Thus changes will occur faster and the effects will be greater if the patient breathes a 7%:93% (carbon dioxide:oxygen) mixture when compared with a 5%:95% mixture. The treatment should be stopped immediately if any of the monitored parameters increase or decrease abruptly or significantly.

CLINICAL ROUNDS 3-3

You are the therapist on call when an asthmatic patient is admitted to the emergency department of the hospital. The attending physician requests that you administer heliox containing 30% oxygen to the patient. While administering the gas from a cylinder labeled 70%:30% (helium:oxygen), the patient becomes progressively more dyspneic and cyanotic. What should you do?

See Appendix A for the answer.

Box 3-3 Clinical Manifestations of Carbon Dioxide Toxicity*

Extrasystole (premature ventricular beats)
Flushed skin
Full and bounding pulse
Hypertension
Muscle twitching

Note that hypercapnia cannot be reliably diagnosed on clinical examination only. Arterial blood gases (measurement of partial pressure of arterial carbon dioxide) should be determined in case of doubt.[46]

Summary

Medical gas therapy is a major responsibility of respiratory care practitioners. The appropriate use of each of the modalities discussed in this chapter requires knowledge of the operational theories of the devices used to administer medical gases and an understanding of the indications and contraindications for each type of therapy. The guidelines for administering oxygen are well-established, but heliox, nitric oxide, and hyperbaric oxygen therapy are relatively new techniques that may provide alternative strategies for the treatment of hypoxia. Our knowledge of the indications, contraindications, and adverse effects of heliox and inhaled nitric oxide continues to grow through cogent clinical studies, thus increasing their use as viable therapeutic interventions. Hyperbaric oxygen therapy has been used quite effectively to treat decompression sickness and other diving disorders. Many studies have demonstrated that it may also be an effective treatment for carbon monoxide and cyanide poisoning, as well as a means of preventing tissue necrosis in certain cases.

Review Questions

See Appendix A for answers.

1. Describe an easy method for determining the number of stages in a multistage regulator.

2. Which of the following devices are considered to be high-flow (fixed performance) oxygen delivery systems?
   I. Nasal cannula
   II. Nasal catheter
   III. Air-entrainment mask
   IV. Partial-rebreathing mask
   a. I and II only
   b. I, II, and III only
   c. III only
   d. I, II, III, and IV

3. True or False? Back-pressure—compensated flowmeters have their needle valves positioned upstream of the indicator tube, whereas non—back-pressure—compensated flowmeters have their needle valves positioned downstream of the indicator tube.

4. Which of the following are advantages of using TTO therapy catheters?
   I. These devices do not require periodic replacement.
   II. The incidence of infections is considerably less than other low flow oxygen devices.
   III. They require lower oxygen flows to achieve a given F_IO_2 compared with standard nasal cannulas.
   IV. They are less obtrusive (i.e., more cosmetically pleasing) than nasal cannulas.
   a. I and III only
   b. II and III only
   c. III and IV only
   d. II, III, and IV only

5. What is the air:oxygen entrainment ratio for delivering 40% oxygen through an oxygen adder?
   a. 1:1
   b. 1:2
   c. 1:3
   d. 3:1

6. Studies have shown that mustache and pendant cannulas can reduce the cost of oxygen therapy by as much as:
   a. 10%
   b. 30%
   c. 50%
   d. 80%

7. What is the approximate partial pressure of inspired oxygen of room air if the barometric pressure is raised to 2 atm?
   a. 150 torr
   b. 300 torr
   c. 200 torr
   d. 1520 torr

8. List five indications and five contraindications for hyperbaric oxygen therapy.

9. Administering heliox can be an effective form of therapy in which of the following situations?
   I. Managing postextubation stridor in pediatric trauma patients
   II. Providing ventilatory support for patients with severe airway obstruction resulting from chronic bronchitis and emphysema
   III. Administering anesthetic gases to patients with small-diameter endotracheal tubes
   IV. Delivering oxygen therapy to asthmatic children
   a. I and II only
   b. I and III only
   c. I, II, and III only
   d. I, II, III, and IV

10. You are asked to administer a helium-oxygen mixture to an asthmatic patient who is admitted to the emergency department with acute respiratory distress. Which of the following devices is the most appropriate method of delivering this form of medical gas therapy?
   a. air-entrainment mask
   b. partial rebreathing mask
   c. nasal cannula
   d. non-rebreathing mask

11. Which of the following is an indication for delivering nitric oxide therapy?
   I. It has been used successfully to treat persistent pulmonary hypertension of the newborn
   II. It can be used as an adjunct to the treatment of congenital cardiac defects
   III. It can be used to reverse pulmonary vasoconstriction associated with adult respiratory distress syndrome
   IV. It can be used to treat refractory croup
   a. I and III only
   b. II and IV only
   c. I, II, and III only
   d. I, II, III, and IV

12. Helium is approximately 1.8 times less dense than oxygen. The gas flow delivered to a patient receiving an 80%:20% (helium:oxygen) mixture is indicated on the standard oxygen flowmeter as 10 L/min. What is the actual gas flow being delivered to the patient?

13. When carbogen is being administered, which of the following vital signs should be monitored?
   I. Pulse
   II. Blood pressure
   III. Respirations
   IV. The patient's mental status
   a. I and II only
   b. I and III only
   c. I, III, and IV only
   d. I, II, III, and IV

14. What are the clinical manifestations of carbon dioxide toxicity?

References

1. Ward JJ: Equipment for mixed gas and oxygen therapy. In Barnes TA, editor: *Core textbook of respiratory care practice*, ed 2, St Louis, 1994, Mosby.

2. Petty, TL: Historical highlights of long-term oxygen therapy. *Respir Care* 45:29, 2000.

3. American Association for Respiratory Care: Clinical practice guideline: oxygen therapy in the home or extended care facility, *Respir Care* 37:918, 1992.

4. American Association for Respiratory Care: Clinical practice guideline: oxygen therapy for adults in the acute care facility—2002 revision and update, *Respir Care* 47:717, 2002.

5. American Association for Respiratory Care: Clinical practice guideline: selection of an oxygen delivery device for neonatal

and pediatric patients—2002 revision and update, *Respir Care* 47, 707, 2002.

6. Eisenberg L: History of inhalation therapy equipment. In International Anesthesiology Clinic: *Ventilators and inhalation therapy*, Boston, 1966, Little, Brown.
7. Vain NE, et al: Regulation of oxygen concentrations delivered to infants by nasal cannulas, *Am J Dis Child* 143:1458, 1989.
8. Heimlich HJ: Respiratory rehabilitation with a transtracheal oxygen system, *Ann Otol Rhinol Laryngol* 91:643, 1982.
9. Saponsnick AB, Hess D: Oxygen therapy: administration and management. In Hess D, MacIntyre N, Adams A, et al: *Respiratory care, principles and practice*, Philadelphia, 2002, WB Saunders.
10. Johnson JT, et al: Transtracheal delivery of oxygen: efficacy and safety for long-term continuous therapy, *Ann Oto Rhinol Laryngol* 100:108, 1991.
11. Tieb BL, Lewis MI: Oxygen conservation and oxygen conserving devices, *Chest* 92(2):263, 1987.
12. Shigeoka JW, Bonnekat HW: The current status of oxygen-conserving devices, *Respir Care* 30(10):833, 1985.
13. Boothby VM, Lovelace WR, Bulbulian AH: I. Oxygen administration: the value of high concentration of oxygen for therapy, II. Oxygen for therapy and aviation: an apparatus for the administration of oxygen or oxygen and helium by inhalation, III. Design and construction of the masks for oxygen inhalation apparatus, *Proc Mayo Clinic* 13:641, 1938.
14. Kacmarek RM: Methods of oxygen delivery in the hospital, *Prob Respir Care* 3:563, 1990.
15. Barach AL, Eckman BS: A physiologically controlled oxygen mask apparatus, *Anesthesiology* 2:421, 1941.
16. Barach AL: Symposium: inhalation therapy historical background, *Anesthesiology* 23:407, 1962.
17. Campbell EJM: A method of controlling oxygen administration which reduces the risk of carbon dioxide retention, *Lancet* 2:12, 1960.
18. Scacci R: Air entrainment masks: jet mixing is how they work; the Bernoulli and Venturi principles are how they don't, *Respir Care* 24:928, 1979.
19. Cohen JL, Demers RR, Sakland M: Air entrainment masks: a performance evaluation, *Respir Care* 22:279, 1977.
20. McPherson S: *Respiratory care equipment*, ed 5, St Louis, 1995, Mosby.
21. Hill SL, et al: Fixed performance oxygen masks: an evaluation, *BMJ* 288:1361, 1984.
22. Cox D, Gilbe C: Fixed performance oxygen masks, *Anesthesiology* 36:958, 1981.
23. Campbell EJM, Minty KB: Controlled oxygen at 60% concentration, *Lancet* 2:1199, 1976.
24. Fourst GN, et al: Shortcomings of using two jet nebulizers in tandem with an aerosol face mask, *Chest* 99:1346, 1991.
25. Kuo CD, Lin SE, Wang JH: Aerosol, humidity, and oxygen levels, *Chest* 99:1325, 1991.
26. Mishoe SC, Brooks CW, Dennison FH, Hill KV, Frye T: Octave waveband analysis to determine sound frequencies and intensities produced by nebulizers and humidifier used with hoods, *Respir Care* 40:1120-1124, 1995.
27. Davis JC, Hunt TK, editors: *Hyperbaric oxygen therapy*, Bethesda, Md, 1977, Undersea Medical Society, Inc.
28. Kindall EP: Clinical hyperbaric oxygen therapy. In Bennett P, Elliott D, editors: *The physiology and medicine of diving*, ed 4, Philadelphia, 1993, WB Saunders.
29. Moon RE, Camporesi EM: Clinical applications of hyperbaric oxygen therapy, *Probl Resp Care* 4:176, 1991.
30. Gallagher TJ, Smith RA, Bell GC: Evaluation of mechanical ventilators in a hyperbaric environment, *Space Environ Med* 49:375, 1978.
31. Lustbader D, Fein A: Other modalities of oxygen therapy: hyperbaric oxygen, nitric oxide, and ECMO, *Resp Care Clin North Am* 6(4):659, 2000.
32. NHLBI workshop summary: Hyperbaric oxygenation therapy, *Am Rev Resp Dis* 144(6):1414, 1991.
33. Myers RAM, et al: Value of hyperbaric oxygen in suspected carbon monoxide poisoning, *JAMA* 246:2478, 1981.
34. Craig J, Mullins D: Nitric oxide inhalation in infants and children: physiologic and clinical implications, *Am J Crit Care* 4(6):43, 1995.
35. Roberts JD, Lang P, Bigatello LM: Inhaled nitric oxide in congenital heart disease, *Circulation* 87:447, 1993.
36. Bone RC: A new therapy for the adult respiratory distress syndrome, *N Engl J Med* 328(6):431, 1993.
37. Bigatello LM, et al: Prolonged inhalation of low concentrations of nitric oxide in patients with severe adult respiratory distress syndrome: effects on pulmonary hemodynamics and oxygenation, *Anesthesiology* 80(4):761, 1994.
38. Brown RH, Zerhouni EA, Hirshman C: Reversal of bronchoconstriction by inhaled nitric oxide: histamine versus methacholine, *Am J Resp Crit Care Med* 150:233, 1994.
39. Hess D, Ritz R, Branson RD: Delivery systems for inhaled nitric oxide, *Resp Care Clin North Am* 3(3):371, 1997.
40. Hess DH, Bigatello LM, Hurford WE: Toxicity and complications of inhaled nitric oxide, *Resp Care Clin North Am* 3(4):487, 1997.
41. Motley HL: Helium-oxygen therapy, *Respir Care* 18:668, 1973.
42. Curtis JL, et al: Helium-oxygen gas therapy: use and availability for the emergency treatment of inoperative airway obstruction, *Chest* 90(3):455, 1986.
43. Scanlan CL, Thalken R: Medical gas therapy. In Scanlan CL, Spearman CB, Sheldon RL, editors: *Egan's fundamentals of respiratory care*, ed 6, St Louis, 1995, Mosby.
44. Stillwell PC, et al: Effectiveness of open-circuit and oxyhood delivery of helium-oxygen, *Chest* 95(6):1222, 1989.
45. Skrinskas GJ, Hyland RH, Hutcheon MA: Using helium-oxygen mixtures in the management of acute upper airway obstruction, *Can Med Assoc J* 128:555, 1983.
46. Kemper KJ, et al: Helium-oxygen mixtures in the treatment of postextubation stridor in pediatric patients, *Crit Care Med* 19(3):356, 1991.
47. Nelson DS, McClellan L: Helium-oxygen mixtures as adjunctive support for refractory viral croup, *Ohio State Med J* 78(10):729, 1982.
48. Emergency Care Research Institute: Cylinders with unmixed helium-oxygen, *Health Devices* 19(4):146, 1990.

Internet Resources

American Association for Respiratory Care (Clinical Practice Guidelines): http://www.aarc.org

The American College of Hyperbaric Medicine: http://www.hyperbaricmedicine.org

American Lung Association: http://www.lungusa.org

Global Anesthesiology Server Network: http://gasnet.med.yale.edu

Joint Commission on Accreditation of Healthcare Organizations: http://www.jcaho.org

Mallinckrodt: http://www.mallinckrodt.com

Medexplorer (Search engine for medicine): http://www.medexplorer.com

The Undersea and Hyperbaric Medical Society: http://www.uhms.org

Virtual Hospital: http://www.vh.org

Chapter 4

Humidity and Aerosol Therapy

Dennis R. Wissing

Chapter Outline

Chapter Learning Objectives

Upon completion of this chapter, the reader should be able to:

1. Define the three types of humidity.
2. Define the terms *evaporation*, *aerosol*, and *humidity deficit*.
3. Describe the natural physiologic humidification process.
4. Identify indications for humidity therapy.
5. Describe factors that affect humidification of a gas.
6. Compare low-flow and high-flow humidifiers.
7. Explain the importance of monitoring and maintaining humidity therapy.
8. Describe the physical characteristics of an aerosol.
9. Discuss factors that influence aerosol deposition.
10. Determine the optimal technique for administering aerosol: small-volume nebulizer, large-volume nebulizer, pressurized metered dose inhaler, or dry powder inhaler.
11. Describe the therapeutic indications for aerosol therapy.
12. Explain how pneumatic aerosol generators work to produce an aerosol.
13. Describe how ultrasonic nebulizers work.
14. Discuss the clinical considerations for aerosol therapy.
15. Determine special considerations for administering aerosol therapy.

Key Terms

Absolute Humidity
Aerosol
Aerosol Mask
Brownian Movement
BTPS
Bubble Humidifier
Cascade Humidifier
Chamber
Condensation
Dry Powder Inhaler (DPI)
Evaporation
Geometric Standard Deviation (GSD)
Heat and Moisture Exchangers (HMEs)
Heated Wire
Humidity
Humidity Deficit
Hygroscopic
Inertial Impaction
Isothermic Saturation Boundary (ISB)
Jet Nebulizer
Kinetic Activity
Large-Volume Nebulizer (LVN)
Mass Median Aerodynamic Diameter (MMAD)
Percent Body Humidity (% BH)
Pressurized Metered Dose Inhaler (pMDI)
Relative Humidity
Sedimentation
Small-Volume Nebulizer (SVN)
Spacer
Wick Humidifier

To safely and effectively administer humidity and aerosol therapy, it is necessary to have a firm understanding of the rationale for instituting this type of therapy. Additionally, it is important to grasp several technical considerations, including the principle of operation and the hazards and limitations of the various devices that are currently available. This chapter describes the various devices that are used to deliver humidity and aerosol therapy and presents information on how these devices may be used in various clinical situations involving general medical and critical care of pediatric and adult patients.

Humidity

Humidity is water that exists as individual molecules in the vaporous or gaseous state. Although it may not be obvious, these molecules of water are present in air that we breathe. Vapor is the presence of individual free molecules of a substance that exist below its critical temperature; so humidity is often described as water vapor. Vapor exerts a pressure as a result of the random, constant movement of water molecules. This pressure, called water-vapor pressure (P_{H2O}), varies with the temperature of the gas. That is, as gas temperature increases, water-vapor pressure increases because gas molecules move faster, increasing molecular collisions and bombardment. This principle is illustrated in Figure 4-1. As temperature increases, the **kinetic activity** of the water molecules also increases, resulting in an increase in pressure. After sufficient kinetic activity is reached, molecules leave the liquid state and enter a vaporous state. This occurs at the boiling point of a substance, which can be defined as the temperature at which the pressure exerted by a substance's molecular activity equals the atmospheric pressure. Critical temperature is defined as the temperature at which a substance's kinetic energy is so high that the substance can only exist as a true gas. Above this temperature, no amount of applied pressure can convert the substance (e.g., water) back to a liquid. Therefore, humidity is not a true gas because our atmosphere is at a temperature below the critical temperature of water (374° C), although the terms gas and vapor are often used interchangeably.

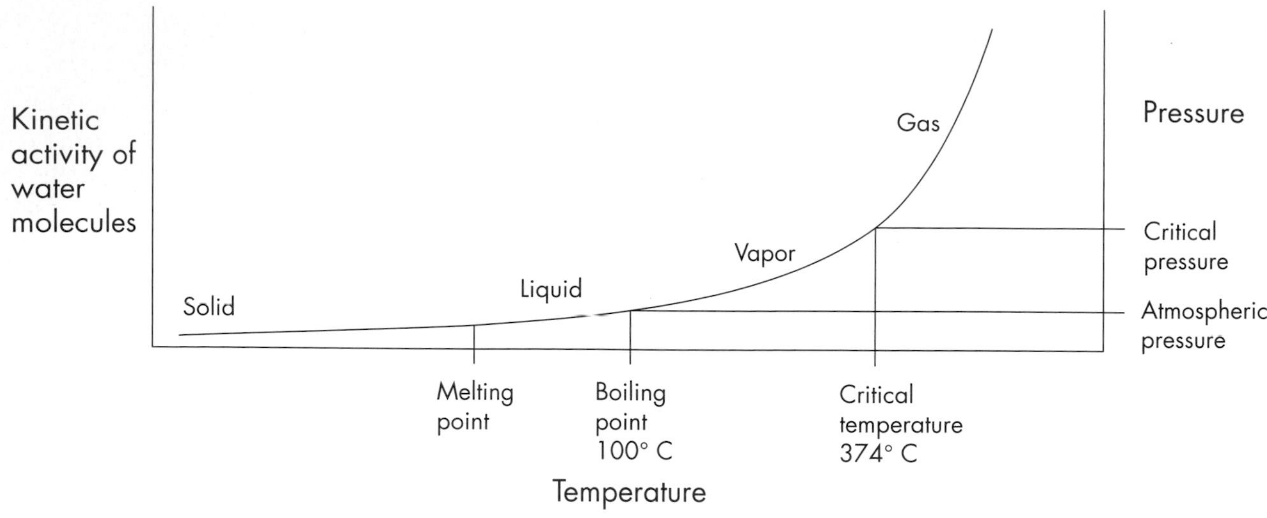

Figure 4-1 The relationship between temperature, pressure, and kinetic activity of water molecules.

As discussed in Chapter 1, vaporization is the result of water changing from a liquid to a vapor, and can result from boiling or evaporation. As water is heated to its boiling point and molecules leave the liquid state and become vapor, water vapor is produced. The boiling point is influenced by the pressure above the water surface. If this pressure increases, the boiling point increases. Likewise, if this pressure decreases, the boiling point decreases. The energy required to vaporize a liquid is called the *latent heat of vaporization*. Vaporization can also result from evaporation, which occurs when a liquid changes to a vapor without reaching its boiling point. Evaporation occurs when liquid molecules near the surface contain enough kinetic energy to break free and enter a vapor state, reducing the volume of the liquid. For example, when a pan of water is left out and exposed to room air, water loss results. Humidity can be measured as **absolute** or **relative humidity.** Absolute humidity is the actual content or weight of water present in a given volume of gas and may be expressed as either grams per cubic meter (g/m^3) or milligrams per liter (mg/L). The term *content* is often substituted for absolute humidity.

Relative humidity (RH) is the ratio of the actual content or weight of the water present in a gas sample relative to the sample's capacity to hold water at that temperature. In other words, RH is a comparison of how much water a gas sample is actually holding with the maximum amount that the gas can hold at a given temperature. RH is calculated by dividing the amount of water in the gas (content) by the amount of water that the gas can hold at that temperature (capacity). This ratio is expressed as a percentage and can be calculated using humidity measurements of weight (mg/L) or partial pressure (P_{H2O}). Box 4-1 shows an example of how to calculate RH.

When the amount of water that a gas contains is equal to the gas's capacity, the RH is 100%. When a gas is at capacity (i.e., it contains the maximum amount of water vapor that it can hold at a given temperature), it is described as saturated (i.e., content equals capacity). The term *saturation* is similar to water-vapor capacity, which refers to a gas at its maximum partial pressure of water vapor. Table 4-1 shows the relationship between partial pressure of water vapor, temperature, and content. It is important to recognize that a gas exerts a partial pressure of water vapor of 47 torr at 37° C and contains 43.9 mg of water per liter of gas. These values are found in gas in the lower respiratory track as a result of an effective upper and lower airway conditioning process for incoming gas from a wide range of ambient conditions. If absolute humidity is held constant, increasing the temperature of the gas will decrease RH because the higher the gas temperature, the greater the gas's capacity to hold water. Likewise, a decrease in temperature will decrease the gas's capacity to hold water, and the RH will remain at 100%. This phenomenon is often encountered by respiratory therapists during heated humidity therapy. When heated humidity is delivered to a patient via large-bore (diameter) corrugated tubing, ambient temperature can cool the gas within the tubing; the absolute humidity remains unchanged, the gas temperature decreases the gas's capacity to hold water, so water vapor is squeezed out of the gas. This excess water, or **condensation,** can accumulate in the delivery tubing and must be removed to eliminate the possibility of the water becoming an obstruction in the gas delivery tube, disrupting gas and humidity delivery to the patient (Figure 4-2).

Percent Body Humidity (% BH) and Humidity Deficit

Percent body humidity (% BH), which is the maximum amount of water that can be held by a gas at body temperature, is often used when discussing RH. Specifically, % BH is gas at BTPS, which is defined as a gas

Box 4-1 Calculating Relative Humidity

The actual water content (absolute humidity) of a sample of room air is measured with a hygrometer and is found to be 12 mg/L. If the room air temperature is 20° C (68° F), what is the relative humidity?

Step 1

Refer to Table 4-1, locate 20°, and note the water content. This refers to the maximum amount of water a gas sample at this temperature can hold, which is 17.30 mg/L.

Step 2

Relative humidity is the ratio of what the gas sample is *actually* holding to what the gas sample can hold when saturated with water vapor. To calculate relative humidity, divide the actual content by the capacity:

$$\frac{\text{measured humidity (content)}}{\text{water capacity}} \times 100 = \text{relative humidity}$$

$$\frac{12\ \text{mg/L}}{17.30\ \text{mg/L}} = 69\%$$

Step 3

Interpret the answer. In this case, the room air is holding 69% of what is capable of holding at 20° C.

Table 4-1 Absolute humidity and water vapor pressure at various temperatures when the gas is saturated with water

Temperature (°C)	Absolute Humidity (mg/L)	Water Vapor Pressure (torr)
19	16.3	16.5
20	17.3	17.5
21	18.4	18.6
22	19.4	19.8
23	20.6	21.0
24	21.8	22.3
25	23.0	23.7
26	24.4	25.1
27	25.8	26.7
28	27.2	28.3
29	28.8	29.9
30	30.4	31.7
31	32.0	33.6
32	33.8	35.5
33	35.6	37.6
34	37.6	39.8
35	39.6	42.0
36	41.7	44.4
37	**43.9**	**46.9**
38	46.2	49.5
39	48.6	52.3
40	51.1	55.1
41	53.7	58.1

at body temperature at the pressure to which the patient is exposed (e.g., atmospheric) and 100% saturated with water vapor. Under normal physiologic conditions, % BH is 43.9 mg/L (see Table 4-1).

A **humidity deficit** is the difference between the amount of water vapor inspired and water vapor contained in the gas in the lungs. In other words, humidity deficit is the difference between % BH and actual ambient humidity. Under most conditions, the upper airway can eliminate a humidity deficit over a wide range of ambient temperatures and humidity levels. Figure 4-3 shows an example of the humidity deficit of a nonintubated patient spontaneously breathing room air. A humidity deficit becomes clinically significant when the deficit is large and maintained for an extended period. A patient breathing a gas that contains little or no humidity may experience pathologic changes in the airways, including drying or retention of secretions, airway plugging, and increased incidence of infection. Most spontaneously breathing, nonintubated patients can adequately humidify inspired gas (see Box 4-2). However, these pathologic changes can occur during other conditions. For example, when the upper airway is bypassed by an artificial airway, there may be systemic dehydration, which can also occur when the patient is breathing low-humidity gas and has a high minute volume of respiration. So that the potential danger of a large humidity deficit and the importance of proper humidification of an anhydrous medical gas are fully understood, a brief review of the physiology of natural humidification is provided.

Physiologic Humidification

The upper and lower respiratory tracts normally provide an effective system for conditioning inspired gas. Besides filtering foreign particles and microbes, the upper airways also warm and humidify inspired gas so that gas traveling beyond the carina enters the lower airways and the alveoli at body temperature, fully saturated with water vapor.[1] As gas enters the upper airway and passes over the nasal turbinates, gas flow becomes turbulent. This turbulence increases the number of gas molecules that come in contact with the nasal mucosa, allowing incoming gas to be more efficiently warmed. This process, called turbulent convection, is an important aspect of normal humidification. As inspired gas is warmed, water is transferred to the incoming gas by evaporation from the mucosa.[2] Therefore, as it flows through the upper airways as a result of inspired gases cooling the

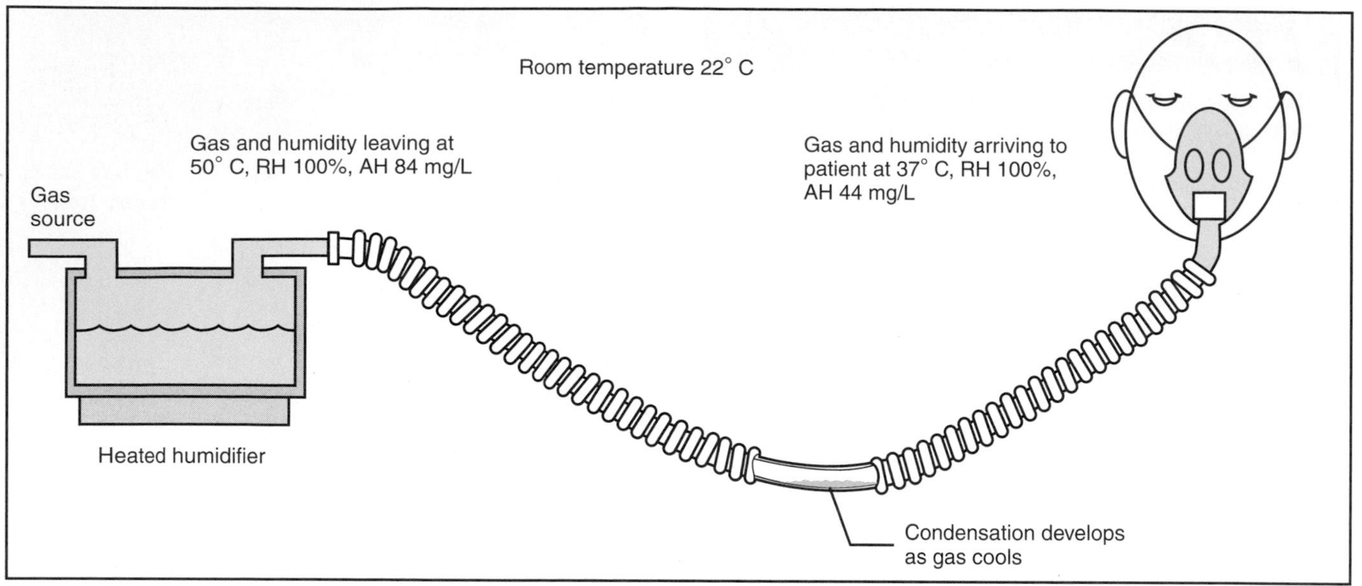

Figure 4-2 Condensation can develop in the gas delivery tube as heated humidity is cooled by ambient conditions. As the temperature of the gas cools, it can hold less water vapor; so excess water leaves the gas and accumulates in gravity-dependent loops of the delivery tubing.

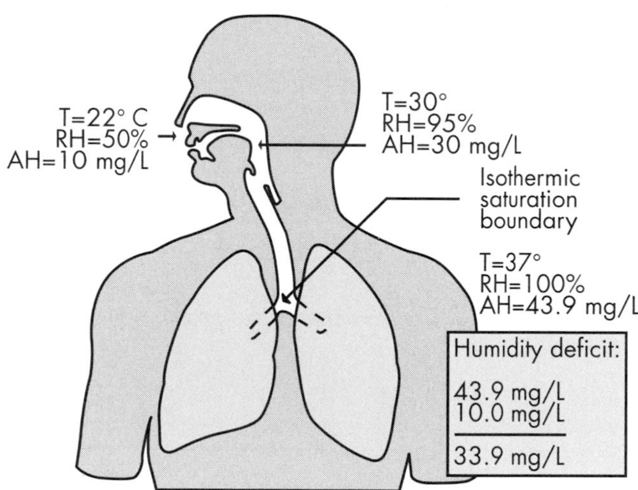

Figure 4-3 This is an example of a spontaneously breathing patient experiencing a humidity deficit. While breathing typical ambient air conditions, a 33.9 mg/L humidity deficit exists, which can be determined by subtracting the ambient absolute humidity from the body humidity (43.9 mg/L).

nasal mucosa, the inspired gas is humidified and warmed through evaporation and convection. This heat energy (previously defined as the latent heat of vaporization) remains in the water vapor until it is released during expiration. As inspiration continues, humidification and warming occur, the mucosa cools, and the incoming gas reaches the **isothermic saturation boundary (ISB).** This boundary is the point at which inspired gas reaches body humidity (at BTPS) and is normally located just below the carina (see Figure 4-3).[3,4]

During exhalation, heat and humidity are transferred back to the nasal mucosa. As gas exits the lower respiratory tract, heat is transferred back to the mucosa by convection. As the expired gas is cooled by this heat loss, the gas's capacity to hold water decreases, and water is released (condensation) onto the airway lining. Thus as expiration occurs, the airway mucosal lining is rewarmed and rehydrated in preparation for the next inspiration. Although some studies report a difference between the gas-conditioning effects of nose vs. mouth breathing, the clinical significance of these differences is minimal. Data suggest that the upper airway can efficiently condition inspired gases from either nasal or mouth breathing.[5,6] As stated previously, the upper airway is an efficient gas conditioner, despite wide fluctuation of ambient temperature and humidity. As ambient temperature increases above body temperature, blood flow to the turbinates increases and heat is lost from the nasal mucosa.[7] At extremely cold temperatures, the upper airway remains capable of providing the lower airways and alveoli with gas at BTPS.

Clinical Indications for Humidity Therapy

Respiratory therapists administer medical gases to a wide variety of patients, from those who are spontaneously breathing (with or without an artificial airway in place) to those who are being mechanically ventilated. To assure effective therapy, an understanding of the indications for humidity therapy is necessary.

Breathing dry or inadequately humidified gas can shift the ISB farther down the lung, compromising the airway's ability to warm and humidify inspired gas. The boundary may move farther into the peripheral airways with endotracheal intubation, large tidal volumes, or inspiration of a cold gas. If the ISB shifts downward, the airway mucosa

Box 4-2 Clinical Signs and Symptoms of Inadequate Airway Humidification

- Atelectasis
- Dry, nonproductive cough
- Increased airway resistance
- Increased incidence of infection
- Increased work of breathing
- Substernal pain
- Thick, dehydrated secretions

is at risk for altered cilia function, a decrease in mucus *rheology* (flow), mucous membrane dehydration, and retention of secretions.[6] Such alterations of mucosal structure may lead to stagnation of secretions, which may lead to partial or complete airway obstruction and increased incidence of infection. If the patient has pulmonary disease, administration of a dry or poorly humidified gas may exacerbate the existing disease and further compromise respiratory function. Such patients may experience partial to complete airway obstruction from mucus plugging and atelectasis and have the potential for ventilatory failure. In an asthmatic a downward shift in the ISB can result in airway constriction and inflammation.[7] Clinical signs and symptoms of inadequate humidification and mucosal damage are listed in Box 4-2.

The goal of humidity therapy is to minimize or eliminate a humidity deficit while the patient is breathing a dry medical gas. Medical gases delivered from a cylinder or central-supply system are delivered at 0% RH. The amount of humidification provided depends on the type of gas-flow system used and the gas's entry point into the respiratory system.

Gas-flow systems can be categorized as either low-flow or high-flow. A low-flow gas system provides a gas flow lower than the patient's inspiratory needs, whereas a high-flow gas system meets the patient's peak inspiratory flow demands. In other words, high-flow systems provide all the gas the patient inspires. Gas from a low-flow system can be humidified, but the patient supplements this humidity with ambient water vapor. An example of a low-flow gas system is a bubble humidifier (Figure 4-4). As oxygen leaves this device, it is humidified to about 40% to 50% RH. As the patient inspires, humidified gas is obtained from the bubble humidifier and ambient air. As the gas enters the respiratory system, it is further humidified by the airway (as previously described) and reaches BTPS at the ISB. With low-flow systems, supplemental humidity may increase patient comfort by minimizing drying of the nasal and oral cavities. Current respiratory care trends include the omission of humidity for dry gases provided to the patient at gas flow rates lower than 4 L/min. Recent data suggest that it is safe to omit supplemental humidity at these flows[8]; however, respiratory therapists should exercise clinical judgment as to when supplemental humidity should be omitted with medical gas delivery from a low-flow system.[9] High-flow gas systems, such as a mechanical ventilator or a properly applied nonrebreathing oxygen mask, provide the entire gas flow to the patient, so adequate humidity must be provided. Official standards for humidity have been established by the American Association for Respiratory Care (AARC).[10] These standards include providing a minimum of 30 mg/L of water at 31° to 35° C with 80% to 100% RH to the airway when the patient is breathing gas through a high-flow gas system and the upper airway is bypassed with an artificial airway (e.g., endotracheal or tracheostomy tube). Humidity at this level can prevent mucosal damage and inspissation or thickening of airway secretions.

It is recommended that the humidity output of any medical gas delivery system match the normal gas conditions at its entry point into the respiratory tract.[9] Box 4-3 lists the humidity and temperature requirements for gases delivered to various points in the respiratory tract.

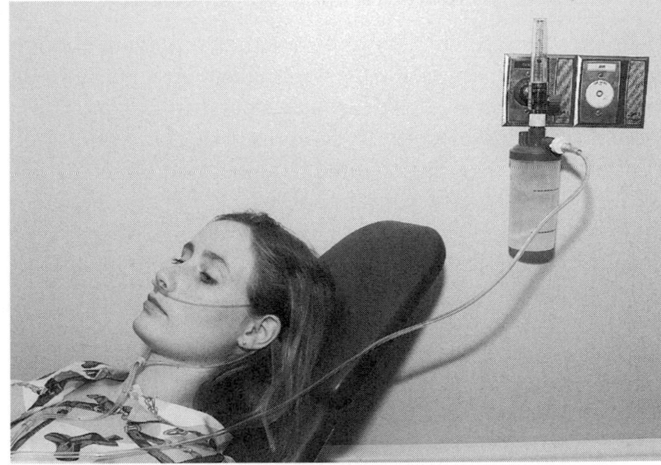

Figure 4-4 A bubble humidifier is a common example of a low-flow humidifier. It humidifies the gas traveling to the patient via nasal cannula to about 40% to 50% of the relative humidity.

Box 4-3 Humidity Requirements for Gas Delivery at Various Sites in the Upper and Lower Airway

Gas Delivered to the Nose or Mouth

50% relative humidity with an absolute humidity level of 10 mg/L at 22° C

Gas Delivered to the Hypopharynx

95% relative humidity with an absolute humidity level of 28 to 34 mg/L at 29° to 32° C

Gas Delivered to the Mid-Trachea

100% relative humidity with an absolute humidity level of 36 to 40 mg/L at 31° to 35° C

Factors that Influence Humidifier Efficiency

Humidity therapy should include either supplying enough water vapor to a dry medical gas to make it equal to ambient conditions in terms of RH and temperature, or providing heated humidity close to body temperature and at 80% to 100% RH when gas is delivered to a bypassed upper airway. Respiratory therapists can choose from a variety of devices to provide humidity therapy. The effectiveness of each type of humidification device depends upon the temperature of the gas being delivered, the ratio of the available water surface area to the gas, and the length of time the gas is exposed to water.

Temperature

As mentioned previously, the higher the temperature of a gas, the more water vapor it can hold. This fundamental concept plays an important role in meeting a patient's humidity needs because heating the humidifier increases the water-carrying capacity of the humidified gas. It is important to recognize that humidified gas delivered to an artificial airway (via endotracheal or tracheostomy tube) must be between 31° and 35° C with a minimum of 30 mg/L of absolute humidity.[10] Therefore, appropriate temperature monitoring at the interface of the patient and the humidifying device is necessary to ensure that temperature and gas humidity levels are within the recommended ranges to avoid mucosal or thermal injury (either because of inadequate humidification and temperature or overheated gas).

Unheated humidifiers are less efficient than heated humidifiers because during operation, an unheated humidifier can lose water temperature in its reservoir as gas flows through it.[11] For example, the temperature of the water reservoir of an unheated bubble humidifier with oxygen flowing through it can decrease to 10° C below room temperature. Even though the gas leaving the unit contains high RH, as it travels to the patient it warms and the RH decreases. After the gas enters the respiratory tract, RH will only be about 30% to 40%.

Surface Area and Time

The greater the ratio of water-surface contact to gas volume, and the longer that the gas is exposed to water, the greater the opportunity for humidification. That is, the greater the water-surface area and the longer the gas is in contact with water, the better the humidification. As gas flows through water, gas molecules are humidified. Typically, during humidity therapy, gas bubbles through or flows across a water reservoir as it travels to the patient. The water-surface area is governed by the amount of water the gas molecules are exposed to, the depth of the water reservoir, and the size of the gas bubbles. The larger the surface area and the greater the depth of the reservoir, the smaller the bubbles, and the longer the gas travels (i.e., a slow gas-flow rate) through the water, the greater the humidification.

As will be described later in this chapter, humidifiers may use either a large water reservoir for gas to flow through (e.g., bubble humidifier) or an adsorbent material or wick to increase gas-to-water contact.

Box 4-4 Types of Humidifiers

Low-Flow Humidifiers
- Bubble humidifiers
- Simple difffuser humidifiers

High-Flow Humidifiers
- Heat and moisture exchangers
- Vapor-phase humidifiers
- Wick type of humidifiers

Humidity-Generating Equipment

Humidifiers can be divided into two categories: low-flow and high-flow. Low-flow humidifiers provide gas and humidity below the inspiratory gas flow needs of the patient, and high-flow humidifiers provide all of the inspiratory gas and humidity flow to the patient. Box 4-4 lists common devices used for each of these categories.

Low-Flow Humidifiers

Low-flow humidifiers are typically classified as bubble type of humidifiers or as bubble-diffuser type of humidifiers. These devices employ a unique physical principle that allows water and gas to come into contact with each other.

Bubble-Type Humidifiers. Of the simple humidifiers, the bubble type of humidifiers are the most widely used devices for humidifying medical gases. Such humidifiers include a water reservoir, a diameter index safety system (DISS) connector for attachment to a gas source (e.g., a flow metering device), a capillary tube that is submerged into the water reservoir, and an outlet for attachment of a delivery device

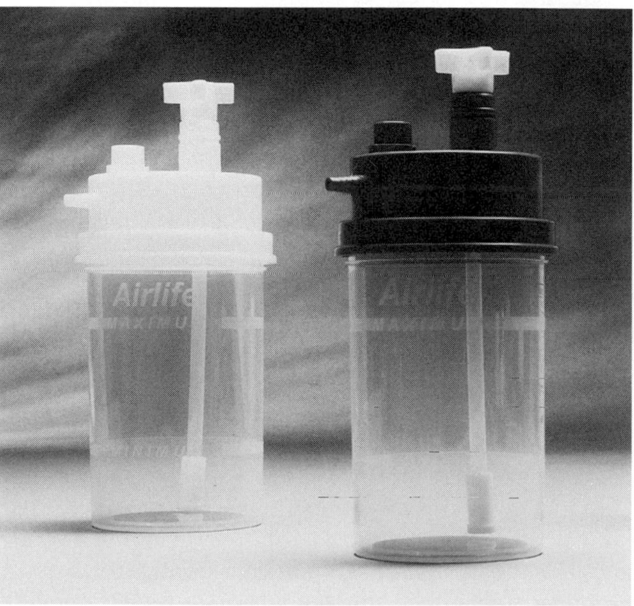

Figure 4-5 A bubble humidifier. (Courtesy Cardinal Health, McGraw Park, Ill.)

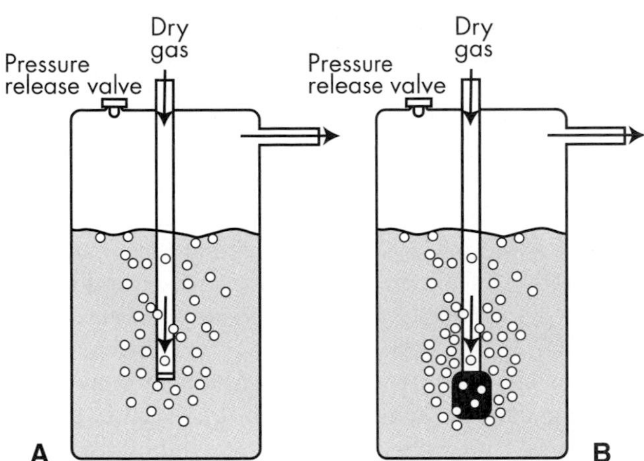

Figure 4-6 Two different types of bubble humidifier capillary tube openings: **A,** an open lumen; **B,** diffuser type of end.

(e.g., an oxygen cannula or mask) (Figure 4-5). A dry gas such as oxygen enters the humidifier through a DISS connector, travels down a capillary type of tube, and exits the tip, breaking up into many small bubbles. Humidification of gas within the bubbles occurs as they rise to the water surface. Once at the surface, the gas bubbles burst, and their water-vapor content is released. The humidifier may also employ a diffuser tip at the distal end of the gas capillary tube to enhance the creation of small gas bubbles. Bubble size is governed by the design of the gas outlet at the bottom of the capillary tube. Some devices have an open lumen, but others employ a diffuser of plastic foam, porous metal, or mesh (Figure 4-6). Diffuser-type of humidifiers are more efficient than capillary tube type of humidifiers because the diffuser creates more small bubbles, allowing a greater surface area for gas and water interaction.[8]

As with other humidifiers, the efficiency of the bubble type of humidifiers depends upon the surface area of the water and gas, the time available for bubbles to remain in contact with the water, and the size of the bubbles. These factors are influenced by the gas flow through the unit (i.e., the faster the gas flow rate, the less time for bubbles and water to stay in contact), the water reservoir level (i.e., the deeper the water, the longer the contact), and the ambient temperature (i.e., the greater the ambient temperature, the lower the RH leaving the device). Bubble humidifiers are more efficient with gas flows of 5 L/min or less. At these flows, absolute humidity is about 10 to 20 mg/L, and RH is 30% to 40% at 37° C.[6,12] At gas flow rates above 5 L/min, delivered humidity decreases because of the reduced temperature of the reservoir and the shorter bubble-to-water contact time.

There are several technical problems with bubble-type humidifiers that should be considered. For example, they can transport water-borne microbes from the unit to the patient when used with high gas flows. At high gas flows an aerosol is created; if microbes are present in the humidifier or delivery tube, water droplets can become contaminated and, if passed onto the patient, an increased opportunity for airway contamination exists. However, typical use of bubble humidifiers are used at flows below 10 L/min, which minimizes this hazard from occurring.

Another problem that may arise with bubble-type humidifiers is the possibility of pressure building up within the humidifier itself. This can occur if the small-bore tubing used to deliver the medical gas becomes kinked or obstructed. If this happens, pressure builds and can possibly rupture the device. To prevent this from occurring, bubble humidifiers use a pressure-relief valve that sounds an audible alarm when pressure builds up within the unit (see Figure 4-6, *B*). The valve can be gravity-operated or spring-loaded and will remain open if the pressure in the unit exceeds 2 psi. After the pressure-relief alarm sounds, corrective actions must be taken to restore medical gas delivery to the patient. Also, maintenance of the water level within the humidifier is critical. Bubble type of humidifiers can be purchased either prefilled (disposable) by the manufacturer as intended for single-patient use (disposable) and permanent (nondisposable). The permanent humidifiers must be filled with sterile water, the level of which must be monitored and maintained; these units must be sterilized between patients.

High-Flow Humidifiers

High-flow humidifiers provide water vapor to the entire gas flow inspired by the patient and include the Passover-type or wick type of humidifiers and heat and moisture exchangers (HMEs). These high-flow humidifiers are commonly used with mechanical ventilation.

Patients receiving mechanical ventilatory support usually require an artificial airway. These airways include endotracheal and tracheostomy tubes, which bypass the patient's natural ability to warm and humidify inspired gases. When an artificial airway is in place, supplemental humidity and heat must be provided to ensure that the gas delivered to the patient contains at least 30 mg/L of water and is at 31° to 35° C. Heated humidity is typically required to prevent hypothermia, dehydration of airway secretions, destruction of airway epithelium, and atelectasis.[8,9,13,14]

Two types of humidifiers are commonly used when an artificial airway is in place: the passover type or HMEs. Each of these humidifiers will be discussed.

Passover Type. A category of high-flow humidifiers is the passover type or more commonly known as wick humidifiers, which employ a cylinder-shaped absorbent paper or sponge that draws water from a reservoir using capillary action. As gas passes through the humidifier, it encounters the large surface area of the wick. Evaporation of water from the wick increases the RH of the gas. Heating the unit allows wick humidifiers to provide up to 100% RH at body temperature. Most wick type of humidifiers offer heated wire technology as an option, which (as discussed later in this chapter) provides heat to the gas-delivery circuit in attempts to maintain desired gas humidity and temperatures as gas travels to the patient. Although there are a number of different manufacturers providing wick-type humidifiers, two examples of models will be discussed. These units that are marketed as using the wick principle include the Hudson RCI Conchapak Humidifier and the Fisher & Paykel Dual Servo Humidifiers.

The Hudson RCI Conchapak humidifiers, which are available in a variety of humidification systems with options for adult, pediatric, and neonatal use, heated wire technology, and servo-controlled heating elements. The Conchapak system has three main components: (1) the servo-controlled heated humidifier (Conchatherm) with or without a heated wire circuit; (2) a humidification column (Conchacolumn); and (3) a sterile water reservoir (Concha sterile water). Hudson provides several different heater units and two unique Conchacolumn designs. The various models available from Hudson include the Conchatherm Heater, the Conchatherm III Plus Heater (16 and 21 volt), the Conchatherm III Humidifier Heater, the Conchatherm IV Heater Humidifier, the pediatric Conchatherm Heater, and the Hi-Flow Conchatherm Heater.

Conchatherm heated humidifiers have a cylindrical heating element (Conchacolumn) that provides a large heating surface area (Figure 4-7). It is made of aluminum with an absorbent paper or wick lining that fits inside and is surrounded by a heating element that maintains an adequate level of heat to ensure that proximal gas temperatures remain at a set level. A side-by-side sterile water reservoir fills the Conchacolumn using a gravity-feed system. A 1650-mL, closed system reservoir continuously feeds the bottom of the column to ensure continuous humidification (Figure 4-8). As the wick is heated and absorbs water, incoming gas is humidified. Gas flow from a mechanical ventilator or gas-flow device enters the top of the column and encounters a heated environment within the chamber. As gas circulates within the column, the heated wick saturates the gas to or near 100% body humidity (based on column temperature).

The Conchatherm III Plus humidifier can be used with or without a heated wire circuit (Figure 4-9). The operator chooses to employ either an intracircuit, heated wire to warm the gas or a conventional circuit with an attached proximal probe to measure the gas temperature delivered to the patient's airway. The servo-controlled heater monitors the heat output of the humidifier. Figure 4-9 depicts the heated wire controller unit as seen on the bottom of the Hudson RCI Conchatherm III Plus. A closer view of the operator's panel for the heated wire is seen in Figure 4-10; this panel regulates the temperature within the breathing circuit to minimize condensation. Use of the heated wire option with the Conchatherm III Plus humidifier allows the operator to control the temperature gradient between the humidifier and the patient. This unit also provides audio and visual alerts to inform the operator when the gradient is not being achieved and an indicator light to show that the wire is being powered. The humidity control adjusts the temperature gradient between the humidifier and the proximal airway or the patient end of the heated wire circuit and can create a temperature difference up to 30° C between the patient and the heater. Adjusting this temperature gradient allows respiratory therapists to compensate for ventilatory gas circuit conditions and ambient variables because this gradient controls the delivered RH. If no gradient occurs, gas temperature will be constant throughout the length of the gas delivery circuit. If the heater temperature is set 3° C cooler than the patient end of the circuit (i.e., positive temperature gradient), additional heat is supplied to the gas-delivery circuit. Notice that this setting will potentially deliver less humidity to the patient with less condensation developing in the delivery circuit. With a cooler heater temperature setting, such as with other types of

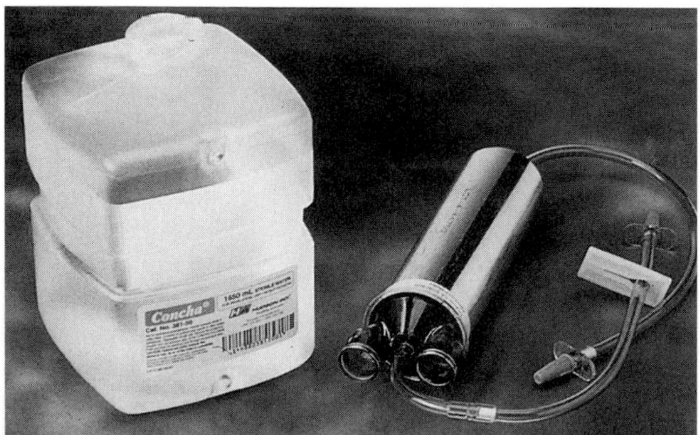

Figure 4-7 The Hudson RCI Conchacolumn. (Courtesy Hudson Respiratory Care, Inc, Temecula, Calif.)

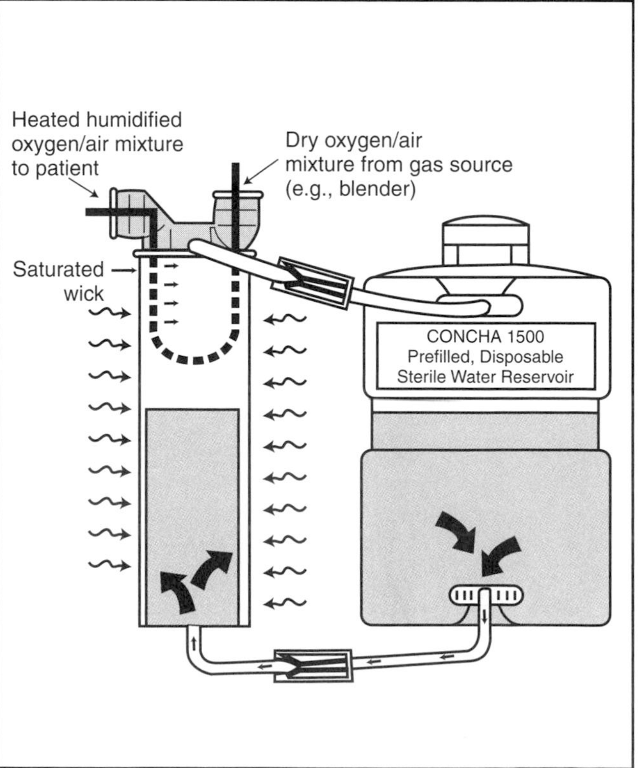

Figure 4-8 The Hudson RCI Conchacolumn and water reservoir assembly. (Redrawn from Hudson Respiratory Care, Inc, Temecula, Calif.)

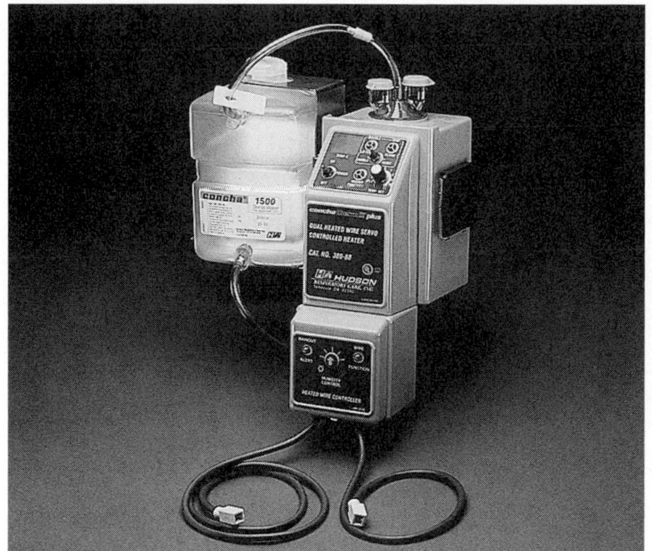

Figure 4-9 The Hudson RCI Conchatherm III Plus Humidifier. (Courtesy Hudson Respiratory Care, Inc, Temecula, Calif.)

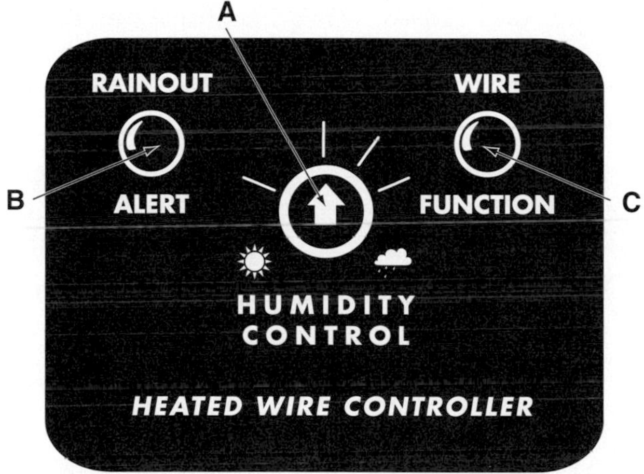

Figure 4-10 The Hudson RCI Conchatherm III Plus Humidifier heated wire control panel. **A,** Humidity control to adjust the temperature gradient between humidifier and patient. **B,** Rain-out alert for showing the operator that the desired temperature gradient is not being achieved. **C,** Wire function light to alert the operator when power is available for the heated wire circuit. (Courtesy Hudson Respiratory Care, Inc, Temecula, Calif.)

heated humidifiers, a humidity deficit may occur, depending upon the operating temperature, the patient's ventilatory parameters, and the airway status (e.g., dehydration). If the humidity control setting is set to allow the heater to be up to 3° C warmer than the patient-end of the circuit (i.e., negative temperature gradient), increased humidity can be delivered. However, this situation may increase the potential for condensation within the gas-delivery circuit.

If a heated wire is not used with the gas circuit tubing, the heated wire controller is automatically disabled, and the heater performs as a conventional wick humidifier. In this case, a temperature probe may be placed at an appropriate location (e.g., proximal airway) and used to measure the gas temperature leaving the humidifier; a light-emitting diode (LED) readout alerts the user of the gas temperature being delivered. The Conchatherm III Plus humidifier can be used with mechanical ventilators, oxygen diluters or blenders, adjustable nebulizer adapters for aerosol therapy, or nonflammable anesthesia gases. This humidifier includes a self-contained water reservoir; audiovisual alarms; a condensation, or rain out, alarm; and probes for adult, pediatric, and neonatal gas circuits.

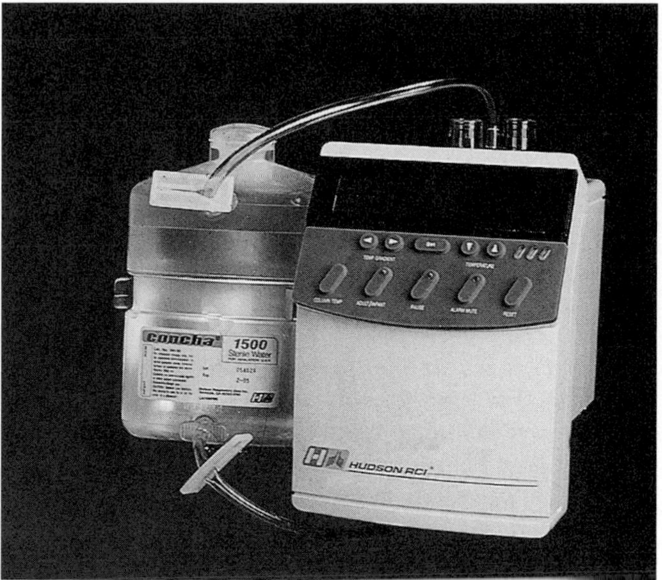

Figure 4-11 The Hudson RCI Conchatherm IV Heater Humidifier. (Courtesy Hudson Respiratory Care, Inc, Temecula, Calif.)

The Conchatherm IV Heater Humidifier (Figure 4-11) for adult or neonatal humidification offers microprocessor technology and uses an interactive control algorithm that provides stable proximal airway temperature and a heated wire function (when used). The LED airway temperature display provides the temperature of gas at the proximal airway or column in whole degrees centigrade. This humidifier provides a 20-minute pause mode to allow time for ventilator circuit changes or delivery of nebulized medications. An advanced alarm package includes tracking alarms for delivered gas temperature, high and low temperatures, probe status, and heated wire disconnects. A unique feature of the Conchatherm IV Heater Humidifier is the bar graph on the front panel showing the difference in gas temperature (temperature gradient) between the Conchacolumn outlet and the patient's proximal airway when the unit is used with a heated wire circuit. During operation, the bar graph displays the actual temperature gradient in the heated wire. Other features of the Conchatherm IV Heater Humidifier include digital temperature selection; adjustable heater-to-patient temperature gradient for control of humidity and condensation; a fixed, high-temperature alarm at 40° C; LCD alarm prompters; and continuous, self-diagnostic evaluations of hardware and software functions.

The humidifiers just discussed use the Conchacolumn to provide humidification. Fluid transferred from the reservoir to the Conchacolumn varies during the ventilatory cycle, depending on the mechanical ventilator settings. Fluid transfer is influenced by several factors, such as peak airway pressure, low respiratory rate, reduced water volume in the water reservoir, increased inspiratory to expiratory ratios, and square pressure waveforms.

The Conchacolumn is available in standard- and low-compliance configurations. The compliance changes are usually not significant for adults on mechanical ventilation; however, changes in compliance are clinically significant for neonatal and pediatric patients on pressure-cycled ventilation. With the smaller tidal volumes associated with neonatal mechanical ventilation, an increase in humidifier compliance can result in a decrease in the actual delivered tidal volume. The compliance of the humidification system is a product of the Conchacolumn compliance and the amount of fluid in both the column and reservoir.[15] It is important to note that as the water level in the column falls, the system's compressible volume increases and compliance changes. In clinical situations in which internal circuit or humidifier compliance must remain constant (e.g., with neonatal patients), a low-compliance Conchacolumn should be used. The low-compliance column contains a beveled sensing tube to control the water level in the column and thus the amount of gas allowed above the water reservoir or column (Figure 4-12). This sensing tube stops gas flow to the reservoir if the column water level is above the bevel of the tube. A one-way valve in the upper reservoir tube allows flow into the reservoir and restricts flow back out, thus preventing the reservoir pressure from being vented back into the column during the expiratory phase of mechanical ventilation. A one-way valve in the lower reservoir tube prevents water flow from the column back into the reservoir during the inspiratory phase of mechanical ventilation.[15]

Fisher & Paykel humidifiers are wick humidifiers that may be used for both adult and neonatal high-flow gas humidification. The servo-controlled MR 850 (Figure 4-13) and 290 humidifiers have inlets, outlets, a wick, and a heating element. Disposable and reusable humidification chambers are available in sizes for both adults and neonatal patients. The MR 850 humidification system allows one button selection for optimal temperature and humidification levels for neonatal, pediatric, and adult patients requiring invasive and noninvasive ventilatory support. This unit employs a continuous digital display of saturated gas temperatures. In addition the unit has an automatic standby feature in the event of gas flow interruption or low reservoir water levels. A limited water *autofeed* system is available with the MR 290 and MR 730 models to maintain water in the reservoir chamber. Temperature is regulated with a dual servo-controlled heater with a range of 30° to 39° C, and the MR

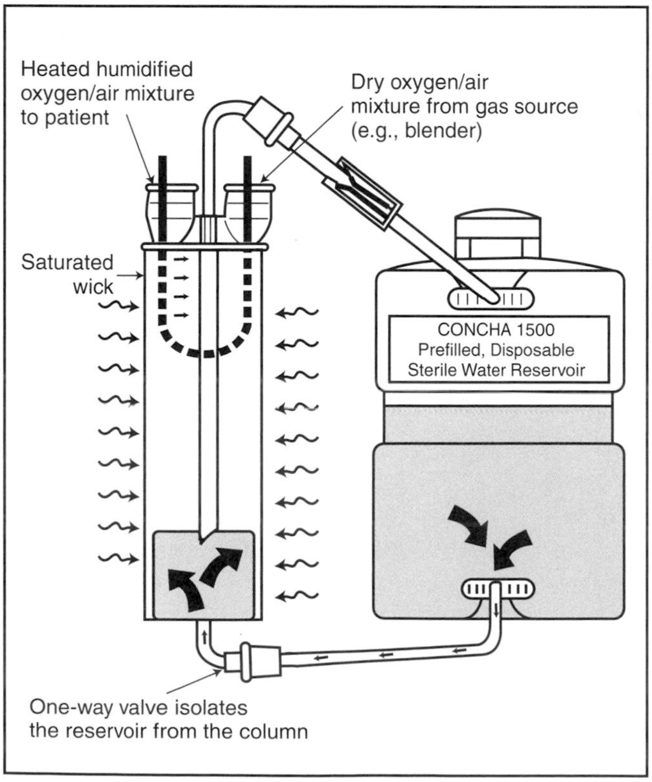

Heated humidified oxygen/air mixture to patient
Dry oxygen/air mixture from gas source (e.g., blender)
Saturated wick
CONCHA 1500
Prefilled, Disposable
Sterile Water Reservoir
One-way valve isolates the reservoir from the column

Figure 4-12 The low-compliance Conchacolumn with water reservoir assembly. (Redrawn from Hudson Respiratory Care, Inc, Temecula, Calif.)

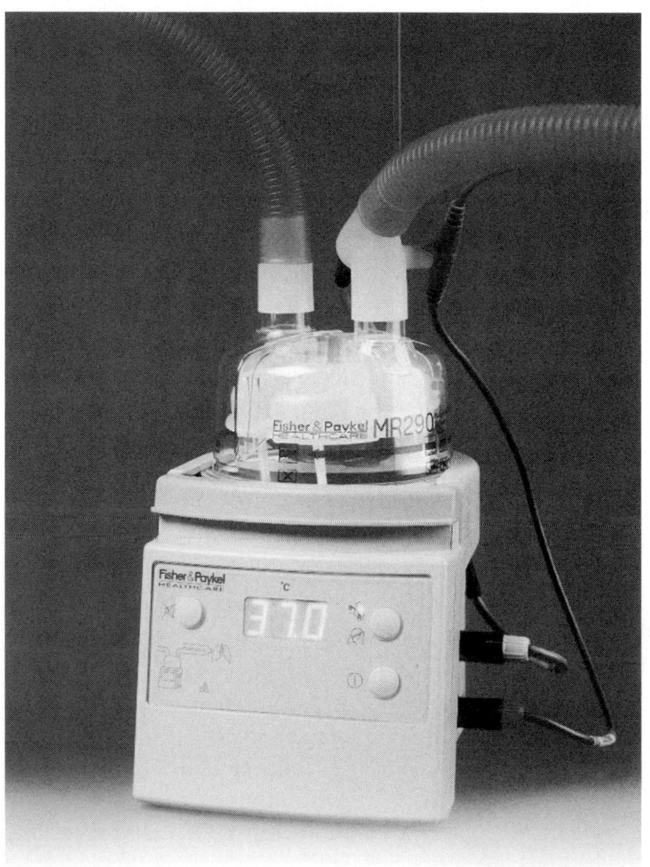

Figure 4-13 The Fisher & Paykel MR 850 heated humidifier. (Courtesy Fisher & Paykel Healthcare, Inc, Irvine, Calif.)

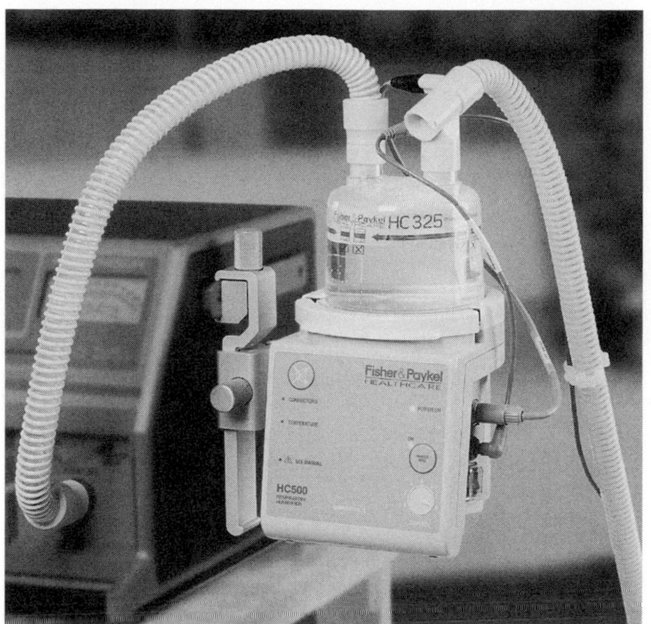

Figure 4-14 The Fisher & Paykel HC 500 Humidification for Home Mechanical Ventilation. (Courtesy Fisher & Paykel Healthcare, Inc, Irvine, Calif.)

730 has a heated wire option. Various alarms are included in these humidifiers, including high- and low-temperature alarms, a probe disconnect alarm, a heated-wire disconnect alarm, and a 3-minute alarm silence option. Fisher & Paykel also provides the HC 500 heated humidifier for home mechanical ventilation (Figure 4-14). This portable unit delivers optimal humidification to the patient's airway along with employing "heated wall" technology to minimize delivery tube condensation.

Heated Wire Circuits

An adjunct to the humidification system often employed to minimize circuit condensation is a heated wire circuit (Figure 4-15). This device is a wire-like structure placed in the lumen of the gas delivery circuit (e.g., ventilator circuit) to maintain a desired gas or temperature gradient throughout the length of the circuit. By maintaining gas temperature at body temperature, condensation (or rain out) can be minimized. Respiratory therapists can choose to provide a heated wire to both the inspiratory and expiratory limbs of the mechanical ventilator circuit or only to the inspiratory side of the circuit. The heated wire system maintains both the temperature within the circuit and the temperature of the heated humidifier, so that as gas flows to the patient, gas temperature is maintained at or near body temperature. If the inspiratory limb does not have a heated wire, a water trap may be used to collect condensation (Figure 4-16).

Heated wire systems are advantageous because they decrease the labor necessary to maintain the medical gas delivery circuit (e.g., less drain time is required for respiratory therapists to remove condensation from the circuit), and they may reduce nosocomial infections resulting from aspiration or lavage of contaminated condensate from circuit movement, and they provide increased absolute humidity.[16] However, heated wire systems may actually decrease RH, resulting in possible inspissation or thickening of secretions. As gas leaves the humidifier with a fixed water content and the temperature increases as a result of the heated wire, RH decreases. Studies suggest that RH may be the dominant factor in drying or thinning of airway secretions in the upper airway, and the use of heated wire circuits may contribute to drying of airway secretions.[16]

New heated humidification devices for home continuous positive airway pressure (CPAP) therapy are available to provide humidity and comfort. The Fisher & Paykel HC 220 provides heated humidification to standard CPAP therapy maintaining mucosal hydration and preventing discomfort. The HC 221 offers a compliance monitor which enables tracking of CPAP usage when humidity is used (Figure 4-17). The HumidAire Heated Humidifier available through ResMed USA (Figure 4-18) is another humidifier for CPAP therapy that effectively warms and humidifies gas with low heat and minimal condensation.

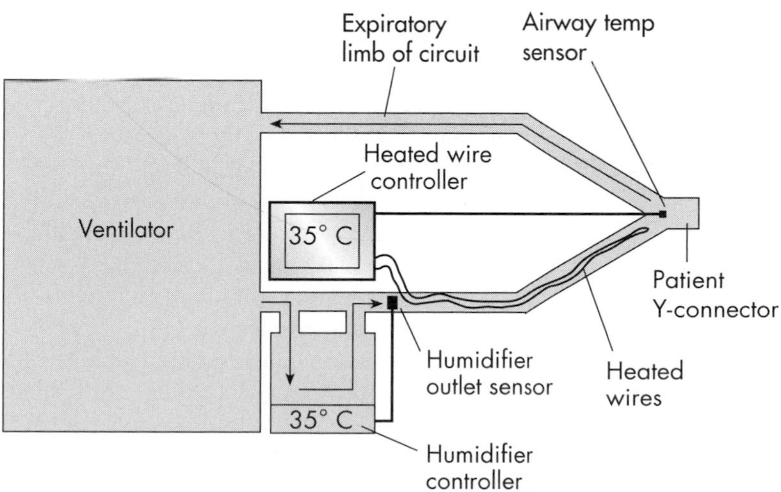

Figure 4-15 A heated wire circuit in the inspiratory limb of the gas delivery tube. (From Scanlan CL, Wilkins RL, Stoller JK: *Egan's fundamentals of respiratory care*, ed 7, St Louis, 1999, Mosby.)

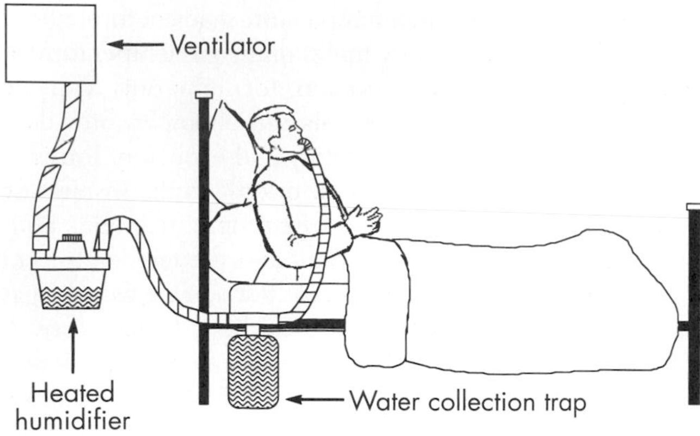

Figure 4-16 Placement of a water trap in a gravity-dependent loop of the heated humidity delivery tube.

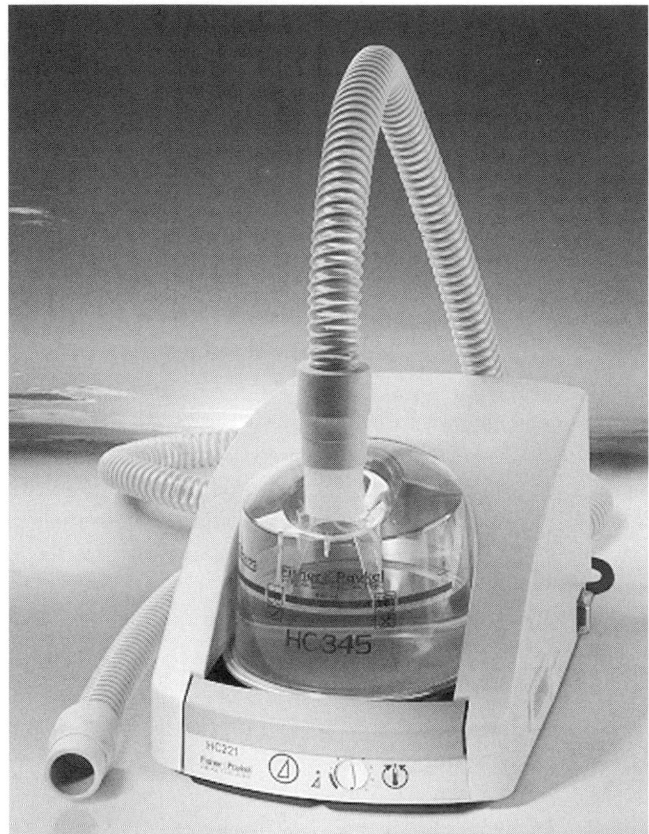

Figure 4-17 The Fisher & Paykel HC Humidification for CPAP. (Courtesy Fisher & Paykel Healthcare, Inc, Irvine, Calif.)

Technical Considerations with Using Humidifiers

Respiratory therapists should be aware of important considerations when using heated humidifiers, such as maintaining an adequate water supply (i.e., replacing the water reservoir with full units as needed), keeping the water at the proper level, and ensuring tight fittings of the temperature probe connection underneath the heated-wire controller. If water collection traps are used they will require monitoring for in the event these traps fill with water added weight can be applied to the delivery tube placing the humidification set-up at risk for being dismantled. In addition, monitoring operating and gas output temperatures are vital. If a heated wire is not used, condensation that gathers within the gas delivery circuit must be removed.

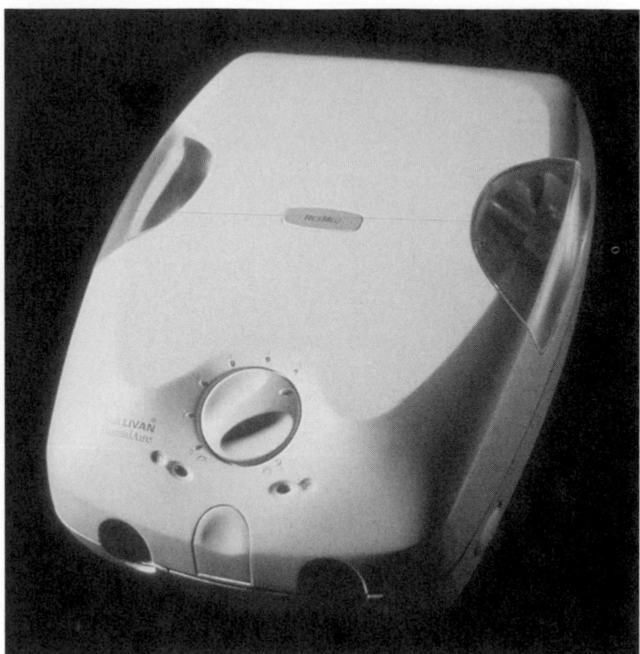

Figure 4-18 The HumidAire Heated Humidifier. (Courtesy ResMed Corp, Poway, Calif.)

Heat and Moisture Exchangers (HME)

An alternative to conventional humidification systems is the use of a heat and moisture exchanger, which is commonly referred to as an artificial nose. HMEs can humidify and warm incoming gases in certain patients receiving mechanical ventilation. HMEs function in a fashion similar to the upper airway by capturing exhaled heat and moisture and using it to heat and humidify the next inhaled or delivered breath. However, these passive, disposable humidifiers do not add heat or water to the patient's airway.

There are many models of HME type of devices available; most have an internal volume of 10 to 98 mL, weigh within the range of 9 to 47 g, and provide a humidity output of 10 to 31 mg/L at a temperature of 30° C. HMEs are best suited for patients undergoing short-term mechanical ventilation (i.e., 96 hours or less), with minute volumes less than 10 L/min, limited secretions, and a normal body temperature.[10] Several physical characteristics influence the overall effectiveness of HME type of humidifiers, including the temperature and humidity levels of the inspired gas, the gas flow through the unit (e.g., faster flows decrease effectiveness), the internal surface area the gas encounters, the dead space volume of the unit, and the outer casing. An ideal HME has low structural compliance and minimal dead space and is lightweight. An HME should also have standard inlet and outlet connections, offer little resistance to gas flow, and operate at least 70% of efficiency.[6] HME efficiency is influenced by the size of the tidal volume, the inspiratory gas flow rate, and the fraction of inspired oxygen (F_IO_2). As each of these factors increases, the overall efficiency of the HME decreases. It has been recommended that clinical use of HMEs be limited to 5 days or less.[17,18]

HME types of humidifiers reduce the accumulation of condensation in the mechanical ventilator gas delivery circuit and may act as a barrier to microbes, thus decreasing the incidence of nosocomial infection. The actual effect of HMEs on infection rates associated with mechanical ventilation remains controversial, and several studies report mixed results. However, studies comparing HMEs with conventional heated humidifiers suggest that HMEs may not be a significant factor in nosocomial infections in patients receiving mechanical ventilation.[17]

Generally, there are four types of HMEs that can be used for short-term humidity therapy: (1) simple HMEs, (2) heat and moisture exchanging filters, (3) hygroscopic condenser humidifiers, and (4) hygroscopic condenser humidifiers with filters.

The simplest HMEs often use layered aluminum with or without a fibrous coating. The use of aluminum casing allows temperatures to be exchanged quickly during gas movement, with moisture accumulating on the aluminum layers. As the patient exhales, heat and moisture are captured by the HME. Then during the inspiration that follows, the captured heat and moisture humidifies inspired gases. These HMEs are the least efficient for providing humidity.[18]

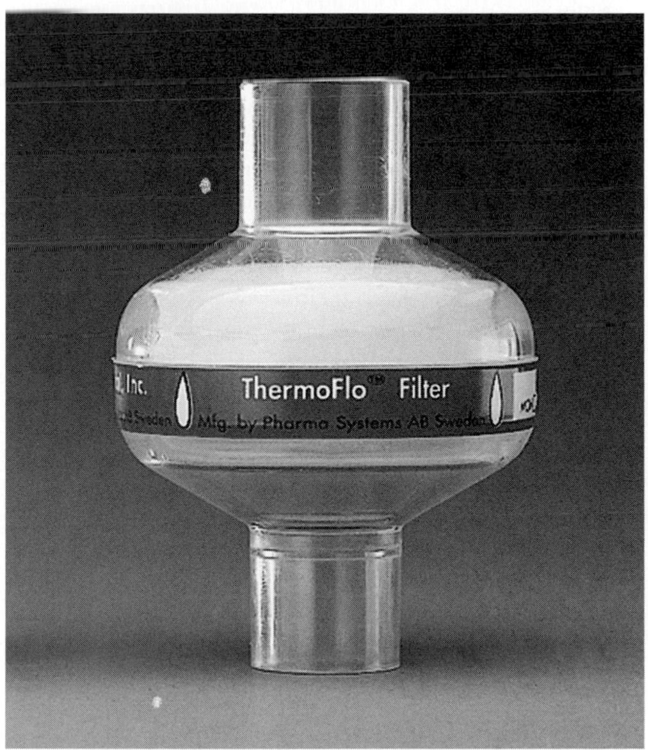

Figure 4-19 The ARC Medical ThermoFlo filter. (Courtesy ARC Medical, Inc. Scottdale, Ga.)

The second type of HMEs are heat and moisture exchanging filters. The ARC Medical ThermoFlo Filter is both an HME and a bacterial filter and can provide up to 30 mg of water with minute volumes up to 20 L/min with no added work of breathing (Figure 4-19). This device is available in a SL model that employs a Luer port on the patient side, allowing for secretion removal and airway pressure monitoring.

The hygroscopic condenser humidifier (HCH) is constructed of a low-thermal conductive material (e.g., corrugated paper, wool, foam) that has been coated with a hygroscopic chemical (calcium chloride or lithium chloride). This special hygroscopic coating increases the retention of exhaled moisture, thus reducing the RH of the expired gas, which results in better humidification of inspired gas when compared with simple HMEs. HCHs capture water particles during expiration as a result of the cool surface area of the condenser element. These water particles become attached to the hygroscopic chemical coating and remain in a liquid state. As inspired gas enters the HCH, water molecules are released from the condensing material to humidify the incoming gas. Most HCH models on the market are capable of providing up to 30 mg of water per liter of gas. Figure 4-20 shows the Hygrolife Mallinckrodt Medical HCH, which provides 30 mg of water per liter of gas at an 800 mL tidal volume and offers low resistance to gas flows up to 90 L/min.

The final category of HME type of devices is hygroscopic condenser humidifiers with filters (HCHFs), which function similarly to the HCHs just described but contain a thin bacterial filter between the condensing material and the incoming gas. Figure 4-21 shows the Gibeck Humid-Vent Compact Filter HCHF, which is composed of corrugated paper coated with calcium chloride and can provide up to 30 mg of water per liter of gas at 30° C.

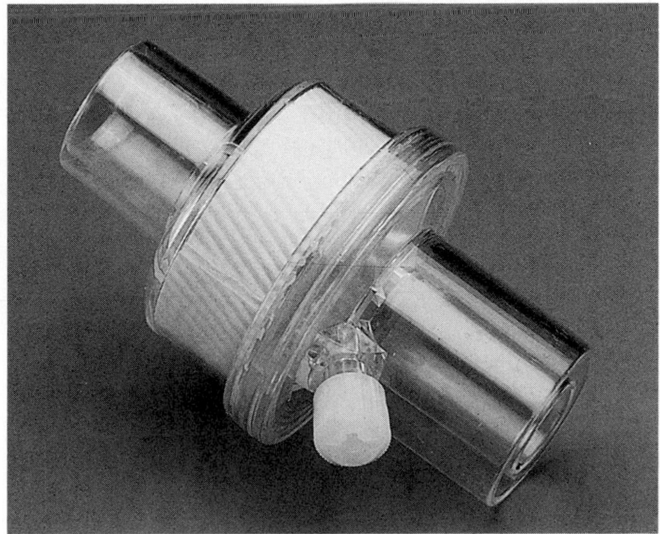

Figure 4-20 The Hygrolife Mallinckrodt Medical HCH. (Courtesy Mallinckrodt Inc, St Louis.)

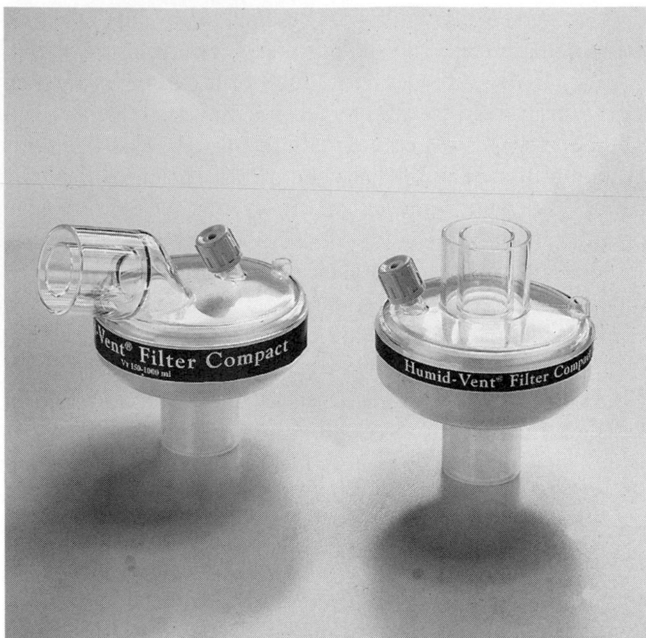

Figure 4-21 The Gibeck Humid-Vent Compact Filter HCHF. (Courtesy Gibeck, Inc, Temecula, Calif.)

Box 4-5 Contraindications for Using a Health and Moisture Exchanger Humidifier

- Increased volume of secretions
- Thick, dehydrated secretions
- Hypothermia
- Large tidal volumes (>1000 mL)
- During aerosol therapy
- Small tidal volume with large-volume HME devices
- With heated humidification
- Airway leaks around artificial airway
- Minute volume >10 L/min

Technical Considerations for HME Type of Humidifiers

Respiratory therapists must be aware of the technical considerations and contraindications of using the HME type of humidifiers. Contraindications for the use of the HME type of humidifiers are listed in Box 4-5. When used during clinical situations, HMEs may aggravate existing pulmonary problems by dehydrating lung secretions. HME use is contraindicated when expired gases do not travel through the HME device (e.g., endotracheal tube cuff leak), when a heated humidifier or small-volume nebulizer is part of the ventilation system, and when there are leaks around the inlet or outlet ports. In addition, the dead space volume of HMEs limits their use with neonatal and pediatric patients.

Maintaining and Monitoring Humidification

Mechanical ventilators provide machine-generated gas flow via a circuit to inflate the lungs. With the exception of noninvasive mechanical ventilation (see Chapter 14), patients on mechanical ventilators will have either an endotracheal or tracheostomy tube in place, which bypass the natural mechanism for conditioning incoming gas. The application of dry medical gases is associated with heat loss, dehydration of the airway lining, epithelial damage, destruction of cilia, disruption of pseudostratified columnar and cuboidal epithelial cells, desquamation of cells, mucosal ulceration, and impaired mucociliary transport of secretions.[4] Consequences of these conditions include secretion retention, atelectasis, and increased incidence of infection. Damage from breathing dry or poorly humidified gas through an artificial airway is proportional to the duration of breathing such a gas mixture.[14] Damaged cilia require several days for repair, and it takes several weeks for the epithelial lining to return to full thickness.[19] With an artificial airway in place, the ISB can shift distally, altering pulmonary mechanics. Altered mechanics may include a decrease in functional residual capacity, lung compliance and hypoxemia.[20-22]

Similarly to insufficient humidification, there are consequences for excessive humidification and overheating. Under normal conditions, heat and moisture exchange occurs within the upper airway via a dynamic equilibrium. The loss and gain of heat and humidity are governed by the physiologic process previously described. This normal equilibrium may be disturbed with the delivery of excess heat and moisture to the airways.

Delivery of gas above body temperature can cause thermal damage to mucosal lining, pulmonary edema, and airway stricture formation. Changes in cilia structure and function have been reported, such as degeneration and adhesion of cilia in smaller airways.[23] In addition, there may be an increase in airway secretions from a decrease in evaporation, which can lead to condensation that may obstruct the airway, leading to atelectasis or an increase in airway resistance.[10] Excessive or overhumidification, just as with underhumidification, may alter lung mechanics by decreasing functional residual capacity and causing hypoxemia and loss of lung compliance.[21] These changes result from atelectasis and intrapulmonary shunting. Excessive humidification may alter or remove surfactant, further encouraging alveolar collapse. Surfactant changes are more prominent with overhydration than underhydration.[23] Some authors report that hyperthermia may occur because the lungs are unable to discard heat.[4,24] In addition, excessive humidification may increase body fluids because of the decrease in insensible water loss from the lungs.[4] This is important to note when providing heated humidity therapy to neonates.

In addition to the physiologic hazards and complications of humidifying the respiratory system, there are technical considerations of humidity therapy that are hazardous. These include the potential for electric shock from heated humidifiers, melting of the circuit by heated wire circuits (possibly burning the patient), increased resistive work while breathing through the humidifier, inadvertent tracheal lavage from unintentional overfilling of the humidifier, and displacement of a condensate bolus. Condensation tends to accumulate within gravity-dependent loops in the gas-delivery circuit while the gas cools as it is delivered to the patient. This condensation can build up and be inadvertently emptied into the patient's airway during patient gas-circuit manipulation (e.g., during routine patient care). Boluses of condensation fluid in the circuit can increase the work of breathing by interfering with the sensing mechanism of the mechanical ventilator or decreasing the diameter of the gas delivery circuit. Under these conditions, the patient must breathe around the bolus to obtain an assisted or spontaneous breath from a mechanical ventilator. This patient-ventilator dyssynchrony can result in altered pulmonary mechanics and an increase in the work of breathing.[10]

Monitoring the humidification device requires the respiratory therapist to frequently inspect the unit. Monitoring and maintenance include checking humidifier and proximal airway temperature to ensure appropriate gas temperatures, removing condensate from loops in the circuit (water traps or heated wires may be used to minimize fluid accumulation), and maintaining alarm settings to be alerted to gas temperature below 31° C or above 40° C (as discussed previously, the recommended range for proximal airway gas temperatures is 31° to 35° C). An increase in humidifier temperature is common when the unit is turned on and there is an absence of gas flowing through it. This can occur, for example, when servo-controlled units are allowed to warm up without gas flowing through the circuit and without a temperature probe inserted into the proximal airway of the ventilator circuit. Non—servo-controlled units can exceed gas temperatures if the thermostat setting is too high.[6] Elevated humidifier temperatures can result in the delivery of excessive gas temperature to the patient upon initial gas flow through the unit.

Additional monitoring includes maintaining humidifier water reservoir level to ensure a water source for humidification. If an HME is substituted for a heated humidifier, it should be inspected regularly for partial or complete obstruction by airway secretions.[10]

Respiratory therapists must document and record the function of the humidification device and the results of therapy. The patient's medical records should include documentation of humidifier settings, proximal airway gas temperature or inspired gas temperature, alarm settings, water level and function of the automatic water feed system, and quantity and quality of airway secretions.[10]

Aerosol Therapy

Aerosols are widely used in the care and treatment of patients with pulmonary disease and play a significant role in respiratory care. This section will address aerosol characteristics, factors that affect deposition, aerosol generation, and hazards of aerosol therapy.

An aerosol is a solid or liquid particle suspended in a gas. Aerosol particles range from submicroscopic to macroscopic (readily visible with the naked eye) and, unlike humidity, they can be measured and counted. Common, nonmedical aerosols include dust, fumes from chemical reactions, smoke from the combustion of various materials, mists and fog from condensation (mists are considered larger than fog particles), and smog and haze, which are broad terms describing atmospheric aerosols from natural and artificial processes. Other examples of aerosols include tobacco smoke, viruses, pollen, and fungal spores.

The human respiratory system has developed an elaborate mechanism for defending itself from most inspired aerosols—both therapeutic and nontherapeutic. This section focuses on therapeutic or medical aerosols, including bland and medicated aerosols, administered to patients with a variety of symptoms associated with pulmonary disease. This section addresses aerosol characteristics, generation of aerosol, and clinical use of aerosol in a variety of settings. Respiratory therapists should carefully select the appropriate aerosol and method of delivery to optimize care of patients with pulmonary disease.

Aerosol therapy may be divided into three broad categories as described by the AARC Clinical Practice Guidelines[25-27]: (1) delivery of bland aerosol, (2) delivery of aerosol to the upper airway, and (3) delivery of medicated aerosol. Each type of aerosol therapy has distinct indications, clinical uses, and hazards. In most cases, they have a common means of generation, but delivery methods can be unique to a particular medical or bland aerosol (Clinical Practice Guidelines 4-1 to 4-3).

Bland aerosols include sterile water and hypotonic, hypertonic, and isotonic saline.[28] Bland aerosols are commonly used in the care of patients in hospitals or at home. Aerosolizing cool, sterile saline or water is primarily indicated for upper airway administration. Use of hypotonic or hypertonic sterile saline is indicated for inducing a cough and expectoration of sputum for obtaining specimens for microbiologic evaluation.

Use of cool, bland aerosol is indicated when there is upper airway edema. Cool aerosol, when applied to the airway mucosa, can result in vasoconstriction, thereby reducing mucosal edema. Indications for cool, bland aerosol include stridor, laryngotracheobronchitis, subglottic edema, postextubation edema, hoarseness, and postoperative care of the upper airway (i.e., discomfort associated with bronchoscopy or other invasive instrumentation of the upper airway).[28,29]

Heated aerosol therapy is only recommended when there is a need to decrease a humidity deficit (i.e., when dry gas is delivered to the lungs and the upper airway has been bypassed by an artificial airway). The delivery of heated aerosol by aerosol mask to a spontaneously breathing patient has not been shown to be effective in promoting secretion hydration and expectoration and, as a result, it is not a very common treatment modality.

Clinical Practice Guidelines 4-1

Selection of an Aerosol Delivery Device

Description

The device selected for administration of pharmacologically active aerosol to the lower airway should produce particles with an MMAD of 2 to 5 μ. These devices include pMDIs, pMDIs with accessory devices (e.g., spacers), DPIs, SVNs, LVNs, and ultrasonic nebulizers (USNs). Note that this guideline does not address bland aerosol administration and sputum induction.

Indications

The need to deliver aerosolized medications, such as beta adrenergic agents, anticholinergic agents (antimuscarinic), anti-inflammatory agents (e.g., corticosteroids), mediator-modifying compounds (e.g., cromolyn sodium), and mucokinetics, to the lower airways.

Contraindications

There are no contraindications to the administration of aerosols by inhalation, although there may be contraindications related to the substances being delivered. Consult the package inserts for product-specific contraindications.

Hazards and Complications

1. Malfunction of device or improper technique may result in the delivery of an incorrect dose of medication.
2. Complications of specific pharmacologic agents may occur.
3. Cardiotoxic effects of freon have been reported as idiosyncratic responses that may be a problem with excessive MDI use.
4. Freon may harm the environment by its effect on the ozone layer.
5. Repeated exposure to aerosols has been reported to produce asthmatic symptoms in some caregivers.

Monitoring

1. Device performance
2. Device application technique
3. Patient response, including changes in vital signs

Infection Control

1. Standard precautions for body substance isolation must be used.
2. SVNs and LVNs are for single-patient use or should be subjected to high-level disinfection between patients.
3. Published data establishing a safe-use period for SVNs and LVNs are lacking; however SVNs and LVNs should probably be changed or subjected to high-level disinfection at about 24-hour intervals.
4. Medications should be handled aseptically. Medications from multidose sources in acute-care facilities must be handled aseptically and discarded after 24 hours, unless manufacturer recommendations specifically state that medications may be stored longer than 24 hours. Tap water should not be used as a diluent.
5. MDI accessory devices are only for single-patient use. There are no documented concerns with contamination of medication in pMDI canisters. Cleaning of accessory devices is based on aesthetic criteria.

For a complete copy of this guideline, see Respir Care *37:891, 1992.*

Contrary to popular belief, the efficacy of using bland aerosol to improve mucus flow or expectoration has not been established. Studies indicate that the physical properties of mucus are only minimally affected by the addition of a bland aerosol.[1,26,28-30] Furthermore, the use of bland aerosol for humidification of the lower airway when the upper airway has been bypassed (i.e., artificial airway) is not as effective as a heated humidifier or HME type of humidifier.[26] Several reasons cited for this finding include difficulty in maintaining the temperature of the aerosol and carrier gas, possible irritation from the aerosol inducing bronchoconstriction, and the risk of cross-contamination. Aerosol particles are capable of transporting microbes, thus becoming a potential source of nosocomial infections.[8]

Medicated aerosol delivery to the upper airway is indicated for upper airway edema and inflammation (e.g., treatment of inflammation associated with laryngotracheobronchitis) when topical anesthesia is required (e.g., to control pain and gagging during placement of invasive upper airway instrumentation) or in the presence of rhinitis (e.g., for relief of seasonal allergy). The administration of a vasoactive aerosol (e.g., steroids, sympathomimetic nose sprays) to the upper airway—especially the nasopharynx—can be effective to decrease nasal congestion and edema associated with allergy or infection. Such agents successfully diminish symptoms such as rhinorrhea, sneezing, and watery discharge.

Medicated aerosol delivery to the lower airway has become the predominant form of medicated aerosol therapy. Inhalation of medicated aerosol allows for rapid onset of effects, is less toxic, and results in fewer side effects than if delivered by mouth or intravenously.[31] The delivery of medicated aerosol focuses on depositing the aerosol of a sufficient dose and at a desired location to produce optimal results. Overall aerosol deposition at specific locations depends upon several factors such as size of the aerosol particle, breathing pattern, and other physical characteristics that will be discussed.

Box 4-6 lists both the diagnostic and therapeutic uses of aerosols. Respiratory therapists should be familiar with the generation, delivery, and hazards of aerosol therapy.

Clinical Practice Guidelines 4-2

Bland Aerosol Administration

Description

For purposes of this guideline, bland aerosol administration includes the delivery of sterile water or hypotonic, isotonic, or hypertonic saline in aerosol form. Bland aerosol administration may be accompanied by oxygen administration.

Indications

Cool, bland aerosol therapy is primarily indicated for upper airway administration; therefore, an MMAD greater than or equal to 5 μ is desirable. The use of hypo- and hypertonic saline is primarily indicated for inducing sputum specimens; therefore an MMAD of 1 to 5 μ is desirable. Heated bland aerosol is primarily indicated for minimizing humidity deficit when the upper airway has been bypassed; therefore an MMAD of 2 to 10 μ is desirable. Specific indications include:

1. The presences of upper airway edema (cool bland aerosol)
2. Laryngotracheobronchitis (LTB)
3. Subglottic edema
4. Postextubation management of the upper airway
5. Postoperative management of the upper airway
6. Bypassed upper airway
7. Need for sputum specimens

Contraindications

1. Bronchoconstriction
2. History of airway hyperresponsiveness

Hazards and Complications

1. Wheezing or bronchospasm
2. Bronchoconstriction when artificial airway is employed
3. Infection
4. Overhydration
5. Patient discomfort
6. Caregiver exposure to droplet nuclei of *Mycobacterium tuberculosis* or other airborne contagion produced as a consequence of coughing, particularly during sputum induction

Assessment of Need

The presence of one or more of the following may be an indication for administration of a water or isotonic or hypotonic saline aerosol:

1. Stridor
2. Brassy, croup-like cough
3. Hoarseness after extubation
4. Diagnosis of LTB or croup
5. Clinical history suggesting upper airway irritation and increased work of breathing (e.g., smoke inhalation)
6. Patient discomfort associated with airway instrumentation or insult
7. Need for sputum induction (e.g., for diagnosis of *Pneumocystis carinii* pneumonia or tuberculosis)

Assessment of Outcome

The desired outcomes for the administration of water, hypotonic, or isotonic saline include:

1. Decreased work of breathing
2. Improved vital signs
3. Decreased stridor
4. Decreased dyspnea
5. Improved arterial blood gas values
6. Improved oxygen saturation as indicated by pulse oximetry (SpO_2)

The desired outcome for the administration of hypertonic saline is a sputum sample adequate for analysis.

Monitoring

The extent of patient monitoring should be determined by the stability and severity of the patient's condition. Monitoring may include:

1. Subjective patient responses of pain, discomfort, dyspnea, or restlessness
2. Heart rate and rhythm
3. Blood pressure
4. Respiratory rate, as well as the breathing pattern and use of accessory respiratory muscles
5. Breath sounds
6. Sputum production quantity, color, consistency, and odor
7. Pulse oximetry (if hypoxemia is suspected)

For a copy of the complete guidelines, see Respir Care *38(11):1196, 1993.*

Aerosol Delivery

The following sections describe the principles of operation, use, and clinical consideration for aerosol delivery devices. These devices include small- and large-volume nebulizers, pressurized metered dose inhalers (pMDIs), dry powder inhalers (DPIs), and ultrasonic nebulizers. The use of large container and chamber-like devices to deliver aerosol, as well as aerosol delivery under special situations (i.e., the delivery of ribavirin) will be discussed later in the chapter.

Clinical Advantages of Aerosol Delivery

Routes for administration of respiratory drugs include enteral (via intestines), parenteral (e.g., intravenously), topical (e.g., directly on skin), and inhalation. For aerosols, inhalation is preferred because it has several advantages. Deposition of aerosols directly onto the respiratory mucosa is a form of topical administration, allowing a drug to be directly administered to the desired location. Aerosolizing medications allows for a high concentration of the drug to be directly

Clinical Practice Guidelines 4-3

Selection of a Device for Aerosol Delivery to the Lung Parenchyma

Description

A device selected for administration of pharmacologically active aerosol to the lung parenchyma should produce particle sizes with an MMAD or 1 to 3 μ. Such devices include ultrasonic nebulizers, some LVNs (e.g., the SPAG unit, which is only intended for ribavirin delivery), and some SVNs (e.g., the Circulaire, Respirgard II, and Pari IS 2).

Indications

The indication for selecting a suitable device is the need to deliver a topical medication (in aerosol form) with a site of action in the lung parenchyma or that is intended for systemic absorption. Such medications may include antibiotics, antivirals, antifungals, surfactants, and enzymes.

Contraindications

There are no contraindications to choosing an appropriate device for parenchymal deposition. Contraindications related to the substances being delivered may exist. Consult the package insert for product-specific contraindications to medication delivery.

Hazards and Complications

1. Device malfunction or improper technique may result in delivery of incorrect medication doses.
2. For mechanically ventilated patients, the nebulizer design and the characteristics of the medication may affect ventilator function (e.g., filter obstruction, altered tidal volume, decreased trigger sensitivity) and medication deposition.
3. Aerosols may cause bronchospasm or airway irritation, and complications related to specific pharmacologic agents can occur.
4. Exposure to medication should be limited to the patient for whom it has been ordered. Nebulizer medication that is released into the atmosphere from the nebulizer or the patient may affect health-care providers and others near the treatment. For example, there has been increased awareness of the possible health effects of aerosols such as ribavirin and pentamidine. Anecdotal reports associate symptoms such as conjunctivitis, decreased tolerance of contact lenses, headaches, bronchospasm, shortness of breath, and rashes in health care workers exposed to secondhand aerosols. Similar concerns have been expressed concerning health care workers who are pregnant or are planning to be pregnant within 8 weeks of administration. The potential exposure effects of aerosolized antibiotics (which may contribute to the development of resistant organisms), steroids, and bronchodilators are less often discussed. Because the data regarding adverse health effects on health care workers and those casually exposed are incomplete, it is wise to minimize exposure in all situations.
5. The Centers for Disease Control and Prevention recommend that:
   a. Warning signs should be posted in an easy-to-see location to apprise all who enter the treatment area of the potential hazards of exposure. Accidental exposures should be documented are reported according to accepted standards.
   b. Staff members who administer medications understand the inherent risks of the medication and the procedures for safely disposing of hazardous wastes. Department administrators should screen staff for adverse effects of aerosol exposure and provide alternative assignments for staff at high risk of adverse effects of exposure (e.g., pregnant women or those with demonstrated sensitivity to the specific agent).
   c. Filters or filtered scavenger systems be used to remove aerosols that cannot be considered.
   d. There should be booths or stalls for sputum induction and aerosolized medication administration in areas where multiple patients are treated. Booths or stalls should be designed to provide adequate air flow to draw aerosol and droplet nuclei from the patient and into an appropriate filtration system with exhaust directed to an appropriate outside vent. Note that filters, nebulizers, and other contaminated components of the aerosol delivery system used with suspect agents (e.g., pentamidine and ribavirin) should be handled as hazardous waste. If scavenger systems or specially designed booths are not available, clinicians administering these treatments should wear personal protection devices to reduce exposure to the medication residues and body substances. These devices may include fitted respirator masks, goggles, gloves, gowns, and splatter shields.

Monitoring

1. Device and scavenging system performance
2. Device application technique
3. Patient response

For a copy of the complete Clinical Practice Guideline see Respir Care *41(7):647, 1996.*

deposited onto the mucosa with local therapeutic effects optimized and side effects minimized. Because of the large surface area of the lung (70 to 80 m^2), absorption and onset of action for aerosolized drugs are rapid. Administration of drugs such as sympathomimetics, anticholinergics, and steroids via inhalation results in fewer side effects than if given systemically.[32] Additionally, gastric, intestinal, and hepatic enzymes are avoided when drugs are given by inhalation so that drug breakdown is less likely to occur.

Aerosol Physics

The depth and effectiveness of an aerosol delivered to the lungs depends upon multiple factors, including the size and physical characteristics of the aerosol particles, the amount

Box 4-6 Common Uses of Nonmedicated and Medicated Aerosols

Nonmedicated Aerosols

Bland Aerosols

Reduce upper airway edema

Induce sputum

Humidify dry medical gases

Hypertonic Saline or Sterile Water

Induce sputum induction

Medicated Aerosols

Sympathomimetic bronchodilators

Antimuscarinic bronchodilators

Mucokinetic agents

Surface-active agents

Antitussive agents

Antimicrobial agents

Glucocorticoids

Antiallergic agents

Local anesthetics

Diagnostic aerosols (for ventilation scans, inhalation challenge for assessing airway response, and dosimetry)

of aerosol produced, the anatomy and geometry of the airways, and the ventilatory pattern. Respiratory therapists should be aware of these factors to provide optimal therapy by choosing an appropriate delivery device, educating the patient in aerosol use, and assuring an effective ventilatory pattern.

Respiratory therapists often attempt to deliver an aerosol to specific locations in the respiratory tract. The size of the aerosol particles is a major determinant in the therapeutic and diagnostic effectiveness within the respiratory system. Therapeutic and diagnostic aerosols are generally heterodispersed; that is, they are composed of a wide range of particle sizes and shapes. Monodispersed aerosols have a narrow range of diameters and are used during special application of aerosol therapy, such as delivery of ribavirin or pentamidine therapy.[33] Terms to describe aerosol particles include: aerosol volume, particle surface area, mass median aerodynamic diameter (MMAD), and geometric standard deviation (GSD). Of these measurements, MMAD is the most common measurement used to describe aerosol particles.

Aerosol Volume

As an aerosol is produced and delivered to the respiratory tract, its density may remain constant. Under this condition, aerosol volume is a product of aerosol particle size. The larger the particle size, the larger the volume of the aerosol. The volume of an aerosol particle is directly proportional to the cube of its radius:

$$\text{Aerosol volume} = 4/3 \times \pi \times (\text{radius}^3).$$

Clinical use of this principle may be appreciated by comparing many small particles with larger particles. Many smaller particles must be administered to the same area of the lung to equal the volume of a few larger ones. Particles that are less than 1 μm have little mass and volume often fail to get deposited in the lung and are usually exhaled. In contrast, particles with larger fluid volume may fail to enter the lower respiratory tract because the upper respiratory tract tends to filter them, thus prohibiting particles larger than 5 μm from entering the lower respiratory tract.

Particle Surface Area

Particle surface area is a function of its diameter (the greater the diameter of an aerosol particle, the greater its surface area), which can be illustrated with the following equation:

$$\text{Particle surface area} = \pi \times (\text{diameter})^2$$

The ratio of surface area to volume increases as particles become smaller and their inertia becomes less. Thus smaller particles are less likely to be deposited by direct impact in the airway and settle more slowly during breath holding.[33]

Mass Median Aerodynamic Diameter

The MMAD is the diameter that divides the range of particle size in half (i.e., 50% of the particles are smaller than the MMAD and 50% are larger).[34] Aerosol particles of equal MMAD have similar deposition patterns in the lung, regardless of their actual size and composition. The concept of MMAD is based on the idea that aerosol particles are created and dispersed in a range of sizes that mimic a typical bell-shaped probability distribution.

Geometric Standard Deviation

The GSD is a measure of how particle diameters vary. As the GSD increases, the wider the range of particle sizes that are present. As the GSD increases, the MMAD increases because larger particles carry a greater mass,[8] which may reduce the amount of aerosol deposited in the lower airway because a greater portion of larger particles are filtered out of the upper airway.

Depth of Penetration

The depth of penetration of an aerosol particle is inversely proportional to particle size. Most therapeutic aerosols have an MMAD from 1 to 10 μm,[33] and aerosols within this range—depending on their size—are deposited in the upper and lower airways. Although particles with a MMAD less than 5 μm tend to get deposited in the lung, most particles greater than 5 μm are trapped in the upper airway. Aerosols with a MMAD of 0.5 to 2.0 μm are generally targeted for delivery into the lower lung—some as far as the 10th generation of the airway. Particles with MMADs of less than 1 μm are so light and stable that many are not deposited. Even if these small particles remain in the lung, they carry little volume, and their effects are minimal. Table 4-2 shows the approximate location of aerosol particle deposition based on size.

Table 4-2 Particle size and deposition site

Particle Size (μm)	Deposition Site
>100	Do not enter respiratory tract
5-100	Mouth, nose, and upper airway
2-5	Bronchi and bronchioles
0.5-2	Can enter alveoli
<0.5	Stable and tend not to become deposited

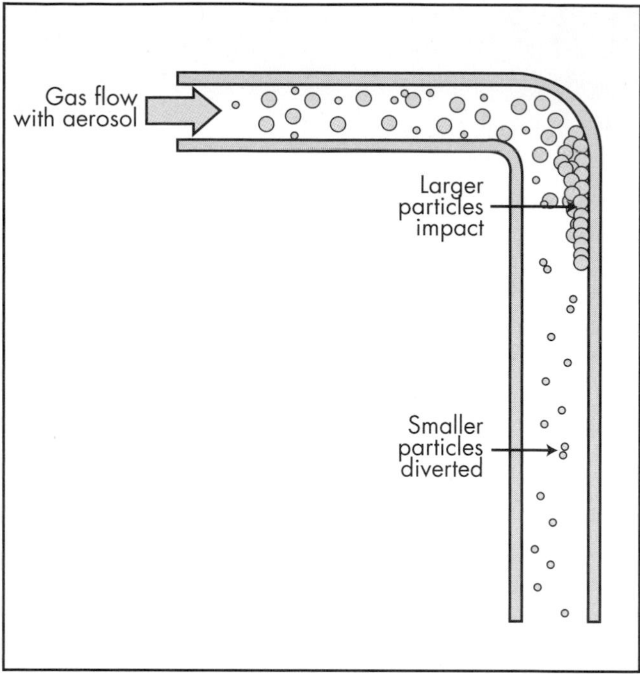

Figure 4-22 Inertial impaction of aerosol particles.

Aerosol Deposition

The goal of aerosol delivery is to deposit a therapeutic or diagnostic aerosol within the respiratory tract, but many factors influence aerosol deposition. Such factors include inertial impaction, gravity or sedimentation, the kinetic activity of the particles, the physical nature of particles, the temperature and humidity of the carrier gas, the patient's ventilatory pattern, and the physical characteristics of the patient's airway.

Inertial Impaction

As a person inspires, gas flow changes direction as the airway changes direction. If particles are suspended in the gas flow inertia may result in these particles not turning with the gas flow and impacting on the upper airway. This is known as inertia impaction (Figure 4-22). This phenomenon often occurs when the patient breathes in an aerosol with a high inspiratory flow resulting in aerosol particles being deposited on the mucosal of the posterior pharynx. High inspiratory gas flows (>1 L/sec) can enhance inertial impaction and cause some particles to impact on the epithelial lining of the upper airway and posterior aspects of the pharynx. It is important, therefore, to use low inspiratory gas flows (<1 L/sec) to ensure effective aerosol therapy; this can be accomplished by instructing the patient to inhale slowly.

Gravity or Sedimentation

As was previously mentioned, the larger the particle, the more likely it will become unstable, fall out of the carrier gas, and be deposited. Small particles (in the 1 to 5 μm range) are deposited by sedimentation resulting from gravity.[35] The actual sedimentation of a particle is governed by Stokes's Law, which states that the sedimentation rate of a particle nearly equals the particle's density multiplied by the square of its diameter. In other words, as particles become larger, gravity has a greater effect on them, and they are more likely to settle out of suspension. Therefore, larger particles are less stable and are deposited before smaller particles.

One factor that opposes gravity and tends to keep particles in suspension is gas density. Note that a suspension of particles in a gas occurs when gas molecules randomly strike the sides of aerosol particles and keep them "floating" in the gas. The denser the gas, the greater the effects of this bombardment because particles are more likely to remain suspended and be transported by the carrier gas than to settle from gravity. On the other hand, the lighter the gas, the less likely it can transport particles. This principle may be better understood by comparing helium with air as a carrier gas for an aerosol. Because helium molecules are smaller than air molecules, aerosol particles are more influenced by gravity than by the molecular collision with the helium carrier gas. Gravity tends to pull particles out of the gas stream, so helium and oxygen mixtures are poor carriers of aerosol particles.

Kinetic Activity

All molecules are continually in motion, colliding with each other and their environment. This phenomenon, kinetic activity, can be seen with submicroscopic aerosol particles that are less than 1 μm. The random movement of these small particles is called Brownian movement (or diffusion). As particles decrease in size, Brownian movement increases. Another way of describing this phenomenon is that the smaller the aerosol particle, the closer it approaches the size of the gas molecules impacting it, thus becoming more susceptible to the Brownian forces. Notice that a particle must be submicroscopic before aerosol deposition is significantly enhanced by kinetic activity. Particles less than 1 μm in diameter are the most stable and tend to be inhaled and exhaled without being deposited on the airway surface. The effects of gravity and kinetic activity on particles in this size range tend to cancel each other. Therefore as aerosol particles increase in size above 1 μm, gravity begins to exert a greater force, affecting particle stability.

Physical Nature of the Particle

The physical nature, or tonicity, of the aerosol particle can also influence deposition. Aerosol particles can either become smaller or increase in size as they travel through the respiratory system. Particles that increase in size within the lungs are called hygroscopic particles. Such particles tend to absorb water and grow in size. As they absorb water and collide with adjacent particles, they consolidate and drop out of the gas stream, which is a key factor to consider when administering solid particles of medication. Hygroscopic tendencies are influenced by the liquid substance (e.g., medication) itself, the tonicity of the particle, the ambient humidity, and the gas temperature, which is discussed in the following section. Hypertonic aerosols have a greater tonicity than body fluids so they tend to absorb water, increase in size, and become unstable earlier than hypotonic aerosols. However, hypotonic aerosols tend to evaporate, decrease in size, and travel further into the respiratory tract. Isotonic aerosol particles have the same tonicity as body fluids and are not likely to change their dimensions.

A clinical example of the principle of tonicity is seen when hypertonic saline aerosol is delivered to enhance expectoration. Hypertonic aerosols are often administered to obtain a sputum sample for microbiological examination because inhalation of a hypertonic aerosol causes larger particles to deposit in the larger airways, thus promoting cough and expectoration.

Temperature and Humidity

The temperature and humidity of the carrier gas also influence aerosol particle size. Particles can either evaporate and get smaller or increase in size, depending on the water content and humidity level of the gas around them. An aerosol that is cooler than room temperature will warm as it travels to the patient via the delivery circuit. As the aerosol warms, particles evaporate and become smaller, so there is potential for deeper deposition in the airways. Heated aerosol cools as it travels to the patient, so particles tend to coalesce and thus become larger, which encourages deposition in the larger airways.[11] When cool aerosol particles are placed in warm, humidified gas (e.g., gas in the respiratory system), they tend to grow as humidity coalesces them. Again, as these particles grow, they are deposited higher in the airway. Dry aerosols (e.g., powdered bronchodilators) tend to clump or aggregate in high humidity environments, thereby reducing their delivered doses.

Ventilatory Pattern and Characteristics of the Patient's Airway

Ventilatory pattern is the most important factor that can be controlled by both the patient and the person administering the aerosol treatment. The ventilatory pattern is influenced by inspiratory gas flow, respiratory rate, and inspiratory pause. High inspiratory gas flow tends to deposit aerosol particles in the upper airways because of inertial impaction. When an aerosol is inhaled at a flow rate higher than 1 L/sec, gas turbulence encourages larger particles to be deposited onto the upper airway lining. Deeper deposition of aerosol particles occurs with slower inspiratory flow. Flow rates lower than 0.5 L/sec result in laminar flow, increasing the chances for deeper deposition.[33] Normal spontaneous inspiratory flows are about 0.5 L/sec (30 L/min).

Tachypnea increases inspiratory flows, which reduces the time the aerosol particle is in the lung and leaves fewer opportunities for deposition.[8] Slower respiratory rates afford the patient improved deposition by allowing more time for aerosol particles to become unstable and fall out of the carrier gas. Slower respiratory rates combined with a breath hold at the end of inspiration have been effective in promoting deeper aerosol deposition.[1,8,33,35] An inspiratory hold of 4 to 10 seconds promotes aerosol deposition. During breath holding, particles have more time to decrease their forward velocity, thus increasing aerosol deposition.[35]

The influence of tidal volume is less predictable. Although larger tidal volumes take in greater amounts of aerosol, the relationship between tidal volume and actual aerosol deposition has not been demonstrated in clinical studies. In a review of the literature, tidal volume was not found to be an important factor in aerosol deposition.[1]

Airway caliber is another factor that influences aerosol deposition. As the caliber of the airway decreases because of bronchoconstriction, edema, or secretions, aerosol deposition is more likely to occur in the upper airway or larger bronchi. Reduced airway diameter may require greater dosages of medicated aerosols to achieve desired effects. Sometimes secretion removal (e.g., airway aspiration or suctioning) can better prepare the respiratory tract for aerosol therapy.

Mouth breathing enhances aerosol deposition in the lower airways more than nose breathing because the nasal cavity can filter out aerosol particles larger than 5 to 10 μm in diameter.[8] Furthermore, aerosol deposition (especially medicated aerosols) by mouthpiece is better than by mask. Patients with an increased work of breathing tend to breathe through their mouth in an attempt to decrease resistance to inspiratory flow. Under these conditions, a medicated aerosol should be administered by mouthpiece whenever possible. Current guidelines recommend that patients younger than 3 years of age should receive aerosol by mask, and patients older than 3 years should receive it by mouthpiece.[27] Other options recommended include using only pMDIs (not nebulizers) for children more than 4 years of age.[36]

Although this is not supported by research data, patients who cannot tolerate an aerosol mask or mouthpiece may benefit from using a blow-by apparatus (Figure 4-23). A blow-by device allows the aerosol spray to be directed right into the patient's oral cavity to promote particle deposition. Note that if the blow-by method is used without close monitoring, aerosol may be directed toward the nasal passages or away from the oral cavity, compromising aerosol deposition. Aerosol by mask or blow-by device may not provide optimal results in infants because they breathe primarily through

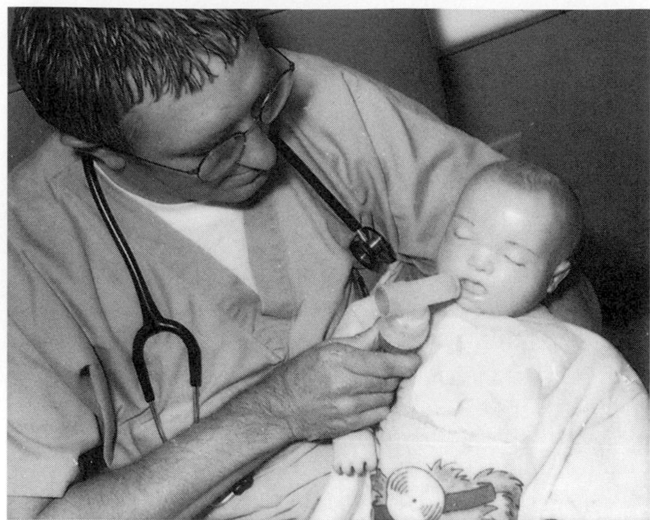

Figure 4-23 A "blow-by" set-up for aerosol administration.

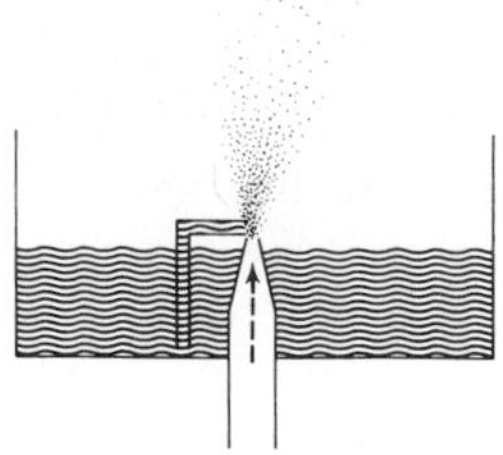

Figure 4-24 The Bernoulli Principle used by jet nebulizers to produce an aerosol. (Modified from Cushing IE, Miller WF: Nebulization therapy. In Safar P: *Respiratory therapy,* Philadelphia, 1965, FA Davis.)

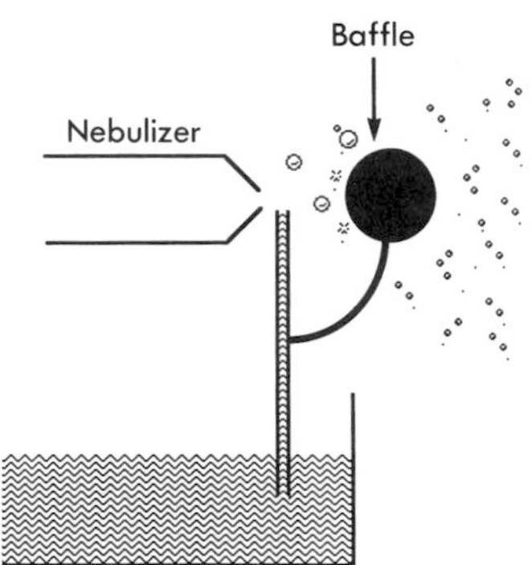

Figure 4-25 Use of a baffle for producing smaller aerosol particles.

their noses. Unfortunately, few controlled studies of nebulized aerosols administered to infants have been completed. For this age group, aerosol therapy is further compromised because of the nonstandardized doses of bronchoactive drugs.

Because of the small tidal volumes of infants and the anatomy of their upper airways, doses recommended for older children or adults cannot be used for infants. Very young children and infants may require relatively higher medication doses to achieve effective results.[36] In summary to optimize aerosol deposition and effectiveness of medicated aerosol therapy a mouthpiece should be used whenever possible with close observation to assure mouth breathing.

Therapeutic Use of Aerosol

Aerosols are administered for various reasons, including for therapeutic and diagnostic effects (see Table 4-6). Major aerosol treatments include bronchodilators, antiinflammatory drugs, antimicrobials, anticholinergics, local anesthetics, and bland aerosols. Safe and effective administration of these treatments requires careful selection of the delivery method and monitoring of patient response. In addition, teaching the patient the proper technique for inspiration during an aerosol treatment is the single most important variable that respiratory therapists can influence. Optimal patient ventilatory pattern, selection of the appropriate aerosol generator, and administration of the correct aerosol solution allows aerosol therapy to remain one of the most effective respiratory care modalities for preventing and treating pulmonary disease.

The following section discusses aerosol generation and equipment, operation, clinical use, and limitations and emphasizes the commonly used aerosol devices including small and large aerosol generators, pMDIs, environmental aerosol units, and special administration of selected aerosols (e.g., pentamidine, ribavirin).

Methods of Aerosol Generation

Aerosols are produced by devices called nebulizers, the most common type of which is the jet nebulizer. Jet nebulizers—regardless of reservoir size—use the Bernoulli principle to produce an aerosol. This principle is based on a decrease in lateral wall pressure to shatter fluid particles into an aerosol at a point where gas flow exits a constriction. As the lateral pressure that surrounds the gas stream decreases below the atmospheric pressure, fluid is drawn up a capillary tube (Figure 4-24). When the fluid reaches the gas stream, it is shattered into small particles, which may encounter baffles. (A baffle reduces aerosol particle size.) Baffles include the fluid surface, sides of the aerosol generator, or structures deliberately placed in the front of the gas stream, such as a plastic ball or a flat device (Figure 4-25). Actually, any object in the path of the aerosol particle can be a baffle, just as can any right-angle bend of the tubing carrying the aerosol. When a large, heavy, aerosol particle hits a baffle, its weight and interrupted forward motion forces it to drop back into the fluid reservoir. Baffles prevent larger particles from being delivered to the patient, so a more uniform aerosol size can be generated. Without baffles, larger particles are delivered.

Nebulizers without a baffle are called atomizers. Because atomizers produce a wide range of particles, they are not commonly used in respiratory care. However, atomizers may be used in clinical conditions that require large aerosol particles to be applied to the upper airway. Such situations

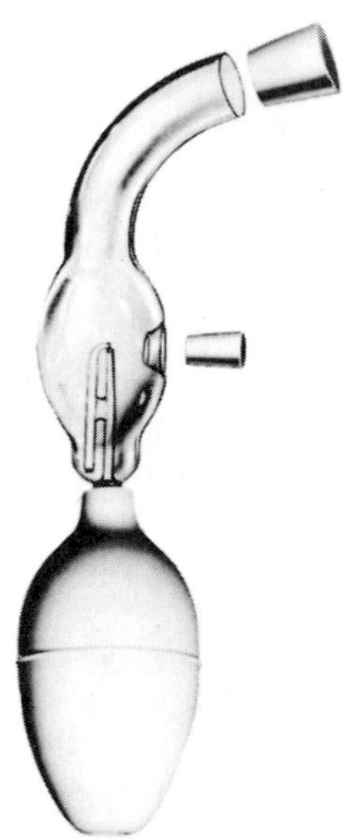

Figure 4-26 The original hand-held bulb type of nebulizer manufactured by DeVilbiss. (Courtesy Sunrise Medical Home Healthcare, Longmont, Colo.)

include administration of topical anesthetics or decongestants to the pharynx and nasal passages for insertion of invasive devices such as bronchoscopes, endotracheal tubes, suction catheters, and nasopharyngeal airways.

Classification of Pneumatic Aerosol Generators

Jet nebulizers require compressed gas to generate an aerosol and therefore are considered pneumatic aerosol generators. These types of nebulizers are generally classified as either small-volume nebulizers (SVNs), pMDIs, or large-volume nebulizers (LVNs).

Small-Volume Nebulizers

One of the first medical nebulizers was the DeVilbiss hand-held type, which incorporated a flexible bulb that when squeezed produced gas flow to a jet, which drew the medication into the gas stream and shattered it into an aerosol (Figure 4-26). Since the development of hand-held, squeeze type of nebulizers, manufacturers have created a variety of SVNs that are employed with gas flow circuits used for intermittent positive-pressure breathing (IPPB) therapy, mechanical ventilation, or as hand-held nebulizers powered by low-flow oxygen or compressed air.

All SVNs used with IPPB therapy or mechanical ventilation are classified as either sidestream nebulizers, in which the aerosol is injected into the gas stream, or as mainstream nebulizers, in which the main flow of gas actually passes through the aerosol generator (Figure 4-27). Several nebulizers with the newer disposable circuits for IPPB or mechanical ventilation can be adapted to either mainstream or sidestream placement, depending on the therapeutic indication or need.

Hand-held nebulizers are a popular version of SVN used to administer medicated aerosols (Figure 4-28). Since the late 1970s, they have become a common modality for providing medicated aerosol to patients for the prevention and treatment of pulmonary disease. As a result of the popularity of SVNs, a variety of models are now available, each with its own characteristics, features, and varying aerosol output. Despite differences in the SVNs available, studies have failed to demonstrate the differences in clinical response based on SVN design.[8]

SVNs employ a jet, which uses the Bernoulli principle, as previously discussed. A high-pressure gas is passed through a constriction, adjacent to which is the open end of a capillary tube. The other end of the tube is immersed in the

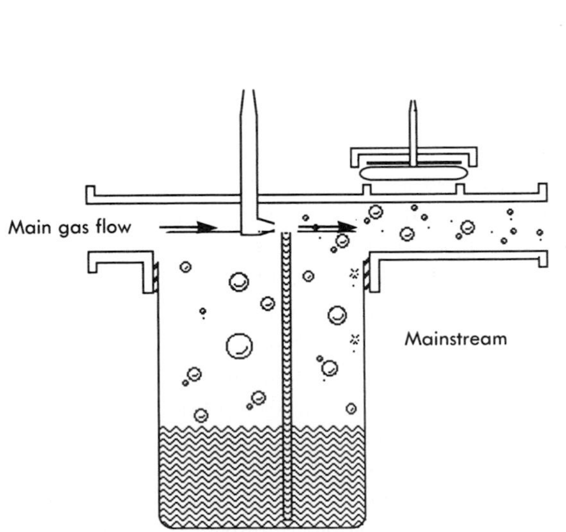

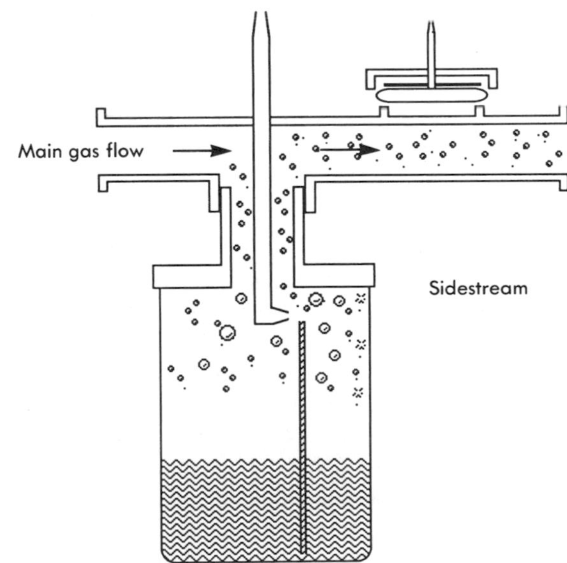

Figure 4-27 Mainstream and sidestream nebulizers.

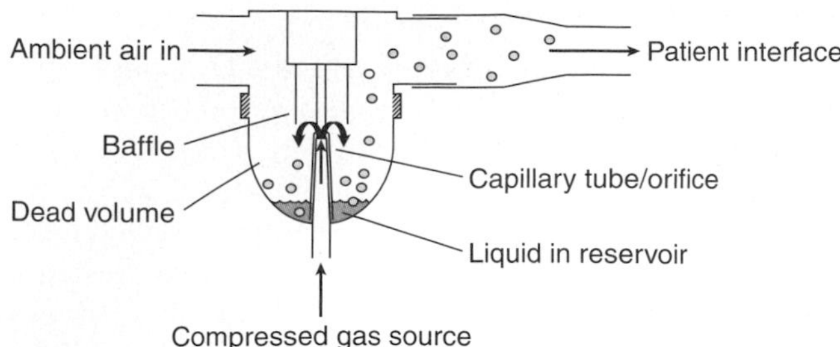

Figure 4-28 Basic components of the design of pneumatic nebulizers. (From Hess DR: Nebulizers: Principles and Performance, *Respir Care* 45[6]:610, 2000.)

fluid (e.g., medication), and, as gas exits the constriction, its forward velocity increases, and the surrounding pressure (i.e., lateral wall pressure) decreases. Liquid is drawn by the subatmospheric pressure and allowed to be shattered by the gas stream. The gas flow and aerosol are allowed to exit the unit via a large-bore outlet, where an adapter fits to accommodate various devices such as a mouthpiece, mask, or gas circuit to a mechanical ventilator. A common SVN set-up is the T-piece (Brigg's adapter) with a mouthpiece and a 50 mL reservoir (Figure 4-29). A reservoir retains additional aerosol for increased deposition. Hand-held SVNs require a gas source, which is usually a portable compressor or flowmeter, to provide flow to generate an aerosol. Typical gas flow rates used with SVNs are 8-10 L/min.

SVN performance is related to the amount of liquid in the unit, the dead space within the unit, and the gas flow rate. Typical SVNs provide more aerosol when the nebulizer volume is 3-4 mL (instead of 2 mL) and when the gas flow rate is 8 L/min.[8] As gas flow through the SVN increases, particle size decreases. Fluid nebulized within the SVN usually consists of a medication and diluent (e.g., sterile saline or water). As the fluid level decreases (as a result of nebulization), the diluent evaporates and the medication concentration increases. The residual volume is the amount of fluid remaining in the SVN at the point when the nebulizer no longer generates an aerosol, which may vary from model to model. A typical residual (dead space) volume ranges from 0.5 to 1 mL. As residual volume increases, less medication is delivered, so the overall efficiency of the unit decreases. It is common to flick the sides of the SVN or shake the unit when it begins to sputter to encourage larger fluid particles adhering to the inside wall of the unit to return to the small fluid reservoir and be nebulized. This action can increase the actual amount of medication delivered. Most SVNs produce a total fluid output of 0.1 to 0.5 mL/min, and a total fluid volume typically placed in an SVN for therapy is 3 to 4 mL. Gas flow rates through the nebulizer are optimal at 6 to 8 L/min, which produces clinically useful aerosol particles. The average aerosol particle MMAD from an SVN is 1 to 5 μm.[33] Above gas flow rates of 10 L/min, treatment time decreases and less medication may actually enter the patient's airway. Gas flow rates below 6 L/min extend treatment time beyond patient tolerance, resulting in the treatment possibly being turned off before all the medication is nebulized. Even with optimal operation and patient technique, SVNs only provide about 10% of the intended medication to the lower airways. Most of the medication (including diluent) is exhaled or remains as dead space volume (Clinical Rounds 4-1).

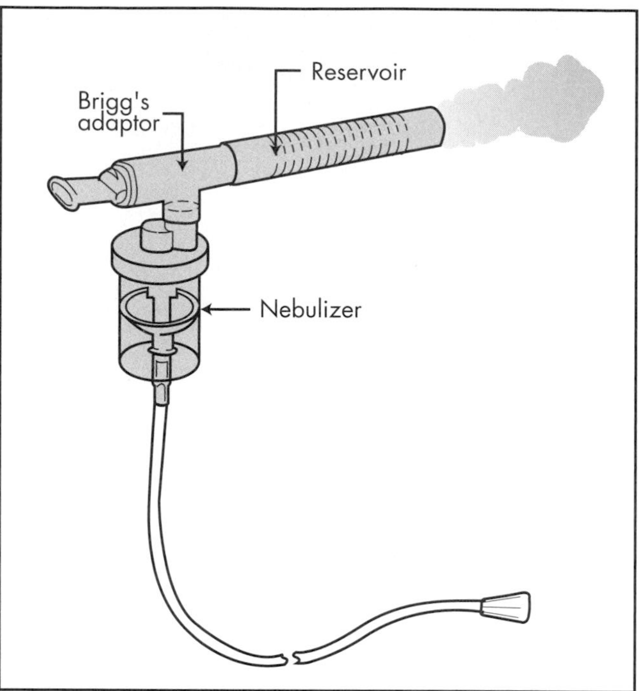

Figure 4-29 A common set-up for an SVN using a Brigg's adapter, reservoir, and mouthpiece.

CLINICAL ROUNDS 4-1

You are called to the emergency department to deliver a medicated aerosol to a 4-year-old child who is alert but restless and complains of shortness of breath. The child's mother says that the child has had several "asthma attacks" since 1 year of age but that all have been mild and this is the first visit to a hospital. The emergency room physician asks you to suggest an appropriate aerosol device. What do you recommend?

See Appendix A for the answer.

The brand or model of SVN, the gas flow rate at which it is operated, and the type of medication affect the unit's overall effectiveness. Most SVNs must remain upright to function, but others can function in a variety of positions. The patient's ability to correctly assemble and operate the SVN should be a major factor when selecting brand and model. The intent of the therapy should also influence the type of SVN used. For example, to treat a lung infection, the smaller

CLINICAL ROUNDS 4-2

A physician requests that you administer an aerosolized antibiotic to a patient with pneumonia. What device could you use, and what MMAD is appropriate?

See Appendix A for the answer.

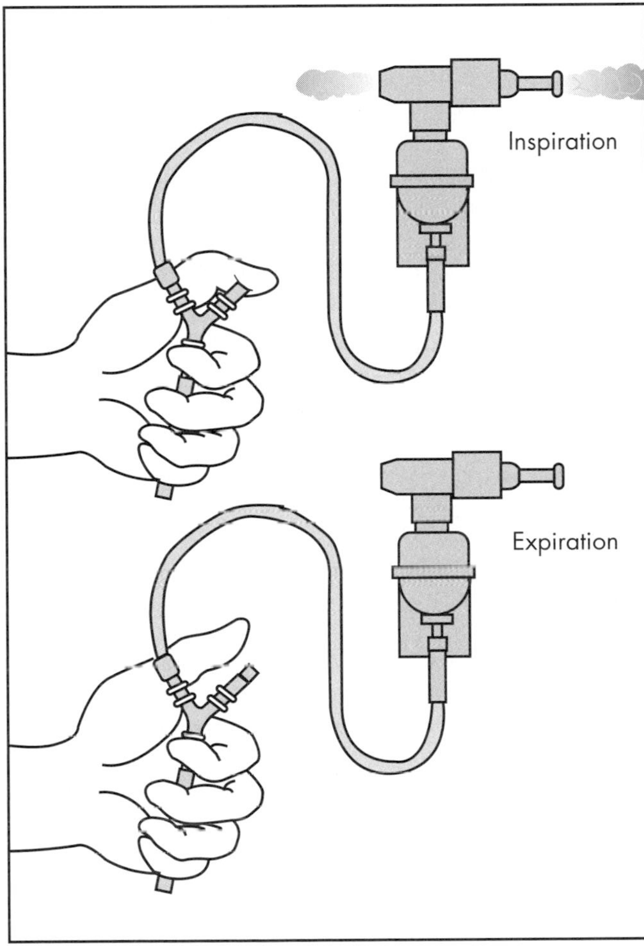

Figure 4-30 Use of a finger control to control aerosol production during inspiration and expiration.

particles generated by Marquest's Respirgard II SVN penetrate more deeply into the lung parenchyma. For home therapy, however, a durable SVN that is easy to clean and maintain should be considered (Clinical Rounds 4-2).

Other specialty nebulizers, such as the Vortran's High Output Extended Aerosol Respiratory Therapy (HEART) and the ICN SPAG-2 units (described later in this chapter), may be used to create more uniform particle sizes. Furthermore, a finger control can be used to create nebulization during inspiration, increase the medication delivered, and reduce waste (Figure 4-30). Although it is popular to use an SVN without finger control, continuous nebulization during both inspiration and expiration can result in a decrease in the dose of the medicated aerosol the medication.

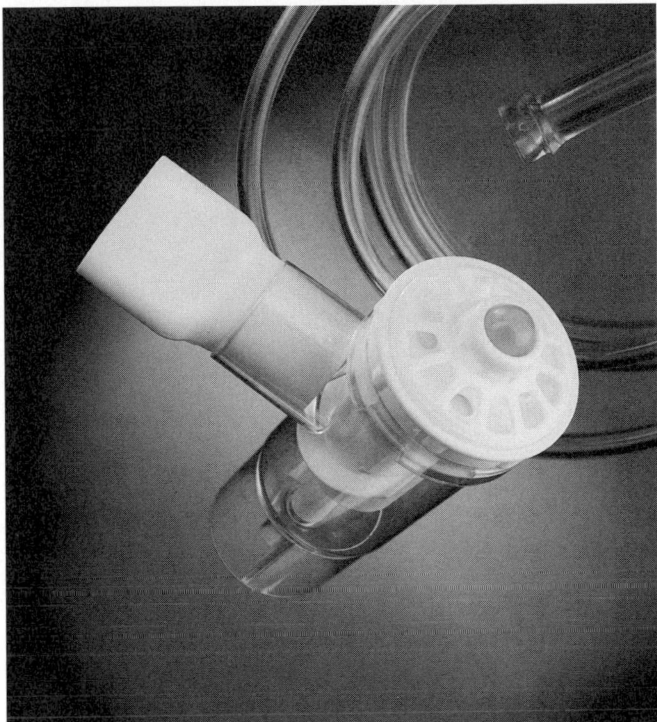

Figure 4-31 The Monaghan AeroEclipse Breath-Actuated Nebulizer. (Courtesy Monaghan Medical Corporation, Syracuse, NY.)

The Monaghan AeroEclipse Breath-Actuated Nebulizer (Figure 4-31) creates aerosol only in precise response to the patient's inspiratory effort. This is often referred to as patient-on-demand therapy. Administering medication during only inspiration means less medication waste and more stable inhaled dosage. This new generation of hand-held nebulizer reduces the risk of exhaled drug aerosol to caregivers because of the aerosol being generated during inspiration only.

The Salter NebuTech HDN SVN is designed to deliver an increased concentration of medication with less residual volume (Figure 4-32). The SVN offers an anti-drool feature, a patented "cone" design to enhance nebulization of medications, and nebulizes 3 milliliters within 7 minutes or less at 7 L/min gas flow rate. The manufacture claims 80% of the aerosol contain particles less than 5 microns. A one-way valve at the inlet and outlet paths reduces the amount of noninhaled aerosol.

Use of a SVN during mechanical ventilation is one method to provide various medications to the lungs of intubated patients. SVN use during neonatal mechanical ventilation has significantly decreased over the past several years. Because of the addition of gas flow from the SVN (if an auxiliary gas source is used instead of nebulizer function from the ventilator) and the potential for an increase in airway

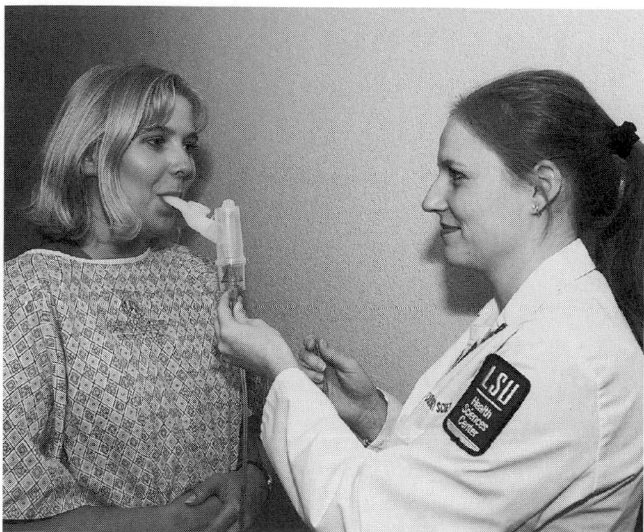

Figure 4-32 Salter NebuTech HDN SVN.

pressures, neonatal SVN therapy has been replaced with alternative methods (i.e., use of a pMDIs, reservoirs, and self-inflating bags). This set-up allows medicated aerosol to be artificially ventilated into the patient's artificial airway.

There are several factors that influence aerosol delivery through the gas delivery circuit and artificial airway that need to be noted, including a baffling effect of the ventilator circuit and artificial airway, and the increased inertial impaction of aerosol particles during high inspiratory gas flow. These factors can decrease deposition of medication in the lung. Several studies demonstrate that only about 1% to 3% of the drug is deposited during mechanical ventilation.[37-40]

In addition to adjusting the medication dose as necessary for delivery to intubated, mechanically ventilated patients, SVN placement is a key to providing effective therapy. Studies have shown that placing the SVN in the inspiratory limb at the manifold of the ventilator circuit about 18 inches from the patient's airway is optimal. The least effective location for an SVN is between the patient and Y-connector of the ventilatory circuit.[8] If an SVN provides continuous nebulization, medicated aerosol can be wasted during the expiratory phase of ventilation, but this can be avoided by using intermittent SVN aerosolization during mechanical ventilation. Box 4-7 summarizes the correct method of SVN use during mechanical ventilation.

Box 4-7 Proper Use of a Small-Volume Nebulizer During Mechanical Ventilation

1. Determine need for therapy.
2. Establish appropriate dose of medication.
3. Assemble the SVN.
4. Place the SVN securely in inspiratory limb of ventilator circuit.
5. Attach a gas source (from either a mechanical ventilator or a flow-metering device) of 6 to 8 L/min to the SVN.
6. Adjust ventilatory parameters (e.g., tidal volume, pressure-limit) to accommodate the excess gas flow from the SVN.
7. Turn off ventilator flow-by or continuous gas flow during SVN therapy.
8. Tap the side of the SVN as needed to nebulize the entire volume of liquid.
9. At the completion of treatment, remove and disassemble SVN and rinse it with *sterile* water or allow it to air dry.
10. Return ventilatory parameters to pretreatment settings.
11. Replace the SVN daily or as indicated.

Pressurized Metered Dose Inhalers (pMDIs)

Portable inhalers or pMDIs are available for delivering various medications, including but not limited to, bronchodilators and antiinflammatory and anticholinergic drugs. The pMDI was originally manufactured by Riker Laboratories, which is now 3M Pharmaceuticals. pMDI therapy has developed into a reliable, efficient, and safe method of providing medicated aerosol to the respiratory tract.[32] Effectiveness and portability make pMDI therapy an important aspect of caring for patients with pulmonary disease. Although pMDIs can be effective, patient instruction and proper use are paramount to optimal delivery. According to the 1994 National Health Interview Survey, 40 million patients use pMDIs. With such widespread use, providing patients education in proper pMDI use and assessing pMDI effectiveness are major tasks of respiratory therapists. Despite the simple appearance of pMDIs and their ease in generating an aerosol puff, studies report that most patients do not use them correctly, resulting in suboptimal therapy.[32,41]

pMDIs (Figure 4-33) are small, pressurized canisters with a mouthpiece that employ pressurized gas propellants. The canisters contain from 80 to 300 doses of a medication, either in liquid or powder form. When the canister is inverted, placed in its mouthpiece adapter, and then depressed, an aerosolized dose of medication is released. Before January 1996, pMDIs used a mixture of two or three chlorofluorocarbon (CFC) propellants with crystals of the medication in suspension. There has since been a total worldwide ban on CFC use and many pMDI manufacturers are now using alternative CFCs or other propellants, such as hydrofluoroalkanes (HFAs).[33] Studies indicate that HFAs have limited impact on the environment and are safe for use in pMDIs.[32]

pMDIs contain vapor pressure from 300 to 500 kPa at 20° C. Each time a pMDI is actuated, a measured amount of propellant carrying medication crystals is delivered. As the propellant emerges from the pMDI, its high vapor pressure causes rapid evaporation and dissipation while the medication is aerosolized and delivered to the patient's open airway. The forward velocity of the aerosol leaving the pMDI is rapid while it is traveling in a forward stream,

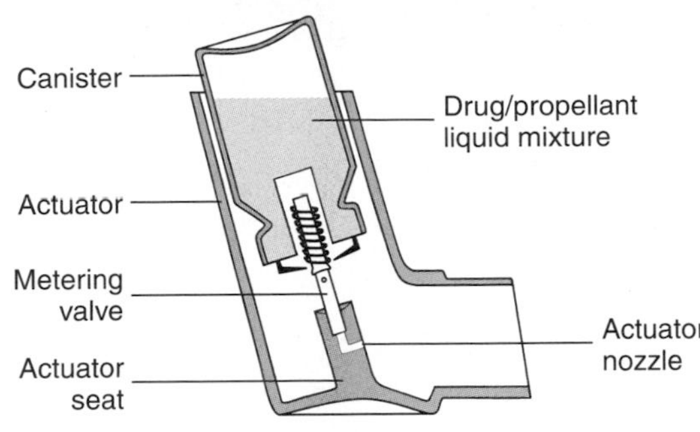

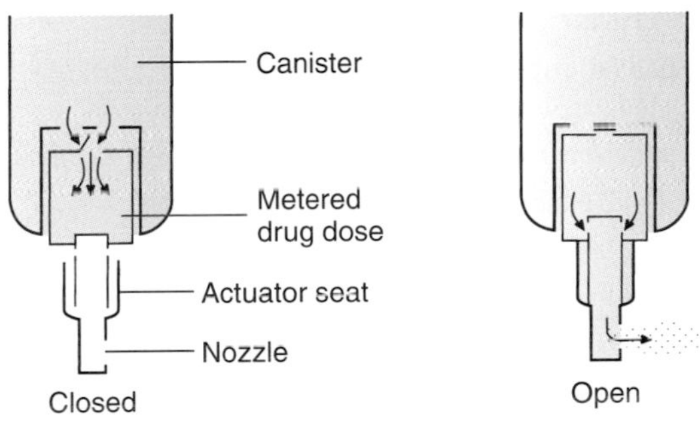

Figure 4-33 A metered dose inhaler. (From Rau JL Jr: *Respiratory care pharmacology*, ed 6, St Louis, 2002, Mosby.)

resulting in a significant amount of medication being deposited in the oropharynx because of inertial impaction. It is estimated that an average of only 10% of the actual medication that leaves the pMDI enters the lower respiratory tract.[42]

The size of the aerosol particle produced by the pMDI is influenced, in part, by the type of drug and the propellant. The temperature of the propellant also influences aerosol size. If the pMDI is placed in a cool environment and the canister becomes cooler than room temperature, vapor pressure within the canister decreases, producing larger aerosol particles. In other words, the cooler the pMDI becomes, the larger the particles released from it. Studies indicate that deeper deposition and smaller particle MMADs occur when canister contents are at 37° C.[43] Patients should be instructed to maintain the pMDI at a warmer temperature in colder climates to preserve its effectiveness.[44] This may be accomplished by having patients carry the pMDI close to their skin or place it in a pocket of clothing near body heat. In addition, proper pMDI preparation before use preserves the intended dosage of medication that leaves the unit when the canister is depressed and the aerosol is produced. Shaking the canister before use allows the medication and propellant to mix. If a pMDI has been not used for several days, the first several puffs may contain suboptimal medication levels, so the patient should be advised to actuate the unit two to three times after shaking it before actually inspiring the aerosol.

Successful delivery of medication with a pMDI depends on the patient's ability to (1) coordinate the actuation of the MDI at the appropriate time during inspiration, (2) create a slow inspiratory gas flow, and (3) hold his or her breath for 4 to 10 seconds at end-inspiration. Actuating the pMDI late or at the end of inspiration (or stopping inhalation) when the cold blast of propellant hits the back of the throat (cold-freon effect) decreases deposition and results in suboptimal therapy. Studies show that inertial impaction of the pMDI aerosol decreases if the patient places the mouthpiece about 4 cm from an open mouth before actuating the MDI.[1,35] If the patient is unable to aim the pMDI mist at the opened mouth, the pMDI mouthpiece should be placed in the entrance to the mouth, or preferably an auxiliary device (discussed later in this chapter) should be used.

Even if the patient demonstrates the correct pMDI technique after initial instruction, a follow-up assessment is usually necessary. Patients tend to alter technique over time (e.g., increase inspiratory flow or poorly coordinate inspiration with pMDI actualization), thus compromising pMDI effectiveness. This is especially true for pediatric and elderly patients.

Another factor that can affect the delivery of the medication is the time between actuations of the pMDI. The initial inspiration of the medication, especially a bronchodilator, increases airway caliber and improves mucus flow. After this happens, subsequent inspirations from the pMDI can be more effective, so it is best to wait from 3 to 10 minutes between actuations.[45] If this length of time is impractical for a particular patient situation (e.g., in cases of severe asthma), waiting at least 1 minute between pMDI inhalations is minimal. These guidelines also apply to pMDI therapy during mechanical ventilation. With the delivery of pMDI medication into the gas delivery circuit with mechanical ventilation, waiting 3 to 10 minutes between breaths enhances the effectiveness of the aerosol. Box 4-8 outlines the correct procedure for use by a spontaneously breathing patient pMDI use (with and without an auxiliary device).

Accessories to Enhance Aerosol Deposition from a pMDI. There are several problems associated with coordinating pMDI use with inspiration. In addition, handling the unit may be difficult for some patients, especially the elderly, younger patients, and the physically challenged. Even if the patient can handle and actuate the pMDI, it is often difficult to coordinate the aerosol with inspiration. The cold-freon effect mentioned previously may also compromise delivery of medication. Respiratory therapists should evaluate each patient's ability to use a pMDI and should implement an auxiliary device designed to enhance medication delivery if a patient is unable to correctly perform therapy. Such devices include spacers and chambers, spring-loaded actuators, and devices to help the patient depress the canister to initiate an aerosol puff from the pMDI.

There are many spacers and chambers available to be attached to a pMDI. (Figure 4-34 shows examples of these devices.) Spacers and chambers may be rigid or collapsible,

Box 4-8 Optimal Technique for Metered-Dose Inhaler Use

Without an Accessory Device

1. Determine the need for therapy
2. Determine number of actuations to be provided
3. Assemble the pMDI and inspect the actuator mouthpiece for foreign matter.
4. Shake the canister vigorously.
5. If it has been more than 24 hours since last use, actuate one puff into the air while holding the pMDI upside down.
6. The patient places the pMDI mouthpiece 4 cm from open mouth.
7. Following a normal exhalation, the patient inspires slowly (<1 L/sec) while depressing the pMDI canister.
8. The patient continues inspiration until total lung capacity is reached.
9. At the end of inspiration, the breath is held for 5 to 10 seconds.
10. Wait 1 to 2 minutes between puffs with the pMDI.

With an Accessory Device (i.e., holding chamber or spacer)

1. Determine the need for therapy.
2. Determine the number of actuations to be provided.
3. Assemble the pMDI and inspect the actuator mouthpiece for foreign matter.
4. Shake the canister vigorously.
5. If it has been more than 24 hours since the last use, deliver one puff into the air while holding the pMDI upside down.
6. Attach accessory device to the pMDI.
   b. Place pMDI mouthpiece into accessory device.
   a. Place valve stem into pMDI canister holding orifice on accessory device.
7. If using mask, attach it to the accessory device.
8. The patient inspires slowly (<1 L/sec) and the pMDI is actuated.
9. The patient continues inspiration until total lung capacity.
10. Wait 1 to 2 minutes between puffs from the pMDI.

based on the model and manufacturer. The goals with these auxiliary devices are as follows: (1) to reduce the velocity of the propelled aerosol from the pMDI, (2) to decrease inertial impaction, (3) to minimize oropharyngeal deposition of the aerosol, and (4) to improve the synchronization of the patient inspiration and generation of the pMDI puff. Studies indicate that use of these devices may increase drug deposition in the lung.[46]

Spacers and Chambers as Partial Reservoirs for Medication. Chambers differ from spacers by employing a one-way valve to hold aerosol particles in the unit until inspiration occurs. Chambers are effective for patients who have problems coordinating inspiration with activation of the pMDI. Spacers and chambers increase the distance for pMDI aerosol to travel, which allows time for evaporation, thus reducing aerosol particle size. The larger the volume of the spacer or chamber, the more likely particles will shrink. These devices also reduce the chance of inertial impaction on inspiration by slowing the aerosol's forward velocity. (This chance decreases independently of spacer or chamber size or shape.)

Those who benefit from spacers or chambers include young children (who cannot coordinate breathing with pMDI use), patients in severe respiratory distress, or any patient who has difficulty coordinating pMDI puffs with inspiration. Some spacers and chambers emit a whistling alarm if the patient inspires too quickly. This audio feedback encourages patients to maintain an appropriate, slow inspiratory flow.

Monaghan Medical Corporation's AeroVent, shown in Figure 4-35, is one of several reservoirs available that is specially designed for pMDIs used with gas delivery circuits for mechanical ventilation and allows improved aerosol deposition to intubated patients. With the AeroVent, the pMDI is actuated 1 to 2 seconds before the inspiratory gas arrives from the mechanical ventilator. An example of a holding chamber for spontaneously breathing older children and adults is Monaghan's AeroChamber (Figure 4-36). The AeroChamber is also available with a mask for administering medication to small children and infants (Figure 4-37).

Additional devices aimed at improving pMDI therapy include actuator aids, such as a spring-loaded Autohaler (3M Pharmaceuticals), which requires an inspiratory effort to actuate the pMDI (Figure 4-38). When the patient flips up a lever on top of the pMDI during an inspiratory effort, a spring-loaded response allows aerosol to leave the pMDI. This device helps the patient to get the pMDI to release its medication but does not aid in controlling the aerosol after it leaves the pMDI.

The Vent-Ease device allows patients with muscular or hand coordination difficulties to actuate the pMDI (Figure 4-39). The Vent-Ease allows the pMDI to be placed within it, and after the extension arm is pressed, the pMDI releases its medication. This device aids in pMDI actualization and does not affect drug delivery.

Dry Powder Inhalers

DPIs are an alternate method for delivering various medications, such as bronchodilators and antiallergic agents. They are practical, small, portable, and do not use CFCs or require a pressurized gas source. DPIs are breath-actuated, so there is no need to coordinate actuation and inspiration. DPIs may better serve patients who have difficulty using pMDIs.

There are several DPIs on the market for treatment of pulmonary disease. GlaxoSmithKline's Advair Diskus (Figure 4-40) provides a powdered form of fluticasone

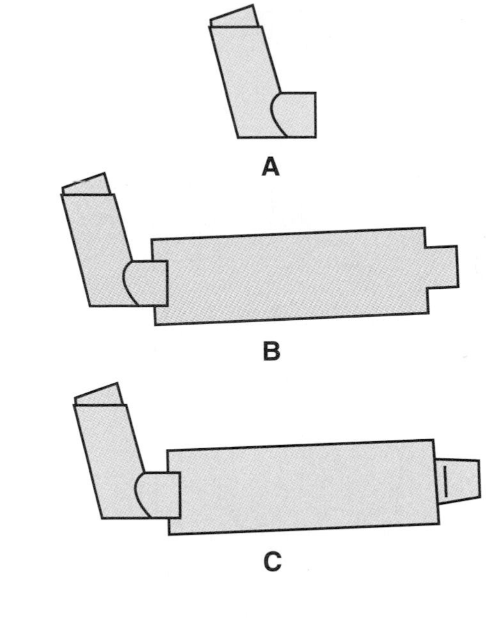

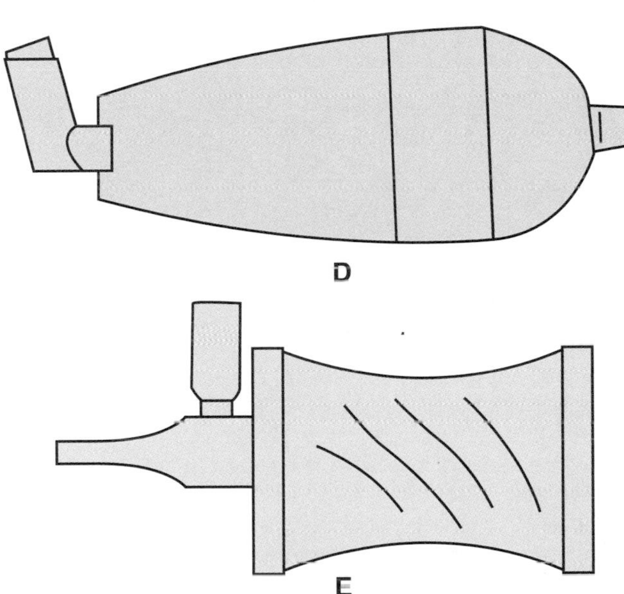

Figure 4-34 Common shapes for reservoirs and chambers used with pMDIs: **A,** pMDI; **B,** elongated reservoir; **C,** elongated chamber; **D,** pear-shaped chamber; and **E,** collapsible reservoir.

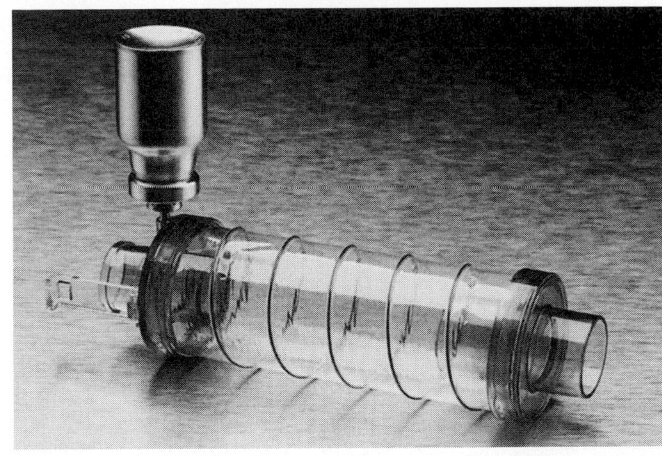

Figure 4-35 The AeroVent reservoir for use with pMDIs and gas flow circuits. (Courtesy Monaghan Medical Corporation, Plattsburgh, NY.)

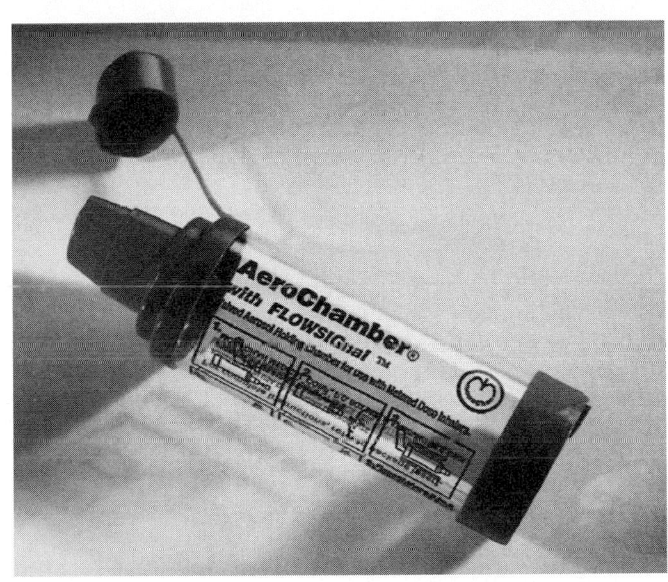

Figure 4-36 The AeroChamber for use with a pMDI. (Courtesy Monaghan Medical Corporation, Plattsburgh, NY.)

propionate and salmeterol and AstraZeneca's Pulmicort Turbuhaler (Figure 4-41) is for delivery of budesonide. Novartis markets a DPI (Foradil Aerolizer) containing a long-acting beta agonist, formoterol fumarate. This unit requires placement of a small capsule into the unit's capsule-chamber (Figure 4-42) followed by depressing the mouthpiece to pierce the capsule. The patient inhales rapidly to distribute the powder into the lungs (Figure 4-43).

Most of the newer DPIs allow patients to see the number of doses remaining. Box 4-9 describes the proper technique for DPIs. Respiratory therapists should give special attention to inspiratory flow rates when inhaling from DPIs. Low-resistant DPIs such as the GlaxoSmithKline's Advair Diskus requires a normal inspiratory flow rate, whereas the Pulmicort Turbuhaler being a high-resistant DPI requires faster inspiratory flows (>1 L/sec). DPIs contain drugs that are either spheronized into agglomerates or mixed with a coarse lactose carrier. Some powdered forms of medications are water-soluble so are affected by humidity. If humidified, the powder clumps, compromising delivery. This characteristic of DPIs prohibits them from being used with mechanical ventilation.

Large-Volume Nebulizers (LVNs)

A variety of nebulizers are available to provide long-term nebulization of solutions, some of which are bland aerosols, bronchodilators, and mucolytics, as well as other medications (e.g., lidocaine). The LVNs available are either pneumatically

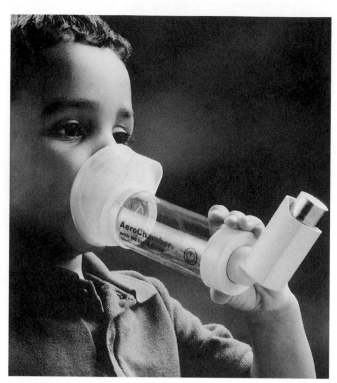

Figure 4-37 The AeroChamber with mask for use with a pMDI. (Courtesy Monaghan Medical Corporation, Plattsburgh, NY.)

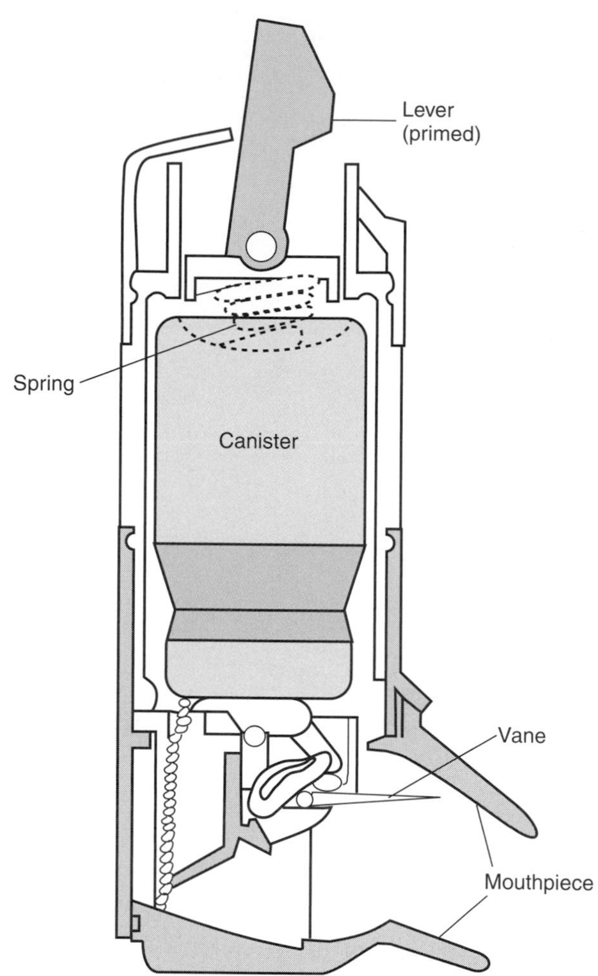

Figure 4-38 The Autohaler MDI. (From Rau JL Jr: *Respiratory care pharmacology*, ed 6, St Louis, 2002, Mosby.)

or electrically powered. Pneumatically powered units are classified as entrainment nebulizers, and electrically powered units are ultrasonic nebulizers, both of which will be discussed along with indications for use, methods of operation, and maintenance.

LVNs can be used to provide long-term nonmedicated and medicated aerosol therapy, but most are used to deliver nonmedicated or bland aerosols (i.e., sterile water or saline). Nonmedicated aerosols are typically delivered to the upper airway to decrease the chances of edema or humidity deficit. As discussed previously, cold-nebulized bland aerosols can result in vasoconstriction of the upper airway, thus reducing mucosal edema. In addition, cold aerosols, especially sterile water, can induce cough and expectoration for obtaining sputum for microbiologic inspection. Heated bland aerosols may be administered with medical gases to patients who have artificial airways in place. Long-term bland aerosols can be delivered by several types of masks (i.e., face, tracheostomy, and face tent) (Figure 4-44), but an aerosol mask is the most common means of bland aerosol therapy.

The use of bland aerosols, whether from pneumatic or electric aerosol generators, has not been shown as an effective means of hydrating secretions or improving mucus flow. Instead, data support the use of parenteral and intravenous fluids to better hydrate the respiratory tract mucosal lining.[1,8] The potential limitations of bland aerosol therapy require respiratory therapists to be selective in its use.

Aggressive care of patients with airway inflammation (asthma) may include frequent or continuous delivery of aerosolized bronchodilators. Continuous delivery of a bronchoactive drugs via LVNs has become a modality for caring for patients with severe asthma.[47,48] LVNs work well for the continuous delivery of bronchodilator solutions (e.g., adrenergic and anticholinergic agents) because they have larger reservoirs for the medication. Special pneumatic nebulizer designs allow titrated doses and optimal aerosol particle size to be delivered to patients via mouthpiece or mask or by mechanical ventilation. Vortran's HEART nebulizer (standard or mini-unit) is an example of an LVN designed to deliver continuous therapy. It has a 240 mL solution reservoir and generates particles between 2.2 and 3.2 μm MMAD. Ultrasonic nebulizers, which are discussed later in this chapter, are another method for aggressive administration of a bronchoactive drugs. They allow respiratory therapists to provide bronchoactive drugs quickly and at effective particle sizes.

Pneumatic Jet LVNs. These units provide large reservoirs for bland aerosols and have a provision for air entrainment. LVNs incorporate the jet venturi principle to entrain fluid and a pressure-relief valve. When operated with oxygen, these aerosol generators can provide a range of oxygen

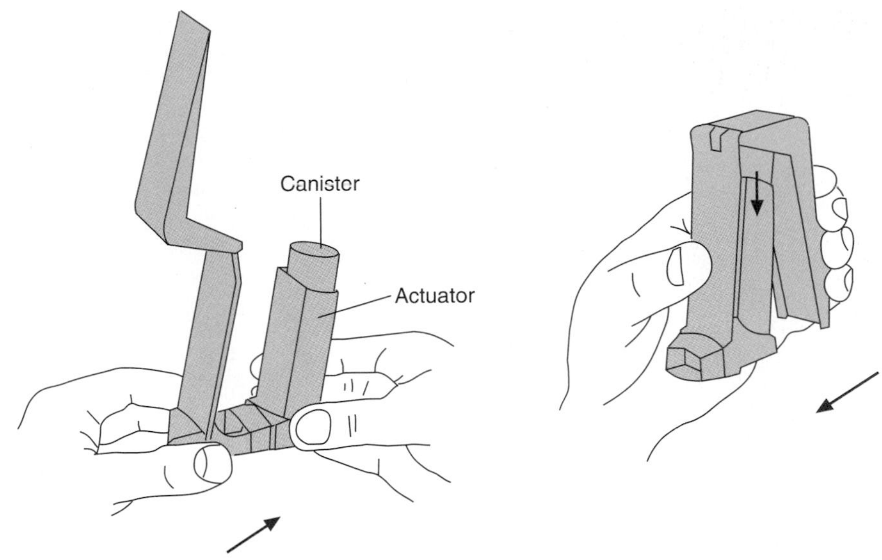

Figure 4-39 The Vent-Ease MDI adapter. (From Rau JL Jr: *Respiratory care pharmacology,* ed 6, St Louis, 2002, Mosby.)

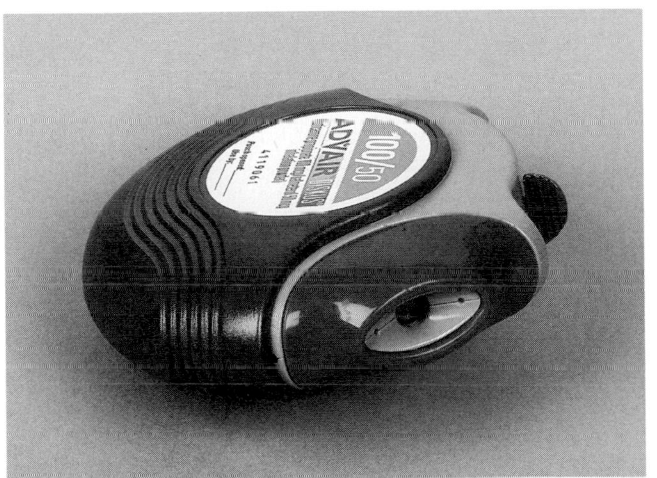

Figure 4-40 GlaxoSmithKline's Advair Diskus.

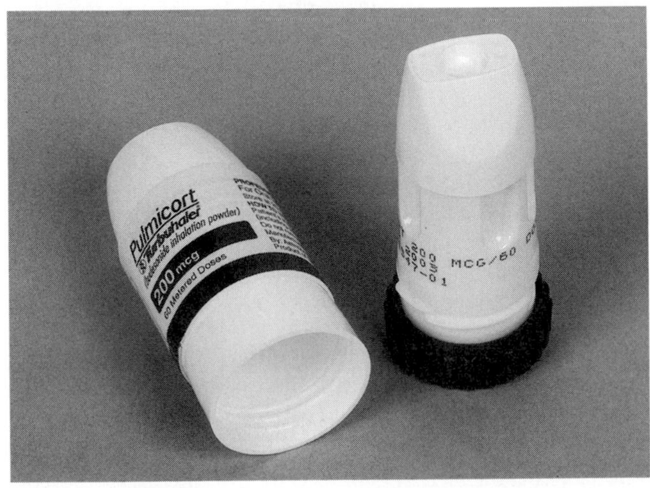

Figure 4-41 AstraZeneca's Pulmicort Turbuhaler.

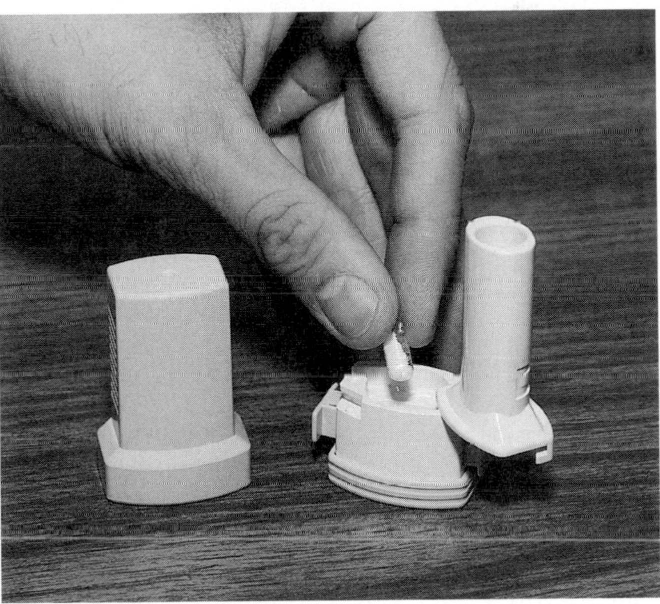

Figure 4-42 The Novartis DPI (Foradil Aerolizer).

percentages. Older units provide a fixed oxygen percentage at three settings: 100%, 70%, and 40% oxygen, but newer units also offer a variable option from about 28% to 100%. A jet venturi allows the entrainment of room air to mix with the oxygen flowing through the unit. This mixing occurs at a fixed ratio of air:oxygen for each oxygen percentage setting. The use of fixed oxygen percentages allows the total gas flow from the unit to the patient to be predicted. Table 4-3 lists total gas flows for two oxygen percentage settings with various flowmeter settings from the Puritan All-Purpose Nebulizer.

Although there are permanent aerosol generators on the market, they all share several features, such as drawing fluid from a reservoir and including a jet for air entrainment. An example of a nondisposable LVN is the Puritan All-Purpose

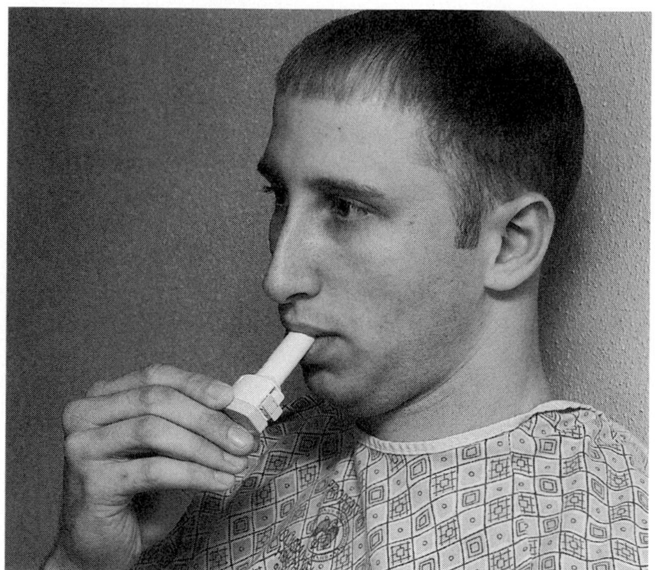

Figure 4-43 Proper use of Novartis's Foradil Aerolizer.

Box 4-9 Optimal Technique for Dry Powder Inhaler Use

1. Determine the need for therapy.
2. Determine the dose of medication to be delivered.
3. Assemble the DPI and inspect the actuator mouthpiece for foreign matter.
4. Load the medication.
5. The patient exhales to normal end-expiration.
6. The DPI mouthpiece is placed in the patient's mouth and lips are closed.
7. The patient inspires rapidly (>1 L/sec).
8. The procedure is repeated until the medication is gone.

Nebulizer (Figure 4-45). These units have optional heating elements for producing heated aerosol (see the following section).

Nondisposable LVNs must be cleaned and sterilized between patients. Although still available, nondisposable LVNs have become less popular in recent years because disposable units are more cost-effective. Respiratory therapists should choose the type of device that best meets patient needs (Clinical Rounds 4-3).

Heated LVNs. Heated aerosol can be administered via several types of heaters (Figure 4-46). The Puritan All-Purpose and the Ohio Deluxe nebulizers can employ an immersion type of heater, which consists of a heating rod that is inserted through a port in the top of the nebulizer and extends into the fluid reservoir. Notice that the immersion heater does not allow temperature to be regulated, so it must be monitored. Also, because the unit is inserted in the solution going to the patient, it must be sterile before use to avoid microbial contamination of the liquid. The immersion heater must be assessed for electrical safety to minimize the chance of electrical shock to the patient or operator during use.

Another option for heated aerosol includes a wraparound, or yolk collar heater (i.e., doughnut heater) (see Figure 4-46). The wraparound heater is placed around the fluid reservoir and plugged into an electrical outlet. As with the immersion

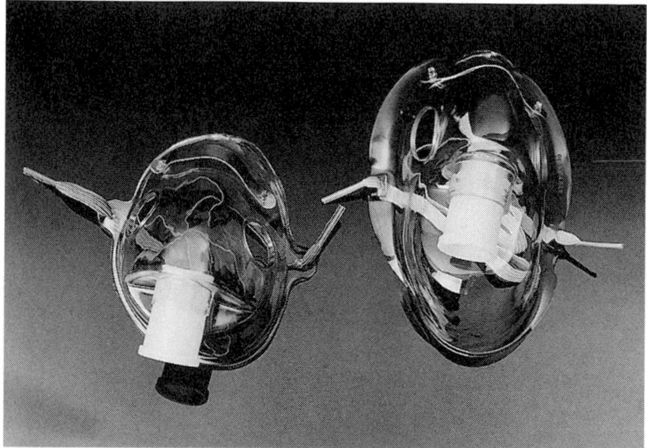

A

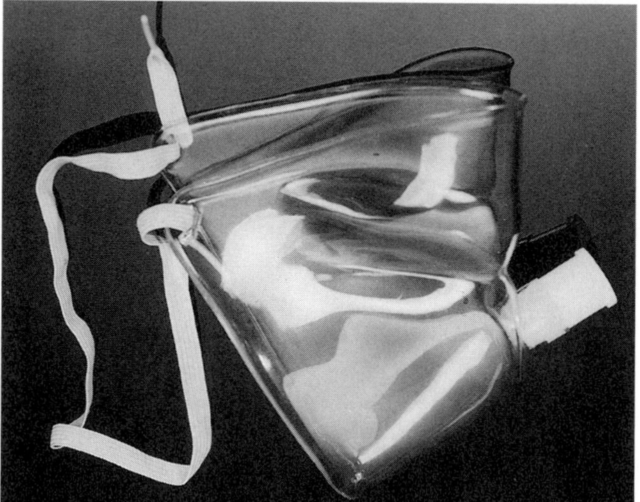

B

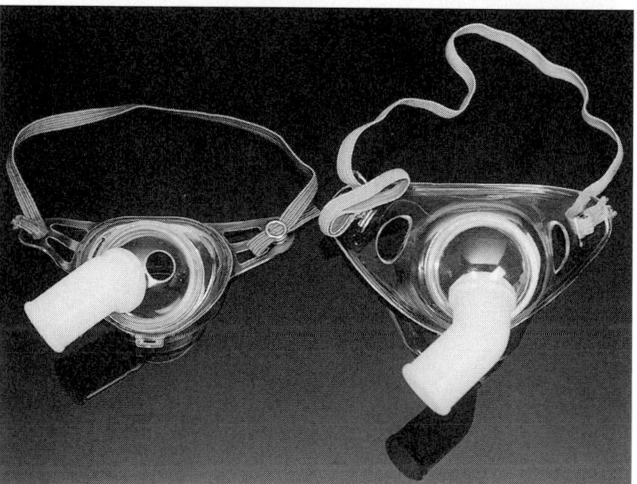

C

Figure 4-44 Aerosol delivery devices. **A,** Aerosol mask; **B,** aerosol face tent; **C,** tracheostomy collar.

Table 4-3 Gas Flow from Puritan All-Purpose Nebulizer*

TOTAL UNRESTRICTED GAS FLOW FROM NEBULIZER (L/MIN)		
Diluted to 40% Oxygen Concentration	70% Oxygen Concentration (L/min)	Flowmeter Setting at Concentration
4	1.6	1
8	3.2	2
12	4.8	3
16	6.4	4
20	8.0	5
24	9.6	6
28	11.2	7
32	12.8	8
36	14.4	9
40	16.0	10
44	17.6	11
48	19.2	12

Courtesy Nellcor Puritan Bennett, Pleasanton, Calif.
**Total gas flow from nebulizer should exceed patient's peak inspiratory flow rate (average 25 to 30 L/min) to achieve maximal aerosol density and stable inspired oxygen concentrations. For accurate flow setting, use a pressure-compensated flowmeter. Newer All-Purpose models have a 35% oxygen setting.*

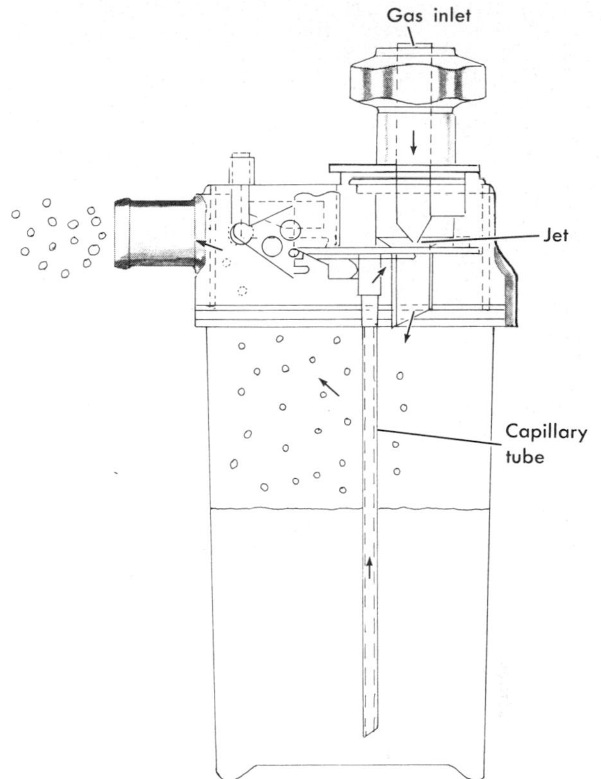

Figure 4-45 The Puritan All-Purpose Nebulizer. (Courtesy Nellcor Puritan Bennett, Mallinckrodt, St Louis, Mo.)

and nonimmersion heaters previously discussed, these units typically do not allow the user to vary operating temperatures and will continue to heat, even if the water level is low or absent, increasing the potential for thermal injury. Conversely, the heating element may stop working and fail to heat without warning, so to ensure proper function the unit should be monitored.

Several nebulizers provide heated aerosol by heating the liquid as it passes through a capillary system. With these devices, the solution to be nebulized in the reservoir does not need to be heated before nebulization. The liquid is heated in smaller amounts right before nebulization. This system allows for a shorter warm-up time than the other types of heaters already discussed. This heating method is found with the Chemetron Heated Nebulizer as well as with several nebulizer models provided by Hudson RCI that are discussed later in this chapter.

Other options for heating aerosols include the servo-control heaters provided by Professional Medical Products' Seamless (Dart) nebulizer, which allows automatic gas and aerosol temperature to be adjusted as it self-monitors gas flow temperature. Continuous temperature feedback with an automatic shut-off safeguard prevents overheating and thermal injury. The ThermaGard Heater is used exclusively with Hudson RCI's Variable Concentration Large Volume

CLINICAL ROUNDS 4-3

A patient is receiving CPAP via an endotracheal tube. What type of humidifying device is appropriate for this patient?

See Appendix A for the answer.

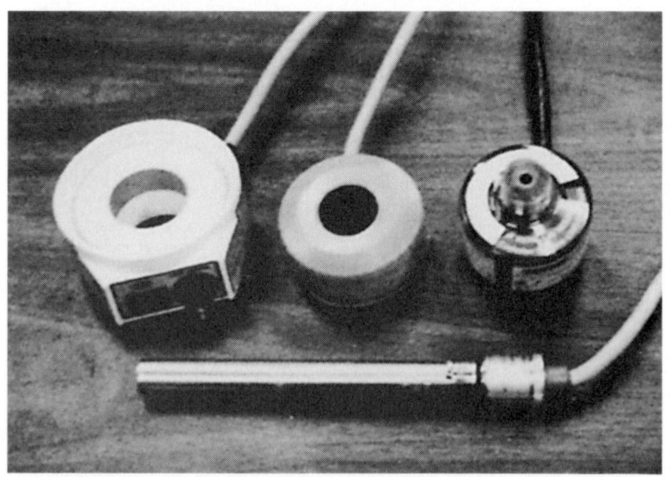

Figure 4-46 Heaters for use with LVNs. (From Scanlan CL, Wilkins RL, Stoller JK: *Egan's fundamentals of respiratory care*, ed 7, St Louis, 1999, Mosby.)

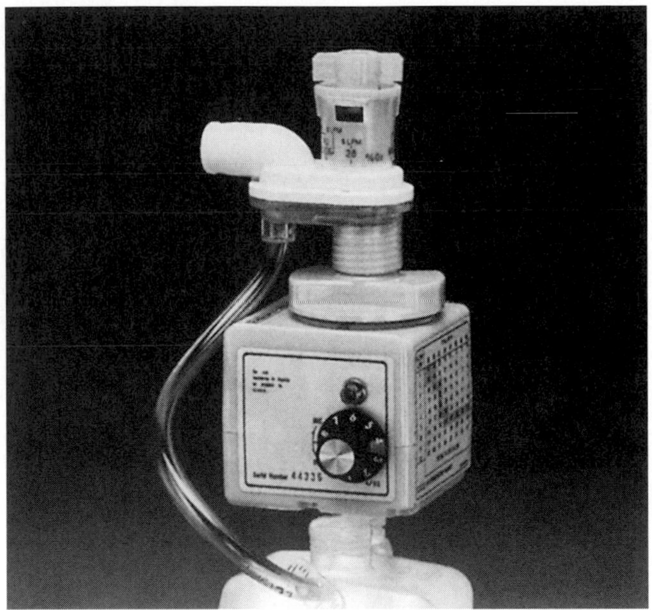

Figure 4-47 The AQUATHERM III External Adjustable Electronic Heater. (Courtesy Hudson Respiratory Care, Inc, Temecula, Calif.)

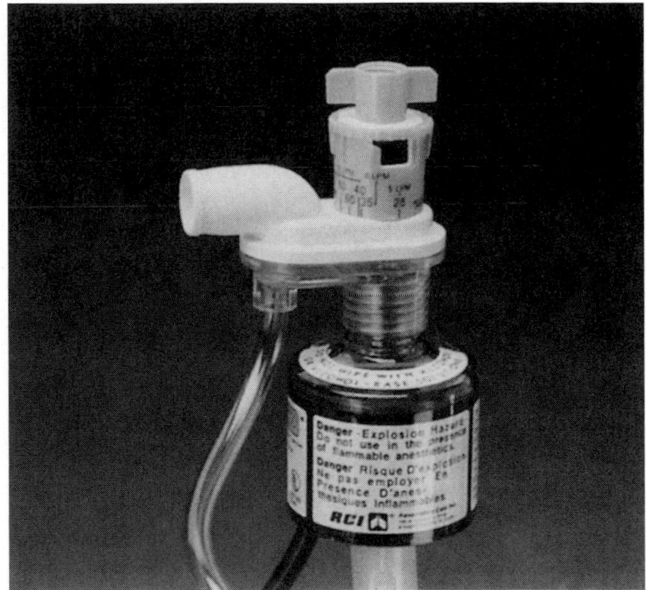

Figure 4-48 The AQUATHERM External Heater. (Courtesy Hudson Respiratory Care, Inc, Temecula, Calif.)

> **CLINICAL ROUNDS 4-4**
>
> After abdominal surgery, a 50-year-old man is brought to the recovery room and started on an aerosol mask at an F_IO_2 of 0.50. While performing your initial assessment of this patient, you notice that his respiratory rate is 20 breaths per minute and he shows signs of respiratory distress. You also note that during inspiration, the aerosol stops flowing from the mask. How would you remedy this situation to ensure the patient 50% oxygen?
>
> *See Appendix A for the answer.*

Nebulizer, which provides continuous, heated aerosol with adjustable temperature settings. The ThermaGard Heater includes a nonreversing thermal fuse to prevent overheating if the control circuit fails and a push-to-turn temperature adjustment to prevent accidental temperature setting changes.

Medical Molding Corporation's Misty Ox Hi-Fi high-flow nebulizer, which is discussed later in this chapter, uses a Turboheater (3M Pharmaceuticals) to heat gas and aerosol and attaches between the reservoir bottle and the nebulizer manifold (i.e., jet assembly). Gas leaves the nebulizer and flows through the heater, where it is warmed before being delivered to the patient. A similar heater, Hudson RCI's AQUATHERM III External Adjustable Electronic Heater, attaches to the nebulizer to heat the aerosol. An adjustable temperature control allows a range of output temperatures (Figure 4-47). Hudson RCI also provides a collar type of heater, the AQUATHERM External Heater, which provides an output temperature from 35° to 38° C at 8 L/min gas flow with full air entrainment (Figure 4-48 and Clinical Rounds 4-4).

As with humidifiers, the output of aerosol generators depends on several factors, including the length of delivery tubing, the total gas flow of carrier gases, the room temperature, and the solution level in the reservoir. For example, the longer the delivery tube, the cooler the gas being delivered becomes; or the faster the gas flow rate, the greater the tendency for gas and aerosol temperature decreases. In contrast, the lower the solution level, the greater the potential of gas and aerosol temperature increases. As the carrier gas temperature decreases en route to the patient, condensation can occur, creating a fluid bolus in the delivery circuit that can obstruct gas flow and alter the delivered oxygen concentration, creating a partial obstruction, which results in back pressure against the jet. This decreases air entrainment and increases the delivered oxygen percentage. This problem can be avoided by intermittently monitoring the aerosol delivery tube patency.

Disposable LVNs. It has become common to provide a variety of therapies using disposable, single-patient-use devices. Disposable LVNs also work by the principle of air entrainment, and there are many available for patient use. The following discussion highlights a sampling of the units on the market.

Practitioners have a choice of either refillable or prefilled disposable nebulizers. Hudson RCI's disposable LVNs provide large reservoirs with an oxygen percentage range from 28% to 98% (Figure 4-50). Tables 4-4 and 4-5 provide data on the performance of Hudson RCI's disposable LVN and also list the aerosol particle size and humidity output at various gas flows and oxygen concentrations. As with other refillable units, the Hudson disposable unit requires monitoring of the fluid level and is designed for single-patient use.

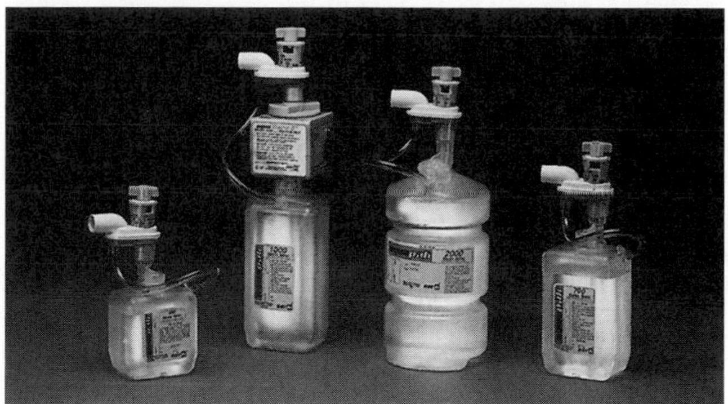

Figure 4-49 Hudson RCI LVNs. (Courtesy Hudson Respiratory Care, Inc, Temecula, Calif.)

Table 4-4 Aerosol particle sizes associated with Hudson RCI disposable nebulizers at different oxygen flows

Flow Rate (L/min)	F_IO_2 (%)	Mean Diameter (μm) Unheated	Mean Diameter (μm) Heated*
5	28	2.3	1.7
8	35	1.7	1.5
10	40	1.6	1.5
10	60	1.6	1.6
10	80	1.7	1.7
10	98	1.8	1.8
10	98	1.8	1.8

*ThermaGard Heater set at a maximum temperature setting.

Table 4-5 Aerosol output of Hudson RCI disposable nebulizers at different oxygen flows

Flow Rate (L/min)	F_IO_2 (%)	Total Output (mL/hour)*	Delivered to Patient (mL/hour)†
5	28	36.16	34.06
10	40	45.04	43.03
10	60	31.04	30.68
10	98	24.96	24.30

*Measures nebulizer outlet.
†Measures at the end of a 72" length of 22-mm tubing.

Prefilled units must be replaced with a new unit before the fluid reservoir reaches a level at which aerosol output is no longer acceptable. The Hudson RCI Prefilled Precision Nebulizer (Figure 4-50) is an example of a prefilled nebulizer that generates high aerosol output and aerosol particles in an effective range of 5 μm or less. The Hudson RCI prefilled

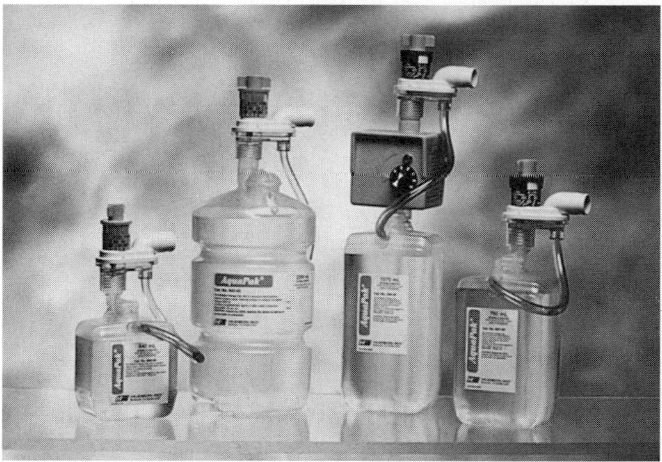

Figure 4-50 The Hudson RCI Prefilled Precision Nebulizer. (Courtesy Hudson Respiratory Care, Inc, Temecula, Calif.)

Table 4-6 Total gas flow developed by large volume air-entrainment nebulizers

		Total flow	
F_IO_2	Air:Oxygen	10 L/minute	15 L/minute
0.24	25:1	260	390
0.30	8.0:1	90	135
0.35	4.6:1	46	69
0.40	3.2:1	32	48
0.60	1.0:1	20	30
0.70	0.6:1	16	24
0.80	0.34:1	13.4	20
0.9	0.14:1	11	16
1.0	0:1	10	15

nebulizer passes aerosol through an offset baffling chamber within the jet assembly where large particles are coalesced and returned to the reservoir. The return tube helps preserve usable water in the reservoir, thus allowing water to be used more times than in other pneumatic nebulizers with similarly sized fluid reservoirs. Because the baffles are efficient, the particles released from the unit are so small that the mist is difficult to see. This unit uses two types of jet manifolds or assemblies. The standard Venturi style of entrainment manifold attaches to the prefilled reservoir with a self-sealing puncture pin, allowing the operator to adjust the diluter ring or entrainment ring for oxygen concentrations from 28% to 98%. The Hudson RCI Critical Care Nebulizer Adapter is an upgrade from the previous jet attachment that also attaches to the reservoir with a self-sealing puncture pin and provides oxygen concentrations from 33% to 98%. Markings on the adjustable entrainment ring are 33%, 35%,

Table 4-7 Total flow rates provided by the Misty Ox Hi-Fi Nebulizer

Entrainment Setting	Oxygen Flow (L/minute)	Total Flow (L/minute)
60%	20-30	40-61
65%	30-40	54-72
75%	30-40	44-58
85%	30-40	37-49
96%	40	42

40%, 50%, 60%, 80%, and 98%. This unit has a special baffling system that reduces the noise associated with nebulization. The screw-on, puncture pin design provides a closed system that may decrease the possibility of microbial contamination of the fluid within the unit.

Average outputs from most disposable pneumatic nebulizers are about 1 to 2 mL of fluid per minute. Prefilled units typically have reservoir capacities ranging from 400 to 2200 mL. Table 4-6 provides air and oxygen entrainment ratios and the total gas flow associated with entrainment type of nebulizers (nondisposable and disposable units).

Several models of pneumatic nebulizers can provide high gas flows at high oxygen concentrations. For example, the Misty Ox Hi-Fi Nebulizer can produce up to 42 L/min with an oxygen concentration of 96% (Table 4-7) and offers a range of oxygen concentrations from 60% to 96%.[12]

The Misty Ox Gas Injector Nebulizer is a specially designed pneumatic (nonentrainment) nebulizer capable of high gas flows. It can provide F_IO_2s from 0.21 to 1.0 at gas flow rates >100 L/min. This high gas flow nebulizer does not depend on entrainment ports to increase the total gas flow or oxygen concentrations to the patient. To produce high gas flow, this unit uses two flowmeters: one operates the jet and can produce up to 40 L/min, and the other feeds into the side of the jet manifold with similar flow rates. This unit can generate over 80 L/min with stable oxygen concentrations.[8] An advantage of this design is that back pressure from other devices will not alter oxygen concentrations.

Ultrasonic Nebulizers

Since their introduction in the 1960s, ultrasonic nebulizers have become an alternative means of providing aerosol therapy. The basic principle of ultrasonic nebulizers is that electric current produces sound waves, which are used to break up fluid into aerosol particles. An electric charge (at a high frequency of vibrations) is applied intermittently to a transducer that has a piezoelectric quality (i.e., the ability to change shape when a charge is applied to it). The electric current creates vibrations at the same frequency as the electric charge applied to the piezoelectric transducer. These ultrasonic vibrations travel through the fluid to the surface, where they produce an aerosol (Figure 4-51).

Ultrasonic nebulizers can employ transducers in various configurations. The transducer is placed within a couplant chamber, which contains tap or sterile water (see Figure 4-52) that serves two purposes: (1) it helps absorb mechanical

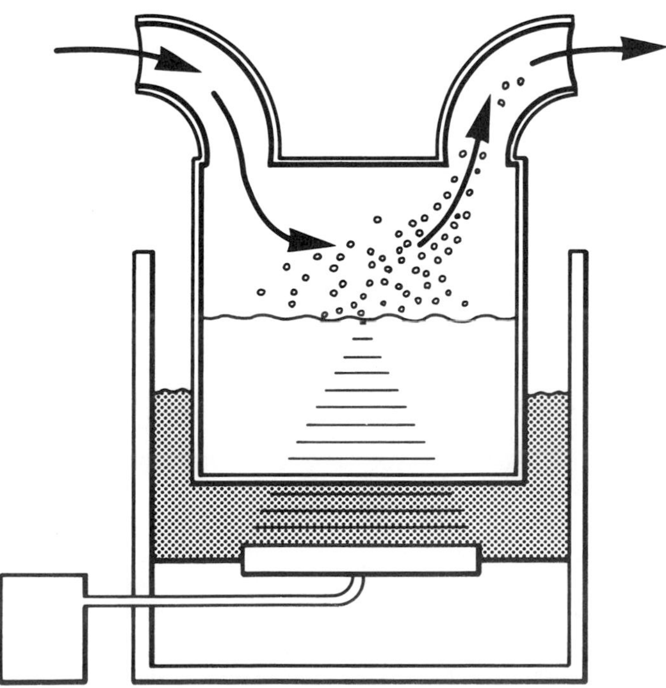

Figure 4-51 The ultrasonic nebulizer. Aerosol is produced when high-frequency sound waves are produced by a transducer and transmitted to the nebulizer compartment, where fluid is broken up into an aerosol. A gas source (e.g., fan) is used to move the aerosol out of the unit. (From Barnes TA: *Core textbook for respiratory care practice*, ed 2, St Louis, 1994, Mosby.)

heat produced by the transducer and (2) acts as a medium for the sound waves to be transferred to a prefilled or refillable container that holds the solution to be nebulized. (Couplant must not contain distilled water because of the need for electrolytes to transfer the ultrasonic waves.) The frequency of the electrical energy supplied to the transducer is typically 1.35 megahertz (Mhz). When this frequency is matched with a transducer that can react optimally to it, a vibration at the same frequency is produced. The frequency determines the particle size of the solution to be nebulized. The amplitude or strength of the sound waves determines the aerosol output. As amplitude is increased with an adjustable dial, aerosol output increases. (Amplitude is adjusted to meet the patient's inspiratory needs.)

Most ultrasonic nebulizers have been constructed so that their particle size range is from 1 to 10 μm, with a mean size of 3 μm. Fluid output averages are higher than those from pneumatic nebulizers (up to 6 mL/minute). A gas-flow source is required to transfer aerosol to the patient; most ultrasonic nebulizers use a fan for this purpose. Supplemental oxygen can be delivered to the unit to provide a range of oxygen concentrations.

Various manufacturers produce ultrasonic nebulizers, such as DeVilbiss (model 800-65 and the 900-35 series), Mistogen (models 142 and 143), and Nellcor Puritan Bennett (model US-1). Each manufacturer uses a differently shaped transducer. Several versions of SVNs that use the ultrasonic nebulizer principle are also available and can be used to nebulize bronchoactive medications during mechanical ventilation or at home. For example, Siemen's Servo Ultra Nebulizer aerosolizes medications during mechanical ventilation with an artificial airway or facemask (Figure 4-52). This is an accessory to the Servo 300/300A and i ventilator series. This ultrasonic nebulizer operates continuously regardless of ventilation mode while adding no additional gas volume to the inspiratory minute volume.

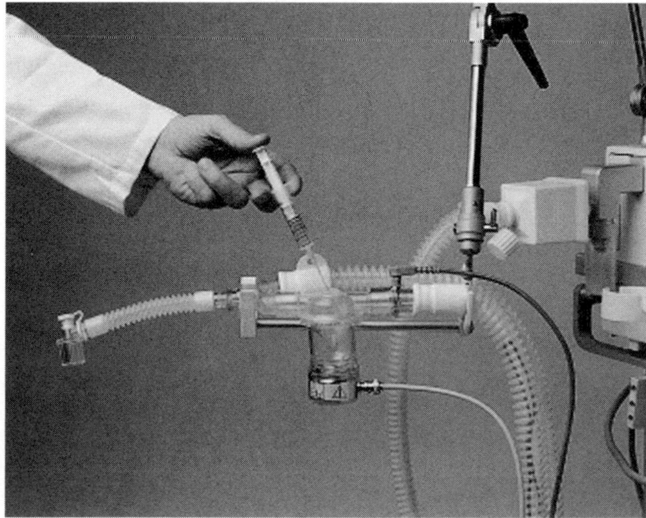

Figure 4-52 Siemen's Servo Ultra Nebulizer. (Siemens-Elma AB, Solna, Sweden.)

Total Flow and F_IO_2

High gas-flow systems, as previously defined, have a total gas and aerosol output from a pneumatic nebulizer that exceeds the patient's inspiratory flow and tidal volume to ensure a fixed oxygen concentration. If the unit fails to provide a total gas flow greater than the patient's inspiratory flow, the delivered oxygen concentration decreases. This reduced inspired oxygen concentration results from the entrainment of room air, which dilutes the gas flow from the LVN. During respiratory distress, peak inspiratory flows can increase substantially, so the total nebulizer output must be assessed. This may be accomplished by adjusting oxygen flow through the flowmeter to ensure continuous flow of aerosol from the large openings on the side of the aerosol mask or at the reservoir end of an aerosol T-piece set up during inspiration and expiration. If a mist is not drifting from the device (e.g., aerosol mask) during inspiration, the patient is inspiring room air and the F_IO_2 will decrease (from the dilution effect of the room air). Figure 4-53 shows a typical set-up for delivering aerosol to a spontaneously breathing patient, and Table 4-6 lists the total gas flows associated with a variety of oxygen concentrations and flow rates. Notice that these gas flows are based on fixed air:oxygen entrainment ratios. In other words, for every liter of oxygen that enters the nebulizer jet, a fixed amount of room air is entrained. Air dilution at the aerosol production site of the nebulizers increases aerosol output (in milliliters per hour) and increases total gas flow to the patient. When adjusting the entrainment ring from a high to a lower oxygen concentration, the total gas flow from the device increases for any flowmeter setting. For example, setting the oxygen flowmeter at 10 L/min and the air-entrainment ring to 60% will make the total flow 20 L/min. Reducing the oxygen concentration to 40% and maintaining the flowmeter at 10 L/min will produce a total gas flow of 32 L/min. In addition, as the oxygen concentration from the unit decreases, the aerosol density or amount of aerosol per liter of gas decreases with increased air entrainment.

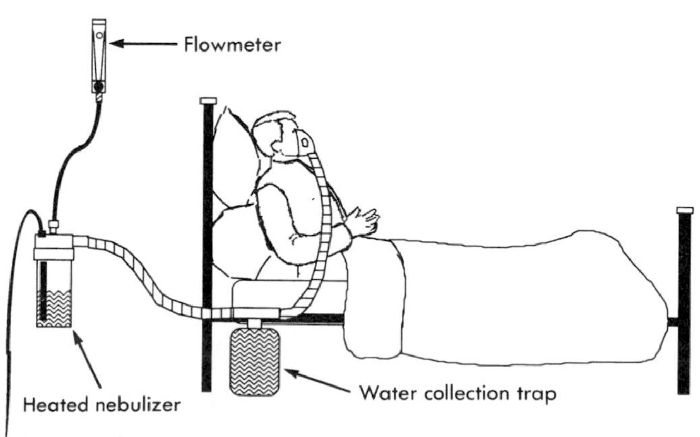

Figure 4-53 A typical set-up for a large volume nebulizer; a water collection bag may be placed in a gravity-dependent loop to collect condensation.

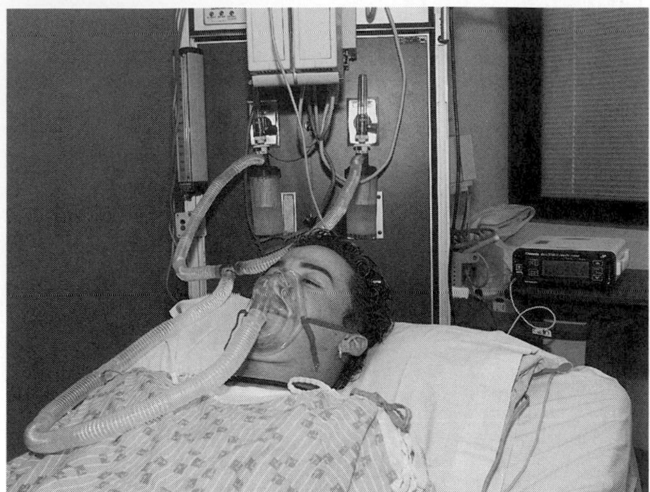

Figure 4-54 Combining multiple nebulizers to create a high-flow system.

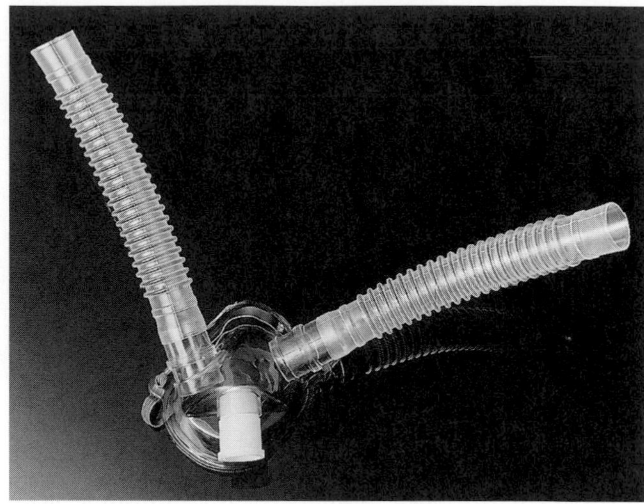

Figure 4-55 Aerosol mask modified with two 50-mL reservoir tubes, which act as possible reservoirs for gas and aerosol.

The actual number of aerosol particles produced at the jet for any given flowmeter setting is fixed, but the number of particles that actually leave the nebulizer is a product of the gas flow. As gas flow increases, more particles are carried out of the unit. There are several ways that high gas flows may be provided to meet the inspiratory demands of a patient with an increased minute volume or inspiratory flow. For example, the high-output nebulizers previously discussed may be used to ensure high-aerosol outputs, but combining several pneumatic nebulizers (attached via a Brigg's adapter) set at the same F_IO_2 will also provide an increased gas flow (Figure 4-54). Extending the size of the reservoir space of an aerosol mask by placing a 50-mL corrugated tube in each of the side ports of the aerosol mask (Figure 4-55) will also increase the amount of gas available to the patient. By adding these tubes, additional aerosol may be trapped, increasing the gas and aerosol available to the patient. However, lack of research on this method lends concern to its appropriateness for clinical use.

Special Considerations for Aerosol Therapy

There are special situations in which a patient may require a unique method of aerosol delivery such as pediatric aerosol tent enclosures, the delivery of toxic medications (e.g., ribavirin), or methods to control environmental contamination.

For years, infants and pediatric patients with upper airway edema (e.g., croup or laryngotracheobronchitis) have been placed in tents designed to contain gas flow and aerosol for the patient to inhale. These containment units provide a cool, dense aerosol and have been effective in the treatment of upper airway edema. The atmosphere within the tent is continuously flushed out to prevent accumulation of exhaled carbon dioxide. In addition, carbon dioxide may leave the tent by diffusion through the plastic canopy and the space between the tent and bed. A cooling source is necessary to keep the temperature inside the tent at a comfortable level. The gas directed into the tent can be cooled with a refrigerator unit such as the one shown in Figure 4-56.

Aerosol containment devices, such as the Ohmeda aerosol tent, allow the child to be placed directly in the tent, providing aerosol and an increased oxygen concentration (if the unit is operated by compressed oxygen). The circulating fan in the tent allows gas to be circulated and cooled. Unit maintenance requires the water reservoir to be monitored, the condensation from the refrigerator drain bottle to be emptied, and the oxygen concentration within the tent to be analyzed to ensure it is appropriate.

Patients receiving ribavirin (Virazole) to treat infections from respiratory syncytial virus (RSV) require a special aerosol-generating device called a small-particle aerosol generator (SPAG). ICN Pharmaceutical's SPAG-2 (Figure 4-57) is a jet-type nebulizer specifically for delivering ribavirin. SPAG units employ a drying chamber with a separate flow control to regulate aerosol particle size, which is 1.2 to 1.4 μm. The SPAG-2 reduces the gas source pressure from 50 to 26 psig and has an adjustable pressure regulator. The regulator has two flowmeters: one to control gas flow into the nebulizer, and the other to feed the drying chamber. As aerosol is generated in the nebulizer, which is in the reservoir chamber, it enters a long, cylindrical drying chamber. The dry flow of gas from the second flowmeter allows aerosol particles to evaporate and reduces the MMAD of the particles going to the patient. The SPAG-2 nebulizer and drying chamber require specific flow rates from the two flowmeters; the nebulizer gas flow rate should be 7 L/min, and the total gas flow from both flowmeters should not to be less than 15 L/min. The SPAG-2 is designed for administering ribavirin via a hoodlike chamber or tent. If allowed to escape and enter the room, aerosolized ribavirin can be harmful to caregivers. Ribavirin may cause bronchoconstriction, rash, conjunctivitis, and can be toxic,[12] so caregivers and women

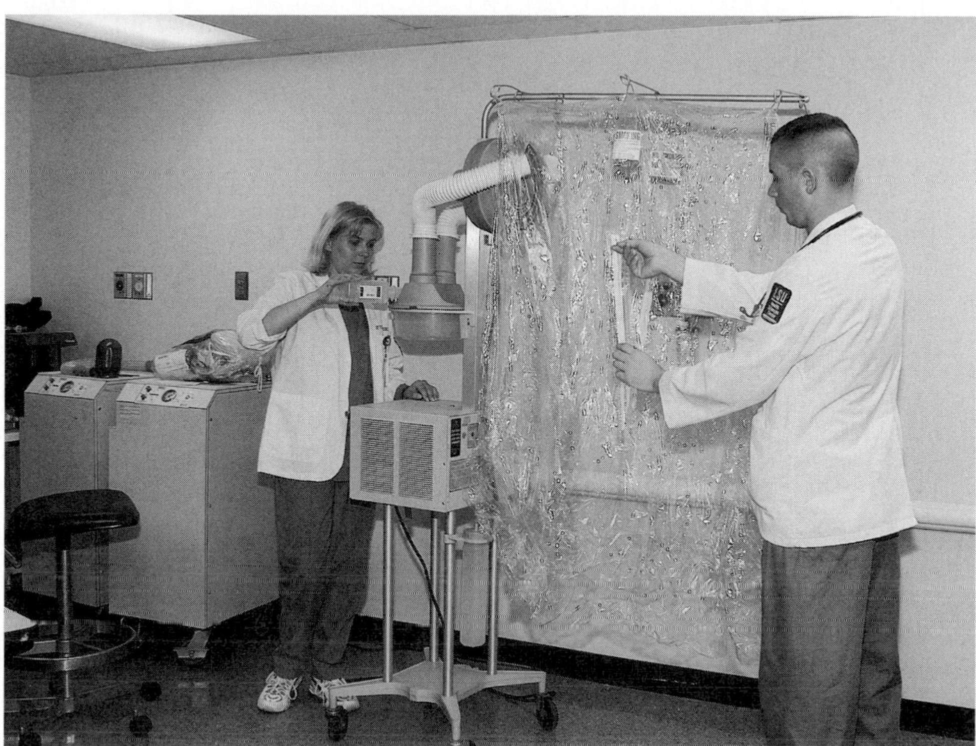

Figure 4-56 Aerosol tent.

who are either pregnant or breast-feeding should especially take precautions to avoid aerosolized ribavirin. Such precautions include placing the patient in a private room with negative pressure ventilation (with a total-room gas exchange at least 6 times per hour) and wearing a high-efficiency particle air (HEPA) mask, gloves, gown, and goggles when administering ribavirin.

The SPAG-2 may be used with gas-delivery circuits and mechanical ventilation. Although drug manufacturers do not recommend aerosolizing ribavirin into a gas circuit associated with mechanical ventilation, it has been shown to be effective when provided to patients with RSV and artificial airways who are receiving mechanical ventilation.[8] However, the ventilator expiratory valve should be protected by filters placed in the expiratory limb of the gas circuit to trap escaping medication. These filters must be changed frequently to avoid increased resistance to expiratory flow.

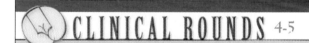

You are administering aerosolized pentamidine to a patient at home. What protective measure should you use?

See Appendix A for the answer.

Hazards of Aerosol Therapy

Hazards associated with aerosol therapy include infection, bronchoconstriction, overhydration, airway thermal injury, and airway obstruction from swollen mucus. This section will briefly address each of these concerns.

Aerosol particles can cross-contaminate the nebulizer, and thus the patient, and the person providing the therapy. Microbes in the solution to be nebulized can be transported via airborne aerosol to the patient and result in nosocomial infection. Guidelines for the care of aerosol generators often change over time, so respiratory therapists should remain aware of current recommendations. The recent guidelines of the Centers for Disease Control and Prevention recommend that humidifiers and aerosol generators be filled with sterile fluids (not tap or distilled water), which should be changed or replaced every 24 hours.[8]

Secondhand exposure to escaped aerosolized toxic medications or microbes exhaled by the patient has become a concern for all caregivers, but especially for respiratory therapists. Contaminated aerosol particles exhaled by patients may become airborne and hazardous to people nearby. This is especially a concern during sputum induction. In addition to exhaled microbes, there are several drugs that can be toxic to health care personnel. Currently, the two drugs that are the greatest risk to practitioners are pentamidine and ribavirin, which have been shown to cause conjunctivitis, headaches, bronchospasm, and rashes to caregivers exposed to them (Clinical Rounds 4-5). Patients who have respiratory tract infections or are

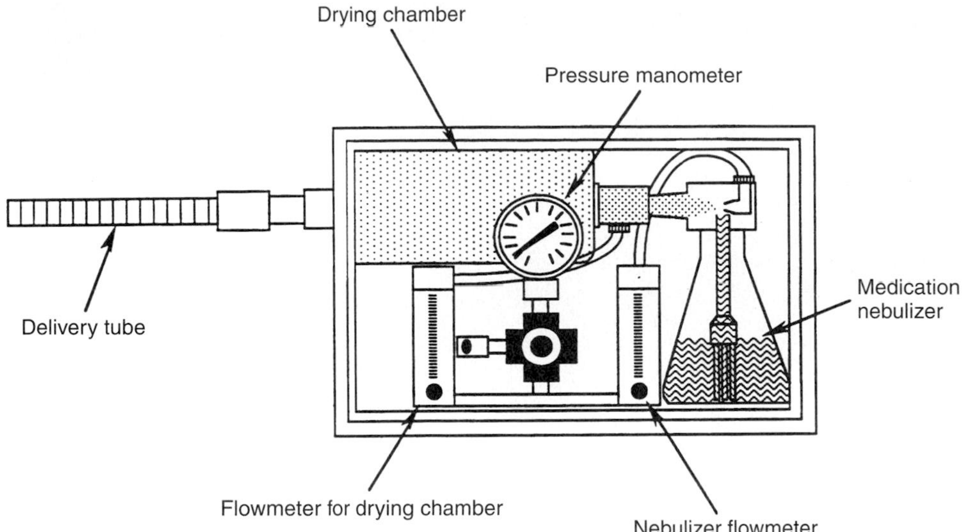

Figure 4-57 A SPAG unit.

receiving potentially toxic medications can be placed in an environmental chamber to reduce caregiver risk. This type of booth (Figure 4-58) provides containment of aerosol during therapy and reduces the risk of secondhand inhalation of aerosol and microbes. These units are cleaned between patients and located in a room with negative ventilation. In addition, these booth-like chambers contain HEPA filtering.

Studies have shown that patients with reactive airway disease (e.g., asthma) may experience bronchoconstriction while inhaling bland aerosols, experiencing an increase in airway resistance and work of breathing.[1] This effect of inhaling aerosol tends to be more common with cool than with heated aerosols, and appropriate administration of a bronchodilator before providing bland aerosol may be indicated. Furthermore, aerosolized mucolytics can induce bronchospasm in some patients, so it is standard practice to provide a bronchodilator with aerosolized mucolytics in addition to assessing patient response.

Long-term continuous administration of bland aerosol may result in overhydration of the patient, which is a more serious consideration with aerosol delivery to infants. Excess water can cause overhydration, and excess aerosolized saline may alter electrolyte concentration, leading to hypernatremia. Although most data published about the potential for overhydration with long-term aerosol (e.g., 72 hours or more) are from canine models, it may be prudent to be cautious when administering bland aerosol. Considering the narrow use of bland aerosols (e.g., treatment of upper airway edema or sputum induction), aerosol therapy should be clinically applied when the indication is clear and patient monitoring by knowledgeable practitioners is available.

Delivering aerosols to patients with an ineffective cough may result in partial or complete airway obstruction, which occurs when the inhaled aerosol mobilizes secretions that are not properly expectorated. In addition, some secretions swell when exposed to aerosol, becoming an obstruction—especially in patients with diminished cough effort or ability.

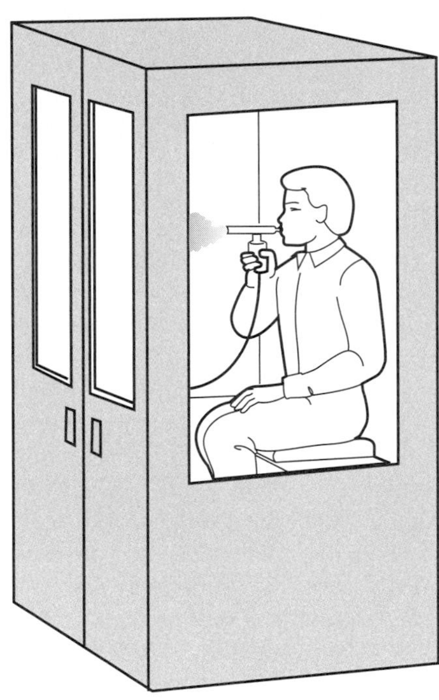

Figure 4-58 An environmental chamber for aerosol delivery to patients.

Appropriate bronchial hygiene techniques and other respiratory care modalities may be necessary with aerosol therapy.

Summary

Supplemental humidity and aerosols are fundamental components of respiratory care. Each type of therapy has a unique set of indications, delivery methods, and hazards. Humidity is water in a vapor state and can be subdivided into absolute humidity, RH, and body humidity states. Under normal physiologic conditions, adequate humidification of inspired atmospheric gases occurs as gas flows through the upper airways. When patients inspire a medical gas through an artificial airway or experience a large humidity deficit by inspiring dry gases, supplemental humidity must be provided. Failure to provide adequate humidity to the lungs can result in drying of secretions and damage to the airway mucosa.

Humidifiers can be classified as either low- or high-flow. A low-flow humidifier does not provide all of the humidity required by the patient and additional humidity is entrained from room air. In contrast, a high-flow humidifier can provide saturated gas near or at body temperature. Bubble humidifiers are examples of low-flow humidifiers; wick humidifiers and HMEs are examples of high-flow humidifiers.

An aerosol is composed of particles suspended in a gas. Aerosols used in respiratory care include bland and medicated aerosols. Bland aerosols are used to humidify medical gas or reduce upper airway edema. Medicated aerosols deliver pharmacologic agents to treat respiratory diseases. Respiratory therapists should be aware of the physical principles governing aerosol particle deposition in the lungs to be able to provide optimal aerosol therapy. Such principles include aerosol particle size, inertial impaction, kinetic activity, physical nature of the particle, temperature and humidity of the delivery gas, and ventilatory pattern.

Aerosols can be delivered by small- and large-volume nebulizers, MDIs, and ultrasonic nebulizers. More specialized aerosol generators include SPAG units and high-flow jet nebulizers. Recent advances in MDI design, including reservoirs or spacers, have made them one of the more popular ways to deliver aerosols. The most common hazards of aerosol therapy include overhydration, mucus swelling, cross-contamination, and bronchoconstriction.

Judicious selection of the type of humidity and aerosol therapy, along with the most appropriate mode of delivery can significantly affect patient outcomes. The effectiveness of the therapy can be monitored by carefully assessing the patient's response (in subjective answers or objective measures [e.g., cardiopulmonary status]) to the treatment.

Review Questions

See Appendix A for answers.

1. As gas temperature increases, its capacity to hold water will:
   a. increase
   b. decrease
   c. remain unchanged

2. If the temperature of a saturated gas decreases, which of the following will occur?
   a. Condensation develops
   b. Absolute humidity increases
   c. Relative humidity decreases
   d. Water-vapor pressure increases

3. With an artificial airway in place, what should be the minimal level of absolute humidity provided to the patient's airways?
   a. 10 mg/L
   b. 20 mg/L
   c. 30 mg/L
   d. 40 mg/L

4. As oxygen leaves a bubble humidifier, it is near or at 100% relative humidity. As it reaches the patient, what is its approximate relative humidity?
   a. 10 to 20 mg/L
   b. 44 mg/L
   c. 47 torr
   d. 100%

5. Based on the AARC Clinical Practice Guideline, the temperature of medical gas delivered through an artificial airway should be:
   a. 30° C
   b. 31° to 35° C
   c. 36° to 42° C
   d. 37° C

6. As aerosol leaves a heated jet nebulizer and travels to the patient through large-bore corrugated tubing, which of the following can occur?
   a. Relative humidity of the delivered aerosol decreases
   b. An increase in absolute humidity is provided to the patient
   c. Condensation occurs and can obstruct the aerosol delivery tube
   d. Aerosol evaporates, and only humidified gas reaches the patient

7. Which of the following is a contraindication for an HME?
   a. Minute volume greater than 10 L/min
   b. Minimal secretions
   c. Small tidal volumes
   d. Short term mechanical ventilation

8. Application of an HME device should be limited to how long?
   a. 96 hours
   b. 120 hours
   c. 20 days
   d. 30 days

9. Name four types of HME devices.

10. Which of the following will result in increased aerosol deposition?
    a. Large tidal volume
    b. Slow inspiratory flow rate
    c. Decrease in expiratory peak flow
    d. Short expiratory times

11. The optimal range of aerosol particle sizes inspired for general deposition through the upper and lower airways is:

a. 0.1 to 1 μm
b. 1 to 5 μm
c. 3 to 10 μm
d. 5 to 15 μm

12. What is the recommended gas flow rate to operate an SVN?
a. 1 L/min
b. 6 to 8 L/min
c. 10 L/min
d. 15 L/min or more

13. What is the most important factor influencing aerosol deposition from an MDI?
a. Tidal volume
b. Inspiratory flow rate
c. Respiratory rate
d. Breath hold

14. While inhaling from a DPI, the patient should be instructed to:
a. breathe in slowly
b. breathe in quickly
c. breathe in normally
d. breathe in deeply and slowly

15. An increase in which of the following can occur if condensation is allowed to accumulate in the large-bore aerosol delivery tubing?
a. Gas flow to the patient
b. Absolute humidity delivered to the patient
c. F_IO_2
d. Total aerosol delivered

References

1. Wissing DR, Boggs PB, George RB: Use of respiratory care procedures in the management of hospitalized asthmatics, *Ann Allergy* 61:407, 1988.
2. Walker JEC, et al: Heat and water exchange in the respiratory tract, *Am J Med* 30:259, 1961.
3. Dery R: The evolution of heat and moisture in the respiratory tract during anesthesia with a non-rebreathing system, *Can J Anesth* 20:296, 1973.
4. Shelley MP, Lloyd GM, Park GR: A review of the mechanisms and the methods of humidification of inspired gases, *Intensive Care Med* 14:1, 1988.
5. Primiano FP Jr, Montague FW Jr, Saidel GM: Measurement system for water vapor and temperature dynamics, *J Appl Physiol* 56:1679, 1984.
6. Eubanks DH, Bone RC, editors: *Principles and applications of cardiorespiratory care equipment*, St Louis, 1994, Mosby.
7. Cohen N, Fink J: Humidity and aerosols. In Eubanks DH, Bone RC, editors: *Principles and applications of cardiorespiratory care equipment*, St Louis, 1994, Mosby.
8. Mani SK, Weidemann HP: Diagnosis and management of asthma, ed 2, 1999, Professional Communications, Inc.
9. Fink J: Humidity and aerosol therapy. In Spearman C, Sheldon RL, editors: *Egan's fundamentals of respiratory care*, St Louis, 1995, Mosby.
10. Chatburn RL, Primiano FP: A rational basis for humidity therapy, *Respir Care* 32:249, 1987.
11. American Association for Respiratory Care: Clinical practice guideline: humidification during mechanical ventilation, *Respir Care* 37:887, 1992.
12. Eubanks DH, Bone RC: *Comprehensive respiratory care: a learning system*, ed 2, St Louis, 1990, Mosby.
13. White GC: *Equipment theory for respiratory care*, ed 2, New York, 1996, Delmar.
14. Dahlby RW: Effect of breathing dry air on structure and function of airways, *J Appl Physiol* 61:312, 1986.
15. Marfatia S, Donahoe PK, Hendren WH: Effect of dry and humidified gases on the respiratory epithelium in rabbits, *J Ped Surg* 10:583, 1975.
16. Hudson RCI: *Conchatherm III Plus operating manual*, Temecula, Calif, 1991, Hudson RCI.
17. Miyao H, et al: Consideration of the international standard for airway humidification using simulated secretions in an artificial airway, *Respir Care* 41:43, 1996.
18. Branson RD, Davis D Jr: Evaluation of 21 passive humidifiers according to the ISO 9360 standard: moisture output, dead space, and flow resistance, *Respir Care* 41:736, 1996.
19. Hess D: Prolonged use of heat and moisture exchangers: Why do we keep changing things? *Crit Care Med* 28:667-1668, 2000.
20. Chalon J, Loew DA, Malebranche J: Effects of dry anesthetic gases on tracheobronchial ciliated epithelium, *Anesthesiol* 37(3):338, 1972.
21. Fonkalsrud EW, et al: A comparative study of the effects of dry vs. humidified ventilation on canine lungs, *Surgery* 78:373, 1975.
22. Noguchi H, Takumi Y, Aochi O: A study of humidification in tracheostomized dogs, *Br J Anaesth* 45:844, 1973.
23. Rashad K, et al: Effect of humidification on anesthetic gases and static compliance, *Anesth Analg* 40:127, 1967.
24. Tsuda T, et al: Optimum humidification of air administered to a tracheostomy in dogs, *Br J Anaesth* 49:965, 1977.
25. Klein EF, Graves SA: "Hot pot" tracheitis, *Chest* 65:225, 1974.
26. American Association for Respiratory Care: Clinical practice guideline: selection of aerosol delivery device, *Respir Care* 37:891, 1992.
27. American Association for Respiratory Care: Clinical practice guideline: bland aerosol administration, *Respir Care* 38:1196, 1993.
28. American Association for Respiratory Care: Clinical practice guideline: delivery of aerosols to the upper airway, *Respir Care* 39:803, 1994.
29. Wanner A, Rao A: Clinical indications for and effects of bland, mucolytic, and antimicrobial aerosols, *Am Rev Respir Dis* 122(5):79, 1980.
30. Brain J: Aerosol and humidity therapy, *Am Rev Respir Dis* 122:17, 1980.
31. Dulfano MJ, Adler K, Wooten O: Physical properties of sputum, IV, effects of 100% humidity and water mist, *Am Rev Resp Dis* 107:130, 1973.

32. Svedmyr N: Clinical advantages of the aerosol route of drug administration, *Respir Care* 36:922, 1991.

33. Cottrell GP, Surkin HB: Pharmacology for respiratory care practitioners, Philadelphia, 1995, FA Davis Co.

34. Ward JJ, Hess D, Helmholz HF Jr: Humidity and aerosol therapy. In Burton CC, Hodgkin JE, Ward JJ, editors: *Respiratory care: a guide to clinical practice,* New York, 1997, JB Lippincott.

35. Dolovich M: Clinical aspects of aerosol therapy, *Respir Care* 36:931, 1991.

36. Rau JL: *Respiratory care pharmacology,* ed 6, 2002, St Louis, Mosby.

37. Pedersen S: Choice of inhalation in paediatrics, *Eur Respir Rev* 18:85, 1994.

38. Alvine GG, Rodgers P, Fitzsimmons KM: Disposable jet nebulizers: how reliable are they? *Chest* 101:316, 1992.

39. Dahlback M, et al: Controlled aerosol delivery during mechanical ventilation, *J Aerosol Med* 4:339, 1989.

40. Fuller HD, et al: Pressurized aerosol versus jet aerosol delivery to mechanically ventilated patients: comparison of dose to the lungs, *Am Rev Respir Dis* 141:440, 1990.

41. McIntyre NR, et al: Aerosol delivery in intubated, mechanically ventilated patients, *Crit Care Med* 13:81, 1985.

42. DeBlaquiere P, et al: Use and misuse of metered-dose inhalers by patients with chronic lung disease, *Am Rev Respir Dis* 140:910, 1989.

43. Newman SP: Aerosol generators and delivery systems, *Respir Care* 36:939, 1991.

44. Wilson AF, Muki DS, Ahdout JJ: Effect of canister temperature on performance of metered dose inhalers, *Am Rev Respir Dis* 143:1034, 1991.

45. Lewis RA, Fleming JS: Fractional deposition from a jet nebulizer: How it differs from a metered dose inhaler, *Br J Dis Chest* 79:361, 1985.

46. Kacmarek RM, Hess D: The interface between the patient and aerosol generator, *Respir Care* 36:952, 1991.

47. Konig P: Spacer devices used with metered dose inhalers: breakthrough or gimmick? *Chest* 88:276, 1985.

48. Moler FW, Hurwitz ME, Custer JR: Improvement in clinical asthma score and $PaCO_2$ in children with severe asthma treated with continuously nebulized terbutaline, *J Allergy Clin Immunol* 81:1101, 1988.

Internet Resources

Humidity

American Association for Respiratory Care: http://www.aarc.org

Humidity and Humidification Lecture: http://www.usyd.edu.au/anaes/lectures/humidity_clt/humidity.html

Infoplease.com: http://www.infoplease.com/ce6/weather/A0824520.html

Relative Humidity Calculator: http://www.esb.act.gov.au/firebreak/humidity.html

Relative Humidity Equations: http://www.uswcl.ars.ag.gov/exper/relhumeq.htm

Virtual Hospital: http://www.vh.org

Aerosol

The Aerosol Society: http://www.aerosol-soc.org.uk/index.asp

Clinical Practice Guideline for aerosol therapy: http://www.hsc.missouri.edu/~shrp/rtwww/rcweb/aarc/saddcpg.html

Mary Ann Lieber, Inc., Publishers: http://www.liebertpub.com/JAM/default1.asp

National AIDS Treatment Information Project: http://www.natip.org/aerosol.html

Total Ozone Mapping Spectrometer: http://toms.gsfc.nasa.gov/aerosols/aerosols.html

Chapter 5

Principles of Infection Control

J.M. Cairo

Chapter Outline

Chapter Learning Objectives

Upon completion of this chapter, the reader should be able to:

1. Identify the major groups of microorganisms associated with nosocomial pneumonia.
2. List four factors that can influence the effectiveness of a germicide.
3. Define *high-level disinfection, intermediate-level disinfection, and low-level disinfection*.
4. Describe the process of pasteurization and its application to the disinfection of respiratory care equipment.
5. Explain how quaternary ammonium compounds, alcohols, acetic acid, phenols, glutaraldehyde, hydrogen peroxide, and iodophors and other halogenated compounds are used as disinfectants.
6. Name the four physical methods commonly used to sterilize medical devices.
7. Discuss the principle of ethylene oxide sterilization.
8. Identify infection-risk devices used in respiratory care.
9. Compare standard precautions with transmission-based precautions.
10. Describe three components of an effective infection surveillance program.

Key Terms

Acid-Fast Bacteria
Aerobes
Airborne
Airborne Precautions
Anaerobes
Autoclave
Bacilli
Bactericide
Chemical Sterilant
Cleaning
Cocci
Contact Precautions
Decontamination
Diplobacilli
Diplococci
Direct Contact
Disinfection
Droplet Precautions
Eukaryotic
Facultative
Fomites
Fungicide
Germicide
Gram-Negative
Gram-Positive
Gram Stain
High-Level Disinfection
Indirect Contact
Infection Surveillance
Intermediate-Level Disinfection
Isolation Techniques
Low-Level Disinfection
Normal Flora
Nosocomial
Pasteurization
Pathogenic
Prokaryotic
Spirochetes
Standard Precautions
Staphylococci
Sterilization
Streptobacilli
Streptococci
Transmission-Based Precautions
Universal Precautions
Vectors
Vehicles
Vibrio
Virucide

Preventing **nosocomial** infections is a formidable task for respiratory therapists. It is particularly challenging because devices used for respiratory care are potential reservoirs and **vehicles** for the transmission of infectious microorganisms. Additionally, many patients receiving respiratory care, especially those of extreme age or who are recovering from thoracoabdominal surgery, have an increased risk of developing nosocomial pneumonia. Underlying diseases, depressed sensorium, and immunosuppression can also add to the risk of developing a nosocomial infection.[1]

This chapter is a review of the aspects of microbiology and infection control that respiratory care practitioners must understand to prevent nosocomial pneumonia. Specifically, the following are described here: (1) the microorganisms that are most often associated with nosocomial pneumonia; (2) the accepted methods for **cleaning, disinfecting,** and **sterilizing** reusable respiratory care equipment; (3) the proper use of **isolation techniques** to prevent person-to-person transmission of microorganisms; and (4) effective methods of **infection surveillance.**

Principles of Clinical Microbiology

Microbiology is the study of microorganisms such as bacteria, viruses, protozoa, fungi, and algae. All of these organisms, with the possible exception of algae, are **pathogenic** and therefore can produce infectious diseases in susceptible hosts.[1] Clinical microbiology is primarily concerned with the isolation, identification, and control of these pathogenic, or disease-producing, organisms.

The active participation of clinical microbiologists in infection control is essential for the identification and treatment of nosocomial infections, as well as for the prevention of these diseases. The process of identifying the infectious agent responsible for the nosocomial infection is fairly straightforward. Diagnosis of an infectious disease requires isolating the suspected pathogen from the site of infection. The specimen is then inoculated onto agar or into a broth containing vital nutrients and incubated for a specified amount of time. In many cases, the organism is allowed to grow at body temperature in a specially designed incubator. It is important that the collection process is performed using aseptic techniques to avoid microbial contamination from adjacent tissue and **normal flora.** Although normal microbial flora, which are microorganisms normally found in or on a particular body site, do not usually cause infectious disease, these organisms can present problems because they can overgrow the pathogen and produce erroneous results.

Identification of microorganisms is most often accomplished by directly examining the specimen through microscopy with the aid of biologic staining techniques. Metabolic and immunologic tests may also help clinical microbiologists discern the nature of the invading microbe, especially as relates to its susceptibility to antibiotics.

Control of pathogenic microorganisms relates to eliminating infections and preventing the spread of infectious diseases through infection control techniques. Infections that overwhelm a person's immune system are usually eradicated by enhancing the host's innate immunity with antibiotics and immunizations. **Decontamination** of diagnostic and therapeutic medical equipment, furniture, and commonly used items and surfaces, and the use of barrier precautions (i.e., isolation precautions) are examples of infection control techniques.

A variety of microorganisms can be isolated from the hospital environment. A brief description of the major groups of pathogenic organisms associated with nosocomial pneumonia follows. More detailed information about the science of microbiology can be found in the references listed at the end of the chapter.[1-3]

Survey of Microorganisms

Bacteria

Bacteria are **prokaryotic,** unicellular organisms that range in size from 0.5 to 50 μm. Bacteria are generally classified according to their morphology (shape) and their staining

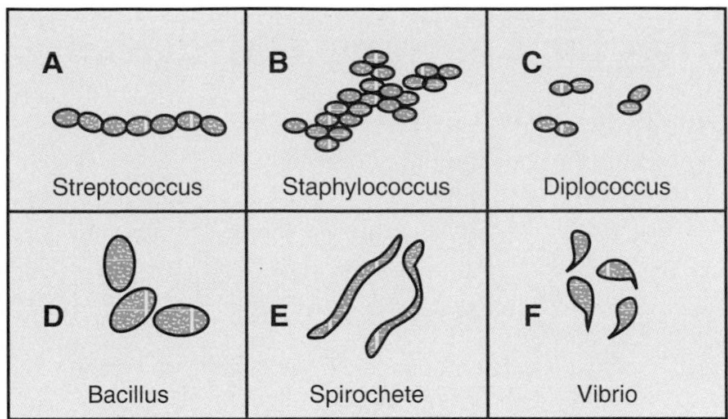

Figure 5-1 The morphology of bacteria: **A,** streptococcus; **B,** staphylococcus; **C,** diplococcus; **D,** bacillus; **E,** spirochete; **F,** vibrio comma.

and metabolic characteristics. Certain bacteria are also capable of producing endospores, which are intermediate bacterial forms that develop in response to adverse condition. As is discussed later in this chapter, bacterial endospores can regenerate to vegetative cells when conditions improve.

As Figure 5-1 shows, the primary bacterial shapes are **cocci** (spherical), **bacilli** (rodlike), and **spirochetes** (spiral). Cocci that occur in irregular clusters are called ***staphylococci.*** Cocci and bacilli that occur in pairs are called ***diplococci*** and ***diplobacilli,*** respectively; chains of cocci and bacilli are called ***streptococci*** and ***streptobacilli,*** respectively.

Classifying bacteria according to their staining characteristics is usually accomplished with simple staining techniques, such as the **Gram stain** and the **acid-fast stain.** A Gram stain separates bacteria into two general classes: those that retain an initial gentian violet stain after an alcohol wash **(gram-positive)** and those that do not retain the initial violet stain **(gram-negative).** Gram-positive organisms appear blue or violet; gram-negative organisms have a red appearance that results from a counterstain of the red dye safranin. Notable gram-positive pathogens are *Bacillus anthracis, Streptococcus pneumoniae, Staphylococcus aureus, Corynebacterium diphtheriae,* and *Clostridium* sp. (e.g., *C. botulinum, C. perfringens, C. tetani*). Gram-negative pathogens include *Pseudomonas aeruginosa, Escherichia coli, Klebsiella pneumoniae, Haemophilus influenzae, Serratia marcescens, Bordetella pertussis, Neisseria meningitidis,* and *Legionella pneumophila.*[3] Clinical Rounds 5-1 provides a clinical scenario that shows how Gram stains can be used in the differential diagnosis of lower respiratory tract infections.

Acid-fast stains (also called Ziehl-Neelsen stains) are used to identify bacteria that belong to the genus Mycobacteria. These microbes retain a red (carbol-fuchsin) dye after an acid wash, thus ***acid-fast bacillus*** is used synonymously with *Mycobacteria. Mycobacteria tuberculosis* organisms are responsible for pulmonary, spinal, and miliary tuberculosis. The incidence of tuberculosis has increased considerably during the past decade, especially in patients infected with the human immunodeficiency virus (HIV; see the following discussion of viruses).

Metabolic characterization of bacteria usually involves identifying the substrate requirements for growth or the production of specific enzymes by the microbe. For example, bacteria that require oxygen for growth are called ***aerobes***, and those that can grow without oxygen are called ***anaerobes***. **Facultative** bacteria can survive with or without oxygen. Other examples of enzyme markers that are commonly quantified include catalase and coagulase.

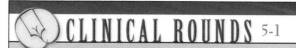

Laboratory examination of a sputum sample from a febrile patient with a productive cough (purulent, blood-streaked sputum) reveals the presence of gram-positive diplococci and many segmented neutrophils. Suggest a possible diagnosis based on these findings.

See Appendix A for the answer.

As mentioned previously, certain bacteria form endospores under adverse conditions. Endospores are metabolically active life forms that can maintain their viability in the presence of dryness, heat, and poor nutrition. Their robust nature makes them especially resistant to disinfectants and a constant source of concern for infection control personnel. The most notable sources of bacterial endospores are from the aerobic *Bacillus* sp. and the anaerobic *Clostridium* sp.

Table 5-1 lists some commonly encountered bacterial genera along with a summary of their morphologic, staining, and metabolic characteristics.

Viruses

Viruses are submicroscopic parasites that consist of a nucleic acid core surrounded by a protein sheath and range in size from 20 to 200 nm. Viruses are typically described as nonliving because they must invade a living organism to replicate. Viruses are generally classified according to their

Table 5-1 Commonly Encountered Bacteria Along with Morphologic, Staining, and Metabolic Characteristics

Genera	Gram Stain	Shape/Configuration	Aerobic/Anaerobic	Species
Bacillus	Positive	Rod, chain	Aerobic	*B. anthracis*
Bordetella	Negative	Rod	Aerobic	*B. pertussis*
Clostridium	Positive	Rod, separate, chain, pairs, palisade	Anaerobic	*C. tetani, C. botulinum, C. perfringens*
Corynebacterium	Positive	Rod, palisade	Aerobic	*C. diphtheriae*
Diplococcus	Positive	Coccus, encapsulated pairs	Aerobic	*D. pneumoniae*
Staphylococcus	Positive	Coccus, clusters	Aerobic	*S. aureus*
Streptococcus	Positive	Coccus, chain	Aerobic	Groups A, B, C, & D
Mycobacterium	Positive	Rod, separate, or "cords"	Aerobic	*M. tuberculosis, M. leprae*
Neisseria	Positive	Coccus, pairs	Aerobic	*N. meningitidis*
Proteus	Negative	Rod, separate	Aerobic	*N. mirabilis, N. vulgaris*
Pseudomonas	Negative	Rod, separate	Aerobic	*P. aeruginosa*
Serratia	Negative	Rod, separate	Aerobic	*S. marcescens*
Escherichia	Negative	Rod, separate	Aerobic, facultatively anaerobic	*E. coli*
Klebsiella	Negative	Rod, separate	Aerobic	*K. pneumoniae*
Haemophilus	Negative	Rod, separate	Aerobic	*H. influenzae, H. haemolyticus, H. parainfluenzae*
Salmonella	Negative	Rod, separate	Aerobic, facultatively anaerobic	*S. typhi, S. enteritidis*

From Kacmarek RM, Mack CW, Dimas S: *The essentials of respiratory care*, ed 3, St Louis, 1990, Mosby.

Table 5-2 Commonly Encountered Viruses

Virus	Transmission Route	Diseases
INFLUENZA	Respiratory tract	Tracheobronchitis Pneumonia Susceptibility to bacterial pneumonia
PARAMYXOVIRUSES		
Mumps	Respiratory tract	Parotitis Orchitis Pancreatitis Encephalitis
Measles (rubeola)	Respiratory tract	Rash, systemic illness Pneumonia Encephalomyelitis
Parainfluenza	Respiratory tract	Upper respiratory disease Croup, pneumonia
Respiratory syncytial	Respiratory tract	Bronchitis Bronchiolitis Pneumonia
ADENOVIRUSES	Respiratory tract Conjunctivae	Tracheobronchitis Pharyngitis Conjunctivitis
RHINOVIRUSES	Respiratory tract	Rhinitis Pharyngitis
ENTEROVIRUSES		
Coxsackie	Respiratory tract Gut	Systemic infections Meningitis Tracheobronchitis Myocarditis
Polio	Gut	Central nervous system damage (including anterior horn cells, paralysis)
HERPESVIRUSES		
Herpes simplex	Oral Genital Eye	Blisters—latent infection Keratoconjunctivitis
Varicella Herpes zoster	Respiratory tract	Vesicles—all ectodermal tissues (skin, mouth, respiratory tract)
Cytomegalovirus	Not known	Usually disseminated disease in newborn and immune deficient
RUBELLA	Respiratory tract	Systemic mild illness, rash, congenital anomalies in embryo
HEPATITIS	Blood, body fluids	Hepatitis Systemic disease
RABIES	Bites, or saliva on cut	Fatal central nervous system damage
HIV	Blood, body fluids	AIDS

From Scanlan CL, Spearman CB, Sheldon RL: *Egan's fundamentals of respiratory care*, ed 6, St Louis, 1995, Mosby.

structure (i.e., icosahedral, helical, or complex) and nucleic acid content (i.e., DNA or RNA). They can also be differentiated by the type of host that they invade (i.e., animal, plant, or bacteria).

The most commonly encountered pathogenic viruses are listed in Table 5-2 and include the influenza viruses, paramyxoviruses, adenoviruses, rhinoviruses, enteroviruses, herpes viruses, rubella viruses, hepatitis virus, and human immunodeficiency viruses. Viruses are responsible for a number of respiratory illnesses, including the common cold, croup, tracheobronchitis, bronchiolitis, and pneumonia. The hepatitis viruses and HIV are particularly important pathogens because they are spread by **direct contact** (i.e., through sexual contact or blood and serum). Universal isolation precautions were designed to prevent the transmission of these types of infections. Isolation precautions for bloodborne pathogens are discussed in detail later in this chapter.

Rickettsiae *and* Chlamydiae *Spp.*

These unusual microorganisms are intracellular parasites. *Rickettsiae* and *Chlamydiae* spp. are both less than 1 μm in diameter. Their complex structures resemble that of bacteria, but they act like viruses because they require a living host to replicate.[4] *Rickettsiae* sp. are transmitted by insects (e.g., lice, fleas, ticks), and *Chlamydiae* sp. are transmitted by contact or the **airborne** route. Common Rickettsial diseases include typhus, Rocky Mountain spotted fever, and Q fever. (Note that Q fever is spread by the aerosol route rather than by insect vectors.) Chlamydial infections are also associated with pneumonia, sinusitis, pharyngitis, and bronchiolitis.[4]

Protozoa

Protozoa are unicellular eukaryotes that occur singly or in colonies. Protozoan infections are common in tropical climates, especially where sanitation is poor or lacking. Common examples of protozoan infections include amebiasis, malaria, and trypanosomiasis.[4] The most important protozoan that can invade the lung and cause pneumonia is *Pneumocystis carinii*. *Pneumocystis* pneumonia is common in immunocompromised patients—particularly those infected with HIV. It is worth noting that although *Pneumocystis* spp. are classified as protozoans, they are more closely related to fungi.[5]

Fungi

Fungi are *eukaryotic* organisms that include molds and yeast. Molds consist of chains of cells or filaments called hyphae and reproduce asexually by forming spores. Yeasts are unicellular fungi that reproduce sexually or asexually by budding. Fungal infections or mycoses can occur in normal healthy individuals, but they are more prevalent in patients with compromised immune function (i.e., opportunistic infections). Fungal infections in otherwise healthy individuals are usually caused by *Histoplasma capsulatum*, *Coccidioides immitis*, and *Blastomyces dermatitidis*. Opportunistic fungal infections are typically caused by *Candida albicans* and *Aspergillus fumigatus*.[3,4]

Transmission of Infectious Diseases

Three elements must be present for infectious material to spread: a source of pathogen, a mode of transmission for the infectious agent, and a susceptible host. Nosocomial pneumonia is most often caused by bacteria; viruses and fungi contribute to a lesser extent. The most common source of pathogenic microorganisms is infected patients, but contaminated water, food, and medications are also sources of infectious material.

Infectious particles can be transmitted by four routes: contact, vehicles, airborne, and vectors (Table 5-3). Direct contact occurs when the infectious organism is physically transferred from a contaminated person to a susceptible host through touching or sexual contact. **Indirect contact** involves transfer of the infectious agent to a susceptible host via a fomite (e.g., clothing, surgical bandages, instruments, equipment).[2] Transfer of infectious materials by vehicles most often occurs through contaminated water and food, although intravenous fluids, blood and blood products, and

Table 5-3 Routes of Infectious Disease Transmission

Mode	Type	Examples
Contact	Direct	Hepatitis A Venereal disease HIV *Staphylococcus* Enteric bacteria
	Indirect	*Pseudomonas* Enteric bacteria Hepatitis B and C HIV
	Droplet	Measles *Streptococcus*
Vehicle	Waterborne	Shigellosis Cholera
	Foodborne	Salmonellosis Hepatitis A
Airborne	Aerosols Droplet nuclei	Legionellosis Tuberculosis Diphtheria
	Dust	Histoplasmosis
Vectorborne	Ticks and mites	Rickettsia, Lyme disease
	Mosquitoes	Malaria
	Fleas	Bubonic plague

From Scanlan CL, Wilkins RL, Stoller JK: *Egan's fundamentals of respiratory care*, ed 7, St Louis, 1999, Mosby.

medications can also occasionally harbor infectious particles.[6] Airborne or respiratory transmission involves the transfer of infectious particles through aerosol droplets and dust particles. Infectious agents are transferred by the vector route when an insect transfers the infectious particle from a host to susceptible individual.[4] Transmission of infections by vectors is rarely associated with nosocomial infections. See Clinical Rounds 5-2 to test your understanding of infection transmission.

CLINICAL ROUNDS 5-2

As previously discussed, infectious agents can be transmitted by a variety of means, including contact, vehicles, airborne, and vector routes. Identify the most probable means of transmission for the following infectious particles:

- *Pseudomonas aeruginosa* organisms
- HIV
- *Mycobacterium tuberculosis* organisms
- *Rickettsiae* sp.

See Appendix A for the answer.

A variety of mechanical and immunological factors usually protect the host from becoming infected with pathogenic organisms.[6] Alterations of mechanical barriers occurring when skin and mucous membranes are breached during surgery, endotracheal intubation, or placement of indwelling catheters can significantly increase an individual's risk of developing a nosocomial infection. Defects in immune function that occur because of an underlying disease or as a result of therapeutic interventions (e.g., radiation therapy, pharmacologic therapies) can also increase the risk for infection. Table 5-4 lists several conditions, possible precipitating causes, and common pathogens associated with hospitalized patients at risk for developing nosocomial infections.

Infection Control Methods

The purpose of any hospital infection control program is to prevent the spread of nosocomial infections. The two most important concepts to understand about infection control are decontamination of patient care items and isolation precautions.

Table 5-4 Medical Conditions and Common Pathogens in Hospitalized Patients with Increased Susceptibility to Nosocomial Infections

Condition	Possible Cause	Common Pathogens
Skin and mucosal barrier disruption	Burns	*Staphylococcus aureus*
	Foley catheter	*Pseudomonas aeruginosa*
	Intravenous catheter	*Enterobacteriaceae* species
	Surgical wound	Candida
	Endotracheal tube	
Neutropenia	Oncochemotherapy	*P. aeruginosa*
	Drug reactions	*Enterobacteriaceae* sp.
	Autoimmune process	*Staphylococcus epidermidis*
	Leukemia	*S. aureus*, *Aspergillus* sp.
Disruption of normal flora	Antibiotic therapy	*Clostridium difficile*
	Oncochemotherapy	Candida
Altered T cells	Cushing's syndrome	*Mycoplasma tuberculosis*
	Corticosteroid therapy	Fungal infections
	Hodgkin's disease	Herpes viruses
	AIDS	*Pneumocystis carinii*
	Organ transplantation	Toxoplasmosis
Hypogammaglobulinemia	Nephrotic syndrome	*Streptococcus pneumoniae*
	Multiple myeloma	*Hemophilus influenzae*
		Enterobacteriaceae sp.
Hypocomplementemia	Systemic lupus erythematosus	*Neisseria meningitidis*
	Liver failure	*Streptococcus pneumoniae*
	Vasculitis	*Enterobacteriaceae* sp.

From Chatburn RL: Decontamination of respiratory care equipment: what can be done, what should be done, *Respir Care* 34(2):98, 1989.

Decontamination, or the removal of pathogenic microorganisms from medical equipment, is accomplished by **cleaning, disinfection,** and **sterilization** with an appropriate **germicide** (i.e., an agent that destroys pathogenic microorganisms). Cleaning is the removal of all foreign material, particularly organic matter (e.g., blood, serum, pus, fecal matter) from objects with hot water, soap, detergent, and enzymatic products. Disinfection is the removal of most pathogenic microorganisms except bacterial endospores. Liquid chemicals and **pasteurization** are the most common disinfection methods used. Sterilization is the elimination of all forms of microbial life. It can be accomplished by either physical or chemical processes.

Factors Influencing the Effectiveness of Germicides

As was previously stated, germicides are agents used to destroy pathogenic microorganisms. They destroy these microorganisms by damaging their cell membranes, denaturing their proteins, or disrupting their cellular processes.[2] **Bactericides** destroy all pathogenic bacteria, **virucides** destroy viruses, and **fungicides** kill fungi. *Germicide* is a general term used to describe agents that destroy pathogenic microorganisms on living tissue and inanimate objects; *disinfectant* is used to describe agents that destroy pathogenic microorganisms on inanimate objects only.[7]

A number of factors can affect disinfection and sterilization, including the number, location, and innate resistance of the microorganisms; the concentration and potency of the germicide; the duration of exposure to the germicide; and the physical and chemical environment in which the germicide is used.[8] A brief discussion of several key points to remember when using germicides follows.

Number and Location of Microorganisms

The amount of time required to kill microorganisms is roughly proportional to the number of microorganisms

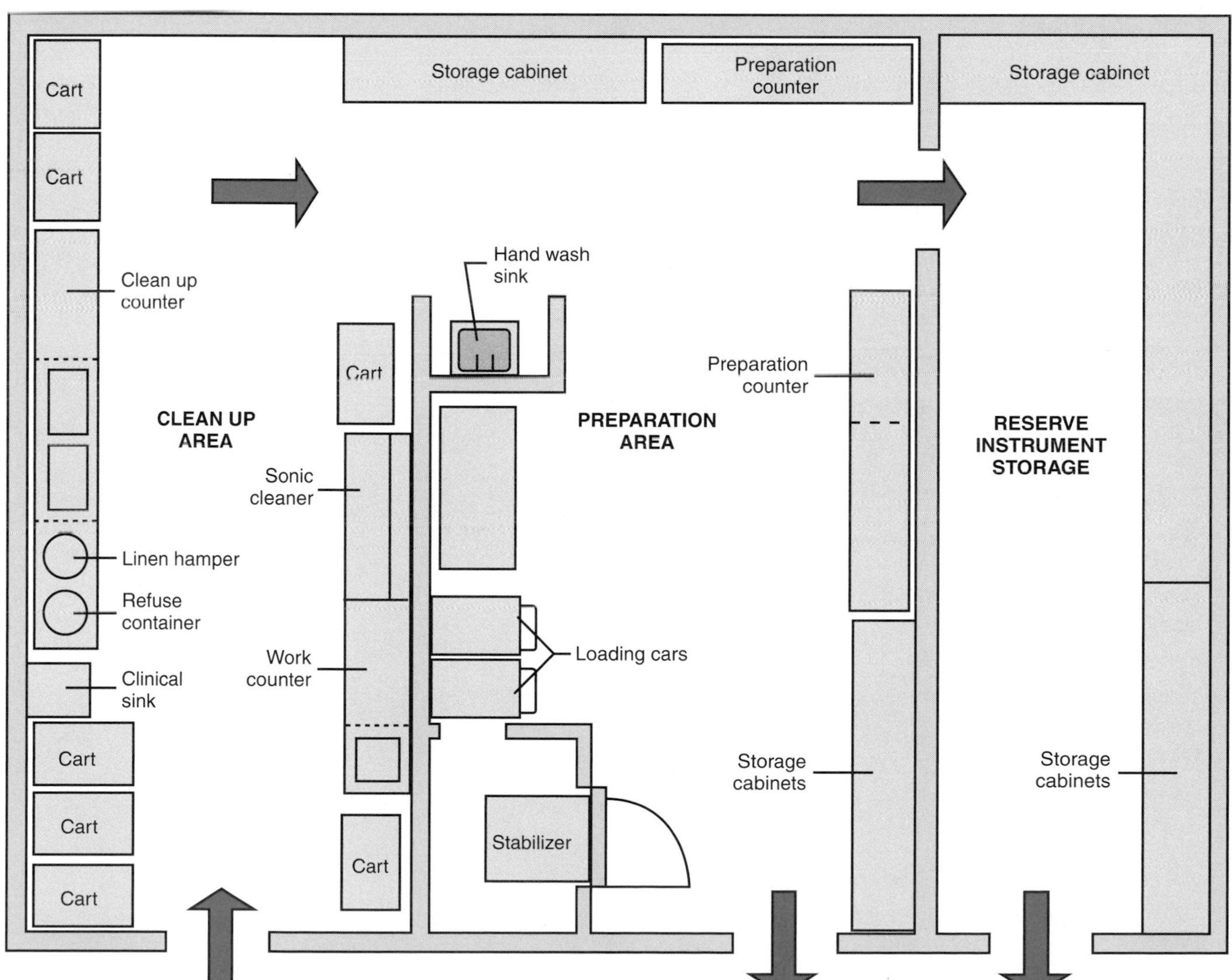

Figure 5-2 Schematic illustrating a typical cleaning area for respiratory care equipment. (Redrawn from Perkins JJ: *Principles and methods of sterilization in health sciences*, Springfield, Ill, 1978, Charles C Thomas.)

present. Cleaning helps to reduce the number of microbes to a manageable number. The location of the microorganisms can also influence the effectiveness of a germicide because physical barriers can prevent contact of the germicide and the microbe. Thus it is imperative that the germicidal agent has direct contact with any part of the device that is exposed to potential pathogens. Therefore, proper disassembly (and assembly) of equipment during the decontamination process can be a limiting factor when assessing the effectiveness of a physical or chemical agent.

Microbial Resistance

The presence of microbial capsules can increase a microorganism's resistance to disinfection and sterilization. This resistance is generally overcome by increasing the exposure time of the microbe to the germicide. Bacterial spores are the most resistant microbes, followed by mycobacterium, nonlipid or small viruses, fungi, lipid or medium viruses, and vegetative bacteria (e.g., *Staphylococcus* and *Pseudomonas* spp.). The resistance of gram-positive and gram-negative microorganisms to disinfection and sterilization is similar, except for *Pseudomonas aeruginosa*, which shows greater resistance to some disinfectants.[9,10]

Concentration and Potency of the Germicide

In general, a disinfectant's potency increases as its concentration increases. (Iodophors are an exception to this statement.) It is important to remember, however, that germicides are affected differently by concentration adjustments. That is, diluting a germicide influences the amount of time required for disinfection or sterilization.

Physical and Chemical Factors

The effectiveness of a germicide depends on the temperature, pH, and relative humidity of the environment in which it is used. Generally, the activity of most germicides increases as the temperature increases. Increasing the pH improves the antimicrobial activity of some disinfectants (e.g., glutaraldehyde and quaternary ammonium compounds); increasing alkalinity of other agents decreases their effectiveness (e.g., phenols, hypochlorites, iodine). Relative humidity is an important determinant of the activity of gaseous disinfectants (e.g., ethylene oxide, formaldehyde).

Cleaning

Cleaning is the first step in the decontamination process. Figure 5-2 is a schematic of a typical cleaning area for respiratory care equipment. Note that the space is divided into dirty and clean areas with separate entries and exits. This design helps to ensure that clean equipment is not mixed or contaminated with soiled items.

The cleaning process usually begins with disassembly of the equipment to help ensure that dirt and organic matter are removed from surfaces that are not necessarily visible when the device is assembled. Ultrasonic systems are sometimes used for cleaning equipment with crevices that are difficult to clean. These ultrasonic devices create small bubbles that can penetrate and dislodge dirt and organic material, particularly in hard-to-reach crevices.

As stated, cleaning is usually done with soaps, detergents, and enzymatic products. Soaps and detergents contain amphipathic molecules that help dissolve fat and grease by reducing surface tension so that water can penetrate the

Table 5-5 Germicidal Properties of Disinfectants and Sterilization Agents

			Inactivates					
Germicide	Use Dilution	Level of Disinfection	Bacteria	Lipophilic Viruses	Hydrophilic Viruses	*M. tuberculosis*	Mycotic Agents	Bacterial Spores
Isopropyl alcohol	60% to 95%	Int	+	+	−	+	+	+
Hydrogen peroxide	3% to 25%	CS/High	+	+	+	+	+	±
Formaldehyde	3% to 8%	High/Int	+	+	+	+	+	±
Quaternary ammonium compounds	0.4% to 1.6% aqueous	Low	+	+	−	−	±	
Phenolic	0.4% to 5% aqueous	Int/Low	+	+	±	+	±	
Chlorine	100 to 1000 ppm free chlorine	High/Low	+	+	+	+	+	±
Iodophors	30 to 50 ppm free iodine	Int	+	+	+	±	±	
Glutaraldehyde	2%	CS/High	+	+	+	+	+	±

organic matter. The amphipathic nature of these agents relates to their ability to dissolve both polar and nonpolar molecules. That is, they can dissolve polar or water-soluble (hydrophilic) substances and nonpolar or water-insoluble (hydrophobic) substances. Soaps are not bactericidal but may be combined with a disinfectant. Detergents are weakly bacteriocidal against Gram-positive organisms but they are not effective against tubercle bacilli and viruses.[4]

Cleaning can be done by hand with a scrub brush or with an automatic system. These automatic systems are similar to dishwashers found in the home. Dirty equipment goes through a series of wash and rinse cycles before automatically undergoing pasteurization or cold disinfection.

After the equipment is cleaned, it should be dried to remove residual water because moisture can alter the effectiveness of disinfectants and sterilizing agents. For example, water can dilute the disinfectant or change its pH.[7] Residual moisture can also combine with ethylene oxide to form ethylene glycol, a toxic chemical that is difficult to remove.[4] To avoid recontamination, equipment should be reassembled in a clean area separate from the area for processing soiled equipment. Clean equipment should never be allowed to sit on open counters for a prolonged time.

Disinfection

By definition, disinfection differs from sterilization because it lacks sporicidal properties.[8] Disinfection can be accomplished by physical and chemical methods. Pasteurization is the most common physical method of disinfection. Quaternary ammonium compounds, alcohols, acetic acid, phenols, iodophores, sodium hypochlorite, glutaraldehyde, and hydrogen peroxide are examples of chemical disinfectants. Table 5-5 lists some commonly used disinfectants and their germicidal properties.

It is important to note that certain disinfectants (e.g., hydrogen peroxide, peracetic acid, glutaraldehyde) can eliminate spores with sufficient exposure time (i.e., 6 to 10 hours). Disinfectants that can eliminate spores are called **chemical sterilants. High-level disinfection** occurs when chemical sterilants are used at reduced exposure times (<45 minutes). High-level disinfectants kill bacteria, fungi, and viruses, but do not kill bacterial spores unless the spores

Table 5-5 Germicidal Properties of Disinfectants and Sterilization Agents—cont'd

Important Characteristics									*Approximate Cost (in dollars)*	
Shelf Life >1 Week	Corrosive/ Deleterious Effects	Residue	Inactivated by Organic Matter	Skin Irritant	Eye Irritant	Respiratory Irritant	Toxic	Easily Obtainable	Purchase ($)/Gal	Cost ($)/Gal at Use Dilution
+	±	−	+	±	+	−	+	+	3.70 (70%)	3.70 (70%)
+	−	−	±	+	+	−	+	+	24.50 (6%)	24.50 (6%)
+	−	+	−	+	+	+	+	+	38.42 (37% wt)	3.84 (3.7% wt)
+	−	−	+	+	+	−	+	+	10.77	0.04 (0.4%)
+	−	+	±	+	+	−	+	+	9.70-15.70	0.06 (0.4%)
+	+	+	+	+	+	+	+	+	1.00 (5.25%)	0.10 (0.5%)
+	±	+	+	±	+	−	+	+	10.10 (110%)	0.05 (0.05%)
+	−	+	−	+	+	+	+	+	6.50-14.00	6.50-14.00

From Rutala WA: Disinfection, sterilization, and waste disposal. In Wenzel RP, editor: Prevention and control of nosocomial infections, Baltimore, 1997, Williams & Wilkins.

*Inactivates all indicated microorganisms with a contact time of 30 minutes or less, except bacterial spores, which require 6- to 10-hour contact time.

Int, Intermediates; CS, chemical sterilant; +, yes; −, no; ±, variable results.

Box 5-1 Properties for an Ideal Disinfectant

Broad Spectrum
Should have a wide antimicrobial spectrum

Fast Acting
Should produce a rapid kill

Not Affected by Environmental Factors
Should be active in the presence of organic matter (e.g., blood, sputum, feces) and compatible with soaps, detergents, and other chemicals encountered in use

Nontoxic
Should not be irritating to user

Surface Compatibility
Should not corrode instruments and metallic surfaces and should not cause the deterioration of cloth, rubber, plastics, and other materials

Residual Effect on Treated Surface
Should leave an antimicrobial film on the treated surface

Easy to Use

Odorless
Should have a pleasant odor or no odor to facilitate its routine use

Economical
Cost should not be prohibitively high

Solubility
Should be soluble in water

Stability
Should be stable in concentrate and use dilution

Cleaner
Should have good cleaning properties

From Rutala WA: Disinfection, sterilization, and waste disposal. In Wenzel RP, editor: *Prevention and control of nosocomial infections*, Baltimore, 1997, Williams & Wilkins.

are exposed to the disinfectant for an extended time. **Intermediate-level disinfectants** remove vegetative bacteria, tubercle bacteria, some viruses, and fungi, but do not necessarily kill spores. **Low-level disinfectants** kill most vegetative bacteria, some fungi, and some viruses. Box 5-1 summarizes the properties of an ideal disinfectant.

Pasteurization

Pasteurization uses moist heat to coagulate cell proteins. The exposure time required to kill vegetative bacteria depends on the temperature. Two techniques are commonly used: the flash process and the batch process. In the flash process, the material to be disinfected is exposed to moist heat at 72° C for 15 seconds. With the batch process, equipment is immersed in a water bath heated to 63° C for 30 minutes. The batch process can kill all vegetative bacteria and some viruses, including HIV. The flash process is used to pasteurize milk and other heat-labile liquids. Most respiratory care equipment can withstand the conditions of the batch process.

Quaternary Ammonium Compounds

Quaternary ammonium compounds (Quats) are organically substituted ammonium compounds that are cationic detergents containing four alkyl or heterocyclic radicals and a halide ion. The halide may be substituted by a sulfate radical. They are thought to interfere with the bacteria's energy-producing enzymes, denature its essential cell proteins, and disrupt the bacterial cell membrane.[8,11,12] Quats are bactericidal, fungicidal, and virucidal against lipophilic viruses. They are not sporicidal or tuberculocidal or virucidal against hydrophilic viruses. They are inactivated by organic material and their effectiveness is reduced by cotton and gauze pads, which may absorb some of their active ingredients.[8] Quats are routinely used to sanitize noncritical surfaces (e.g., floors, walls, furniture) and can generally retain their activity for as long as 2 weeks if they are kept free of organic material.[7]

Alcohols

Ethyl and isopropyl alcohol are the two most common alcohols used for disinfection. Both are bactericidal, fungicidal, and virucidal and do not kill bacterial spores. The optimum concentrations of both alcohols range from 60% to 90%. Their ability to disinfect decreases significantly at concentrations below 50%.[8]

It is thought that alcohols kill microorganisms by denaturing proteins. This is a reasonable hypothesis considering that absolute ethyl alcohol, a dehydrating agent, is less bactericidal than an ethyl alcohol and water mixture because proteins are denatured more quickly in the presence of water.[13] Although alcohols have been shown to be effective in fairly short periods (<5 minutes), the Centers for Disease Control and Prevention (CDC) recommend that exposure times of 15 minutes be required for 70% ethanol.[7]

Alcohols are used to disinfect rubber stoppers of multiple-use medication vials, oral and rectal thermometers, stethoscopes, and fiberoptic endoscopes. They can also be used to clean the surfaces of mechanical ventilators and areas used for medication preparation.[8] Alcohols are good solvents, and therefore can remove shellac from equipment surfaces. They can cause swelling and hardening of rubber and plastic tubes after prolonged and repeated use.

Acetic Acid

Acetic acid (white household vinegar) is used extensively as a method for decontaminating home-care respiratory care equipment. It is also used in hospitals, but on a limited basis. Because of its acidic nature (pH ~2), its presumed mechanism of bactericidal action is lowering a microbe's intracellular pH, thus inactivating its energy-producing enzymes.

The optimum concentration of acetic acid is 1.25%, which is the equivalent of one part 5% white household vinegar and three parts water. It has been shown to be an effective bactericidal agent (particularly against *P. aeruginosa*), but its sporicidal and virucidal activity has not been documented.[14]

Peracetic acid, or peroxyacetic acid, is acetic acid to which an oxygen atom has been added. It has been shown to be an excellent disinfectant with sterilization capabilities.[4] Peracetic acid is a strong oxidizing agent that kills microbes by denaturing proteins, disrupting cell wall permeability, and oxidizing cellular metabolites.[15] Its strong oxidizing action is also a shortcoming because it can corrode brass, iron, copper, and steel.[8]

Phenols

Carbolic acid, the prototype of these six-carbon aromatic compounds, was first used as a germicide by Lister in his pioneering work on antiseptic surgery.[8] Although carbolic acid is no longer used as a disinfectant, chemical manufacturers have synthesized numerous phenol derivatives that have been shown to be effective bactericidal, fungicidal, virucidal, and tuberculocidal agents. (Note that these derivatives are not sporicidal.) Phenol derivatives contain an alkyl, phenyl, benzyl, or halogen substituted for one of the hydrogen atoms attached to the aromatic ring. Commonly used phenols include orthophenylphenol and orthobenzylparachlorophenol.

Phenols kill microbes by denaturing proteins and injuring the cell wall. They are primarily used as surface disinfectants for floors, walls, and countertops. Phenols are readily absorbed by porous material, and residual disinfectant can cause skin irritation. They have been associated with hyperbilirubinemia in neonates when used as disinfectants in nurseries.[16]

Iodophors and Other Halogenated Compounds

An iodophor is a solution that contains iodine and a solubilizing agent or carrier. This combination results in a chemical that provides a sustained release of free iodine in an aqueous solution.[8] The best known iodophor is povidone-iodine, which is used as an antiseptic and disinfectant.

Iodophors penetrate the cell wall of microorganisms, and their mode of action is thought to be disruption of protein and nucleic metabolisms. They are bactericidal, tuberculocidal, fungicidal, and virucidal, but are not effective against bacterial spores. Note that solutions formulated for antiseptic use are not suitable for disinfectant use because antiseptic solutions contain significantly less free iodine than those formulated as disinfectants.

Sodium hypochlorite contains free available chlorine in an aqueous solution. Three forms of chlorine are present in the sodium hypochlorite mixture: free chlorine (Cl_2), hypochlorite anion (OCl^-), and hypochlorous acid (HOCl). It has been suggested that these forms of chlorine kill microbes by interfering with cellular metabolism, denaturing proteins, and inactivating nucleic acids.[8,17,18] Sodium hypochlorite (household bleach) demonstrates a range of "-cidal" activities. A 1:100 dilution is bactericidal, tuberculocidal, and virucidal in 10 minutes, and fungicidal in 1 hour. The CDC recommends that a 1:10 dilution is used to clean blood spills.[4,19] It is not, however, sporicidal. Although sodium hypochlorite is inexpensive and relatively fast-acting, it is corrosive to metals. It forms bischloromethyl ether (a carcinogen) when it comes in contact with formaldehyde and trihalomethane when hot water is hyperchlorinated. It has a limited shelf life and is inactivated by organic matter.

Glutaraldehyde

Glutaraldehyde solutions have been some of the most common disinfectants used in respiratory care departments. As stated, these solutions can be used as chemical sterilants if exposure time is extended. They kill microbes by alkylating hydroxyl, sulfhydryl, carboxy, and amino groups of microorganisms, which ultimately interfere with protein synthesis.[8] Alkaline and acid glutaraldehyde solutions are commercially available.

Alkaline glutaraldehyde is packaged as a mildly acidic solution (2% glutaraldehyde) that is activated with a bicarbonate solution, yielding a solution with a pH of 7.5 to 8.5. It is bactericidal, fungicidal, tuberculocidal, and virucidal with an exposure time of 10 minutes. It is sporicidal with an exposure time of 6 to 10 hours. The average shelf life of alkaline glutaraldehyde is 14 days to 1 month. It is irritating to skin and mucous membranes (particularly the eyes). The Occupational Safety and Health Administration (OSHA), therefore, limits exposure of workers to 0.2 ppm airborne alkaline glutaraldehyde. Union Carbide, a manufacturer of glutaraldehyde, has recently suggested that the threshold for exposure should be lowered to 0.1 ppm. Individuals working with glutaraldehyde should wear protective eyewear, masks, gloves, and splash gowns or aprons.[20,21] Ideally, glutaraldehyde should be used under a fume hood or in a room that is under negative pressure.

Acid glutaraldehyde, which has a pH of 2.7 to 3.7, is available as a 2% solution that does not require activation and comes ready to use. Acid glutaraldehyde is similar to alkaline glutaraldehyde in its -cidal activity—it is bactericidal, tuberculocidal, and fungicidal; however, exposure time must be extended to 20 minutes for acid glutaraldehyde to be tuberculocidal. The activity of an acid glutaraldehyde solution can be enhanced by warming it to 60° C. At this temperature, acid glutaraldehyde is bactericidal, fungicidal, and virucidal in 5 minutes, tuberculocidal in 20 minutes, and sporicidal in 60 minutes.[4] Acid glutaraldehyde is not irritating to skin and mucous membranes as is alkaline glutaraldehyde. Its shelf life is approximately 30 days.

Hydrogen Peroxide

Commercially available 3% solutions of hydrogen peroxide are effective disinfectants of bacteria (including *Mycobacteria* sp.), fungi, and viruses, and are active within 10 minutes at room temperature. Higher concentrations (6% to 25%) and prolonged exposure are required for sterilization. Hydrogen peroxide is sporicidal in 6 hours at 20° C; it is effective against spores in 20 minutes at 50° C.[8]

Hydrogen peroxide kills microorganisms by forming hydroxyl radicals that can attack membrane lipids, nucleic acids, and other essential compounds. Note that catalase-positive aerobes and facultative anaerobic bacteria can inactivate metabolically produced hydrogen peroxide by degrading it into water and oxygen.

Sterilization

As with disinfection, sterilization techniques are generally divided into physical and chemical methods. Physical methods most often rely on heat, specifically dry heat, boiling water, steam under pressure **(autoclave),** and incineration. Ionizing radiation (i.e., gamma and x-rays) has also been shown to be an effective method of sterilization; however, this method is used on a limited basis in the hospitals. The most commonly used chemical for sterilization is ethylene oxide. See Table 5-5 for a comparison of the advantages and disadvantages of various sterilization methods.

Heat

Probably the simplest and surest means of destroying microorganisms is burning or incineration. This method is reserved for items that are disposable or are so contaminated that their reuse is prohibited.[4] Besides destroying the material that is being sterilized, it should be recognized that incineration creates air pollution.

Dry heat is another effective method of heat sterilization. Its use is limited to items that are not heat-sensitive. Temperatures must be maintained between 160° to 180° C for 1 to 2 hours for sterilization. Dry heat is routinely used to sterilize

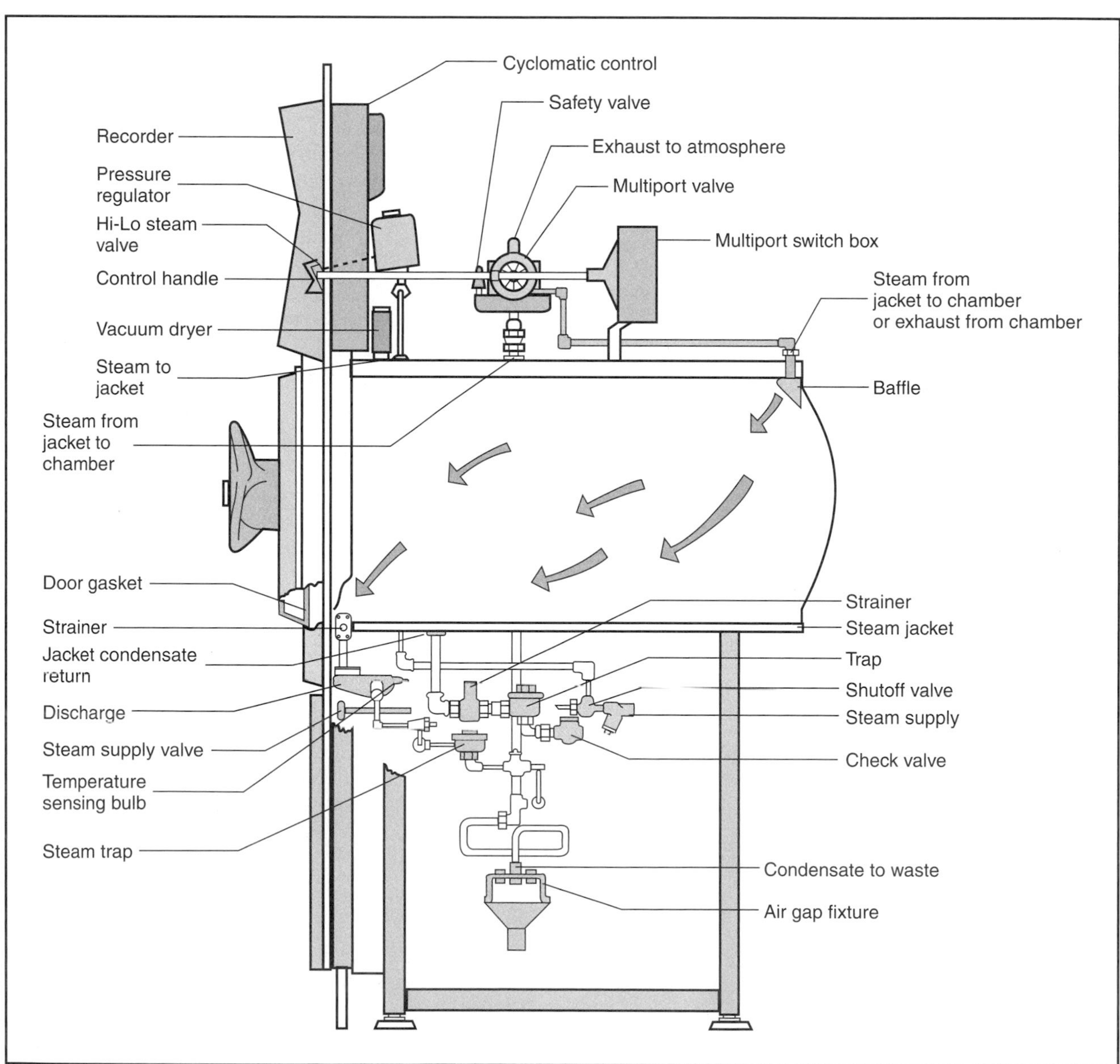

Figure 5-3 Components of an autoclave. (From Perkins JJ: *Principles and methods of sterilization in health sciences*, Springfield, Ill, 1978, Charles C Thomas.)

laboratory glassware and surgical instruments, but cannot be used for heat-sensitive items made of rubber or plastic.

Boiling water kills vegetative bacteria and most viruses in 30 minutes; but its effectiveness against spores, especially those of thermophilic organisms, is somewhat questionable. Boiling water is commonly used to sterilize metal surgical instruments. As with dry heat, its use is prohibited with heat-sensitive equipment. Because water boils at a lower temperature at high altitudes, exposure time must be prolonged when using this form of sterilization at high elevations.[4,6] Steam under pressure, or autoclaving, is a highly effective and inexpensive method of sterilization. Of the aforementioned techniques, autoclaving is probably the most versatile. It is routinely used on laboratory glassware, surgical instruments, liquids, linens, and other heat- and moisture-resistant materials.

The technique of autoclaving is fairly simple. Items to be autoclaved are cleaned and wrapped in linen, gauze, or paper. They are then placed in a chamber like the one shown in Figure 5-3, which is closed and secured. It is evacuated of air, moisture is added (100% humidity), and the pressure inside is raised to 15 to 20 psig. Air is evacuated from the chamber because residual air prolongs the penetration time of steam, thus increasing the total autoclave cycle time. Pressure is used to raise the temperature of the steam, which is critical because the amount of time required to achieve sterilization depends on the temperature inside of the autoclave. For example, at atmospheric pressure, steam has a temperature of 100° C. At 15 psig it has a temperature of 121° C, and at 20 psig it has a temperature of 132° C. At 121° C, all microbes and spores are killed within 15 minutes; at 132° C, killing occurs in 10 minutes.

Because the process of autoclaving depends on several factors, heat-sensitive and biologic indicators are routinely used to ensure quality control during the process. Heat-sensitive tape that is used for packaging materials for autoclaving changes color when it is exposed to a given temperature for a prescribed amount of time. The most common biologic indicators for autoclaving are strips of paper that are impregnated with *Bacillus stearothermophilus* spores. These strips should be used weekly (at a minimum) to ensure that the autoclave is working properly.

Ethylene Oxide

Ethylene oxide (ETO) is a sterilant that has been used since the 1950s. It is a colorless gas that is flammable and explosive. It kills microorganisms by alkylating proteins, DNA, and RNA, thus interfering with cellular metabolism.[11] ETO was originally combined with chlorofluorocarbons (CFCs), which acted as a stabilizing agent. Under provisions of the Clean Air Act of 1993, CFCs were phased out in 1995 because of their detrimental effect on the ozone layer. Currently, ETO is used alone or in combination with different stabilizing agents, such as carbon dioxide or hydrochlorofluorocarbons.

ETO kills all microorganisms and spores, with bacterial spores being more resistant than vegetative microbes. The effectiveness of ETO depends on the gas concentration (450 to 1200 mg/L), the temperature (29° C to 65° C), the humidity (45% to 85% relative humidity), and the exposure time (2 to 5 hours).[8] Generally, increases in ETO concentration and temperature shorten sterilization time.

All equipment to be sterilized with ETO must be free of water because water interferes with the sterilization process. Additionally, equipment must be packaged in ETO-permeable materials, such as paper, muslin, or plastic bags made of polyethylene or polypropylene. The actual process of automated ETO sterilization consists of several stages: a preconditioning phase and a gas-injection phase, exposure of the item to the ETO, evacuation of gas from the chamber, and an air-washing period.[8] After sterilization, all equipment exposed to ETO must be aerated before use. Note that the aeration time is usually not considered part of the sterilization time and is usually accomplished by mechanical aeration for 8 to 12 hours at 50° to 60° C. Aeration at room temperature is considered dangerous because of ETO's toxicity.

Biologic indicators, similar to those used for autoclaving, must be used to monitor the effectiveness of the ETO. *Bacillus subtilis* spores are generally used for this purpose. Figure 5-4 shows a typical device for monitoring sterilization. *B. subtilis* organisms imbedded in a paper strip are housed within a plastic capsule inside of a glass ampule containing

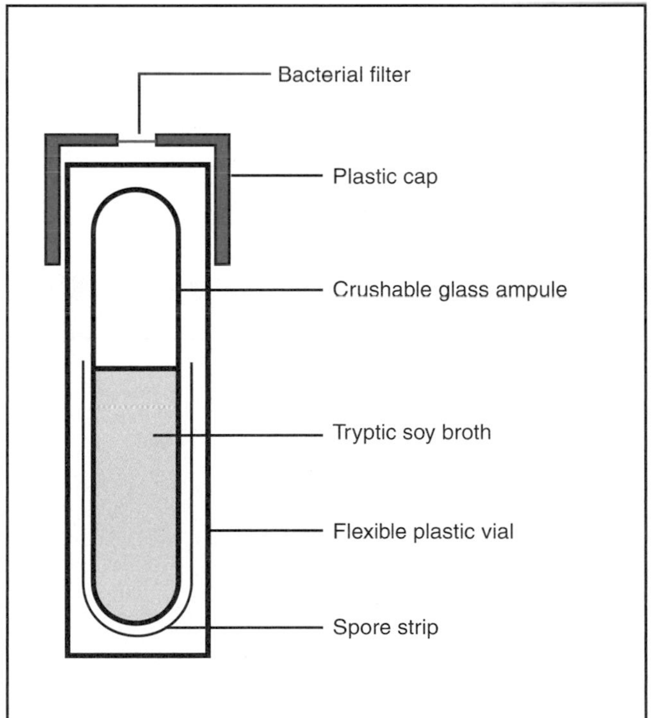

Figure 5-4 Biologic sterilization indicators: the capsule contains a strip impregnated with bacterial spores, a pH indicator, and a culture medium (e.g., tryptic soy broth). After sterilization, the ampule is crushed, releasing culture medium onto the strip containing the spores. Incomplete sterilization is indicated if the capsule turns yellow. (Redrawn from Boyd RF, Hoerl BG: *Basic medical microbiology*, ed 3, Boston, 1986, Little, Brown.)

a growth medium (e.g., tryptic soy broth).[8] The ampule is placed among the materials to be sterilized. After the sterilization cycle, the ampule is crushed and the paper strip is immersed in the liquid. The strip is then incubated according to manufacturer directions. Microbe growth is indicated by changes in the turbidity of the growth medium after incubation.[2]

Inhalation of ETO has been associated with nose and eye irritation, dyspnea, headache, nausea, vomiting, dizziness, and convulsions.[22] Direct contact with ETO causes skin irritation and burns. The OSHA and the Joint Commission for Accreditation of Hospital Organizations provide general guidelines for the safe use of ETO. The current OSHA standard for ETO exposure is 1 ppm in 8 hours, with a maximum short-term exposure of 5 to 10 ppm for 15 minutes.[23,24]

Identifying Infection-Risk Devices

It is unnecessary to sterilize all patient-care items. Whether a medical device should be cleaned and disinfected or sterilized depends on its intended use. In 1968, E.H. Spaulding[25a] devised a classification scheme that could be used by infection-control professionals in the planning of disinfection and sterilization methods for patient-care items and equipment. Spaulding's classification system placed devices into three categories based on the degree of risk of infection involved in their use. The categories are critical, semicritical, and noncritical. Critical items must be sterilized because they are introduced into sterile tissue or the vascular system (e.g., surgical instruments, implants, cardiac and urinary catheters, heart-lung and hemodialysis equipment, needles). Because semicritical items (e.g., ventilator tubing) come in contact with intact mucous membranes, a minimum of high-level disinfection is recommended. Respiratory care and anesthesia equipment, endoscopes, and thermometers are semicritical items. High-level disinfection is effective against bloodborne pathogens (i.e., HIV, hepatitis B virus) and *Mycobacteria tuberculosis.* Noncritical items come in contact with intact skin, but not mucous membranes. Intact skin acts as an effective barrier to most microorganisms, so sterility is not critical. Common examples of noncritical items are face masks, ventilators, stethoscopes, and blood pressure cuffs. Table 5-6 lists examples of medical devices and how they are classified by Spaulding's system. Box 5-2 contains a summary of the guidelines for processing reusable respiratory care equipment. Box 5-3 describes several strategies for preventing the spread of pathogenic organisms by in-use respiratory care equipment (e.g., nebulizers, ventilator circuits, manual resuscitators, oxygen therapy apparatuses). Clinical Rounds 5-3 provides a test of your understanding of the principles of infection control techniques.

Isolation Precautions

In 1996, the CDC, in cooperation with the Hospital Infection Control Practices Advisory Committee, revised its guideline for isolation precautions in hospitals.[26] The revised guideline contains information on the history of isolation practices, along with recommendations for isolation precautions in hospitals. The recommendations for isolation techniques are intended for acute-care hospitals, although some of the precautions are applicable to subacute or extended-care facilities.

The revised recommendations contain two levels of precautions: **standard precautions** and **transmission-based precautions.** Standard precautions are to be used with all hospitalized patients, regardless of their diagnosis or presumed infection status.[26] Standard precautions represent a

Table 5-6 Infection-risk categories for medical equipment

Category	Description	Examples	Processing
Critical	Devices introduced into the blood stream or other parts of the body	Surgical devices Cardiac catheters Implants Heart-lung and hemodialysis components	Sterilization
Semicritical	Devices that contact intact mucus membranes	Endoscopes Tracheal tubes Ventilator tubing Face masks Blood-pressure cuffs Ventilators	High-level disinfection
Noncritical	Devices that touch only intact skin or do not contact patient	Face masks Blood-pressure cuffs Ventilators	Detergent washing Low-intermediate level disinfection

Modified from Chatburn RL: Decontamination of respiratory care equipment: what can be done, what should be done, *Respir Care* 34(2):98, 1989. In Scanlan CL, Spearman CB, Sheldon RL: *Egan's fundamentals of respiratory care*, ed 6, St Louis, 1995, Mosby.

Box 5-2 Guidelines for Processing Reusable Respiratory Care Equipment

- All reusable respiratory care equipment should undergo low- or intermediate-level disinfection as part of the initial cleaning.
- All reusable breathing circuit components (including tubing and exhalation valves, medication nebulizers and their reservoirs, large-volume jet nebulizers and their reservoirs) should be considered semicritical items.
- Semicritical items should be sterilized between patient use; heat-stable items should be autoclaved, and heat-labile items should undergo ETO sterilization.
- If sterilization is not feasible, semicritical items should undergo high-level disinfection or pasteurization.
- The internal machinery of ventilators and breathing machines need not be routinely sterilized or disinfected between patients.
- Respirometers and other equipment used to monitor multiple patients should not directly touch any part of a ventilator circuit or a patient's mucus membranes. Rather, disposable extension pieces and low-resistance HEPA filters should be used to isolate the device. If the device cannot be isolated from the patient or circuit, it must be sterilized or receive high-level disinfection before use on other patients.
- After they have been used on one patient, nondisposable resuscitation bags should be sterilized or receive high-level disinfection before use on other patients.

From Scanlan CL, Wilkins RL, Stoller JK: *Egan's fundamentals of respiratory care*, ed 7, St Louis, 1999, Mosby. Data from Chatburn RL: Decontamination of respiratory care equipment: what can be done, what should be done, *Respir Care* 34(2)98, 1989; AARC Technical Standards and Safety Committee: Recommendations for respiratory therapy equipment: processing, handling, and surveillance, *Respir Care* 22:928, 1977.

Box 5-3 Strategies for Preventing the Spread of Pathogenic Organisms by In-Use Respiratory Care Equipment[2,6,34,36]

- Nebulizers should always be filled with sterile distilled water. Large-volume nebulizers should be filled completely before initial use. When replenishing fluid, any fluid remaining in the nebulizer should be emptied, and the reservoir filled completely.
- Large-volume jet nebulizers and medication nebulizers and their reservoirs and tubing should be changed or replaced every 24 hours with equipment that has undergone high-level disinfection.
- Avoid using humidifiers and nebulizers that create droplets for purposes of room humidification.
- In-use ventilator circuits, including their humidifiers and nebulizers, should be changed every second or third day (48 to 72 hours). If a heat-moisture exchanger bacterial filter (i.e., artificial nose) is used instead of water humidifier, changing the circuit between patients may be satisfactory.
- Water condensation in ventilator and nebulizer tubing should be discarded and not drained back into the reservoir.

CLINICAL ROUNDS 5-3

The hospital infection control committee notifies your department that the incidence of nosocomial pneumonia in the recovery room increases significantly during the month of December. It has been suggested that the source of the pneumonia could be reusable large-volume jet nebulizers. How would you determine if in-use large volume jet nebulizers are responsible for this outbreak of pneumonia? How could you monitor the effectiveness of the sterilization of these devices?

See Appendix A for the answer.

combination of **universal precautions** and body substance isolation precautions, and apply to blood, all body fluids (secretions and excretions [except sweat]), nonintact skin, and mucous membranes. Standard precautions are designed to reduce the risk of transmission of microorganisms from both recognized and unrecognized sources of infection in hospitals.[26]

Transmission-based precautions are designed to interrupt transmission of known or suspected pathogens that can be transmitted by airborne or droplet routes or by direct contact with skin and contaminated surfaces. Transmission-based precautions are for the care of patients with highly transmissible or epidemiologically important pathogens that necessitate additional precautions to stop their transmission. Box 5-4 gives a synopsis of the various types of isolation precautions and a list of conditions requiring each type of precaution. Table 5-7 lists clinical syndromes or conditions warranting additional precautions to prevent the transmission of epidemiologically important pathogens upon confirmation of diagnosis.

Fundamentals of Isolation Protection

Hand washing is the most important prevention strategy to protect health care workers from being infected by contacting infected patients. It also reduces the risk of health care workers transmitting infectious microorganisms from one patient to another or from a contaminated to a clean site on the same patient.[27-29] Routine hand washing should comprise a soap and water wash with a rubbing action to create a lather over both hands for longer than

Box 5-4 Infection Control Precautions and Patients Requiring Them

Standard Precautions

Use standard precautions for the care of all patients.

Airborne Precautions

In addition to standard precautions, use airborne precautions for patients known or suspected to have serious illnesses transmitted by airborne droplet nuclei. Examples of such illnesses include:

- Measles
- Varicella (including disseminated zoster)*
- Tuberculosis†

Droplet Precautions

In addition to standard precautions, use droplet precautions for patients known or suspected to have serious illnesses transmitted by large particle droplets. Examples of such illnesses include:

Invasive *Haemophilus influenza* type b disease (meningitis, pneumonia, epiglottis, and sepsis)

Invasive *Neisseria meningitidis* disease (meningitis, pneumonia, and sepsis)

Other serious bacterial respiratory infections spread by droplet transmission, including:

- Diphtheria (pharyngeal)
- Mycoplasma pneumonia
- Pertussis
- Pneumonic plague
- Streptococcal pharyngitis, pneumonia, or scarlet fever in infants and young children

Serious viral infections spread by droplet transmission, including:

- Adenovirus*
- Influenza
- Mumps
- Parvovirus B19
- Rubella

Contact Precautions

In addition to standard precautions, use contact precautions for patients known or suspected to have serious illnesses easily transmitted by direct patient contact or by contact with items in the patient's environment. Examples of such illnesses include: gastrointestinal, respiratory, skin, or wound infections or colonization with multidrug-resistant bacteria (judged by the infection control program based on current state, regional, or national recommendations to be of special clinical and epidemiologic significance).

Enteric infections with a low infectious dose or prolonged environmental survival, including: *Clostridium difficile* organisms.

For diapered or incontinent patients: enterohemorrhagic *Escherichia coli, Shigella*, hepatitis A, or rotavirus.

Respiratory syncytial virus, parainfluenza virus, or enteroviral infections in infants and young children.

Skin infections that are highly contagious or that may occur on dry skin, including:

- Diphtheria (cutaneous)
- Herpes simplex-virus (neonatal or mucocutaneous)
- Impetigo
- Noncontained abscesses, cellulitis, or decubiti
- Pediculosis
- Scabies
- Staphylococcal furunculosis in infants and young children
- Zoster (disseminated or in the immunocompromised host)*

Viral/hemorrhagic conjunctivitis

Viral hemorrhagic infections (Ebola, Lassa, or Marburg)

From Garner JS: Guideline for isolation precautions in hospitals, *Infect Control Hosp Epidemiol* 17:53, 1996.
*Certain infections require more than one type of precaution.
†See *CDC Guidelines for Preventing the Transmission of Tuberculosis in Health-Care Settings.*[35]

10 seconds. Hands should be rinsed thoroughly and dried with disposable or single-use towels or an air drier.[30] The Centers for Disease Control and Prevention updated its recommendations for hand washing technique ion October 25, 2002. These updated guidelines specify that alcohol-based hand rubs should be used in conjunction with traditional soap and water to protect patients in health care settings. Note that hands should be washed before caring for any patient, but it is particularly important that hands are washed before and after performing invasive procedures or touching wounds or patients at a high risk of infection.

Gloves are worn for several reasons: (1) to protect the health care worker from contact with blood and body fluids (i.e., bloodborne pathogens); (2) to be a barrier so that resident and transient microorganisms on the hands of health care workers are not transferred to patients during patient care or medical or surgical procedures; and (3) to prevent health care workers from indirectly transmitting pathogens from an infected patient to another patient.[27,32] It is important to remember that hand washing is essential after removing gloves after each patient contact because hands can be contaminated during glove removal. Defects or tears in gloves can also contaminate the hands.[33,34]

Gowns and other protective apparel (e.g., shoe covers) are worn to prevent contamination of clothing and protect the skin of personnel from blood and body fluid exposure.[26] This protective apparel should be impermeable to liquids and worn only once, then discarded. Wearing gowns and protective apparel is mandated by OSHA's final rule on bloodborne pathogens.[31]

Face shields or masks with protective eyewear should be worn whenever there is a possibility of blood or body fluid being splashed or sprayed. They may also be mandated in special circumstances stated in the OSHA Bloodborne

Table 5-7 Clinical Syndromes and Conditions Warranting Additional Empiric Precautions to Prevent the Transmission of Infectious Disease*

Clinical Syndrome or Condition†	Potential Pathogens‡	Empiric Precautions
Diarrhea		
Acute diarrhea with a likely infectious cause in an incontinent or diapered patient	Enteric pathogens§	Contact
Diarrhea in an adult with a history of recent antibiotic use	*Clostridium difficile*	Contact
Meningitis	*Neisseria meningitides*	Droplet
Rash or exanthems, generalized, etiology unknown Petechial/ecchymotic with fever Vesicular	*Neisseria meningitidis* Varicella	Droplet Airborne contact
Maculopapular with coryza fever	Rubeola (measles)	Airborne
Respiratory infections Cough/fever/upper lobe pulmonary infiltrate in an HIV-negative patient or a patient at low risk for HIV infection	*Mycobacterium tuberculosis*	Airborne
Cough/fever/pulmonary infiltrate in an HIV-negative patient or a patient at high risk for HIV infection	*Mycobacterium tuberculosis*	Airborne
Paroxysmal or severe persistent cough during periods of pertussis activity	*Bordetella pertussis*	Droplet
Respiratory infections, particularly bronchiolitis croup, in infants and young children	Respiratory syncytial or parainfluenza virus	Contact
Risk of multidrug-resistant microorganisms History if infection or colonization with multidrug-resistant organisms	Resistant bacteria‖	Contact
Skin, wound, urinary tract infection in a patient with a recent hospital or nursing home stay in a facility where multidrug-resistant organisms are prevalent	Resistant bacteria‖	Contact
Skin or wound infection Abscess or draining wound that cannot be covered	*Staphylococcus aureus* Group A streptococcus	Contact

From Garner JS: Guideline for isolation precautions in hospitals, *Infect Control Hosp Epidemiol* 17:52, 1996.

*Infection control professionals are encouraged to modify or adapt this table according to local conditions. To ensure that appropriate empiric precautions are always implemented, hospitals must have systems in place to evaluate patients routinely according to these criteria as part of their preadmission and admission care.

†Patients with the syndromes or conditions listed below may present with atypical signs or symptoms (e.g., pertussis in neonates and adults may not have paroxysmal or severe cough). The clinician's index of suspicion should be guided by the prevalence of specific conditions in the community, as well as clinical judgment.

‡The organisms listed under this column are not intended to represent the complete, or even most likely, diagnosis, but rather are possible etiologic agents that require additional precautions until they can be ruled out.

§These pathogens include enterohemorrhagic *Escherichia coli*, *Shigella* sp., hepatitis A, and rotavirus.

‖Resistant bacteria judged by the infection control program, based on current state, regional, or national recommendations, to be of special clinical or epidemiologic significance.

Pathogen Final Rule.[31] Face masks are used to prevent the spread of large particle droplets that are transmitted by close contact (e.g., when working with patients who are coughing or sneezing), although the efficacy of wearing a mask to prevent transmitting *Mycobacterium tuberculosis* organisms has been questioned.[35] Respiratory protective devices are now required to prevent the inhalation of airborne droplet nuclei. A wide range of respirators that meet National Institute of Occupational Safety and Health standards are available to prevent the inhalation of droplet nuclei. Face shields or protective eyewear should be worn during all invasive procedures (i.e., when obtaining arterial blood gas samples and inserting intravascular catheters).

Patient care equipment and articles that can potentially be **fomites** for transmitting infectious particles (e.g., needles, scalpels, other sharp objects) should be disposed in specially designated containers. Disposable medical gas therapy devices, such as nebulizers and tubing, should be disposed of by being placed in a sturdy bag or container. Reusable items should be sterilized or disinfected by standard procedures to avoid transmitting infectious microorganisms from patient to patient. Disposable items should be disposed of according to hospital and applicable government regulations. Take care not to contaminate the outside of the bag when it is being handled or transported.

Fluids and medications that are used to treat patients should be sterile. Thus only sterile water should be used to fill nebulizers and humidifiers. Unused portions of large bottles of sterile water should be discarded within 24 hours. Single-dose ampules of sterile water and normal saline are ideal for small-volume nebulizers. Multidose vials should be stored according to manufacturer's specifications (e.g., refrigerated after opening). Single-dose and multidose vials should not be used beyond the date on the label.[2]

Standard Precautions

As was stated previously, standard precautions are a synthesis of previous CDC guidelines for universal precautions and body substance isolation techniques. Hands should be washed between tasks and procedures on the same patient to prevent cross-contamination of different body sites.[26] Gloves, masks, protective eyewear, and gowns should be worn when there is a chance of splashing blood, body fluids, secretions, excretions, and contacting contaminated items. Needles and other sharp objects should be handled with care to prevent injuries. Needles should not be recapped; when it is necessary to recap a syringe, both hands should never be used, instead use the one-hand "scoop" technique or a mechanical device to recap syringe needles safely.[27]

Airborne Precautions

Airborne precautions have two major components: (1) placement of the infected patient in an area with appropriate air handling and ventilation and (2) use of respiratory protective devices by health care workers and visitors entering the patient's room.[26,27] Measles, chickenpox (primary Varicella zoster), and tuberculosis are illnesses that require airborne precautions. Because Varicella zoster organisms can also be transmitted by direct contact, infected patients may also require contact isolation.

Droplet Precautions

Droplet precautions are designed to prevent the transmission of microorganisms contained in droplets that are generated by sneezing, coughing, or talking, or during procedures such as bronchoscopy and suctioning.[26] Precautions include gloves, masks, and protective eyewear. Special air handling and ventilation are not required. *Haemophilus influenzae* type b organisms and *Neisseria meningitidis* organisms are transmitted by this route. Other serious infections are adenovirus, influenza, parvovirus B19, pertussis, streptococcal pharyngitis, pneumonia, and scarlet fever.[27]

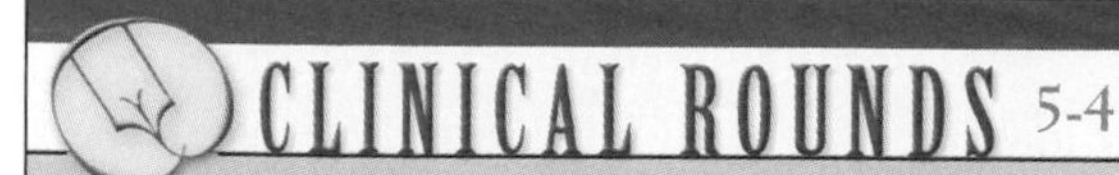

You are on call in the emergency room when one adult and two children are admitted after a house fire. The children incurred only minor cuts and bruises, but the adult sustained third-degree burns over 60% of his body. What precautions should you take when treating burn patients?

See Appendix A for the answer.

Contact Precautions

Contact precautions are recommended for patients infected with pathogenic organisms that can be spread by direct patient contact or through contact with items in the patient's environment.[26] Contact precautions require the patient to be isolated in a private room with a bath. Masks, gloves, and gowns should be used when caring for these patients. Illnesses requiring contact isolation include gastrointestinal, respiratory, and skin infections. Some of the organisms responsible for these illnesses are *Clostridium difficile*, *Shigella* sp., hepatitis A, respiratory syncytial virus, and the parainfluenza virus. Patients colonized with multidrug-resistant organisms of special clinical and epidemiologic significance also require contact isolation. Clinical Rounds 5-4 provides a problem-solving exercise on isolation precautions typically required in the clinical setting.

Surveillance

Ongoing surveillance is required to ensure that an infection control program is providing adequate protection for patients and health care providers. Surveillance typically consists of three components: monitoring equipment-processing procedures, sampling in-use equipment routinely, and microbiologically identifying suspected pathogens.[4] Equipment processing is monitored using the aforementioned chemical and biologic indicators. In-use equipment can be routinely sampled with sterile cotton swabs, liquid broth, and aerosol impaction. Swabs can be used to obtain samples from easily accessible surfaces of respiratory care equipment. Liquid broth can be used to obtain samples when cotton swabs cannot reach many parts of the equipment (e.g., inside tubing). Aerosol impaction is used to sample the particulate output of nebulizers.

Microbiologic identification requires the hospital's clinical laboratory staff to work with clinicians to identify infectious organisms. Clinical microbiologists can provide information about nosocomial infections from direct smears and stains, cultures, serologic tests, and antibiotic susceptibility testing. Identifying the cause of a nosocomial infection is essential to prevent and minimize hospital epidemics.[4]

Summary

Three elements must be present for an infectious disease to spread: a source of pathogens, a mode of transmission of the infectious agent, and a susceptible host. Nosocomial pneumonia is most often the result of bacteria, but viruses, protozoa, and fungi contribute to a lesser extent. Most nosocomial bacterial pneumonias are described as polymicrobial, with Gram-negative bacilli being the predominant microbes identified.

There are four routes of transmission of infectious materials: contact, vehicles, airborne, and vectors. Nosocomial pneumonia can be spread by any of these routes. Contact, vehicle, and airborne transmission are the most common routes in hospital settings. Infection-control methods involve cleaning, disinfecting, and sterilizing respiratory care equipment, along with isolation precautions, which are the primary means of stopping the spread of nosocomial pneumonia.

The effectiveness of an infection control program should be monitored routinely with mechanical, chemical, and biologic indicators. These indicators are readily available, easy to use, and ultimate proof that patients are not being exposed to microorganisms that can cause hospital-acquired infections.

Review Questions

See Appendix A for the answers.

1. Which of the following organisms are gram-negative bacteria often associated with nosocomial pneumonia?
   a. *Pseudomonas aeruginosa*
   b. *Diplococcus pneumoniae*
   c. *Clostridium botulinum*
   d. *Staphylococcus aureus*

2. *Mycobacterium tuberculosis* organisms are:
   a. Gram-negative bacilli
   b. Anaerobic infection
   c. Acid-fast bacteria
   d. Spore-producing bacteria

3. All of the following are transmitted through the respiratory route except:
   a. Rubella
   b. Rhinoviruses
   c. Varicella
   d. HIV

4. Briefly describe the most recent CDC guidelines for proper hand hygiene.

5. Which of the following disinfectants can be used as a chemical sterilant?
   a. Povidone-iodine
   b. Acetic acid
   c. Glutaraldehyde
   d. Isopropyl alcohol

6. Indicate whether each of the following presents a critical, semicritical, or noncritical risk of infection.
   a. Ventilator tubing
   b. Swan-Ganz catheter
   c. Blood pressure cuff
   d. Endoscope (bronchoscope)
   e. Endotracheal tubes

7. Which of these clinical conditions warrants additional precautions to prevent the spread of epidemiologically significant pathogens?
   a. Meningitis
   b. Pertussis
   c. Measles
   d. Diarrhea in an adult with a history of recent antibiotic use

8. The best method to sterilize a bronchoscope is:
   a. Ethylene oxide
   b. Soaking in 2% glutaraldehyde for 10 hours
   c. Soaking in 70% isopropyl alcohol for 20 minutes
   d. Steam autoclave

9. Which of the following methods should not be used to sterilize plastic oxygen masks?
   a. Ethylene oxide
   b. Steam autoclave
   c. 70% isopropyl alcohol
   d. 2% alkaline glutaraldehyde

10. Which of the following conditions requires the application of contact precautions?
    a. Legionellosis
    b. Diphtheria
    c. Hepatitis
    d. Rubella

11. Which of the following are potential causes of skin and mucosal barrier disruption?
    I. Foley catheters
    II. Intravenous catheters
    III. Endotracheal tubes
    IV. Burns
       a. I and II only
       b. II and III only
       c. I, II, and IV only
       d. I, II, III, and IV

12. *Bacillus anthracis* is a(n):
    a. gram-negative bacterium
    b. anaerobic infection
    c. acid-fast bacterium
    d. spore-producing bacterium

13. Name three elements that must be present for the spread of infectious materials.

14. Describe various techniques that are routinely used to determine the effectiveness of sterilization.

15. Which of the following precautions should be taken with a patient with respiratory isolation?
    I. Private room.
    II. Gowns should be worn by all persons entering the room.
    III. Articles contaminated with secretions must be disinfected or discarded.
    IV. Masks must be worn by all persons who will be in close contact with the patient.
        a. II and III only
        b. III and IV only
        c. I, II, and III only
        d. I, III, and IV only

16. Define *standard precautions.*

17. Match the following:

1. _______ HIV	a. Bronchitis, bronchiolitis
2. _______ Respiratory syncytial virus	b. Fungal infection
3. _______ Parainfluenza	c. Croup, pneumonia
4. _______ Influenza	d. Tracheobronchitis
5. _______ Histoplasmosis	e. AIDS

18. Give an example of a disease that is transmitted for each of the following routes of transmission:
    a. Contact (direct)
    b. Vehicle (foodborne)
    c. Airborne (droplet nuclei)
    d. Vectorborne (fleas)

References

1. Delost MD: *Introduction to diagnostic microbiology,* St Louis, 1997, Mosby.
2. Scanlan CL, Spearman CB, Sheldon RL: *Egan's fundamentals of respiratory care,* ed 6, St Louis, 1995, Mosby.
3. Niederman MS, Sarosi GA, Glassroth J: *Respiratory infections: a scientific basis for management,* Philadelphia, 1994, WB Saunders.
4. Pilbeam SM: Microbiology. In Kacmarek RM, Mack CW, Dimas S, editors: *The essentials of respiratory care,* St Louis, 1990, Mosby.
5. Zimmerman PE, Martin WJ: Pneumocystis carinii. In Niederman MS, Sarosi GA, Glassroth J, editors: *Respiratory infections: a scientific basis for management,* Philadelphia, 1994, WB Saunders.
6. Schaberg DR: How infections spread in the hospital, *Respir Care* 34(2):81, 1989.
7. Chatburn RL: Decontamination of respiratory care equipment: what can be done, what should be done, *Respir Care* 34(2):8, 1989.
8. Rutala WA: Disinfection, sterilization, and waste disposal. In Wenzel RP, editor: *Prevention and control of nosocomial infections,* Baltimore, 1997, Williams & Wilkins.
9. Favero MS, et al: Gram-negative water bacteria in hemodialysis systems, *Health Lab Sci* 12:321, 1987.
10. Rutala WA, Cole EC: Ineffectiveness of hospital disinfectants against bacteria: a collaborative study, *Infect Control* 8:501, 1987.
11. Sykes G: *Disinfection and sterilization,* ed 2, London, 1965, E & FN Spon, Ltd.
12. Petrocci AN: Surface active agents: quaternary ammonium compounds. In Block SS, editor: *Disinfection, sterilization, and preservation,* ed 3, Philadelphia, 1983, Lea & Febiger.
13. Morton HE: Alcohols. In Block SS, editor: *Disinfection, sterilization, and preservation,* ed 3, Philadelphia, 1983, Lea & Febiger.
14. Chatburn RE, Kallstrom TJ, Bajaksouzian MS: A comparison of acetic acid with a quaternary ammonium compound for the disinfection of hand-held nebulizers, *Respir Care* 33:179, 1988.
15. Block SS: Peroxygen compounds. In Block SS, editor: *Disinfection, sterilization, and preservation,* ed 3, Philadelphia, 1983, Lea & Febiger.
16. Rutala WA: APIC guideline for selection and use of disinfectants, *Am J Infect Control* 18(2):99, 1990.
17. Bloomfield SF, Uso EE: The antibacterial properties of sodium hypochlorite and sodium dichloroisocyanurate as hospital disinfectants, *J Hosp Infect* 6:20, 1985.
18. Favero MS, Bond WW: Chemical disinfection of medical and surgical materials. In Block SS, editor: *Disinfection, sterilization, and preservation,* ed 3, Philadelphia, 1983, Lea & Febiger.
19. United States Department of Labor: Bloodborne pathogens and acute care facilities, *OSHA* 3128, 1992.
20. Gorman SP, Scott EM, Russell AD: A review: antimicrobial activity, uses, and mechanisms of action of glutaraldehyde, *J Appl Bacteriol* 48:161, 1980.
21. Association for the Advancement of Medical Instrumentation: American National Standard, *Safe use and handling of glutaraldehyde-based products in health care settings,* ANSI/AAMI ST58, 1996.
22. Gross JA, Haas MI, Swift TR: Ethylene oxide neurotoxicity: report of four cases and review of the literature, *Neurology* 29:978, 1979.
23. Occupation Safety and Health Administration: Occupational exposure to ethylene oxide—OSHA, Final standard, *Fed Register* 49(122):25734, 1984.
24. Kruger DA: What is 5 ppm? Understanding and complying with the new ETO STEL (short-term exposure limit) regulation, *J Health Material Manage* 7(2):34, 1989.
25. Garner JS: Guideline for isolation precautions in hospitals, *Infect Control Hosp Epidemiol* 17:53, 1996.

25a. Spaulding EH: Chemical disinfection of medical and surgical materials. In Lawrence CA, Block SS, editors: *Disinfection, sterilization, and preservation,* ed 3, Philadelphia, 1968, Lea & Febiger.

26. Beekman SE, Henderson DK: Controversies in isolation policies and practices. In Wenzel RP, editor: *Prevention and control of nosocomial infections,* Baltimore, 1997, Williams & Wilkins.
27. Larson E: APIC guideline for handwashing and hand antisepsis in health care settings, *Am J Infect Control* 23:251, 1995.

28. Garner J, Favero M: *Guideline for handwashing and hospital environmental control,* United States Department of Health and Human Services Public Health Service, Centers for Disease Control, 7:59, 1986.

29. Donowitz LG: *Infection control for the health care worker,* Baltimore, 1994, Williams & Wilkins.

30. Garner JS, Favero MS: Guideline for handwashing and hospital environmental control, *Infect Control* 7:231, 1986.

31. Department of Labor, Occupational Safety and Health Administration: Occupational exposure to bloodborne pathogens: final rule, *Federal Register* 56:64175, 1991.

32. Olsen R, et al: Examination gloves as barriers to hand contamination and clinical practice, *JAMA* 350, 1993.

33. Doebbeling B, et al: Removal of nosocomial pathogens from the contaminated glove: implications for glove reuse and handwashing, *Ann Inter Med* 109:394, 1988.

34. Cadwallader HL, Bradley CR, Ayliffe GA: Bacterial contamination and frequency of changing ventilator circuits, *J Hosp Infect* 5(1):65, 1990.

35. Centers for Disease Control and Prevention: Guidelines for preventing the transmission of tuberculosis in health-care settings, with special focus on HIV-related issues, *MMWR* 39(RR-17):1, 1990.

36. Gallagher J, Stangeways JE, Allt-Graham J: Contamination control in long term ventilation: a clinical study using a heat and moisture exchanging filter, *Anesthesia* 42(5):476, 1987.

Bibliography

Bartlett JG, et al: Bacteriology of hospital-acquired pneumonia, *Arch Intern Med* 146:868, 1986.

Boucher RM: Cidex and sonacide compared, *Respir Care* 22:790, 1977.

Centers for Disease Control and Prevention: Guidelines for preventing the transmission of tuberculosis in health-care settings, with special focus on HIV-related issues, *MMWR* 39(RR-17):1, 1990.

Fagon JY, et al: Nosocomial pneumonia in patients receiving continuous mechanical ventilation: prospective analysis of 52 episodes with use of a protected specimen brush and quantitative culture techniques, *Am Rev Respir Dis* 139:877, 1989.

Hierholzer WJ: Guideline for prevention of nosocomial pneumonia, *Respir Care* 39(12):1191, 1994.

Centers for Disease Control and Prevention: Guideline for hand hygiene in health-care settings, *MMWR* 51(RR16):1-44, 2002.

Internet Resources

National Center for Infectious Disease: http://www.cdc.gov/ncidod

Centers for Disease Control and Prevention: http://www.cdc.gov

Joint Commission on Accreditation of Health Care Organizations: http://www.jcaho.org

Health Resources and Services Administration (HRSA): http://www.hrsa.gov

Federation of American Scientists: http://www.fas.org/promed

Office of the United States Surgeon General: http://www.surgeongeneral.gov

AIDS Clinical Trials Information Service: http://www.actis.org

Chapter 6

Airway Management

Charles G. Durbin, Jr.

Chapter Outline

Chapter Learning Objectives

Upon completion of this chapter, the reader should be able to:

1. Describe ways to displace the tongue to improve gas exchange in unconscious patients.
2. List several complications from improper placement of oral and nasopharyngeal airways.
3. Describe how to place the laryngeal mask airway and the Combitube (Sheridan Catheter Corp.) in unconscious patients.
4. List the appropriate sequence of steps to insert an endotracheal tube to provide a secure airway.
5. Identify at least three ways to confirm that an endotracheal tube lies in the trachea.
6. List the equipment necessary to perform invasive ventilation (transtracheal or surgical airway) and describe a procedure for airway entry.
7. Describe various types of manual resuscitators and discuss common hazards associated with using these devices.
8. List the complications related to invasive airway access and the treatment of each.
9. Review the equipment and steps necessary for obtaining sputum samples from patients with tracheostomy tubes.
10. Describe three ways to wean patients from tracheostomy tubes.
11. List three methods to allow patients with tracheostomy tubes to speak.
12. Identify the airway risks facing intubated patients and identify strategies and equipment for the prevention of each.

Key Terms

Berman Airway
Cardiopulmonary Resuscitation
Combitube
Double-Lumen Endotracheal Tube (DLET)
Duckbill Valve
Endotracheal Tube (ET)
Fastrack LMA
Fishmouth Valve
French Sizes
Guedel Airway
Laryngeal Mask Airway (LMA)
Laryngoscope
Leaf-Type Valve
Luer-Loc
Lukens Sputum Trap
Macintosh Blade
Miller Blade
Nasopharyngeal Airway
Nasotracheal Intubation
Nonrebreathing Valve
Oropharyngeal Airway
Resuscitation Devices
Sniffer's Position
Spring-loaded
Translaryngeal Intubation

One of the most dramatic and rapidly fatal medical emergencies occurs when a person loses the ability to breathe spontaneously. This can be caused by upper airway obstruction, as with foreign body aspiration; lower airway obstruction, as with severe bronchospasm or a tension pneumothorax; or from an altered respiratory drive, as with depressant drug overdose or after a stroke. Failure to restore adequate respiratory gas exchange can result in hypoxic brain injury or death within minutes. These serious consequences have led to universal acceptance of the "ABCs of resuscitation" (Airway, Breathing, and Circulation), with establishment of an adequate airway as the first and highest priority.

This chapter reviews the devices and techniques used to establish and maintain a patent upper airway, including tongue-displacement devices and endotracheal (ET) and tracheostomy tubes (TT). Table 6-1 briefly describes some of these devices. Additional equipment used for patients with artificial airways, and some of the risks and problems encountered in their use, will be described. Many devices and pieces of equipment for airway management have been developed over the years, with some only fitting a small, clinical niche. Some of these airway devices have passed into history, never gaining widespread popularity. Only devices that are widely in use are described in detail in this chapter.

Opening the Upper Airway—Displacing the Tongue

Simple maneuvers are often effective to restore breathing to patients with obstructed airways. In the supine position, when the pharyngeal and tongue muscles lose tone, the tongue falls backward, often occluding the pharynx. Elevating and extending the head advances the jaw and moves the tongue forward, helping to open a closed airway. This so-called "sniffer's position," shown in Figure 6-1, opens the upper airway and places the long axes of the mouth, pharynx, and larynx in alignment. This head position is also optimal for endotracheal intubation with direct vision. By forcing the jaw anteriorly with a jaw thrust or a chin lift maneuver (Figures 6-2 and 6-3), the tongue is moved farther from the

Table 6-1 Devices and Techniques Used to Establish and Maintain a Patent Upper Airway

Device or Maneuver	Description	Concerns and Contraindications
Extreme extension, or "sniffer's position"	Extension of the occiput with head extent	Unstable cervical spine
Jaw thrust or chin lift	Anterior displacement of the mandible with or without dislocation of the temporomandibular joints	Temporomandibular joint disease or a fractured mandible
Oropharyngeal airways	Rigid, curved device with an air passage, placed through the mouth with end resting distal to the tongue above the glottic opening	Gagging or vomiting, improper size, incorrect placement
Nasopharyngeal airways	Soft or semirigid hollow tube placed through the nares, the tip lying distal to the tongue above the glottic opening	Gagging or vomiting (usually better tolerated in noncomatose patients); posterior pharyngeal wall dissection; severe bleeding
Laryngeal mask airways	Custom-formed, soft mask with a hollow tube fitting into the pyriform sinuses directly above the larynx	Confirmation of correct placement difficult, mask may fold, epiglottis may obstruct laryngeal opening, trachea not protected from aspiration
Endotracheal tubes	Semirigid, hollow tube placed into the trachea with or without an inflatable cuff	Usually requires special devices (e.g., laryngoscopy) and technical skill for consistent correct placement, tracheal placement must be objectively confirmed, and esophageal placement and ET displacement avoided
Transtracheal invasive airway	Emergent, direct entry into the trachea below the larynx by a large-bore needle, or surgical incision with endotracheal tube	Hypoxia, bleeding, nerve or esophageal injury, failure to establish an airway, gas dissection
Tracheostomy tubes	A hollow tube, with or without a cuff, electively inserted directly into the trachea through a surgical incision or with a wire-guided progressive dilation technique	Hypoxia, bleeding, nerve or esophageal injury, failure to establish the airway due to nontracheal placement, the airway due to nontracheal placement, displacement

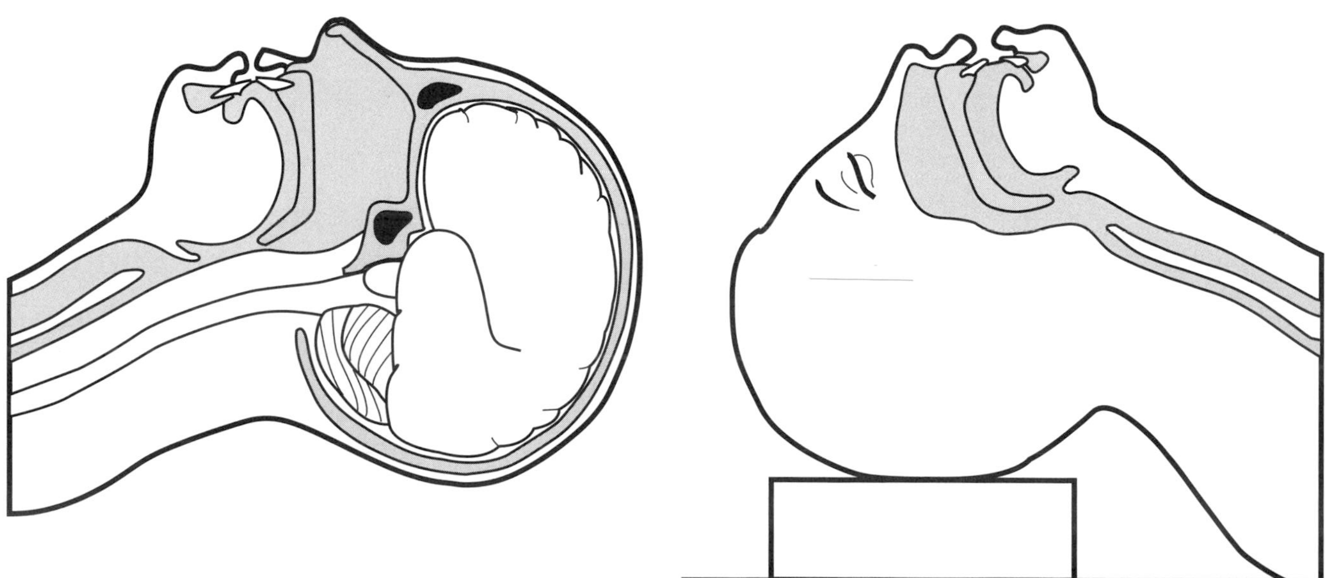

Figure 6-1 "Sniffer's position," the optimal position for opening the upper airway, can be obtained by supporting the occiput of the head on a solid surface and extending the head. This is also the optimal position for oral intubation using a curved laryngoscope blade.

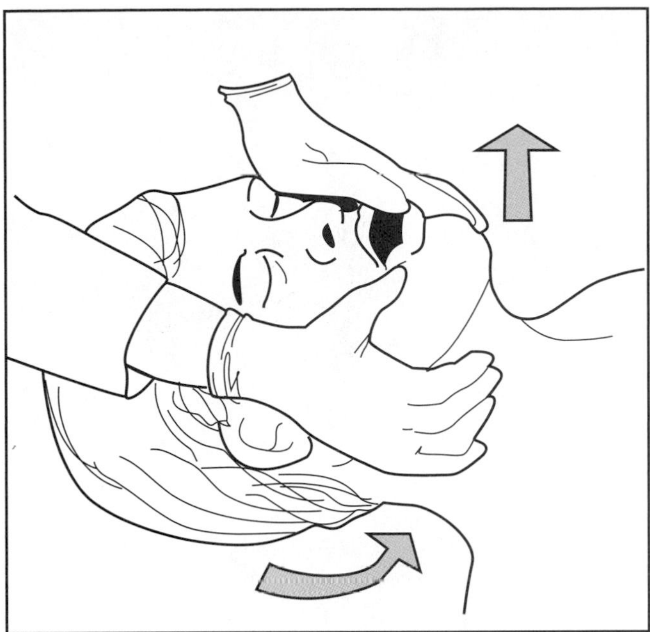

Figure 6-2 The index fingers of both hands are used to perform a jaw thrust, which displaces the temporomandibular joints anteriorly, achieving a patent airway without neck extension. This is particularly useful for patients with cervical injuries.

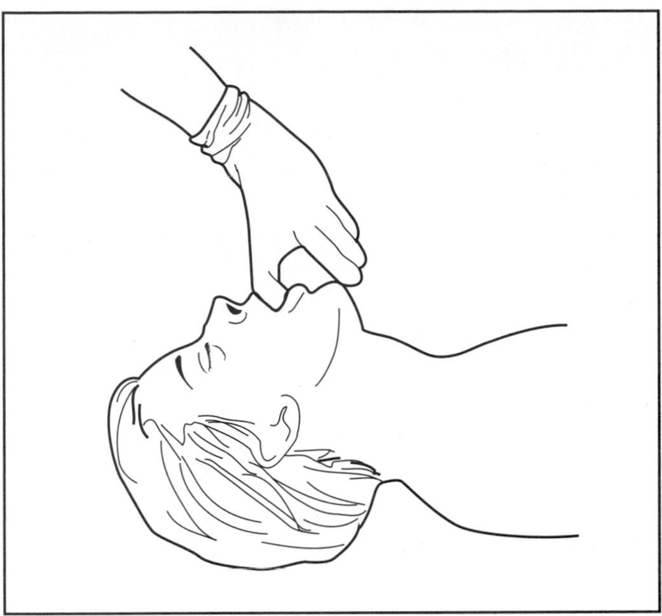

Figure 6-3 A chin lift is another method for opening the upper airway by moving the tongue anteriorly and can be successful without extending the cervical spine.

hard and soft palates, so a patent upper airway allowing spontaneous ventilation may be achieved. In some patients, these simple manual maneuvers are ineffective for opening air passages past an obstructing tongue, so mechanical devices must be used.

The most common device for this purpose is the oral pharyngeal airway. A **Guedel airway** consists of a hollow, central channel for air passage, a buccal flange, a bite portion, and a curved portion that follows the contour of the hard palate. The airway must extend past the posterior part of the tongue to allow air to pass. A **Berman airway** is shaped similarly to the Guedel airway but has a different cross-section profile without a protected central channel (Figure 6-4). Available in a variety of lengths, the American National Standards Institute (ANSI) standard for oral airways is that the size is the "nominal" length in millimeters. This measurement convention is shown in Figure 6-5. Because jaw sizes differ markedly among individuals, the correct-size oropharyngeal airway can be estimated as one that reaches from the angle of the jaw or the earlobe to the lips. It is safer to choose an airway that is too large rather than one even slightly too small because the tongue will not be bypassed by an airway that is too short, so no air will pass into the lungs. If the airway is too long, the excess length will protrude from the mouth, but the air passage will be patent.

An oropharyngeal airway may be inserted into an unconscious person in several ways. Using a tongue blade or gloved fingers, the mouth can be opened and the airway inserted following the curve of the hard palate and seated with the tip past the back of the tongue. Getting the tip past the flaccid tongue is sometimes difficult, but it is essential for success. To reduce the likelihood of the airway tip getting hung up on the back of the tongue, the airway can be inserted upside down with the tip riding along the hard palate until past the tongue, when it is rotated 180 degrees. A modification of this technique that may be less traumatic to the palate is to insert the airway rotated 90 degrees from the side of the mouth, using it like a tongue blade to move the tongue out of the way, and then rotate it back 90 degrees to seat it. These three insertion techniques are illustrated in Figures 6-6, 6-7, and 6-8.

Correct size and proper seating are essential to creating an open air passage with an oropharyngeal airway. An important sign that the distal airway tip may not have passed the back of the tongue is if the flange protrudes from the patient's mouth. If attempts to push the airway farther in just bounce it back out, it is probably catching on the back of the tongue and should be removed and replaced immediately using one of the previously described methods of insertion in this chapter. An alternative technique for seating an airway that has failed to pass the tongue is to perform a jaw thrust and push (with the thumbs) the airway in past the anteriorly displaced tongue. This technique is shown in Figure 6-9.

Specialized oral airways, some of which are shown in Figure 6-10, have been developed to allow blind and fiberoptic-directed endotracheal intubation. The simplest of these is a hollow bite block that protects the endoscope from damage if the patient reflexively bites down during the procedure. Airways that facilitate intubation either have open channels or are split devices that can be removed, leaving the ET in place.

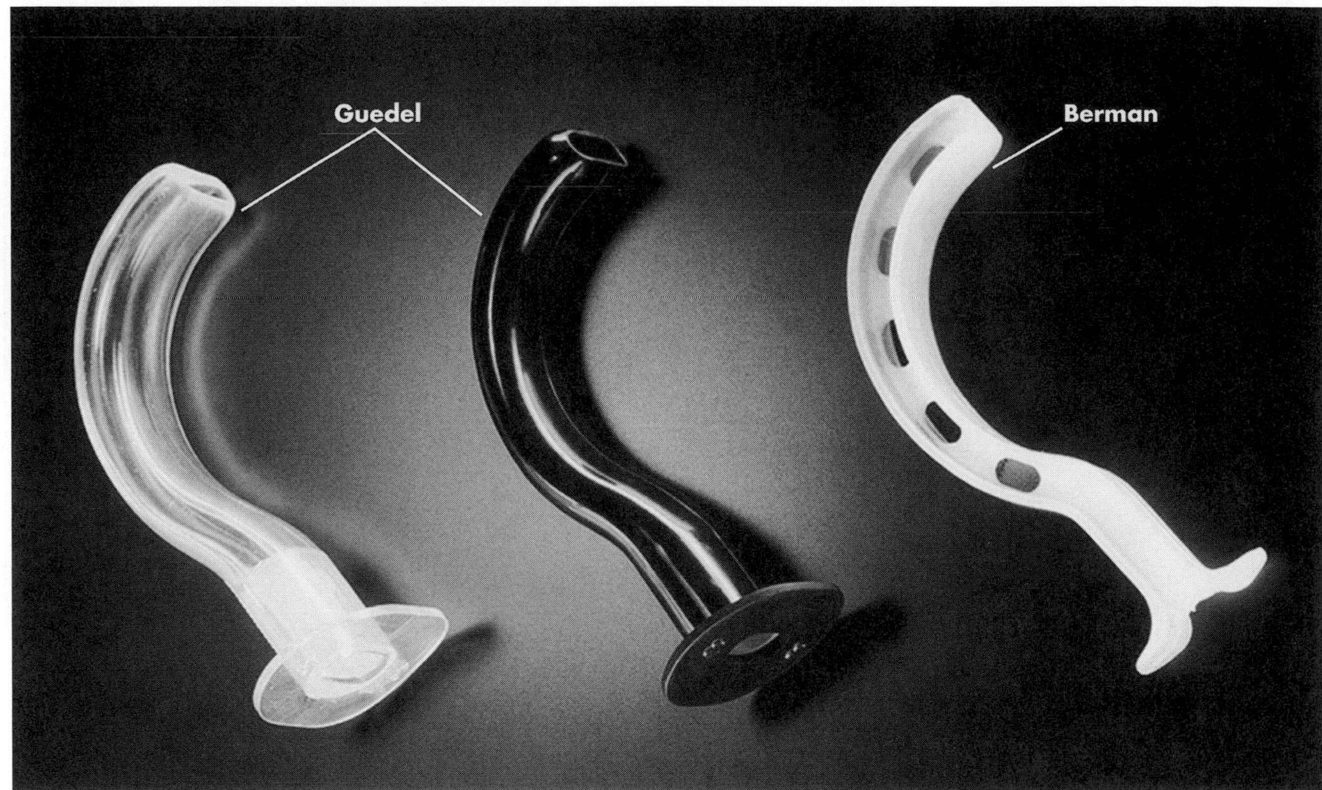

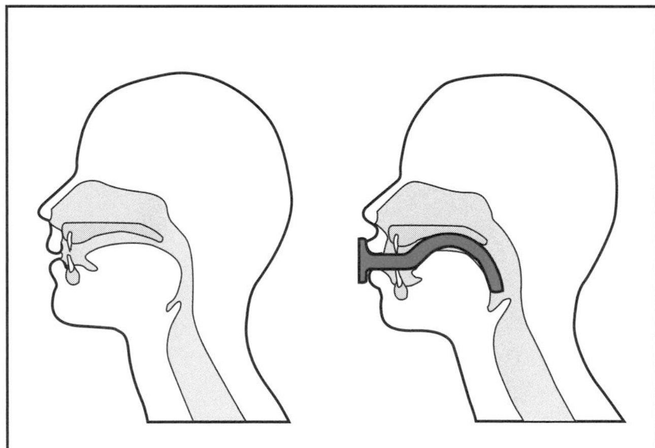

Figure 6-4 Guedel and Berman airways are upper airway devices used to provide air passage distal to an obstructing tongue. (Courtesy Cardinal Health, Respiratory Care Products and Services, McGaw Park, Ill.)

Nasopharyngeal Airways

Oropharyngeal airways are contraindicated in patients who retain airway protective reflexes, because gagging or vomiting may result. Such airways can cause dental damage if the patient forcibly bites the hard plastic or metal airway. If the patient struggles to expel the airway, attempts at insertion should be abandoned, and an improved head position or a nasopharyngeal airway should be used to open the upper airway. **Nasopharyngeal airways,** which are also called nasal trumpets or nasal airways, are better tolerated than are oral airways in semi-awake patients who retain some airway protective reflexes.

Nasopharyngeal airways resemble shortened, uncuffed endotracheal tubes and are made of soft latex or polyethylene. The end is flared to prevent airway loss through the nose. The ANSI sizing system gives the internal diameter in millimeters, although **French sizes** (i.e., the external circumference in millimeters) are also frequently used. The critical size, however, is related to the airway length, which must be long enough to pass to a position beyond the tongue base but not enter the esophagus. Each manufacturer uses a different length: diameter ratio, so the proper airway for a certain patient may be a matter of trial and error. The correct length of the nasopharyngeal airway can be estimated by positioning the airway along the side of the head. For proper function, the tip should extend past the angle of the jaw. An airway that is too long may enter the esophagus and not provide an air passage. Unlike oropharyngeal airways, nasopharyngeal airways that are too short will not make a bad airway worse, they just will not improve the problem.

Nasal bleeding can complicate insertion of the nasopharyngeal airway. Correct insertion technique, generous lubrication, and vasoconstrictive agents can reduce the frequency of this complication. A mixture of local anesthetic solution (i.e., 4% lidocaine) and phenylephrine (Neo-Synephrine) or oxymetazoline (Afrin) is effective in this regard. In emergency situations, the airway should only be well-lubricated to avoid delay for drug effects to occur.

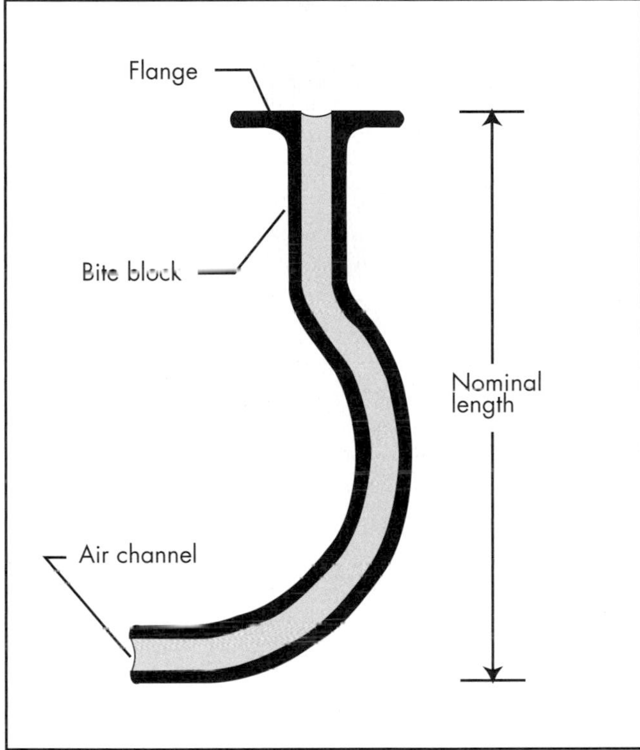

Figure 6-5 Oral airway components.

The airway is inserted parallel to the floor of the nasal pharynx and slightly medially (Figure 6-11). Mistakenly, clinicians often attempt to insert the airway "up the nose" (parallel to the long axis of the nose), which increases the likelihood of bleeding and fails to secure placement. The nasal pharyngeal opening is usually directly posterior to the anterior nares. The size of the external nares is unrelated to the room between the nasal turbinates. If undue resistance is met on one side of the nose, airway insertion should be attempted on the other side. Softer airways are less likely to cause bleeding and will conform to a distorted passageway as they pass through a narrow nasal channel. They are also more likely to obstruct and not allow passage of a suction catheter. The airway should be inserted with gentle, continuous pressure unless significant resistance is encountered. An airway that is smaller in diameter may be used if a larger one cannot be inserted. If only a small airway can be passed through the external nasal passage, it may not function because of its concomitant short length.

Uncuffed ETs can be used as nasopharyngeal airways (Figure 6-12). Tube length can be customized to fit individual patient anatomy. A long, thin tube can be created by trimming the tube to proper length. The tube connector can be used to prevent the tube from disappearing into the nose; however, the friction fit may be inadequate to prevent accidental separation. Also, the connector's internal diameter is smaller than the tube and may prevent suction catheter passage and limit gas flow rates during ventilation. Leaving extra length so that the tube can be taped at the correct distance is another solution, but it may reduce the efficiency of mask ventilation. Cut endotracheal tubes for nasopharyngeal

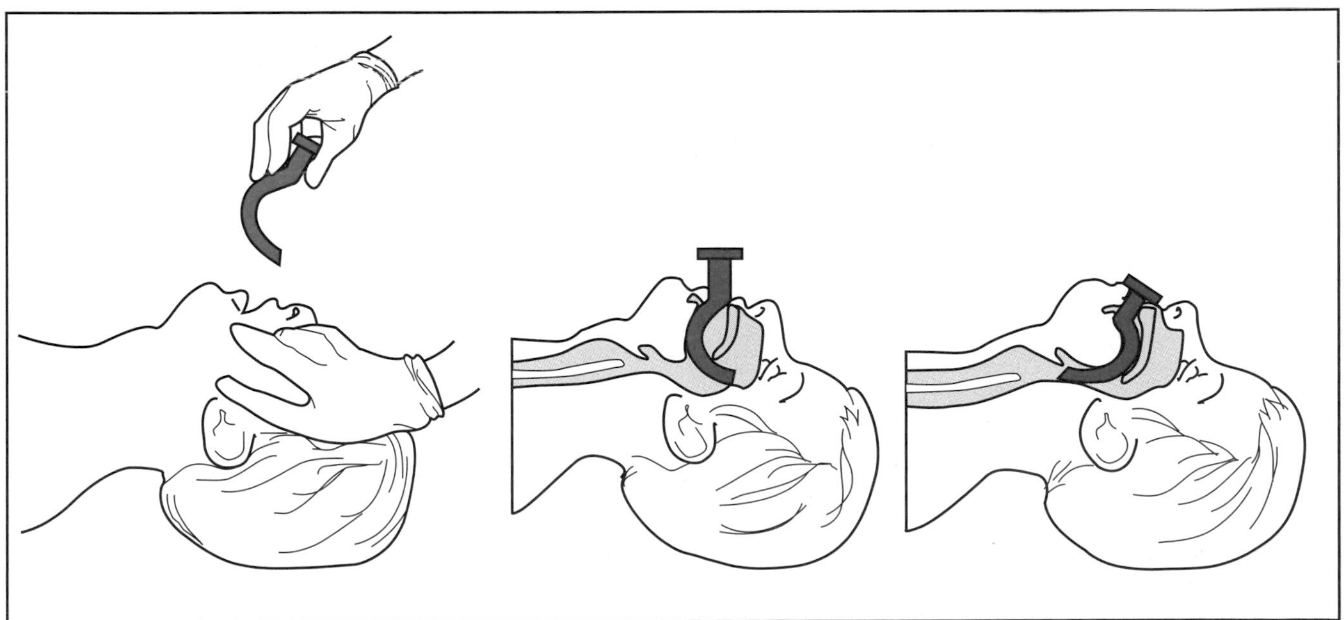

Figure 6-6 Antianatomical insertion of an oral airway.

airways are often used for infants and children. Accidental movement can be prevented by placing a safety pin through the side of the tube, avoiding compromise of the center lumen with the tube secured with tape (Figure 6-13).

As mentioned previously, nasal bleeding is a real concern, so nasopharyngeal airways should be used with caution in patients prone to uncontrollable bleeding. If bleeding occurs, use topical vasoconstrictors and directly tamponade the bleeding source by leaving the device in place. Significant hemorrhage may necessitate a transfusion. A relative contraindication for nasopharyngeal airway use is a basal skull fracture. Penetration of the brain by the airway is possible, although unlikely, so this risk must be weighed against the urgency of the airway need and the failure of other techniques. Sinus infection is a long-term risk of nasopharyngeal tube placement.

As with oral airways, fiberoptic or blind tracheal entry can be facilitated with a nasopharyngeal airway. Removal of the device after intubation is more difficult because split devices are not commercially available. Nasopharyngeal airways are useful for protecting the nose from trauma during blind nasotracheal suctioning. Once securely in place, they are usually well-tolerated—even in individuals who are awake.

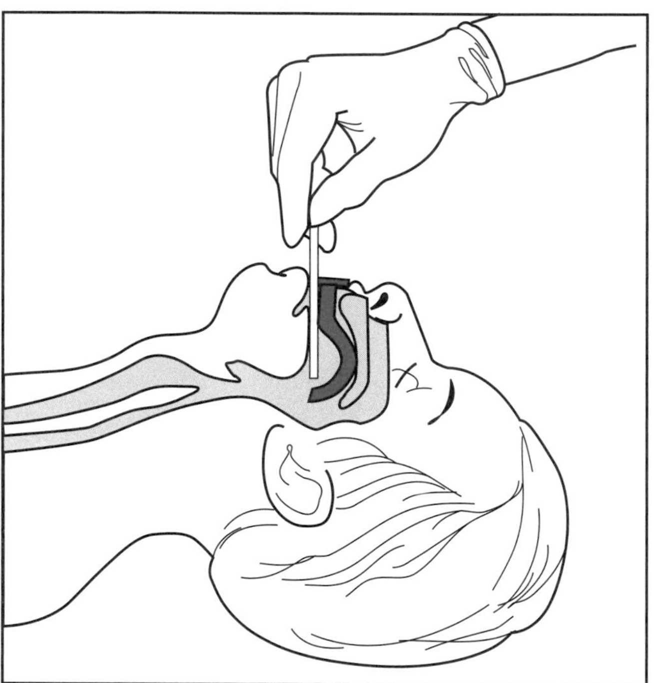

Figure 6-7 Anatomical insertion of an oral airway with a tongue blade.

Laryngeal Mask Airway (LMA)

Recently becoming popular, the LMA, or "mask on a tube," is designed to form a low-pressure seal in the laryngeal inlet by means of an inflated cuff. It is placed blindly and bypasses the upper airway structures. Its tip rests against the upper esophageal sphincter (cricopharyngeus muscle), and the cuff seats laterally in the pyriform fossa. It is equipped with a standard 15-mm slip fitting, and positive-pressure ventilation can be delivered. Pressures exceeding 20 cm of water usually result in ventilation volume loss and gas leakage around the cuff. This device does not replace endotracheal intubation because the lung is not protected from aspiration, although the quantity of aspirated material may be reduced compared to an unprotected airway. The LMA is a useful emergency airway device for several reasons: (1) insertion is simple and easy to teach and learn; (2) it provides a patent airway that is usually superior to that with an oral or nasopharyngeal device; (3) it does not require airway manipulation or extreme head positioning; and (4) once in place, it frees the user's hands for other tasks. Its major drawbacks are: (1) the expense; reusable models are handmade from silicone rubber and cost about $200, and disposable models cost about $36; (2) choosing the correct size is difficult because

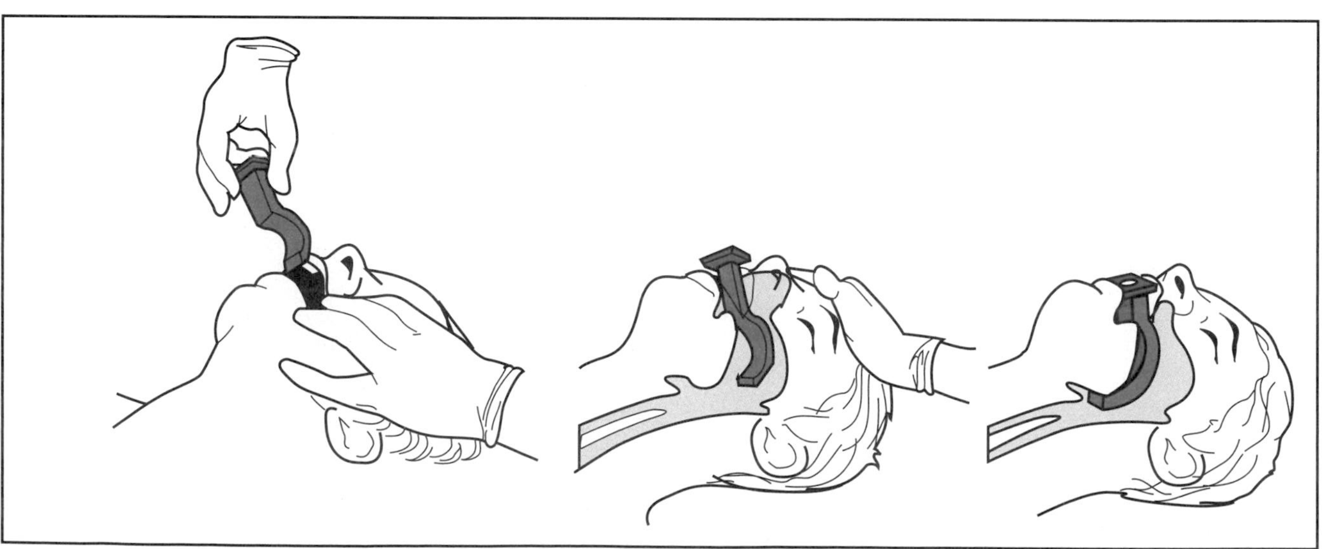

Figure 6-8 Insertion of an oral airway from the side of the mouth. The airway itself can be used as a tongue blade to displace the tongue while inserting the airway.

the larynx is not seen, so standard sizes are used but may not fit correctly, requiring a different-sized replacement; and (3) aspiration is not prevented. Sizes for neonates (size 1); children (sizes 2 and $2\frac{1}{2}$); and small, normal, and large adults (sizes 3, 4, and 5) are available in the reusable form, but only adult sizes (3, 4, and 5) are available as single-use devices.

The cuff is inflated and examined for discoloration and its ability to maintain inflation, then it is deflated completely and everted (Figure 6-14). A water-soluble lubricant is used on the back side of the cuff to help slide it past the hard and soft palates. Insertion of the LMA is easily accomplished. The insertion technique is shown in Figure 6-15. A black line along the length of the tube marks the center of the device and is used to prevent rotation after the placement. The head may be extended and a finger used to guide the deflated cuff past the tongue and pharynx. The tube is held in place with the other hand while the guiding fingers are withdrawn. The tube is then advanced until it is fully seated, and resistance to further insertion is felt. With the tube free in the mouth, the cuff is inflated. If it is seated correctly in the pyriform sinuses, the tube will move back about 1 cm out of the mouth. This should be done "hands free" and without any ventilation equipment attached to the tube. If the mask is too small, it may pass down the esophagus, and no backward movement will occur on cuff inflation. The final test of correct placement is that adequate breath sounds are present over both lung fields and not over the stomach with positive-pressure ventilation. If ventilation fails, the head position may be altered (further extension is usually helpful), the LMA inserted farther, or the device removed and reinserted. A size change may also be necessary. After the device is properly placed and a patent airway obtained, the tube is secured with tape; then either spontaneous or positive-pressure ventilation can be used. Attention must still to be paid to the airway when it is secured with the LMA because loss of airway patency, which can be due to device dislodgment or twisting, foreign body aspiration, or LMA obstruction, has been reported.

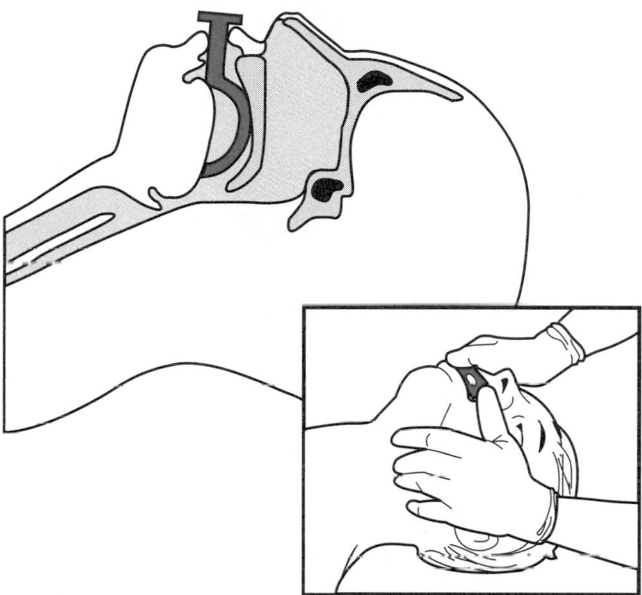

Figure 6-9 A jaw thrust is performed to seat the oropharyngeal airway, which has become blocked by the tongue. When the correct-size oropharyngeal airway fails to seat properly and protrudes from the mouth, performing a jaw thrust and using the thumbs to insert the airway will provide proper placement.

Blind (or fiberoptic) intubation with a cuffed endotracheal tube can be performed through an LMA to establish a definitive or secure airway, as shown in Figure 6-16. Occasionally the epiglottis is trapped under the LMA (it usually lies on top of the mask cuff), but this seems to have

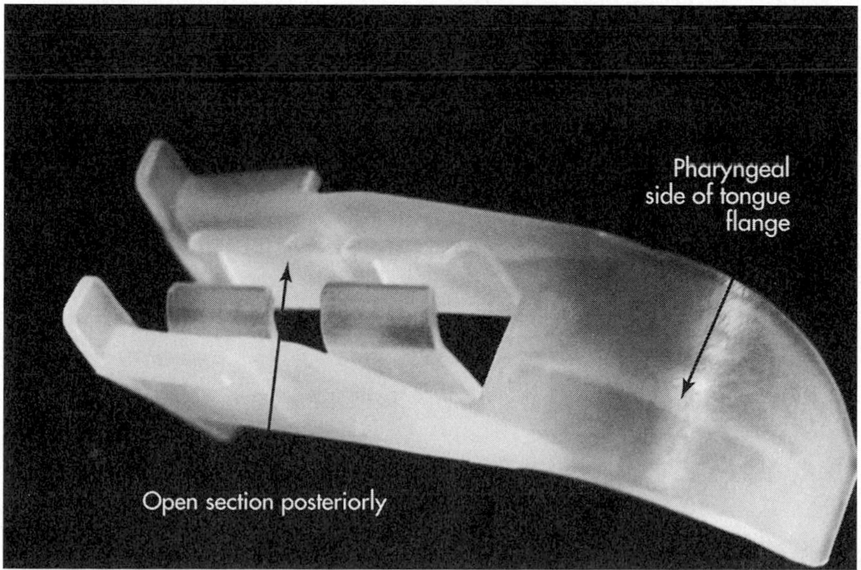

Figure 6-10 Intubating airways can be used to support and direct a fiberoptic bronchoscope and ET into the trachea with direct vision. The incomplete channel allows separation of the scope from the airway after tracheal intubation. (From Benumof JL: *Airway management: principles and practice*, St Louis, 1996, Mosby.)

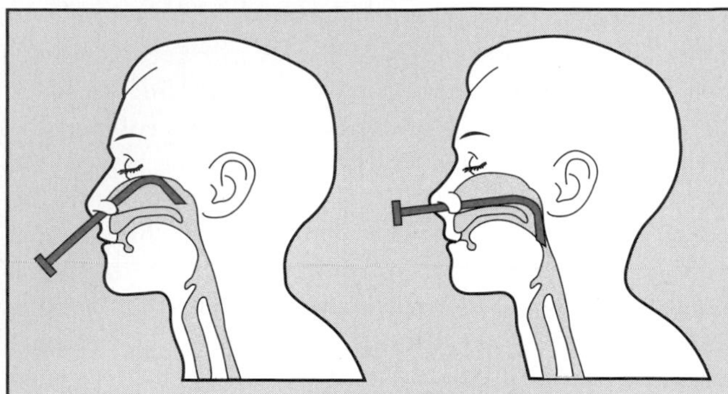

Figure 6-11 Placement of a nasopharyngeal airway. The correct way to insert the device is to advance the tip directly posteriorly–not upward–because the nasopharynx lies directly behind the external nares.

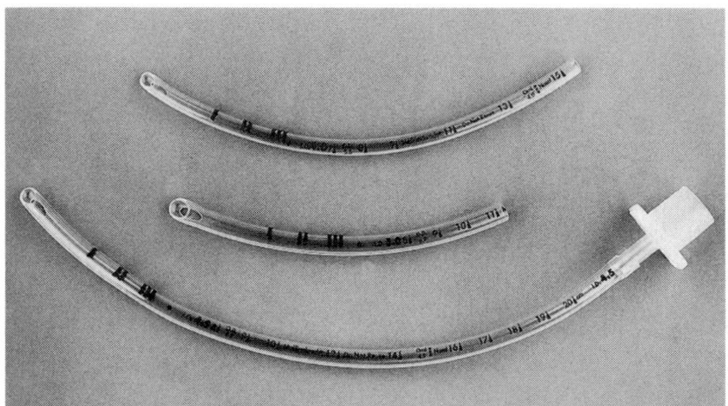

Figure 6-12 Uncuffed ETs can be used as nasopharyngeal airways.

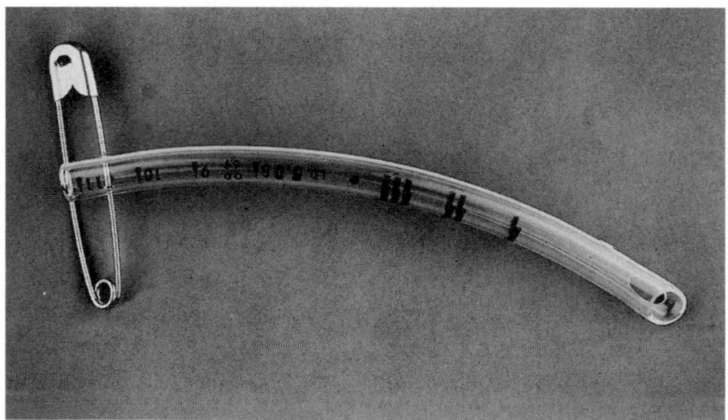

Figure 6-13 Use of a safety pin just through the tube wall helps secure a custom-cut ET used as a nasopharyngeal airway.

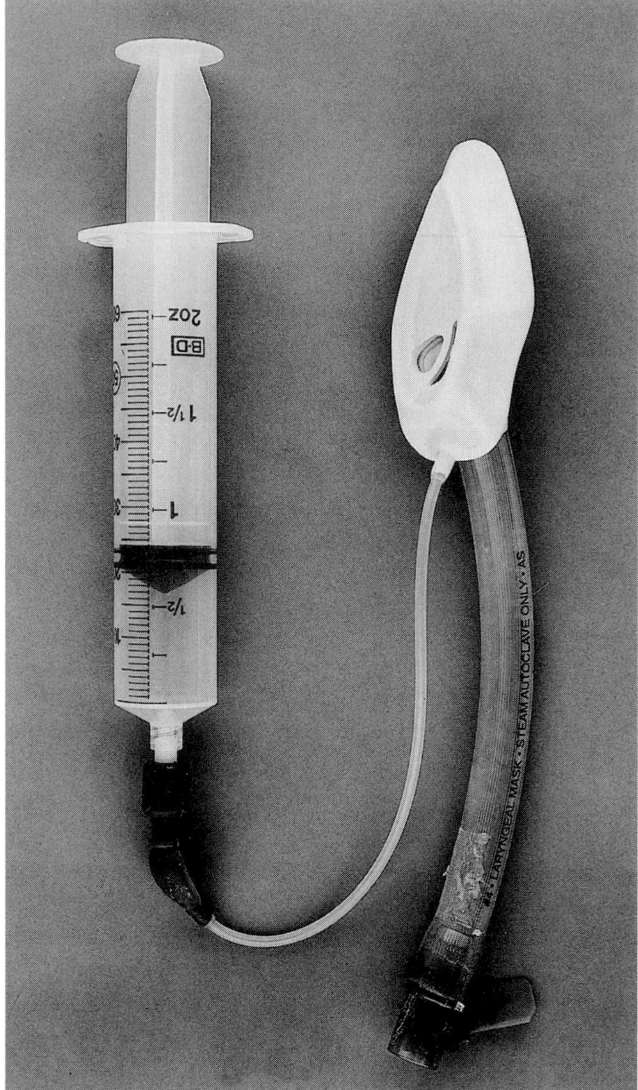

Figure 6-14 For correct LMA insertion, the cuff should be completely deflated with the mask forming an upward, open-bowl configuration. This minimizes risk of oral damage and helps prevent the mask from folding over during insertion.

little effect on its function. The LMA is of particular use in patients with a known or anticipated difficult airway. Pregnant and obese patients predictably have improved ventilation with an LMA when compared with other upper airway control devices. The LMA is potentially life-saving when intubation has failed.

LMA use is becoming widespread outside of operating rooms because it is easier to master the necessary LMA skills than those needed for effective mask ventilation or endotracheal intubation. Emergency personnel are reporting excellent results in field trials. Infant and pediatric use is especially encouraging because the skills necessary for other airway techniques for these patients are difficult to learn and maintain.

After use, LMAs should be mechanically washed with a mild soap solution and autoclaved at 134° C or less. The cuff must be completely evacuated or it will rupture during the sterilization process. Glutaraldehyde should not be used because it is quite toxic to the laryngeal mucosa. LMAs may be resterilized 100 to 200 times, but marked discoloration and failure of the pilot tube and cuff to hold pressure are indications that the tube should be discarded. Disposable, single-use LMAs in adult sizes have been produced and are available for clinical use. They are less reliable but are useful in emergencies and in areas where a central processing and control system is unavailable.

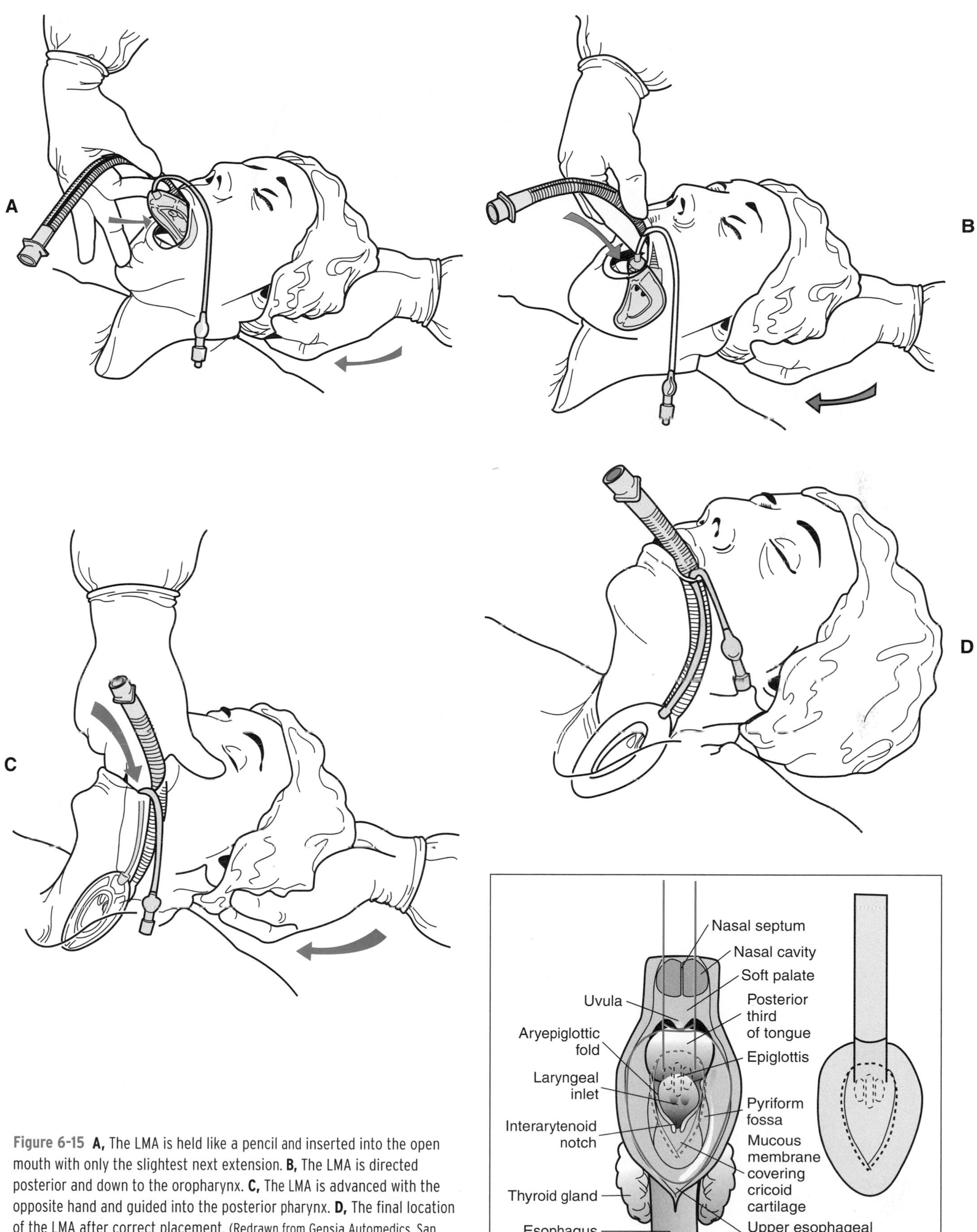

Figure 6-15 **A,** The LMA is held like a pencil and inserted into the open mouth with only the slightest next extension. **B,** The LMA is directed posterior and down to the oropharynx. **C,** The LMA is advanced with the opposite hand and guided into the posterior pharynx. **D,** The final location of the LMA after correct placement. (Redrawn from Gensia Automedics, San Diego, Brain Medical Limited, 1992.)

Fastrack LMA

Taking advantage of the fact that the LMA is simple to place and rests directly in front the larynx, a modification of the device has been developed to facilitate intubation in the patient with a difficult airway. Called the Fastrack (Figure 6-17), this device consists of a curved, hollow metal shaft, preformed to fit the average airway. The Fastrack tube is large enough to pass a special cuffed, Silastic wire—wrapped ET tube through the larynx and into the trachea. The Fastrack has a metal handle allowing control and manipulation of the mask orientation, improving the chances of blind intubation. After intubation, the Fastrack is removed using a "pusher" to maintain the endotracheal tube in place. The Fastrack device is an important part of any emergency or difficult airway cart.

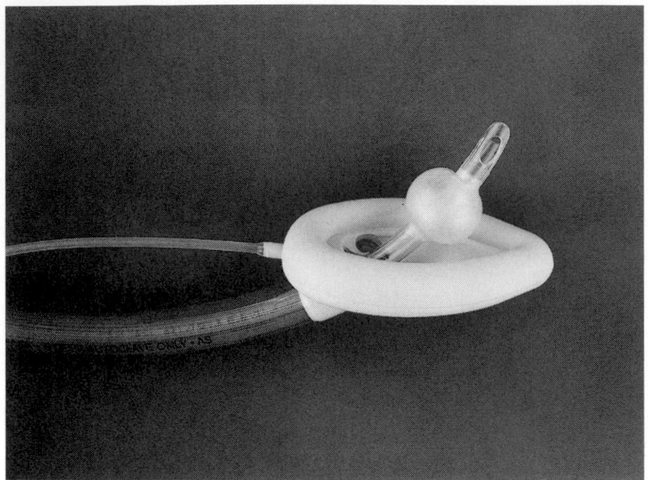

Figure 6-16 The intubating LMA is show with its special Silastic ET and tube pusher which is used to help remove the LMA and leave the ET tube in place.

Combitube

The **Combitube** is a double-lumen device designed to provide a patent upper airway when inserted blindly in comatose patients with airway difficulties or after failed intubation. It has two cuffs designed to seal in the esophagus and the pharynx (Figure 6-18). The tube is lubricated and inserted through the mouth, following the contour to the pharynx. Insertion continues until the depth marks reach the lips or significant resistance is encountered. The cuffs are then inflated, the esophageal cuff with 15 mL and the pharyngeal cuff with 100 mL. The esophageal lumen may occasionally enter the trachea, and because it has an opening at its end, it can be used as a conventional ET. Ventilation is normally provided through the other lumen, which opens in a series of holes into the hypopharynx. The

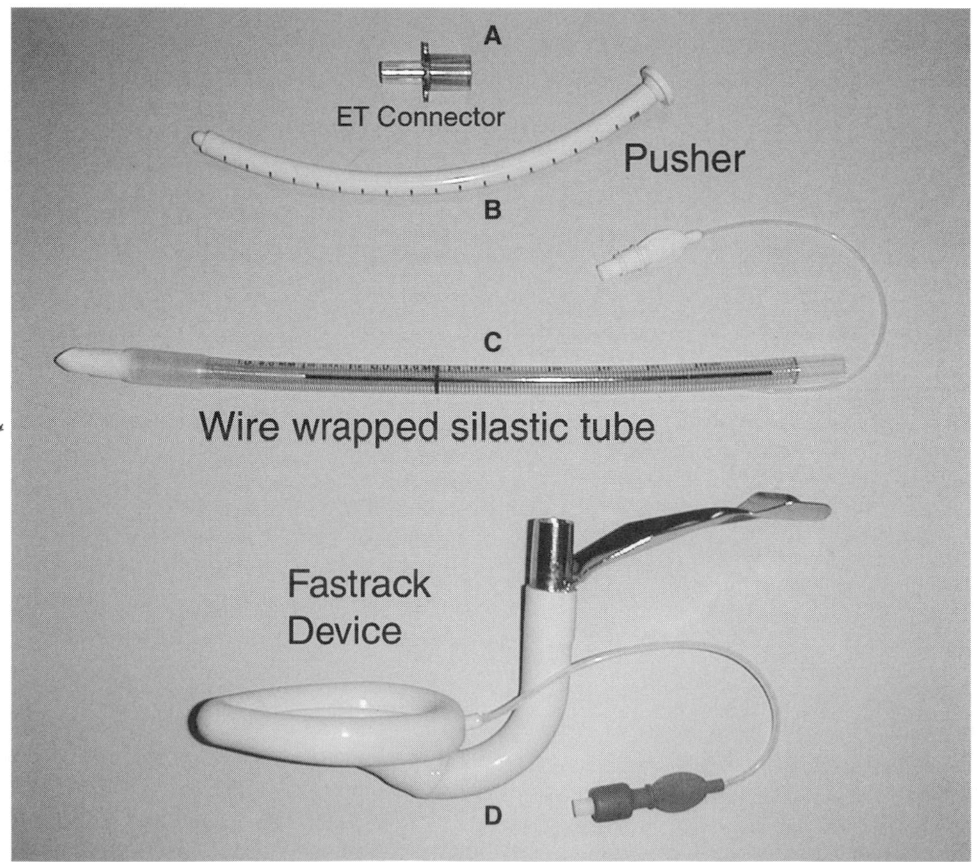

Figure 6-17 The Fastrack Tube.

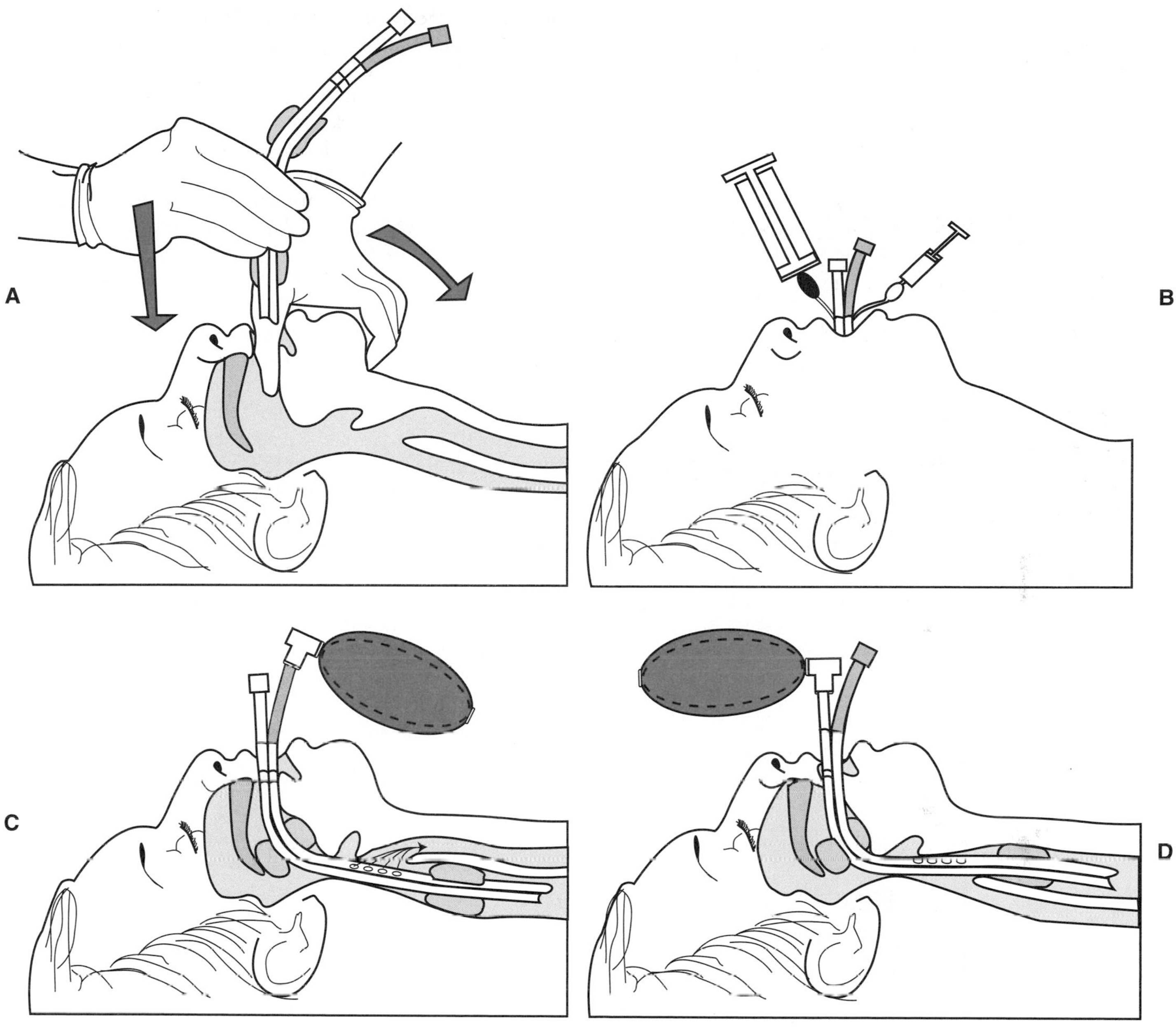

Figure 6-18 The Combitube is inserted with the head in the neutral position **(A)** and both cuffs inflated **(B).** The two possible locations of the distal lumen are the usual, esophageal **(C)** and rarely, the trachea **(D).**

esophageal cuff affords some protection from regurgitation, but as with the LMA, the Combitube is not considered a secure airway device. A nasogastric tube can be inserted through the esophageal lumen into the stomach for decompression; unfortunately, only one size (for average adults) is available.

Endotracheal Tubes

The definitive device for airway management is a cuffed ET. ETs allow ventilation with high levels of positive pressure, provide direct access to the lower airway for secretion removal and drug delivery, prevent aspiration of foreign material into the lung, and permit bronchoscopic examination of the peripheral airways. Placing an ET requires a high degree of skill and specialized equipment (i.e., **laryngoscopes**) and risks hypoxia and hypercarbia and attendant cardiovascular changes during attempted placement. Before ET placement, adequate gas exchange must be established using other airway devices or maneuvers. Intubation may be an urgent procedure but should rarely be performed in a patient without a previously established patent airway and at least reasonable gas exchange. If a patent airway cannot be established by a simple means, an invasive airway (needle or surgical cricothyrotomy)—not insertion of an ET through the mouth or nose—should be performed quickly. Therefore, endotracheal intubation should be an elective procedure.

The conventional, or Murphy type, of ET consists of a round, plastic tube with a beveled tip, a sidehole (Murphy eye) opposite the bevel, a cuff attached to a pilot balloon with a spring-loaded valve, and a 15-mm standard connector. These components are shown in Figure 6-19. The tube should have distance markers indicated and a radiopaque marker imbedded along its length. The Murphy eye allows gas flow if the bevel tip becomes occluded. ETs lacking Murphy eyes are called Magill type of tubes. ETs are sized by internal diameter (in millimeters), although occasionally French sizes are reported (outer circumference in millimeters). Uncuffed tubes are generally used for children because the smaller lumen necessary to accommodate a cuff would further compromise an airway that is already small in diameter. Also, the narrowest part of an infant's airway is below the larynx at the cricoid ring, and a snug fit at this level will permit positive-pressure ventilation. The correct size tube for an infant or child can only be determined during actual intubation; a tube that will not pass easily down the trachea should be changed for a smaller diameter tube. To avoid postintubation croup or subglottic stenosis, an air leak at about 20 cm H_2O should be obtained in children intubated with an uncuffed ET.

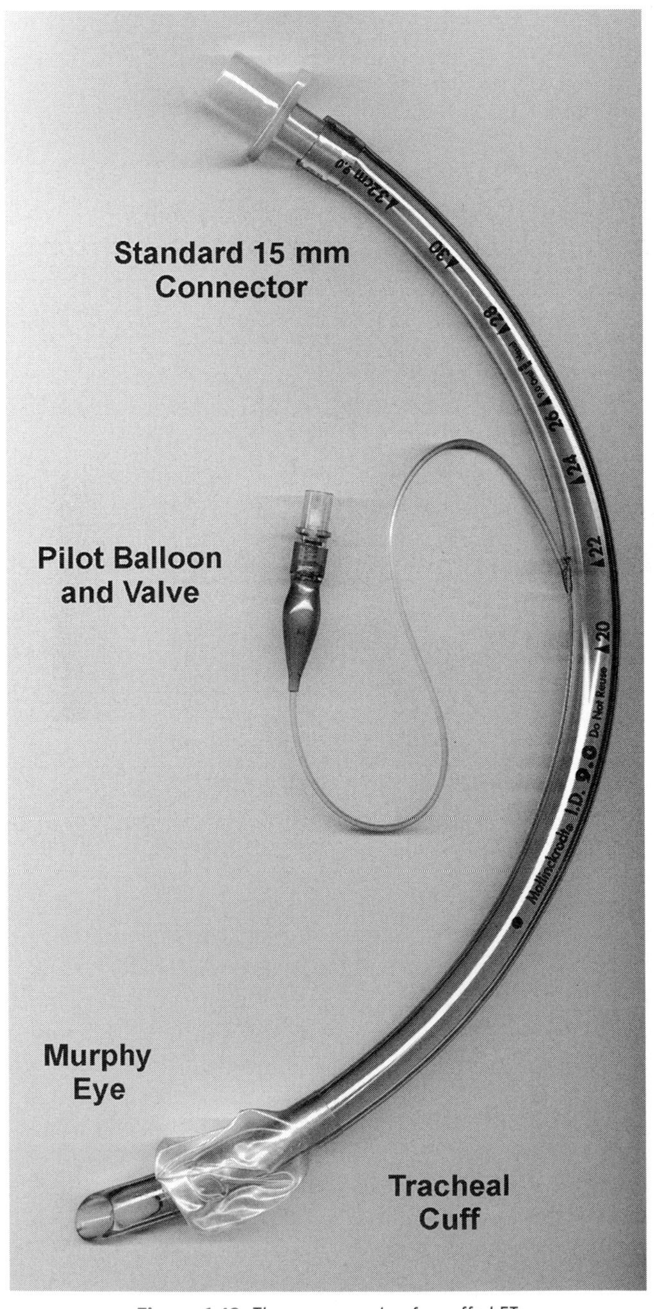

Figure 6-19 The components of a cuffed ET.

Many variants of the basic ET design have been developed to solve clinical problems. The plastic tube tends to collapse and obstruct when bent at an angle, which frequently occurs in the posterior pharynx with a nasally placed ET. Spiral wire-embedded tubes (Figure 6-20) help prevent this problem, but these tubes are flimsy, do not hold a preformed arch shape, and are often difficult to place in the trachea. Another solution to the bending/kinking problem is the RAE tube (Ring-Adair-Elwin), which has a preformed bend for oral or nasal intubation, as shown in Figures 6-21 and 6-22. Because bend placement is based on tube diameter and "average" patient dimensions, these tubes may not be the correct shape for certain patients and should be used with caution. During laser surgery in the airway, problems with ET fires have been reported. Flexible, corrugated metal tubes without cuffs, foil-wrapped tubes, and water-filled double-cuffed tubes have helped overcome this problem. Several of these devices are shown in Figure 6-23.

Aids to Endotracheal Intubation

The ET is placed through the mouth or nose into the trachea, and the cuff forms a seal against the tracheal wall. Placement of the ET is usually performed using a laryngoscope, which allows direct vision of the larynx and control of the supraglottic structures. Laryngoscopes consist of a handle that also contains batteries and a detachable blade with a light. There are two basic types of laryngoscope blades: straight (**Miller** type) and curved (**Macintosh** type). Laryngoscopy is performed slightly differently with each type of blade. With either blade attached, the handle is held like a hammer in the left hand (although "left-handed" models have been made, which are to be held in the right hand) with the blade down and the long axis directed forward (Figure 6-24). The mouth is opened and the blade is inserted along the right side of the tongue. After it is past the base of the tongue, the blade is brought back to the midline of the oral cavity, moving the tongue completely to the left. With the straight blade, the epiglottis is identified and hooked with the tip of the blade, the jaw and epiglottis are lifted forward and upward (not rocked backward, which would cause trauma to the upper teeth), and the light then shines on the larynx and down the trachea. With a curved blade, the epiglottis is identified and the tip inserted above it into the vallecula. With the same forward and upward lift, the larynx is illuminated, and the ET can be passed into the trachea. The light is farther down toward the blade tip on

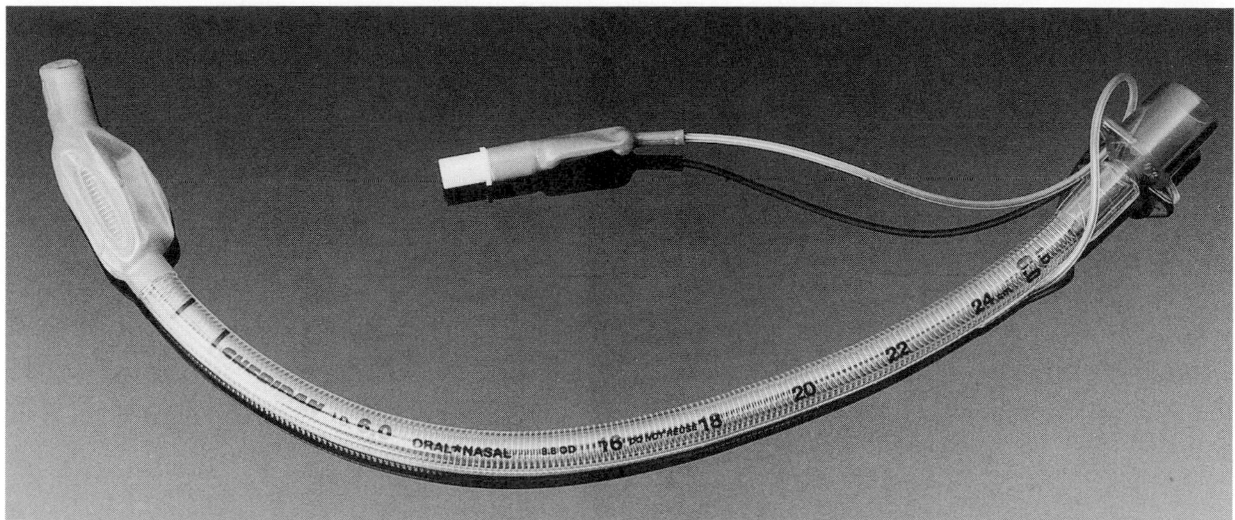

Figure 6-20 Spiral wire-reinforced ET.

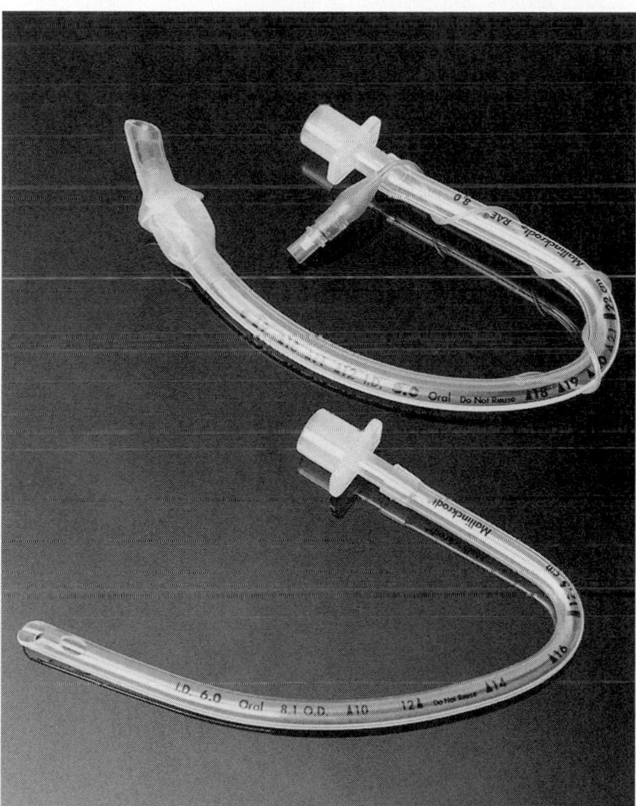

Figure 6-21 Cuffed and uncuffed oral RAE ETs in various sizes with preformed curves.

straight blades and brightly illuminates the larynx, whereas the light on curved blades is about midway down the blade and illuminates the pharynx and supraglottic area. The broad flange (Figure 6-25) of the curved blade gives better tongue control and more working room for tube insertion than does the straight blade. In children, the epiglottis is less rigid than in adults, and often a straight-blade technique (i.e., lifting the epiglottis) is necessary, even if a curved blade is used.

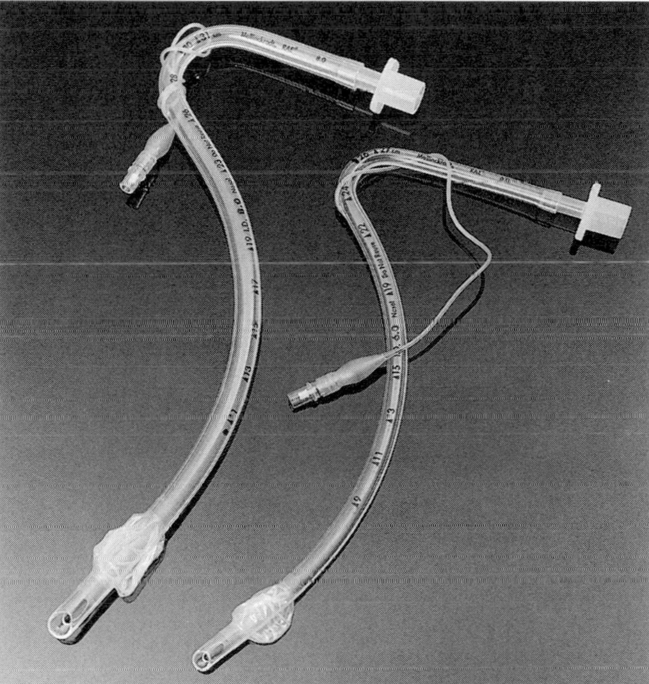

Figure 6-22 Nasal RAE ETs in various sizes with nasal curves.

The basic laryngoscope blades have been modified over the years. The size and shape of the flange and the location of the light on the curved blade are common places for innovation. Ports for suction or oxygen insufflation have been added. Straight blades have had modifications of cross-sectional shape to give better tongue control or working room during ET insertion. No standardized size equivalency is represented in blade numbers, but a #0 or #1 blade is generally correct for infants, and a #3 is usually appropriate for average adults. The angle the blade leaves the handle is another area of modification. An acute angle may improve visualization, and an obtuse or offset angle may allow insertion

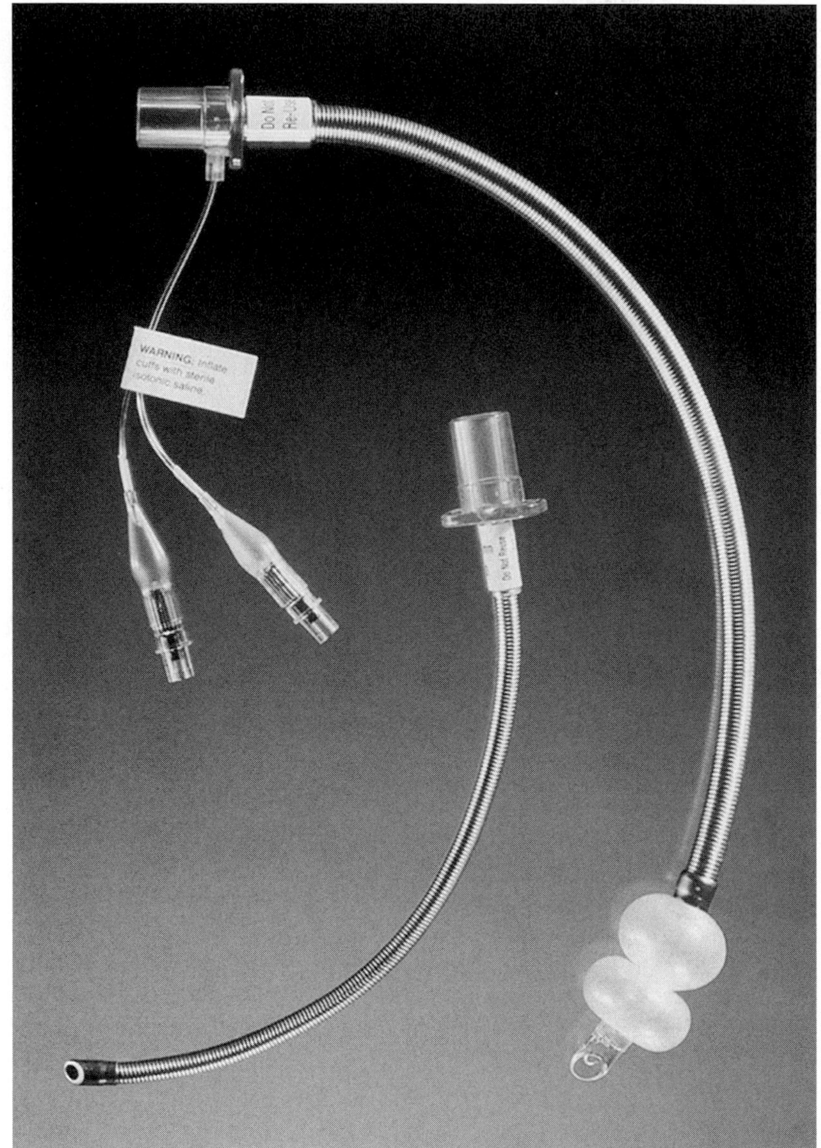

Figure 6-23 Flammable materials cause problem during laser surgery. Metal tubes and water-filled cuffs are solutions to this problem. (Courtesy Cardinal Health, Respiratory Care Products and Services, McGaw Park, Ill.)

of the blade when pendulous breasts or an orthopedic apparatus is in the way. An angled blade tip, a mirror, or a prism may allow the intubator to see "around the corner" into the larynx. These specialized devices are expensive and require considerable practice to master their use.

Although being able to see the laryngeal structures is useful, a good view does not guarantee ET insertion. Manipulating the ET into the trachea can be facilitated in several ways. The first is proper head position. As shown in Figure 6-1, the sniffer's position is ideal for opening up the upper airway and aligning the trachea for intubation. The next consideration is the position of the intubator's head. The intubator's head should be far enough away from the patient's mouth to allow binocular vision (Figure 6-26, *A* and *B*). In *B*, the intubator is too close to the airway, and depth perception is compromised. In general, if the laryngoscope arm is 90 degrees or more at the elbow, eye distance will be correct. In difficult intubations, the larynx is often described as being anteriorly placed, which means that the laryngeal opening is above the field of vision with the laryngoscope. A malleable stylette can be inserted into the ET to provide stiffness and be bent to give the tube an upward hook at its end. This so-called "hockey stick curve" is very useful if the problem is an anterior location of the larynx. Intubation can often be accomplished with this curved tip, even if a direct laryngeal view is not possible. So that it can be easily withdrawn, the stylette should be lubricated before it is placed into the ET. Another solution to controlling the ET tip is the Endotrol Tube (Mallinckrodt Medical, Inc.). With this device, an implanted string with a pull-ring turns the tip anterior when pulled (Figure 6-27). This device is particularly well-suited for blind nasotracheal intubation.

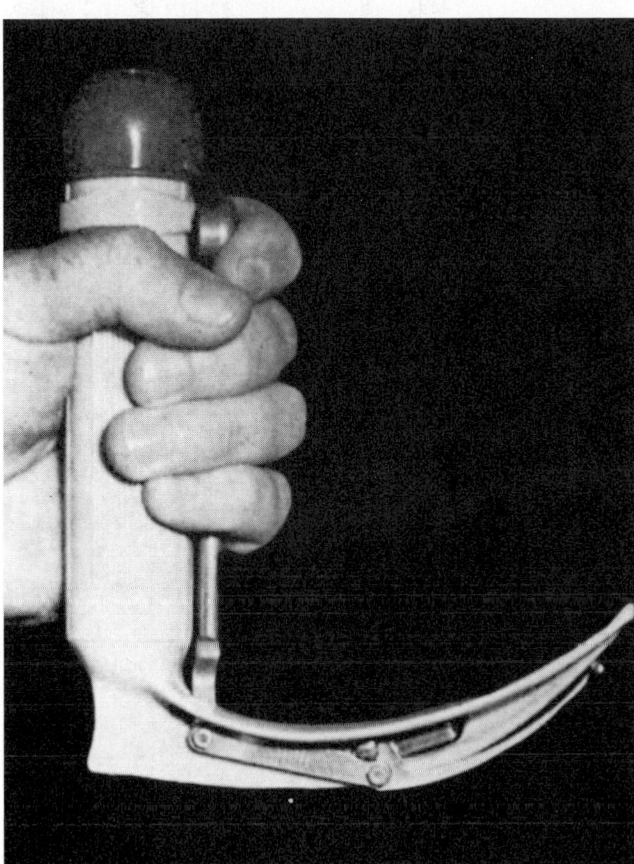

Figure 6-24 The laryngoscope is held like a hammer in the left hand. (From Grant GC: A new laryngoscope, *Anesthes Intens Care* V(3):263, 1977.)

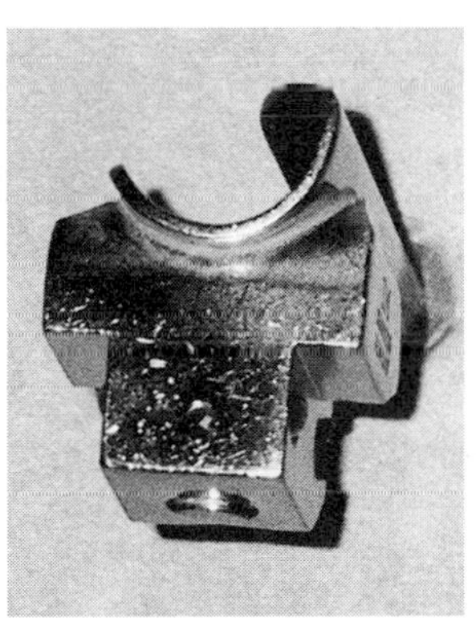

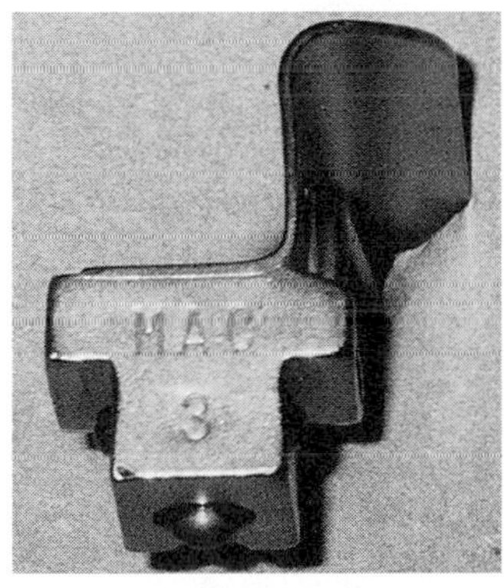

A B

Figure 6-25 Cross-section of straight and curved blades. The broad flange of the curved blade gives better tongue control and working room during intubation.

When the larynx cannot be seen, it may be possible to pass a rigid stylette blindly into the trachea. The Eschmann stylette or the gum elastic bougie is such a device. A characteristic washboard feeling is obtained when the device is advancing down the trachea over the tracheal rings. An ET can be threaded over the stylette to obtain intubation.

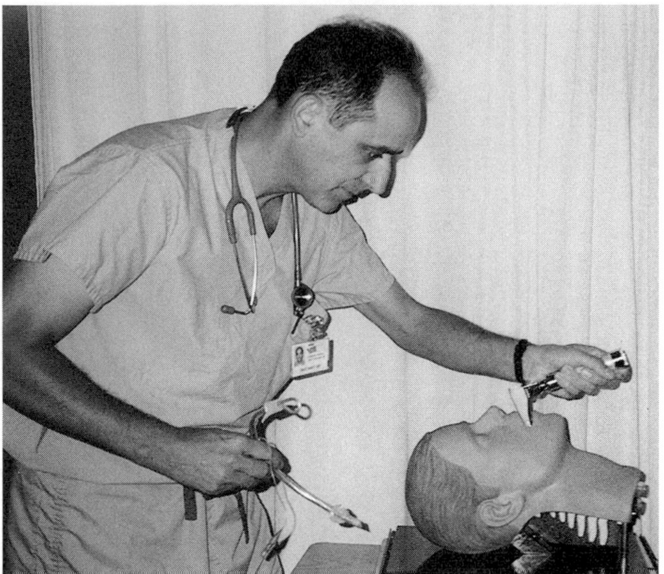

A

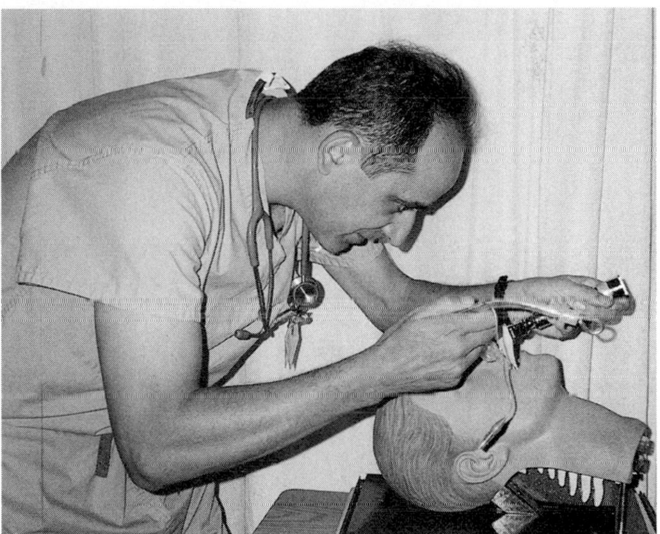

B

Figure 6-26 **A,** The correct head to trachea distance during intubation allows depth perception to be maintained. **B,** Being too close to the airway does not allow the proper distance to be perceived, so intubation is more difficult.

Lighted stylettes can be used to blindly place ETs in spontaneously breathing patients. In a darkened room, the light at the tip of the ET can be seen through the tissues of the neck. A characteristic V-shaped shadow is seen when the tube is directly in front of the trachea. The ET is then slid off the stylette into the trachea.

Another approach to tracheal intubation is through the nasal passage. Nasotracheal intubation is usually performed in spontaneously breathing, semiconscious individuals. As with nasopharyngeal airway insertion, a well-lubricated ET is inserted posteriorly, directly through the nasopharynx. Topical local anesthetics and vasoconstrictors should reduce patient discomfort and bleeding. Instead of the sniffing

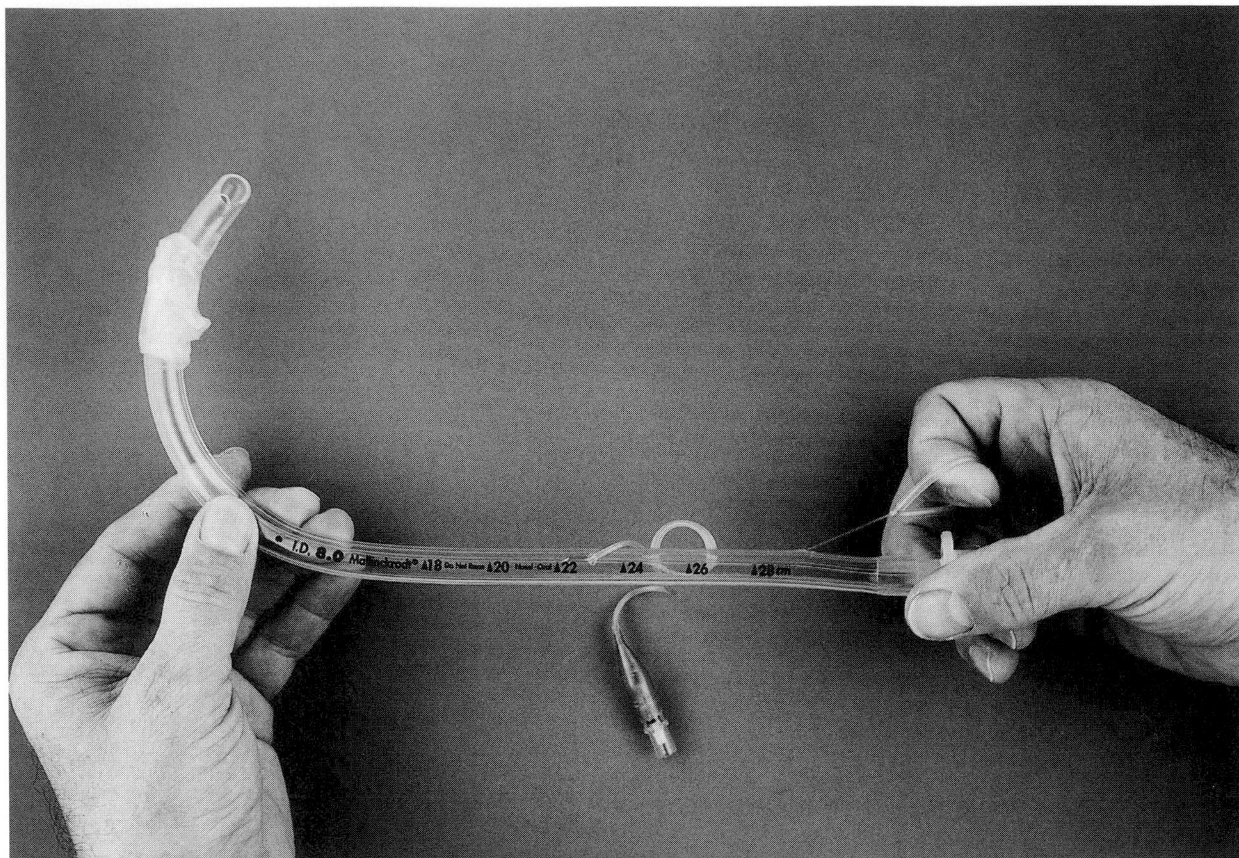

Figure 6-27 The Endotrol Tube has a string that when pulled directs the tip anteriorly during intubation attempts.

position, a neutral or slightly flexed head position is optimal for blind nasal intubation. Breath sounds or moisture in the tube is used to identify the tip location and the timing of tube advancement. Breath sounds or moisture disappears when the tube enters the esophagus. ETs are placed just above the larynx and rapidly advanced 1 to 2 cm during inspiration when the cords are maximally abducted. If tracheal topical anesthesia is not used, a vigorous cough will follow successful tracheal intubation. Turning the head to one side or the other or flexing it further or pushing the thyroid cartilage posteriorly may lead to success. Use of the fiberoptic bronchoscope may be necessary to complete nasotracheal intubation in some difficult settings. A nasally inserted ET tube can be directed anteriorly into the trachea using a laryngoscope in the mouth and Magill forceps, although care must be taken not to rip the cuff with the sharp teeth of the Magill forceps.

Fiberoptic laryngoscopy allows ET insertion by using the scope as a guide. The ET is threaded over the scope before endoscopy, but the standard ET connector needs to be removed first. After the airway is entered, the tube can be guided over the scope and into the trachea. This technique can be used for oral or nasal intubation. Skill in fiberoptic examination of the unintubated patient is a prerequisite for this technique (Clinical Rounds 6-1).

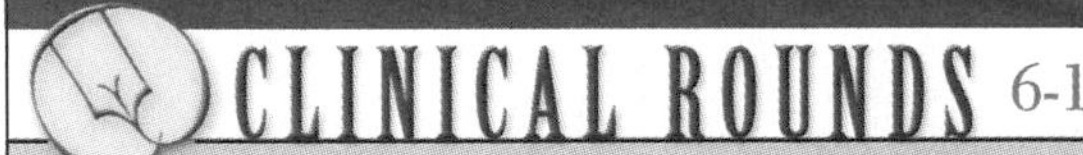

A 56-year-old man who has experienced cardiopulmonary arrest is admitted to the emergency department. Several attempts to insert an ET have not established a definitive and secure airway. What alternative methods could be used to establish a secure airway for this patient?

See Appendix A for the answer.

Blind oral ET insertion techniques have been described. Using two fingers to retract the epiglottis and direct the tube tip anteriorly can result in proper placement. The Berman intubating airway (Berman II) is an oropharyngeal airway with a hooked end and an open channel for an ET. The ET is placed through the channel while the tip is used to lift the vallecula. The tube can be passed into the trachea blindly and then separated from the open channel of the airway.

After the ET is in place in the trachea, the cuff can be used to form a seal with the tracheal wall. Usually, air is inflated through the one-way valve in the pilot balloon until a seal forms or high pressure develops. Most ET cuffs are

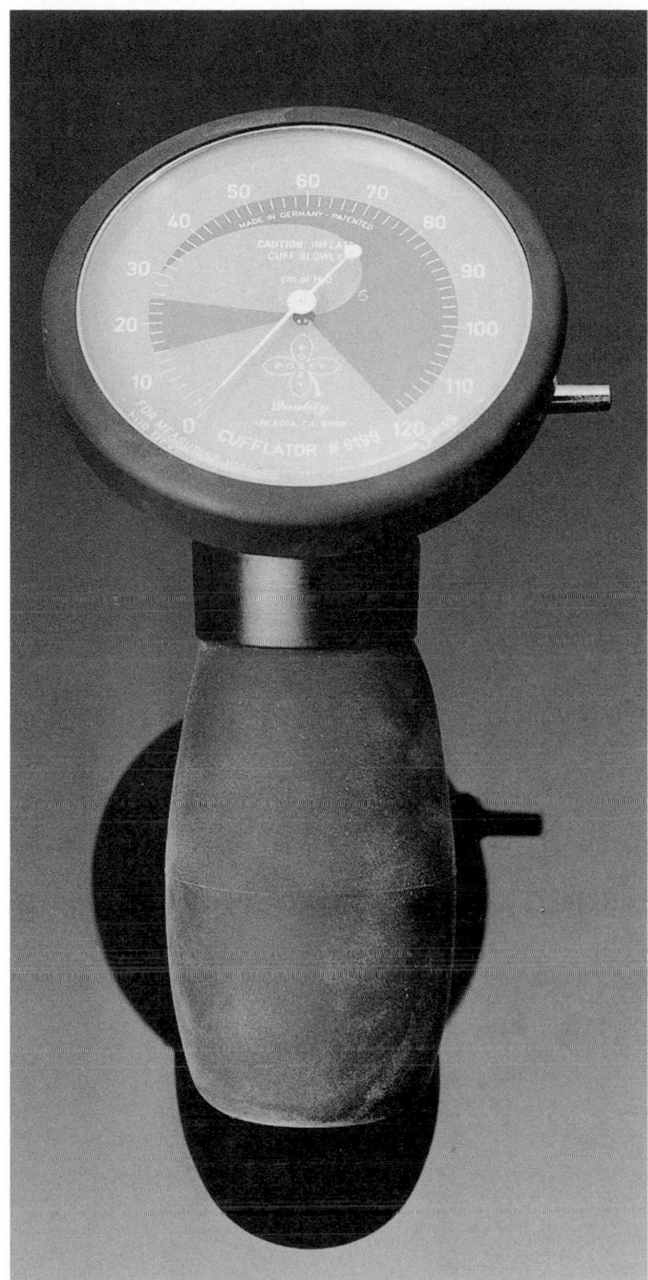

Figure 6-28 A device for measuring ET cuff pressure.

large-volume, low-pressure devices meant to contact a large portion of the tracheal wall with a low pressure. Because of tracheal mucosal blood pressure-flow characteristics, cuff pressure should be below 25 cm Hg to prevent tracheal damage. A manometer for determining and regulating cuff pressure is shown in Figure 6-28. If a manometer is not available, a "just seal" or "minimal seal" technique can be used to minimize the lateral tracheal wall pressure from the inflated cuff. For some patients who require high airway pressure for mechanical ventilation, cuff pressure cannot be kept below 25 cm Hg without significant volume loss. Whatever pressure is needed should be used to guarantee adequate ventilation and protection from aspiration. An

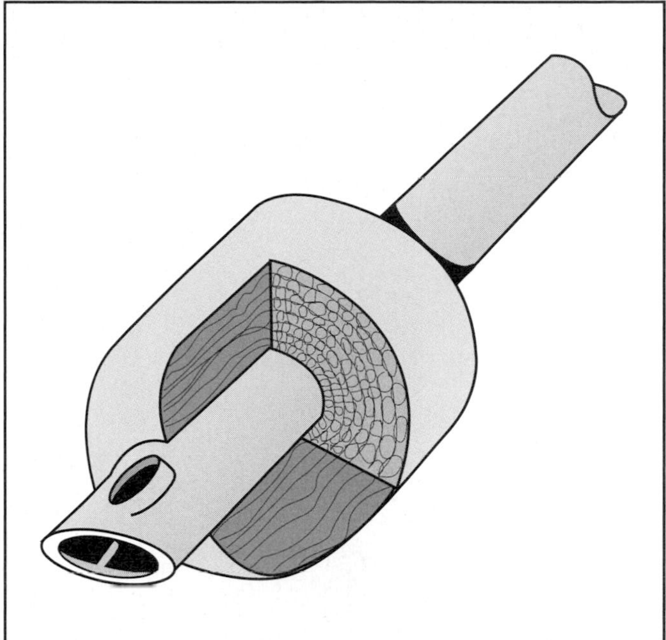

Figure 6-29 An ET tube with a self-inflating, foam-filled cuff.

alternative to an inflatable cuff is a self-inflating one that is filled with foam (Figure 6-29). Before insertion, this type of cuff must be actively deflated and clamped, then the clamp is removed and the cuff is allowed to expand to form a seal. There is no valve in the pilot port of foam-filled cuffs. A common problem with ETs is that they are inserted or migrate too far into the trachea, so the cuff may obstruct a bronchus or only one lung may be ventilated. Right mainstem intubation is most common, especially in children, because the angle of take-off of the right main bronchus is less than that of the left.

Confirmation of Tracheal Intubation

Objective confirmation of tracheal placement, rather than esophageal intubation, is imperative. This is especially true after intubating with a blind technique. The best way to confirm correct placement is to detect expired carbon dioxide with a capnograph or a color-change device; however, these devices will not detect carbon dioxide when cardiac output is profoundly depressed (e.g., during chest compressions for cardiac arrest). The esophageal detection device (a rubber bulb attached to the ET) will rapidly reinflate if the ET is in the trachea, but will remain collapsed if the ET is in the esophagus (Figure 6-30). This device does not depend on cardiac function to confirm correct tube placement. False-positive and false-negative results have been reported by this device in obese and pregnant patients. Auscultation should be performed in at least three areas after intubation. This examination should evidence bilateral thoracic breath sounds, but no audible sounds over the gastric area. Sounds

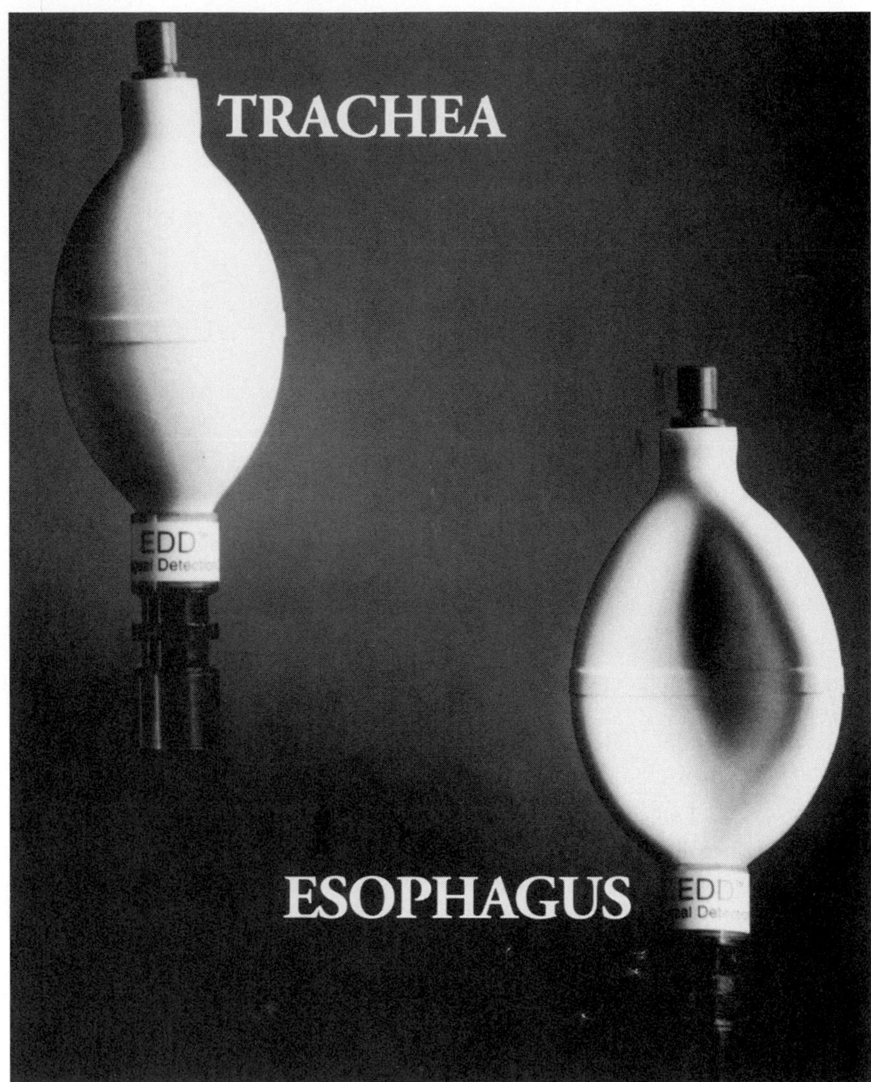

Figure 6-30 Esophageal detection device. (Courtesy ARC Medical, Inc.)

from esophageal and gastric ventilation can be heard transmitted to the chest. Directly viewing the trachea with a bronchoscope passed through the ET is another way to confirm correct placement. Chest radiography (anterior-posterior view) is useful for confirming the tube depth in the chest relative to the carina—but not the correct location within the trachea. A lateral film can identify tracheal rather than esophageal placement, but the other techniques described give quick feedback of incorrect placement in enough time to prevent disaster (Clinical Rounds 6-2).

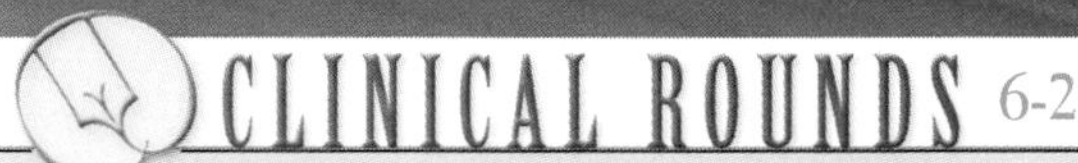

After an emergency intubation of a patient in the surgical intensive care unit, a capnometer is attached to the ET to confirm its placement. The indicator shows a carbon dioxide level of zero. How would you interpret this finding?

See Appendix A for the answer.

Manual Resuscitators

Manual resuscitators (or resuscitator bags) are portable, hand-held devices that provide a means of delivering positive pressure to a patient's airway. These devices incorporate a self-inflating bag, an air-intake valve, a **nonrebreathing valve** mechanism, an oxygen-inlet nipple, and an oxygen reservoir, which may be a tube or a bag.[1,2] Manual resuscitators can deliver room air, oxygen, or air/oxygen mixtures via a mask or through an adaptor that attaches directly to a patient's ET.

As their name implies, manual resuscitators were originally designed to ventilate patients during **cardiopulmonary resuscitation (CPR),** but they have become an indispensable part of managing mechanically ventilated patients. They can be used to hyperinflate patients with enriched oxygen mixtures before and after suctioning procedures and to ventilate bradypneic or apneic (ventilator-dependent) patients while they are being transported from one area of the hospital to another.

Types of Manual Resuscitators (Bag-Valve Units)

Manual resuscitators are generally classified by the type of nonrebreathing valve used.[3] Therefore, two classes of resuscitators are usually described: those using a spring-loaded mechanism and those relying on diaphragm valves. Diaphragm valves can be further subdivided into **duckbill** or **fishmouth** and **leaf-type valves.**

Spring-Loaded Valves

Spring-loaded devices use a nonrebreathing valve that consists of a disk or ball attached to a spring. When the operator compresses the self-inflating bag, a spring pushes a disk or ball against the exhalation port, occluding it, and gas is directed to the patient's airway. After the flow from the bag stops, the exhalation port opens, and gas exhaled by the patient is vented to the atmosphere. Simultaneously, as gas enters the self-inflating bag through the one-way air inlet valve (which is attached to a reservoir), the bag inflates. The air-inlet valve can be attached directly to the nonrebreathing valve or located separately at the bottom of the bag.

The most common examples of this type of manual resuscitator are the early Ambu (Air-Mask-Bag Unit) system, the Ohio Hope II Bag, the Air Viva, and the Vital Signs Stat Blue Resuscitator. Early versions of the Ambu system used a spring-loaded, disk type of nonrebreathing valve that is no longer produced. The Hope II (Figure 6-31) and the Vital Signs Stat Blue (Figure 6-32) resuscitators both rely on the spring-disk type of nonrebreathing valve. Notice that the reservoir of the Hope II resuscitator, which allows for oxygen accumulation and potential delivery of 100% oxygen, is located on the bottom of the self-inflating bag. This reservoir is designed so that the angle of the oxygen inlet valve allows for oxygen flows in excess of 30 L/min to be used without interrupting normal function. The Vital Signs Stat Blue Resuscitator differs from the Ohio Hope II bag because oxygen is drawn in through the neck, where a reservoir is attached.

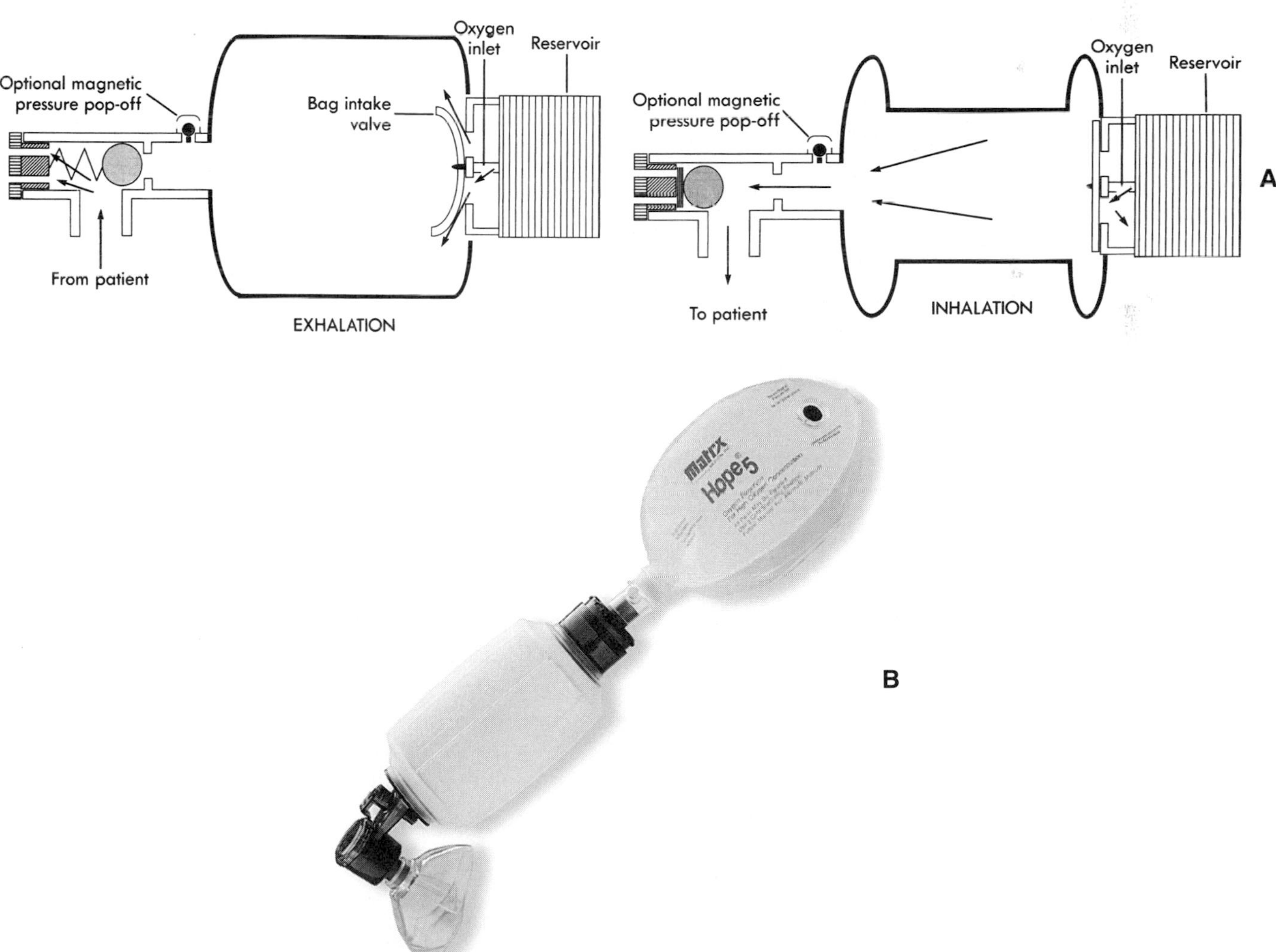

Figure 6-31 **A,** Valves for the Ohio Hope II resuscitator. **B,** The adult model of the Hope II with an oxygen reservoir. (**B,** Courtesy MDS Matrx, Orchard Park, NY.)

Diaphragm Valves

Duckbill Valves

This second class of resuscitators incorporates diaphragm type of nonrebreathing valves in place of spring-loaded mechanisms. The Laerdal Silicone Resuscitator, the Laerdal Adult Resuscitator, the Laerdal Infant and Child Resuscitators (Figure 6-33), the Hudson Life Saver II resuscitator (Figure 6-34), and the Life Design Systems disposable resuscitators are examples of devices that use the duckbill/diaphragm valves.

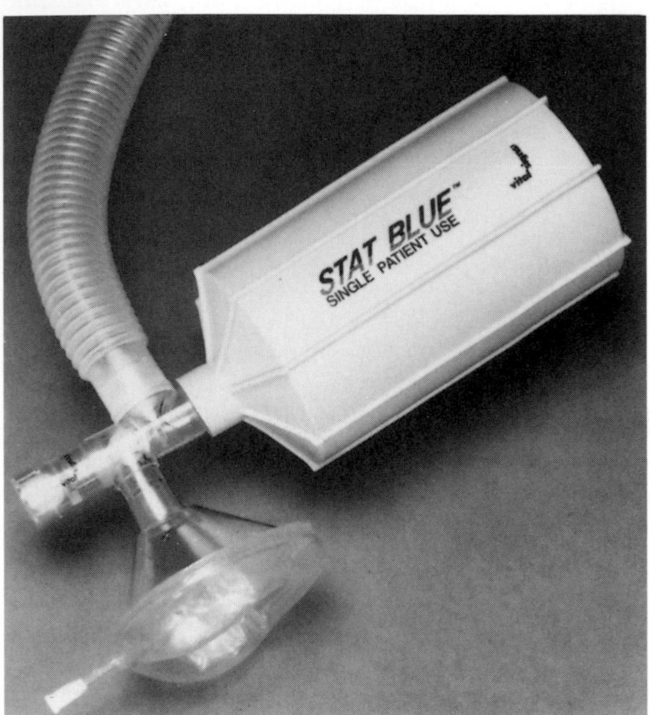

Figure 6-32 Vital Signs Stat Blue Resuscitator. (Courtesy Vital Signs, Totowa, N.J.)

The operational principle of these devices is comparable to that of spring-loaded resuscitators. Compression of the bag pushes a diaphragm against the exhalation ports. At the same time, the duckbill valve opens and gas flows to the patient. After the flow from the bag ceases, the duckbill valve closes, and the diaphragm is pushed away from the exhalation port. Exhaled gas can then exit through the exhalation ports. During reexpansion of the bag, the bag inlet valve allows air or oxygen from the reservoir to enter the self-inflating bag. Notice that the inlet valve is a simple, one-way leaf valve that closes when the bag is compressed to prevent gas leakage. The one-way valve opens when the bag reexpands as a result of subatmospheric pressure within the bag.

Leaf Valves

Resuscitators that use leaf-type valves operate similarly to duckbill resuscitators. As shown in Figure 6-35, when the bag is compressed, a diaphragm swells and occludes the exhalation ports. The leaf valve in the middle of the diaphragm is pushed open, and gas is directed to the patient. During exhalation, the bag reexpands, creating a negative pressure that causes the diaphragm to move away from the exhalation ports. The leaf then closes and prevents exhaled gas from leaking into the bag. The bag inlet valve is opened, and the bag reinflates. The Respironics disposable resuscitator, the Hudson Lifesaver, and the Robertshaw Resuscitators are examples of devices that use leaf valves.

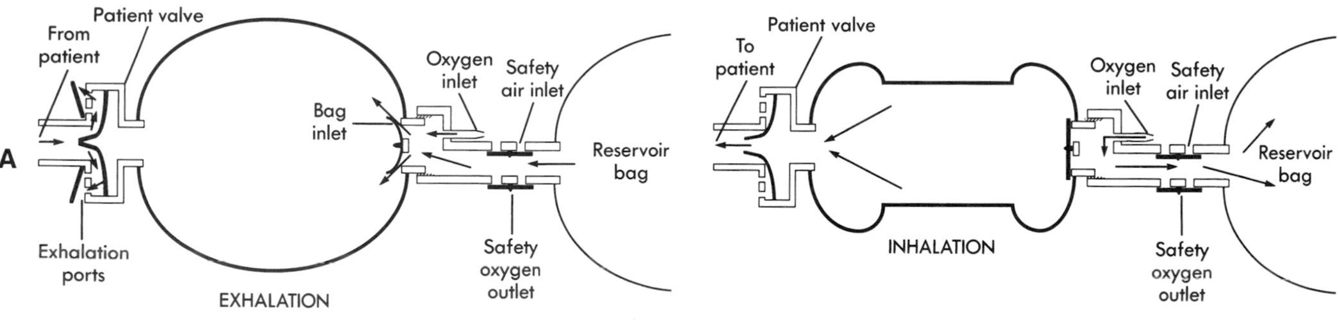

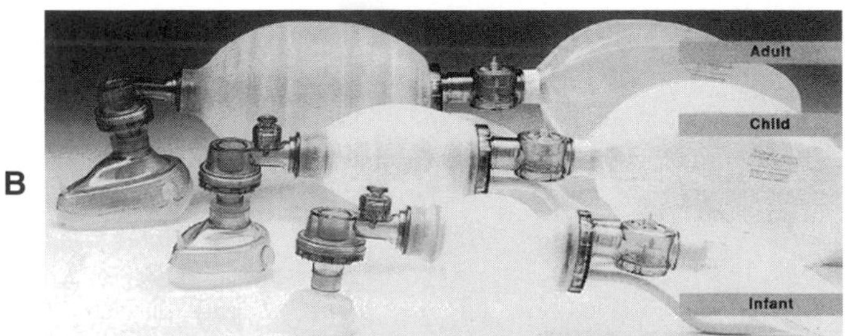

Figure 6-33 **A,** Valves for the adult and child with an oxygen reservoir system for adults. **B,** The Laerdal adult and infant resuscitators with oxygen reservoir systems. (**B,** Courtesy Laerdal Medical Corp, Wappingers Falls, NY.)

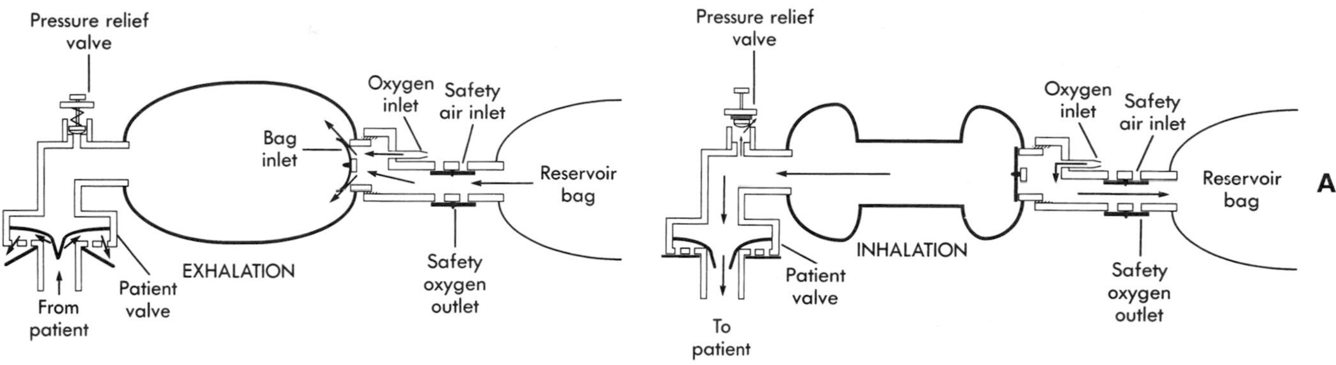

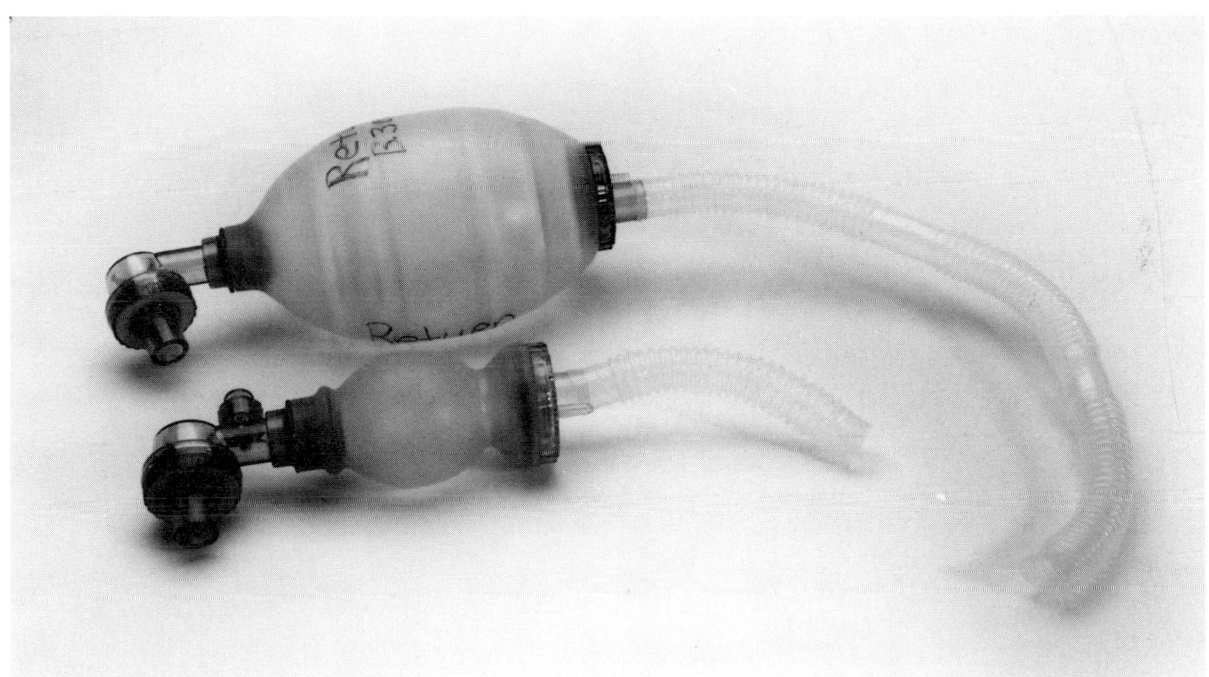

Figure 6-34 **A,** Valves for the Laerdal Child and Infant Resuscitators with oxygen reservoir systems. **B,** Laerdal Silicone Resuscitators with oxygen reservoir systems.

Standards for Manual Resuscitators

Standards for the design, construction, and use of manual resuscitators are published by the American Society for Testing and Materials (ASTM) and the International Standards Organization (ISO).[4,5] The ECRI (formerly Emergency Care Research Institute) and the American Heart Association (AHA) also provide standards for the use and evaluation of manual resuscitators, specifically relating to the level and timing of ventilation during CPR.[6] (Box 6-1 summarizes these standards.)

Table 6-2 compares the performance patterns required by the ASTM, ISO, and AHA standards—although it may not be possible to deliver a tidal volume of 800 mL (as specified by the AHA) unless a patient is intubated. Figure 6-36 shows the results of several studies in which investigators measured the average tidal volumes delivered by one-handed compression of the bag.[7-12] It has been suggested that the lower tidal volumes could have resulted from either an inability to maintain an adequate mask seal while ensuring a patent airway, or from gastric expansion. Another consideration is that the operator may be unable to deliver an appropriate tidal volume unless the bag is compressed with both hands. Although manual resuscitators may differ in design, it is generally agreed that ideal manual resuscitators should possess certain characteristics.[13-15] Box 6-2 lists the characteristics of ideal manual resuscitators.

Oxygen-Powered Resuscitators

Oxygen-powered resuscitators are pressure-limited devices that work similarly to reducing valves. A typical oxygen-powered resuscitator consists of a demand valve that can be manually operated or patient-triggered.[2] Oxygen-powered

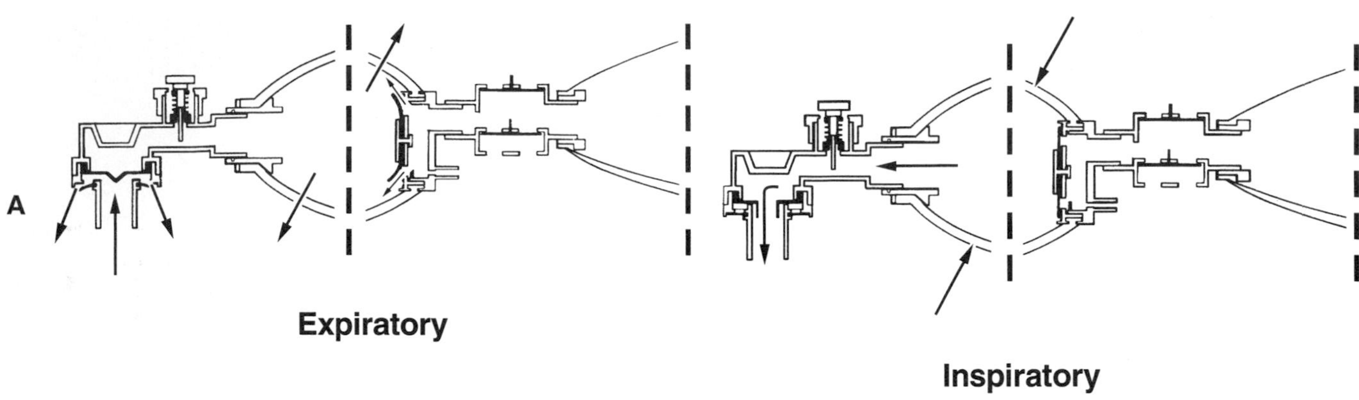

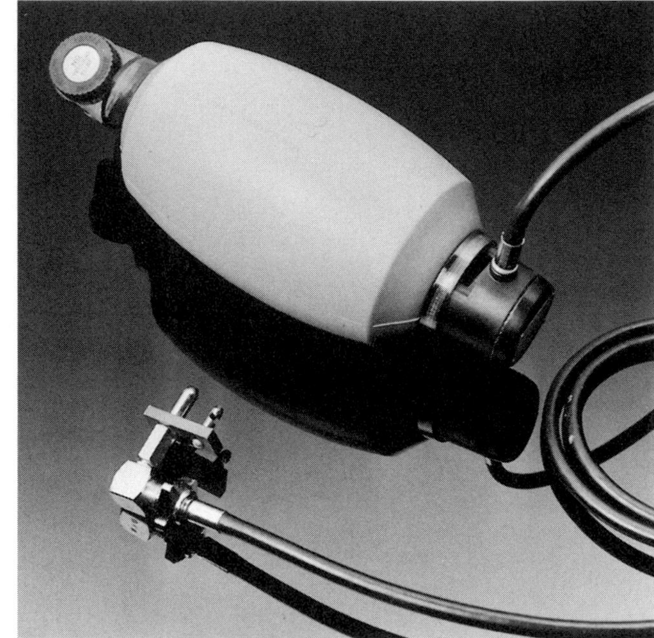

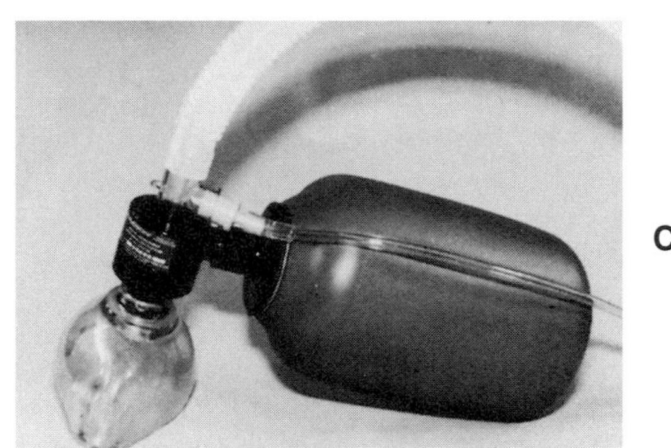

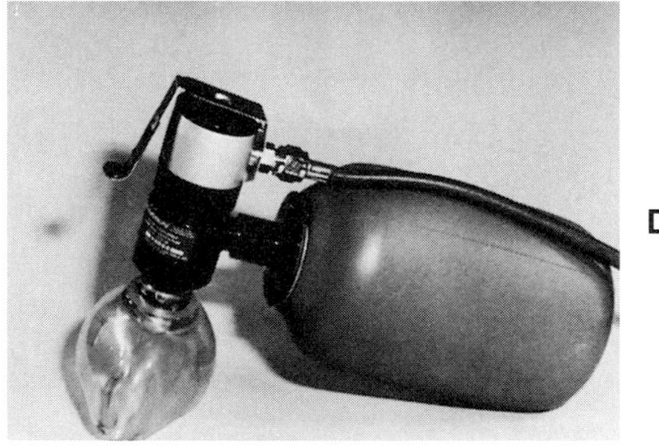

Figure 6-35 **A,** Operations of the leaf and diagram valves for a Hudson Manual Resuscitator (as well as for a Robertshaw Bag Resuscitator). **B,** Hudson Lifesaver Manual Resuscitator with a manufacturer-supplied reservoir system attached. **C,** A modified reservoir system with 22-mm T-connection used for attaching the oxygen inlet at a right angle to the bag-inlet valve. **D,** Robertshaw Demand Valve attached to the bag inlet for providing 100% oxygen or other source gas to bag. (**A,** Courtesy Hudson Oxygen Therapy Sales Co, Temecula, Calif.)

resuscitators can deliver 100% oxygen at flows of less than 40 L/min. Inspiratory pressures are generally limited to 60 cm H_2O, but the pressure-relief valve may be set to 80 cm H_2O, if necessary.

Figure 6-37 is an example of an oxygen-powered resuscitator. When the manual control actuator is depressed, oxygen enters the device from a 50 psig gas source and flows to the patient through a standard 15:22 mm (inner diameter [ID]:outer diameter [OD]) connector. The connector can be coupled to a mask, an ET, a TT, or an esophageal obturator airway.

Hazards Associated with Manual Resuscitators

The most common hazards encountered with these devices include delivery of excessively high airway pressures, a defective or malfunctioning nonrebreathing valve, and faulty pressure-relief valves.[16] Excessively high airway pressures are more likely in patients who are intubated compared with patients being ventilated with a bag-mask-valve device. Having the nonrebreathing valve stuck in the inspiratory position because of improper assembly, inadvertently squeezing the bag while the patient exhales,

Box 6-1 Standards for the Design and Construction of Manual Resuscitators

1. The ASTM and the ISO recommend that manual resuscitators must be capable of delivering an FiO_2 of 0.85 with an oxygen flow of 15 L/min. Recognize that these are minimum requirements and may not be optimal for treating patients during cardiopulmonary resuscitation. It is therefore prudent to choose a device that can deliver $FiO_2 \geq 0.95$.
2. Manual resuscitators must be able to operate at extreme temperatures (−180° to 600° C) and at a relative humidity of 40% to 96%.
3. Adult resuscitators shall deliver a tidal volume of at least 600 mL into a test lung set at a compliance of 0.02 L/cm H_2O and a resistance of 20 cm H_2O/L/sec.
4. The resuscitator's nonrebreathing valve must be designed so that the valve will not jam at oxygen flow rates up to 30 L/min.
5. If the resuscitator valve malfunctions because of a foreign obstruction (e.g., vomitus), the valve must be restored to proper function within 20 seconds.
6. Patient connectors of the resuscitator valve must have a 15:22-mm (ID:OD) fitting.
7. Resuscitators used for adults should not have a pressure-limiting system. Bag-valve devices used for children must incorporate a pressure-release valve that limits peak inspiratory pressure to 40 ± 10 cm H_2O; devices used for infants may incorporate a pressure-release valve that limits peak inspiratory pressure to 40 ± 5 cm H_2O.
8. When a pressure-limiting system is incorporated into a resuscitator, an override capability must exist that is readily apparent to the operator (i.e., it should be visible that the valve is on or off), and an audible signal should indicate that the gas is being vented. The override mechanism should be provided for times when lung impedance is high and the patient has an ET in place.
9. The resuscitator must be able to operate after being dropped from a height of 1 meter onto a concrete floor.

Table 6-2 Ventilation Patterns Specified by Standards for FDO_2 and Ventilation for Bag-Valve Devices

	Ventilation pattern (mL × cycles/min)					
Specification	ASTM[4]	ISO[5]	AHA[6]	O_2 Flow (L/min)	Compliance L/cm H_2O	Resistance cm H_2O/L/sec
FDO_2						
Adult	600 × 12	600 × 12	800 × 12	15	0.020	20
Child	300 × 20	15/kg × 20	N/A	15	0.010	200
Infant	20 × 60	20 × 60	6-8 kg × 40	15	0.001	400
VENTILATION						
Adult	600 × 20	600 × 20	800 × 12		0.020	20
Child 1	300 × 20	15/kg × 20	N/A		0.010	20
Child 2	70 × 30	150 × 25	N/A		0.010	20
Infant 1	70 × 30	20 × 60	6-8/kg × 40		0.010	20
Infant 2	20 × 60	N/A	N/A		0.010	400

From Barnes TA: *Core textbook of respiratory care practice*, ed 2, St Louis, 1994, Mosby.
ASTM, American Society for Testing and Materials; *ISO*, International Standards Organization; *AHA*, American Heart Association; *FDO_2*, fraction of delivered oxygen; *N/A*, not available.

or obstruction of the exhalation port (e.g., mucus plug) will result in dramatic increases in airway pressure. Defective nonrebreathing valves may cause an inspiratory leak resulting in part of the tidal volume escaping through the exhalation port and not being delivered to the patient. Low tidal volumes can also occur with using an inappropriately sized mask or failure to maintain an adequate seal between the mask and the patient's face. Improper setting of the pressure-relief valve can also be a problem when dealing with these devices. This type of malfunction can cause gas delivery at excessively high pressures, and increase the risk of barotrauma.

Surgical Airway Devices

On rare occasions, the establishment of a patent airway with the previously described techniques (i.e., head position, oral and nasal airways, LMA, and Combitube) is unsuccessful, and the patient becomes hypoxic. Invasive airway access should be quickly established to prevent death or severe brain injury. In experienced hands, one brief intubation trial may be attempted before transtracheal needle or tube placement in such circumstances. The simplest invasive airway device is a large-bore intravenous catheter inserted percutaneously through the cricothyroid membrane. This

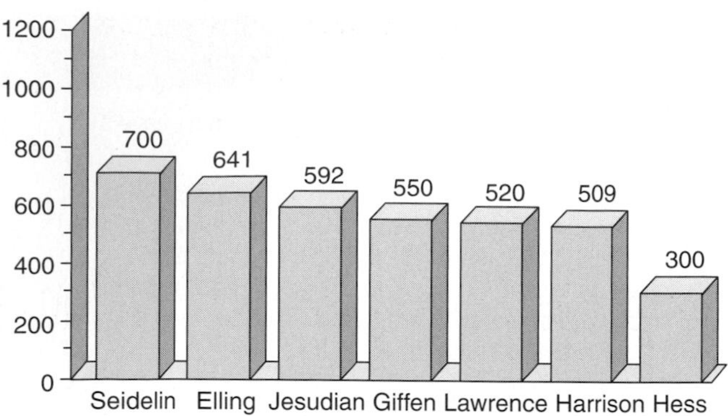

Figure 6-36 Tidal volume by bag-valve mask devices from published studies. (From Barnes TA: *Core textbook of respiratory care practice*, ed 2, St Louis, 1994, Mosby.)

Box 6-2 Properties of an Ideal Manual Resuscitator

1. It should be lightweight and held easily in one hand.
2. It should have standard 15:22 mm (ID:OD) patient adaptors.
3. The bag-valve device should be easy to disassemble, clean, and reassemble.
4. It should be constructed of durable materials (e.g., rubber, silicone, polyvinyl chloride).
5. The nonrebreathing valve should prevent back leaking of patient-exhaled gases into the bag. It should have a low resistance to inspiratory and expiratory airflow and a small dead space volume (< 30 mL for adult models). The nonrebreathing valve should be transparent to allow detection of vomitus or any other obstruction.
6. A manual resuscitator should be able to deliver oxygen concentrations of 0.40 when oxygen in available.
7. The bag construction should allow rapid refill so faster respiratory rates can be achieved as necessary.
8. The volume of the self-inflating bad should be at least twice the volume to be delivered because not all of the bag volume will be delivered when the bag is compressed. For example, adult resuscitators should have a volume of 1600 mL or more to be able to deliver a tidal volume of 800 mL. Resuscitation bags used for children should have a volume of at least 500 mL, and infant bags should hold at least 240 mL.
9. The bag-valve device should allow a positive end expiratory pressure valve or spirometer attachments to measure exhaled volumes. It should be equipped with a tap for monitoring airway pressure with an aneroid manometer.
10. Every manual resuscitator should be supplied with a face mask that attaches to the standard patient connector of the resuscitator. The mask should provide an effective seal when applied to the patient's face.

easily identified space is between the thyroid cartilage and the cricoid ring. A 14-gauge or larger catheter over a needle intravenous device is attached to a syringe and inserted through the cricothyroid membrane. Continuous aspiration is applied until air returns, then the catheter is passed over the needle into the trachea (Figure 6-38). To provide adequate gas delivery through a tracheal needle, a high-pressure gas source (50 psi) must be used. A pressure interrupter or Saunders valve (Figure 6-39) must be attached to the catheter with a Luer-Lok system to prevent disconnection from the catheter during ventilation. Expiration is passive and occurs through the upper airway. With brief jets of gas, normal ventilation and oxygenation can be maintained with this technique. To be successful in an emergency, the proper equipment must be assembled and ready for use ahead of time. Complications of needle-jet ventilation include formation of a false passage, development of subcutaneous emphysema, creation of a pneumothorax, bleeding, failure to ventilate, and damage to neck structures.

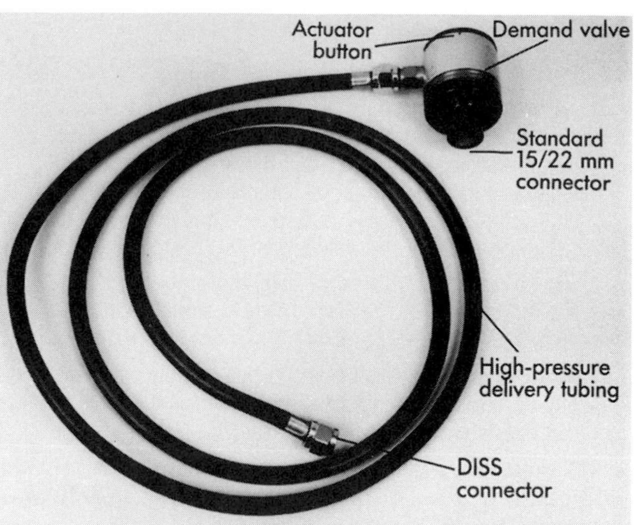

Figure 6-37 Gas-powered resuscitator. (From Scanlan CL, Wilkins RL, Stoller JK: *Egan's fundamentals of respiratory care*, ed 7, St Louis, 1998, Mosby.)

A cricothyroidotomy is a surgical incision in the trachea that passes through the cricothyroid membrane. A conventional ET or tracheostomy tube can be placed through the incision. Routine airway equipment can be used to provide ventilation and oxygen delivery with the tube in place. A single, horizontal slash incision through the skin to the trachea is performed. Bleeding is usually minimal because no large vascular structures lie in the area of the incision. Complications include false placement and failure to provide adequate gas exchange, bleeding, and damage to other neck structures. Subglottic or laryngeal stenosis may be a long-term problem after cricothyroidotomy. Most authorities suggest elective conversion of an emergency cricothyroidotomy to a formal tracheostomy within 24 hours to reduce the likelihood of these severe problems.

Tracheostomy Tubes

Similar to an ET, a TT consists of a round, plastic tube—with or without a cuff, pilot balloon, and valve—with a standard 15-mm connector (Figure 6-40). Metal TTs (Jackson tubes) are occasionally used to maintain a patent

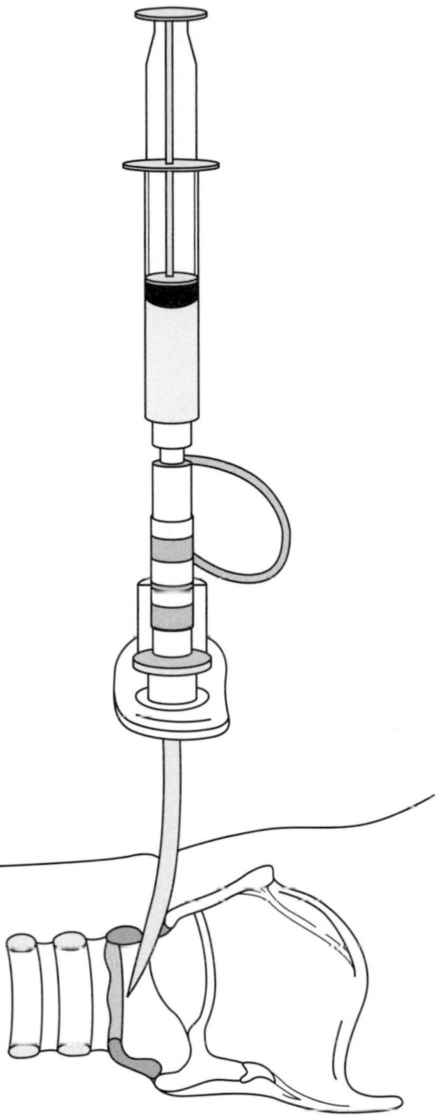

Figure 6-38 Transtracheal jet ventilation can be performed through a large-bore intravenous catheter placed through the cricothyroid membrane.

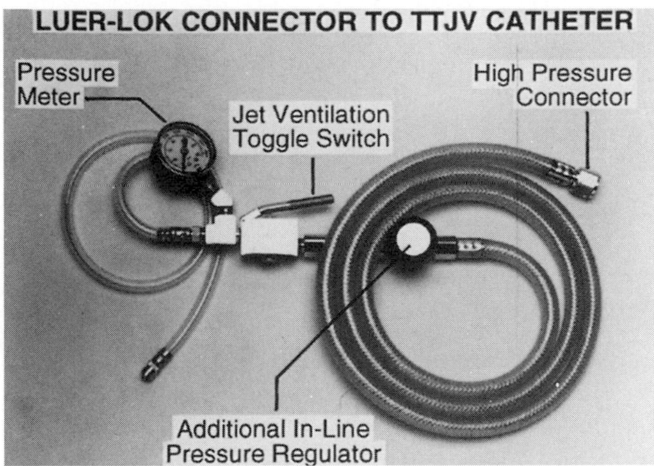

Figure 6-39 A high-pressure jet ventilator system. (From Benumof JL: *Airway management: principles and practice*, St Louis, 1996, Mosby.)

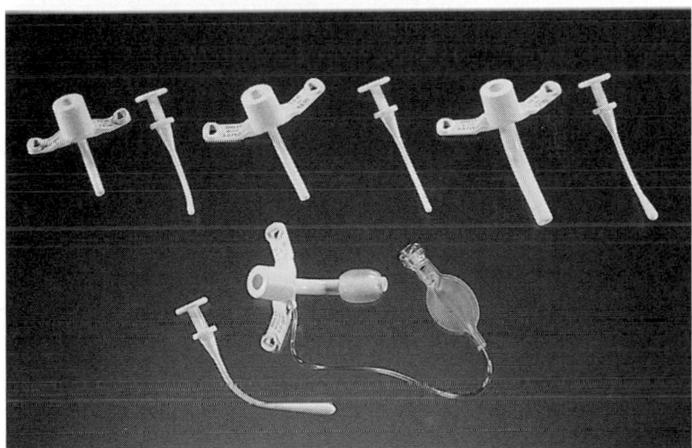

Figure 6-40 A conventional cuffed TT and general uncuffed TTs. Obstructors are used to occlude the TT end during replacement or change of the tube. (Courtesy Shiley, Mallinckrodt, St Louis.)

stoma, allow for suctioning, or gradually reduce the stoma size. These tubes are rarely equipped with a cuff and need adapters to be mated with standard airway equipment. TTs are bent at a 90-degree angle to fit flat against the skin and lie parallel to the axis of the trachea. As with ETs, TT sizes are assigned as the internal diameter in millimeters, although the use of French sizes is still popular. TTs are generally more rigid than ETs, although more flexible TTs are now available that are less likely to kink and must be carefully selected to fit the patient correctly. TTs typically have a collar that is used to secure the tube. The distance from the collar to the bend, the length of the tube distal to the bend (Figure 6-41), and the size and shape of the cuff vary by manufacturer and may be quite different. Some tubes have movable collars that accommodate different skin-to-tracheal distances. The standard fitting may be part of a removable connector or inner cannula. TTs are usually placed occluded with a blunt, solid obturator that makes passage through the tissues less traumatic and less difficult. The obturator is removed after the tube is in place but should remain with the patient and be conveniently available to reinsert the TT if it is accidentally dislodged. Some surgeons place strong, tagging sutures at the corners of the tracheal incision that can be grasped and pulled forward to expose the tract and facilitate reinserting a displaced TT. If ventilation is difficult after urgent replacement of a dislodged TT, it may not lie in the trachea, and manual ventilation through the upper airway should be initiated without delay. TT cuffs are various sizes and, as with ET cuffs, can cause mucosal ischemia if overpressurized. Cuff pressure monitoring and pressure reduction are methods of reducing complications associated with maintenance of TTs.

Although modern materials are less toxic than the hard rubber from which ETs and TTs were originally made, these artificial airways can damage the structures through which they pass. Translaryngeal airways can damage the nasal

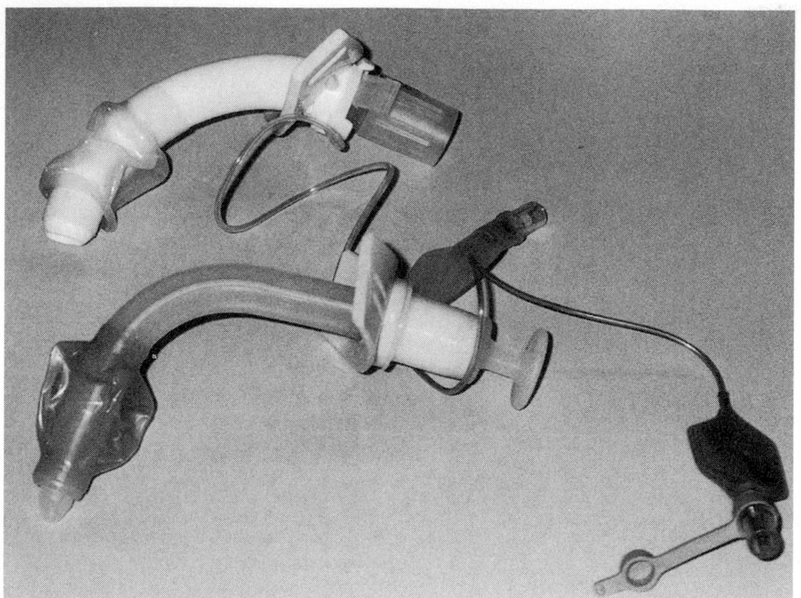

Figure 6-41 TTs come in preformed shapes with lengths that are not standardized.

septum, the tongue, and the larynx, as well as the trachea from cuff pressure and tip trauma. TTs can cause damage at cuff and tip locations and at the stoma. Severe vocal cord damage and laryngeal stenosis are dreaded complications from **translaryngeal intubation.** They are difficult to treat and may permanently disable the patient. These complications increase with the duration of intubation and the larger diameter of the tube. If the need for tracheal intubation exceeds 2 to 3 weeks in adults, a tracheostomy is usually performed to decrease laryngeal complications. Trauma to the trachea from the tube cuff or tip can result in ulcers, cartilage loss, tracheomalacia, or rupture, which are complications of both TTs and ETs. Granulation tissue may form at the TT stoma; and after removal of the TT, stenosis at the stomal site may occur in up to 10% of patients. Treatment of these complications is difficult and often requires resecting of tracheal segments or placement of a stent.

With intubation, the patient's ability to speak is lost. This loss of control can lead to psychological stress. Several methods for allowing seminormal speech with a tracheostomy have been developed. A fenestrated TT is one in which there is a hole in the curved portion of the tube above the cuff that can be used to allow air to pass into the upper airway through the larynx so that normal speech is possible (Figure 6-42). When positive-pressure ventilation is needed, an inner, nonfenestrated cannula can be inserted. A one-way valve attached to the TT will allow inspiration from the TT and exhalation upward through the larynx. Two of the available devices are the Passy-Muir valve and the Olympic Trach-Talk (Figure 6-43). These devices can only be used in patients capable of initiating and maintaining spontaneous ventilation. Obviously, without an open upper airway, unobstructed

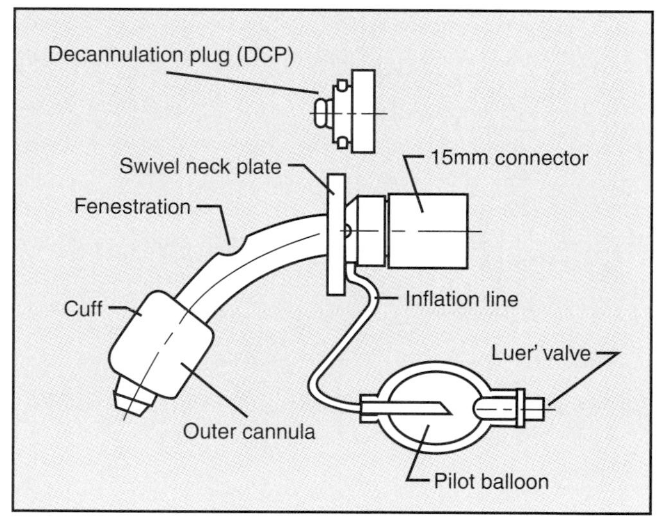

Figure 6-42 A fenestrated TT.

fenestration, or a deflated TT cuff, a lethal, closed system with no portal for exhalation would exist. When attaching one-way valves to patients with artificial airways, careful observation for immediate problems with exhalation is essential (Clinical Rounds 6-3). In patients unable to sustain unaided ventilation, an extra port on the TT can be used to provide gas flow through the larynx. The Pitt Speaking TT in Figure 6-44 was designed for this purpose, although speech with it is usually only a whisper. Vibrating devices can be used in the mouth or on the neck to produce audible speech when mouthing words. Restoration of the ability to speak in patients with artificial airways can improve the patient's mood, increase cooperation with caregivers, and accelerate recovery.

A

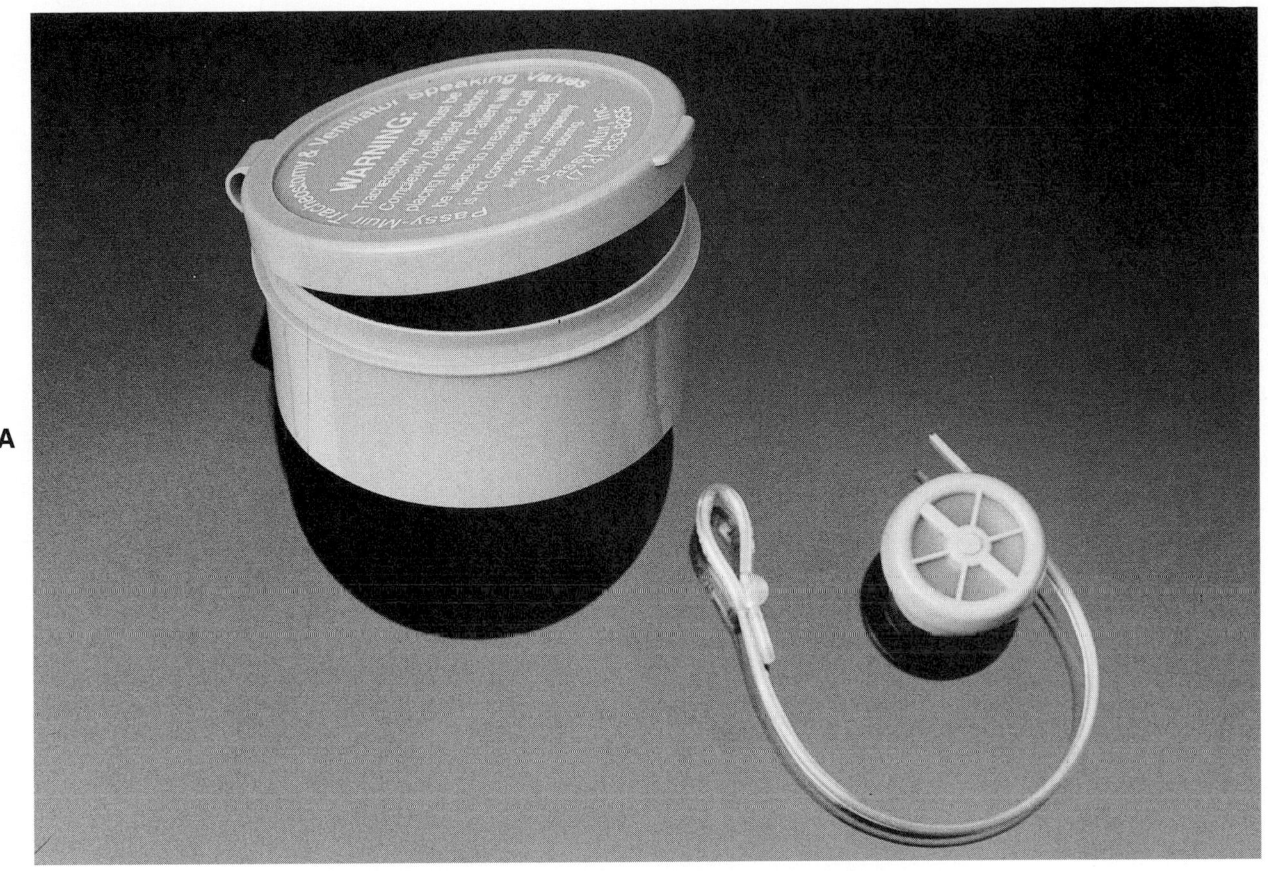

B

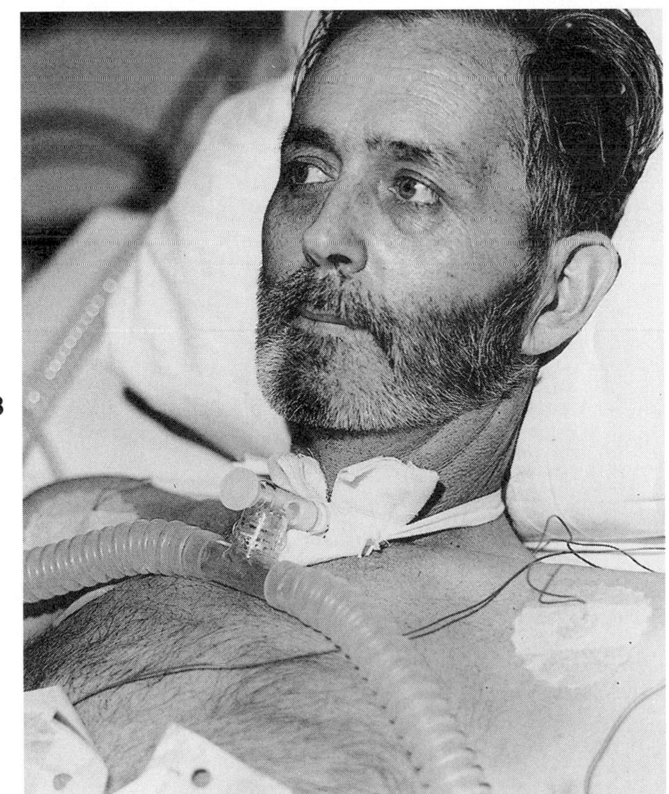

Figure 6-43 **A,** A Passy-Muir speaking valve. **B,** An Olympic Trach-Talk speaking device.

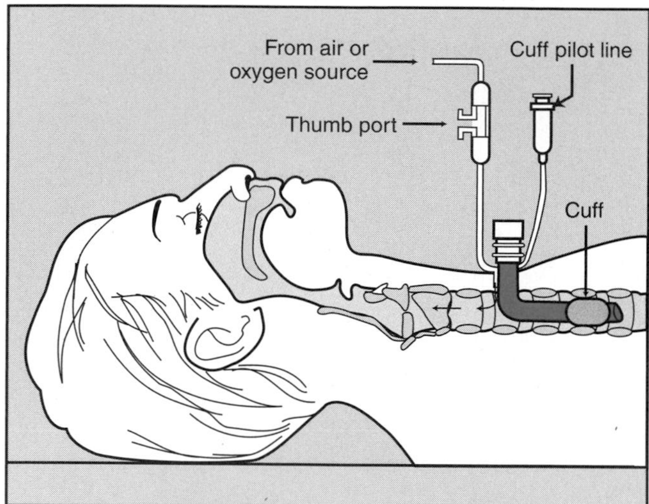

Figure 6-44 A Pittsburgh speaking TT.

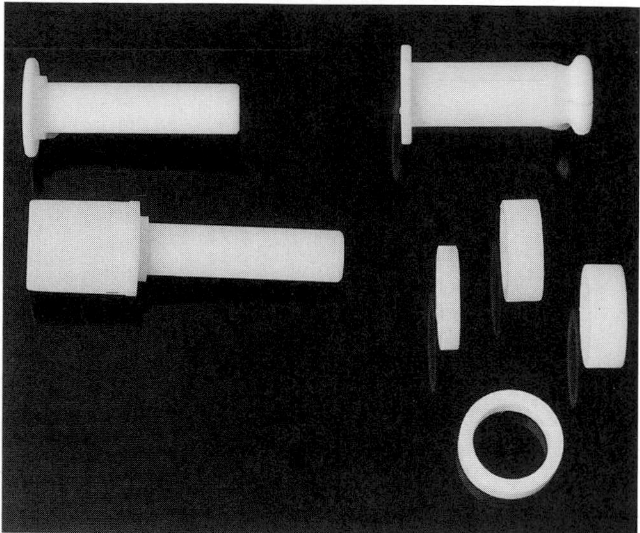

Figure 6-45 An Olympic tracheostomy button.

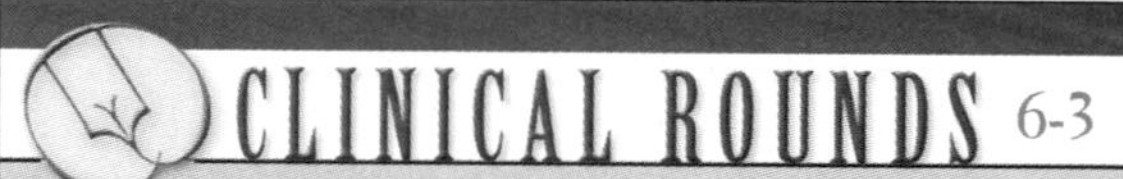

A patient has a fenestrated TT in place. To evaluate the patient's ability to move air around the tube and into the upper airway, what procedure should the respiratory therapist perform?

See Appendix A for the answer.

After the need for a TT no longer exists, the patient should be weaned from his or her tracheostomy. If the tube is simply removed and the stoma covered with an occlusive dressing, the stoma will close in several days. Some clinicians prefer to gradually reduce the TT size every few days until only a small tube is in place. If direct tracheal access—but not ventilation—is needed for a longer time, several devices can be used to keep a stoma patent. A 4-mm, uncuffed metal or silastic TT allows tracheal suctioning and causes very little airway obstruction in most adult patients. If reinsertion of a larger, cuffed tube is later needed, the tract can be easily dilated to accommodate a larger tube. Another device used to maintain a tracheostomy stoma is the Olympic button shown in Figure 6-45. It protrudes slightly into the airway but is usually less obstructive than a small TT. It is usually kept capped or plugged unless airway access is needed; it cannot be effectively used to provide positive-pressure ventilation but can be exchanged for a cuffed TT if necessary.

Specialized Endotracheal Tubes

Occasionally, it is desirable to provide a different kind of ventilatory support to each lung, and specialized ETs that allow independent lung ventilation are available. These tubes were developed for bronchoalveolar lavage (to treat alveolar proteinosis) and performing differential lung function tests before a pneumonectomy. They have been refined and are frequently used to improve surgical exposure and reduce risk during anesthesia for lung resection. Sometimes **double-lumen ETs (DLETs)** are used outside the operating room to protect the "good" lung from blood contamination in patients with massive hemoptysis. Probably the most common use of these devices outside the operating room is after single-lung transplant when the compliance of the native lung and that of the transplanted lung are very different. Two ventilator systems can be used to titrate appropriate support for each lung independently. DLETs consist of two separate semicircular lumens fused together. At the tip, one lumen terminates in a right or left main bronchial tube with a small cuff. The other terminates in the trachea below the tracheal cuff to provide ventilation to the other lung. Two standard adapters and pilot balloons are present (Figure 6-46).

If possible, only left-sided DLETs should be used. They seat more easily (with less of an acute angle of take-off from the left main bronchus), and the bronchial cuff will not occlude the upper lobe bronchus. The right upper lobe bronchial take-off is only 1 to 2 cm from the carina, and it is likely that the bronchial cuff will occlude the upper lobe bronchus if a right-sided tube is placed. A recent modification of right-side cuff design (i.e., placing the cuff diagonally on the bronchial lumen) may decrease this problem (Figure 6-47).

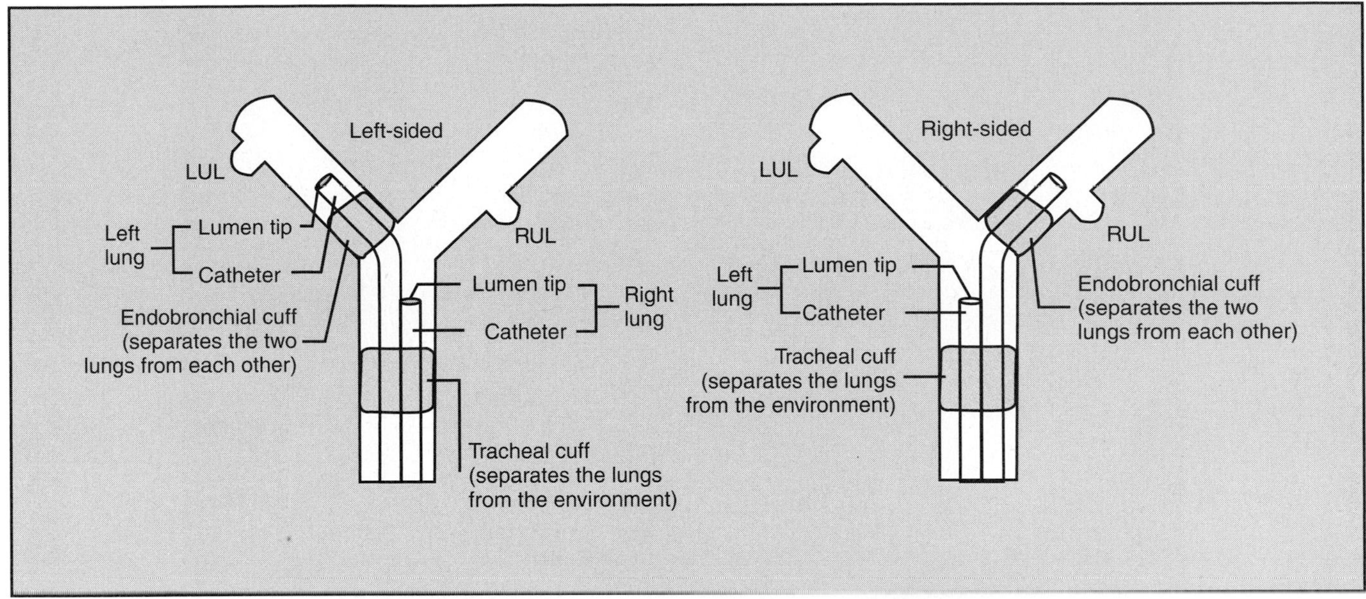

Figure 6-46 A double lumen endotracheal tube used for lung isolation.

Although physical examination with sequential occlusion of individual lumens can be used to confirm proper seating of DLETs, direct visualization with a small fiberoptic bronchoscope passed through the tracheal lumen is a more reliable method of confirming correct placement. The bronchial cuff should be just visible below the carina. Tubes are in French sizes: 35 and 37 are usually used for average women; 39 and 41 for average men. The bronchial cuff should take from 1 to 3 mL of air to seal if the correct size tube has been chosen and the cuff is properly seated. A high-pressure bronchial seal should be avoided because bronchial stenosis, a devastating injury, may result.

Because of their bulk and rigidity, DLETs are often difficult to place through the larynx. Prolonged intubation attempts may be necessary. This is especially true with an airway full of blood in a patient with massive hemoptysis. Although the idea of using a DLET in patients with massive hemoptysis is appealing, the technical issues of placement can be daunting.

Other specialized ETs may have distal airway channels. One is the Hi-Lo Jet ET (Mallinckrodt Medical Inc.), in which the additional lumen can be used for distal airway pressure monitoring during jet ventilation (Figure 6-48). Another specialized ET has lumens designed for tracheal drug delivery (Figure 6-49). Recognition of the role of aspiration of small amounts of infective oral secretions into the lung around the ET tube cuff in developing ventilator-associated pneumonia (VAP) has led to the production of a specialized ET with a large suction port located above the cuff (Figure 6-50). Removal of subglottic secretions with continuous or intermittent aspiration through the suction lumen reduces the risk of development of VAP. Use of this specialized ET tube is recommended as part of a strategy to reduce nosocomial pneumonia in patients requiring prolonged supraglottic intubation.

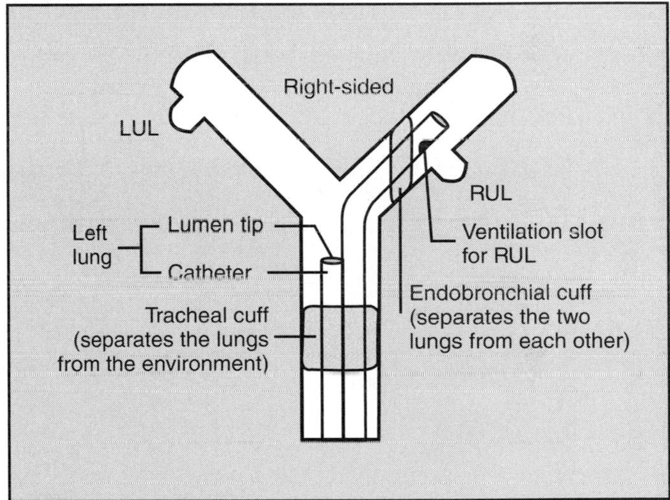

Figure 6-47 A diagonal cuff on the endobronchial lumen may decrease incidence of obstruction of the right upper lobe bronchus.

Equipment Used to Manage Artificial Airways

Intubated patients have their upper airways bypassed. Humidifying and warming inspired gases are primary functions of the upper airway. Active or passive humidification systems should be used in patients using ETs for a prolonged period. Even with these devices, airway secretions may be increased because of tracheal irritation and thickened from inadequate humidification or infection. The ability to cough is severely compromised because the glottis cannot be closed when the patient is intubated. Secretions must be aspirated from the lung in most intubated patients. Suction

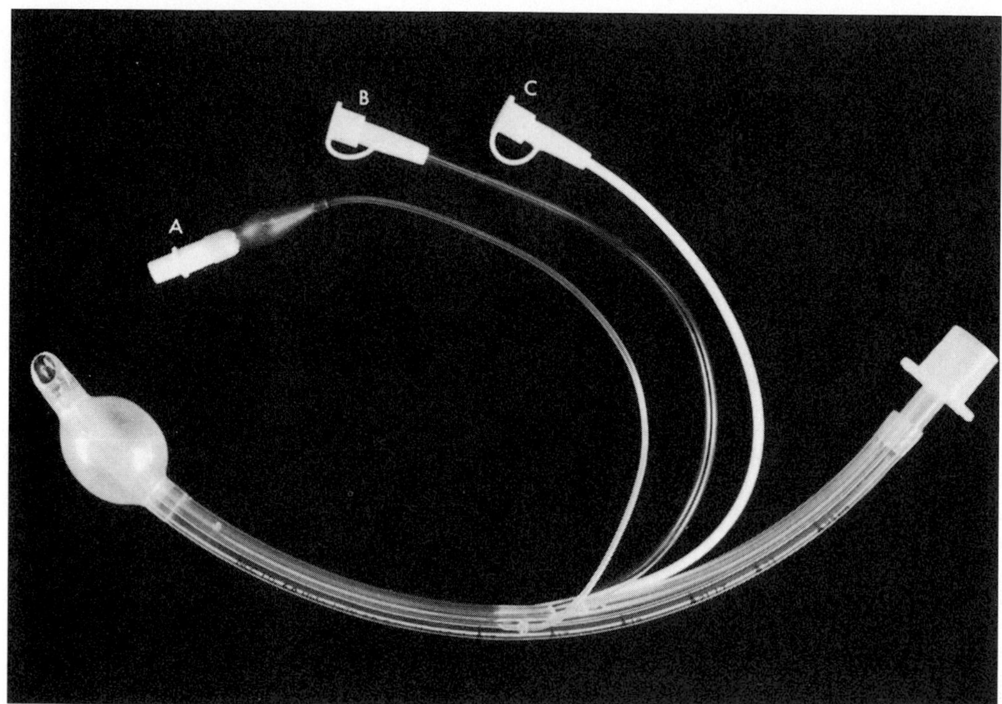

Figure 6-48 An ET with multiple lumens for jet ventilation and airway pressure measurement. (Courtesy Cardinal Health, Respiratory Care Products and Services, McGaw Park, Ill.)

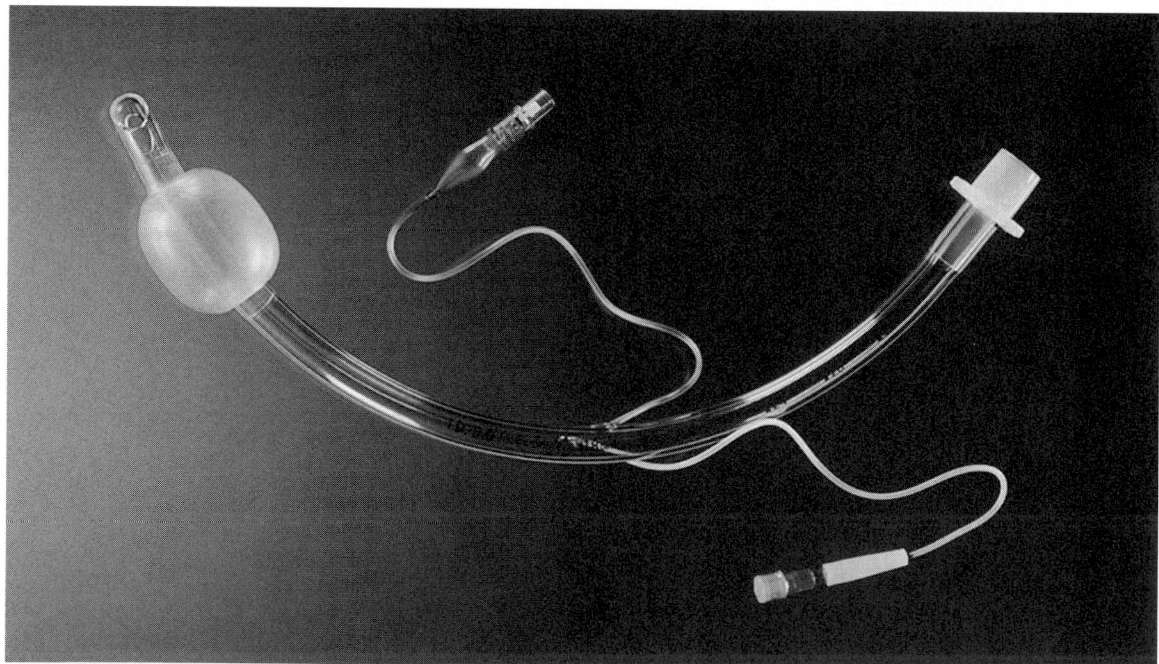

Figure 6-49 An ET with an additional port to be used for instillation of medications. (Courtesy Cardinal Health, Respiratory Care Products and Services, McGaw Park, Ill.)

catheters are illustrated in Figure 6-51. Suction catheters are available in a variety of sizes and designs, but it is generally recommended that the catheter diameter should be less than half of the internal diameter of the artificial airway. It is important to recognize that suction catheters are sized according to the tube's outer diameter (i.e., French size). Conversion from inner to outer diameter can be accomplished by multiplying the internal diameter by 3 and then dividing the product by 2. For example, a size 8.0 (inner diameter) TT requires a 12 French catheter.

$$(8.0 \times 3) \div 2 = 12 \text{ Fr}$$

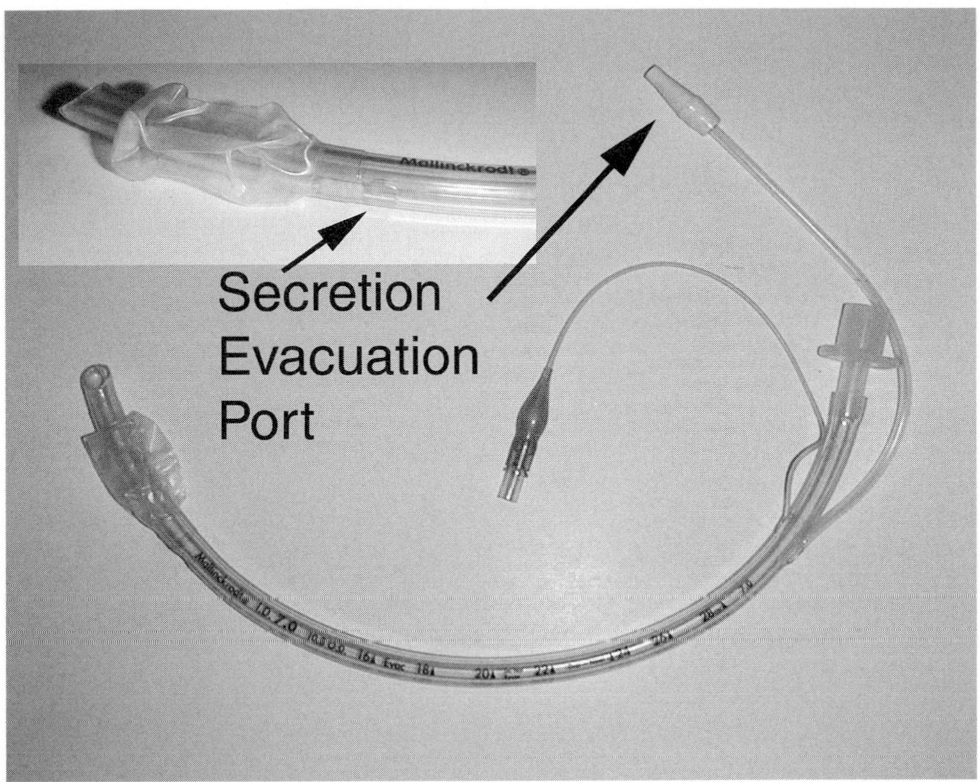

Figure 6-50 The Hi-Low Evac tube has a portal for suctioning subglottic secretions and is used as part of a program to reduce the incidence of ventilator associated pneumonia in intubated patients.

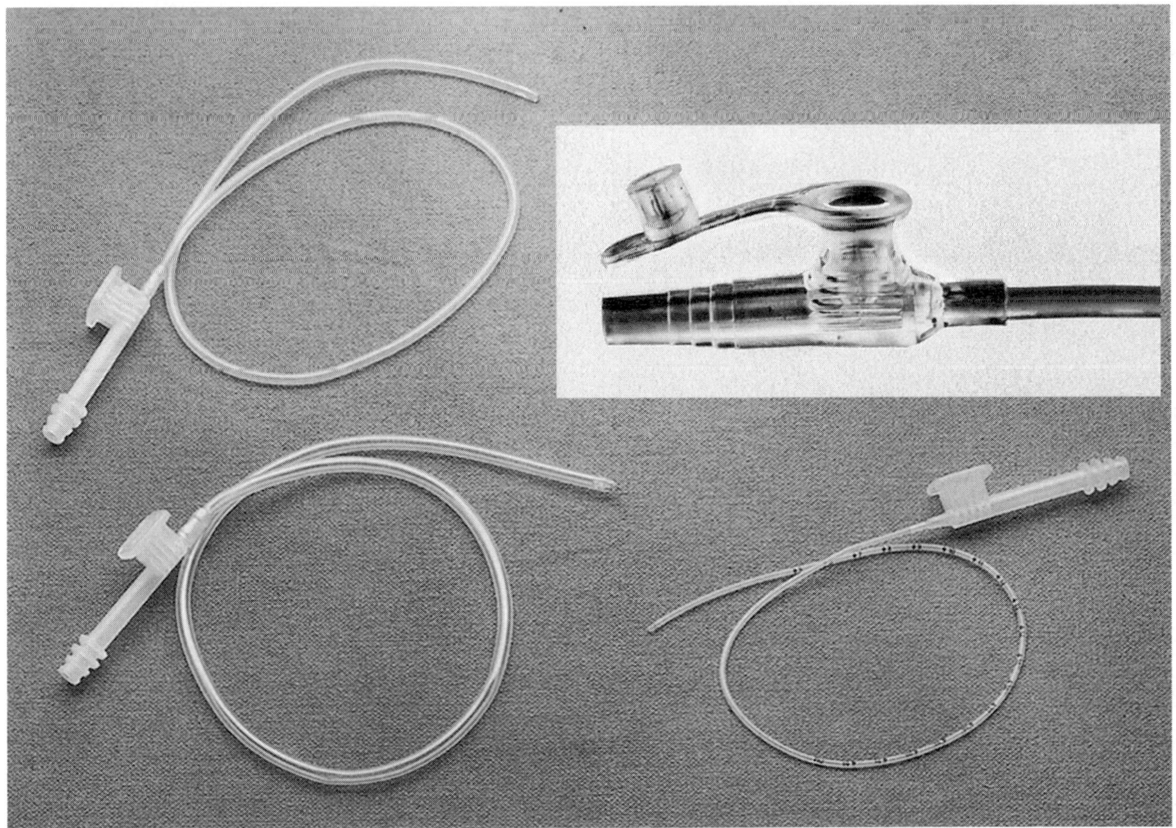

Figure 6-51 Suction catheters of various types. (Courtesy Cardinal Health, Respiratory Care Products and Services, McGaw Park, Ill.)

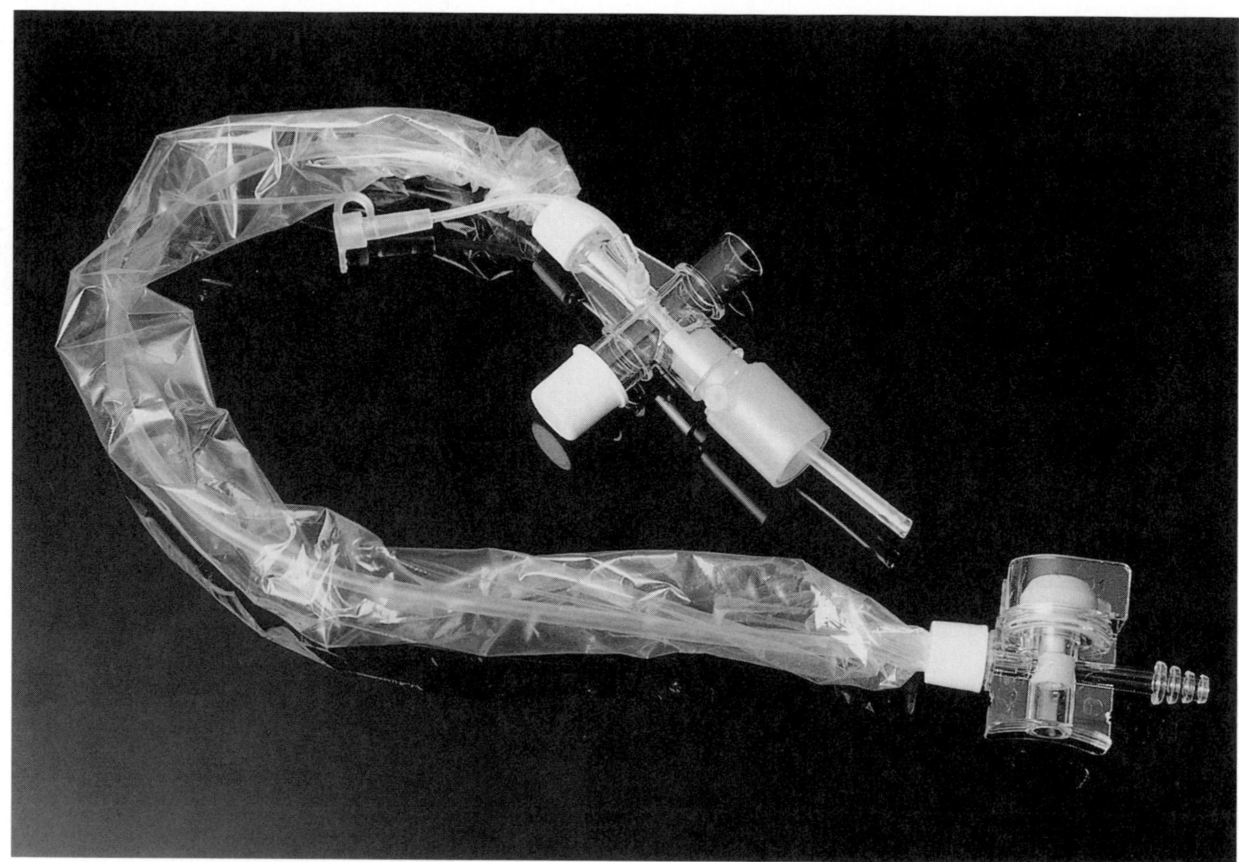

Figure 6-52 A closed-system suction catheter system.

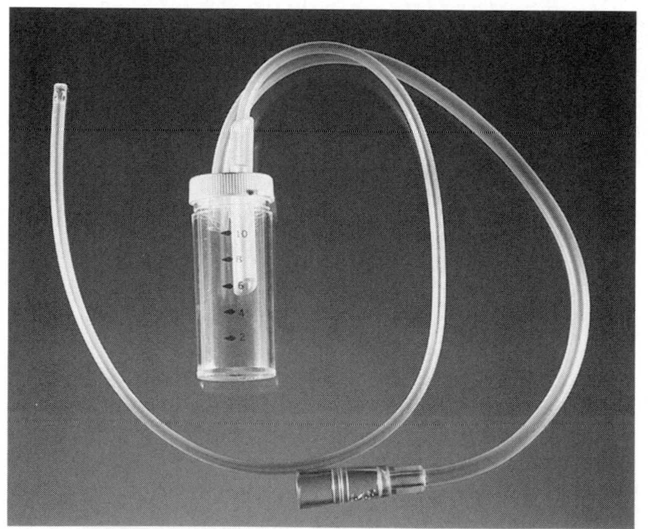

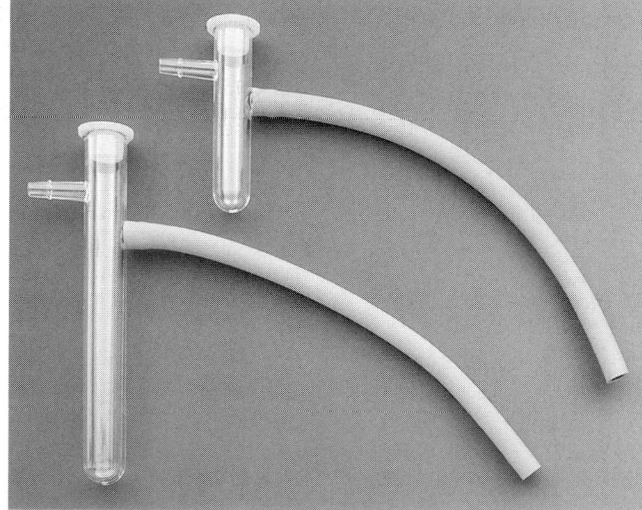

Figure 6-53 Uncontaminated sputum samples may be collected with a Lukens sputum trap. (Courtesy Cardinal Health, Respiratory Care Products and Services. McGaw Park, Ill.)

Preoxygenation, sterile preparation, and standard precautions should be used during endotracheal suctioning. In-line closed-system suction devices (Figure 6-52) may reduce caregiver and patient risk of infectious disease exposure, lower costs, and compromise ventilation less during suctioning. Sterile sputum samples can be obtained using a **Lukens sputum trap** (Figure 6-53). Box 6-3 provides a sample protocol for suctioning patients with artificial airways.

Many devices have been developed to help secure ETs. Effective methods of securing these tubes are especially important in children. Judicious use of sedation and physical restraint are important for the comfort and safety of the intubated patient.

Changing an ET may pose significant risk to critically ill patients. A catheter designed specifically for this purpose is shown in Figure 6-54. The tube changer is inserted through

Box 6-3 Protocol for Suctioning Patients with Endotracheal Tubes

1. The following equipment should be available:
   a. Functional vacuum system that can generate pressures from 100 to 150 mm Hg.
   b. Suction catheter and sterile water or saline for instillation.
   c. Protective equipment, including gloves, masks, and eye protection.
   d. Pulse oximeter
2. Explain the procedure to the patient.
3. Wash your hands with antibacterial soap. Glove both hands and attach the catheter to the vacuum system using aseptic technique.
4. Preoxygenate the patient with 100% oxygen for a minimum of 30 to 60 seconds before suctioning. Note the baseline heart rate, electrocardiogram (ECG) rhythm, and pulse oximeter saturation.
5. Advance the catheter without suctioning until an obstruction is detected. Apply suction and gently withdraw the catheter. Limit the suctioning time to 10 to 15 seconds or less if indicated by ECG and pulse oximeter readings. Instillation of several milliliters (1 to 3 mL) of sterile saline (0.9% NaCl) may help to decrease the viscosity of the secretions in patient with thick tenacious mucus.
6. Allow the patient to rest and provide postsuctioning oxygenation and hyperinflation.
7. Repeat the procedure only as needed. Note that the patient's mouth or trachea should not be suctioned after the nose.

From Ptevak DJ, Ward JJ: Airway management. In Burton GC, Hodgkin JE, Ward J, editors: *Respiratory care: a guide to clinical practice*, ed 4, Philadelphia, 1997, JB Lippincott.

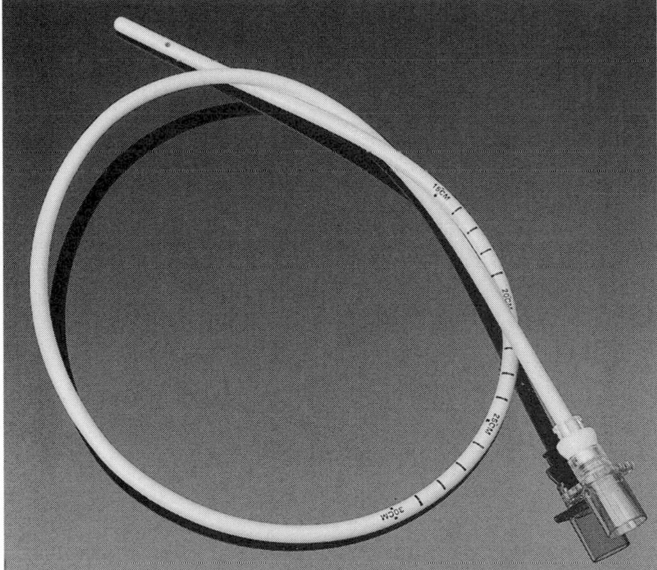

Figure 6-54 An ET tube changer.

the ET, and the tube is withdrawn and removed. Oxygen can be insufflated through the tube changer during the procedure. A new ET can be slipped over the tube changer and threaded down it into the lung. Occasionally, the new tube catches on the larynx and needs to be gently rotated into position, but this method is not always successful, so equipment for reintubation must be at hand.

A common indication for changing a tube is failure of the cuff to hold pressure. If the pilot balloon remains inflated, and the tube transiently seals when more air is added but quickly develops a leak again, the cuff has probably herniated through the vocal cords. This can be remedied by deflating the cuff completely, advancing the ET 2 to 3 cm, and reinflating the cuff. If the pilot balloon holds pressure while the syringe is attached but deflates when it is disconnected, the pilot-tube valve is probably defective. This can be overcome by inserting a stopcock into the valve, inflating the cuff, and turning the stopcock off toward the cuff. The pilot balloon and valve can be replaced with a

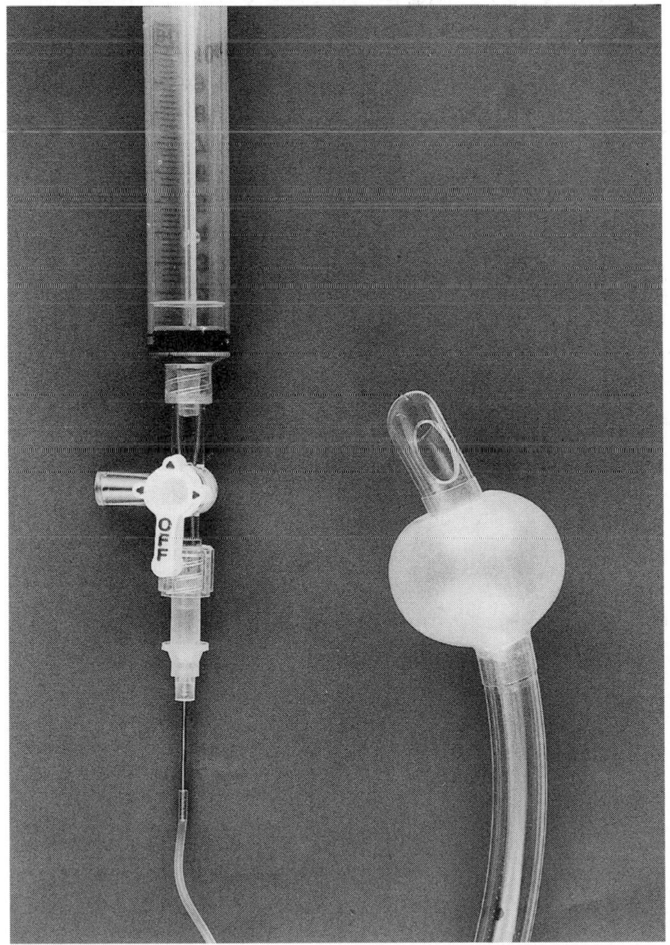

Figure 6-55 If the pilot balloon or pilot balloon valve fails to hold air, the entire assembly may be temporarily replaced by inserting a cut-off 19-gauge needle with a stopcock into the pilot tubing.

blunt needle, and the stopcock inserted into the pilot tube after the balloon has been cut off (Figure 6-55). These methods of valve and pilot balloon repair may save patients the risk and trauma of reintubation.

Summary

Inadequate gas exchange is an acute emergency. Failure to restore adequate respiratory gas exchange can result in hypoxic brain injury or death within minutes. Various devices, such as oral and nasopharyngeal airways, laryngeal mask airways, and Combitube, can be used in emergency situations to improve the patency of the upper airway and permit manual ventilation.

ETs and TTs are definitive devices for airway management, allowing for ventilation with high levels of positive pressure as well as directing access to the lower airways for secretion removal and drug delivery. These devices also prevent aspiration of foreign materials into the lung and allow bronchoscopic examination of the peripheral airways. Correct sizing, proper placement, and securing of ETs and TTs are essential for creating and maintaining an open airway.

Providing adequate, routine bronchial hygiene should be a primary concern of respiratory therapists caring for patients with ETs or TTs in place. Proper airway management can reduce caregiver and patient risk of infectious disease exposure and prevent many of the complications associated with artificial airways.

Review Questions

See Appendix A for the answers.

1. The most important concern in an unconscious person is:
   a. establishing a patent airway
   b. calling for help
   c. administering oxygen by mask
   d. preventing aspiration

2. The laryngeal mask airway:
   a. is a definitive, secure airway
   b. can be easily inserted in a conscious patient
   c. bypasses upper airway obstructions
   d. can be used to provide positive-pressure ventilation in patients with reduced pulmonary compliance

3. A patient with a foam cuff tracheostomy tube:
   a. should have a syringe to inflate the cuff
   b. will need a stopcock on the pilot balloon to form a tracheal seal
   c. will have the pilot balloon valve "open" to seal the cuff
   d. should have the pilot balloon "tense" to guarantee a good seal

4. Which of the following is the preferred artificial airway for a liver patient who is vomiting blood?
   a. nasotracheal intubation with a cuffed tube
   b. oral intubation with a cuffed tube
   c. laryngeal mask airway
   d. cricothyroidotomy with a cuffed tube

5. A Combitube is placed in an unconscious patient. If breath sounds are clearly heard when ventilating through the pharyngeal lumen with both cuffs inflated, which of the following is true?
   a. a gastric tube should not be passed through the esophageal lumen
   b. the lung is not protected from aspiration
   c. oxygen should be added to the esophageal lumen
   d. more air should be placed in the pharyngeal cuff

6. When placing an appropriately sized oral pharyngeal airway, the flange protrudes out of the mouth. Attempts to insert it result in the device popping back out. This could be caused by:
   a. the airway catching on the back of the tongue
   b. using too small of an airway
   c. a foreign body in the pharynx
   d. false teeth

7. Which of the following is a complication of performing a cricothyroidotomy?
   a. gas embolism syndrome
   b. cervical spinal cord injury
   c. stroke
   d. subcutaneous emphysema

8. The most important concern with blind nasal intubation is:
   a. failure to recognize esophageal intubation
   b. nasal hemorrhage
   c. sinusitis
   d. loss of ability to speak

9. After oral intubation, there is no carbon dioxide during exhalation. This could be due to:
   a. esophageal intubation
   b. cardiac arrest
   c. low cardiac output
   d. all of the above

10. A patient has a 7.0 (inner diameter) TT in the trachea. What size suction tube should be used?
    a. 10 Fr
    b. 12 Fr
    c. 14 Fr
    d. 16 Fr

11. List three methods that can be used to confirm placement of an ET in the trachea rather than the esophagus.

12. A ______ laryngoscope blade should be used when attempting intubation of an average adult.
    a. #0
    b. #1
    c. #3
    d. #6

13. Which of the following are complications associated with TT placement?
    I. Hypoxia
    II. Hemorrhage
    III. Nerve injury
    IV. Gas dissection of the tissues surrounding the tracheotomy site
    a. I and II only
    b. II and III only
    c. I, II, and IV only
    d. I, II, III, and IV

14. Trauma from overinflation of an endotracheal tube cuff can result in:
    I. Tracheal ulcers
    II. Tracheal cartilage loss
    III. Tracheal malacia
    IV. Tracheal rupture
    a. I only
    b. I and II only
    c. II, III, and IV only
    d. I, II, III, and IV

15. The proper ET size for a premature infant is:
    a. 2.5-mm inner diameter
    b. 3.5-mm inner diameter
    c. 4.0-mm inner diameter
    d. 4.5-mm inner diameter

16. A large, adult, male patient has a 7-mm (inner diameter) ET in place and is being mechanically ventilated. Cuff pressures of 35 cm H_2O are required to maintain an adequate cuff seal. Which of the following strategies would you suggest to correct this problem?
    a. lower cuff pressures to no more than 25 cm H_2O
    b. change the ET tube to an 8.5-mm (inner diameter) tube
    c. request placement of a TT
    d. periodically deflate and inflate the cuff

17. A patient who has undergone a single-lung transplant is to be ventilated with two ventilators connected in tandem. What is the most appropriate type of airway to use?
    a. Magill type of ET
    b. Murphy type of ET
    c. DLET
    d. combination of TT and oral ET

18. What is the minimum FiO_2 that a manual resuscitator with a reservoir should deliver according to ASTM and ISO recommendations?
    a. 0.40 with an oxygen flow of 8 L/min
    b. 0.70 with an oxygen flow of 10 L/min
    c. 0.85 with an oxygen flow of 15 L/min
    d. 1.0 with an oxygen flow of 6 L/min

19. Which of the following are standards recommended for the design and construction of manual resuscitators?
    I. Manual resuscitators must be able to operate at relative humidities of 40% to 96%.
    II. Adult resuscitators must deliver a tidal volume of at least 600 mL into a test lung set at a compliance of 0.02 L/cm H_2O.
    III. The resuscitator's nonrebreathing valve must be designed so that the valve will not jam at oxygen flows up to 40 L/min.
    IV. Resuscitators that are used for adults should have a pressure-limiting system.
    a. I only
    b. I and II only
    c. I, II, and III only
    d. I, II, III, and IV

References

1. Fink JB: Volume expansion therapy. In Burton GC, Hodgkin JE, Ward JJ, editors: *Respiratory care, a guide to clinical practice*, ed 4, Philadelphia, 1997, JB Lippincott.
2. McPherson SP: *Respiratory care equipment*, ed 5, St Louis, 1995, Mosby.
3. Barnes TA, Watson ME: Cardiopulmonary resuscitation and emergency cardiac care. In Barnes TA, editor: *Core textbook of respiratory care practice*, ed 2, St Louis, 1994, Mosby.
4. Standard specification for performance and safety requirements for resuscitators intended for use with humans, Designation F-920-985, Philadelphia, American Society for Testing and Materials.
5. ISO Technical Committee ISO/TC 121: *Anesthetic and Respiratory Equipment: International Standard ISO 8382: resuscitators intended for use with humans*, Switzerland, 1988, International Organization for Standardization.
6. Emergency Cardiac Care Committee, American Heart Association: *Textbook on advanced cardiac care*, ed 4, Dallas, 1996, American Heart Association.
7. Eiling R, Plitis J: An evaluation of emergency medical technicians' ability to use manual ventilation devices, *Ann Emerg Med* 12:765, 1983.
8. Giffen PR, Hope CE: Preliminary evaluation of a prototype tube-valve-mask ventilator for emergency artificial ventilation, *Ann Emerg Med* 20:262, 1991.
9. Harrison RR, et al: Mouth-to-mask ventilation: a superior method of rescue breathing, *Ann Emerg Med* 11:74, 1982.
10. Hess D, Baran C: Ventilatory volumes using mouth-to-mouth, mouth-to-mask, and bag-valve-mask techniques at various resistances and compliances, *Respir Care* 32:1025, 1987.
11. Jesudian MC, et al: Bag-valve-mask ventilation two rescuers are better than one: preliminary report, *Crit Care Med* 13:122, 1985.
12. Seidelin PH, Stolarek IH, Littlewood DG: Comparison of six methods of emergency ventilation, *Lancet* 2:1274, 1986.
13. Hess D, Goff G, Johnson K: The effects of hand size, resuscitator brand, and the use of two hand on volume delivered during adult bag-valve ventilation, *Respir Care* 34:805, 1989.
14. Barnes TA: Emergency ventilation techniques and related equipment, *Respir Care* 37:673, 1992.
15. Melker RJ, Banner MJ: Ventilation during CPR: two rescuer standards reappraised, *Ann Emerg Med* 14:397, 1985.
16. Dorsch JA, Dorsch SE: *Understanding anesthesia equipment*, ed 4, Philadelphia, Lippincott, Williams & Wilkins, 1998.

Bibliography

Asai T, Morris S: The laryngeal mask airway: its features, effects and role, *Can J Anesth* 41:930, 1994.

Benumof JL, Scheller MS: The importance of transtracheal jet ventilation in the management of the difficult airway, *Anesthesiol* 71:769, 1989.

Branson RD, Hess DR, Chatburn RL: *Respiratory care equipment*, Philadelphia, 1995, JB Lippincott.

Burkey B, Esclamado R, Morganroth M: The role of cricothyroidotomy in airway management, *Clin Chest Med* 12:561, 1991.

Dorsch JA, Dorsch SE: *Understanding anesthesia equipment: construction, care and complications*, ed 3, Baltimore, 1994, Williams & Wilkins.

Hastings RH, Marks JD: Airway management for trauma patients with potential cervical spine injuries, *Anesth Analg* 73:471, 1991.

Josephson GD, et al: Airway obstruction: new modalities in treatment, *Med Clin North Am* 77:539, 1993.

Schwartz DE, Wiener-Kronish JP: Management of the difficult airway, *Clin Chest Med* 12:483, 1991.

Tobias JD: Airway management for pediatric emergencies, *Ped Ann* 25:317, 1996.

Todres ID: Pediatric airway control and ventilation, *Ann Em Med* 22:440, 1993.

Internet Resources

Airway images from the University of Miami: http://umdas.med.miami.edu

American Association for Respiratory Care: http://www.aarc.org

American Society of Anesthesiologists: http://www.asahq.org

Healthcare Professionals Resources: http://www.healthanswers.com

The Internet Journal of Anesthesiology: http://www.ispub.com/journals/ija.htm

The Internet Journal of Emergency and Intensive Care Medicine: http://www.ispub.com/journals/ijeicm.htm

The Internet Journal of Pulmonary Medicine: http://www.ispub.com/journals/ijpm.htm

Mallinckrodt Corporation: http://www.mallinckrodt.com

National Library of Medicine (Medline/Grateful Med Services): http://www.nlm.nih.gov/databases/freemedl.html

Chapter 7

Lung Expansion Devices

J.M. Cairo

Chapter Outline

Chapter Learning Objectives

Upon completion of this chapter, the reader should be able to:

1. Compare volume-displacement and flow-dependent incentive spirometers.
2. Describe two types of machines used to administer IPPB therapy.
3. Discuss how EPAP, CPAP, and PEP therapies are used to mobilize secretions and treat atelectasis.
4. Identify the major components of pneumatically and electrically powered percussors.
5. Describe the theory of operation of four devices that enhance clearance of airway secretions by producing high-frequency oscillations to the lungs and chest wall.

Key Terms

Bennett Valve
Diluter Regulator
Flow-Dependent Incentive Spirometers
Flutter Valve
Gas-Collector Exhalation Valve
High-Frequency Percussive Breaths
Leaf Type of Valve
Magnetic Valve Resistors
Mainstream Nebulizer
Negative End-Expiratory Pressure (NEEP)
Nonrebreathing Valve
PEP Therapy
Phasitron
Sidestream Nebulizer
Spring-Loaded Resistors
Sustained Maximum Inspiration (SMI)
Volume-Displacement Incentive Spirometers
Underwater Seal Resistors
Weighted Ball Resistors

Lung expansion therapy is an integral part of respiratory care. Various strategies and devices are used to help patients achieve and maintain optimal lung function. The most common strategies include deep breathing exercises, directed coughing, postural drainage, endotracheal suctioning, and medical aerosol therapy. Some of the devices used in lung expansion therapy are incentive spirometers, intermittent positive pressure breathing (IPPB) devices, chest wall percussors, and high-frequency oscillation devices.

The primary indication for lung expansion therapy is to prevent atelectasis. If it is untreated, atelectasis can result in pulmonary shunting, hypoxemia, hypercapnia, and, ultimately, respiratory failure. Factors that contribute to the development of atelectasis include retained secretions, altered breathing patterns, pain associated with surgery and trauma, chronic obstructive and restrictive pulmonary diseases, prolonged immobilization in a supine position, and increased intraabdominal pressure.[1]

The most common devices used by respiratory care practitioners to perform lung expansion therapy are described in this chapter. Selection of the appropriate device should be based on the patient's ability to perform the assigned therapy. Continuation of or changes in therapeutic goals should be determined by frequent assessment of patient status through physical assessment and review of laboratory tests.

Incentive Spirometers

Incentive spirometry (IS) is a lung expansion technique designed to mimic natural sighing or yawning by encouraging patients to take slow, deep breaths.[2] It is a simple and relatively safe method of preventing atelectasis in alert patients who are predisposed to shallow breathing (e.g., patients recovering from thoracic or upper abdominal surgery, chronic obstructive pulmonary distress [COPD] patients recovering from other surgery, patients immobilized or confined to bed).[3] The only contraindication of IS involves patients who are confused, uncooperative, or unable to effectively deep breathe (i.e., vital capacity <10 mL/kg, or inspiratory capacity less than one-third predicted value).[2,3]

Although commercially produced incentive spirometers have been available for about two decades, the concept of sustained maximum inspiration (SMI) has been used since the latter part of the 19th century. Blow-bottles, blow-gloves, and carbon dioxide—induced hyperventilation are examples of devices and techniques that were used by clinicians before the introduction of incentive spirometers to accomplish the goal of having patients take deep breaths to prevent atelectasis.[1]

The principle of incentive spirometry is based on the idea that the patient is encouraged to achieve a preset volume or flow, which is determined from predicted values or baseline measurements. Commercially available incentive spirometers are classified as either volume-displacement or flow-dependent devices. With volume-displacement devices, the volume of air that the patient inspires during a sustained maximum inspiration is measured and displayed. In contrast, flow-dependent devices measure the inspiratory flow that the patient achieves during a maximum sustained inspiratory effort. Volume displacement can be derived with these latter devices by multiplying the flow achieved by the amount of time the flow is maintained.

CLINICAL ROUNDS 7-1

You are asked to assess a 50-year-old postoperative woman recovering from abdominal surgery. A physical examination revealed no acute distress, but the patient is having problems clearing secretions. Auscultation of the chest indicates retention of secretions, particularly in the right lower lung; the patient has no history of lung disease. Suggest a therapeutic plan for her.

See Appendix A for the answer.

We are not aware of any prospective studies that have demonstrated that incentive spirometry is superior to other hyperexpansion methods relying on natural deep breathing exercises. Indeed, evidence suggests that deep breathing alone—without an incentive spirometer—can be beneficial in preventing or reversing pulmonary complications in some postoperative patients.[4-6] The advantage of using an incentive spirometer may be related to the fact that patients receive immediate visual feedback about whether they are achieving the prescribed goal (Clinical Rounds 7-1). Furthermore, patients can perform the treatment regimen without the direct supervision of a respiratory therapist after they have demonstrated mastery of the technique, thus providing a cost-effective approach to lung expansion therapy.[5] CPG 7-1 summarizes the American Association for Respiratory Care (AARC) Clinical Practice Guideline for incentive spirometry.

Volume-Displacement Devices

Figure 7-1 is a schematic of a prototype of a volume-displacement incentive spirometer. The operational principle is simple: the patients inhale air through a mouthpiece and corrugated tubing attached to a flexible plastic bellows. The volume of air displaced is indicated on a scale, which is located on the device enclosure. After patients have achieved the maximum volume, they are instructed to hold this volume constant for 3 to 5 seconds. They can then remove the mouthpiece and exhale, while the bellows expand to the starting position. Some authors have suggested that patients should perform a minimum of 5 to 10 breaths per session every hour while awake.[2] Note that the respiratory therapist does not have to be present for each performance, and patients should be encouraged to perform this therapy independently.

Incentive spirometers used for adult patients typically have a total volume capacity of about 4 L, and those used for children have a volume capacity of about 2 L. DHD Medical

Clinical Practice Guidelines 7-1

Incentive Spirometry (IS)

Indications

1. Conditions predisposed to the development of pulmonary atelectasis, such as upper-abdominal surgery, thoracic surgery, and surgery in patients with chronic obstructive pulmonary disease (COPD).
2. Pulmonary atelectasis
3. Restrictive lung defects associated with quadriplegia or dysfunctional diaphragm

Contraindications

1. Patient cannot be instructed or supervised to ensure appropriate use of the device
2. Patient is unable to deep breathe effectively (e.g., vital capacity <10 mL/kg, or inspiratory capacity is less than one third of that predicted).

Complications

1. Must be closely supervised or performed as ordered
2. Inappropriate as the only treatment for major lung collapse or consolidation
3. Hyperventilation
4. Barotrauma (emphysematous lungs)
5. Discomfort secondary to inadequate pain control
6. Hypoxia secondary to interruption of oxygen therapy if face mask or shield is being used
7. Exacerbation of bronchospasm
8. Fatigue

Assessment of Outcome

Absence of or improvement in signs of atelectasis:

a. Decreased respiratory rate
b. Resolution of fever
c. Normal pulse rate
d. No crackles on auscultation, or improvement in previously absent or diminished breath sounds
e. Normal chest radiograph
f. Improved arterial oxygenation
g. Increased vital capacity and peak expiratory flows
h. Return of functional residual capacity or vital capacity to preoperative values without lung resection
i. Improved inspiratory muscle performance

Monitoring

Direct patient supervision is not necessary once the patient has demonstrated mastery of the technique; however, preoperative instruction, volume goals, and feedback are essential to optimal performance.

AARC Clinical Practice Guideline: Incentive spirometry, *Respir Care* 36:1402, 1991.

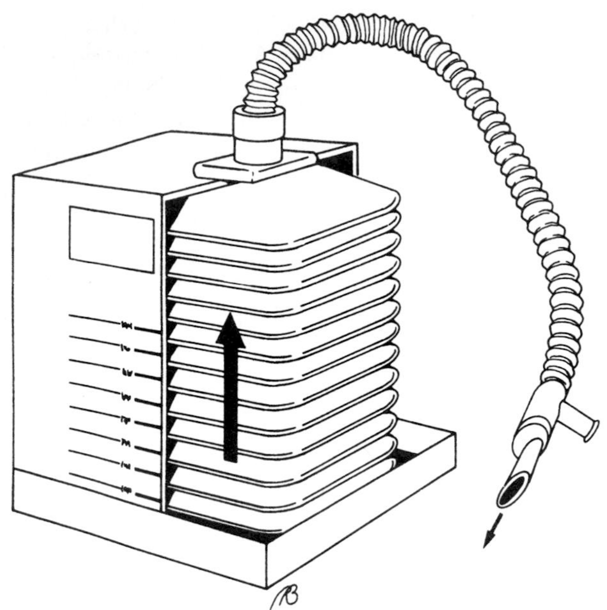

Figure 7-1 Volume-incentive breathing exerciser. (From Eubanks DH, Bone RC: *Comprehensive respiratory care, a learning system*, ed 2, St Louis, 1990, Mosby.)

Products' Volurex incentive spirometer (Figure 7-2, *A*) is a disposable device that operates similarly to the prototype unit described previously. It is slightly more sophisticated, however, in that after the patient inhales, the plastic bellows must be released by the push of a button before it returns to its starting position. Sherwood Medical's Voldyne Exerciser (Figure 7-2, *B*) and DHD's Coach 2300 (Figure 7-2, *C*) and Coach Jr consist of a movable piston in a clear cylinder. As the patient inhales, the piston rises and the inspired volume is indicated on a scale engraved on the side of the cylinder. A flow indicator is also included as a visual aid encouraging the patient to take slow, deep breaths.

Although most incentive spirometers are designed for single-patient use, multiple-use devices are available even though these latter devices are rarely used anymore. Single-patient devices are usually made of plastic and can be discarded after the patient has completed the course of therapy. (Actually, patients should be encouraged to keep these devices and use them if similar respiratory illnesses are incurred.) Multiple-use incentive spirometers are usually electrically powered devices that use disposable mouthpieces and flow tubes and typically require that a respiratory therapist is available during treatment.

Flow-Dependent Devices

Figure 7-3 shows a typical flow-dependent incentive spirometer, which consists of a mouthpiece and corrugated tubing connected to a manifold that is composed of three flow tubes containing lightweight plastic balls. As the patient inhales through the mouthpiece, a negative pressure is created within the tubes, causing them to rise. The device is designed so that the number of balls and the level that the balls rise depends on the flow achieved. At lower flows, the first ball rises to a level that depends on the magnitude of the flow. As the inspiratory flow increases, the second ball rises, followed by the third ball. The flow achieved by the patient can be estimated based on the manufacturer's specifications. For example, with Sherwood Medical's Triflo incentive spirometer, the patient must achieve a flow of 600 mL/sec to raise the first ball. A flow of 900 mL/sec is required to raise the second ball, and a flow of 1200 mL/sec must be generated to raise the third ball. As with volume-displacement incentive spirometers, it is important that the patient perform a maximum sustained inspiration.

The DHD Respirex incentive spirometer (Figure 7-4) consists of a single tube containing a plastic ball. An adjustable volume selector can be used to vary the patient effort necessary to attain the desired inspiratory capacity. The Intertech incentive spirometer uses a similar design but can also display the number of successful efforts and the maximum flow achieved.[3] The Hudson incentive spirometer (Figure 7-5) uses a different type of design: the patient inhales through a mouthpiece and corrugated tubing connected to a dual-chamber device. The two chambers of this device are arranged in series. The ball in the inner chamber rises when the patient achieves a flow that equals the inspiratory flow selected by the operator. Inspiratory flows vary from 200 mL/sec to 1200 mL/sec.

Intermittent Positive Pressure Breathing (IPPB) Devices

IPPB is a short-term therapeutic modality that involves the delivery of inspiratory positive pressure to spontaneously breathing patients. Since its introduction in 1947, IPPB has been used for a variety of reasons, including short-term ventilatory support and lung expansion therapy, and as an aid in delivering aerosolized medications.[7,8] During the past two decades, the effectiveness of IPPB as a therapeutic modality has been questioned rigorously, resulting in a reassessment of the indications for its prescription. In 1993, the AARC produced a Clinical Practice Guideline providing a rational basis for prescribing and administering IPPB treatments (see CPG 7-2 for a summary of this guideline).[8] It should be recognized that although IPPB is not the therapy of choice when other modalities can be used for aerosol delivery or lung expansion in spontaneously breathing patients, it can be potentially beneficial when incentive spirometry, chest physiotherapy, deep breathing exercises, and positive airway pressure (PAP) techniques have been unsuccessful (Clinical Rounds 7-2).[8]

IPPB can be administered with any device that can deliver intermittent positive pressure to the airway (e.g., conventional mechanical ventilators or manual resuscitators), but it is most often performed with specially designed electrically and pneumatically powered ventilators. These specially designed IPPB machines are usually categorized as patient-triggered, pressure-cycled mechanical ventilators.

A

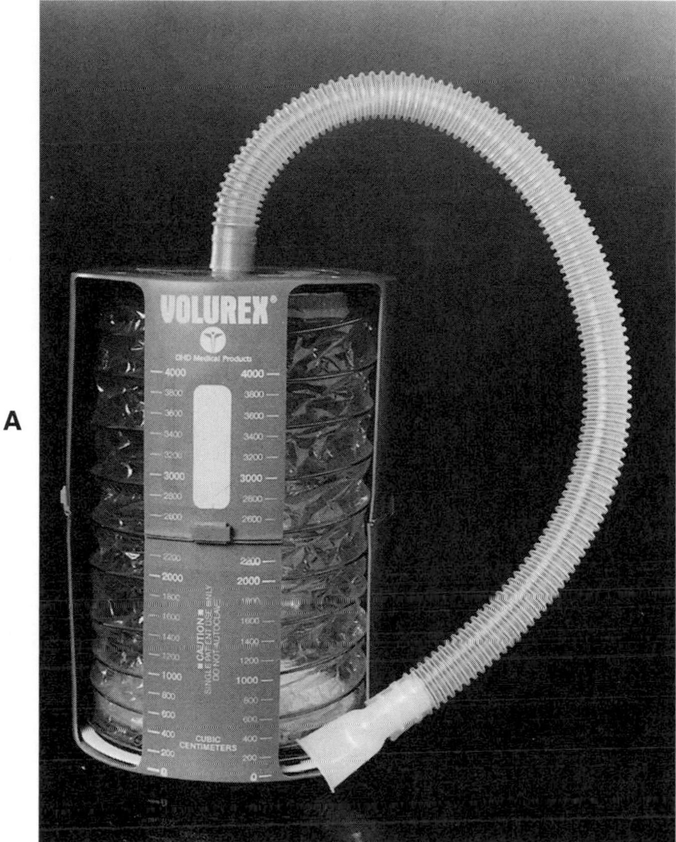

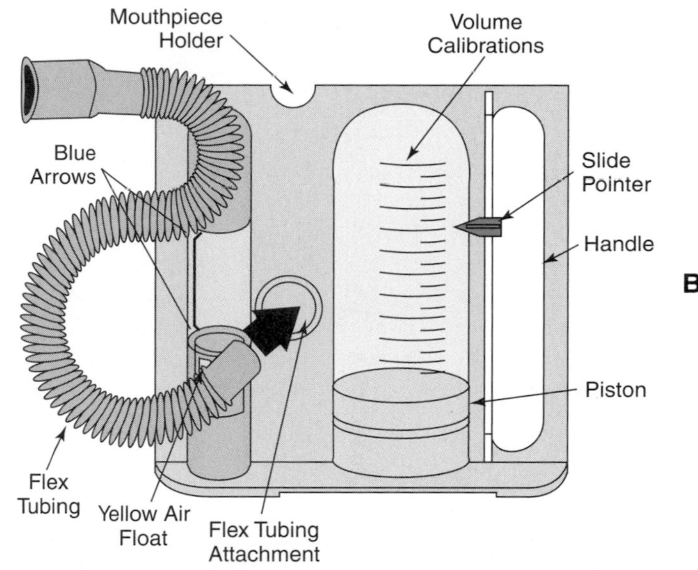

B

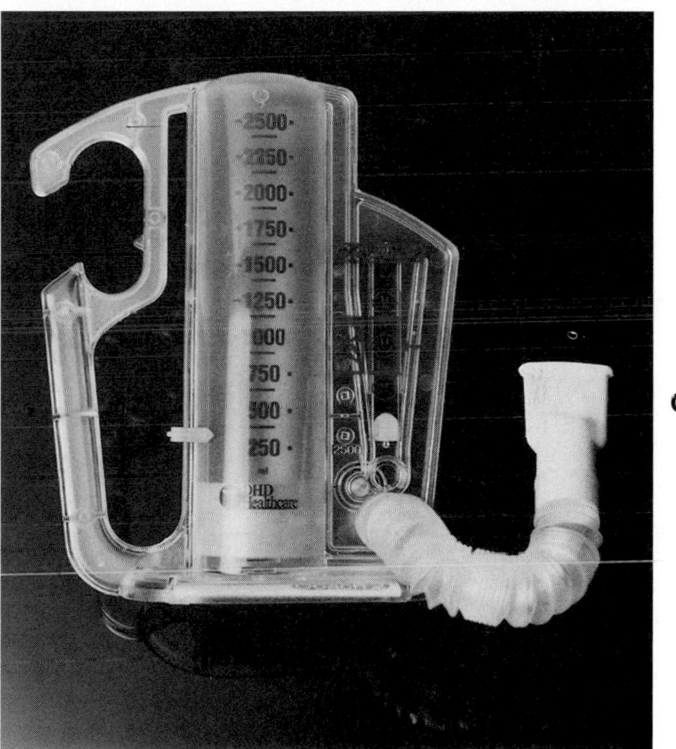

C

Figure 7-2 **A,** Volurex incentive spirometer. **B,** Picture Voldyne Exerciser. **C,** DHD Coach 2300. (**B** courtesy Sherwood Medical, St Louis.)

Regardless of the manufacturer, all IPPB machines require a 45 to 55 psig gas pressure source, such as a compressed gas cylinder, a bulk air or oxygen system, or an air compressor. Furthermore, they all incorporate control valves that begin inspiration when a negative pressure is generated by the patient and terminate it when a preset pressure is achieved. The amount of negative pressure (i.e., patient effort) required to initiate inspiration depends on the sensitivity of the device, which may be fixed or adjustable. The pressure that must be achieved to end inspiration, and thus initiate exhalation, can typically be adjusted to as high as 60 cm H_2O.[8]

Machines manufactured by Puritan Bennett (Tyco Healthcare) and the Bird Products Corporation (Viasys Healthcare) are still the most widely used devices for IPPB therapy.[9] A brief description of the most commonly used IPPB units produced by these companies follows.

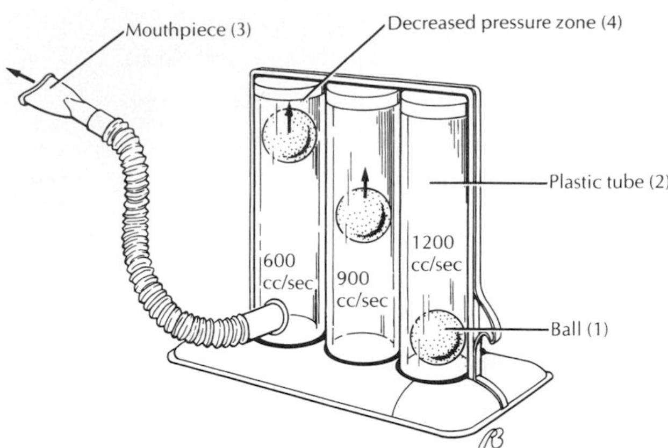

Figure 7-3 Flow-oriented incentive spirometer. (From Eubanks DH, Bone RC: *Comprehensive respiratory care,* St Louis, 1985, Mosby.)

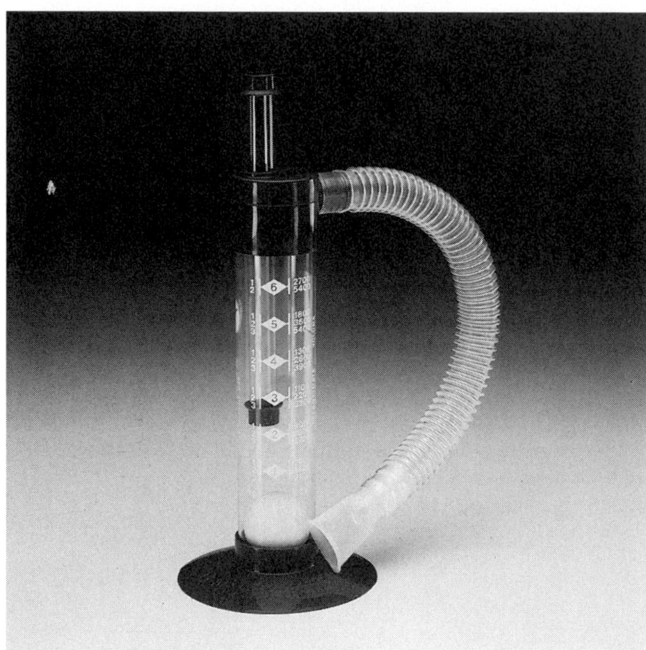

Figure 7-4 DHD Respirex incentive spirometer. (Courtesy DHD Medical Products, Wampsville, New York.)

Puritan Bennett Devices

Puritan Bennett manufactures pneumatically and electrically powered IPPB machines. The tank ventilator (TV), the pedestal ventilator (PV), and the pedestal respirator (PR) series are pneumatically powered IPPB machines; the air-powered (AP) series of ventilators are electrically powered. The PR-1 and PR-2 models are the most commonly used pneumatically powered IPPB devices. The AP-4 and AP-5 models are the most commonly used electrically powered IPPB machines.

Puritan Bennett PR Series

The PR-1 (Figure 7-6) and PR-2 (Figure 7-7) ventilators are pneumatically powered devices that can be time- or pressure-triggered, but both are flow-cycled and pressure-

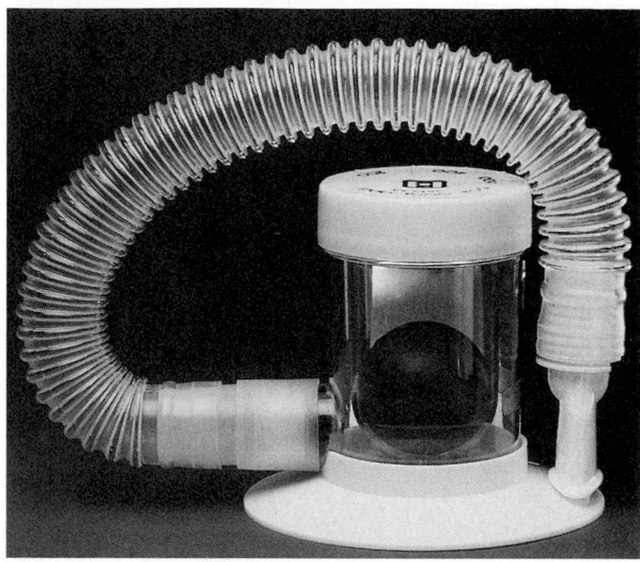

Figure 7-5 Hudson incentive spirometer. (Courtesy Hudson RCI, Temecula, Calif.)

limited. (Note that time cycling allows these devices to provide controlled, short-term ventilatory support.) They can deliver either 100% source gas or air-diluted source gas.

The PR-2 has adjustable controls for setting the pressure limit and the sensitivity or level of negative pressure that must be achieved to initiate inspiration. It also has controls for adjusting the peak flow, inspiratory and expiratory nebulizer gas flows, and negative end-expiratory pressure (NEEP). A terminal flow control is provided for minor leak compensation. In contrast, the PR-1 does not have a peak flow control or the capability of providing NEEP. The PR-1 does not have separate controls for inspiratory and expiratory nebulization; instead, the inspiratory nebulization is a composite of continuous nebulization and the inspiratory nebulizer flow. The PR-1 does not have an expiratory time control.

Gas flow through the PR-2 ventilator is shown in Figure 7-8. (Note that gas flow through the PR-1 is comparable.) Compressed gas from a 50 psig gas source enters the ventilator through a brass filter. It is directed to a diluter regulator, to the nebulizer pressure switch, and to a low-pressure regulator. The diluter regulator (Figure 7-9) is an adjustable reducing valve that regulates the gas pressure delivered to the patient. It can be set from 0 to 30 cm H_2O using a control knob on the front panel of the machine. Gas flow to nebulizer switch controls the flow of gas to the nebulizer during inspiration and expiration. Nebulizer flow can be adjusted with two knobs on the lower part of the machine's side panel. (Note that the nebulizer is powered by 100% source gas; therefore, use of the nebulizer affects the delivered fractionated inspired oxygen [F_IO_2] when the PR-2 is set to air-dilution mode.) Gas flow to the nebulizer also controls a Venturi that allows the application of NEEP from 0 to –6 cm H_2O. The NEEP level can be adjusted with a knob just above the inspiratory nebulizer control on

Clinical Practice Guidelines 7-2

Intermittent Positive Pressure Breathing (IPPB)

Indications

1. The need to improve lung expansion, particularly for those patients who demonstrate clinically important atelectasis when other forms of therapy, such as incentive spirometry, CPT, deep breathing exercises, and PAP are unsuccessful. It may also be useful for patients who cannot cooperate with standard lung expansion techniques.
2. Inability to adequately clear secretions because of pathology that severely limits the patient's ability to ventilate or cough effectively
3. As an alternative to endotracheal intubation and continuous ventilatory support for patients requiring short-term ventilatory support
4. To deliver aerosolized medications to patients fatigued as a result of respiratory muscle weakness. It can also be used to deliver aerosolized medications to patients not able to use an MDI.

Contraindications

1. Elevated intracranial pressure (>15 mm Hg)
2. Hemodynamic instability
3. Recent facial, oral, or skull surgery
4. Tracheoesophageal fistula
5. Recent esophageal surgery
6. Active hemoptysis
7. Nausea
8. Air swallowing
9. Active, untreated tuberculosis
10. Radiographic evidence of bleb
11. Hiccups

Hazards

1. Barotrauma, pneumothorax
2. Hemoptysis
3. Hypocarbia (hypocapnia)
4. Increased airway resistance
5. Gastric distension
6. Impeded venous return
7. $\dot{V}/\dot{Q}$ mismatch
8. Air trapping, auto-PEEP, overdistended alveoli
9. Psychological dependence
10. Impaction of secretions resulting from inadequate humidification

Assessment of Need

1. Presence of atelectasis
2. Reduced pulmonary function: FVC <70% of predicted; MVV <50% of predicted; or VC <10 mL/kg of predicted, precluding an effective cough
3. Neuromuscular disorders (e.g., kyphoscoliosis) associated with reduced lung volumes
4. Fatigue or respiratory muscle weakness with impending respiratory failure
5. If effective, the patient preference for a positive-pressure device should be honored

Assessment of Outcomes

1. Tidal volume during IPPB is greater than during spontaneous breathing by at least 25%
2. Increase in forced expiratory volume in one second ($FEV_{1.0}$) or peak expiratory flow (PEF)
3. Improved cough with treatment, leading to better clearance of secretions
4. Improvements in chest radiographs
5. Improved breath sounds
6. Favorable patient response

AARC Clinical Practice Guideline: Intermittent positive pressure breathing (IPPB), *Respir Care* 38:1189, 1993.

the side panel. NEEP was originally proposed as a means of reducing the level of airtrapping experienced by some patients during IPPB. Because it was subsequently found that applying NEEP actually increased the level of airtrapping, this therapeutic mode is no longer used.

From the diluter regulator, gas flows to the Bennett valve, which consists of a counterweighted, hollow drum with attached vanes (Figure 7-10). (It is called a Bennett valve for Dr. Ray Bennett, who invented it in 1945 for use in high-altitude aircraft breathing apparatuses. After World War II, the valve was adapted for medical applications.[9]) The drum rotates in a special housing on the front and rear jeweled bearings.* As Figure 7-10, A, shows, the drum vane creates a barrier between atmospheric and circuit pressures. Inspiration is triggered when the patient removes enough volume from the tubing to create a pressure gradient of 0.5 cm H_2O across the valve, thus causing it to rotate counterclockwise *(B)*. (Note that the manufacturer presets the sensitivity of the machine at 0.5 cm H_2O, but the sensitivity [or amount of patient effort] that must be exerted to trigger inspiration can be changed by rotating the sensitivity knob counterclockwise.) The sensitivity of this valve is ultimately controlled by gas that flows to the low-pressure regulator mentioned previously. Gas flow from the low-pressure regulator is directed to the Bennett valve via a port located just above the upper drum vane. As the sensitivity is increased, the gas flow through the port rotates the drum counterclockwise toward inspiration, making it easier for the patient to trigger the ventilator (i.e., the patient can trigger inspiration with less effort). A small flow of gas

**It is important to recognize that the bearing and housing have serial numbers that must match. These components are specially machined, and mismatching of the serial numbers or damage to the bearing will impair the function of the valve.[9]*

CLINICAL ROUNDS 7-2

A 38-year-old man is admitted to the hospital from a rehabilitation center with a diagnosis of pneumonia. He has quadriplegia and permanent brain damage as a result of a motor vehicle accident. He also has a permanent tracheostomy but does not require ventilatory support. Current evaluation reveals the following: temperature 103° F; respiratory rate = 28 breaths/min; heart rate = 100 beats/min; pulse oximetry saturation (SpO_2) on 30% heated tracheostomy collar is 93%. Copious amounts of thick, green secretions are present, and the patient coughs only when stimulated with suctioning. Crackles are present in both bases. Based on these findings, what form of respiratory care would you recommend?

See Appendix A for the answer.

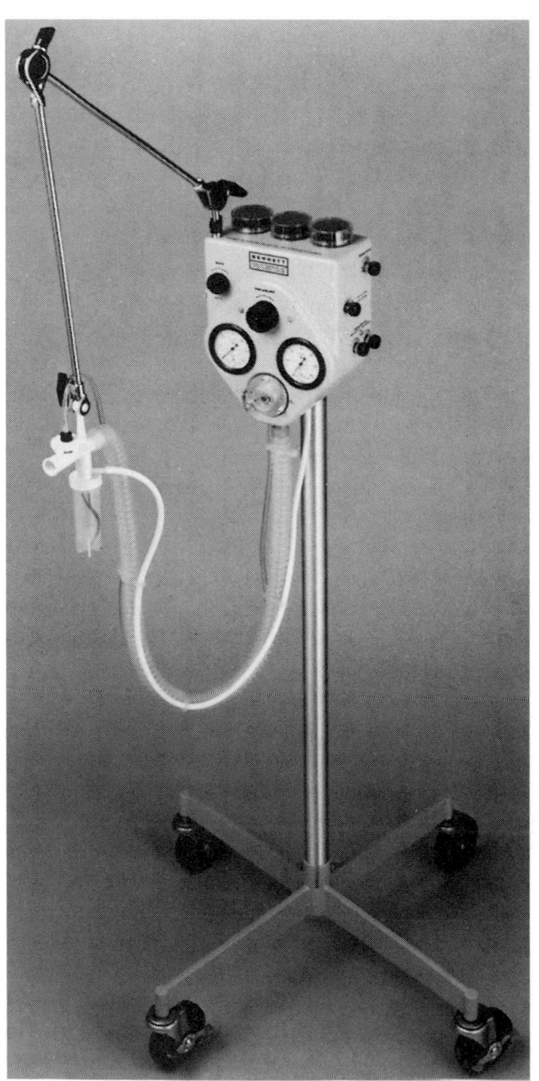

Figure 7-6 Bennett PR-1 ventilator. (Courtesy Tyco Healthcare, Puritan Bennett, Pleasanton, Calif.)

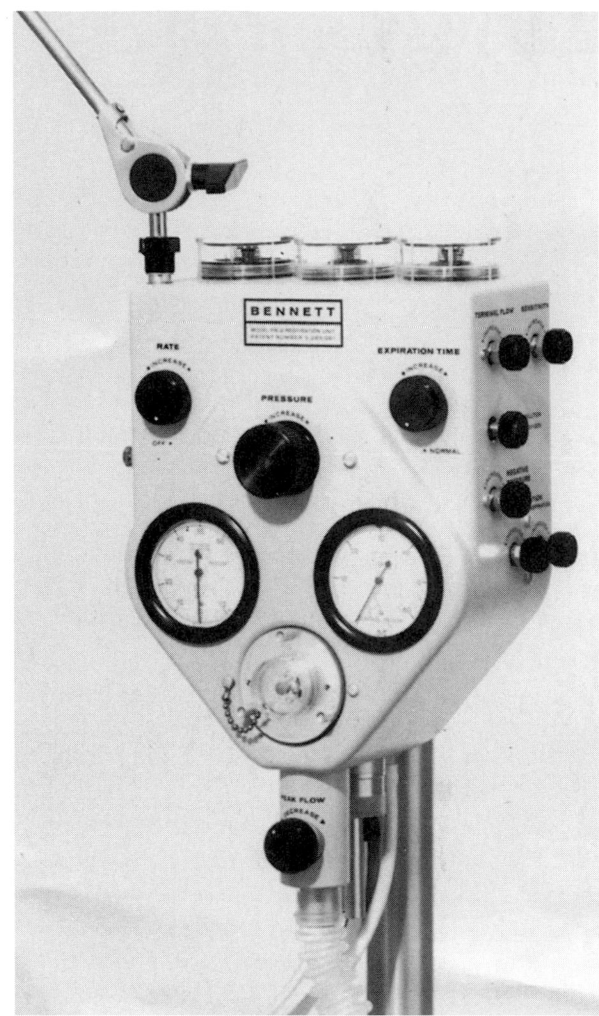

Figure 7-7 Bennett PR-2 ventilator. (Courtesy Tyco Healthcare, Puritan Bennett, Pleasanton, Calif.)

from the valve travels out of the exhalation valve line and inflates an exhalation diaphragm, preventing gas from escaping through the exhalation port during the inspiratory phase. Gas, which is directed into the breathing circuit and to the patient, flows through the valve, holding it open. As the pressure proximal to the valve is kept constant, the pressure gradient decreases, allowing gravity to cause a counterweight to slowly rotate the valve clockwise, back toward the closed position *(C)*. When the flow through the valve decreases to 1 to 3 L/min, the force of gravity is sufficient to swing the valve completely closed, thus terminating inspiration *(D)*. After the valve is closed, gas flow to the exhalation diaphragm is halted and the diaphragm deflates, allowing gas from the patient circuit to flow into the room.

Notice that the Bennett valve also includes a port (which releases gas from within the drum to atmospheric pressure [exhalation]), a bleed hole (which allows a small leak when the valve opens to prevent it from recoiling or fluttering), and two manometer ports (see Figure 7-10, *A*). One of these manometer ports is for controlling pressure from the diluter

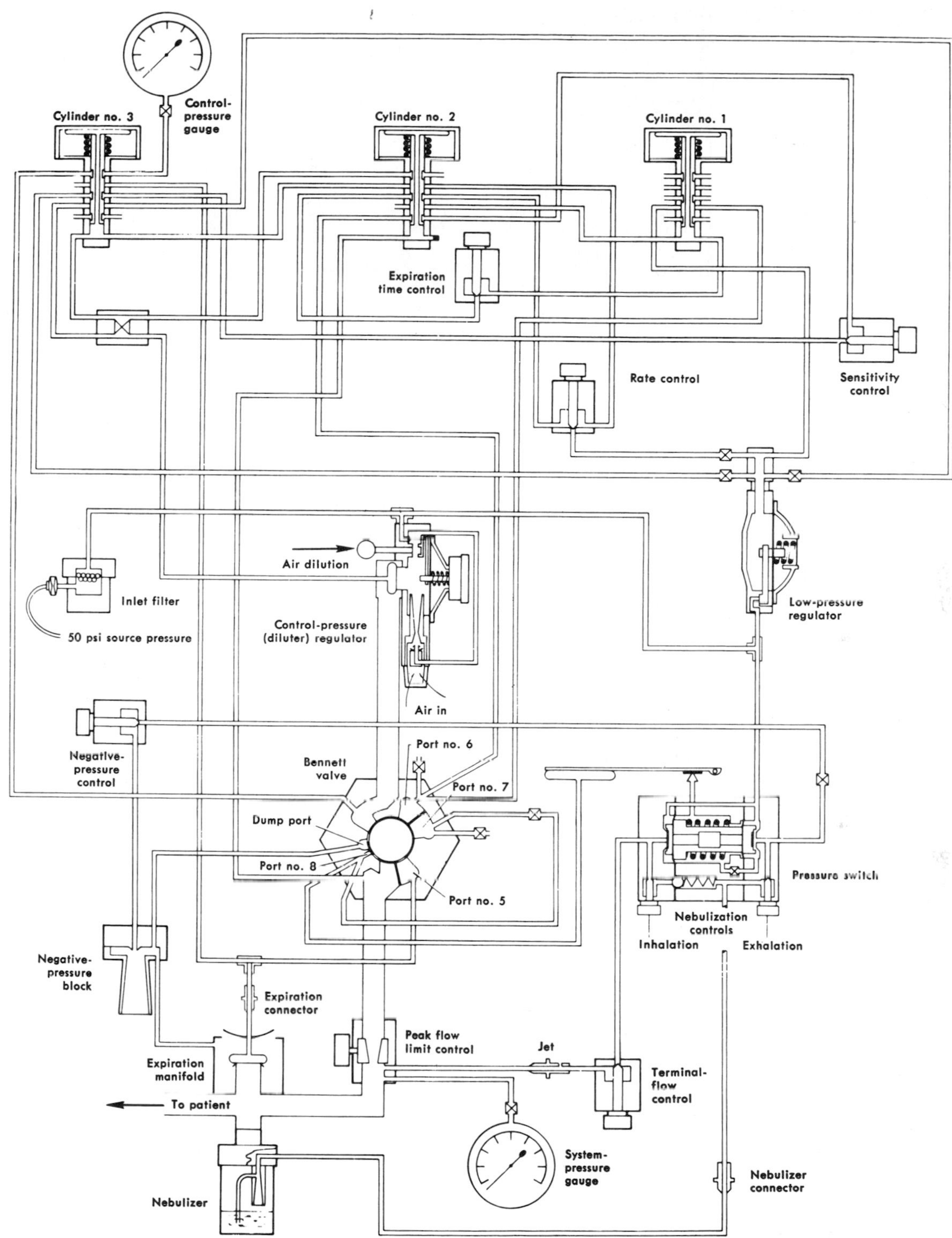

Figure 7-8 Flow schematic of a PR-2 ventilator as shown from behind the device. (Courtesy Tyco Healthcare, Puritan Bennett, Pleasanton, Calif.)

regulator, and the other monitors pressure in the patient circuit.

Puritan Bennett AP Series

The AP-4 and AP-5 units (Figure 7-11) are electrically powered, pressure-limited ventilators. Unlike the PR series, these devices are only patient-triggered, so they can be used for IPPB therapy but not for providing short-term ventilatory support of apneic patients. As shown in Figure 7-12, air from the unit's compressor passes through a filter and flows to the Venturi jet in the pressure control and then to a needle valve that controls the level of nebulization. The

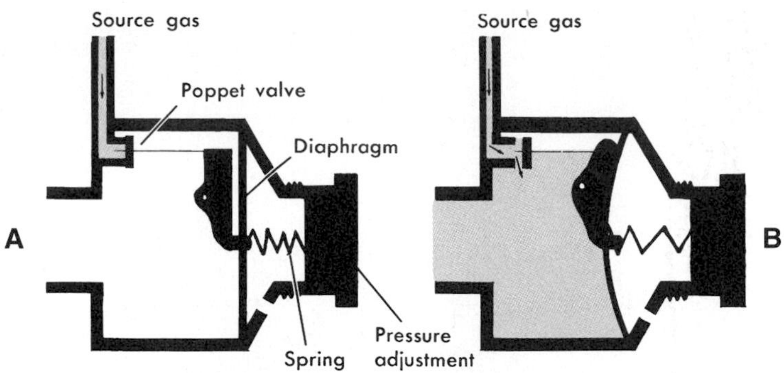

Figure 7-9 Bennett diluter regulator. **A,** Pressure equals spring tension. **B,** Pressure is below spring tension. This product is no longer manufactured by Neller Puritan Bennett.

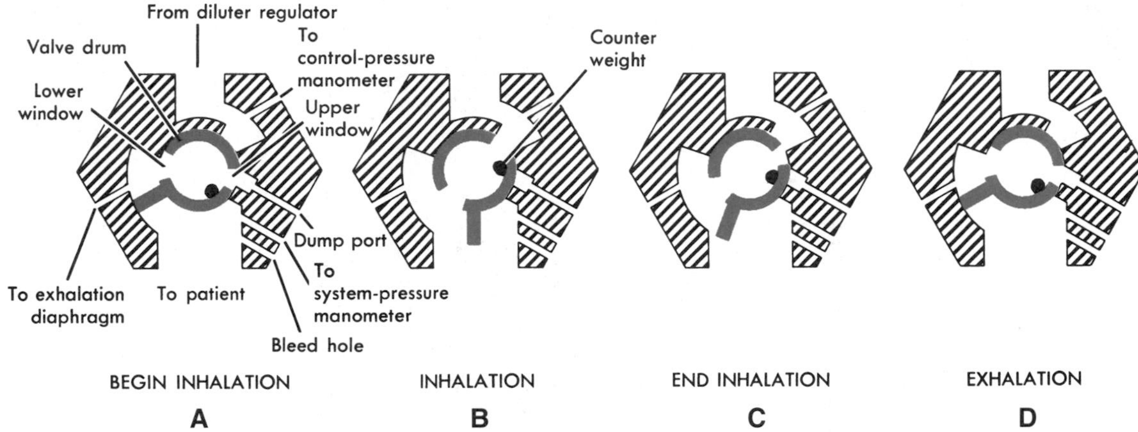

Figure 7-10 The Bennett Valve: a function diagram. (Courtesy Tyco Healthcare, Puritan Bennett, Pleasanton, Calif.)

Venturi jet entrains additional air through an intake filter, and there is a spring-disk release valve instead of the diluter regulator of the PR series. When the pressure in the system control unit exceeds that of the spring tension, the pressure pushes the disk to the left, allowing the excess pressure to vent to ambient pressure. Note that the spring tension on the disk, and thus the peak pressure, can be adjusted to values of 0 to 30 cm H_2O. With all gas venting through the release valve, the Bennett valve rotates shut, starting exhalation. When the Bennett valve opens, gas flows from the control unit to the patient.

Puritan Bennett Circuits

The basic components of the Puritan Bennett breathing circuit comprise large-bore corrugated tubing, a nebulizer, and an exhalation valve. Two types of nebulizers are available: mainstream (Bennett slip/stream) and sidestream (Bennett Twin) nebulizers (Figure 7-13).

The Bennett retard exhalation valve consists of a spring that is compressed as the diaphragm nut is tightened (Figure 7-14). When the nut is loosened, the spring pushes the diaphragm closer to the shoulder of the exhalation valve, causing a resistance to expiratory gas flow. The gas-collector exhalation valve (Figure 7-15) allows expired gases to be measured through one directional port.

Bird Devices

The prototype Bird ventilator is the Mark 7, which was designed and developed by Forrest M. Bird, founder of the Bird Corporation. Bird subsequently introduced the Mark 8, which functions similarly to the Mark 7, but can provide a flow of source gas during the expiratory phase, thus allowing the operator to apply a negative expiratory pressure. A second generation of Bird ventilators were introduced in the late 1970s and provided additional capabilities. These latter units, however, also used the same ceramic control valve and ambient and pressure compartments as the first generation of Bird ventilators.

Before the components of the various Bird IPPB ventilators are described, their basic operational principle should be discussed. This principle has been referred as magnetism versus gas pressure and can be described using the schematic in Figure 7-16. Notice that the schematic includes a series of boxes. Each box is divided into two compartments by a diaphragm, which has metal clutch plates attached to either side. Permanent magnets, which are aligned with the clutch plates, are located in each compartment. The left compartment is exposed to atmospheric pressure through a port in the lower left corner of box. The pressure on the right side of each box can be

A

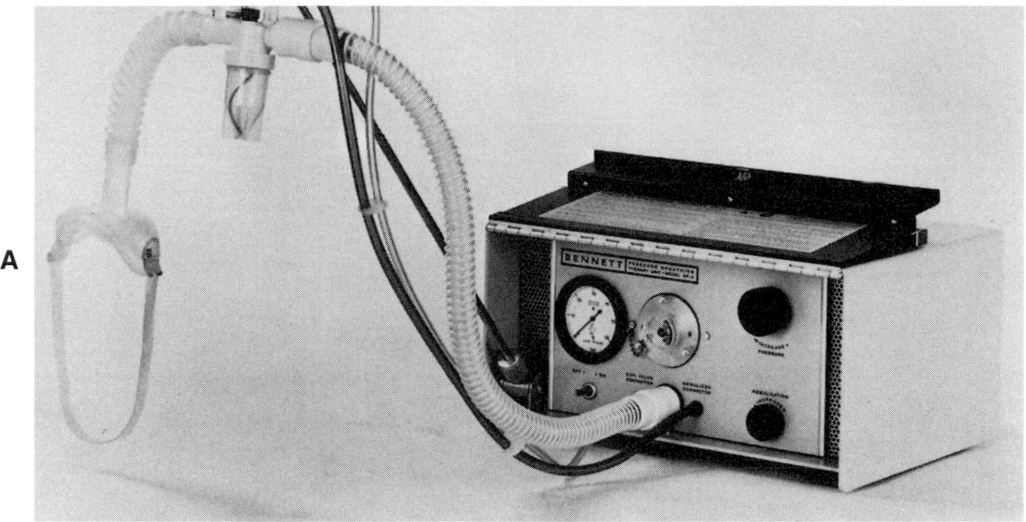

B

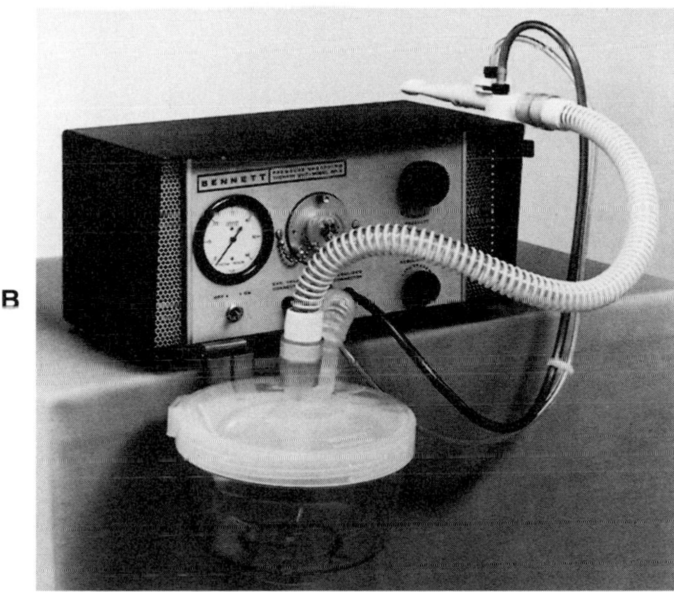

Figure 7-11 **A,** Bennett AP-4. **B,** Bennett AP-5. Both units are air compressor-driven ventilators. (Courtesy Tyco Healthcare, Puritan Bennett, Pleasanton, Calif.)

varied by moving gas into and out of a port in the lower right corner of the box.

If the two compartments are subjected to atmospheric pressure (see Figure 7-16, A), there is no pressure difference between them, and the diaphragm remains straight. But when a pressure gradient is created between the right and left compartments, the diaphragm flexes. In Figure 7-16, *B*, as gas volume is removed from the right compartment, the pressure inside the compartment decreases to below atmospheric, causing the diaphragm and the attached metal plates to flex to the right. The clutch plate on the right is now close to the magnet on the right, and the plate and magnet are attracted to each other. Although the pressure on the right may return to atmospheric pressure (Figure 7-16, C), the diaphragm will remain attracted to the right magnet until sufficient gas volume and pressure are added to the right side to overcome the magnetic attraction (Figure 7-16, *D*). After there is sufficient positive pressure to overcome the magnetic attraction, the diaphragm will be pushed to the left where it will remain.

Bird Mark 7 Series

The Mark 7 is a pneumatically powered ventilator, which can be time-, pressure-, or manually triggered and time- or pressure-cycled. Similar to the Puritan Bennett PR series, the Mark 7 can be used to provide short-term ventilatory support, but it is primarily used as a means of delivering IPPB therapy.

Figure 7-17 shows the major components of the Bird Mark 7 ventilator. Gas flow through the Mark 7 is shown in

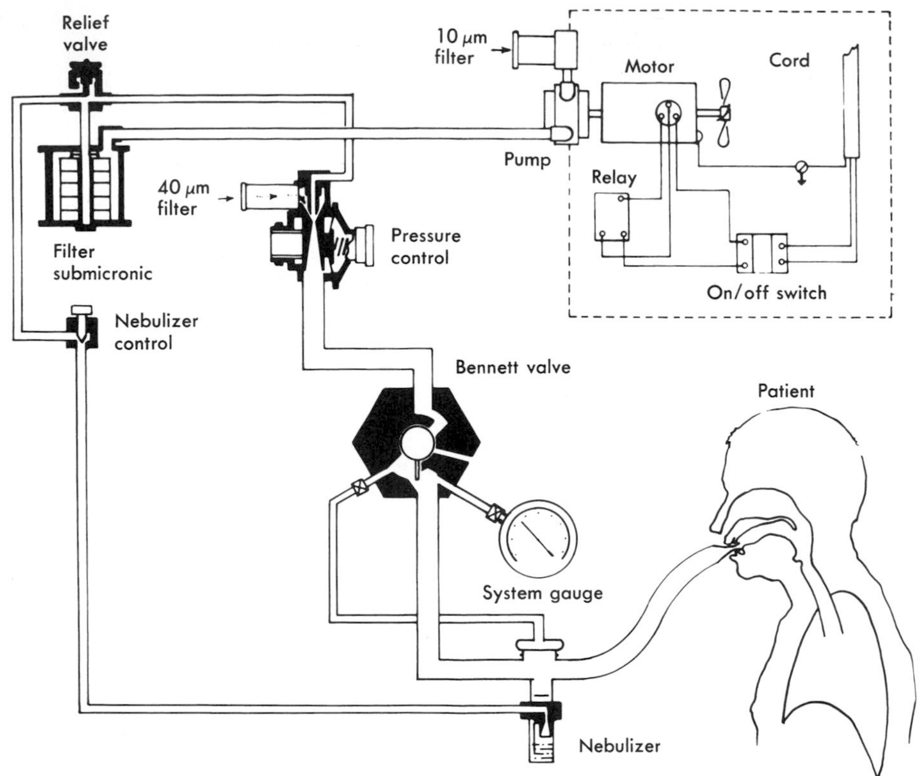

Figure 7-12 Functional diagram of AP series ventilators. (Courtesy Tyco Healthcare, Puritan Bennett, Pleasanton, Calif.)

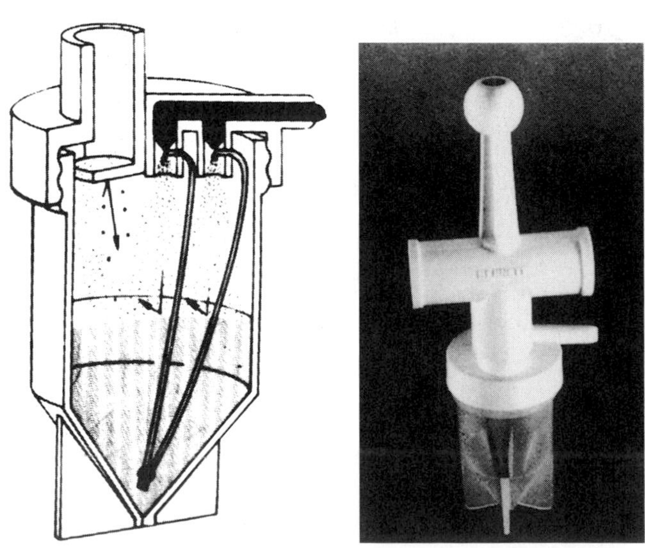

Figure 7-13 Bennet Twin jet nebulizer. (Courtesy Tyco Healthcare, Puritan Bennett, Pleasanton, Calif.)

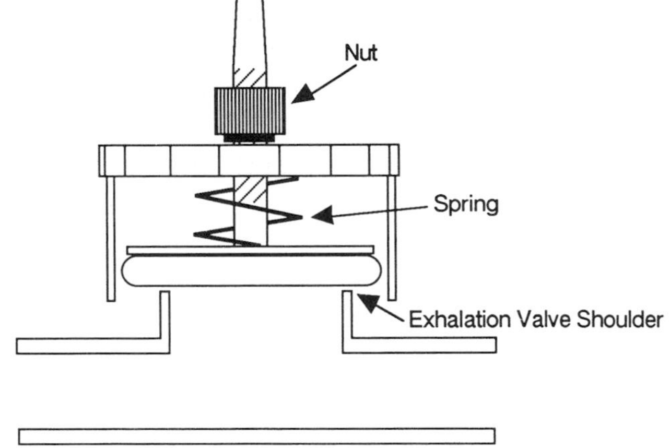

Figure 7-14 Bennett retard exhalation valve.

Figure 7-18. During inspiration *(A)*, negative pressure generated by the patient (along with atmospheric pressure in the left compartment) causes the diaphragm to move toward the right, away from the left compartment. Gas flow is allowed to pass through the ceramic control switch and then splits, traveling in the left side to the Venturi jet and passing to the line powering the nebulizer and exhalation valve. The Venturi jet then entrains air, and gas moves

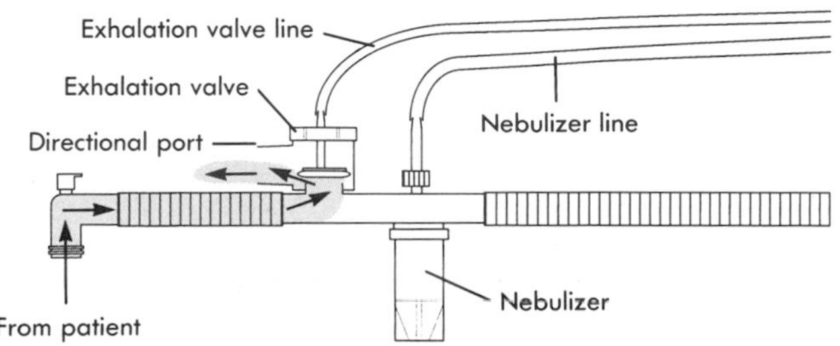

Figure 7-15 Bennett gas collector exhalation valve.

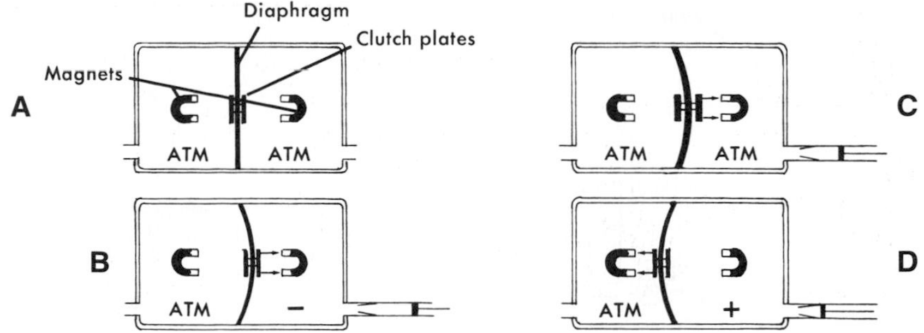

Figure 7-16 Pressure changes across the diaphragm with magnetic force (see text for explanation). *ATM,* Atmospheric pressure. (Modified from Viasys Healthcare, Critical Care Division, Palm Springs, Calif.)

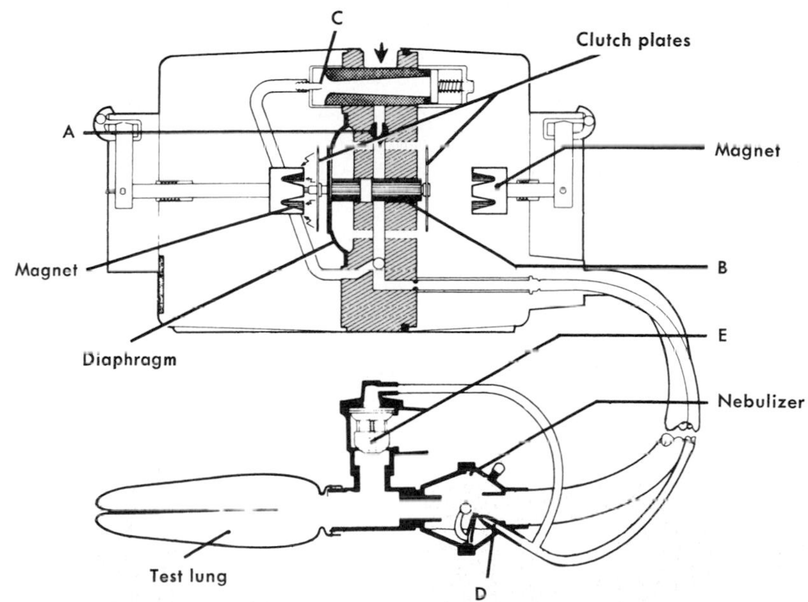

Figure 7-17 Structure of a Bird Mark 7. (Modified from Viasys Healthcare, Critical Care Division, Palm Springs, Calif.)

through the Venturi gate to the patient. This gas then enters the patient's lungs, and the pressure begins to build in the right compartment. Thus at the beginning of inspiration, gas flow into the circuit comes from three sources: (1) the Venturi, (2) the air the Venturi entrains, and (3) the nebulizer jet. As end-inspiration is approached, the pressure in the right compartment equals the forward pressure through the Venturi, and the Venturi gate closes. The gas from the Venturi jet is then forced into the left side of the machine, flushing that compartment with source gas. After the Venturi gate closes, the only gas flowing into the patient's system during the remainder of inspiration comes from source gas through the nebulizer jet. Eventually, this jet adds enough gas to make the pressure exceed the magnetic attraction of the right (pressure-controlled) magnet. The diaphragm, clutch plate, and ceramic switch are then forced to the left, occluding gas flow into the respirator and starting exhalation. The amount of pressure needed to end inspiration depends on the magnetic attraction between the right clutch plate and the corresponding magnet. As with the left clutch plate and magnet, the amount of attraction is related to the distance between the right plate and its magnet. The distance, and thus the peak inspiratory pressure, can be set with the pressure adjustment lever on the right side of the machine. Because gas is no longer flowing into the flow control valve, the gas in the lines below the ceramic switch exits through the jets. The diaphragm and exhalation valve are now uncharged, and the existing positive pressure in the patient circuit simply pushes the exhalation valve gate open, allowing the patient to exhale passively (see Figure 7-19, *B*).

The Mark 7 contains a pneumatic expiratory timing device that can be used to provide pressure-cycled ventilation. The timer is a pneumatic cartridge with an adjustable leak (Figure 7-19). On inspiration, the cartridge is charged by source gas, which enters via a one-way valve. The gas pushes the diaphragm to the left, depressing the spring and moving the plunger and arm to the left. The leak from the cartridge around the needle valve control is small when compared with the incoming gas flow. Thus after inspiration has begun, the unit is completely charged until inhalation ends. At

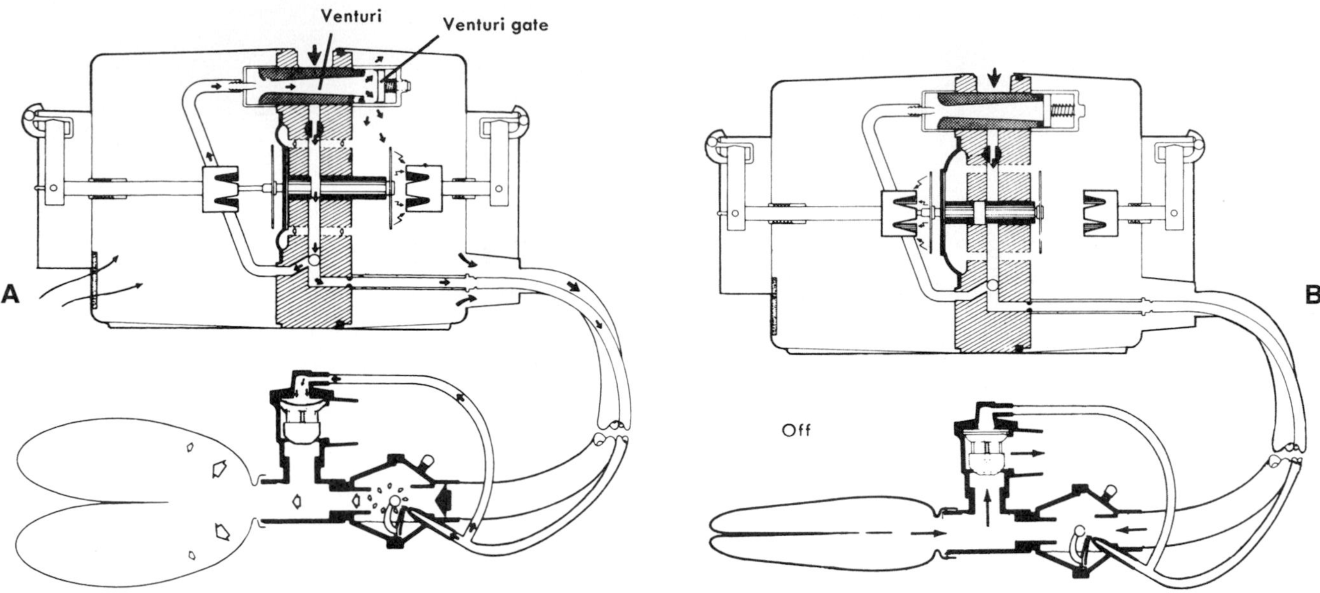

Figure 7-18 **A,** Inhalation. **B,** Exhalation. (Modified from Viasys Healthcare, Critical Care Division, Palm Springs, Calif.)

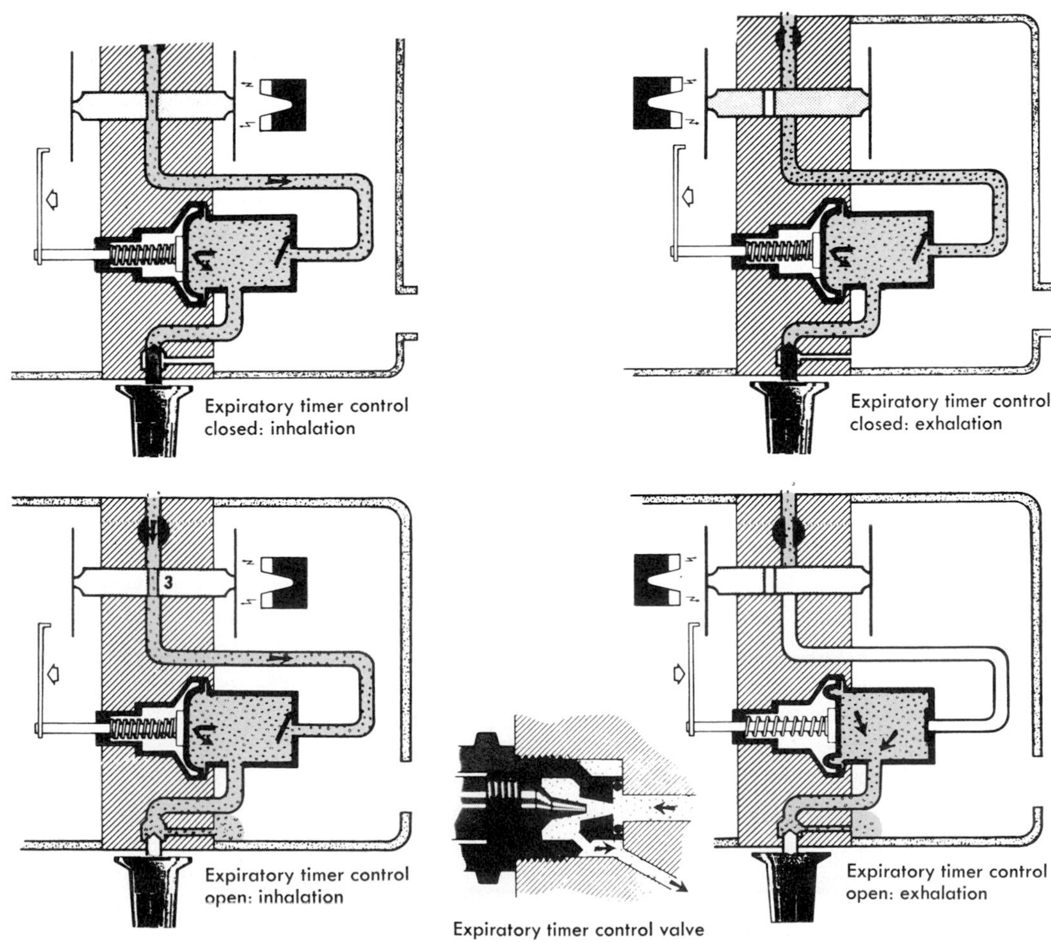

Figure 7-19 Exhalation timer and control. (Modified from Viasys Healthcare, Critical Care Division, Palm Springs, Calif.)

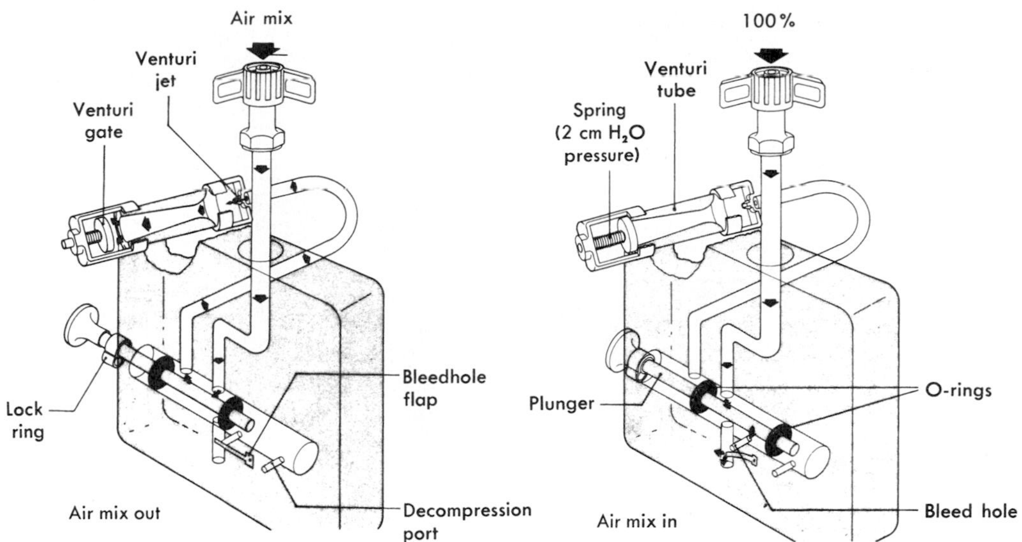

Figure 7-20 Air-Mix control for Bird Mark 7. The schematics show typical patterns for flow and pressure during Air-Mix *(left)* and 100% oxygen *(right)*. (Modified from Viasys Healthcare, Critical Care Division, Palm Springs, Calif.)

end-inspiration, no source gas is supplied to the cartridge, and the one-way entrance valve closes. The only way for gas to leave the cartridge is the leak past the needle valve on the outflow track. As gas leaks out, pressure decreases, and the diaphragm is pushed to the right by the spring. Concurrently, the plunger and its attached arm are moved slowly to the right. After the arm touches the clutch plate, the clutch plate is pushed away from the magnet, and the ceramic switch is moved into the "on" position. Thus the length of expiratory time is controlled by the needle valve; and the greater the leak past the needle valve, the faster the cartridge will discharge and the shorter the exhalation time.

Notice that directly below the ceramic switch is the air-mix control. As shown in Figure 7-19, it is a two-position switch, allowing for delivery of either an air-mixed gas (varying F_IO_2) or a gas with an F_IO_2 of 1.0. When this switch is pushed in, the O rings seal the incoming source gas and direct it out the reed-covered bleed hole in the center body, providing a constant flow during the inspiratory phase. When the air-mix control switch is pulled out, the top O ring blocks the bleed hole, and gas is directed to the jet of the air-mix Venturi. The decompression port above the bleed hole allows the plunger to be pushed in without compressing the gas behind it, so functionally it plays no part in the air-mix control. In the air-mix (switch pulled out) setting (Figure 7-20, A), source gas is from: (1) the Venturi jet, (2) the air entrained by the Venturi system, and (3) the nebulizer jet. In the air-mix position, the Venturi is activated, producing a descending flow pattern and an irregular pressure waveform that ranges from ascending to rectangular, depending on the compliance and resistance of the patient's respiratory system. In the 100% setting (i.e., switch pushed in; *B*), there are two sources of gas flow throughout inspiration, producing a square-wave or constant flow pattern and an ascending pressure waveform.

The Mark 7A Respirator, which is an updated version of the Mark 7 Respirator, is available from Viasys Healthcare. It features Apneustic Flowtime, which is a mechanical means of simulating a dynamic (time-cycled) postinspiratory breath hold for increased distribution and retention of inspired aerosols. In addition to the Apneustic Flowtime device, the device contains an independent flow control that permits precise regulation of gas flow.

Bird Mark 8 Series

The Bird Mark 8 (Figure 7-21) is functionally similar to the Mark 7, but it can provide a constant flow of source gas during the expiratory phase. The knob for adjusting the level of flow is on top of the machine, connected to a needle valve and a flow interrupter switch. The switch is a pneumatic cartridge containing a plunger, spring, and diaphragm. During inspiration, gas flows through the ceramic switch, which charges the cartridge and blocks the flow of 50 psig source gas to the Venturi. During expiration, gas flowing through the Venturi entrains expired gases from the circuit and the patient and directs them out the exhalation valve.

The Bird Mark 8 was originally designed to allow for the application of NEEP. As previously stated, NEEP has been shown to be ineffective in reducing airtrapping and is no longer used.

Bird Mark 10 and 14 Series

The Mark 10 and Mark 14 ventilators are similar to the Mark 7 series, except that they do not have an air-mix control, which means that they can only operate in the air-dilution mode. Additionally, they include a control for providing inspiratory flow acceleration, which can be used to compensate for leaks in the system. The primary difference between the Mark 14 series and the Mark 10 series is that Mark 14 ventilators can produce pressures as high as 200 cm H_2O.[9]

A

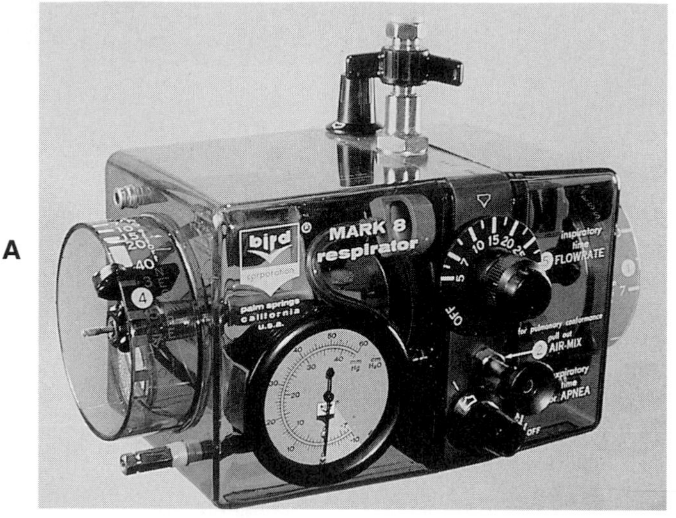

B

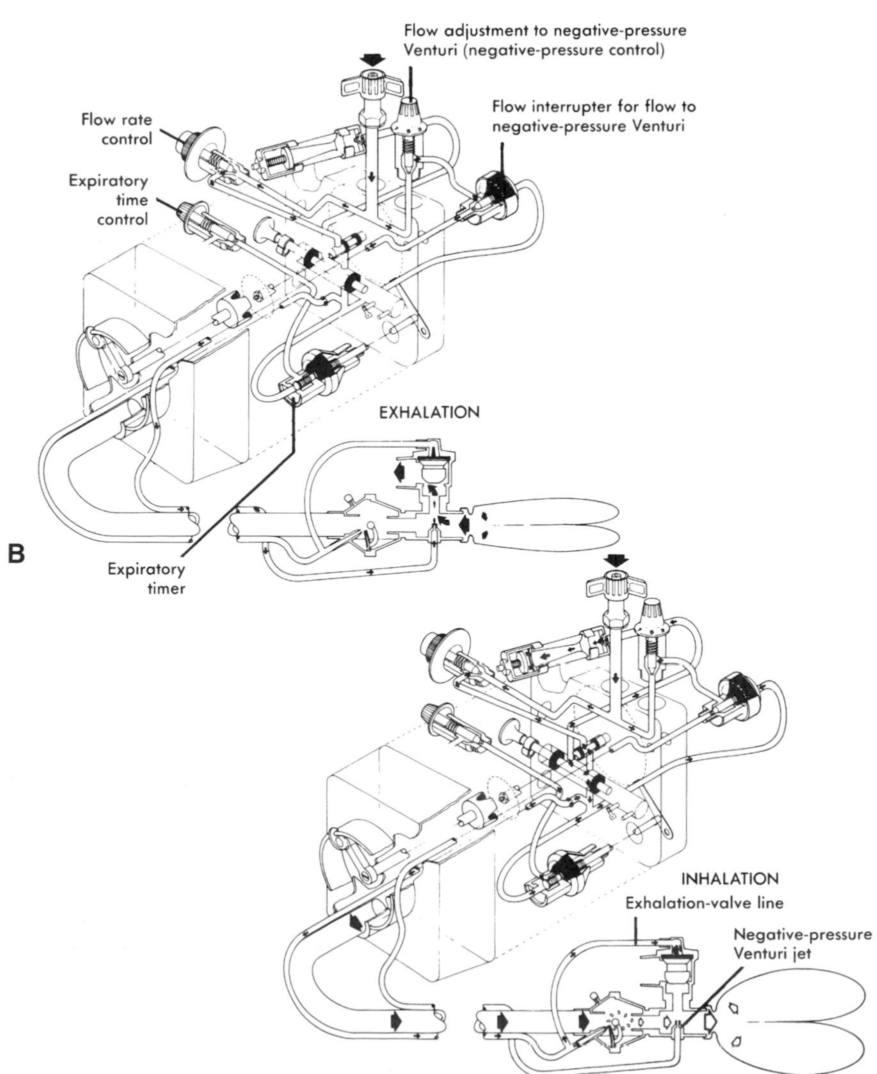

Figure 7-21 **A,** Bird Mark 8. **B,** Bird Mark 8 flow diagram. (Modified from Viasys Healthcare, Critical Care Division, Palm Springs, Calif.)

Clinical Practice Guidelines 7-3

Use of Positive Airway Pressure Adjuncts to Bronchial Hygiene Therapy

Indications

1. To reduce air trapping in patients with asthma or COPD
2. To help mobilize retained secretions in patients with cystic fibrosis or chronic bronchitis
3. To prevent or reverse atelectasis
4. To optimize bronchodilator delivery in patients receiving bronchial hygiene therapy

Contraindications

1. Patients unable to tolerate the increased work of breathing (acute asthma, COPD)
2. Intracranial pressure >20 mm Hg
3. Hemodynamic instability
4. Recent facial, oral, or skull surgery
5. Acute sinusitis
6. Epistaxis
7. Esophageal surgery
8. Active hemoptysis
9. Nausea
10. Known or suspected tympanic membrane rupture or other middle ear pathology
11. Untreated pneumothorax

Assessment of Outcome

1. Increased sputum production in patient producing >30 mL/day of sputum without PEP suggests that therapy should be continues
2. Improved breath sounds (i.e., diminished breath sounds change to adventitious breath sounds) that can be auscultated over the larger airways, demonstrating that therapy is indicated
3. Patient response to therapy
4. Changes in vital signs: moderate changes in respiratory rate or pulse rate are expected, but bradycardia, tachycardia, an increasingly irregular pulse, or a drop or dramatic increase in blood pressure are indications to stop therapy
5. Changes in arterial blood gases or oxygen saturation should improve as atelectasis resolves

Monitoring

1. Patient response to pain, discomfort, dyspnea, and therapy in general
2. Pulse rate and cardiac rhythm (if electrocardiogram is available)
3. Breathing pattern and rate
4. Sputum production (quantity, color, consistency, and odor)
5. Mental function
6. Cyanosis or pallor
7. Breath sounds
8. Blood pressure
9. Pulse oximetry (if hypoxemia with the procedure has been previously demonstrated or is suspected)
10. Blood gas analysis (if indicated)
11. Intracranial pressure in patients for whom this value is of critical importance

AARC Clinical Practice Guideline: Use of positive airway pressure adjuncts to bronchial hygiene therapy, *Respir Care* 38:516, 1993.

Positive Airway Pressure (PAP) Devices

PAP techniques, which include continuous positive airway pressure (CPAP), expiratory positive airway pressure (EPAP), and positive expiratory pressure (PEP), are airway adjuncts that can be used to enhance bronchial hygiene therapy by reducing airtrapping in susceptible patients.[10] As such, these techniques have been shown to be quite effective in mobilizing retained secretions, preventing or reversing atelectasis, and optimizing the delivery of bronchodilators for patients with cystic fibrosis and chronic bronchitis. The AARC has produced a Clinical Practice Guideline for PAP adjuncts to bronchial hygiene therapy, which should be read before PAP therapy is performed on patients.[10] CPG 7-3 summarizes several important points from this guideline.

Continuous Positive Airway Pressure

This form of PAP therapy involves the application of positive pressure to a patient's airways throughout the respiratory cycle (i.e., the airway pressure is consistently maintained between 5 and 20 cm H_2O during both inspiration and expiration). It is accomplished by having the patient breathe from a pressurized circuit that incorporates a threshold resistor in the expiratory limb.

Figure 7-22 shows four types of threshold resistors: underwater seal resistors, weighted-ball resistors, spring-loaded valve resistors, and magnetic valve resistors.[11] With underwater seal resistors, tubing attached to the expiratory port of the circuit is submerged under a column of water. The level of CPAP is determined by the height of the column. Weighted-ball resistors consist of a specially milled steel ball placed over a calibrated orifice, which is attached directly above the expiratory port of the circuit. It is important that the balls are maintained in a vertical position to ensure consistent pressure.[1] Spring-loaded resistors rely on a spring to hold a disc or diaphragm down over the expiratory port of the circuit. Magnetic valve resistors contain a bar magnet that attracts a ferromagnetic disc seated on the expiratory port of the circuit. The amount of pressure required to separate the disc from the magnet is determined by the distance between them (i.e., the greater the distance between the magnet and the disc, the lower the pressure required to open the expiratory port, and thus the lower the level of CPAP). All of these valves operate on the principle that the

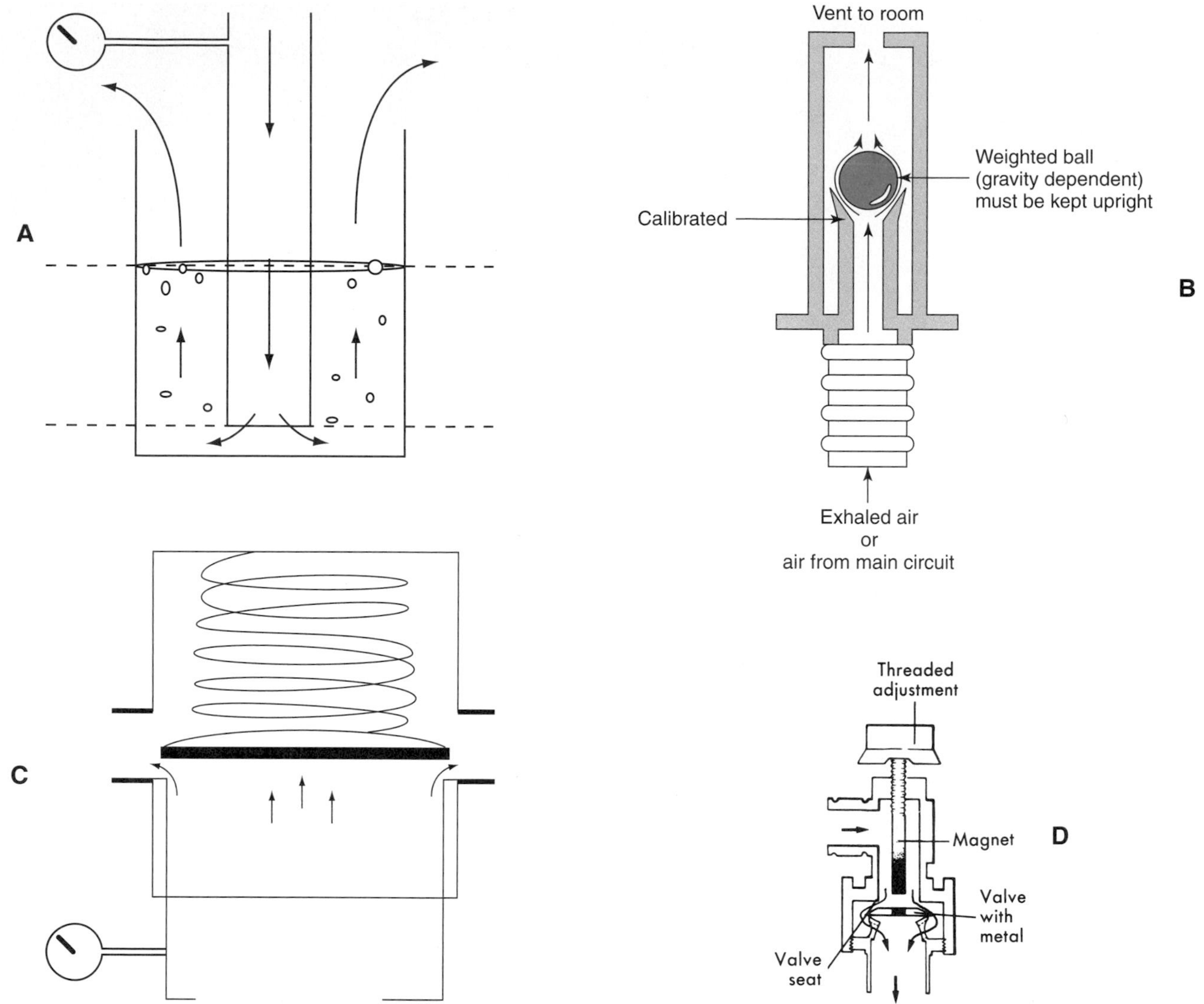

Figure 7-22 Four types of threshold resistors. **A,** Underwater seal resistor; **B,** weighted-ball resistor; **C,** spring-loaded valve resistor; **D,** magnetic valve resistor. (**A** and **C** Redrawn from Burton GG, Hodkin JE, Ward JJ: *Respiratory care: a guide to clinical practice*, ed 4, Philadelphia, 1997, JB Lippincott; **B** Redrawn from Pilbeam SP: *Mechanical ventilation: physiological and clinical applications*, ed 2, St Louis, 1992, Mosby; **D** From Spearman CB, Sanders GH: Physical principles and functional designs of ventilators. In Kirby RR, Smith RA, Desautels DA, editors: *Mechanical ventilation*, New York, 1985, Churchill-Livingstone.)

level of PAP generated within the circuit depends on the amount of resistance that must be overcome to allow gas to exit the exhalation valve. The main advantage of threshold resistors is that they provide predictable, quantifiable, and constant force during expiration that is independent of the flow achieved by the patient during exhalation.[1]

Expiratory Positive Airway Pressure

EPAP is another method of delivering PAP to spontaneously breathing patients and differs from CPAP because it involves the creation of PAP only during expiration. With EPAP, the patient generates a subatmospheric pressure on inspiration, and then exhales against a threshold expiratory resistance similar to those described for CPAP devices. Airway pressures during EPAP can be set at 10 to 20 cm H_2O.

Positive Expiratory Pressure

This form of PAP has received considerable attention during the past 10 years, especially in the management of patients with cystic fibrosis. The rationale for performing PEP therapy is similar to that for using CPAP and EPAP, except that PEP seems to be less cumbersome and more manageable for patients.

Figure 7-23 shows the equipment required for PEP therapy, which includes a mouthpiece (or ventilation mask), a T-piece assembly with a one-way valve, a series of fixed orifice resistors (or an adjustable orifice resistor), and a pressure manometer. Two examples of PEP devices that are currently available include the Resistex (Mercury Medical, Clearwater, Fla.) and the TheraPEP (DHD Healthcare,

A

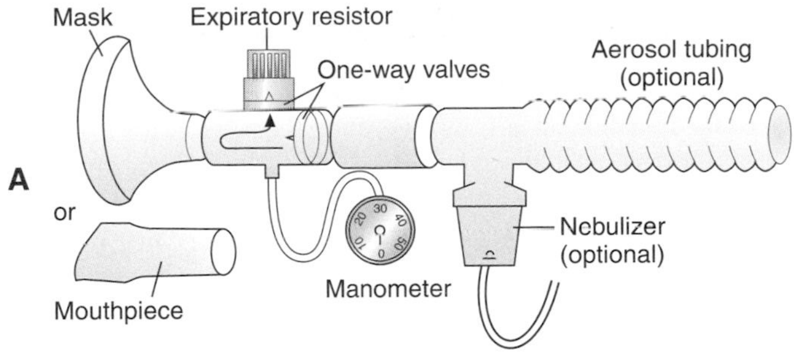

B

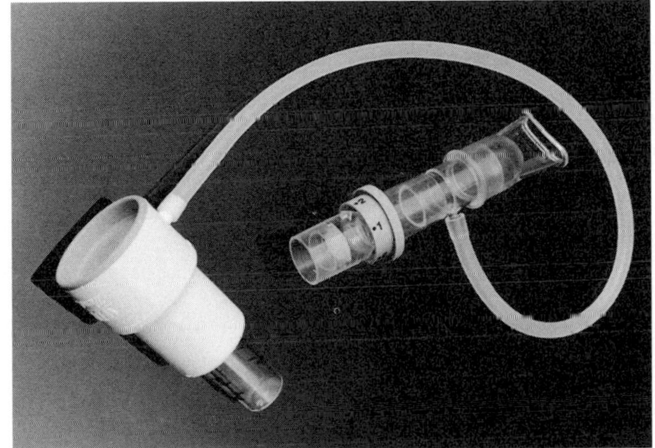

Figure 7-23 Equipment used during PEP therapy.

Wampsville, NY). Notice that bronchodilator therapy with an metered-dose inhaler (MDI) or small volume nebulizer (SVN) can be performed simultaneously by attaching these devices to the inspiratory port of the mask or mouthpiece. The AeroPEP (Monaghan Medical, Plattsburg, NY) is a specially designed device with pressurized MDI, a valved holding chamber, and a fixed orifice resistor for simultaneously administering aerosol therapy and PEP.

The amount of PAP generated with the fixed-orifice resistor varies with the size of the orifice and the level of expiratory flow produced by the patient. For example, for any given expiratory flow, the smaller the resistor's orifice, the greater the expiratory pressure generated. Conversely, for a given orifice size, the higher the expiratory flow, the greater the expiratory pressure generated.[1] For this reason, the patient must be encouraged to achieve a flow high enough to maintain expiratory pressure at 10 to 20 cm H_2O.

The procedure for performing PEP therapy is shown in Box 7-1. Several factors should be considered when creating a therapeutic regimen using these devices. The level of resistance chosen should allow the patient to achieve the therapeutic goal of generating PEP of 10 to 20 cm H_2O

Box 7-1 Procedure for Performing PEP Therapy

1. The mask is applied tightly but comfortably over the patient's nose and mouth. When a mouthpiece is used, patients are instructed to form a tight seal around the mouthpiece.
2. Patients are instructed to inspire through the one-way valve to a volume that is greater than their normal tidal volume—but not their total lung capacity.
3. At the end of inspiration, patients are encouraged to actively but not forcefully exhale to FRC to achieve an airway pressure of 10 to 20 cm H_2O.
4. Patients should perform 10 to 20 breaths through the device, then perform a series of two to three huff coughs to clear loosened secretions.
5. This cycle should be repeated 5 to 10 times during a 15- to 20-minute session

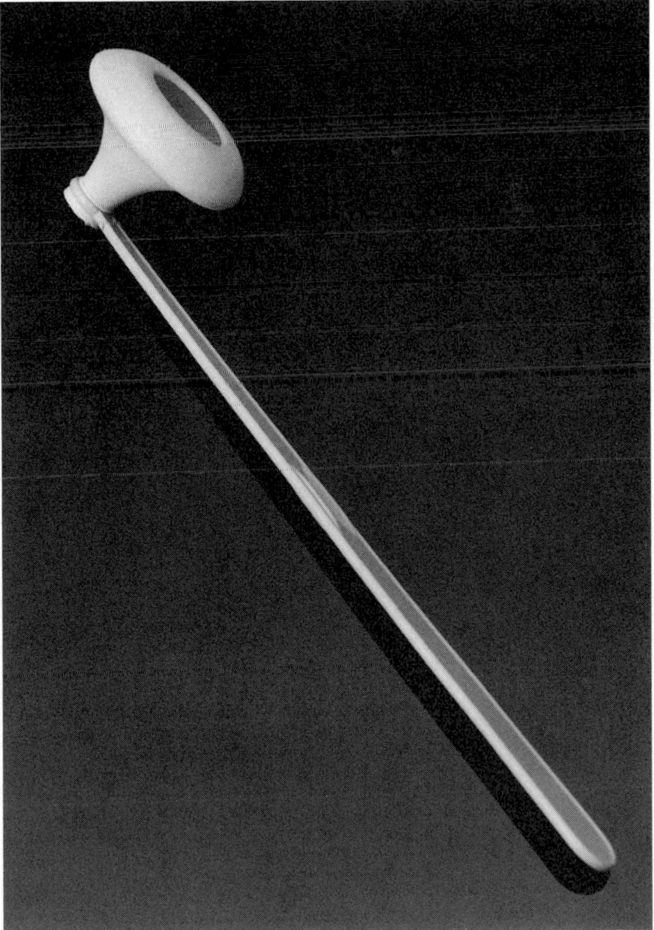

Figure 7-24 Manual percussor.

with an inspiratory to expiratory ratio (I:E) of 1:3 or 1:4. The patient should perform 10 to 20 breaths through the device, then perform a series of two to three huff coughs to clear loosened secretions. This cycle should be repeated 5 to 10 times during a 15- to 20-minute session. Finally, the patient should be encouraged to learn how to self-administer this therapy, though more than one session may be required to ensure patient proficiency in using these devices.

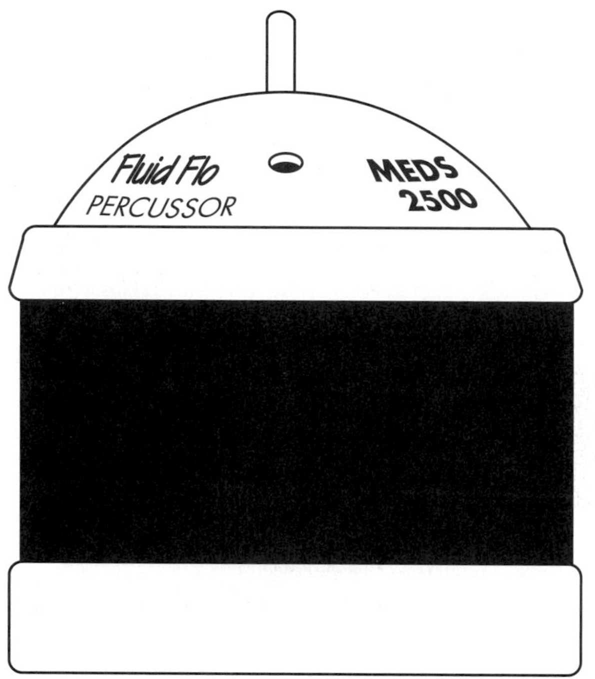

Figure 7-25 Fluid Flo pneumatic percussor. (Courtesy Med Systems, Inc, San Diego, Calif.)

Chest Physiotherapy Devices

Chest physiotherapy (CPT) is a collection of techniques used to help clear airway secretions and improve the distribution of ventilation. Historically these techniques have included breathing exercises, directed coughing, postural drainage, and chest percussion. Newer techniques involving the delivery of high-frequency oscillations to the lungs and chest wall are receiving increased interest as alternative methods for clearance of airway secretions.

Percussion and vibration, both of which involve the application of mechanical energy to the chest wall and lungs, provide a means of loosening retained secretions from the walls of the tracheobronchial tract. After they are loosened, the secretions can be coughed up and expectorated or be removed by suctioning.

Percussion can be accomplished using either the hands or various mechanical or electrical devices. For this discussion, chest percussors have been divided into three categories: manual percussors, pneumatically powered devices, and electrically powered devices. Devices that produce vibrations to the lungs and chest wall will be discussed separately in the section on high-frequency oscillation devices.

Manual Percussors

The traditional method of administering CPT involves cupping the hand (as if scooping water from a basin) and clapping on the patient's chest wall. Although this technique is quite effective in most cases, it can be tiring for the person administering the therapy and somewhat painful for the patient (if performed by someone inexperienced in CPT). As a result of these potential problems, several companies have produced some simple manual percussors that are

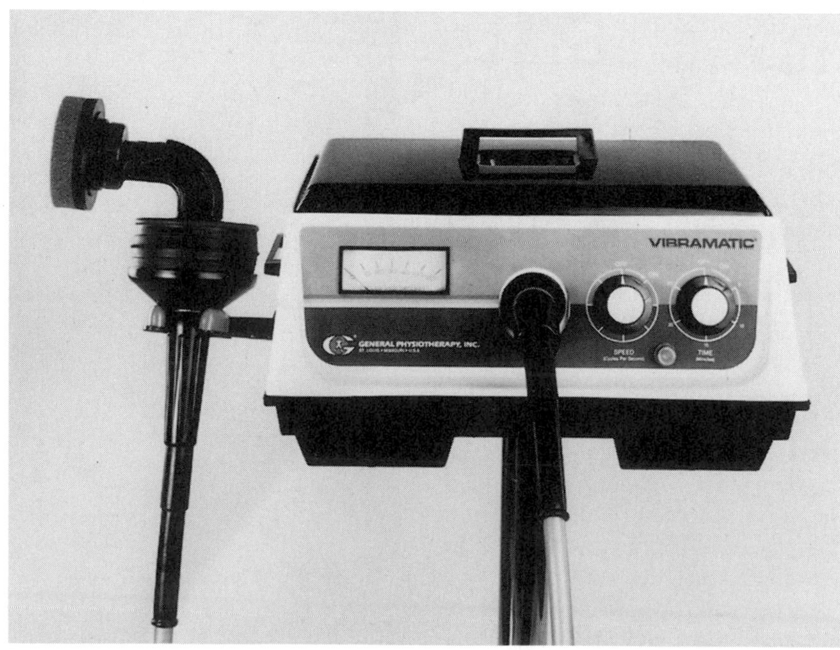

Figure 7-26 Vibramatic/Multimatic electrically powered percussor. (Courtesy General Physiotherapy, Inc, St Louis.)

fairly inexpensive and easy to use. Figure 7-24 shows a typical manual percussor marketed by DHD Medical Products. This device is made of soft vinyl and is formed to the shape of the palm. It is available in neonatal, pediatric, and adult sizes.

Pneumatically Powered Devices

These percussors are powered by a compressed-air or oxygen source that operates at 45 to 55 psig. Although devices may differ in the number of accessories provided, each device usually comprises a high-pressure hose, a body with controls for varying the frequency and force of percussive strokes, and a remote head with a concave applicator. Several common examples of pneumatically powered percussors are the Fluid Flo (Figure 7-25), the Hudson Pediatric, the Mercury MJ, and the Fluid Flo percussors. The Strom PPS3, the Mercury MJ, and the Fluid Flo are designed for pediatric and adult patients. The Fluid Flo is only for adult patients.

CLINICAL ROUNDS 7-3

A 22-year-old man previously diagnosed with cystic fibrosis is admitted to the emergency department after a recent history of upper respiratory infection. A physical examination reveals that the patient is alert and cooperative, his respiratory rate is 40 breaths/min. Coarse, wet breath sounds are heard over all lung fields. He reports producing copious amounts of purulent, foul-smelling sputum for the past 3 days. His heart rate is 110 beats/min, and his oral temperature is 102° F. Arterial blood pressure is 150/100; MIP is –50 cm H_2O; and SpO_2 is 90%. Chest radiographs show bilateral pneumonia. The pulmonology resident suggests using IPPB treatments. Do you agree with this suggestion?

See Appendix A for the answer.

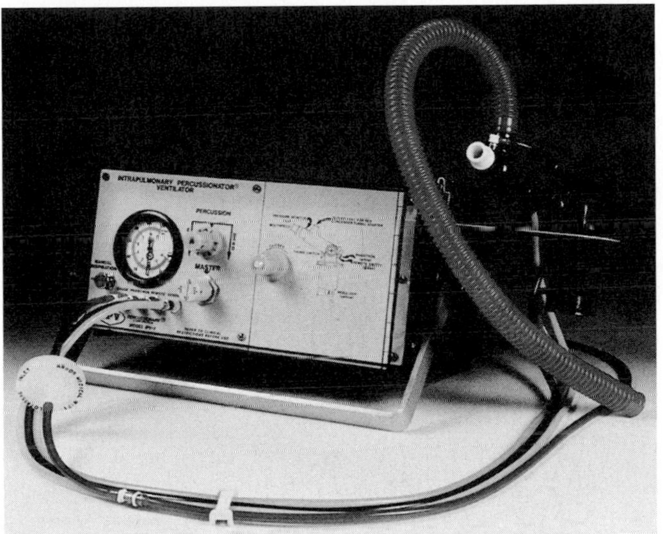

Figure 7-27 Percussionaire Intrapulmonary Percussive Ventilator (IPV-1). (Courtesy Percussionaire Corp, Sandpoint, Idaho.)

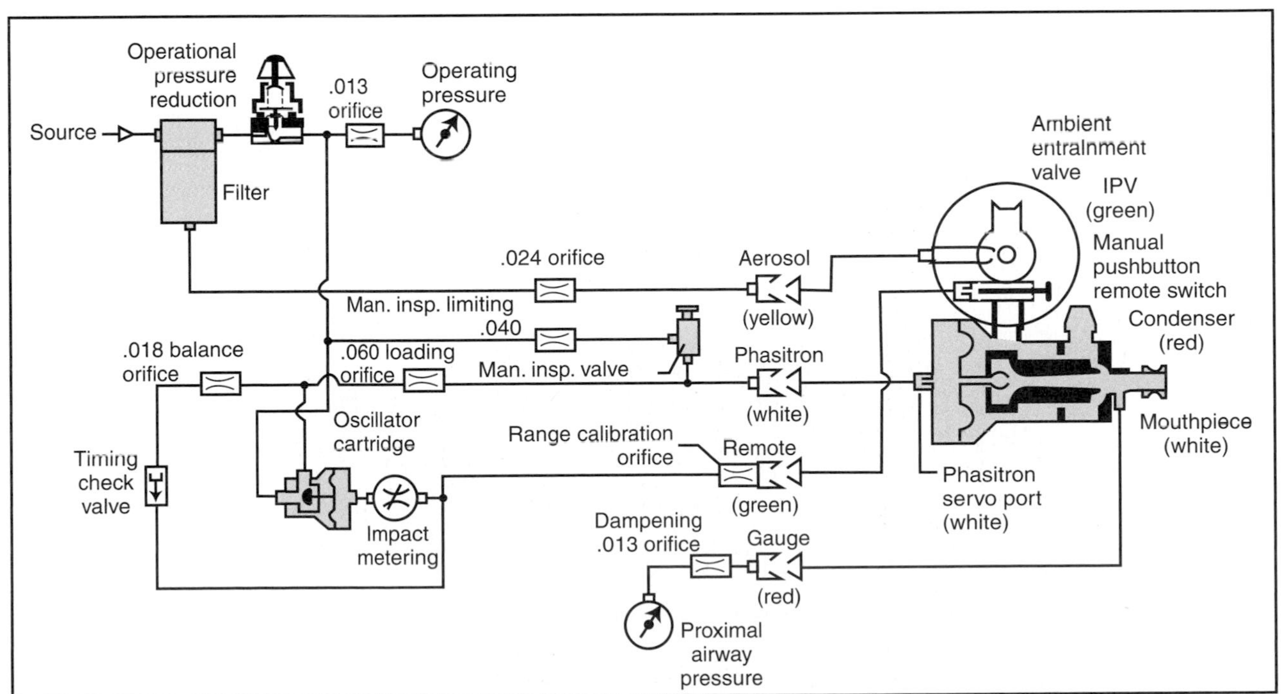

Figure 7-28 Gas flow through the IPV-1. (Courtesy Percussionaire, Sandpoint, Idaho.)

Electrically Powered Percussors

Most of these devices are powered by electrical outputs of 110 V of alternating current, although some units are battery-powered. Several of the more common units available in the United States are produced by General Physiotherapy (the Vibramatic/Multimatic, the Flimm Fighter, and the Neo-Cussor), Strom, and Nellcor Puritan Bennett (Vibrator/Percussor). Most units typically have a variable control switch for setting the frequency of percussions and can be used for both adult and pediatric patients.

Each system, however, has unique features. The Vibramatic/Multimatic (Figure 7-26) produces two directional forces: one produces a stroking action that operates perpendicular to the chest wall to loosen mucus attached to the tracheobronchial tubes, and the other operates parallel to the chest wall and moves the mucus toward the central airways. The Flimm Fighter is designed primarily for home use—it comes with a foam pad and a Velcro (Velcro USA, Inc., Manchester, NH) belt to allow for self-application of the device. The Neo-Cussor is a battery-operated device that uses a disposable applicator and is specifically designed for use with neonates and pediatric patients. The Nellcor Puritan Bennett Vibrator/Percussor allows for independent control of frequency and stroke intensity.

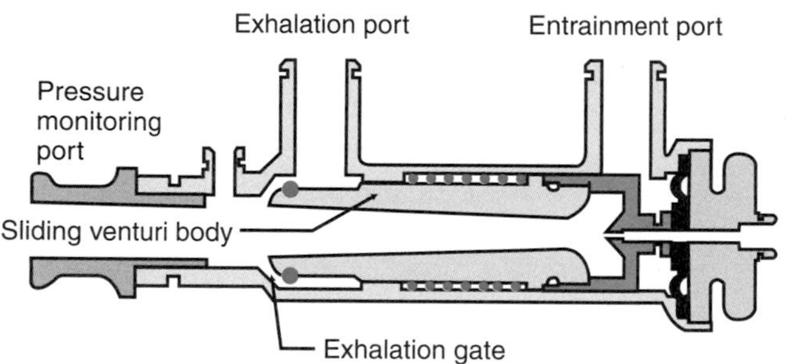

Figure 7-29 Phasitron unit used in the IPV-1. (Courtesy Percussionaire, Sandpoint, Idaho.)

High-Frequency Oscillation Devices

Administering high-frequency oscillations to the lungs via the airway opening or through the chest wall has been shown to be quite effective in mobilizing secretions in select patient groups. Although the mechanism of action of these devices is uncertain, several factors are thought to enhance clearance of airway secretions. Some of these factors may include reducing the viscoelasticity of sputum through sheering forces generated during the oscillations, transient changes in airflow that occur during the inspiratory and expiratory phases of each oscillation, and redistribution of lung volume to airways partially obstructed with mucus.[12,13]

The most commonly used devices for delivering high-frequency oscillation therapy include the Percussionaire intermittent percussive ventilation (IPV) device, the Flutter valve, The Vest and the Hayek Oscillator IPV and Flutter valves transmit high-frequency oscillation via the airway opening whereas The Vest and the Hayek Oscillator produce vibration of the chest wall by delivering high-frequency oscillations to the external chest wall.

Intrapulmonary Percussive Ventilation (IPV)

This form of oscillator therapy was introduced by Forrest Bird in 1979 as an adjunct technique for mobilizing airway secretions.[14] It involves the delivery of high-frequency percussive breaths into the patient's airways instead of applying percussions to the outside of the chest wall as in standard CPT techniques (Clinical Rounds 7-3).

The Percussionaire Intrapulmonary Percussive Ventilator (IPV-1), which is the prototype IPV device, is shown in Figure 7-27. It is manually cycled and can provide pressure- or flow-targeted breaths. Inspiration can be triggered manually by selecting a push-button control on the nebulizer (i.e., the patient is typically instructed to trigger inspiration by

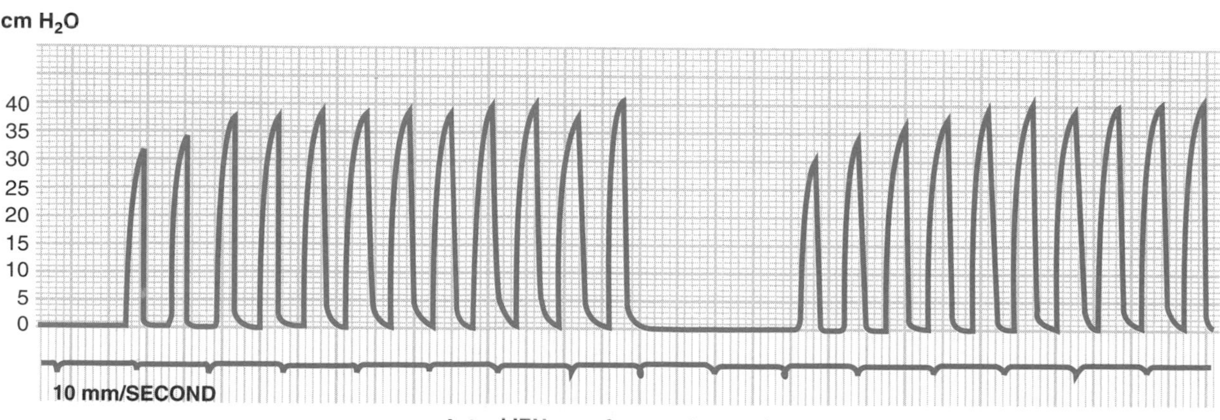

Figure 7-30 Pressure waveform generated during operation of the IPV-1. (Courtesy Percussionaire, Sandpoint, Idaho.)

Box 7-2 Procedure for Administration of Flutter Therapy

1. Assess whether Flutter therapy is indicated and design a treatment program.
   a. Bring equipment to the bedside and provide initial therapy, adjusting pressure settings to meet patient need.
   b. After initial treatment or patient training, communicate the treatment plan to the physician(s) and nurse(s) and provide instruction to the nursing staff, if required.
2. Explain that Flutter therapy is used to re-expand lung tissue and help mobilize secretions. Patients should be taught to huff.
3. Instruct the patient to:
   a. Sit comfortably
   b. Take in a breath that is larger than normal, but not to fill the lungs completely
   c. Seal the lips firmly around the Flutter device mouthpiece and exhale actively, but not forcefully, holding the Flutter valve at an angle that produces maximum oscillation
   d. Perform 10 to 20 breaths
   e. Remove the Flutter mouthpiece and perform two to three huffs and then rest as needed
   f. Repeat above cycle 4-8 times, not to exceed 20 minutes
4. Evaluate the patient for ability to self-administer.
5. When appropriate, teach the patient to self-administer Flutter therapy. Observe the patient conduct the self-administration on several occasions to ensure proper uncoached Flutter technique before allowing the patient to self-administer without supervision.
6. When patients are also receiving bronchodilator aerosol, administer in conjunction with Flutter by administering bronchodilator immediately preceding the Flutter breaths.
7. When visibly soiled, rinse Flutter device with sterile water and shake/air dry. Leave the device within reach at patient bedside.
8. Send the Flutter device home with the patient.
9. Document, in the patient's medical record, procedures performed (including device, number of breaths per treatment, and frequency), patient response to therapy, patient teaching provided, and patient ability to self-administer.

From Fink JB: High-frequency oscillation of the airway and chest wall, *Respir Care* 47(7):799, 2002.

depressing the button for 5 to 10 seconds). Alternately, the therapist can trigger the percussive cycle by pressing the inspiration button on the control panel. Expiration is manually cycled by releasing the inspiratory control button.

The Percussionaire is powered by a 25 to 50 psi compressed-gas source. Figure 7-28 shows gas flow through the IPV-1 unit.[14] Gas enters the unit and passes through a filter before flowing into a pressure regulator, which reduces the pressure to a value preset by the operator. From there, gas flows to: (1) an oscillator cartridge and a Phasitron, which increases and decreases air pressures; (2) a nebulizer; and (3) a remote control. Gas travels from the Phasitron outlet through small-bore tubing to the Phasitron unit, which contains a sliding Venturi (Figure 7-29). The Venturi slides forward during the impact phase, and a burst of air travels into the Venturi orifice, which in turn entrains room air (i.e., for each unit of gas that passes through the Venturi, 4 units of air are entrained). This enhanced burst of gas then passes through the mouthpiece to the patient. After the injection phase, the Venturi slides back, and the expiratory valve simultaneously opens, allowing the patient to passively exhale.

The nebulizer receives high-pressure gas from the internal regulator via the small-bore tubing connected to the front of the unit. Air flows through the jet, past the nebulizer, creating an area of reduced pressure that draws medication from the reservoir. A high-pressure gas at the top of the jet meets the stream of medication, creating a mist that is delivered to the circuit. Note that the entrainment post of the Venturi is connected to the nebulizer by large-bore aerosol tubing, thus allowing the patient to receive the mist during the percussive phase of operation.

The Percussionaire can deliver percussive pressures of 25 to 40 cm H_2O at about 100 to 300 cycles per minute, or 1.7 to 5.0 Hz (Figure 7-30). The effectiveness of IPV therapy, compared with that of traditional chest physiotherapy techniques, is still under investigation. It has been suggested that IPV may provide another potentially useful method of improving sputum mobilization in certain patients (e.g., those with cystic fibrosis or chronic bronchitis). Although a study by Deakins and Chatburn[15] provided encouraging results for this type of therapy for the treatment of atelectasis in pediatric patients when compared with conventional chest physiotherapy techniques, additional studies are needed to more clearly define the appropriate indications and contraindications for IPV therapy.

Flutter Valve

The concept for the Flutter mucus clearance device or Flutter valve (Scandipharm, Birmingham, Ala.) was first introduced by Freitag et al.[16] The appeal for this device is undoubtedly influenced by it simplicity of design and by the fact that it is relatively easy for patients to use. As shown in Figure 7-31, the Flutter valve consists of a pipe-shaped apparatus with a steel ball in a bowl that is covered by a perforated cap.[16] The steel ball creates a positive expiratory pressure (similar to a PEP device) that helps to prevent early airway closure, whereas the internal dimensions of the pipe allow the steel ball to "flutter," resulting in the creation of a series of high-frequency oscillations that are transmitted the lung through the airway opening.

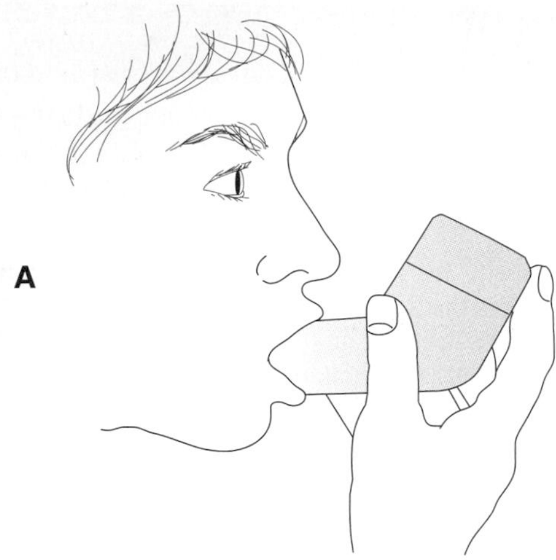

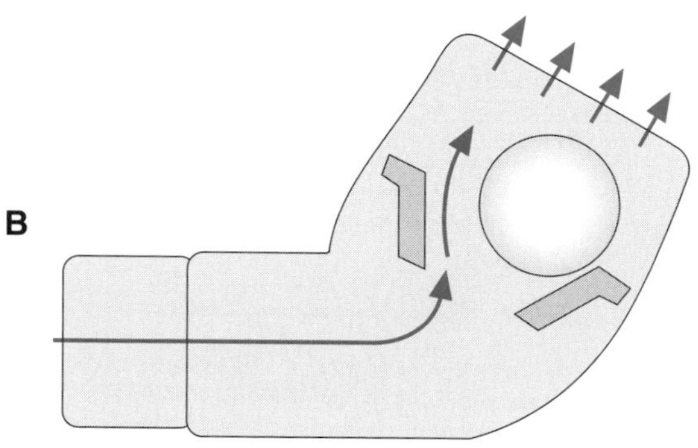

Figure 7-31 **A,** Position of flutter valve in patient's mouth. **B,** During exhalation, the position of the steel ball is the result of an equilibrium between the pressure of the exhaled gas, the force of gravity on the ball, and the angle of the cone where the contact with the ball occurs. As the steel ball rolls and bounces up and down, it creates oscillation in the airway. (From Hess DR et al: *Respiratory care: principles and practice*, St Louis, 2002, WB Saunders.)

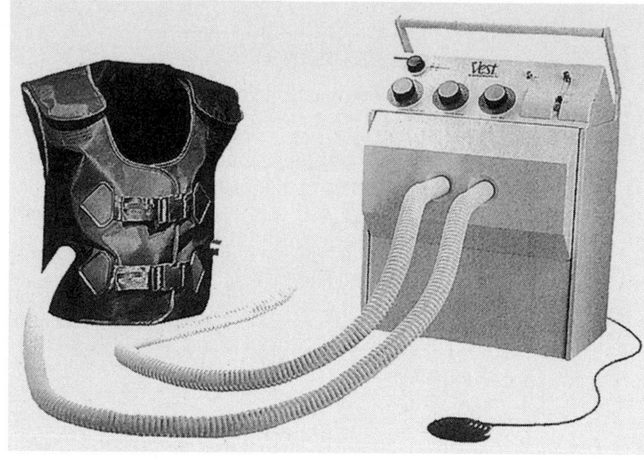

Figure 7-32 The Vest airway clearance system. (Courtesy Advanced Respiratory, St Paul, Minn.)

Box 7-2 summarizes the protocol for administering Flutter therapy.[13] A number of studies have demonstrated that Flutter therapy is a viable alternative to standard chest physiotherapy techniques in select patient populations. Further in vivo studies involving greater numbers and more diverse patient groups will be required to better determine the effectiveness of Flutter therapy devices compared to other airway clearance techniques involving positive airway pressure.

High-Frequency Chest Wall Oscillation Devices

The Vest (Advanced Respiratory, St Paul, Minn.) and the Hayek Oscillator (Breasy Medical Equipment Ltd, London, UK) are devices that can be used to deliver high-frequency external chest wall oscillations. The Vest was developed by Warwick and colleagues. As Figure 7-32 shows, it consists of a nonstretchable, inflatable vest that extends over the entire torso area down to the iliac crest.[12] Chest wall vibrations are delivered to the vest through a series of pressure pulses that are produced by an air compressor connected to the vest via a vacuum hose. The timing of the pulse delivery (i.e., during expiration or throughout the respiratory cycle) can be manually controlled by the patient using a foot pedal. The intensity and frequency of the pressure pulses can be adjusted by the patient to achieve pressures ranging from approximately 25 to 40 mm Hg over a frequency range of 5 to 25 Hz, respectively.

The Hayek Oscillator (Figure 7-33), which is technically classified as an electrically powered noninvasive ventilator, consists of a flexible chest cuirass that is applied over the chest wall. Its unique design characteristics allow for delivery of both negative and positive pressures to the chest wall during the respiratory cycle. Thus negative pressure is delivered during the inspiratory portion of the cycle causing the chest wall and lungs to expand and positive pressure is delivered while the patient exhales to produce a forced expiration. The frequency of oscillations, the inspiratory-expiratory ratio, and the inspiratory pressure are controlled by a microprocessor, which can be programmed by the respiratory therapist depending on the patient's needs. The frequency of oscillations can range from 8 to 999 oscillations/min and the I:E ratio can be varied from 6:1 to 1:6. Inspiratory and expiratory pressures of –70 to +70 cm H_2O can be achieved.[13] Although several therapeutic regiments have been suggested to improve the efficacy of using high-frequency oscillations for clearing airway secretions, more studies will be required to determine the best method for using these devices.[12,17]

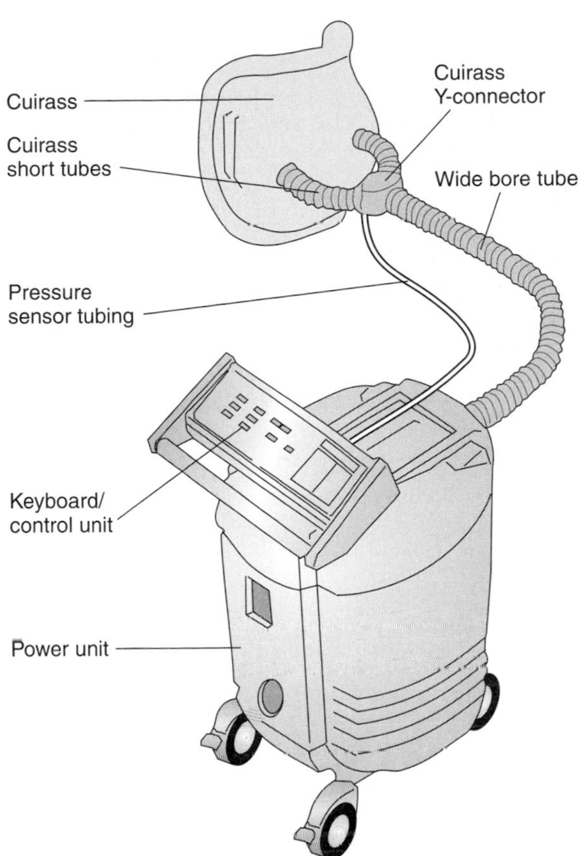

Figure 7-33 Schematic drawing of the Hayek Oscillator. (From Hess DR et al: *Respiratory care: principles and practice*, St Louis, 2002, WB Saunders. Modified from materials courtesy of Breasy Medical Equipment, Stanford, Conn.)

Summary

The primary indications for lung expansion therapy are to prevent and treat atelectasis. One of the most important ways to accomplish this goal is to maintain effective clearance of airway secretions with lung inflation therapy. Various strategies and devices are available to accomplish this goal. Incentive spirometry, IPPB, PAP techniques, and CPT have all been shown to be effective lung hyperexpansion methods. Newer devices that provide high-frequency oscillations to the lungs and chest wall are receiving considerable attention as viable alternatives to these techniques. Selection of the appropriate device and therapeutic modality should be based on the patient's ability to perform the procedure and on the therapeutic goals. Evaluation of the effectiveness of therapy should be based on history and physical findings, chest radiographs, and a review of laboratory tests (i.e., arterial blood gases).

Review Questions

See Appendix A for the answers.

1. What is the primary indication for lung inflation therapy?
   I. Prevent atelectasis
   II. Prevent hypoxemia
   III. Reverse hypercapnia
   IV. Reduce pulmonary shunting
   a. I only
   b. I and II only
   c. II and III only
   d. I, II, III, and IV

2. Incentive spirometry is indicated for patients who are predisposed to develop atelectasis. List four medical conditions where incentive spirometry is indicated.

3. You are asked to show an adult patient how to properly use a Triflo incentive spirometer. Although the patient appears to be following your instructions, she is unable to achieve the prescribed goal that you established for this patient. Briefly describe several factors that could cause this problem.

4. Which of these parameters is used to set the therapeutic goal for a patient using a volume-displacement incentive spirometer?
   a. Total lung capacity
   b. Inspiratory capacity
   c. Inspiratory reserve volume
   d. Expiratory reserve volume

5. You are asked to suggest a lung inflation therapy for a 55-year-old man who is 72 inches tall and weighs 85 kg. He has just undergone a cholecystectomy and his chest radiograph shows right middle lobe atelectasis. He has a 10 pack-per-year history of smoking cigarettes, and his preoperative pulmonary function studies showed that his vital capacity was 20 mL/kg. He is alert and cooperative but complains of some upper abdominal pain when taking a deep breath. What modality would you suggest?

6. Which of the following are contraindications for administering IPPB?
   I. Active hemoptysis
   II. Nausea
   III. Intracranial pressure >15 mm Hg
   IV. Recent esophageal surgery
   a. I and III only
   b. II and III only
   c. I, II, and III only
   d. I, II, III, and IV

7. The AARC Clinical Practice Guideline for IPPB states that this form of therapy is a viable lung expansion technique for patients with reduced lung function. Which of the following findings from a patient suggest that IPPB is warranted?

I. FVC = 50% predicted
II. $FEV_{1.0}$ = 70% predicted
III. MVV <50% predicted
IV. VC = 15 mL/kg
a. I only
b. IV only
c. II and III only
d. I and III only

8. You can set the tidal volume delivered by a Bennett PR-2 ventilator by adjusting which of these parameters?
a. Inspiratory time
b. Inspiratory flow
c. Peak inspiratory pressure
d. Trigger sensitivity

9. What F_IO_2 will a patient receive if the air-mix control on the Bird Mark 7 is pushed in?

10. What types of percussive pressure does the Percussionaire IPV device deliver?
a. 10 to 20 cm H_2O
b. 25 to 40 cm H_2O
c. 50 to 100 cm H_2O
d. >200 cm H_2O

11. Name four types of threshold resistors used to administer CPAP.

12. Which of the following are considered positive outcomes to PEP therapy?
I. Increased sputum production
II. Increased respiratory rate
III. Resolution of hypoxemia
IV. Diminished breath sounds become adventitious sounds that can be auscultated over the larger airways
a. I only
b. I and III only
c. II and III only
d. I, III, and IV only

13. The function of the steel ball in the flutter device is to:
a. help prevent early airway closure.
b. provide high frequency oscillation.
c. create a positive expiratory pressure.
d. all of the above.

14. The Vest is used to:
a. provide positive pressure on exhalation.
b. keep infants core temperature stable.
c. oscillate the chest wall to promote secretion clearance.
d. give biofeedback in teaching diaphragmatic breathing.

References

1. Fink JB: Volume expansion therapy. In Burton GC, Hodgkin JE, Ward JL (editors): *Respiratory care: a guide to clinical practice*, ed 4, Philadelphia, 1997, JB Lippincott.
2. AARC Clinical Practice Guideline: Incentive spirometry, *Respir Care* 36:1402, 1991.
3. Scanlan CL, Wilkins, RL, Stoller JK: *Egan's fundamentals of respiratory care*, ed 7, St Louis, 1998, Mosby.
4. Gooselink R, Schever K, Cops P, et al: Incentive spirometry does not enhance recover after thoracic surgery, *Crit Care Med* 29: 679-683, 2000.
5. Rau JL, Thomas L, Haynes RL: The effect of method of administering incentive spirometry on postoperative pulmonary complications in coronary bypass patients, *Respir Care* 33:771-778, 1988.
6. Craven JL, et al: The evaluation of incentive spirometry in the management of postoperative pulmonary complications, *Br J Surg* 61:793, 1974.
7. Petz TJ: Physiologic effects of IPPB, blow bottles, and incentive spirometry, *Curr Rev Respir Ther* 1:107, 1979.
8. AARC Clinical Practice Guideline: Intermittent positive pressure breathing (IPPB), *Respir Care* 38:1189, 1993.
9. McPherson SP: *Respiratory care equipment*, ed 5, St Louis, 1995, Mosby.
10. AARC Clinical Practice Guideline: Use of positive airway pressure adjuncts to bronchial hygiene therapy, *Respir Care* 38:516, 1993.
11. Pilbeam SP: *Mechanical ventilation*, ed 3, St Louis, 1998, Mosby.
12. Fink JB, Hess DR: Secretion clearance techniques. In Hess DR, MacIntyre NR, Mishoe SC, et al (editors): *Respiratory care, principles and practice*, Philadelphia, 2002, WB Saunders.
13. Fink JB, Mahlmeister MJ: High-frequency oscillation of the airway and chest wall, *Respir Care* 47(7):797, 2002.
14. Operator's Manual of the Percussionaire Intrapulmonary Percussive Ventilation (IPV-1) unit, Percussionaire, Sandpoint, Idaho.
15. Deakins K, Chatburn R: A comparison of intrapulmonary percussive ventilation and conventional chest physiotherapy for the treatment of atelectasis in the pediatric patient, *Respir Care* 47(10):1162, 2002.
16. Freitag L, Long WM, Kim CS, Wanner A: Removal of excessive bronchial secretions by asymmetrical high-frequency oscillations, *J Appl Physiol* 67(2):614, 1989.
17. Scherer TA, Barandun J, Martinez E, et al: Effect of high-frequency oral airway and chest wall oscillations and conventional chest physical therapy on expectoration in patients with stable cystic fibrosis, *Chest* 113:1019, 1998.

Internet Resources

1. American Association for Respiratory Care: http://www.aarc.org
2. Viasys Healthcare Products: http://www.birdprod.com
3. American Society of Anesthesiologists: http://www.asahq.org
4. American College of Chest Physicians: http://www.chestnet.org
5. American Thoracic Society: http://www.thoracic.org
6. National Library of Medicine (free access to Medline): http://www.nlm.nih.gov/medlineplus/
7. DHD Healthcare: http://www.dhd.com
8. Medscape: http://www.medscape.com
9. Medical Business Search Engine: http://www.infomedical.com
10. Tyco Healthcare/Puritan Bennett: http://www.puritanbennett.com

Chapter 8

Assessment of Pulmonary Function

J.M. Cairo

Chapter Outline

Chapter Learning Objectives

After reading this chapter, the reader should be able to:

1. Identify three types of volume-collecting spirometers.
2. Explain the operational theory of thermal flowmeters.
3. Name three types of pneumotachometers.
4. Discuss the ATS standards for spirometry.
5. Describe three types of body plethysmographs.
6. Compare the nitrogen washout and the helium dilution techniques for measuring functional residual capacity (FRC) and residual volume.
7. Explain the operational theories of strain gauge, variable inductance, and variable capacitance pressure transducers.
8. Describe various conditions that interfere with the operation of impedance pneumographs.
9. List and describe measured and derived variables that are commonly used to assess respiratory mechanics.
10. Compare the operational principles of the two types of oxygen analyzers used in the clinical setting.
11. Describe two techniques for monitoring nitrogen oxides in the clinical setting.
12. Identify the components of a normal capnogram.
13. Assess an abnormal capnogram and suggest possible pathophysiologic processes that could contribute to the contour of the carbon dioxide waveform.
14. Compare closed-circuit and open-circuit indirect calorimeters.
15. Calculate energy expenditure using measurements obtained during indirect calorimetry.
16. Explain how indirect calorimetry can be used to determine substrate utilization patterns in healthy subjects and in those with cardiopulmonary dysfunctions.

Key Terms

Accuracy
Airways Resistance (R_{aw})
Alveolar Ventilation
Anemometer
Aneroid Manometer
Auto-PEEP
Bell Factor
Body Plethysmography
Capnogram
Chemiluminescence Monitoring
Closed-Circuit Calorimeters
Dead Space Ventilation
Doppler Effect
Dry-Rolling Seal Spirometer
Electrical Impedance
Electrochemical
Electrochemical Monitoring
Electromechanical Transducer
Energy Expenditure (EE)
Fleisch Pneumotachograph
Functional Residual Capacity (FRC)
Galvanic Analyzer
Haldane Transformation
Indirect Calorimetry
Inert Gas Techniques
Kymograph
Lung and Chest Wall Compliance
Mainstream Capnograph
Maximal Voluntary Ventilation (MVV)
Metabolic Carts
Minute Ventilation ($\dot{V}_E$)
Monel
Open-Circuit Calorimeters
$P_{0.1}$
Paramagnetic
Peak Flow Meter
Peak Inspiratory Pressure (PIP)
Plateau Pressure
Polarographic Oxygen Analyzers
Pneumotachograph
Precision
Quenching
Residual Volume (RV)
Respiratory System Compliance
Sidestream Capnograph
Spirogram
Stead-Wells Spirometer
Thermal Flowmeter
Thoracic Gas Volume (TGV)
Total Lung Capacity (TLC)
Vital Capacity (VC)
Wheatstone Bridge
Work of Breathing

Respiration is the exchange of oxygen and carbon dioxide between an organism and its environment. Normal gas exchange in humans requires efficiently operating chest bellows and lungs, an alveolar-capillary network in which ventilation and blood flow are evenly matched, intact systemic circulation for transporting oxygen from the lungs to the tissues and carbon dioxide from the tissues to the lungs, and integrated neural and chemical control mechanisms that regulate pH, oxygen, and carbon dioxide levels in the blood.[1] If any of these processes fail, hypoxia, hypercapnia, and, ultimately, respiratory and cardiovascular failure may result.

Advances in microprocessor technology have significantly improved our ability to evaluate patient respiratory function, both in the laboratory and at the bedside. This chapter discusses the devices and techniques commonly used by respiratory therapists to assess respiratory system mechanics, gas exchange, and metabolic function of patients with cardiopulmonary disease.

Respiratory System Mechanics

Ventilation can be defined as the movement of air between the atmosphere and the lungs. Gas flow into and out of the respiratory system is influenced by the pressure gradient that exists between the airway opening and the alveoli and the impedance offered by the lungs and the chest wall. Respiratory muscular effort or the force generated by a mechanical ventilator establishes the pressure gradient between the atmosphere and the alveoli. The impedance to airflow results from the elastic and frictional forces that are offered by the lungs and thorax.[2]

The mechanics of breathing can be assessed by measuring the air volume exchanged during ventilation, the gas flow into and out of the lungs, and the pressure that must be generated to achieve a given volume or flow during breathing. Derived variables (e.g., **airway resistance, lung and chest wall compliance**, and **work of breathing**) can be calculated using the three measurements previously mentioned.

The usefulness of respiratory mechanics measurements ultimately depends on the accuracy and precision of the equipment used. **Accuracy** can be explained as how closely a measured value is related to the true (correct) value of the quantity measured. The accuracy of any instrument depends on its linearity and frequency response, its sensitivity to environmental conditions, and how well it is calibrated.[3] Accuracy of mechanics measurements is also influenced by patient cooperation while performing the test. In most cases, patient cooperation depends on a firm understanding of how to perform the test. If the technologist does not properly instruct patients how to perform the test, the results can be severely affected. **Precision** is the expression of an instrument's ability to reproduce a measurement (i.e., repeatability). The precision of a measuring device can be quantified by calculating the standard deviation of repeated measurements made by the device.[3]

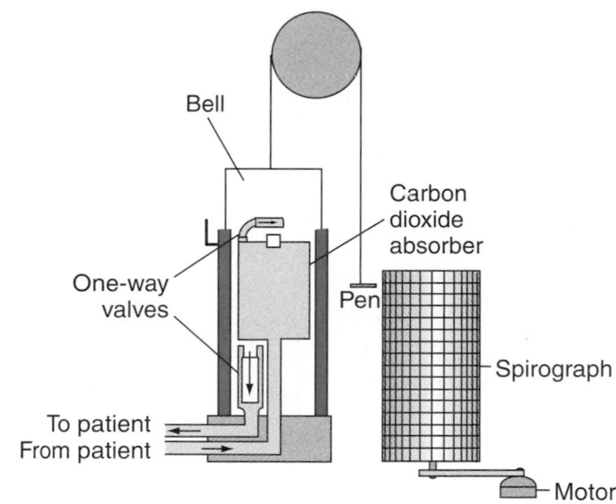

Figure 8-1 Water-sealed spirometer. (Modified from Collins Medical, Inc., Braintree, Mass.)

Volume and Flow Measurements

A spirometer is a device for measuring volume or flow changes at the airway opening. Therefore spirometers are generally classified by whether they measure lung-volume changes or airflow. Volume-displacement devices measure lung-volume changes by collecting exhaled gas into an expandable container and noting the amount of displacement that occurs. Typical examples of volume-collecting devices include water-sealed spirometers, bellows spirometers, and **dry-rolling seal spirometers.** Flow-sensing devices measure airflow by using thermal or hot wire **anemometers,** turbine flowmeters, and differential pressure **pneumotachographs.**

Water-Sealed Spirometers

As Figure 8-1 shows, a water-sealed spirometer consists of a bell that is sealed from the atmosphere by water. The patient is connected to the bell in rebreathing fashion by a breathing circuit, which consists of tubing with one-way valves and a carbon dioxide absorber. The bell, which is made of metal (usually aluminum), is suspended by a chain and pulley mechanism with a weight that counterbalances the weight of the bell.* A pen attached to the chain-and-pulley mechanism records bell movements on a separate motor-driven rotating drum called a **kymograph.** As patients exhale into the system, the bell moves upward and the attached pen moves proportionately downward on graph paper, creating a **spirogram.** Inhalation causes the bell to move downward and the pen to move upward. The rotating drum can move at a constant speed (32, 160, or 1920 mm/min), allowing the operator to measure volume changes relative to time. The slower speeds (32 and 160 mm/min) are used for measuring tidal volume, **minute ventilation ($\dot{V}_E$),** and **maximum voluntary ventilation (MVV).** The slower speeds are also used for specialized measurements (e.g., the diffusion capacity of carbon monoxide [D_LCO]). The fastest speed

The counterweight minimizes the effects of gravity acting on the metal bell.

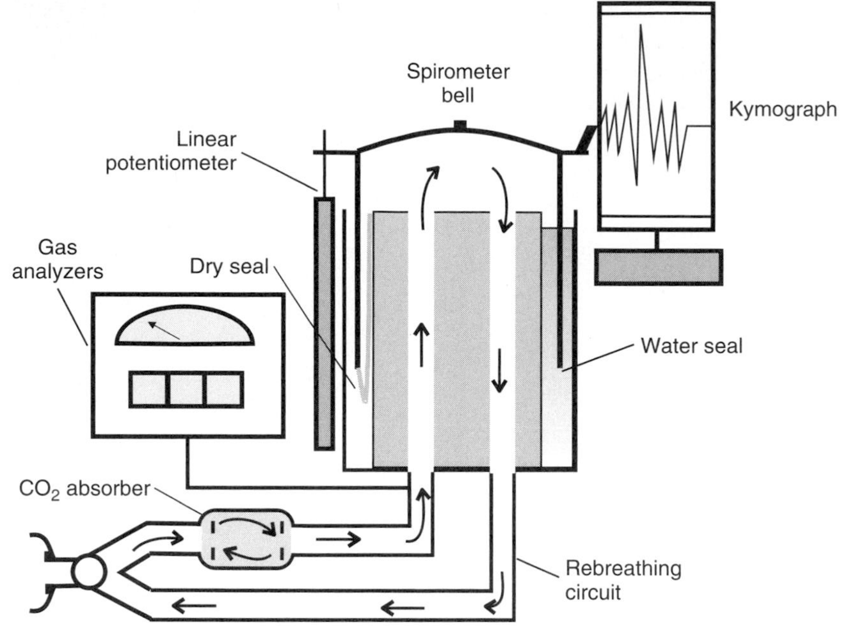

Figure 8-2 Stead-Wells spirometer. (From Ruppel G: Manual of pulmonary function testing, ed 7, St Louis, 1998, Mosby.)

(1920 mm/min) is used for recording volume changes during forced vital capacity (FVC) maneuvers.

Two bell sizes are available: 9 L and 13.5 L. The volume of the bell determines how many millimeters the pen moves when a given volume is displaced. For example, a 9 L bell will move 1 mm for every 20.93 mL of gas displaced, and a 13.5 L bell will move 1 mm for every 41.73 mL of gas displaced. (Note that the number of milliliters of gas that must be displaced to cause the kymograph pen to move 1 mm is called the **bell factor.**) The total gas volume displaced during a breath is calculated by multiplying the number of millimeters the pen is displaced on the spirogram by the bell factor for the spirometer.

The **Stead-Wells spirometer** (Figure 8-2) is similar in design to the original Collins water-sealed spirometer, except that a plastic bell is used instead of the metal one, eliminating the need for a counterweight because the bell weighs less. Stead-Wells spirometers show excellent frequency response characteristics, especially when recording rapid breathing maneuvers, such as FVC, timed expiratory volume measurements (e.g., forced expiratory volume in 1 second, or $FEV_{1.0}$), and MVV. Stead-Wells spirometers are available in 7-, 10-, and 14-L bell sizes. The pen recorder for the Stead-Wells spirometer is attached directly to the bell, so as the bell moves upward during exhalation, the pen inscribes on the spirogram in an upward motion. Conversely, the bell and pen move downward during inhalation.

Bellows Spirometers

With this type of spirometer, exhaled gases are collected into an expandable bellows (Figure 8-3). Air entering the bellows causes the free wall of the bellows to move outward, and its displacement is directly related to the volume of air exhaled. Volume changes can be recorded by attaching a pen recorder or a potentiometer to the free wall of the bellows.

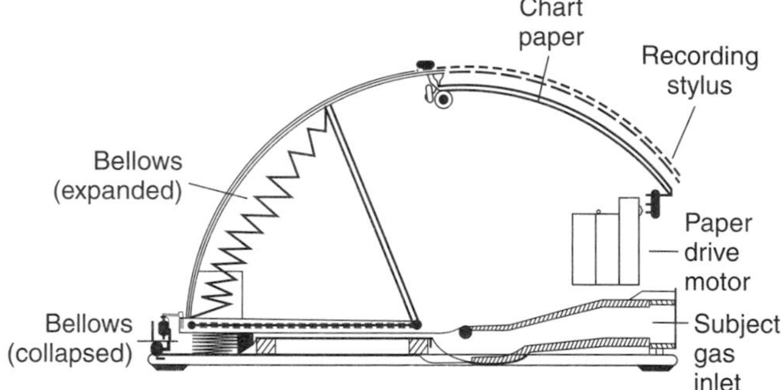

Figure 8-3 Wedge-bellows spirometer. (Modified from Vitalograph, Shawnee Mission, Kan.)

The bellows is usually constructed of silicon rubber or plastic, and several different designs are currently available. These designs differ in that the free wall can move horizontally, vertically, and/or diagonally. The frequency response of these devices is good, so they can be used to measure lung-volume changes during rapid breathing maneuvers (e.g., FVC, FEV_1, and MVV).

Dry-Rolling Seal Spirometers

These devices consist of a canister containing a piston that is sealed to it with a rolling diaphragmlike seal. As Figure 8-4 shows, gas entering the cylinder displaces the piston. The large surface area of the piston minimizes the mechanical resistance to movement and gives these devices good frequency response characteristics. A pen recorder or potentiometer

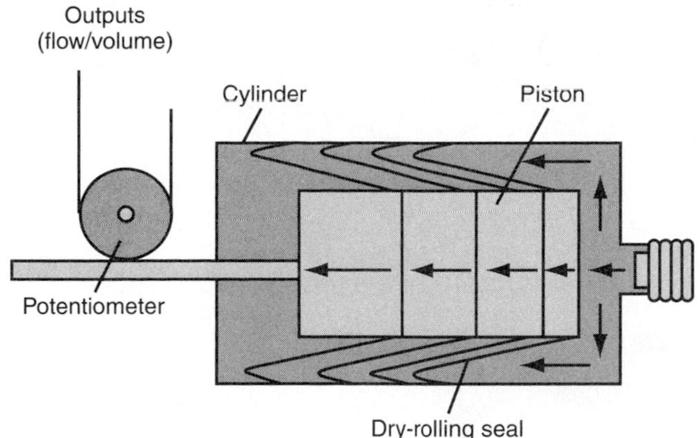

Figure 8-4 Dry-rolling seal spirometer. (From Datex-Ohmeda, Madison, Wis.)

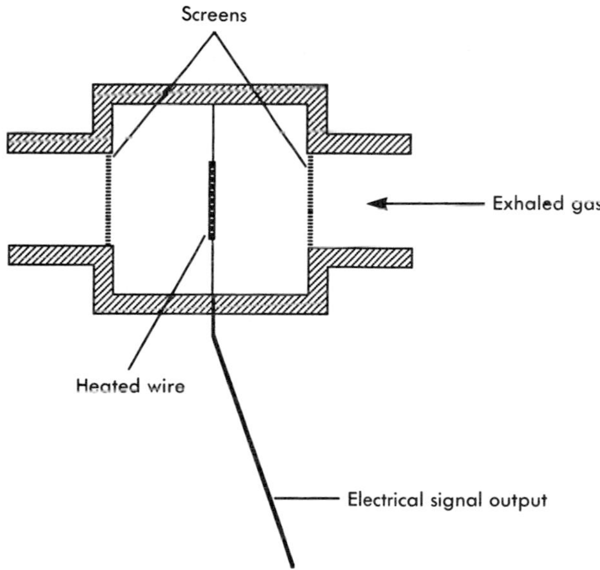

Figure 8-5 Thermal ("hot wire") anemometer.

attached to the cylinder shaft detects the piston's movement and registers the signal on an output display (e.g., graph paper or an oscilloscope).

Thermal Flowmeters

Figure 8-5 is a schematic of a thermal or "hot wire" anemometer. These devices use sensors that are temperature-sensitive, resistive elements (e.g., thermistor beads or heated wires). **Thermal flowmeters** operate on the principle that as gas passes over the thermistor bead or the heated wire, the sensor cools and changes its resistance, which in turn is proportional to the gas flow past it.* With thermistor beads, cooling increases resistance, whereas with a heated wire, cooling decreases resistance. Gas flow can be calculated because the amount of power needed to maintain the temperature of the heating element above the ambient temperature is

**The amount of cooling depends on the gas viscosity and the thermal conductivity of the gas being measured.*

> **CLINICAL ROUNDS 8-1**
>
> You are asked to perform bedside spirometry on a patient receiving bronchodilator therapy. You connect the mouthpiece to the measuring device (a heated-wire or thermal flowmeter) and instruct the patient to breathe in deeply and exhale forcefully into the mouthpiece. When the patient does this you notice that the digital display fails to register a reading of estimated volume. What could cause this type of problem?
>
> See Appendix A for the answer.

related to the velocity of the gas flow. Actually, the signal is related to the log of the velocity of gas flow, and therefore must be linearized.[3] Thermal flowmeters are unidirectional devices and cannot be used for measuring bidirectional flows during breathing. Clinical Rounds 8-1 presents a decision-making problem involving a thermal flowmeter spirometer.

Turbine Flowmeters

Turbine flowmeters (Figure 8-6) use a rotating vane or turbine to measure gas flow. As gas flows through the device, the vane turns at a rate dependent on the flow rate of the gas. The flow rate can be measured by counting the number of times the vane turns, which can be done mechanically (by linking the vane to a needle attached to a calibrated display) or electronically (by using a light beam that is interrupted each time the vane turns).

Turbine flowmeters, such as hand-held respirometers, are usually accurate for flows between 3 and 300 L/min. They are portable and easy to use, but they are slow to respond to flow changes because of inertia (low-frequency response). Some turbine devices, such as those found in commercially available **metabolic carts** use a bias flow of gas to keep the turbine constantly turning, thus reducing the inertia of the vane.[3] These devices are good for measuring unidirectional flow, but they are inaccurate for measuring bidirectional flows.[2]

Some **peak flow meters** operate by measuring the gas flow against a rotating vane. The operating mechanism consists of a pivoted vane with an attached needle indicator. The rotation of the vane is opposed by air resistance and a calibrated spring. During a forced exhalation, the vane and the indicator needle rotate until the maximum available flow is reached. The indicator needle attached to the vane is spring-loaded, and therefore maintains the measurement of peak expiratory flow (PEF) until it is mechanically reset.

Peak flow meters are typically calibrated in liters per minute. The Wright Peak Flow Meter (Figure 8-7, A), designed by B.M. Wright, can measure flows between 60 and 1000 L/min with an accuracy of ±10 L/min. Its reproducibility is within ±2 L/min. Because of its wide range,

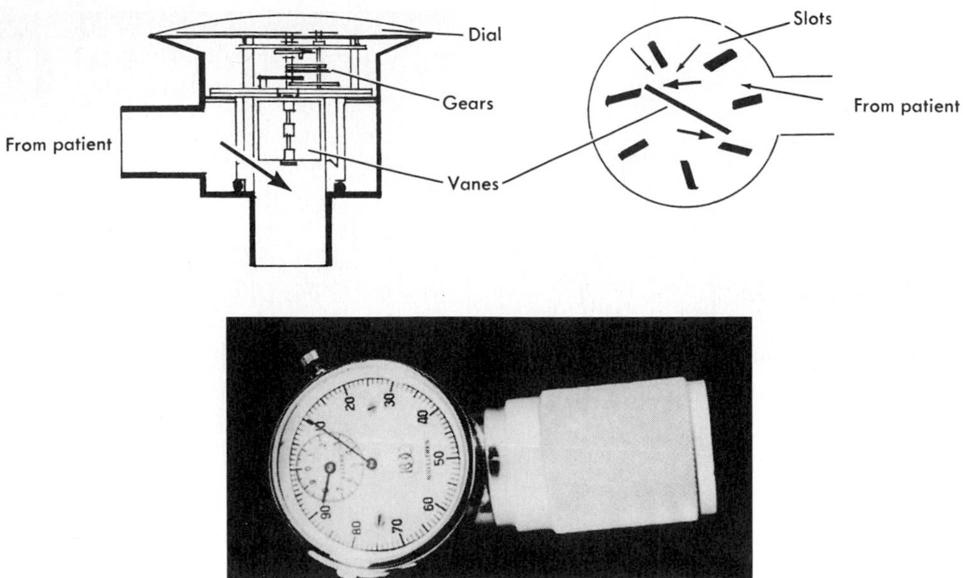

Figure 8-6 Turbine flowmeter.

it can be used to measure peak flows for both pediatric and adult patients. Reusable and disposable mouthpieces are available in pediatric and adult sizes, so these devices can be used for multiple patients.

Increased use of peak flow meters in the management of asthmatics has prompted many medical device manufacturers to market inexpensive peak flow meters that are durable and easy to use (see Figure 8-7, *B*). These expendable units are constructed of plastic and operate with a piston and spring mechanism. Exhaled air pushes against the piston, causing the needle to move on a calibrated scale. Although these devices possess accuracy and reproducibility similar to non-expendable peak flow meters, they typically operate over a slightly narrower range of flows (80 to 800 L/min).

Pneumotachographs

Several different types of pneumotachographs are shown in Figure 8-8, including a Fleisch type of pneumotachograph, a screen pneumotachograph, a variable orifice pneumotachograph, and an ultrasonic pneumotachograph. All of these devices except the ultrasonic pneumotachograph operate on the principle that gas flow through them is proportional to the pressure drop that occurs as the gas flows across a known resistance. Ultrasonic pneumotachographs rely on the **Doppler effect** to quantify the airflow velocity.

The **Fleisch pneumotachograph** (see Figure 8-8, *A*) uses a bundle of brass capillary tubes arranged in a parallel manner to create the known resistance.[4] A differential pressure transducer monitors the pressures before and after the resistance and converts the difference into a flow signal. (With unidirectional flow, a single pressure measurement is required.) A heater is attached to raise the temperature of the entering gas and prevent moisture condensation on the capillary tubes.*

**The accumulation of moisture on the capillary tubes can change their resistance and thus alter the accuracy of the device.*

Fleisch pneumotachographs are most accurate when the gas flow is smooth or laminar. Turbulent airflow, which occurs at high flows or with obstructions or bends in the breathing circuit, can adversely affect the accuracy of airflow measurements. Turbulent airflow can also be caused by increases in the gas viscosity. Therefore it is important to compensate for different viscosities either mathematically or by calibrating the instrument with the gas mixture breathed during measurement. For example, room air has a viscosity of 184 poise (P), and 100% oxygen has a viscosity of 206 P. A pneumotachograph calibrated with room air will show an error of 12% if it used to measure airflow in a patient breathing 100% oxygen.[5]

Ceramic pneumotachographs are similar in design to Fleisch pneumotachographs, except that they use ceramic material containing a number of parallel channels to create the fixed resistance. The ceramic channels smooth the air flowing through them and provide a constant resistance to airflow. A heating element is incorporated into the design. The temperature of the gas mixture flowing through these devices tends to equilibrate with the temperature of the ceramic material because of the high heat capacity of the ceramic. Additionally, moisture that condenses during breathing tends to be absorbed by the porous ceramic material, rather than occluding the tubes.[5]

Screen pneumotachographs (see Figure 8-8, *B*) use a series of fine-mesh screens to create a fixed resistance. Most of these devices use a stainless-steel (**Monel**) screen with a mesh size of 400 wires/in.[5] When a triple screen configuration is used, the center screen acts as the main resistive element, and the two outer screens smooth the airflow and protect the inner screen from particulate matter.[5] Similar to Fleisch type of devices, a heating element is incorporated to prevent water condensation on the metal screens.

A

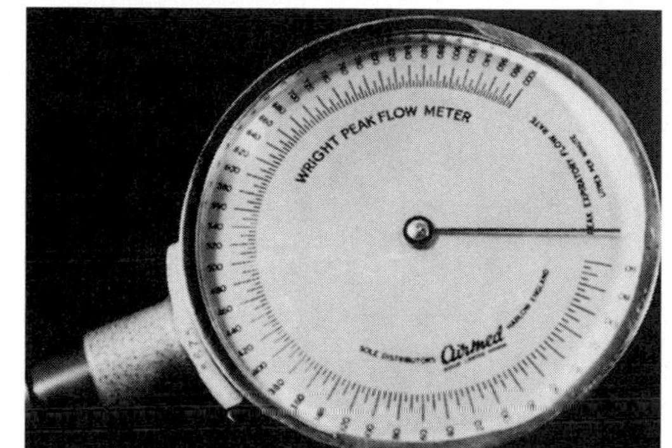

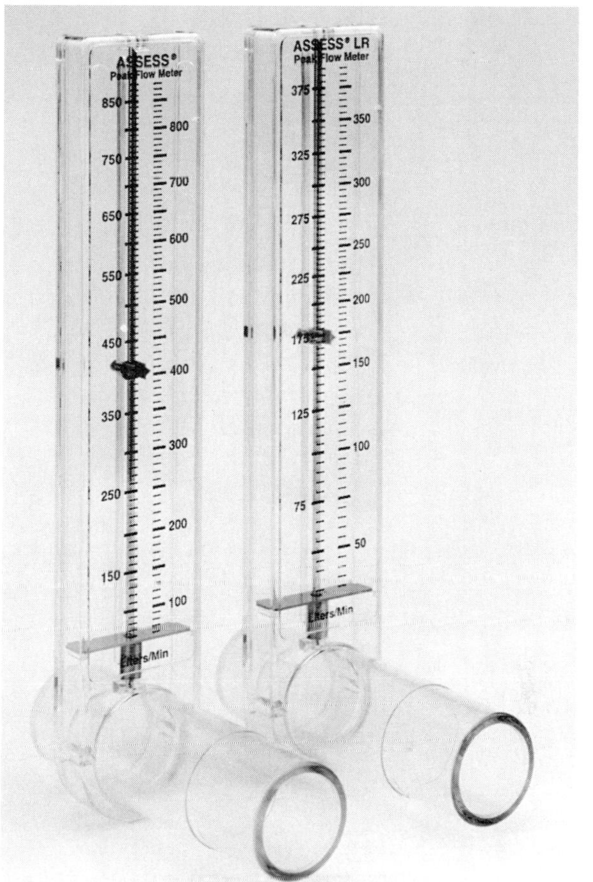

B

Figure 8-7 **A,** Wright Peak Flow Meter; **B,** commercially available disposable peak flow meter (**B,** Courtesy Respironics/HealthScan, Inc, Cedar Grove, NJ. In Ruppel GL: *Manual of pulmonary function testing*, ed 7, St Louis, 1998, Mosby.)

Some screen type of devices use fibrous material, which looks like a paper filter, instead of metal screens to create the known resistance. These devices operate at ambient temperature, and therefore do not require a heating element. The main advantage of using them is that they are inexpensive and disposable, allowing patients to have their own peak flow meter, which reduces the risk of cross-contamination. The disadvantages of using these devices are that they are unidirectional devices, and the accuracy varies by device.[5] Additionally, moisture absorbed by the paper filter can severely affect device accuracy.

Variable orifice pneumotachographs (see Figure 8-8, *C*) are disposable, bidirectional, flow-measuring devices that use a variable area, flexible obstruction for measuring flow as a function of the pressure differential generated by the obstruction. They contain minimum dead space (about 10 mL) and can measure flows from 1.2 to 180 L/min.[2] Although the flow-pressure characteristics of variable orifice pneumotachographs are nonlinear, this discrepancy can be compensated for electronically.

Vortex ultrasonic flowmeters (see Figure 8-8, *D*) use struts to create a partial obstruction to gas flow. As gases flow past these struts, whirlpools or vortices are produced. The frequency at which these whirlpools are produced is related to gas flow through the struts. An ultrasonic transmitter perpendicular to the flow produces sound waves that are modulated by the frequency of the vortices. The extent of modulation related to actual flow is then determined.[6] Vortex ultrasonic flowmeters are not affected by the viscosity, density, or temperature of the gas being measured. They are unidirectional devices, and therefore cannot measure inspiratory or expiratory flow simultaneously.[2]

Non–vortex ultrasonic flow meters (see Figure 8-8, *E*) estimate airflow by projecting pulsed sound waves along the longitudinal axis of the flow meter (i.e., parallel to the gas flow instead of across it). The theory is that the speed of the ultrasonic wave transmission is influenced by the rate of gas flow through the device.[4] Non–vortex ultrasonic flowmeters are not affected by moisture or the viscosity of the gas being breathed, and can be used to measure bidirectional flows.

American Thoracic Society (ATS) Standards for Spirometry

In 1979, ATS members met in Snowbird, Utah, to discuss standardization of the instruments and techniques used during spirometric testing. A statement was subsequently released providing recommendations for the standardization of spirometry.[7] (Table 8-1 gives a summary of these

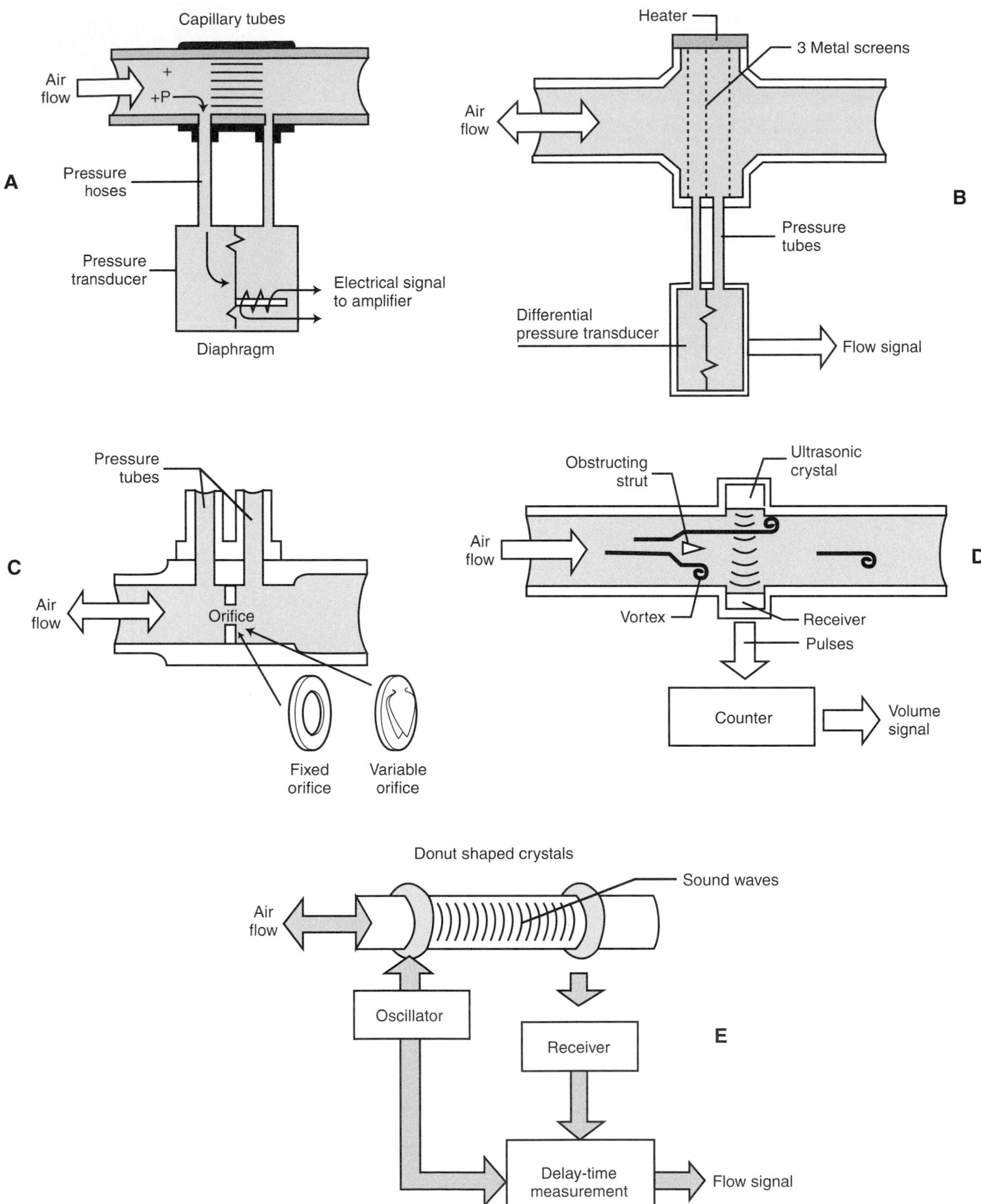

Figure 8-8 Pneumotachographs. **A,** Fleish type of device; **B,** screen type of device; **C,** variable orifice device; **D,** vortex ultrasonic device; **E,** non-vortex device. (Redrawn from Sullivan WJ, Peters GM, Enright PL: Pneumotachography: theory and clinical application, *Respir Care* 29:736, 1984.)

Table 8-1 Minimal recommendations for diagnostic spirometry*

Test	Range/Accuracy (*BTPS*)	Flow Range (*L/s*)	Time (*s*)	Resistance and Back Pressure	Test Signal
VC	0.5 to 8 L ±3% of reading or ±0.050 L, whichever is greater	0 to 14	30		3-L Cal Syringe
FVC	0.5 to 8 L ±3% of reading or ±0.050 L, whichever is greater	0 to 14	15	<1.5 cm H_2O/L/s	24 standard waveforms
$FEV_{1.0}$	0.5 to 8 L ±3% of reading or ±0.050 L, whichever is greater	0 to 14	1	<1.5 cm H_2O/L/s	3-L Cal Syringe
Time zero	The time point from which all $FEV_{1.0}$ measurements are taken			Back extrapolation	24 standard waveforms
PEF	Accuracy: ±10% of reading or ±0.400 L/s, whichever is greater Precision: ±5% of reading or ±0.200 L/s, whichever is greater	0 to 14		Same as $FEV_{1.0}$	26 flow standard waveforms
$FEF_{25-75\%}$	7.0 L/s ±5% of reading or ±0.200 L/s, whichever is greater	±14	15	Same as $FEV_{1.0}$	24 standard waveforms
$\dot{V}$	± 14 L/s ±5% of reading or ±0.200 L/s, whichever is greater	0 to 14	15	Same as $FEV_{1.0}$	Proof from manufacturer
MVV	250 L/min at V_t of 2 L within (10% of reading or ±15 L/min, whichever is greater	±14 ±3%	12 to 15	Pressure <±10 cm H_2O at 2-L TV at 2.0 Hz	Sine wave pump

*Unless specifically stated, precision requirements are the same as the accuracy requirements.

From American Thoracic Society: *Standardization of spirometry,* 1994 update, *Am Rev Dis* 152:1107, 1995.

recommendations.) The central goal of this and another document published in 1987 was to improve performance characteristics of spirometers and decrease variability of laboratory testing.[8] To date, most spirometer manufacturers have complied with the standards suggested by the ATS, and as a result, spirometry results are not only consistent within a laboratory but also between laboratories.

As was previously stated, the recommendations of the 1979 ATS Conference and the subsequent document published in 1987 focused on instrumentation. In 1991 and again in 1995, the ATS widened the scope of its recommendations to include guidelines for the selection of reference values, the performance of spirometry, and the quality control of spirometers, as well as minimal recommendations for monitoring devices.[9,10] Guidelines for the selection of reference values, along with guidelines for the calibration and quality control of spirometers, have been presented by the ATS.[9,10] Table 8-2 lists the recommendations for monitoring devices.

The impetus for establishing standards for monitoring devices was the increased use of portable peak flow meters in the management of asthmatic patients. Note that the standards for monitoring devices are different from those recommended for spirometry because they only address FVC, FEV_1, and PEF. They also have wider ranges of accuracy (±5% for monitoring devices vs. ±3% for diagnostic spirometry) and a requirement of a 3% precision (or 0.050 mL, whichever is greater). For these reasons, the ATS "does not recommend the use of monitoring devices for diagnostic purposes in the traditional diagnostic setting where one is comparing a measured value with a reference values."[10]

In 1996, the AARC produced a Clinical Practice Guideline for Spirometry,[11] which updates prior ATS statements on spirometry. It includes indications and contraindications, hazards and complications, and limitations of methodology. It also provides recommended times for withholding commonly used bronchodilators before testing when bronchodilator response is to be assessed. A separate statement on assessing patient response to bronchodilator therapy at the point of care is also available.[12]

Measurement of Residual Volume

Vital capacity (VC) and its subdivisions can be measured in the pulmonary function laboratory with any of the aforementioned spirometers. Measurements of **residual volume** (RV), **functional residual capacity** (FRC), and **total lung capacity** (TLC) are obtained using **body plethysmography** and **inert gas techniques,** such as nitrogen washout and helium dilution.[13,14,15]

Table 8-2 Minimal recommendations for monitoring devices

Requirement	FVC & FEV_t (*BTPS*)	PEF (*BTPS*)
Range	High: 0.50 to 8 L	High: 100 L/min to ≥700 L/min but ≤850 L/min
	Low: 0.5 to 6 L	Low: 60 L/min to ≥275 L/min but ≤400 L/min
Accuracy	±5% of reading or ±0.100 L, whichever is greater	±10% of reading or ±20 L/min, whichever is greater
Precision	±3% of reading or ±0.050 L, whichever is greater	Intradevice: ≤5% of reading or ≤10 L/min, whichever is greater
		Interdevice: ≤10% of reading or ≤20 L/min, whichever is greater
Linearity	Within 3% over range	Within 5% over range
Graduations	Constant over entire range	Constant over entire range
	High: 0.100 L	High: 20 L/min
	Low: 0.050 L	Low: 10 L/min
Resolution	High: 0.050 L	High: 10 L/min
	Low: 0.025 L	Low: 5 L/min
Resistance	<2.5 cm H_2O/L/s, from 0 to 14 L/s	<2.5 cm H_2O/L/s, from 0 to 14 L/s
Minimal detectable volume	0.030 L	–
Test signal	24 standard volume-time waveforms	26 standard flow-time waveforms

From American Thoracic Society: *Standardization of spirometry,* 1994 Update, *Am Rev Respir Dis* 152:1107, 1995.

High, High-range devices; *low,* low-range devices.

Body Plethysmography

A body plethysmograph (or "body box") is a rigidly walled, airtight enclosure, as shown in Figure 8-9. A number of variables can be measured with the body plethysmography but **thoracic gas volume (VTG)** and **airways resistance (R_{aw})** are by far the most common measurements obtained with these devices. Airways conductance (G_{aw}), which is the reciprocal of R_{aw} and specific airways conductance (sG_{aw} = conductance/unit of lung volume) are calculated variables that are also routinely reported. Two types of body plethysmographs are usually described: constant-volume pressure plethysmographs and variable pressure and volume flow plethysmographs. Constant-volume pressure devices are the most common plethysmographs used. With these devices, the patient sits within the enclosure, which contains a pressure transducer within the wall of the device, and breathes through a mouthpiece connected to an assembly containing an electronic shutter and a differential pressure pneumotachometer. Mouth pressure and box pressure changes measured during tidal breathing and panting maneuvers performed by the patient at the end of a quiet expiration are displayed on an oscilloscope and directed to a microprocessor unit that calculates thoracic gas volume from empirically derived pressure-volume relationships.[13,14] (Note that the reference pressure-volume relationships are empirically derived using an electronically driven piston to deliver known volumes into the enclosure. Pressure changes associated with a known volume change are recorded in the system's microprocessor and used to calculate the thoracic gas volume.) The microprocessor corrects for variations in ambient temperature and pressure from data entered manually by the technologist.

The FRC is calculated using the following relationship:

$$V_{FRC} = \Delta V \div \Delta P \times P_B - P_{H2O},$$

where ΔV and ΔP are the box volume and alveolar pressure changes measured during the panting maneuver, P_B is the ambient barometric pressure, and P_{H2O} is the water vapor pressure (assume 47 mm Hg for 37° C). The resultant thoracic gas volume measured at FRC (V_{FRC}) is then corrected for the volume displaced from the box by the patient (Clinical Rounds 8-2).[14]

Airways resistance is derived from two separate maneuvers. In the first maneuver, the subject pants while the mouth shutter is open so that flow changes ($\dot{V}$) can be measured. In the second part of the measurement, the mouth shutter is closed at subject's end expiratory or FRC level and the subject is instructed to continue panting while maintaining an open glottis. This maneuver provides a measure of the driving pressure that is used to move air into the lungs (i.e.,

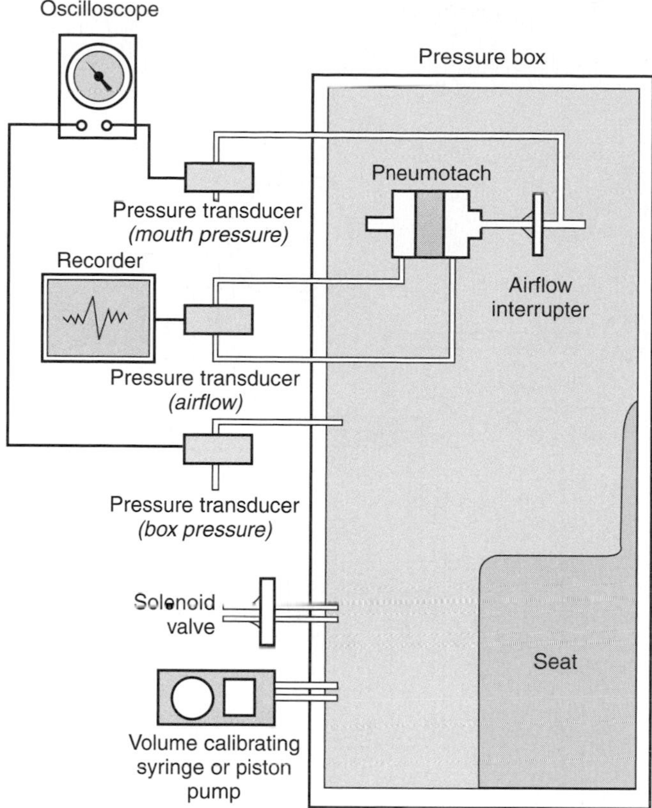

Figure 8-9 Schematic of a contrast volume (pressure) plethysmograph. (Redrawn from Miller WF, Scacci R, Gast LR: *Laboratory evaluation of pulmonary function*, Philadelphia, 1987, JB Lippincott.)

P_{mo}). It is important to recognize that airflow and mouth pressure measurements are recorded separately and must therefore be related to changes in the plethysmograph or box pressure to insure accurate readings. R_{aw} is ultimately derived using the following relationship:

$$R_{aw} = P_{mo} \div \dot{V}$$

Inert Gas Techniques

Nitrogen washout tests are performed using the equipment shown in Figure 8-10, including a spirometer with a rapidly responding nitrogen analyzer, a source of 100% oxygen, a nonrebreathing valve, and the appropriate tubing.[14] The FRC is determined by initiating the test at the end of a quiet expiration. The patient inspires 100% oxygen and exhales into the spirometer through the nonrebreathing valve. The patient continues to breathe the 100% oxygen until the exhaled nitrogen concentration is less than 1.5%. The nitrogen volume present in the lungs at the beginning of the test (i.e., FRC) can be determined by first measuring the total volume of exhaled gas and then multiplying this volume by the percentage of nitrogen in the mixed expired air, which is measured with the nitrogen analyzer.[15] This resultant volume represents the nitrogen volume in the lungs at the beginning of the test. Multiplying this volume by 1.25 allows the lung volume at the beginning of the test to be determined.* Remember that the resultant volume is measured under ambient conditions (ATPS) and must be converted to BTPS (body temperature, ambient pressure and saturated with water vapor).

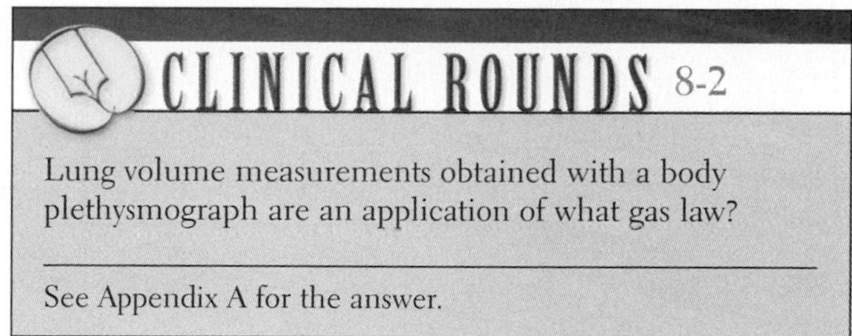

Lung volume measurements obtained with a body plethysmograph are an application of what gas law?

See Appendix A for the answer.

Helium dilution tests can be performed using an apparatus such as the one illustrated in Figure 8-11. Note that this type of device contains a spirometer with a thermal conductivity analyzer (for measuring helium), a mixing fan, a source of helium and oxygen, and the appropriate tubing for a rebreathing breathing circuit.[14,15] The FRC is measured while patients breathe into and out of a reservoir containing known concentrations of helium and oxygen. As patients breathe into and out of the system, the added volume of air from the patient's lungs dilutes the helium concentration. The end point of the test is reached when the helium percentage remains steady for 2 minutes, indicating that the helium is equilibrated between the spirometer and the patient's lungs. The FRC volume is calculated as:

$$FRC = (He_{mL} \div He_{final}) - (He_{mL} \div He_{initial}) - Vrb - Vcorr,$$

where He_{mL} is the number of milliliters of helium added to the system, $He_{initial}$ is the helium concentration at the beginning of the test, He_{final} is the helium concentration at the end of the test, *Vrb* is the apparatus dead space, and *Vcorr* is a correction volume for the amount of helium that is theoretically absorbed by the body, respiratory quotient (RQ) changes, and changes in nitrogen in the circuit.[15]

It is important to recognize that the inert gas techniques can only measure gas volumes in communicating airways (i.e., airways that are open between the mouth and the alveoli), whereas body plethysmography measures all of the volume in the thorax (i.e., thoracic lung volume). Therefore inert gas measurements of FRC for patients with chronic obstructive pulmonary disorder and severe air trapping are lower than FRC (i.e., VTG) measurements from body plethysmography.

Pressure Measurements

In Chapter 1, several simple devices that can be used to measure pressure (e.g., U-shaped tubes and mercury barometers) were described. These devices were effective in

**The correction factor of 1.25 is used because the room air that filled the patient's lungs before the test began contains approximately 80% nitrogen.*

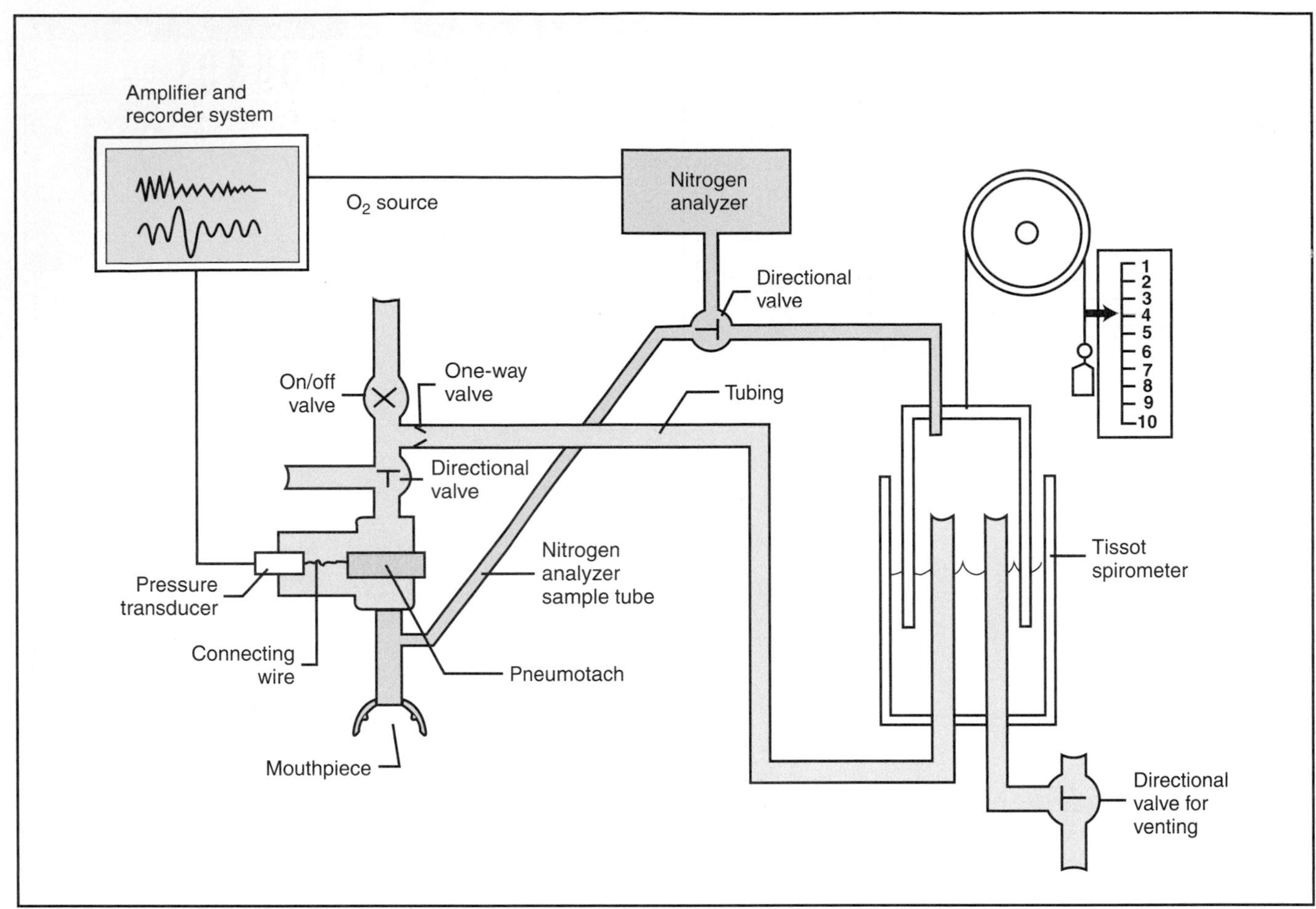

Figure 8-10 Breathing circuit for performing nitrogen washout test. (Redrawn from Miller WF, Scacci R, Gast LR: *Laboratory evaluation of pulmonary function*, Philadelphia, 1987, JB Lippincott.)

measuring constant or slowly changing pressures (e.g., atmospheric pressure) but limited in their ability to measure dynamic pressures. Pressure changes, such as those occurring during breathing, can be measured with an **aneroid manometer** or an **electromechanical transducer.**

An aneroid manometer (Figure 8-12) consists of a vacuum chamber with a flexible cover or diaphragm that flexes when pressure is applied to it. This flexing motion is translated into a pressure measurement via a lever system that is attached to a calibrated scale. The Bourdon gauge, which consists of a coiled tube with a needle attached to a calibrated scale by a gear mechanism (see Chapter 1), is a variation of this concept. As the pressure within the Bourdon tube increases, its force tends to straighten the tube, causing the attached needle to become displaced. The amount of displacement is measured on the calibrated scale.

Aneroid manometers are used extensively in mechanical ventilators and as independent units for instantaneous pressure measurements, such as maximum inspiratory and expiratory pressures. The pressure is displayed relative to atmospheric pressure or as gauge pressure (psig). Thus a gauge pressure of 5 mm Hg measured at sea level (1 atmosphere = 760 mm Hg) corresponds to an absolute pressure of 765 mm Hg. Although aneroid manometers can measure a wide range of pressures, their frequency response is low.

Electromechanical transducers are generally classified as strain gauge devices, variable inductance devices, or variable capacitance devices.[3] Strain gauge pressure transducers (Figure 8-13, A) use sensors that consist of a metal wire or semiconductor incorporated into a **Wheatstone bridge** circuit. When pressure is applied to the sensor, the wire or semiconductor elongates, causing its electrical resistance to increase. The increased resistance decreases the output voltage by an amount that is proportional to the applied pressure.

The variable inductance transducer (see Figure 8-13, *B*) consists of a stainless steel diaphragm that is positioned between two coils. When the diaphragm is not flexed, the inductance of the two coils is equal. The diaphragm flexes when pressure is applied, changing the inductance between the two coils by an amount that is proportional to the applied pressure. The variable capacitance transducer (see Figure 8-13, C) operates similarly to variable inductance

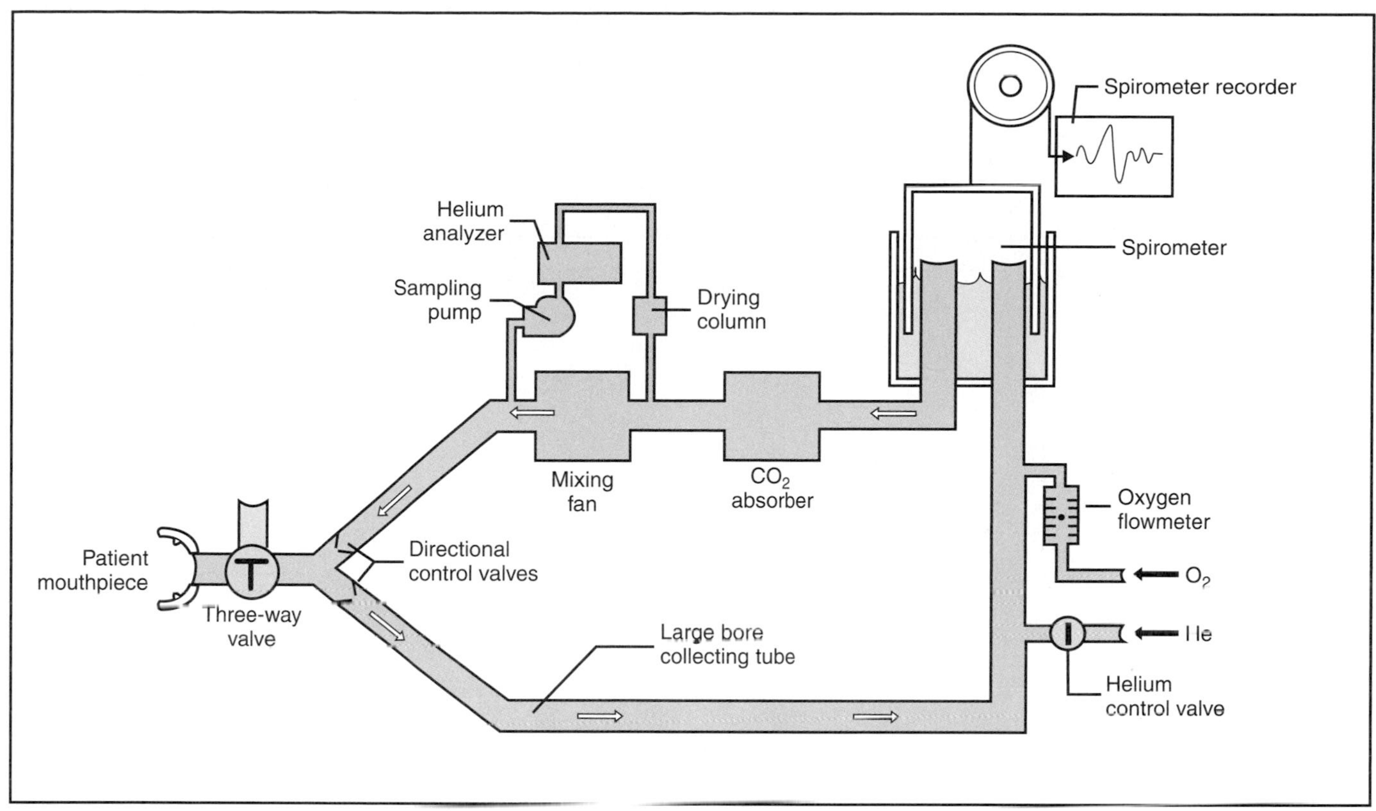

Figure 8-11 Breathing circuit for performing helium dilution tests. (Redrawn from Miller WF, Scacci R, Gast LR: *Laboratory evaluation of pulmonary function*, Philadelphia, 1987, JB Lippincott.)

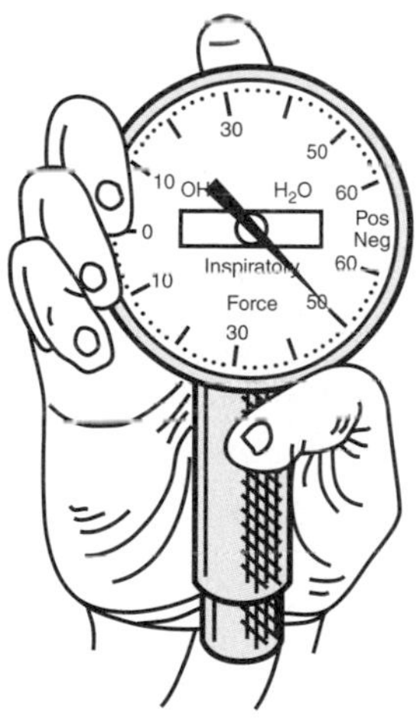

Figure 8-12 Aneroid manometer. (From Pilbeam SP: *Mechanical ventilation: physiological and clinical applications*, St Louis, Mosby.)

devices, except that the diaphragm of the capacitance device constitutes one plate of a capacitor. The other half of the plate is a stationery electrode. Displacement of the diaphragm alters the capacitance of the device and changes the output voltage in a manner that is proportional to the applied pressure.[3]

Strain gauge and variable inductance pressure transducers are commonly used for measuring respiratory and cardiovascular pressures. These devices respond quickly to pressure changes, and thus have good frequency response characteristics over a wide range of pressures. These devices are usually quite stable, being relatively insensitive to vibration and shock.[3] Variable capacitance transducers are large, bulky, very sensitive to vibration, and have poor frequency response compared with strain gauge and variable inductance types of transducers.

Bedside Measurement of Respiratory Mechanics

A number of commercial systems are now available for measuring bedside respiratory mechanics, especially during artificial ventilation. These include "stand alone" units, such as the BICORE CP-100 Pulmonary Monitoring System and Novametrix Medical Systems' Ventrac system, as well as microprocessor units that are incorporated into some ventilators (e.g., Siemens Servo 300 and Drager E4 ventilators).

The BICORE CP-100 Pulmonary Monitor (Figure 8-14) and the Ventrac system use variable orifice pneumotachographs to measure airflow and airway pressures and an electronic transducer attached to a triple-lumen esophageal catheter to measure esophageal pressures (i.e., esophageal pressure ~ intrapleural pressure). These catheters are multifunctional and may be used for gastric suctioning and feeding. The catheter can be positioned by noting the pressure recorded as the catheter is inserted. Its ideal position is the lower third of the esophagus, which is easily detected because when the catheter enters into the stomach, a positive

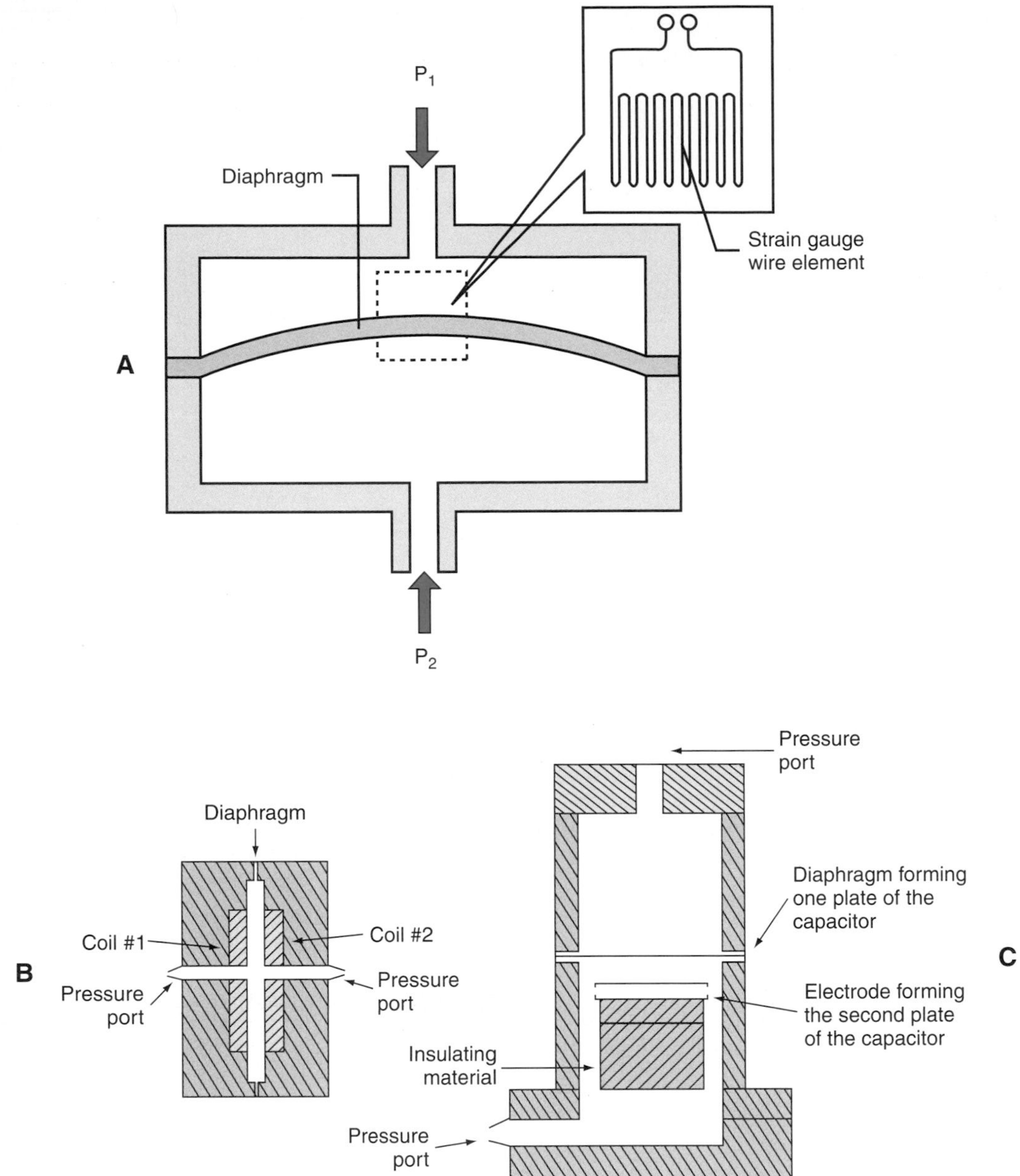

Figure 8-13 Electromechanical transducers. **A,** Strain gauge device; **B,** variable inductance device; **C,** variable capacitance device. (**B** and **C,** Courtesy Snow M: Instrumentation. In Clause JL, editor: *Pulmonary function testing guidelines and controversies*, New York, 1992, Academic Press.)

pressure is recorded. Thus after the pressure becomes positive, the catheter can be correctly positioned by retracting it until the pressure returns to a negative value. The catheter can be anchored to the nose with surgical tape.

Airflow and pressure measurements are relayed to the system's microprocessor and displayed on a cathode ray tube (CRT). The system can display real time tracings of airway pressure, tidal volume, and airflow measured at the mouth (Figure 8-15). The microprocessor unit can also provide flow-volume, pressure-volume, and pressure-flow plots, along with calculations of airway resistance, patient-ventilator compliance, intrinsic or **auto-positive end expiratory pressure (auto-PEEP), $P_{0.1}$,** and work of breathing. Although both the BICORE CP-100 and Ventrak systems can be used with spontaneously breathing patients, they are almost exclusively used by clinicians to monitor the respiratory system mechanics of mechanically ventilated patients.

As was previously mentioned, many of the new ventilators can also provide respiratory mechanics measurements. These ventilators contain pressure and airflow transducers for measuring airway pressures and airflow,

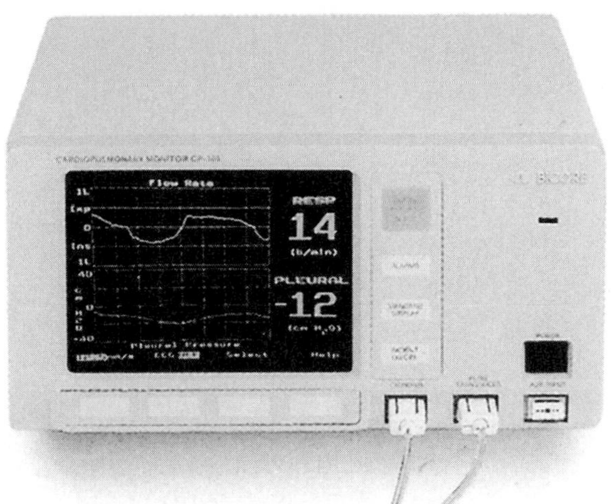

Figure 8-14 The Bicore pulmonary monitor. (Courtesy Viasys, Conshohocken, Pa.)

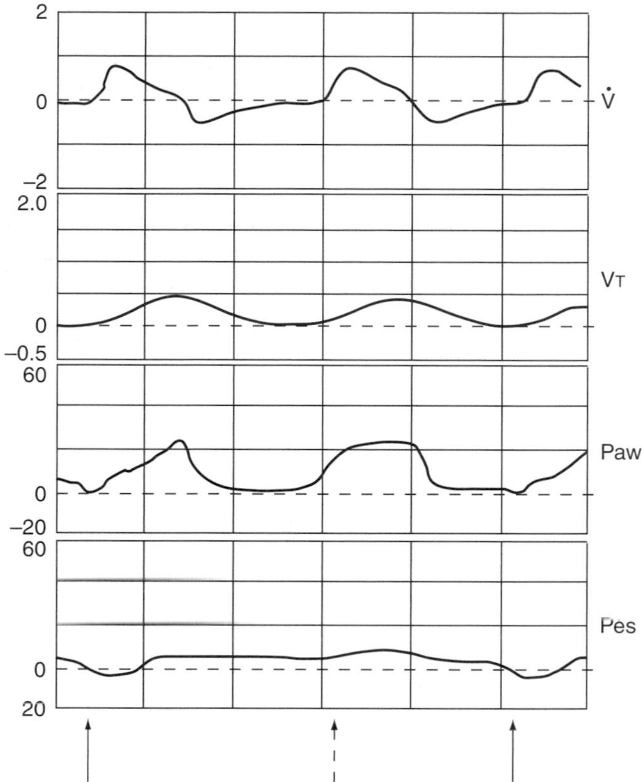

Figure 8-15 Real-time tracings of airway pressure, tidal volume, and airflow at the mouth recorded during mechanical ventilation. (From MacIntyre NR, Gropper C: Monitoring ventilatory function II: respiratory system mechanics and muscle function. In Levine RL, Fromm RE, editors: *Critical care monitoring: from prehospital to ICU*, St Louis, 1995, Mosby.)

which can be displayed in real time. A microprocessor incorporated into the system's hardware provides calculations of airway resistance, lung compliance, and intrinsic PEEP. (See Chapter 11 for a discussion of intrinsic or auto-PEEP.)

Impedance Plethysmography

These devices estimate lung-volume changes by measuring the changes in electrical impedance between two electrodes placed on the chest wall. **Electrical impedance,** which is opposition to the flow of an alternating current, is determined by the resistance and capacitance of the circuit through which the current must pass. In the case of lung-volume measurements, changes in chest wall impedance are caused by variations in the amount of blood, bone, and tissue present. Thus as the chest wall expands during inspiration, thoracic blood volume increases. Conversely, as the lungs deflate during expiration, thoracic blood volume decreases, and its electrical impedance decrease. Note that the contributions of air to electrical impedance are minimal.

The electrodes used in impedance plethysmography are similar to the standard electrocardiograph electrodes and are placed in the midclavicular line at the level of the manubrium. A constant high-frequency (100 kHz), low-amplitude, electrical current is passed between the two electrodes, and the return voltage is used to calculate the impedance. Variations in impedance measured during the respiratory cycle are demodulated and displayed as a waveform. The respiratory rate is extrapolated from a 4- to 6-breath average.[16]

Impedance pneumography is most often used in home apnea monitoring units, like the one shown in Figure 8-16. Each unit contains adjustable low and high respiratory rate alarms. The sensitivity of the monitor can be adjusted by the operator to avoid false alarms because of changes in impedance caused by movement instead of by changes in respiration.

Recent evidence suggests that bradycardia and upper airway obstruction may cause these monitors to fail to recognize apnea.[17,18] In the case of bradycardia, cardiac oscillations and intrathoracic blood-volume changes cause an increase in impedance, which is sensed as part of the respiratory cycle. Continued respiratory efforts in the presence of upper airway obstructions are sensed as normal respiratory efforts.

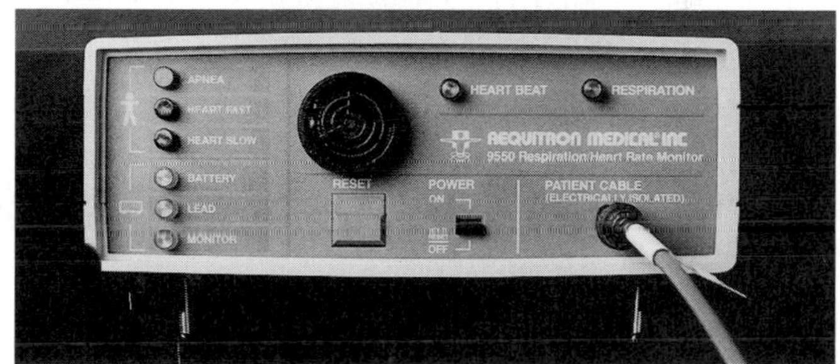

Figure 8-16 Apnea monitor.

Respiratory Inductive Plethysmography

This technique is based on the principle developed by Konno and Mead[19] that the respiratory system moves with two degrees of freedom. That is, it consists of two moving parts: the rib cage and the abdomen. During inspiration,

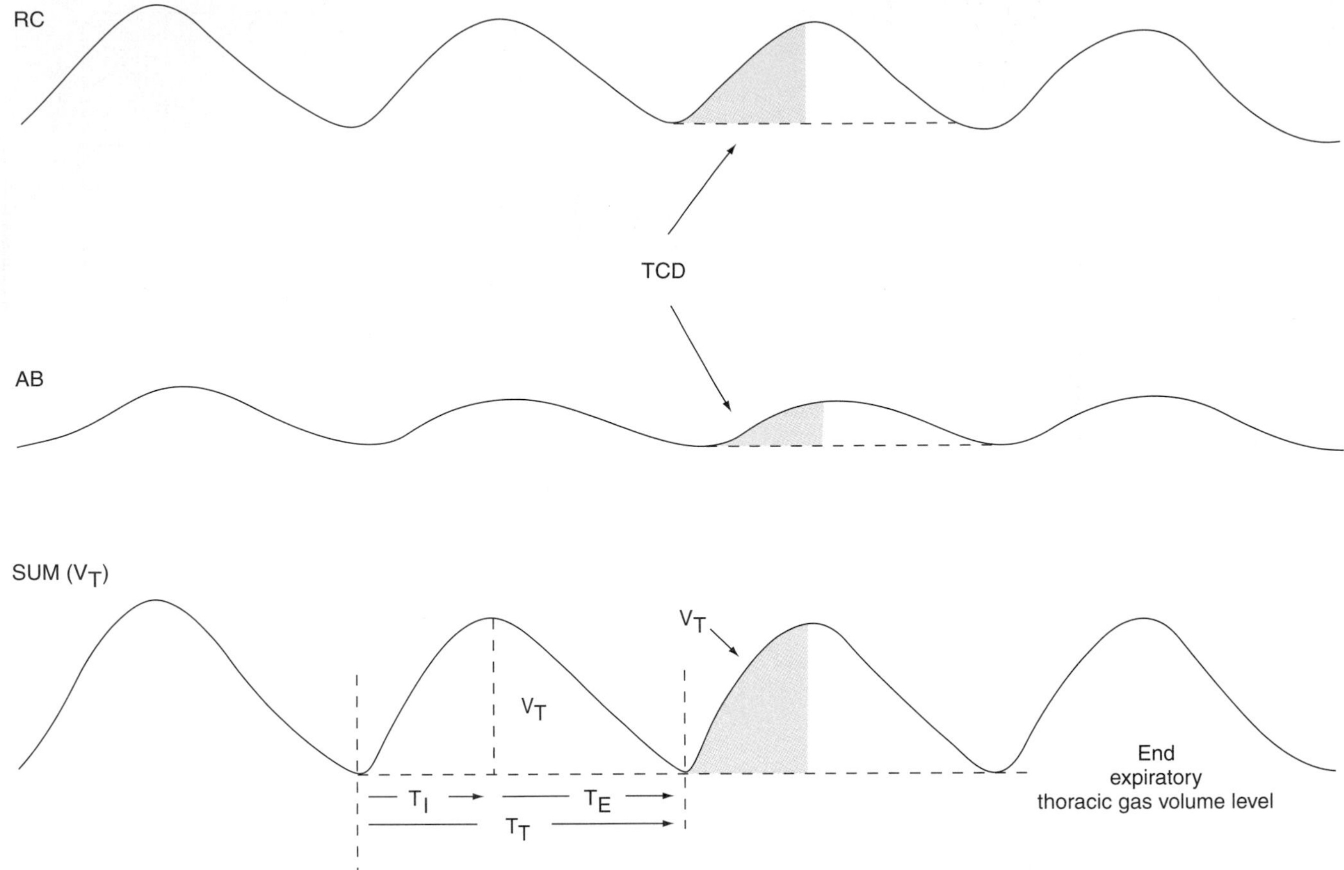

Figure 8-17 Idealized respiratory inductive plethysmography tracing showing ribcage *(RC)*, abdominal *(AB)*, and total compartment displacement *(TCD)*. Note that RC and AB motions are in synchrony. TCD equals the sum of RC and AB. Inspiratory time *(T_I)*, expiratory time *(T_E)*, and total respiratory time *(T_T)* are marked on the TCD tracing. (From Branson R, Campbell RS: Impedance pneumography, apnea monitoring, and respiratory inductive plethysmography. In Kacmarek RM, Hess D, Stoller JK: *Monitoring in respiratory care*, St Louis, 1993, Mosby.)

the rib cage moves outward as the lungs expand in the thorax. Simultaneously, the abdomen is displaced outward by the downward movement of the diaphragm. Because the two compartments are arranged in a series, the sum of the two displacements can be used to calculate the air volume inspired (Figure 8-17).

The respiratory inductive plethysmograph consists of two elastic cloth bands into which insulated polytetrafluoroethylene wire has been sewn in a sinusoidal pattern.[20] One band is placed around the rib cage, and the other is placed around the abdomen. The wires of the two bands are connected to an oscillator, which provides a 20 mV, alternating current voltage at a frequency of 300 kHz. Changes in the cross-sectional diameter of the wire caused by changes in the ribcage or abdominal diameter alter the oscillatory frequencies as a function of changes in self-inductance.[20] The frequency alterations are processed and converted to analog voltages that are then displayed on an oscilloscope or with a pen recorder.

Clinical indices that are most often reported from respiratory inductive plethysmography include tidal volume and respiratory rate. The total compartmental displacement (TCD, or the sum of rib cage plus abdominal movements) can be expressed as TCD/V_T. The percentage of the total displacement (i.e., tidal volume) contributed by ribcage movement is expressed as %RC/V_T.

Respiratory inductive plethysmography has been used extensively in research on respiratory muscle function. It has also been used clinically as a means of monitoring breathing patterns of patients in sleep laboratories, in pulmonary function laboratories, and in intensive care units (ICUs). In the ICU, it has been primarily used to identify uncoordinated thoracoabdominal movements that are associated with respiratory muscle fatigue or failure.[20]

Clinical Applications of Respiratory Mechanics Measurements

Respiratory system mechanics data can provide valuable information about the ventilatory capacity of a patient with cardiopulmonary disease. These data are generally divided into two categories: measured and derived variables. Measured variables include lung volumes and capacities, airflow, and airway and intrapleural pressures. Airway resistance,

Box 8-1 Respiratory Mechanics Measurements

Standard Lung Volumes and Capacities
- Tidal volume (TV or V_T)
- Inspiratory reserve volume (IRV)
- Residual volume (RV)
- Total lung capacity (TLC)
- Vital capacity (VC)
- Functional residual capacity (FRC)
- Inspiratory capacity (IC)

Dynamic Lung Volumes (Flows)
- Forced vital capacity (FVC)
- Forced expiratory volume in 1 second ($FEV_{1.0}$)
- Forced expiratory flow from 25% to 75% of the vital capacity (FEF_{25-75})
- Peak expiratory flow (PEF)

Minute ventilation
- Minute volume (MV, $\dot{V}_E$ or $\dot{V}I$)
- Breathing frequency (f_B)

Respiratory Pressures
- Maximum inspiratory pressure (MIP)
- Maximum expiratory pressure (MEP)
- Peak airway inspiratory pressure (PIP)
- Plateau pressure ($P_{plateau}$)

respiratory system compliance, and work of breathing are derived variables that can be calculated from volume, flow, and pressure measurements.

Box 8-1 contains a list of some of the more common respiratory mechanics measurements that are used by clinicians.

Lung Volumes and Airflow

Laboratory measurements of lung volumes focus on the standard subdivisions shown in Figure 8-18. As was previously stated, simple spirometers can measure three of the four standard lung volumes (i.e., tidal volume [V_T], inspiratory reserve volume [IRV], and expiratory reserve volume [ERV]) and therefore the VC and IC. They can also measure all of the dynamic lung volumes, including FVC, FEV_1, FEF_{25-75}, and peak flows. RV, FRC, and TLC cannot be measured with simple spirometry; they require specialized equipment and procedures, such as body plethysmography and inert gas techniques. Simple spirometry is used as a screening technique, and full lung-volume tests are usually reserved for patients demonstrating abnormal spirometric results.[15] Table 8-3 describes the characteristic lung-volume changes associated with obstructive and restrictive pulmonary disorders; and Clinical Rounds 8-3 presents a case related to lung volume measurements in chronic obstructive pulmonary disease (COPD) patients.

At the bedside, the most commonly measured lung volume is the expired minute volume. In spontaneously breathing patients, the minute volume is usually measured with a hand-held respirometer. For mechanically ventilated patients, minute volume can be measured by attaching a spirometer to the exhalation valve of the ventilator. In most newer ventilators, a flow transducer is incorporated into the system design to give continual updates of tidal and minute volume. (Note that minute volume is calculated based on 5 to 10 breaths and extrapolated to a minute volume value.)

Minute ventilation expresses patient ventilatory needs in liters per minute. It is influenced by the metabolic demands of the tissues and the level of **alveolar ventilation.** For example, elevated minute volumes are associated with increased metabolic rates and/or reductions in effective ventilation (decreased alveolar ventilation or increased **dead space ventilation**).

Monitoring dynamic lung volumes can also alert the clinician to significant changes in a patient's airway resistance. PEF measurements are routinely monitored at the bedside to assess the effectiveness of bronchodilator therapy. These same devices can be used at home by asthmatic patients to monitor daily variations in airway resistance and thus guide therapeutic interventions.[12] (Clinical Practice Guideline 8-1 summarizes the AARC Clinical Practice Guideline for assessing response to bronchodilator at point of care.)

Airflow measurements during mechanical ventilation can signal changes in the resistance and compliance of the patient-ventilator system. For example, high-frequency ripples on the inspiratory flow tracing can indicate turbulent flow caused by secretions in the airway or water in the ventilator circuit.[21] Expiratory flow limitations should be suspected if the decay in expiratory flow is linear instead of exponential.[15]

Airway Pressures

The most common airway pressure measurements made on spontaneously breathing patients are the maximum inspiratory and expiratory pressures (MIP and MEP), **peak inspiratory pressure (PIP),** and static, or **plateau pressure ($P_{plateau}$).**

MIP is obtained by measuring the maximum sustained pressure that patients achieve while making a forceful inspiration starting at the residual volume. The MEP is recorded while the patient makes a forceful effort starting at TLC. MIP and MEP are easily obtained from spontaneously breathing patients with an apparatus such as the one in Figure 8-12. MIP is normally –60 to –100 cm H_2O, and MEP is +80 to +100 cm H_2O.

PIP is the maximum inspiratory pressure generated during a tidal breath. PIP is influenced by the gas flow into the patient's lungs and by the resistance and compliance of the patient's lungs and chest wall. The static or plateau pressure represents the amount of pressure required to maintain the tidal volume within the patient's lungs during a period of no gas flow. It is determined by the compliance of the lungs and chest wall.[21,22]

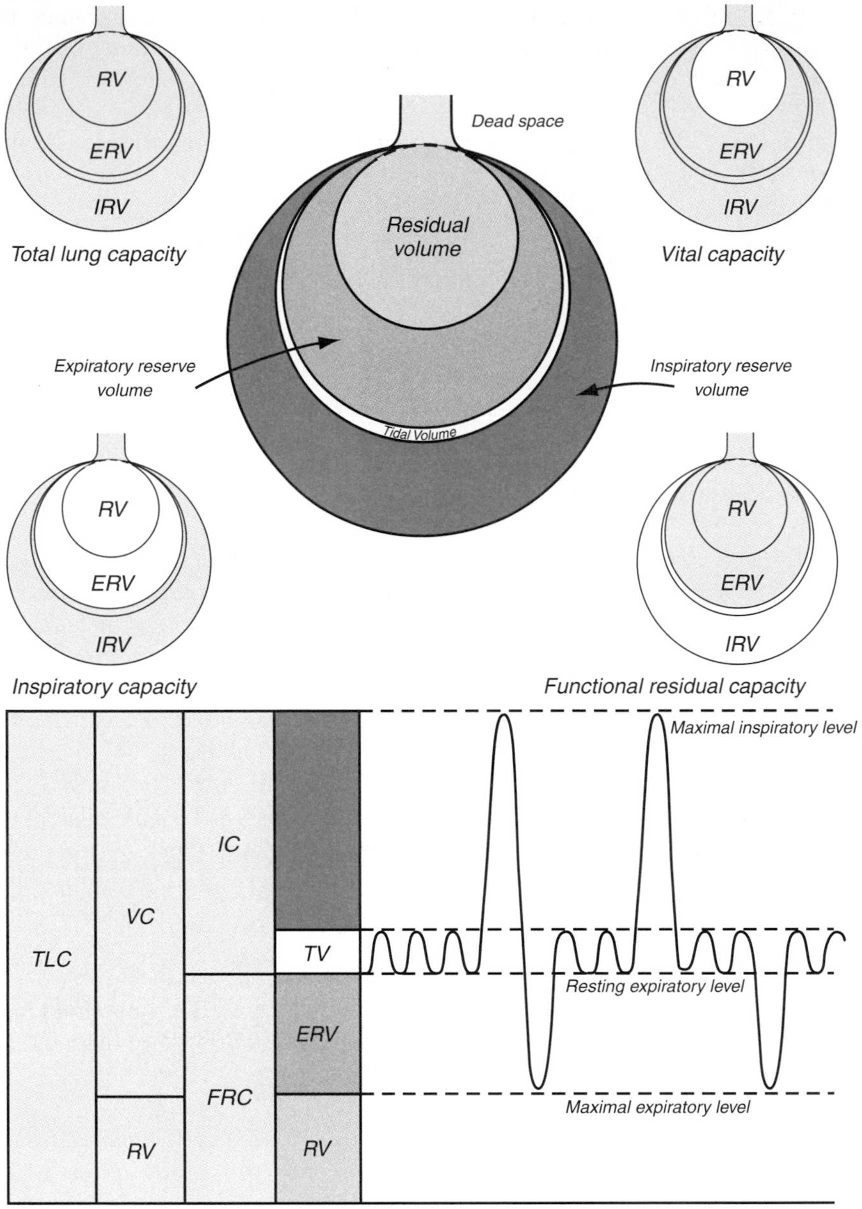

Figure 8-18 Standard lung volumes and capacities. (From Comroe J: *The lung*, ed 3, Chicago, 1986, Mosby.)

Table 8-3 Static and dynamic lung volume changes associated with obstructive and restrictive pulmonary diseases

	Obstructive Pulmonary Disease	Restrictive Pulmonary Disease
TLC	Increased	Decreased
FRC	Increased	Normal or decreased
VC	Normal or decreased	Decreased
$FEV_{1.0}$	Decreased	Decreased
$FEV_{1.0}/VC$	Decreased	Normal
FEF_{25-75}	Decreased	Normal
MVV	Decreased	Decreased in severe disease

PIP and $P_{plateau}$ are measured during mechanical ventilation. Instantaneous PIP can be measured with an aneroid manometer that is incorporated into the ventilator (see Chapter 11). PIP can be derived from continuous recordings of airway pressure that can be made during the breathing cycle using a strain-gauge transducer. $P_{plateau}$ is measured during mechanical ventilation by occluding the expiratory valve of the ventilator at the end of a tidal inspiration and noting the new pressure level. Most newer ventilators have a manual control incorporated into the ventilator circuit that operates an inflation-hold shutter valve that closes at the end of inspiration.[21,22]

Figure 8-19 is a tracing that shows the measurement of PIP and $P_{plateau}$. Note that PIP is greater than $P_{plateau}$, but remember that PIP is a dynamic measurement and $P_{plateau}$ is measured under static conditions. The PIP represents the total force that must be applied to overcome the elastic and frictional forces offered by the patient-ventilator system, whereas $P_{plateau}$ represents that portion of the total pressure required to overcome only elastic forces.

Increases in the elastance of the respiratory system (i.e., decreases in compliance of the lung or chest wall) increase both PIP and $P_{plateau}$. Elevated airway resistance increases peak airway pressure but does not affect $P_{plateau}$.

Airway Resistance

Airway resistance is the opposition to airflow from nonelastic forces of the lung. It can be calculated by subtracting $P_{plateau}$

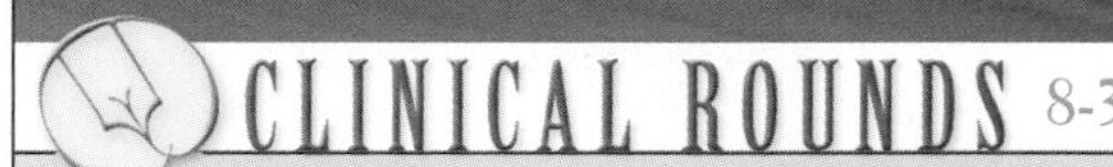

The following lung volume measurements were obtained from a 65-year-old man whose chief complaint is shortness of breath on exertion, which has increased significantly during the past year. He has a 40-pack-per-year history of cigarette smoking (i.e., he smoked 2 packs of cigarettes per day for 20 years). FVC is 60% of predicted, FEV_1 is 50% of predicted, FEF_{25-75} is 40% of predicted, $FEV_{1.0}$/VC is 60% of predicted, RV is 140% of predicted, and FRC is 150% of predicted. Interpret these results.

See Appendix A for the answer.

Clinical Practice Guidelines 8-1

Assessing Response to Bronchodilator Therapy at Point of Care

Indications:

1. To confirm appropriateness of therapy.
2. To individualize patient's dose per treatment or frequency of administration.
3. To help determine patient status during acute and long-term pharmacological therapy.
4. To determine a need for change of therapy.

Contraindications:

In cases of acute severe distress, some assessment maneuvers may be contraindicated or should be postponed until therapy and supportive measures have been instituted.

Hazards/Complications

Forced exhalations may be associated with bronchoconstriction, airway collapse, and paroxysmal coughing with or without syncope.

Limitations of Methodology

1. Cost and accessibility.
2. Patient inability to perform FVC or PEF maneuvers.
3. Accuracy and reproducibility of peak flow meters vary among models and units, so results from the same device should be compared for consistency and accuracy.
4. The measurement of peak flows is an effort-dependent test. The patient should be encouraged to perform the maneuver vigorously. Three trials are desirable; report the best of the three peak flows measured.
5. An artificial airway will increase resistance and may limit inspiratory and expiratory flows.

Resources

1. Equipment may include portable laboratory spirometer, peak flow meter, stethoscope, and pulse oximeter. Spirometers and peak flow meters should adhere to ATS standards.
2. Personnel performing the tests should be licensed or credentialed respiratory care practitioners or people with equivalent knowledge.
3. The patient or family caregiver providing maintenance therapy must demonstrate an ability to monitor and measure response to bronchodilator, use proper technique for administering medication and using the devices, modify doses and frequency as prescribed and instructed in response to adverse reactions or increased severity of symptoms, and appropriately communicate the severity of symptoms to the physician.

Monitoring

The following observations will assist the clinician in assessing the response to bronchodilator therapy.

1. Patient's general appearance, use of accessory muscles, and sputum volume and consistency.
2. Patient's vital signs and measurement of FVC, FEV1, PEF, and pulse oximetry.
3. In ventilator patients, PIP, $P_{plateau}$, increased inspiratory/expiratory flows (F-V loops), and decreased autoPEEP.

For a copy of the complete text, see *Resp Care* 40(12):1300, 1995.

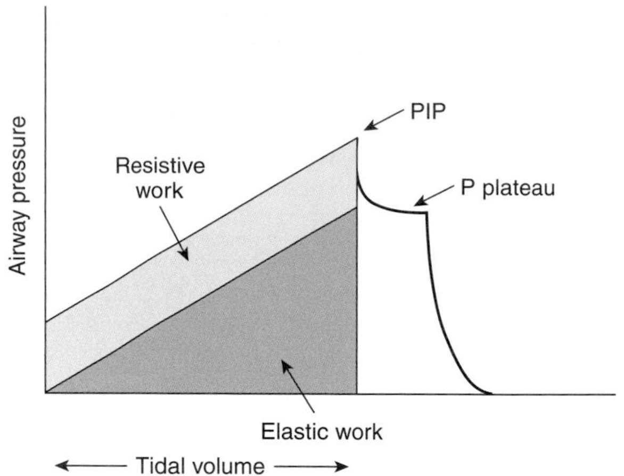

Figure 8-19 Airway pressure tracing showing peak airway pressure and plateau pressure. (From Pilbeam SP: *Mechanical ventilation*, ed 3, St Louis, 1998, Mosby.)

from PIP and dividing the resultant pressure by the airflow. Airway resistance averages 2 to 5 cm H_2O/L/sec. It is primarily determined by the caliber of the airway (according to Poiseuille's law, a twofold decrease in airway diameter results in a sixteenfold increase in airway resistance). Thus retention of secretions, peribronchiolar edema, and bronchoconstriction associated with asthma result in increased airway resistance. Smoke inhalation can also cause severe bronchoconstriction. Conversely, bronchodilation causes a reduction in airway resistance, such as occurs after the administration of a bronchodilator (see Clinical Practice Guideline 8-1).

Respiratory System Compliance

Respiratory system compliance can be simply defined as the distensibility of the lungs and chest wall. Lung-thorax compliance can be determined by dividing the tidal volume by $P_{plateau}$. The normal compliance of the respiratory system averages 0.1 L/cm H_2O.

Pathologic conditions (e.g., pulmonary interstitial fibrosis, atelectasis, and pulmonary vascular engorgement) decrease the compliance of the pulmonary parenchyma, resulting in increases in both $P_{plateau}$ and PIP (i.e., decreasing lung compliance). Conditions such as kyphoscoliosis and myasthenia gravis increase PIP and $P_{plateau}$ by reducing chest wall compliance.[22]

Work of Breathing

In normal healthy individuals, work of breathing only constitutes about 2% to 5% of total oxygen consumption, but this value can rise sharply with a pathologic pulmonary condition. Therefore increases in airway resistance or decreases in respiratory system compliance can lead to considerable increases in work of breathing, and thus oxygen consumption.

Although there is considerable interest in using work of breathing measurements in clinical practice, the technique is somewhat difficult to master and limited in use. Its most practical uses have been in establishing optimum levels of pressure-support ventilation and determining the work of breathing for various forms of ventilatory support.

Table 8-4 summarizes the lung mechanics measurements used to assess patients receiving ventilatory support.

Measurement of Inspired Oxygen

Oxygen Analyzers

Two types of analyzers are generally used for measuring the oxygen concentration in inspired gases: (1) **electrochemical** analyzers (including **polarographic** and galvanic devices), and (2) electric analyzers. A brief discussion of paramagnetic analyzers is included for historical purposes. See Historical Note 8-1.

Electrochemical Analyzers

These are the most commonly used oxygen analyzers. They are generally classified as galvanic or polarographic devices.

Galvanic analyzers use an oxygen-mediated chemical reaction to generate an electrical current. As shown in Figure 8-20, A, a gold cathode and a lead anode are immersed in a potassium hydroxide bath. The gas sample to be analyzed is separated from the bath by a semipermeable membrane that is usually made of polytetrafluoroethylene (Teflon). As oxygen diffuses across the membrane into the hydroxide solution, it reacts with water and free electrons from the gold cathode to form hydroxyl ions (OH^-). The OH^- ions diffuse toward the lead (Pb) anode, forming lead oxide (PbO_2), water, and free electrons. The flow of the electrons produces a current that can be measured with an ammeter, and the amount of current flow detected is directly related to oxygen concentration. (Note that galvanic oxygen analyzers do not have to be "turned on." They continually read 21% oxygen when the sensor is exposed to room air, so it is important to keep the sensor capped to prolong its life.)

Polarographic analyzers also use an oxygen-mediated chemical reaction to create current flow, but they differ slightly in design from galvanic type of devices (see Figure 8-20, *B*). Polarographic analyzers contain a platinum cathode and a silver anode immersed in a potassium hydroxide bath. Additionally, they typically use a 9 V battery to polarize the silver anode, resulting in an improved response time because the OH^- ions are attracted to the difference in electrical charge. The reaction formula is basically similar to that of galvanic analyzers, but the reaction time is faster.

Galvanic and polarographic analyzers can be used for intermittent or continuous monitoring of fractional inspired oxygen (F_IO_2) and can be used with flammable gases during anesthesia. Because they respond to changes in partial pressure, readings can be affected by changes in ambient pressure, as may occur during mechanical ventilation or at high altitudes. Although galvanic analyzers have a slower response time than that of polarographic analyzers, they do

Table 8-4 Measurements of lung mechanics used to assess ventilatory function in mechanically ventilated patients

Variable	Description	Measuring Technique
Effective compliance (C_{eff})	The reciprocal of the elastic property of the patient-ventilator system (mL/cm H_2O)	Mandatory (i.e., passive inspiration expiration) breath (V_T); end-inspiratory pause of at least 1 sec ($P_{plateau}$); corrected for tubing compression. Calculation: $C_{eff} = V_T/(P_{plateau} - \text{total PEEP})$.
Inspiratory resistance	Inspiratory resistive component of patient-ventilator system impedance (cm $H_2O \times sec \times L^{-1}$)	Mandatory (i.e., passive inspiration and expiration) breath (V_T) with fixed constant flow over fixed time (T_i); end-inspiratory pause as described for C_{eff}. Calculation: $R_I = \frac{P_{peak} - P_{plateau}}{V_T/T_i}$
Expiratory resistance	Expiratory resistive component of the patient-ventilator system (cm $H_2O \times sec \times L^{-1}$)	Mandatory (i.e., passive inspiration and expiration) breath (VT); end-inspiratory pause as described for C_{eff}. Calculation: $R_E = \frac{P_{plateau} - \text{total } PEEP_{tot}}{\text{Flow at onset of exhalation}}$
Mean airway pressure	Average airway pressure over a respiratory cycle	Mean airway pressure should be reported over a time period that includes a representative number of machine- and patient-cycled breaths.
Negative inspiratory force (NIF)	Maximal negative inspiratory pressure generated by patient, against closed circuit	One-way valve allowing expiration; expiratory hold of 15 to 20 seconds.
Intrinsic positive end-expiratory pressure (auto-PEEP)	Positive end-expiratory alveolar pressure resulting from inadequate expiratory time, dynamic airway collapse, or both	Auto-PEEP measurement is clinically important but may be difficult during spontaneous or assisted breathing. It is recommended that the ventilator be equipped with an expiratory hold control to facilitate manual determination of auto-PEEP by airway occlusion as close to the proximal airway as possible; circuit pressures should stabilize during the expiratory hold. Measurement reflects total PEEP but tends to underestimate the intrinsic component because of pressure equilibration in compliant circuitry.

From MacIntyre NR, Gropper C: Monitoring ventilatory function II: respiratory system mechanics and muscle function. In Levine RL, Fromm RE, editors: *Critical care monitoring: from prehospital to ICU*, St Louis, 1995, Mosby.

not require an external power supply, and their electrodes may last longer.

Commercially available galvanic analyzers are available from Teledyne, Hudson, Biomarine, and Ohmeda. Polarographic oxygen analyzers are available from SensorMedics/Viasys Healthcare, Hudson-Ventronics, IL, IMI, Teledyne, and Critikon.

Electrical Analyzers

These analyzers operate on the principle of thermal conductivity and use an electronic device called a Wheatstone bridge. Figure 8-21 shows how these devices operate. Two parallel wires receive current flow from an external power source, usually a battery. One of these wires, which serves as the reference, is exposed to room air. The other wire is located in the sample chamber and is exposed to the gas being analyzed. If the sample gas contains a higher oxygen:nitrogen ratio than room air, the sample wire cools, and its resistance decreases because oxygen is a better conductor of heat than is nitrogen. Consequently, current flow increases through the sample wire when compared with the reference wire. An ammeter detects the change in current flow and relates it to oxygen concentration.

The primary advantage of using an electrical analyzer is that it compares the oxygen concentration of an unknown gas with ambient air. Therefore it is responsive to changes in the percent of oxygen instead of partial pressure, and it is unaffected by changes in pressure (e.g., those that occur with altitude changes). Several problems can occur when using these devices. For example, the Wheatstone bridge can generate significant amounts of heat and therefore is dangerous to use in the presence of flammable gases. Also, because contaminant gases can dissipate heat at different rates than oxygen and nitrogen, if gases other than oxygen and nitrogen are present, it can lead to erroneous F_IO_2 levels.

Measurement of Nitrogen Oxides

As discussed in Chapter 3, nitric oxide (NO) is a simple, diatomic molecule that can cause vasodilation, macrophage cytotoxicity, and platelet adhesion.[24] It has been used to successfully treat pulmonary hypertension

HISTORICAL NOTE 8-1
Paramagnetic Oxygen Analyzers

The paramagnetic oxygen analyzer was first described by Pauling, Wood, and Sturdivant[23] in 1946 and relies on the fact that oxygen is a paramagnetic gas and the other respired gases (e.g., nitrogen and carbon dioxide) are diamagnetic. Thus the paramagnetic oxygen molecules align themselves with the strongest part of a heterogenous magnetic field. The diamagnetic nitrogen and carbon dioxide molecules are repelled by the magnetic field, so they tend to be found in the weaker part of a magnetic field.

The Beckman D-2 oxygen analyzer is an example of a device that uses the physical principle of paramagnetism to measure oxygen concentration. With this device, a glass dumbbell filled with nitrogen is suspended on a quartz string and held in place by two magnets. The dumbbell and the magnets are enclosed within a sample chamber. When oxygen is introduced into this chamber, it is attracted to the magnetic field, which causes the dumbbell to rotate slightly. The amount of rotation depends on the concentration of the oxygen introduced into the chamber. The oxygen concentration can be measured because a mirror attached to the dumbbell reflects a light focused on it onto a translucent scale. The scale is calibrated to display both partial pressures (in mm Hg) and the percent of oxygen concentration.

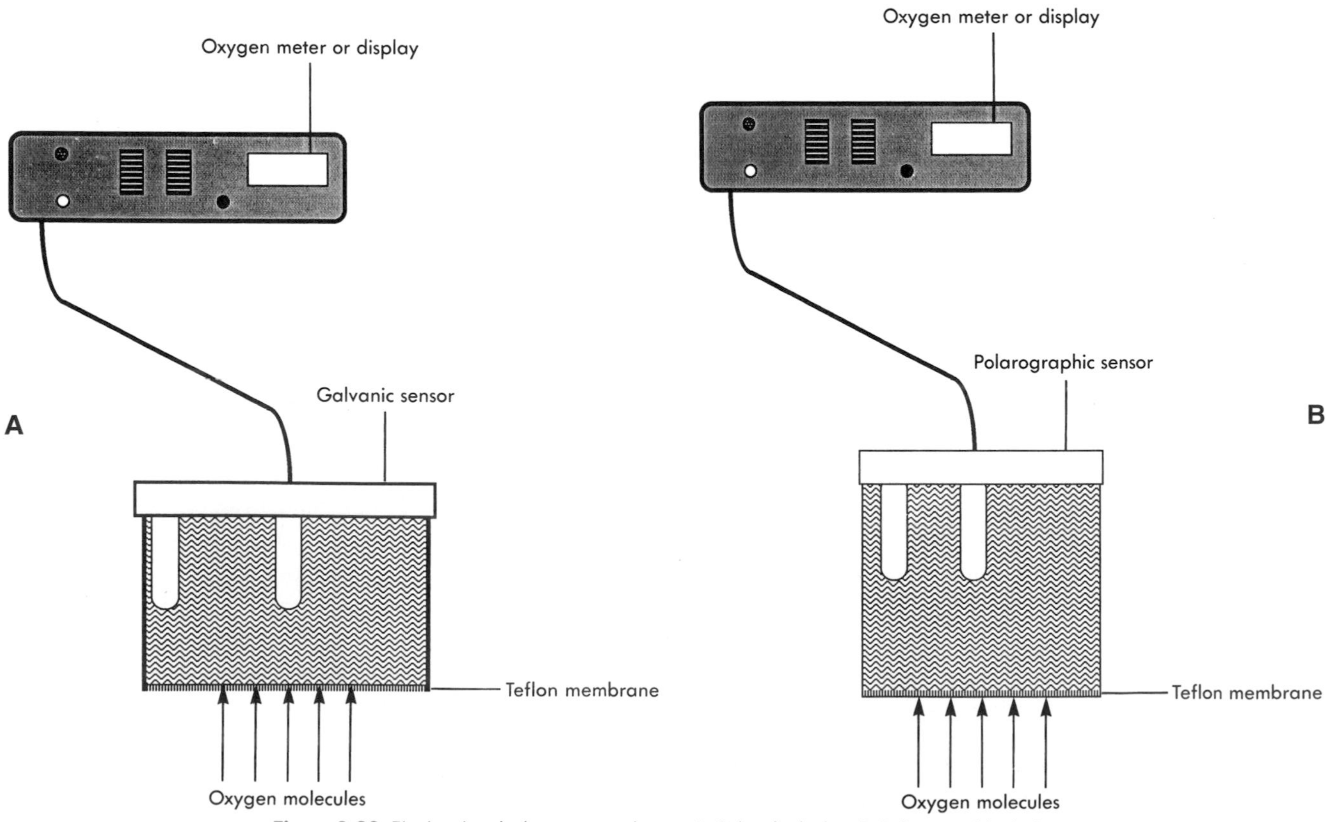

Figure 8-20 Electrochemical oxygen analyzers. **A,** Galvanic device. **B,** Polarographic device.

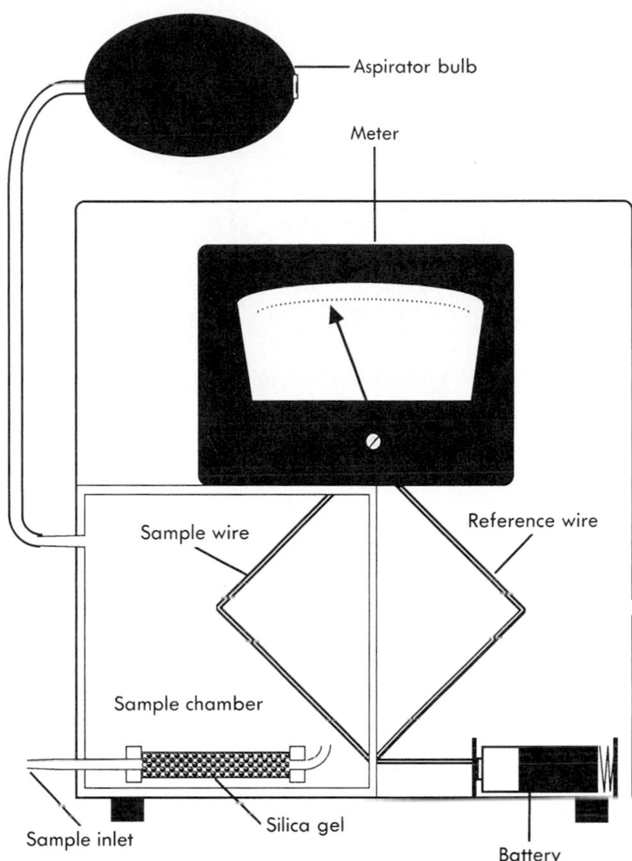

Figure 8-21 Electrical oxygen analyzer showing Wheatstone bridge circuit.

in neonates and to improve gas exchange in critically ill patients.[25,26]

Because of the potential for pulmonary toxicity induced by high levels of NO and nitrogen dioxide (NO_2), it is important to monitor the concentration of these molecules when nitric oxide is used clinically. Body and Hartigan[26] have recently written an excellent review of nitrogen oxide measurement. Two types of monitoring systems are routinely used when administering nitric oxide: **chemiluminescence monitoring** and **electrochemical monitoring.**[26] A brief discussion of each follows.

Chemiluminescence Monitoring

Chemiluminescence monitoring involves the quantification of gas-specific photoemission.[24] Gases sampled by the chemiluminescence monitor react with ozone (O_3) to produce nitrogen dioxide with an electron in an unstable excited state (NO_2^*). Because this unstable molecule decays to its lower energy (ground) state, photons are emitted with energies in the 600 to 3000 nanometer (nm) wavelength range.[24] Photon emissions are measured by photomultiplier tubes and electronically converted into a displayable signal.

Nitrogen dioxide levels can be measured indirectly by converting NO_2 to NO with a catalytic or chemical converter, and then measuring the NO concentration as described previously.[26] Thermal catalytic converters, which are made of stainless steel, operate at temperatures of 600° to 800° C.[24] Chemical converters rely on molybdenum and carbon to convert NO_2 to NO. Although chemical converters must be periodically replenished, they can be used at lower temperatures and are more stable than catalytic converters. They are also less affected by interference from other gases.

The NO_2 concentration is determined by measuring the total concentration of nitrogen oxides and subtracting the NO concentration. Figure 8-22 contains schematics of two different types of commercially available chemiluminescence nitrogen oxide monitors. In A, one reaction chamber is used to measure NO and NO_2. This system operates on the principle that the NO_2 converter is switched into the sample line at 10- to 30-second intervals. *B* shows a system that uses two separate chambers for measuring NO and NO_2, with a single photomultiplier tube for measuring the outputs from both chambers.

The accuracy of a chemiluminescence monitor can be altered either by variations in the sample gas composition or by interference with the operation of the photomultiplier tubes. Variations in the composition of the sample gas can result from **quenching** of excited states of nitrogen dioxide, false identification of contaminant gases, such as NO_2, and alterations in the viscosity of the sample gas by background gases. Quenching occurs when NO_2 is converted to ground state NO_2 by inadvertent collisions of the former gases with other background gases like oxygen, carbon dioxide, and water.[24] **Ammonia** (NH_2) and N_2O are two gases that can be falsely identified as NO_2. Increases in the viscosity of the sample gas (such as can occur with high percentages of oxygen) decrease the gas flow into the reaction chamber, thus reducing the number of NO molecules entering the chamber. Inaccuracies caused by photomultiplier tube interference are generally associated with photon emissions from contaminating gases in the sample reaction chamber and with thermal fluctuations.

Electrochemical Monitoring

This technique is based on a principle similar to that used with polarographic (Clark) electrodes. That is, gases diffusing across a semipermeable membrane react with an electrolyte solution, generating a current flow between two polarized electrodes as electrons are liberated or consumed.[24]

Figure 8-23 shows an example of an electrochemical NO analyzer. It consists of three electrodes (a sensing electrode, a counter electrode, and a reference electrode) immersed in an electrolyte solution that contains a highly conductive concentrated acid or alkali solution. The electrodes are separated from the gas sample to be analyzed by a semipermeable membrane. NO and NO_2 from the unknown gas sample diffuse across a semipermeable membrane and react with the electrolyte solution near the sensing electrode, generating electrons in the following oxidation reaction:

$$NO + 2H_2O \rightarrow HNO_3 + 3H^+ + 3e^-.$$

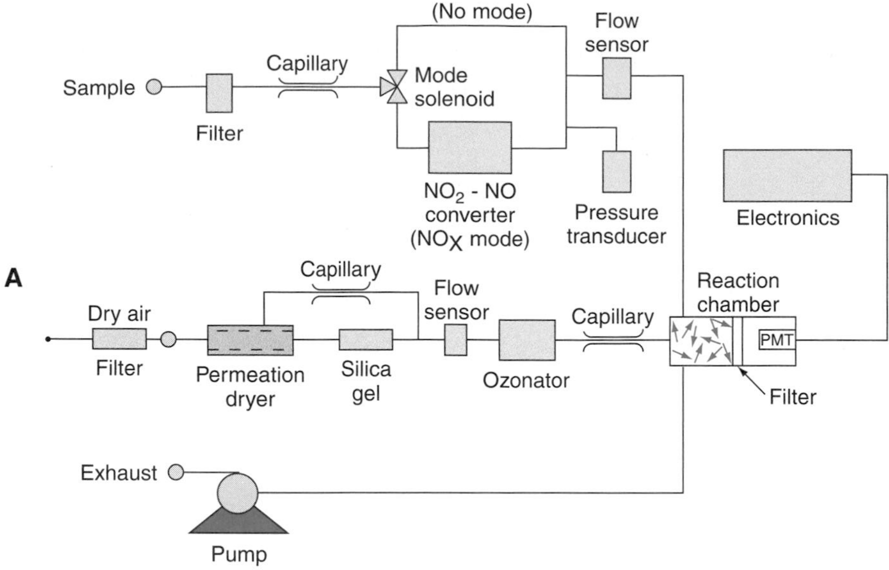

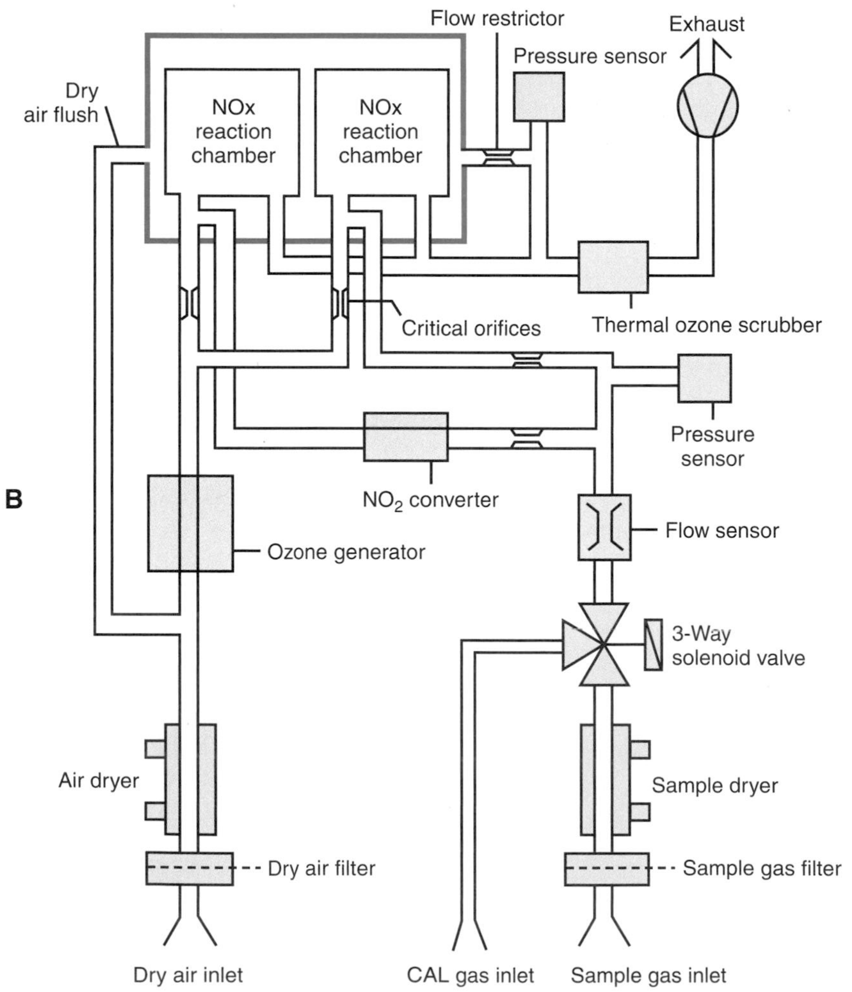

Figure 8-22 Schematic illustrating two types of chemiluminescence nitrogen oxide monitors. **A,** A single-reaction chamber chemiluminescence device; **B,** a dual-reaction chamber chemiluminescence device. (From Body S, et al: Nitric oxide: delivery, measurement, and clinical application, *J Cardiothoracic Vasc Anesth* 9(6):748, 1995.)

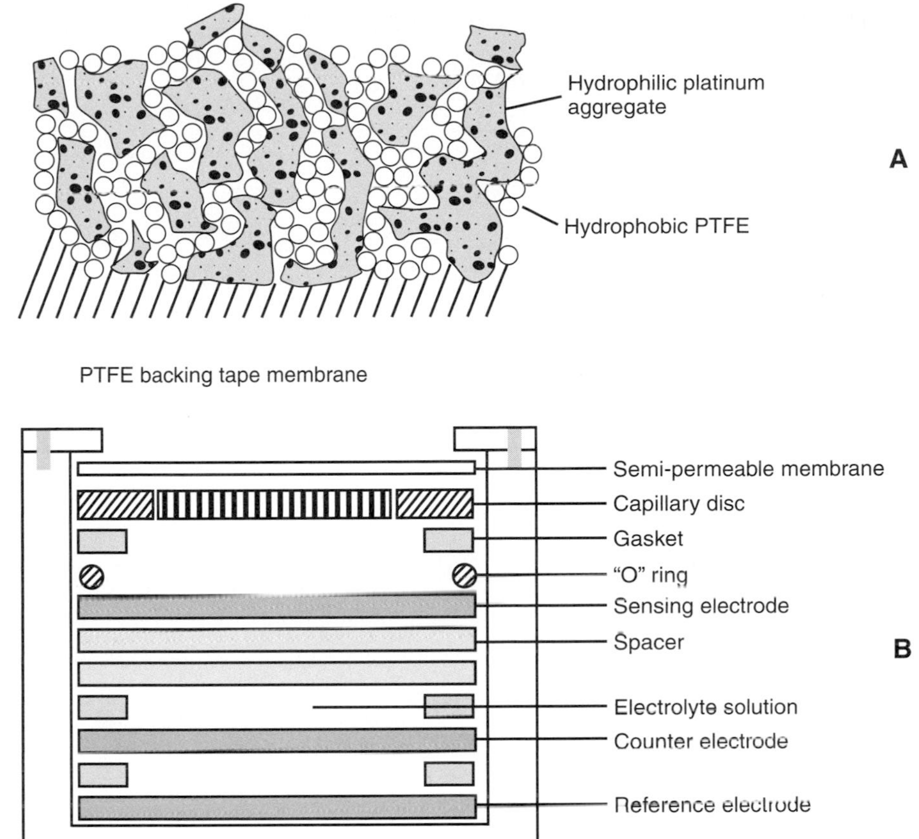

Figure 8-23 Schematic of an electrochemical nitrogen oxide monitor. (From Body S, et al: Nitric oxide: delivery, measurement, and clinical application, *J Cardiothoracic Vasc Anesth* 9(6):748, 1995.)

Box 8-2 Proposed FDA Standards for Nitric Oxide and Nitrogen Dioxide Monitoring Devices

Monitoring Range

1 ppm NO lower limit. No upper limit specified.

1 to 5 ppm NO_2.

Accuracy*

≤20 ppm NO; ±20% of NO concentration, or 0.5 ppm—whichever is greater.

>20 ppm NO; ±10% of NO concentration.

NO_2; ±20% of NO_2 concentration.

Response Time

10% to 90% of full signal response time <30 seconds.

Alarms

Audible and visual alarms: for NO, an upper level alarm able to be sent from 2 ppm NO to maximum signal; for NO_2, an upper level alarm able to be sent from 2 ppm NO_2 to maximum signal.

Other Considerations

Electrical safety (IEC601-1)

Electromagnetic compatibility and immunity (IEC601-1-2)

Environmental protection (temperature, humidity, and spill resistance)

Environmental pollution

Software safety (IEC601-1-4)

From Body SC, Hartigan PM: Manufacture and measurement of nitrogen oxides. In Hess D, Hurford WE, editors: Inhaled nitric oxide I, *Respir Care Clin North Am* 3(3):414, 1997.

*The stated accuracy must be present in the following background gases: 0 and 5 ppm NO_2 (for NO monitoring); 0, 10, and 40 ppm NO (for NO_2 monitoring); 21%, 60%, and 95% oxygen and 0%, 50%, and 100% relative humidity. If the monitoring device is placed within the ventilator circuit and subject to lung inflation pressures, the accuracy must be maintained over a pressure range of $^{-}15$ to $^{+}100$ cm H_2O.

Table 8-5 Comparison of chemiluminescence and electrochemical monitoring devices

Factor	Electrochemical	Chemiluminescence
Cost	$2500-$5800	$11,00-23,000
Ease of use	+ + +	+
Ease of servicing	+ + +	+
Ease of setup	+ + +	+
Accuracy	+	+ + +
Response time	10-30 seconds	0.15-20 seconds
Measurement range	+ +	+ + +
Size	+ + +	+
O_2% correction required	No	Yes
Ozone production	No	Yes

Modified from Body S et al: Nitric oxide: delivery, measurement, and clinical application, *J Cardiothorac Vasc Anesth* 9(6):748, 1995.

The electrons generated are consumed at the counter electrode through the reduction of oxygen, or:

$$O_2 + 4H^+ + 4e^- \rightarrow 2H_2O.$$

Balancing the equations at both electrodes yields the following equation,

$$4NO + 2H_2O + 3O_2 \rightarrow 4HNO_3.$$

NO_2 can be measured by electrochemical analysis using a similar principle. In this series of reactions, NO_2 is reduced to NO at the sensing electrode, and H_2O is oxidized at the counter electrode, or:

$$NO_2 + 2H^+ + 2e^- \rightarrow NO + H_2O$$
$$2H_2O \rightarrow 4H^+ + 4e^- + O_2.$$

The accuracy of NO/NO_2 electrochemical monitors can be altered by increases in ambient pressure (as occur with positive-pressure ventilation) and also by the presence of background gases, such as CO_2, CO, and NH_2, that have lower oxidation potentials than the sensor potential. The accuracy of these electrochemical monitors is also limited in the clinical setting for NO concentrations less than 0.1 ppm.[27]

Box 8-2 lists the Food and Drug Administration (FDA) standards for NO and NO_2 monitoring devices. Table 8-5 shows a comparison of chemiluminescence and electrochemical nitrogen oxide analyzers.

Capnography (Capnometry)

Capnography, or capnometry, is the continuous measurement of carbon dioxide concentrations at the airway opening during respiration. The term capnography is used to describe the technique in which carbon dioxide concentration is displayed as a graphic waveform called a **capnogram;** capnometry is the technique in which carbon dioxide concentration is displayed as a numeric reading.[28] In both cases, the carbon dioxide concentration can be displayed in millimeters of mercury (i.e., mm Hg), representing the partial pressure, or as a percentage of carbon dioxide.[28]

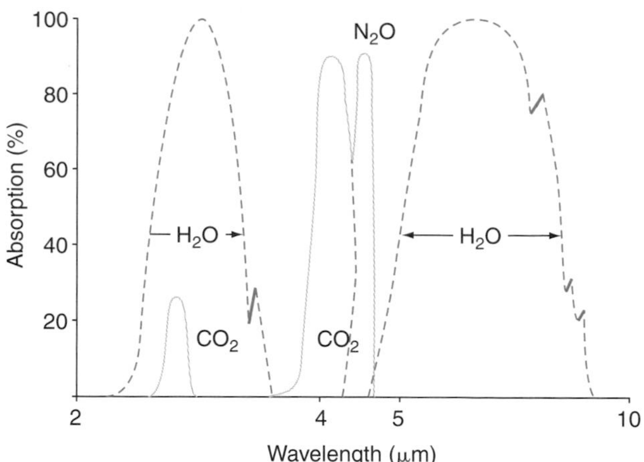

Figure 8-24 Infrared absorption spectra for carbon dioxide, nitrous oxide, and water. (From Hess D: Capnometry and capnography: technical aspects, physiologic aspects, and clinical applications, *Respir Care* 35:558, 1990.)

Several methods are used to measure carbon dioxide, including infrared (IR) spectroscopy, mass spectroscopy, and Raman spectroscopy. IR and Raman spectrometers are portable devices used by individual patients. Mass spectrometers are shared devices that can sample gases from 10 to 12 patients. IR spectroscopy is currently the method of choice in critical-care settings, and mass spectroscopy is most often used in surgical suites. The use of Raman spectroscopy for capnography is limited.

Infrared Spectroscopy

IR spectroscopy is based on the principle that molecules containing more than one element absorb IR light in a characteristic manner.[29] Normally, carbon dioxide maximally absorbs infrared radiation at 4.26 μm. The carbon dioxide concentration of a gas sample can be estimated because the amount of carbon dioxide in a gas sample is directly related to the amount of infrared light absorbed.[30]

As Figure 8-24 shows, the peak carbon dioxide absorption is very close to the absorption peaks for water and nitrous oxide. Thus if water or nitrous oxide are present, the carbon dioxide readings during IR monitoring can be erroneous. The effects of water vapor can be eliminated by passing the gas sample through an absorbent (i.e., drying the sample) before it is analyzed. Nitrous oxide artifacts can be removed with filters or by using correction factors.[31]

Figure 8-25 shows two types of infrared capnographs: A is a single-beam, negative filter device, and B is a double-beam, positive filter capnograph. With the single-beam

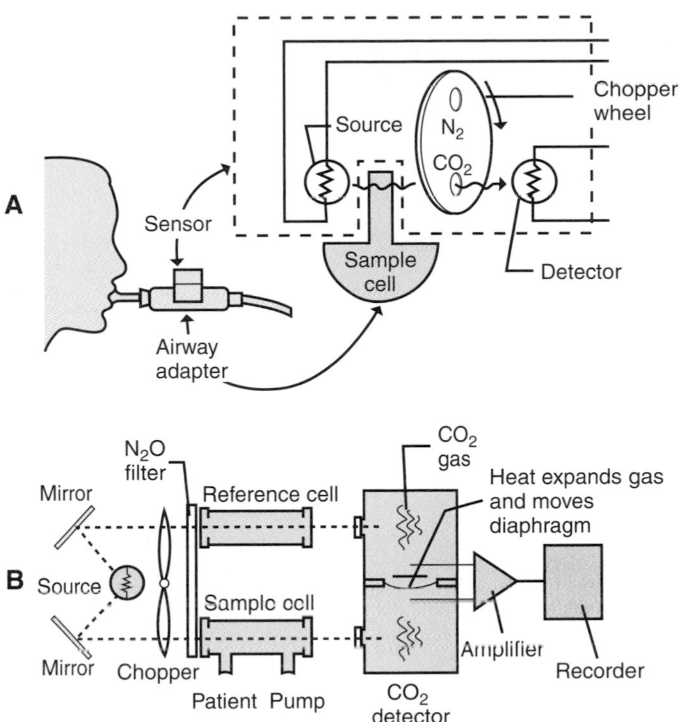

Figure 8-25 **A,** Single-beam nondispersive infrared capnograph; **B,** double-beam, nondispersive infrared capnograph. (Redrawn from Gravenstein JS, Paulus DA, Hayes TJ: *Capnography in clinical practice*, Boston, 1989, Butterworth.)

device, the sample gas is directed to a sample chamber that lies between the IR radiation source and a detection chamber. A chopper blade with two transparent cells (one containing carbon dioxide and the other containing nitrogen) is positioned between the sample chamber and the detector. Gas passing through the sample must pass through the circulating chopper cells before reaching the detection chamber. As the blade turns, two signals are generated, the ratio of which is detected and used to calculate the carbon dioxide concentration.

In the double-beam type of analyzer, gas is drawn into a sample chamber that contains a cuvette made of sodium chloride and sodium bromide.[29] IR radiation is beamed through the cuvette containing the sample of gas to be analyzed and through a reference chamber containing gas free of carbon dioxide. The carbon dioxide in the sample chamber absorbs some of the radiation, therefore decreasing the amount of radiation reaching the detector. The difference between the radiation transmitted through the sample cell and the radiation transmitted through the reference causes a diaphragm within the detector chamber to move. This diaphragm movement is converted into an electrical signal that is amplified and displayed in millimeters of mercury, representing the partial pressure or a percentage of carbon dioxide.[33]

Clinicians generally classify infrared analyzers by the method used to sample gases at the airway. Figure 8-26 shows a sidestream and a mainstream device. With the sidestream devices, the gas to be analyzed is aspirated from the airway at a flow rate of approximately 500 mL/min through a narrow bore polyethylene tube and transferred to the sample chamber, which is located in a separate console. With mainstream devices, analysis is performed at the airway, and gas passes into the sampling chamber that is attached directly to the endotracheal tube (ET).

Although sidestream devices are quite reliable, they show a slight delay between sampling and reporting times because of the time required to transport the sample from the airway to the sample chamber. Consequently, these devices may not be appropriate for patients breathing at high rates (e.g., neonates). The plastic tube that transports sample gas from the airway to the analyzer is prone to plugging by water and secretions, and therefore can lead to erroneous readings. Contamination with ambient air from leaks in the sample line is also a concern. Clinical Rounds 8-4 illustrates a common problem that occurs with **sidestream capnographs.**

Mainstream devices do not show a delay between sampling and reporting times because the analyzer is attached directly to the ET. However, these devices add dead space to the airway, which must be quantified to prevent erroneous readings of the partial pressure of carbon dioxide. The additional weight placed on the artificial airway by this type of analyzer increases the possibility of dislodgment or complete extubation. It should also be recognized that because this type of analyzer is directly attached to the airway, it is subject to damage from mishandling (i.e., dropping the device on the floor).

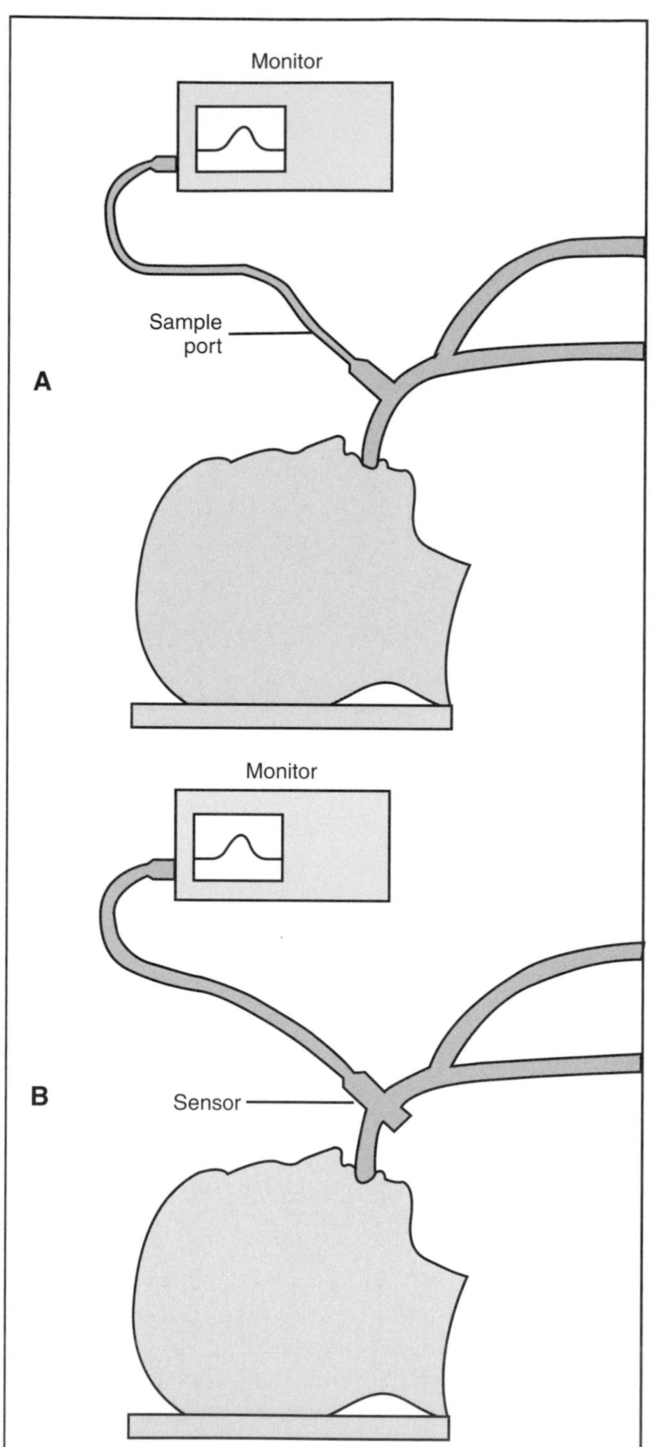

Figure 8-26 Capnographs can be classified by sampling technique. **A,** Sidestream capnograph: exhaled gas is extracted through small-bore tubing and transported to a console containing the infrared sensor; **B,** mainstream capnograph: exhaled gas in measured at the airway.

Mass Spectroscopy

Mass spectroscopy is based on the principle that a gas molecules can be identified by their mass:charge ratio when they are passed through a magnetic field. Figure 8-27 is a schematic that shows this principle. The gas to be analyzed is aspirated into a chamber and ionized by a stream of electrons emitted from a filament. The ionized gas molecules are accelerated and deflected by a magnetic field onto a collector plate. The amount of deflection depends on their mass:charge ratio. The gas molecules are then separated according to their mass:charge ratio, and as they reach the collector plate, they generate a signal that is picked up by a detector. The strength of the signal, which depends on the number of particles detected, can then be amplified and displayed.[32]

Although mass spectrometers are expensive, they can be used for several patients (i.e., multiplexing in the surgical suite) and can be used to measure gases other than carbon dioxide, including oxygen, nitrogen, and nitrous oxide. This added capacity does have drawbacks, however, because carbon dioxide and nitrous oxide have the same molecular weight. Therefore separation of the basis of weight alone can lead to erroneous readings. This problem is overcome by ionizing N_2O to N_2O^+ and CO_2 to C^+.[30,32]

> **CLINICAL ROUNDS 8-4**
>
> A patient is being monitored with a sidestream capnograph. Although no problems were noted during the initial period of monitoring, the capnograph now shows an irregular waveform because the percentage of carbon dioxide does not rise above 1%. What could cause this?
>
> See Appendix A for the answer.

Raman Spectroscopy

This type of spectroscopy relies on the **Raman effect,** which occurs when light interacts with gas molecules to cause rotational or vibrational energy changes in the gas molecules. The light that is emitted from a gas molecule as it relaxes to its original state results in a shift in the wavelength that is characteristic of the molecule being analyzed. For example, monochromatic radiation that is passed through a gas mixture will demonstrate a spectral change that depends on the structure of the individual molecules present in the gas mixture.[32]

Although Raman spectroscopy has been available for some time, its use in clinical medicine is still somewhat limited. Because the accuracy of these devices has been shown to be similar to mass spectroscopy, the future use of this technology remains promising.

Physiologic Basis of Capnography

Under normal circumstances, inspired air contains virtually no carbon dioxide (actually it contains about 0.3%). Expired air, on the other hand, contains about 4% to 6% carbon dioxide. Figure 8-28 is an idealized capnogram of a resting

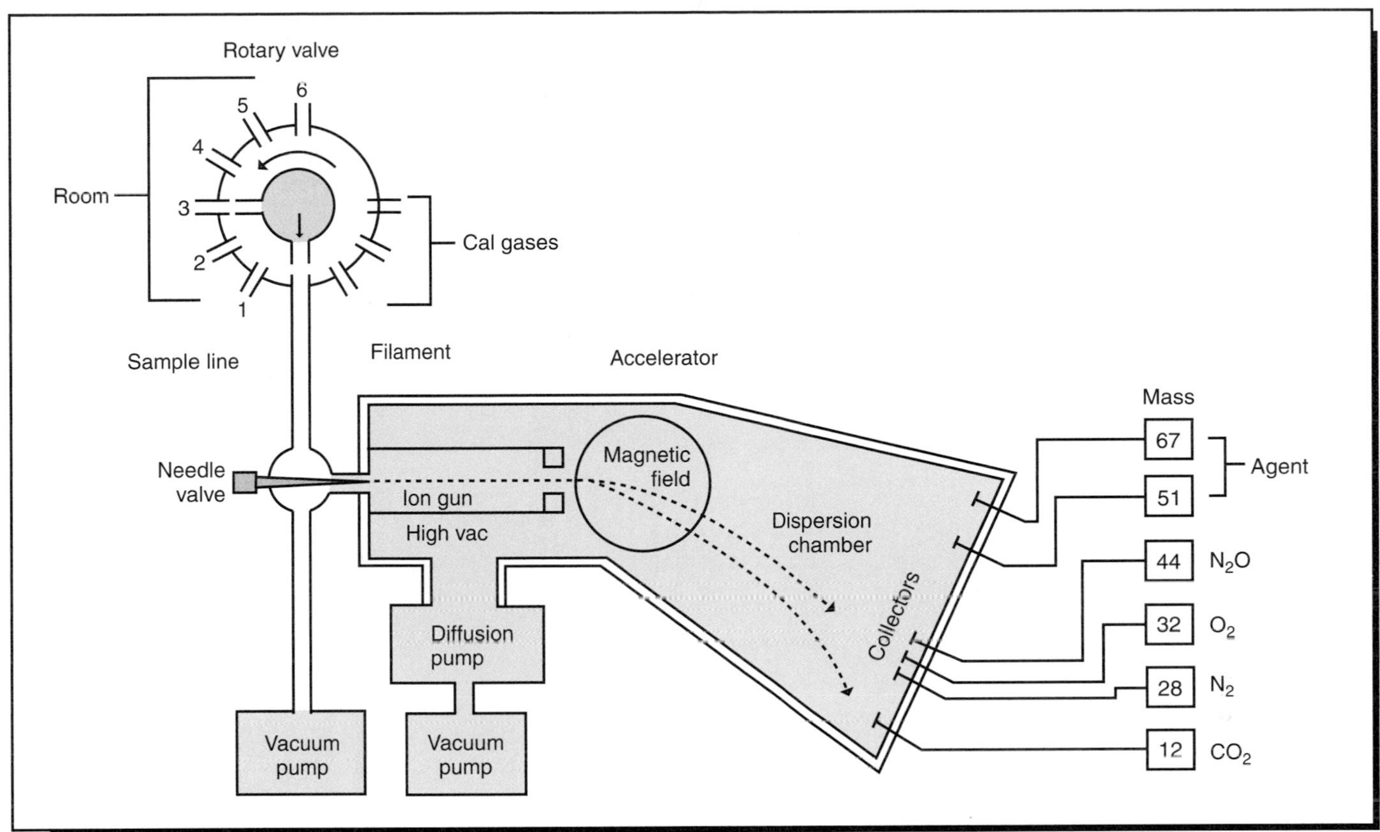

Figure 8-27 Schematic of a mass spectrometer. (Redrawn from Gravenstein JS, Paulus DA, Hayes TJ: *Capnography in clinical practice*, Boston, 1989, Butterworth.)

individual who is quietly breathing room air. This waveform, which is divided into four phases, reflects the elimination of carbon dioxide from the lungs during respiration. During Phase 1, gas is exhaled from the large conducting airways, which contain essentially no carbon dioxide. In Phase 2, some alveolar gas containing carbon dioxide mixes with gas from the smaller conducting airways, and the carbon dioxide concentration rises. During Phase 3, the carbon dioxide concentration curve remains relatively constant, as primarily alveolar gas is exhaled (alveolar plateau).* On inspiration (Phase 4), the concentration falls to 0.

The amount of carbon dioxide in exhaled air depends on a balance between carbon dioxide production and elimination. Production is primarily determined by the metabolic rate, but elimination is dependent upon alveolar ventilation, which is ultimately influenced by the ventilation/perfusion ($\dot{V}/\dot{Q}$) ratio of the lungs.

The relationship between $\dot{V}/\dot{Q}$ and gas exchange (i.e., the partial pressure of alveolar carbon dioxide [P_ACO_2]) can therefore be expressed with $\dot{V}/\dot{Q}$ relationships. Figure 8-29 shows three $\dot{V}/\dot{Q}$ relationships that can potentially affect the level of partial pressure of arterial carbon dioxide (P_aCO_2). In A, ventilation and perfusion are equally matched. P_aCO_2 and P_ACO_2 are nearly equal. Note that although the partial pressure of end-tidal carbon dioxide ($P_{ET}CO_2$) should equal P_aCO_2, it is actually about 4 to 6 mm Hg lower than the P_aCO_2. In *B*, ventilation decreases relative to perfusion (low $\dot{V}/\dot{Q}$ or shunt). The P_ACO_2 eventually equilibrates with the partial pressure of carbon dioxide in mixed venous blood. Clinical situations when this type of $\dot{V}/\dot{Q}$ relationship can exist throughout the lung, leading to higher than normal

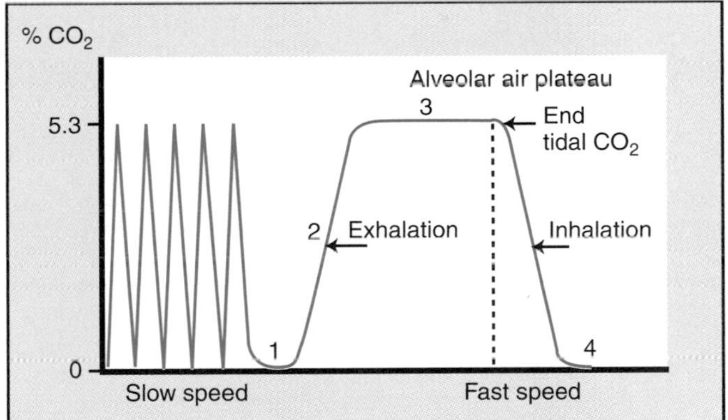

Figure 8-28 A normal capnogram *1*, exhaled gas from conducting airways; *2*, a mixture of conducting airways and alveolar air; *3*, alveolar plateau; *4*, inspired air (0.3% CO_2).

**The concentration of carbon dioxide at the end of the alveolar phase (just before inspiration begins) is called the end-tidal* P_{CO_2} ($P_{ET}CO_2$).

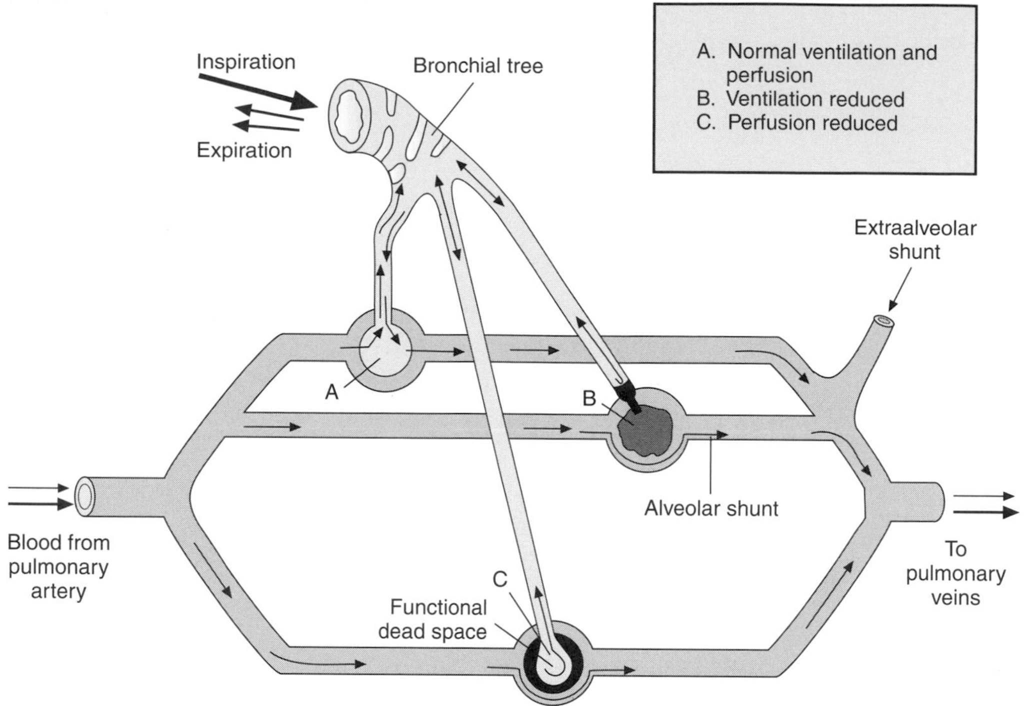

Figure 8-29 Ventilation/perfusion relationships: **A,** normal; **B,** low $\dot{V}/\dot{Q}$. (In Pilbeam SP: *Mechanical ventilation: physiological and clinical applications*, ed 3, St. Louis, 1998, Mosby. Modified from Despopoulos A, Sibernagl S: *Color atlas of physiology*, ed 4, New York, 1991, Thieme Medical Publishers.)

Clinical Practice Guidelines 8-2

Capnography/Capnometry during Mechanical Ventilation

Indications

Based on current evidence, capnography is useful for:

1. Monitoring the severity of pulmonary disease and evaluating the response to therapy, especially therapy intended to improve VD/VT and $\dot{V}/\dot{Q}$ relationships. It may also provide valuable information about therapy for improving coronary blood flow.
2. Determining that tracheal rather than esophageal intubation has taken place.
3. Monitoring the integrity of the mechanical ventilatory circuit and artificial airway.
4. Evaluating the efficiency of mechanical ventilatory support.
5. Monitoring the adequacy of pulmonary and coronary blood flow.
6. Monitoring carbon dioxide production.

Contraindications

There are no absolute contraindications to capnography in mechanical ventilated adult patients.

Monitoring

During capnography, the following should be recorded:

1. Ventilatory variables, including tidal volume, respiratory rate, positive end-expiratory pressure, inspiratory:expiratory ratio, peak airway pressure, and respiratory gas concentrations.
2. Hemodynamic variables, including systemic and pulmonary pressures, cardiac output, shunt, and $\dot{V}/\dot{Q}$ imbalances.

For a copy of the complete text, see *Resp Care* 40(12):1321, 1995.

$P_{ET}CO_2$s include respiratory center depression, muscular paralysis, and COPD. In *C*, ventilation is higher than perfusion (high $\dot{V}/\dot{Q}$, or dead space ventilation). Physiologic dead space ventilation increases, and the P_ACO_2 approaches inspired air (0 torr). Decreased $P_{ET}CO_2$s are found with this type of $\dot{V}/\dot{Q}$ relationship in patients with pulmonary embolism, excessive PEEP (mechanical or intrinsic), and any disorder with pulmonary hypoperfusion.

Clinical Applications of Capnography

Capnography can be used for both spontaneously breathing and mechanically ventilated patients. Because it has been

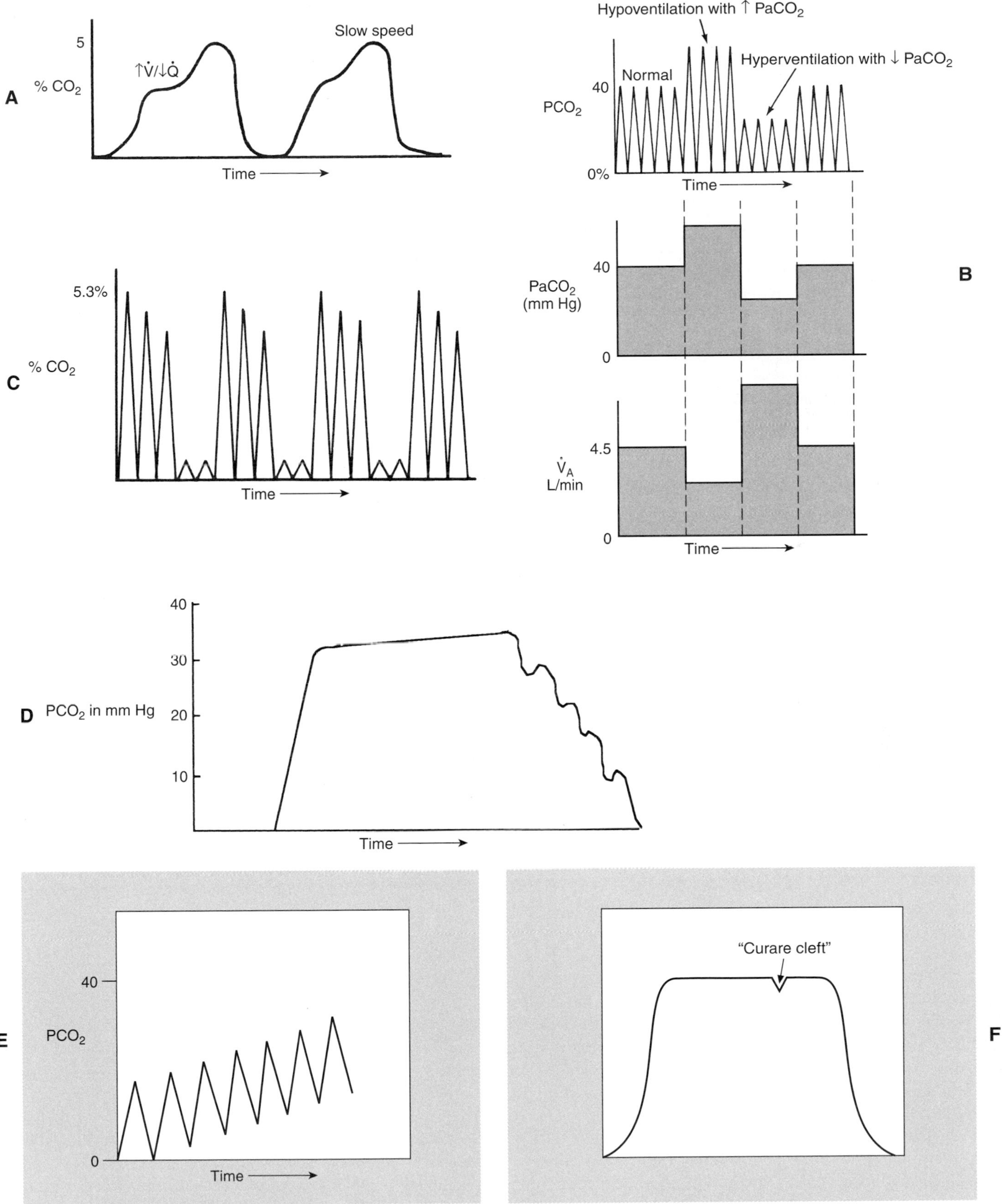

Figure 8-30 Capnogram contours associated with various breathing patterns: **A,** COPD; **B,** hyperventilation and hypoventilation; **C,** Cheyne-Stokes breathing; **D,** cardiac oscillations; **E,** rebreathing exhaled gases; **F,** curare cleft. (From Pilbeam SP: *Mechanical ventilation: physiological and clinical applications*, ed 3, St Louis, 1998, Mosby.)

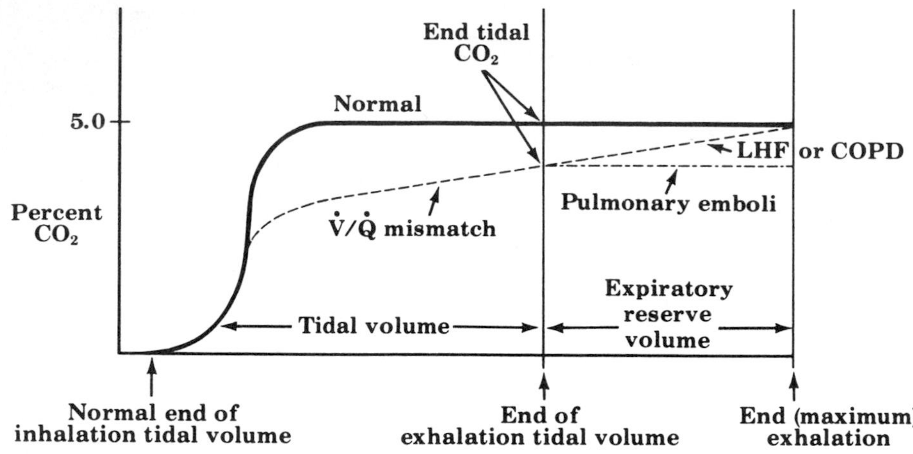

Figure 8-31 Capnogram illustrating exhaled carbon dioxide at the end of a quiet expiration and following a maximum expiration. The difference between these two values can be used to assess $\dot{V}/\dot{Q}$ relationships. A patient with COPD will typically show an end-tidal carbon dioxide less than that measured after a maximum expiration. For patients suspected to have pulmonary embolus, the end-tidal and maximum expiratory carbon dioxide measurements and nearly equal. (From Pilbeam SP: *Mechanical ventilation: physiological and clinical applications*, ed 3, St Louis, 1998, Mosby.)

primarily used with mechanically ventilated patients, the AARC has prepared a guideline for using capnography to monitor such patients.[28] CPG 8-2 summarizes the key points of this guideline. A discussion of how capnography can be used in the management of mechanically ventilated patients follows.

Capnograph Contours

Capnography can be used to detect increases in dead space ventilation, hyper- and hypoventilation, apnea or periodic breathing, inadequate neuromuscular blockade in pharmacologically paralyzed patients, and the presence of carbon dioxide rebreathing. It can also be used to effectively monitor gas exchange during cardiopulmonary resuscitation (CPR). Figure 8-30 shows various capnogram contours that are characteristic of several common situations.

In cases when physiologic dead space increases, as in COPD, Phase 3 becomes indistinguishable (see Figure 8-30, *A*). Hyperventilation is characterized by a reduction in P_aCO_2 and therefore in $P_{ET}CO_2$ *(B)*. Conversely, hypoventilation is associated with elevated P_aCO_2s and $P_{ET}CO_2$s *(B)*. *C* is a capnogram from a patient demonstrating Cheyne-Stokes breathing. During bradypnea, Phase 3 typically shows cardiac oscillations that result from the transferal of the beating heart motion to the conducting airways *(D)*. Rebreathing exhaled gas is recognized because the capnogram does not return to baseline *(E)*. F is a capnogram demonstrating the characteristic Phase 3 "curare cleft" that can occur when a patient is receiving insufficient neuromuscular blockade.[30,32]

Capnography can be used to detect cessation of pulmonary blood flow, as occurs with pulmonary embolism or during cardiac arrest.[28,30,32] Indeed, a number of investigators have advocated use of capnography as an adjunct to CPR. Laboratory studies suggest that capnography can be used as an indication of the progress and success of CPR, and demonstrated that $P_{ET}CO_2$ increases as $\dot{V}/\dot{Q}$ is restored to normal.[29,30]

Capnography can also be used during CPR to detect accidental esophageal intubation.[28,32] Gastric PCO_2 is generally equal to room air. Thus failure to detect the characteristic changes in carbon dioxide concentration during ventilation might indicate esophageal intubation. Although, low perfusion of the lungs is also associated with low $P_{ET}CO_2$ and should not be confused with esophageal intubation. Also, gastric PCO_2 may be elevated after

Box 8-3 Formulae Used During Indirect Calorimetry

Energy Expenditure

Weir Equation[39]

$EE = [3.941 (\dot{V}O_2) + 1.106 (\dot{V}CO_2)]\ 1.44 - 12.17\ (UN)$

Modified Weir Equations

$EE = [3.9 (\dot{V}O_2) + 1.1 (\dot{V}CO_2)] \times 1.44$

Substrate Utilization[40]

Carbohydrates

$dS = 4.115 (\dot{V}CO_2) - 2.909 (\dot{V}O_2) - 2.539\ (UN)$

Fats

$dF = 1.689 (\dot{V}O_2 - \dot{V}CO_2) - 1.943\ (UN)$

Proteins

$dP = 6.25\ (UN)$

dS, dF, and dP represent grams of carbohydrate, fat, and protein, respectively, for a fasting individual.

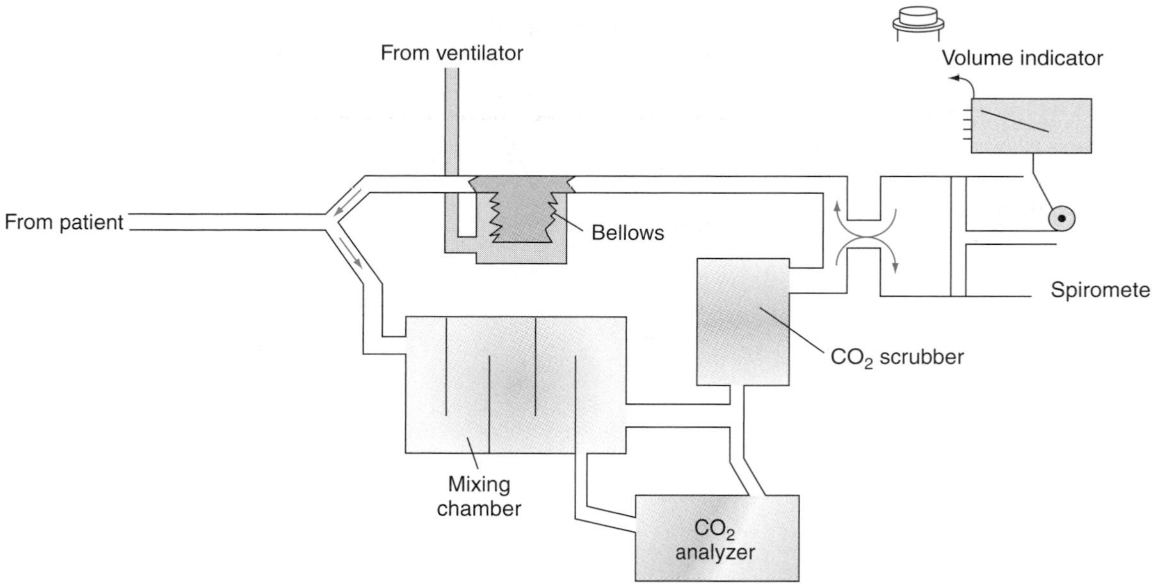

Figure 8-32 Closed-circuit indirect calorimeters. Oxygen consumption is estimated by measuring the amount of oxygen used from a reservoir. (From Branson RD: The measurement of energy expenditure: instrumentation, practical considerations, and clinical applications, *Respir Care* 35:640, 1990.)

mouth-to-mouth breathing or ingestion of a carbonated beverage.

Arterial-to-Maximum End-Expiratory PCO_2 Difference

As was previously mentioned, arterial-to-end-tidal partial pressure of carbon dioxide (a-et PCO_2) for tidal breathing should be negligible (essentially zero). It becomes elevated in patients with COPD, left heart failure, and pulmonary embolism due to an increase in their physiologic dead space.[28-30,32]

Another technique that can be used to further evaluate the severity of the disease is to compare the arterial PCO_2 measurements with the maximum expired PCO_2 measurements (the arterial to maximum expiratory PCO_2 gradient).[33,34] With this technique, the expired PCO_2 recorded at the end of a maximum exhalation to residual volume is compared with the P_aCO_2. Normally, the difference between these two values is minimal. Interestingly, patients with COPD and left heart failure do not show an arterial-to-maximum expiration PCO_2 difference, whereas patients with pulmonary embolism do show an increased gradient. These differences are shown in Figure 8-31.

Indirect Calorimetry and Metabolic Monitoring

Most clinicians rely on equations derived by Harris and Benedict[35] in 1919 to estimate patient energy requirements. Although these formulae can be quite useful for normal subjects and non-critically ill patients, they may be limited for some critically ill patients. Kinney and associates[36] derived correction factors to compensate for the increased energy demands in critically ill patients (e.g., burns, bone fractures), but these factors are limited in their ability to account for situations in which multiple conditions may exist simultaneously in a patient (e.g., sepsis, adult respiratory distress syndrome).

Recent advances in microprocessor technology have made it relatively easy for respiratory therapists to accurately measure energy needs and substrate utilization patterns in hospitalized patients. The technique used to accomplish this task is called **indirect calorimetry.**

Indirect Calorimetry

Indirect calorimetry is based on the theory that all of a person's energy is derived from the oxidation of carbohydrates, fats, and proteins, and that the ratio of carbon dioxide produced to oxygen consumed (i.e., the respiratory quotient, or $\dot{V}CO_2/\dot{V}O_2$) is characteristic of the fuel being burned.[37] **Energy expenditure (EE)** is calculated from $\dot{V}O_2$ and $\dot{V}CO_2$ measurements using the Weir equation, and substrate utilization patterns can be determined using equations like those derived by Burszein et al and Consolazio.[38-40] Box 8-3 summarizes these equations.

Indirect calorimeters are generally classified by their method of determining $\dot{V}O_2$. Thus two methods are usually described: the **closed-circuit** and the **open-circuit** methods. With the closed-circuit method, the patient breathes into and out of a container prefilled with oxygen. Oxygen consumption is determined by measuring the oxygen volume used by the patient. With the open-circuit method, $\dot{V}O_2$ is determined by measuring the volume of inspired and expired gases, as well as the fractional concentrations of oxygen in the each. The $\dot{V}O_2$ is then determined by

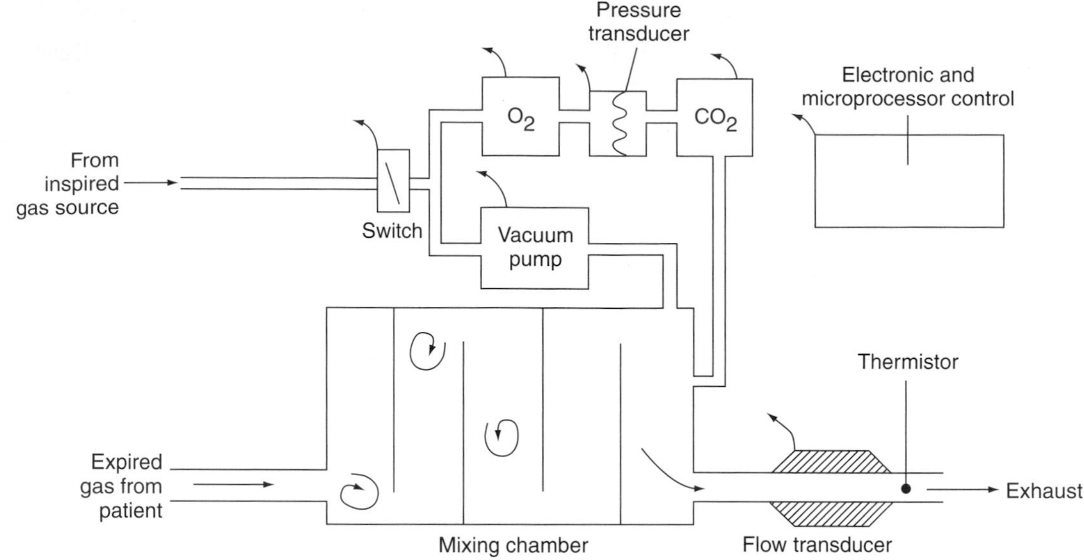

Figure 8-33 Open circuit indirect calorimeter. Oxygen consumption and carbon dioxide production are estimated by multiplying the minute ventilation by the fractional concentration of oxygen and carbon dioxide during inspiration and expiration. (From Branson RD: The measurement of energy expenditure: instrumentation, practical considerations, and clinical applications, *Respir Care* 35:640, 1990.)

calculating the difference between the amount of oxygen in inspired gas ($\dot{V}_I \times F_IO_2$) and the amount of oxygen in expired gas ($\dot{V}_E \times F_EO_2$).

Closed-Circuit Calorimeters

With closed-circuit devices, oxygen consumption can be determined by measuring either the oxygen volume removed from the device or by measuring the oxygen volume that must added to the system to maintain the original oxygen volume.

Figure 8-32 illustrates a closed-circuit system in which $\dot{V}O_2$ is determined by measuring the amount of oxygen removed from a reservoir over time. The system consists of a breathing circuit connected to a spirometer that is prefilled with oxygen. The patient's exhaled gases are directed to a mixing chamber, then through a carbon dioxide absorber, and back to the spirometer. Carbon dioxide production ($\dot{V}CO_2$) can be measured by incorporating the carbon dioxide analyzer positioned between the mixing chamber and the carbon dioxide absorber. Closed-circuit calorimeters can be used for both spontaneously breathing and mechanically ventilated patients.

Oxygen consumption is determined by measuring the oxygen volume removed from the spirometer. The volume of oxygen removed can be determined by measuring the change in the end-expiratory level. (Oxygen consumption is expressed in milliliters/minute.) The fractional concentration of mixed expired carbon dioxide (F_ECO_2) is determined by aspirating a sample of the mixed expired gas (from the mixing chamber) into the carbon dioxide analyzer located between the mixing chamber and the spirometer. Carbon dioxide production is calculated by multiplying the fractional concentration of mixed expired carbon dioxide by the minute ventilation, and is expressed in milliliters/minute.

Another variation of the closed-circuit technique for estimating oxygen consumption involves measuring the oxygen volume that must be replenished while the patient removes oxygen from the reservoir. This system consists of a breathing circuit, a bellows containing oxygen, a carbon dioxide absorber, and an ultrasonic transducer to monitor the bellows position. As the patient breathes into and out of the bellows, oxygen that is used by the patient is replaced on demand by an external oxygen supply. The amount of oxygen that must be added back to the system is a measure of the oxygen consumption. These systems can be used for spontaneously breathing and mechanically ventilated patients.

Open-Circuit Calorimeters

Open-circuit calorimeters use mixing chambers, dilution techniques, and breath-by-breath measurements to determine oxygen consumption. With mixing chambers, expired gases are directed into a collecting chamber containing baffles to ensure adequate mixing of gases. A vacuum attached to the chamber aspirates a sample of the mixed-expired gas and directs it into the oxygen and carbon dioxide analyzers. After they are analyzed, the gases are returned to the mixing chamber, and the entire volume of the mixing chamber is routed through a volume- or flow-sensing device.

Dilution systems also use a mixing chamber, but they use a bias flow of room air to dilute the gas sample and move it through the system. The amounts of oxygen and carbon dioxide exhaled are calculated by multiplying the fractional concentrations of oxygen and carbon dioxide by the total flow through the system, which is usually about 40 L/min.

Breath-by-breath devices measure the volume and fractional concentrations of oxygen and carbon dioxide in each breath. The amount of oxygen and carbon dioxide in inspired and mixed expired gases is actually determined by averaging the volumes and concentrations of several breaths. The number of breaths to be averaged can be preselected by the technologist or preset by the manufacturer.

Figure 8-33 is a schematic of an open-circuit, indirect calorimeter. A flow- or volume-sensing device is used to measure the inspired and expired gas volumes; a polarographic analyzer is used to measure the fractional concentrations of oxygen; and a nondispersive infrared analyzer is used to measure the fractional concentration of carbon dioxide.

Box 8-4 Conditions for Obtaining Indirect Calorimetry Measurements

1. The patient should be at rest and in a supine position for at least 30 minutes before the measurement is made.
2. Room temperature should be from 20° to 25° C.
3. The patient should remain relaxed during the measurement (i.e., no voluntary physical activity).
4. Measurements should be recorded for 15 to 30 minutes, or until there is less than a 5% variation in $\dot{V}O_2$ and $\dot{V}CO_2$.

Because changes in ambient temperature and pressure can affect gas concentrations, a sensor for measuring the ambient temperature and barometric pressure of the gases being analyzed is also incorporated into the system design.

Although open-circuit devices can be used for both spontaneously breathing and mechanically ventilated patients, special problems can arise when these systems are used with mechanically ventilated patients. Some of these problems include fluctuations in F_IO_2, separation of the patient's inspired and expired gases from the continuous gas flow from the ventilator, and handling of water vapor.[41] Problems with fluctuations in F_IO_2 can be alleviated to some extent by using air/oxygen blenders or premixed gases.* Beyond F_IO_2s of 0.50 to 0.60, most systems are unreliable because of the **Haldane transformation** and should be viewed skeptically. Inspired and expired gases can be separated using isolation valves supplied by the manufacturer of the metabolic monitor. Water vapor is always a problem when performing continuous measurements on ventilator patients, but is accentuated when cascade humidifiers are used to

The latter solution is expensive considering the amount of gas that would be used during the measurement.

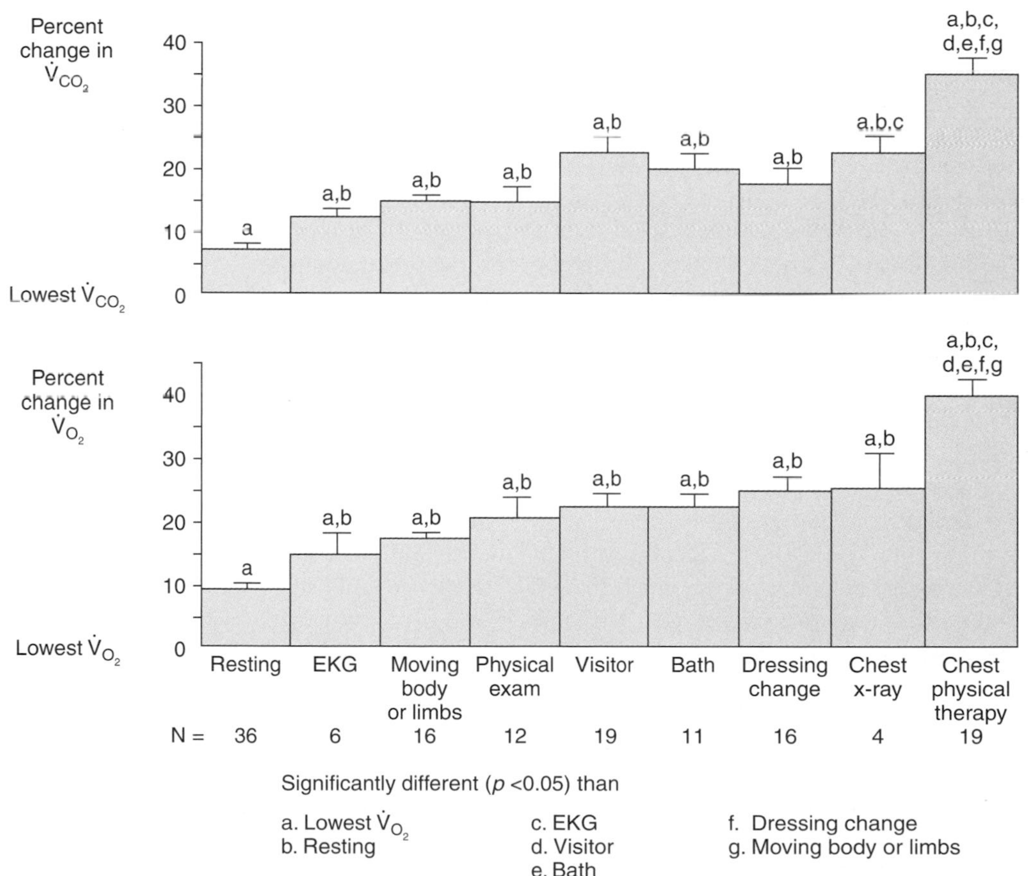

Figure 8-34 Variations in oxygen consumption and carbon dioxide production (expressed as percent change) associated with diagnostic and therapeutic interactions in an ICU patient. (From Weismann C, Kemper MC, Damask M: The effects of routine interactions on metabolic rate, *Chest* 86(6):815, 1984.)

Table 8-6 Variations in respiratory quotient

Substrate	RQ
Carbohydrates oxidation	1.0
Fats oxidation	0.7
Protein oxidation	0.8
Lipogenesis	>1.0

supply humidity to the patient. Replacing these humidifiers with artificial noses may help to minimize the problem.

Practical Applications of Indirect Calorimetry

Spontaneously breathing patients who are breathing room air can be connected to the system by breathing through a mouthpiece or mask attached to a nonrebreathing valve. Specially designed canopies and hoods can also be used for spontaneously breathing patients who are not receiving ventilatory support.

Patients with ETs or tracheostomy tubes (TTs) can be connected to the system if the nonrebreathing valve is placed directly onto the airway opening and expired gases are routed into the system. It is important to inflate the cuffs of ETs and TTs when measuring inspired and exhaled gases, because failure to do so will result in loss of expired air around the tube and erroneous measurements of $\dot{V}O_2$ and $\dot{V}CO_2$. For patients receiving a continuous flow of gas during ventilatory support, such as occurs when a bias flow is present, an isolation valve must be used to ensure that only the patient's exhaled gases are delivered to the system.

As was previously stated, oxygen consumption and carbon dioxide production are calculated by comparing the fractional concentrations of oxygen and carbon dioxide of inspired and expired air. When the patient is breathing room air, however, it is reasonable to assume that the fractional concentration of inspired oxygen is 20.9%, and the fractional concentration of inspired carbon dioxide is 0.3%. For patients receiving enriched oxygen mixtures, the fractional concentration of inspired oxygen must be measured by the system. Fluctuations in F_IO_2 can be caused by air leaks in the patient-ventilator/metabolic monitor system and also by varying gas volumes and pressure demands, as occur during intermittent mandatory ventilation. Unstable air-oxygen blending systems within the ventilator circuit may also contribute to unstable F_IO_2s. Additionally, clinical studies have demonstrated that currently available systems cannot provide accurate and reproducible $\dot{V}O_2$ measurements for patients breathing F_IO_2s greater than 0.5. Box 8-4 contains a summary of conditions that should be observed when making indirect calorimetry measurements.

Metabolic Monitoring

The main advantage of using indirect calorimetry instead of prediction equations like those of Harris and Benedict is that indirect calorimetry can provide actual measurements of patient caloric needs. When combined with measurements of nitrogen excretion, indirect calorimetry can also provide information about substrate utilization, thus giving the clinician valuable insight into the types of substrates that are being used by the patient to generate energy.

Energy Expenditure

Energy expenditure is typically expressed in kilocalories per day (kcal/day) or relative to an individual's body surface area (kcal/hr/m^2). A normal, healthy adult uses from 1500 to 3000 kcal/day, or about 30 to 40 kcal/hr/m.[2,41]

Many factors can influence the metabolic rate, including the type and rate of food ingested, the time of day of the measurement, the patient activity level, and if the patient is recovering from infection, surgery, or trauma.

Prolonged starvation is associated with a decreased metabolic rate. Feeding raises metabolic rate through a mechanism called specific dynamic action. It is thought that specific dynamic action is related to the digestion and absorption of food.[41] Energy expenditure shows diurnal variation (i.e., it is usually higher in the morning than in the evening), which may be related to the variations in hormone levels that naturally occur daily.[41] It is well-recognized that changes in activity can alter metabolic rate. Figure 8-34 shows how changes in physical activity can affect energy expenditure in a hospitalized patient. Note that sleep is associated with a reduction in metabolic rate, and even the slightest exertion is associated an increase in metabolic rate. Fever, as can occur with bacterial and viral infection, can also have a profound effect on metabolic rate. For example, an increase in body temperature of 1° F will cause a 10% increase in metabolic rate. Burns, long-bone fractures, and surgery can increase the metabolic rate by as much as 200%.[36]

Substrate Utilization Patterns

The substrate utilization pattern is the proportion of carbohydrates, fats, and proteins that is contributing to the total energy metabolism. As was previously stated, the percentage of the total energy that a substrate contributes can be determined using the RQ. Remember that the RQ is the ratio of $\dot{V}CO_2$ to $\dot{V}O_2$. The RQs for various foods are shown in Table 8-6. When pure fat is burned, the RQ is 0.7. The RQ for pure carbohydrate is 1.0, and the RQ for protein is approximately 0.8. RQs greater than 1.0 are associated with lipogenesis (fat synthesis), metabolic acidosis, and hyperventilation. RQs less than 0.7 are associated with ketosis.

Healthy adults consuming a typical American diet derive 45% to 50% of their calories from carbohydrates, 35% to 40% from lipids, and 10% to 15% from proteins. The resultant RQ ranges from 0.80 to 0.85. Under normal conditions, proteins normally contribute only minor amounts to energy metabolism. Note that the percentage of protein used represents the normal turnover rate for replenishing structural and functional proteins in the body. Proteins may contribute significantly to EE, however, in cases of starvation. For this reason, a nonprotein RQ is usually reported to indicate the contribution to RQ made by carbohydrates and lipids.

Substrate utilization is determined by the types of substrates ingested and the ability of an individual to use various types of foods. For example, eating a large amount of glucose raises the RQ to about 1.0, suggesting that carbohydrates are providing most of the energy expenditure. Prolonged starvation lowers the RQ to about 0.7, indicating that the individual is relying almost completely on fats for energy. Many systemic diseases adversely affect an individual's ability to use various types of substrates. For example, several studies have shown that patients with severe sepsis have RQs of approximately 0.7 because of their reliance on lipid metabolism for energy and an inability to use carbohydrates.

Summary

Recent developments in microprocessor technology have significantly improved our ability to monitor the physiologic functions of patients with cardiopulmonary dysfunctions. Devices and techniques designed to assess respiratory system mechanics, inspired and exhaled gases, and metabolic function can provide valuable information for the clinician. Oxygen analyzers, capnographs, and indirect calorimeters are examples of devices that are routinely used by respiratory therapists in both the general and critical care settings. Chemiluminescence and electrochemical monitoring of nitrogen oxides are relatively newer techniques that are becoming common in the care of critically ill patients. Proper use of these devices requires an understanding of the operational theory of each, as well as how and when these devices can be used most effectively.

Review Questions

See Appendix A for the answers.

1. Which of the following spirometers are classified as flow-sensing devices?
   I. Wright respirometers
   II. Hot wire anemometers
   III. Dry-rolling seal spirometers
   IV. Stead-Wells spirometers
   a. I and II only
   b. II and III only
   c. II and IV only
   d. I, II, and III only

2. Which of the following can influence the accuracy of spirometer measurements?
   I. The linearity and frequency response of the device
   II. The device's sensitivity to environmental condition
   III. Frequency of calibration
   IV. The presence of an obstructive or restrictive pulmonary disease
   a. I and II only
   b. II and III only
   c. I, II, and III only
   d. I, II, III, and IV

3. According to ATS standards, spirometers used to measure vital capacity should have an accuracy range (in BTPS) of:
   a. 5 liters ±10% of the reading, or 50 mL—whichever is greater
   b. 6 liters ±5% of the reading, or 50 mL—whichever is greater
   c. 7 liters ±3% of the reading, or 50 mL—whichever is greater
   d. 12 liters ±3% of the reading, or 50 mL—whichever is greater

4. Which of the following is considered the primary criteria for identifying the end of a successful nitrogen washout test?
   a. Patient becomes fatigued
   b. Exhaled nitrogen concentration is <1.5%
   c. Nitrogen percentage remains stable for 2 minutes
   d. Exhaled volume equals the FRC

5. Which of the following can cause erroneous measurements with impedance pneumography?
   I. Sinus tachycardia
   II. Upper airway obstruction
   III. Central apnea
   IV. Tachypnea
   a. I only
   b. II only
   c. II and III only
   d. I, II, and III only

6. Which of the following lung volumes cannot be measured by simple spirometry?
   I. VC
   II. RV
   III. TLC
   IV. IC
   a. I and II only
   b. II and III only
   c. III and IV only
   d. I, III, and IV only

7. Maximum inspiratory pressures are normally:
   a. –20 to –40 cm H_2O
   b. –50 to –80 cm H_2O
   c. –60 to –100 cm H_2O
   d. –150 to –200 cm H_2O

8. The Beckman D2 oxygen analyzer is an example of a:
   a. paramagnetic oxygen analyzer
   b. polarographic oxygen analyzer
   c. galvanic oxygen analyzer
   d. electric (thermal conductivity) oxygen analyzer

9. Lack of a definitive Phase 3 on a capnogram is most often associated with:

a. insufficient neuromuscular blockade
b. cardiac oscillations
c. $\dot{V}/\dot{Q}$ imbalances, such as occur with patients with emphysema or chronic bronchitis
d. rebreathing exhaled gases

10. How many kilocalories of energy per day should a typical healthy adult ingest to maintain energy balance?
a. 500 to 1000
b. 900 to 1200
c. 1200 to 1800
d. 1500 to 3000

11. You notice that the FRC measured on a patient with COPD with the nitrogen washout technique is different than that measured with body plethysmography. In fact, the volume measured with the body box is approximately 500 mL greater than the FRC measured with nitrogen washout. Why might this difference exist?

12. Which of the following analyzers can be used to measure nitric oxide?
I. Chemiluminescence analyzer
II. Polarographic analyzer
III. Electrochemical analyzer
IV. Capnography
a. I only
b. II only
c. I and III only
d. I, II, and III only

13. A patient receiving mechanical ventilatory support via an ET is being monitored for oxygen consumption. Which of the following could lead to an erroneous measurement?
I. The patient appears agitated.
II. The measurement is performed immediately after the patient received a physical therapy treatment.
III. The F_IO_2 is 0.8.
IV. The patient's ET cuff is inflated to seal the airway.
a. I and II only
b. II and III only
c. I, II, and III only
d. I, II, III, and IV

14. The only source of nutrition administered to a patient is D_5W (i.e., 5% dextrose in water). What would you expect to find when measuring RQ?
a. 0.7 to 0.75
b. 0.8 to 0.85
c. 0.9 to 0.95
d. 1.0

15. Which of the following patient conditions would you expect to be hypermetabolic (elevated $\dot{V}O_2$)?
a. Starvation
b. Fever
c. Sedation
d. Hypothermia

References

1. Wasserman K, et al: *Principles of exercise testing and interpretation*, Philadelphia, 1994, Lea & Febiger.
2. East TD: What makes noninvasive monitoring tick? A review of basic engineering principles, *Respir Care* 35:500, 1990.
3. Snow M: Instrumentation. In Clausen JL, editor: *Pulmonary function testing: guidelines and controversies*, New York, 1882, Academic Press.
4. Fleisch A: Der pneumotachograph: ein apparacat zur beischwindig-kertregstrier der ateniluft, *Arch Ges Physiol* 209:713, 1925.
5. Sullivan WJ, Peters GM, Enright PL: Pneumotachography: theory and clinical application, *Respir Care* 29:736, 1984.
6. Kacmarek RM, Hess D, Stoller JK: *Monitoring in respiratory care*, St Louis, 1993, Mosby.
7. American Thoracic Society: Snowbird workshop on standardization of spirometry, *Am Rev Respir Dis* 119:831, 1979.
8. American Thoracic Society: Standardization of spirometry, 1987 update, *Am Rev Respir Dis* 136:1285, 1987.
9. American Thoracic Society: Lung function testing: selection of reference values and interpretation, *Am Rev Respir Dis* 144:1202, 1991.
10. American Thoracic Society: Standardization of spirometry, 1994 update, *Am Rev Respir Dis* 152:1107, 1995.
11. American Association for Respiratory Care: Clinical practice guideline: spirometry, 1996 update, *Respir Care* 41:629, 1996.
12. American Association for Respiratory Care: Clinical practice guideline: assessing response to bronchodilator therapy at point of care, *Respir Care* 40:1300, 1995.
13. American Association for Respiratory Care: Clinical practice guideline: body plethysmography, *Respir Care* 46(5):506-513, 2001.
14. Ruppel GL: Manual of pulmonary function testing, ed 7, St Louis, 1997, Mosby.
15. American Association for Respiratory Care: Clinical practice guideline: static lung volumes, 2001 Revision and Update, *Respir Care* 46(5):531-539, 2001.
16. Branson RD and Campbell RS: Impedance pneumography, apnea monitoring, and respiratory inductive plethysmography. In Kacmarek RM, Hess D, and Stoller JK, editors: Monitoring in respiratory care, St Louis, 1993, Mosby.
17. Southhall DP, et al: Undetected episodes of prolonged apnea and severe bradycardia in preterm infants, *Pediatrics* 72:541, 1983.
18. Wayburton D, Stork AR, Taeusch HW: Apnea monitoring in infants with upper airway obstruction, *Pediatrics* 60:742, 1967.
19. Konno K, Mead J: Measurement of the separate changes of rib cage and abdomen during breathing, *J Appl Physiol* 22:407, 1967.
20. Krieger BP: Ventilatory pattern monitoring: instrumentation and application, *Respir Care* 35:697, 1990.
21. Marini JJ: Lung mechanics determination at the bedside: instrumentation and clinical application, *Respir Care* 35:669, 1990.

22. Osborne JJ, Wilson RM: Monitoring the mechanical properties of the lung. In Spence AA, editor: *Respiratory monitoring in the intensive care*, New York, 1980, Churchill-Livingstone.

23. Pauling L, Wood RE, and Sturdivant JH: Oxygen meter, *J Am Chem Soc* 68:795, 1946.

24. Etches PC, et al: Clinical monitoring of inhaled nitric oxide: comparison of chemiluminescence and electrochemical sensors, *Biomed Instrum Technol* 29:134, 1995.

25. Miller CC: Chemiluminescence analysis and nitrogen dioxide measurement, *Lancet* 34(3):300, 1994.

26. Body S, et al: Nitric oxide: delivery, measurement, and clinical application, *J Cardiothoracic Vasc Anesth* 9:748, 1995.

27. Purtz E, Hess D, Kacmarek R: Evaluation of electrochemical nitric oxide and nitrogen dioxide analyzers suitable for use during mechanical ventilation, *J Clin Monit* 13:25, 1997.

28. American Association for Respiratory Care: Clinical practice guideline: capnography, *Respir Care* 40:1321, 1995.

29. Stock MC: Capnography for adults, *Critical Care Clin* 11:219, 1995.

30. Hess D: Capnometry and capnography: technical aspects, physiologic aspects, and clinical applications, *Respir Care* 35:557, 1990.

31. Kennel EM, Andrews RW, Wollman H: Correction factors for nitrous oxide in the infrared analysis of carbon dioxide, *Anesthesiology* 39:441, 1973.

32. Gravenstein JS, Paulus DA, Hayes TJ: *Capnography in clinical practice*, Boston, 1989, Butterworth.

33. Pilbeam SP: *Mechanical ventilation*, ed 3, St Louis, 1997, Mosby.

34. Davis PD, Parbrook GD, Kenny GNC: *Basic physics and measurement in anesthesia*, ed 4, Oxford, 1995, Butterworth-Heinemann.

35. Harris JA, Benedict F: *Standard basal metabolism constants for physiologists and clinicians: a biometric study of basal metabolism in man*, Philadelphia, 1919, JB Lippincott.

36. Kinney JM: The application of indirect calorimetry in clinical studies: assessment of energy metabolism in health and disease. In Kinney JM, editor: *Report of the first Ross conference on medical research*, Columbus, Ohio, 1980, Ross Laboratories.

37. Ferrannini E: The theoretical basis of indirect calorimetry: a review, *Metabolism* 37:287, 1987.

38. Weir JB: New method for calculating metabolic rate with special reference to protein metabolism, *J Physiology* 109:1, 1949.

39. Burszein P, et al: Utilization of protein, carbohydrate, and fat in fasting and postabsorptive subjects, *Am J Clin Nutr* 33:998, 1980.

40. Consolazio CJ, Johnson RE, Pecora LJ: *Physiological measurements of metabolic function in man*, New York, 1963, McGraw-Hill.

41. Branson RD, Lacey J, Berry S: Indirect calorimetry and nutritional monitoring. In Levine RL, Fromm RE, editors: *Critical care monitoring*, St Louis, 1995, Mosby.

Internet Resources

1. American Association for Respiratory Care: http://www.aarc.org
2. Critical Care Medicine: http://www.pitt.edu/~crippen/index.html
3. American Association of Cardiovascular and Pulmonary Rehabilitation: http://www.aacvpr.org
4. Canadian Journal of Respiratory Therapy: http://www.csrt.com/CJRT/index.htm
5. Virtual Hospital: http://www.vh.org
6. Gasnet, Global Anesthesiology Server Network: http://gasnet.med.yale.edu
7. Medline Search Engine: http://medline.cos.com
8. National Library of Medicine: http://www.nlm.nih.gov

Chapter 9

Cardiovascular Diagnostic Testing

J.M. Cairo

Chapter Outline

Chapter Learning Objectives

After reading this chapter, the reader should be able to:

1. Discuss the electrophysiologic properties of the heart.
2. Explain the principles of electrocardiography.
3. Identify the major components of an electrocardiograph.
4. Demonstrate the correct placement of electrodes on a patient to obtain a 12-lead electrocardiogram.
5. Explain the various waves, complexes and intervals that appear on a normal electrocardiogram.
6. List and describe the most common dysrhythmias encountered in clinical electrocardiography.
7. Describe the pressure, volume, and flow events that occur in the heart and major blood vessels during a typical cardiac cycle.
8. Explain the principle of operation of various noninvasive and invasive devices that are routinely used to obtain blood pressure measurements.
9. Describe various methods that are used to measure cardiac output.
10. Interpret hemodynamic measurements that are obtained from patients in a critical care setting.

Key Terms

Absolute Refractory Period
Action Potential
Atrial Diastole
Atrial Fibrillation
Atrial Flutter
Atrial Premature Depolarizations
Atrial Systole
Automaticity
Cardiac Cycle
Cardiac Work
Conductivity
Diastasis
Diastolic Depolarization
Effective Refractory Period
Excitability
Floating Electrodes
Heart Blocks
Heart Sounds
Impedance Cardiography
Impedance Plethysmography
Incisura
Isovolumetric Contraction
Isovolumetric Relaxation
Junctional Escape Rhythm
Korotkoff Sounds
Murmurs
Myocyte
Normal Sinus Rhythm
Paroxysmal Atrial Tachycardia
Phonocardiogram
Premature Ventricular Beats
Premature Ventricular Depolarizations
Pulmonary Vascular Resistance
Relative Refractory Period
Rhythmicity
Sinus Arrhythmia
Sinus Bradycardia
Sinus Tachycardia
Sphygmomanometer
Systemic Vascular Resistance
Ventricular Asystole
Ventricular Diastole
Ventricular Fibrillation
Ventricular Systole
Ventricular Tachycardia
Volume Conductor
Wolff-Parkinson-White Syndrome

Successful management of patients with cardiovascular and pulmonary dysfunctions requires a working knowledge of cardiovascular physiology. This knowledge can be applied clinically to quantify various aspects of cardiovascular function with techniques such as electrocardiography and hemodynamic monitoring. This chapter provides an overview of the most common devices and techniques that are used by respiratory therapists to assess cardiovascular function.

Electrocardiography

Electrophysiology of Cardiac Cells

Contraction of cardiac muscle provides the energy required to propel blood through the circulation. Under normal circumstances, each heartbeat is initiated by specialized pacemaker cells of the heart, which have the property of rhythmic spontaneous electrical activity. When these specialized pacemaker cells depolarize (i.e., become electrically activated), they cause other electrically excitable cells of the heart to depolarize, resulting in simultaneous activation of the right and left atria followed by a simultaneous activation of the right and left ventricles.[1,2]

To fully appreciate this ability of cardiac cells to initiate and conduct electrical impulses, we must consider three important aspects of the electrophysiology of the heart: **excitability, automaticity,** and **conductivity.** Excitability may be defined as the ability of a cell to respond to an electrical stimulus. Automaticity is the ability of certain specialized cells of the heart to depolarize spontaneously. These specialized cells, which are located at the sinoatrial (SA) and atrioventricular (AV) nodes, can initiate action potentials in the absence of nerve impulses from the central nervous system. Conductivity is the ability of cardiac tissue to propagate an action potential.

Understanding the cellular events that occur during a heartbeat provides a foundation for studying electrocardiography and for identifying abnormalities of the electrical activity of the heart. We will therefore begin our discussion of electrocardiography with a brief description of the basic electrophysiologic properties of the heart.

Resting Membrane Potentials

Cardiac cells, as with other cells of the human body, are *polarized,* that is, the inside of a cardiac cell has a negative electrical charge relative to the outside of the cell. This property of polarization can be explained by the selective permeability of the cell membrane to various types of molecules and ions.[2] Large molecules, such as proteins, normally possess a negative charge at physiologic pH. These negatively charged macromolecules are trapped within cells because they are too large to pass freely through pores within the membrane. Smaller ions, such as potassium, sodium, and calcium, are also influenced by the selective permeability characteristics of the cell membrane albeit that their movements across the membrane are primarily governed by chemical and electrical gradients rather than particle size. For example, under normal resting conditions there is a higher concentration of potassium ions in the intracellular fluid than in the extracellular fluid. Conversely, there are higher concentrations of sodium and calcium ions in the extracellular fluid compared to the intracellular fluid. If the membrane were freely permeable to all ions it is reasonable to assume that there would be an equal exchange of positive ions across the membrane. In fact, the resting cell membrane is much more permeable to potassium ions than it is to sodium and calcium ions, causing more potassium ions to leak from the cell than sodium or calcium ions to leak into the cell. Thus under resting conditions, the greater efflux of potassium out of the cell compared to influx of sodium and calcium into the cell results in the cell membrane being polarized with the intracellular charge being more negative than the extracellular charge. It is important to mention that electrical gradients can also influence the movement of these small ions across the cell membrane. In the situation described here, potassium movement out of the cell is promoted by the chemical concentration gradient and opposed by the electrical gradient between the inside and outside of the cell; sodium movement into the cell is promoted by both gradients. Table 9-1 shows the chemical composition of intracellular and extracellular fluid.[1]

Another factor that must be considered when discussing the origin of the resting membrane potential is the *sodium-potassium ATPase pump,* which is an enzyme located within the cell membrane. This pump functions to move excess sodium that leaks into the cell out of the cell and excess potassium that leaks out of the cell back into the intracellular compartment. It is important to recognize that the sodium-potassium pump moves more sodium out of the cell than it moves potassium back into the cell, thus adding to the potential difference across the cell membrane.[2] It is also worth noting that this pump represents an active (i.e., energy dependent) mechanism to move ions across the cell membrane compared with the passive electrochemical forces that were previously discussed.

Cardiac Action Potentials

Cardiac cells, as with other excitable tissue, can depolarize, rapidly initiating an **action potential,** and then repolarize. In muscle cells, action potentials are responsible for the initiation of muscle contraction. If an excitable cell is depolarized either by a propagated wave of excitation originally initiated by pacemaker cells or by artificial stimulation, it may reach a critical level called its *threshold potential,* and an action potential will occur.[2]

Most of the excitable cardiac cells, including atrial and ventricular muscle cells, and the specialized conducting cells, such as Purkinje fibers, have action potentials like the one shown in Figure 9-1, *A.* Pacemaker cells, including those of the SA node and AV node possess a slightly different type of action potential, as illustrated in Figure 9-1, *B.* We will discuss these latter action potentials in the section on pacemaker cell action potentials.

As Figure 9-1, *A,* illustrates, the action potential begins when the cell membrane of the excitable cell is exposed to a depolarizing current and eventually reaches its excitation threshold potential. The initial phase of this type of action potential (at the point where the cell reaches its threshold potential), referred to as phase 0, consists of a rapid upstroke or depolarization. This change in membrane potential to a more positive value occurs because of a rapid influx of sodium ions into the cell. (At the peak of phase 0, the inside of the cell will actually become positive relative to the

Table 9-1 Chemical composition of intracellular and extracellular spaces

	Extracellular Fluid	Intracellular Fluid
Na^+	142 mEq/L	10 mEq/L
K^+	4 mEq/L	140 mEq/L
Ca^{++}	2.4 mEq/L	0.0001 mEq/L
Mg^{++}	1.2 mEq/L	58 mEq/L
Cl^-	103 mEq/L	4 mEq/L
HCO_3^-	24 mEq/L	10 mEq/L
Phosphates	4 mEq/L	75 mEq/L
SO_4^-	1 mEq/L	2 mEq/L
Glucose	90 mg/dL	0-20 mg/dL
Proteins	2 gm/dL	5 gm/dL

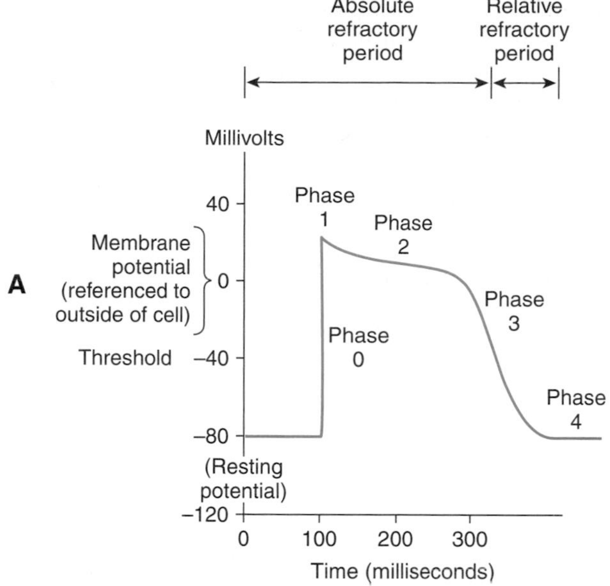

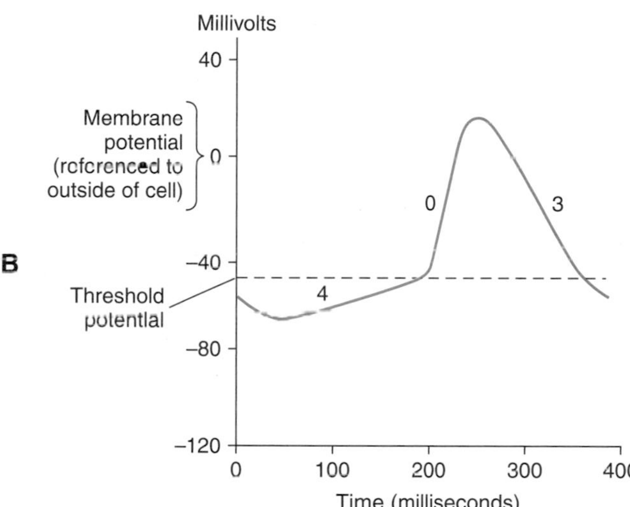

Figure 9-1 Cardiac action potentials. **A,** Fast type action potentials, such as those seen in atrial and ventricular muscle, and His-Purkinje fibers; **B,** slow type action potentials characteristic of nodal tissue, such as the SA node and AV node.

outside of the cell.) The increased conductance of sodium into the cell during this phase of the action potential is thought to occur as a result of activation of the so-called *fast* sodium channels located within the cell membrane.[1,2] After several milliseconds, these sodium channels become inactivated and close. They remain closed until the cell reaches its resting membrane potential. As we will discuss shortly, when these fast sodium channels are closed, the cell is refractory to additional stimuli. During phase 1, the cell undergoes a partial repolarization, in which the membrane potential falls from a value of about +20 mV to a value of about 0 mV. It is thought that this partial repolarization results from a countercurrent flow of potassium out of the cell and to a decrease in sodium conductance into the cell with closure of the fast sodium gates. At this time, a series of *slow* calcium and sodium channels open and a plateau phase 2 is established. Phase 2 lasts approximately 200 to 300 milliseconds. Phase 3 of the action potential begins when the myocardial cell starts to repolarize and return toward the negative resting membrane potential or phase 4 of the action potential. This repolarization occurs because the membrane becomes more permeable to potassium ions, allowing a greater number of these charged ions to move outside of the cell, and inactivation of the slow channels for calcium and sodium. The increased efflux of positive potassium ions occurring at the same time as the decreased influx of sodium and calcium ions results in restoration of the negative resting membrane potential.[1,2]

The period from the beginning of phase 0 to the middle of phase 3 is referred to as the **absolute** or **effective refractory period** because, regardless of the strength of the stimulus, the myocyte cannot be depolarized again. A **relative refractory period** follows immediately after the absolute refractory period (this period begins during the middle of phase 3 and lasts until to the beginning of phase 4). During the relative refractory period, the myocyte can be depolarized again by a stronger than normal stimulus; however, the amplitude and duration of these action potentials are considerably reduced.

Pacemaker Action Potentials (Rhythmicity)

As mentioned previously, pacemaker cells of the SA and AV nodes normally have action potentials that differ from those of other excitable cells of the heart. As shown in Figure 9-1, *B*, the resting membrane potential and threshold potential of pacemaker cells are less negative than other excitable myocardial cells. Phase 0 of pacemaker cells is slower than the action potentials atrial, ventricular, and Purkinje fiber myocardial cells. (Because the slope of phase 0 of the pacemaker cell's action potential is less than those of the atrial, ventricular, and Purkinje fiber action potentials, the former are often referred to as a *slow* action potential, whereas the latter is called a *fast* action potential.) Additionally, pacemaker cells demonstrate the absence of a prolonged phase 2 or plateau (i.e., the action potential for these cells therefore include phases 0, 3, and 4 only). The most important difference between these *slow* versus *fast* action potentials is the rate at which pacemaker cells can elicit a spontaneous action potential during phase 4. It is thought that this ability of pacemaker cells to discharge automatically results from a progressive decrease in permeability of the cell membrane to potassium ions while the permeability of the membrane to sodium remains unchanged. The result is that the inside of the cell progressively depolarizes (i.e., phase 4 **diastolic depolarization**). When the threshold is reached, the action potential occurs. Although the frequency of discharge (i.e., heart rate) is influenced primarily by the decrease in permeability of the membrane to potassium, the amplitude of the slow action potential is determined by the influx of calcium into the cell. Under normal conditions the SA node discharges approximately 60 to 100 times per minute,

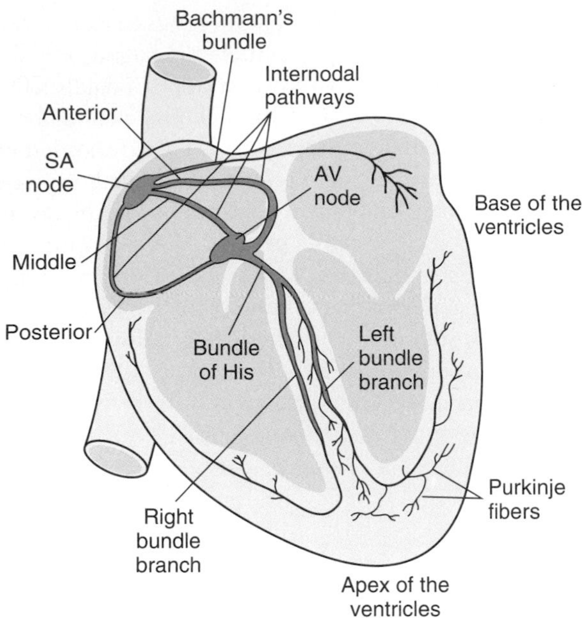

Figure 9-2 Electrical conduction system of the heart.

whereas the AV node discharges 40 to 60 times per minute. Although other myocardial cells, such as Purkinje fiber cells, can also discharge spontaneously, their discharge rate is so low (15 to 40 times per minute) that they do not normally act as pacemaker cells.

The heart rate can be increased by anything that increases the rate of spontaneous depolarization. That is, anything that increases the slope of the phase 4 diastolic depolarization, raises the resting membrane potential (make it less negative), or decreases the threshold potential. Conversely, heart rate is decreased by anything that would decrease the rate of spontaneous phase 4 depolarization, whether by decreasing the slope of phase 4, hyperpolarizing the resting membrane potential (making the resting membrane potential more negative), or raising the threshold potential.

Although it has been stated that the heart can initiate impulses in the absence of inputs from the central nervous system, it should be apparent that an individual's heart rate changes dramatically with alterations in the level of activation of the autonomic nervous system (i.e., sympathetic versus parasympathetic control). Norepinephrine and epinephrine, which mediate sympathetic control, can increase heart rate by increasing the slope of the phase 4 diastolic depolarization, decreasing the threshold potential, or hypopolarizing the resting membrane potential; acetylcholine, which mediates parasympathetic control, can decrease heart rate by decreasing the slope of the phase 4 depolarization, increasing the threshold potential, or hyperpolarizing the resting membrane potential. It is important to understand that pacemaker cells receive continuous input from both divisions of the autonomic nervous system. Thus heart rate can be increased by an increase in sympathetic stimulation or a decrease in parasympathetic activity. Conversely, heart rate can be decreased by an increase in parasympathetic stimulation or by decreasing sympathetic tone.

Conduction Pathways of the Heart

As stated previously, conductivity is defined as the ability of the heart to propagate impulses throughout the heart. This property of conductivity is remarkably consistent under normal circumstances. Depolarization of the SA node, which is located at the bifurcation of the superior vena cava and the right atrium, initiates the heart beat by triggering a wave of excitation that spreads throughout the right and left atria as it moves toward the AV node. (*Note:* The SA node is normally considered to be the pacemaker of the heart because it has the highest rate of automatic discharge.) As shown in Figure 9-2, the movement of electrical impulses between the SA and AV node occurs through a series of high-speed internodal conduction pathways, referred to as the anterior, middle, and posterior internodal pathways. Impulses travel to the left atrium via a branch of the anterior internodal pathway, which is called *Bachmann's bundle.*[2]

As the impulse travels through the AV node, there is a 100-ms delay in the conduction. This important delay allows the atria to become fully depolarized and contract before ventricular excitation begins, thus allowing the atrial contraction and emptying (i.e., "atrial kick") to contribute optimally to ventricular filling. (The AV node is divided into three distinct regions: (1) an A-N region, which is a transitional zone between the atria and the AV nodal tissue, (2) an N region, which represents the middle of the AV node, and (3) an N-H region, in which nodal fibers gradually merge with the bundle of His and enter into the Purkinje fiber system.) Following the delay and depolarization of the AV node, the excitation wave spreads to the muscle cells of the ventricles via a specialized high-speed conduction system that starts at the *bundle of His* and then splits into the right and left bundle branches. The bundle branches ultimately divide into a complex network of specialized conducting fibers, the *Purkinje fibers,* located beneath the surface of the endocardium. Excitation of the ventricular muscle cells finally occurs as impulses travel cell to cell from the inner endocardial surface to the outer epicardial surface and from apex to the base of the heart. Repolarization of the ventricles normally occurs from epicardium to endocardium, that is, in the opposite direction of depolarization. Repolarization of the ventricles also usually begins in the apex of the heart and travels toward the base.

Principles of Electrocardiography

The electrocardiogram (ECG) is a graphic representation of electrical voltages generated by cardiac tissue. Because the heart can be considered to be as an electrical generator located within a **volume conductor,** electrical potentials measured at various points on the body surface can be related to electrical impulses traveling through the heart. (Although the term *volume conductor* is sometimes difficult to understand, it can be best explained in the following manner. The heart is surrounded by tissues that contain ions that can conduct electrical impulses generated in the heart to the body surface where these electrical signals can be detected by electrodes placed on the skin.) The electrical activity measured by the ECG is not directly comparable to the action potentials of any individual cell but rather represents *summed* information from many cells at any instant. Thus the potential difference determined actually shows the resolved direction or vector, with respect to a particular frame of reference, of the movement of a wave of depolarization as it travels within the heart.[2] The electrocardiograph is wired in such a way that a wave or vector of depolarization traveling toward the sensing or positive electrode results in an upward deflection on the recording paper or monitor. Conversely, a wave of depolarization moving away from the sensing electrode will result in a downward deflection on the recording paper or monitor.

The contour of ECG waveforms remain relatively constant, although the heart rate may vary considerably.[2,3] For patients with heart disease, pathologic alterations in the excitability, **rhythmicity,** and conductivity of the heart can result in significant changes in the amplitude and duration of the ECG waveforms. In the following sections, we will consider several aspects of electrocardiography, including standard methods for recording electrocardiograms along with selective criteria that can be used to define a "normal" electrocardiogram. Finally, a clinically relevant approach to the analysis of ECGs will be provided for recognizing the presence of abnormalities in the cardiac electrical activity.

The Electrocardiograph

The major components of an electrocardiograph are illustrated in Figure 9-3. Electrodes placed on the skin of the patient act as transducers to convert ionic potentials into electrical impulses. These electrical impulses are then transmitted to an amplifier before being registered on an output display, such as a graphic recorder or a cathode ray tube (CRT).

Electrodes

A variety of electrodes have been used in clinical electrocardiography, including plate, suction-cup, and **floating electrodes.** Plate and suction-cup electrodes are made of silver, nickel, or a similar alloy with high conductivity. A thin coat of conduction jelly or electrolyte paste, which reduces the impedance of the skin-electrode interface, is applied evenly to the electrode before it is attached to the body surface. Although both plate and suction-cup electrodes

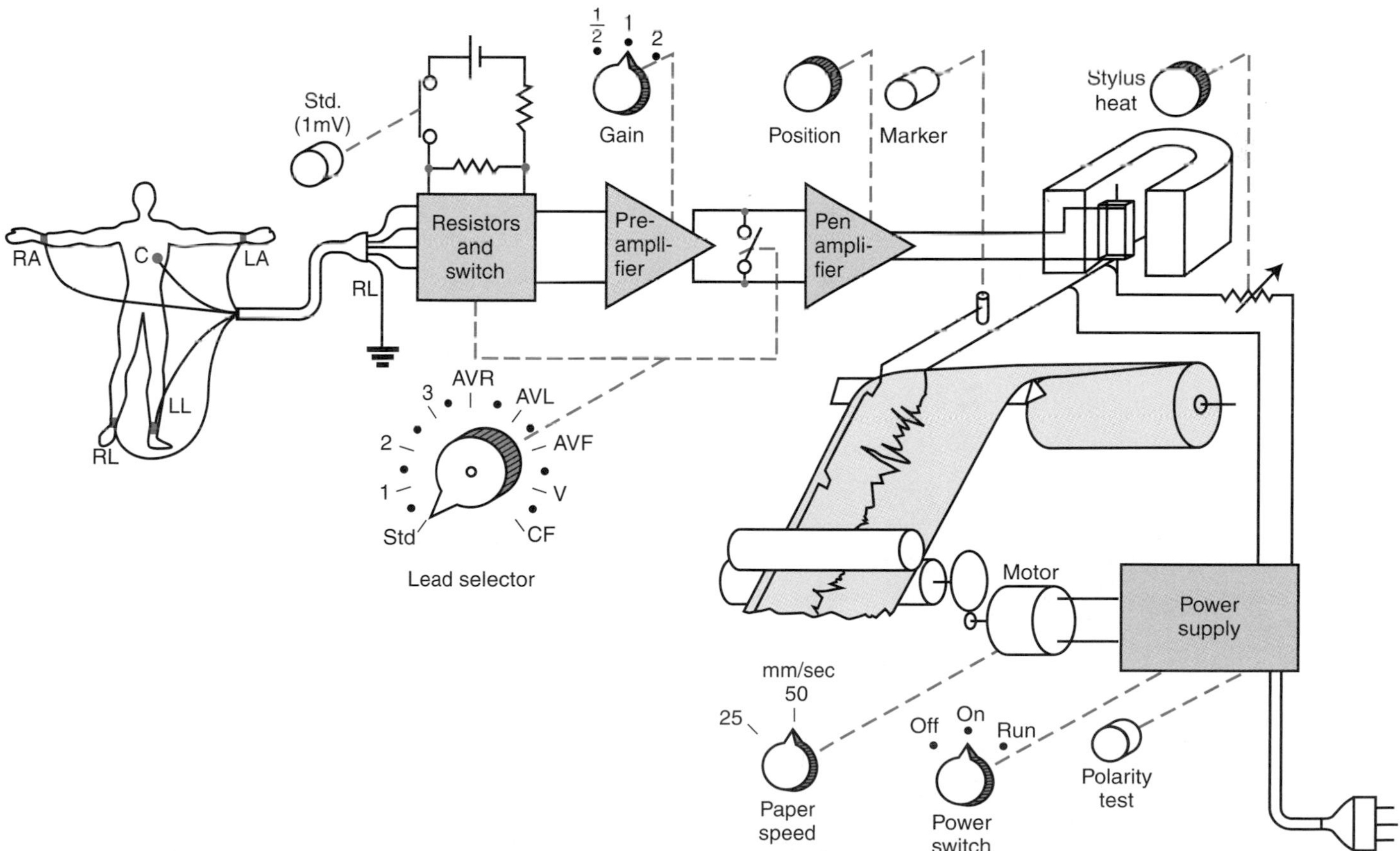

Figure 9-3 Major components of an electrocardiograph. (Modified from Cromwell L, Weibell FJ, Pfeiffer EA: *Biomedical instrumentation and measurements*, Englewood Cliffs, NJ, 1980, Prentice-Hall.)

provide accurate and reliable results, their use in clinical electrocardiography has waned since the introduction of disposable floating electrodes. Floating electrodes consist of a silver-silver chloride electrode that is encased within a plastic housing. The surface of the electrode is covered with a conductive gel or paste. The entire electrode assembly can be attached to the skin with a double-sided ring, which adheres to the patient's skin and to the plastic housing of the electrode. These electrodes are referred to as "floating" electrodes because the only conductive path between the electrode and the patient's skin is the electrolyte gel or paste.

Lead Configurations

The standard electrocardiogram includes 12 leads: 3 standard limb leads, 3 augmented limb leads, and 6 precordial or chest leads. The standard limb leads plus the augmented limb leads are oriented in a hexaxial arrangement that gives

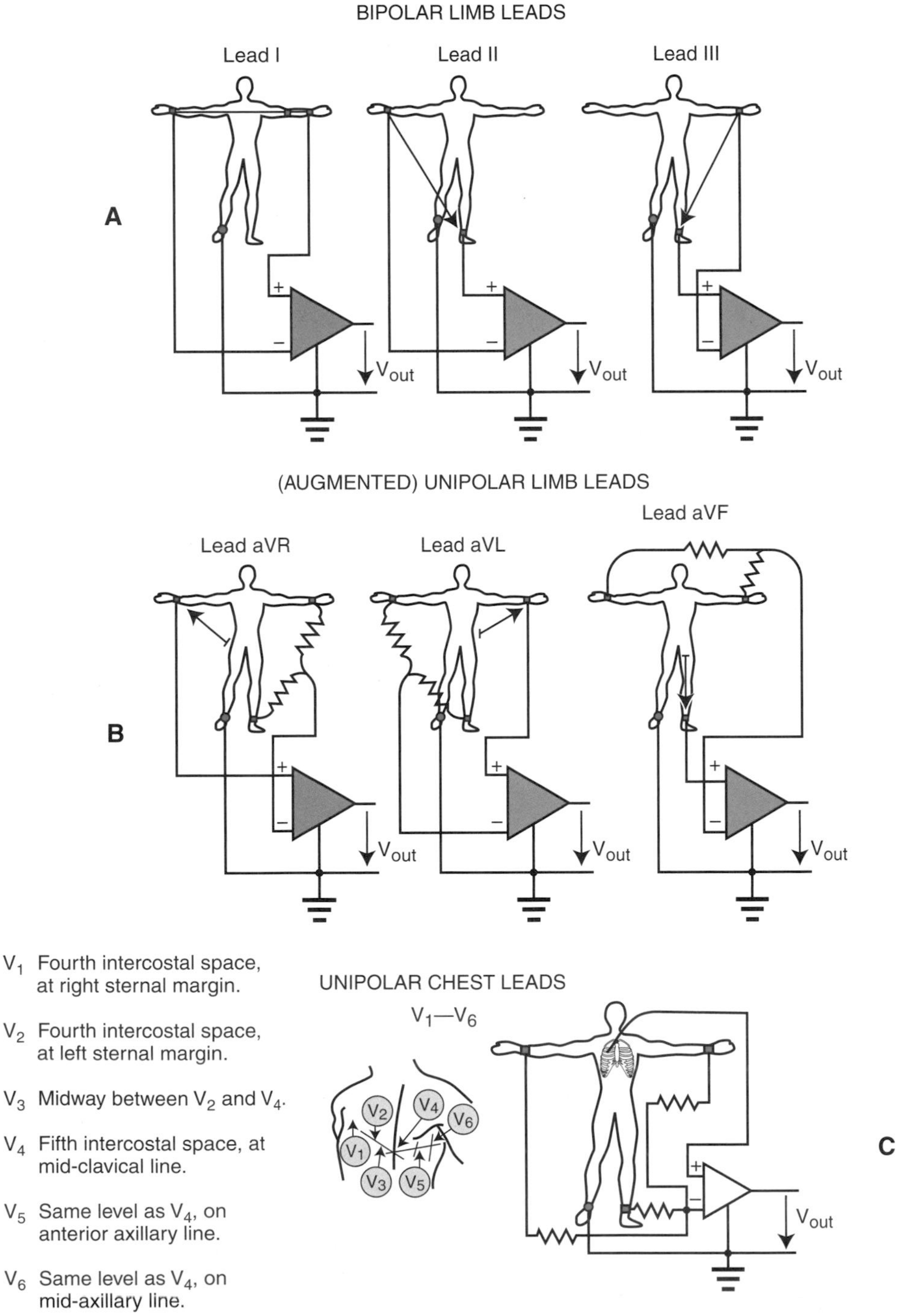
BIPOLAR LIMB LEADS
Lead I
Lead II
Lead III
A
V_{out}
(AUGMENTED) UNIPOLAR LIMB LEADS
Lead aVR
Lead aVL
Lead aVF
B
V_1 Fourth intercostal space, at right sternal margin.
V_2 Fourth intercostal space, at left sternal margin.
V_3 Midway between V_2 and V_4.
V_4 Fifth intercostal space, at mid-clavical line.
V_5 Same level as V_4, on anterior axillary line.
V_6 Same level as V_4, on mid-axillary line.
UNIPOLAR CHEST LEADS
V_1—V_6
C

Figure 9-4 ECG lead systems. **A,** Standard limb leads; **B,** augmented limb leads; **C,** precordial (chest) leads. (Modified from Cromwell L, Weibell FJ, Pfeiffer EA: *Biomedical instrumentation and measurements*, Englewood Cliffs, NJ, 1980, Prentice-Hall.)

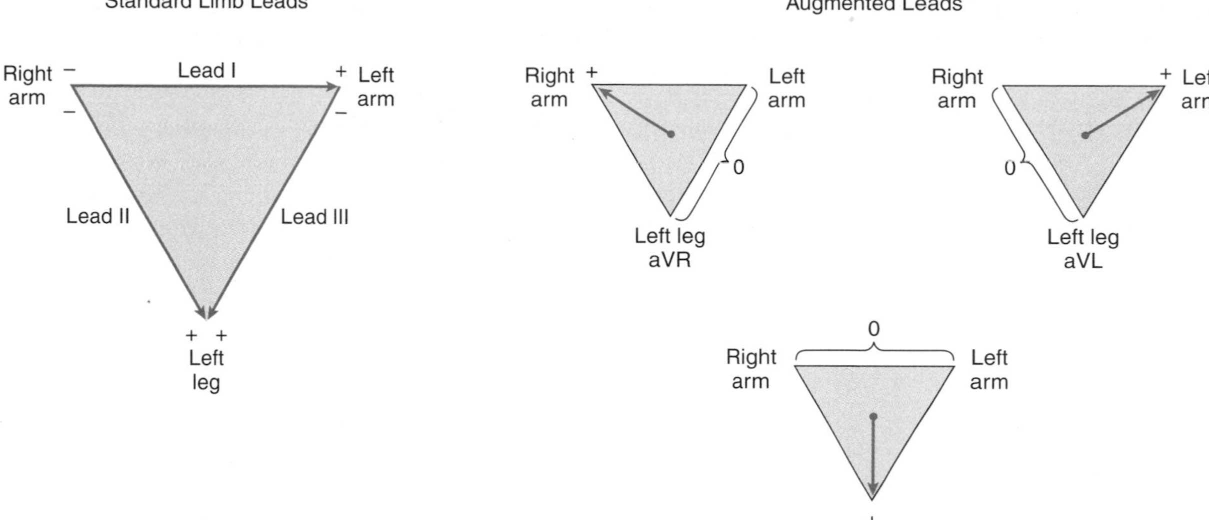

Figure 9-5 Einthoven's triangle.

information about the frontal plane of the heart (i.e., the frontal plane of the heart is divided into six different angles). The chest leads provide information about electrical activity of the heart when it is observed in the horizontal plane. Figure 9-4 shows electrode placement for a standard 12-lead ECG.

The standard limb leads, which are designated leads I, II, and III form an equilateral triangle or as it is often referred to as *Einthoven's triangle* (Figure 9-5). These leads are bipolar with one positive electrode and one negative electrode. In lead I, the right arm is negative and the left arm is positive. In lead II, the right arm is negative and the left leg is positive. In lead III, the left arm is negative and the left leg is positive. In all of the standard limb leads, the right leg electrode serves as a ground. Notice that the limb electrodes may be attached to the torso rather than on the arms (i.e., *Mason-Liker* lead configurations).[4]

The augmented leads, which are designated leads aVR, aVL, and aVF are all unipolar, that is, each lead is arranged such that each one of the three limb electrodes is designated as the positive electrode whereas the other two are taken together to be zero or the reference electrode. For example, in lead aVR the right arm is the positive electrode whereas the left arm and left leg electrodes compose the zero reference. In lead aVL, the left arm is positive and the right arm and left leg taken together are the zero reference. For lead aVF, the left leg is positive and the right arm and left arm taken together are the reference. The term augmented is applied to these electrodes because the waveforms generated with these lead configurations are typically electronically amplified one and one-half times the recorded amplitude before being displayed.[3]

The precordial or chest leads V_1 to V_6 are unipolar leads arranged around the chest. In these leads, the positive or exploring electrode is located at a standard position on the chest as shown in Figure 9-4; the three limb electrodes are averaged together to create a reference or the central terminal. In special cases, additional precordial leads may be used, including leads V_7, V_8, V_9, and V_3R, V_4R, V_5R, V_6R, V_7R, V_8R, and V_9R. Note that V_7 is located in the fifth intercostal space at the posterior axillary line.[4] Leads V_8 and V_9 are located at the angle of the scapula, over the spine at the level of V_3 and V_4. V_3R through V_9R are placed on the right side of the chest in the position oriented similarly to those of V_3 through V_9.[4]

During clinical exercise testing, modified chest leads (MCL) are often used to monitor patients with suspected dysrhythmias. These leads include a positive electrode in the V_3 or V_5 position and a negative electrode placed on the left shoulder or forehead. For example, with the mcL3 lead the positive electrode is at the V_3 position.[5] Figure 9-6 illustrates electrode placement for mcL3.

ECG Recorders

The typical ECG recorder includes a differential amplifier with filtering circuits and an output display, such as a strip chart recorder or a CRT (Figure 9-7). The differential amplifier and filtering circuits serve to increase the power output of the electrical signals detected by the surface electrodes and to remove extraneous electrical interference. Electrical interference or "noise" can be caused by action potentials generated by skeletal muscle (electromyographic interference), fluorescent lights, and television and radio signals, as well as by other electrical monitoring devices that are attached to the patient. A special circuit that allows for a 1 mV standardization voltage to be introduced into the system is also included in the central processing unit so that the output display can be calibrated. In older ECG systems, a lead selector switch is used to access information from each of the 12 standard leads. Newer systems contain microprocessors that automatically access each of the standard 12 leads in sequence.

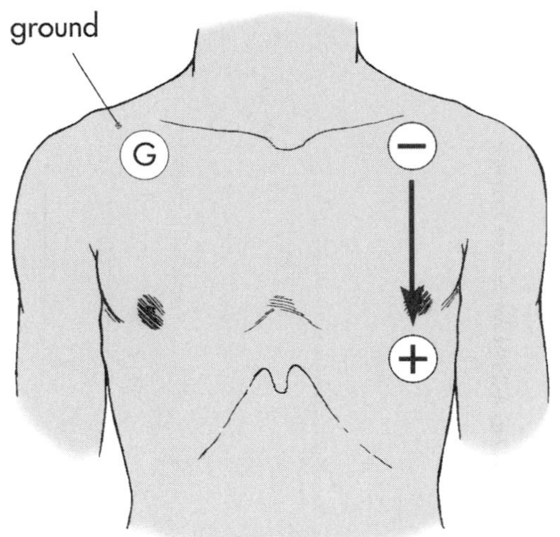

Figure 9-6 Electrode placement for modified chest leads (MCL3)

Most electrocardiographs contain direct-writing recorders for providing a permanent ECG records, as well as a CRT for long-term monitoring. For direct-writing strip chart recorders, the ECG is inscribed on a moving sheet of heat-sensitive paper with an electrically heated stylus. The paper upon which the ECG is recorded is ruled in lines 1 mm apart, both vertically and horizontally. As discussed in the next section, when properly standardized, the amplitude and duration of waves, complexes, and intervals can be determined from the electrocardiogram.

The Normal Electrocardiogram

Figure 9-8 illustrates the main waves, complexes and intervals normally seen on an electrocardiogram.[2,6] (The ECG waveform shown in this figure is derived from lead II. Note that the amplitude of each of the waves will vary depending on the lead being examined and the vectors of depolarization and repolarization.) It is important to understand that all ECGs are standardized, that is, ECGs are recorded on paper that is ruled in millimeters in the horizontal and vertical planes. Notice that there are heavy lines every fifth millimeter, both in the horizontal and vertical directions. When recording an ECG, the paper speed is set so that it moves at a speed of 25 mm per second, which is equal to 1500 mm per minute. As such, time is recorded on the x-axis, with each millimeter representing 0.04 seconds and 0.2 seconds between each heavy vertical line. Marks are

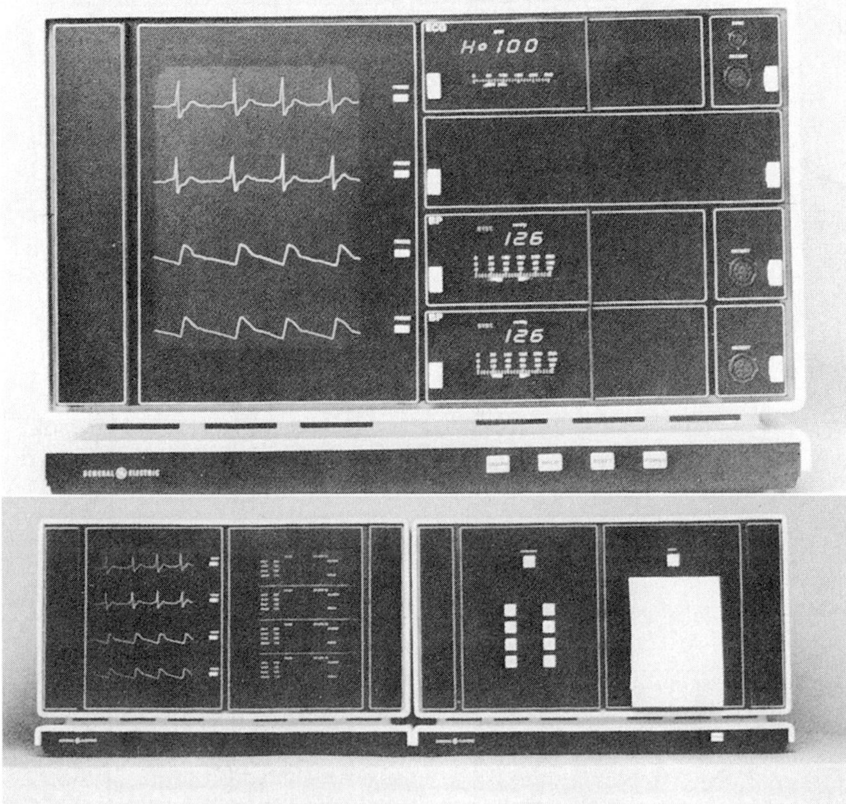

Figure 9-7 Typical electrocardiogram monitor used in a critical care unit. (Courtesy General Electric Company, Medical Systems Division, Milwaukee, Wis.)

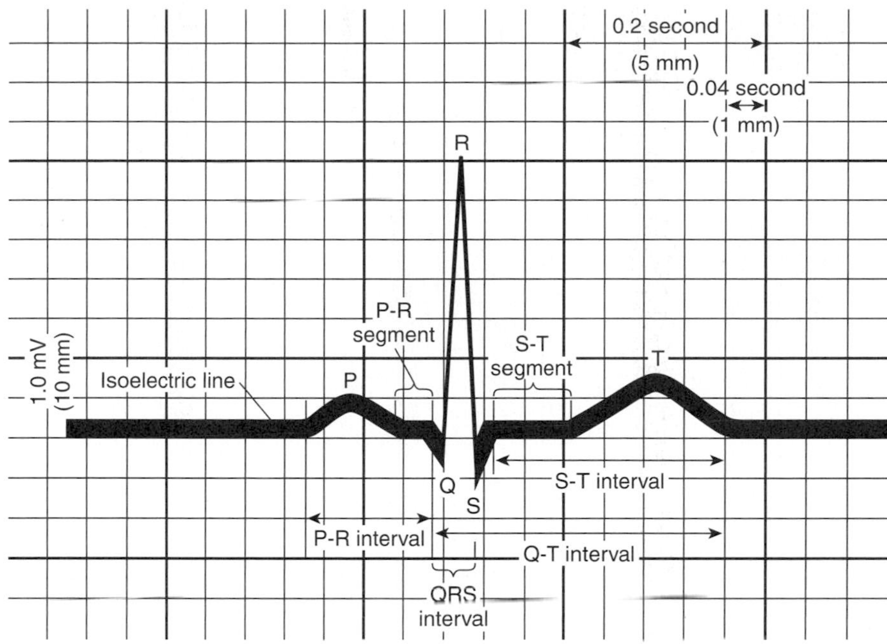

Figure 9-8 Normal electrocardiogram showing waves, complexes, and intervals.

often seen at 75-mm intervals along the top of the strip, corresponding to 3-second intervals. ECGs are also calibrated so that each millimeter on the y-axis is equal to 0.1 mV. Therefore, a 10-mm deflection vertically equals 1 mV.

Waves, Complexes, and Intervals

P wave

The P wave represents depolarization of the atria. As previously discussed, atrial depolarization normally begins at the SA node and travels from right to left and toward the AV node. The P wave is upward in leads I, II, aVF, and V_3 to V_6. It is usually inverted in leads aVR, V_1, and sometimes V_2. The P wave is normally 0.1 to 0.3 mV in amplitude and 0.06 to 0.10 seconds in duration. Atrial disease is associated with a prolongation of the P wave to greater than 0.1 second.

PR Interval

The PR interval, which is the time interval between the beginning of the P wave and the beginning of the QRS complex, represents the conduction time required for an impulse that is initiated in the atria to travel through the AV node. It normally ranges from 0.12 to 0.20 seconds in duration. The PR segment, which occurs between the end of the P wave and the beginning of the QRS complex, corresponds to the 0.1-second delay that occurs as the cardiac impulse travels through the AV node. Because the delay occurs after the atrial muscle mass has depolarized completely, the PR segment is on the line of zero potential, which is called the *isoelectric* line. Blocks in conduction through the AV node, which are discussed in greater detail later, may result in either prolonged PR intervals or P waves not followed by QRS complexes. These are called first-degree, second-degree, and third-degree AV blocks. Shortening of the PR interval is associated with pre-excitation syndrome (see Wolff-Parkinson-White Syndrome in this chapter) and with atrial impulses initiated low in the atria near the AV node.

QRS Complexes

The QRS complex represents ventricular depolarization. A Q wave is defined as a downward deflection that precedes the upward deflection of an R wave; an S wave is a downward deflection following an R wave. Figure 9-9 illustrates several different types of QRS complexes that may be observed in ECGs. Under normal circumstances, the QRS duration is approximately 0.1 second because the high-speed conduction system of the bundle of His, left and right bundle branches, and the Purkinje fiber system allow rapid and complete depolarization of the ventricles. Prolonged QRS durations with abnormal appearing QRS complexes indicate ventricular muscle cell to muscle cell conduction caused by either blocks in the high-speed conduction pathway or initiation of ventricular depolarization by an ectopic focus. An ectopic beat is typically defined as electrical activation of the heart outside of the normal pacemaker cells (i.e., SA node). The QRS vector is normally upward in leads I, II, aVL, and V_5 and V_6. It is usually downward in leads aVR and V_1.

ST Segment

After the ventricles are completely depolarized, an ST segment appears on the ECG. The ventricles stay completely depolarized for a substantial interval, as noted in the discussion of the phase II plateau in the section on cardiac action potentials. The ST segment, which is measured from the

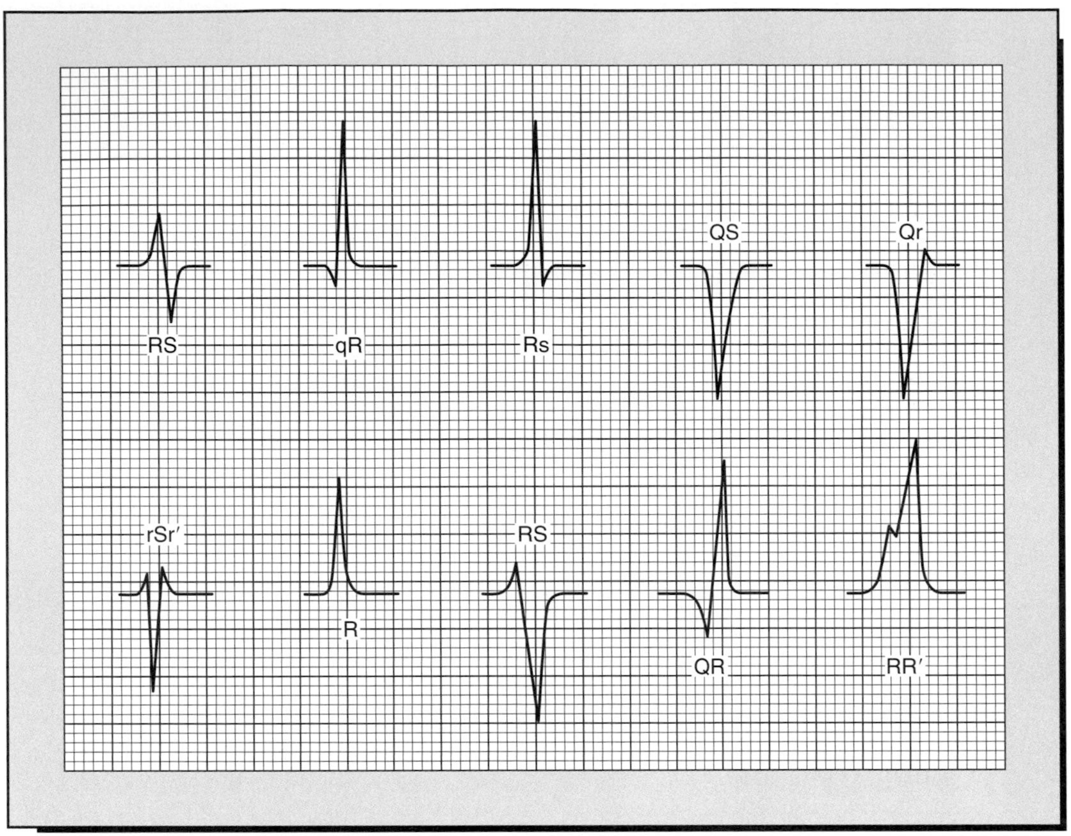

Figure 9-9 Different types of QRS complexes. (Modified from Graver K: *A practical guide to ECG interpretation*, St Louis, 1991, Mosby.)

end of the QRS complex to the beginning of the T wave, falls on the isoelectric line. ST segments above and below the isoelectric line may be seen during myocardial injury as a result of "currents of injury" caused by ions moving into and out of injured cardiac cells. The *J point*, which is the junction between the QRS complex and ST segment, is often used as a reference for describing alterations in the ST segment.

T Wave

The T wave represents ventricular repolarization. It is usually upright in all leads except aVR. At first this may seem odd because repolarization is the opposite of depolarization, but as noted previously, repolarization usually occurs in a direction opposite to that of depolarization. The T wave is usually rounded and its amplitude is less than 0.5 mV in the limb leads and less than 1.0 mV in the precordial leads. It is typically 0.1 to 0.2 seconds in duration.

Repolarization is an energy-dependent phenomenon that is mainly a function of the movement of potassium ions. Any situation compromising the energy state, such as myocardial ischemia, injury, or infarction can therefore affect this potassium balance of the heart, resulting in altered T waves. Tall T waves may suggest myocardial infarction, potassium excess, coronary ischemia, or ventricular overload. Inversion of T waves is related to coronary ischemia and injury. T-wave inversion will occur in these situations if the T wave was originally upright. If the individuals initially demonstrated inverted T waves, ischemia and injury will produce an upright T wave. This is sometimes referred to as *pseudonormalization* of the T wave.[6]

Atrial repolarization is not usually visible in the ECG because it does not represent much electrical activity and it usually occurs during ventricular depolarization.

QT Interval

This interval is measured from the beginning of the QRS complex to the end of the T wave. It represents the time required for ventricular depolarization and repolarization to occur and also approximates the time of ventricular systole. For heart rates of 60 to 100 beats per minute, the QT interval is approximately 0.4 seconds. Note that the QT interval varies inversely with the heart rate. Slowing the heart rate lengthens the QT interval while increasing the heart rate shortens the QT interval. The QT interval can be prolonged with congestive heart failure, myocardial infarction, procainamide administration, hypocalcemia, and hypomagnesemia. The QT interval is shortened by digitalis, hypocalcemia, and hyperkalemia.[7]

U Wave

The U wave follows the T wave and precedes the succeeding P wave. It is thought to represent remnants of ventricular repolarization or repolarization of the papillary muscles.

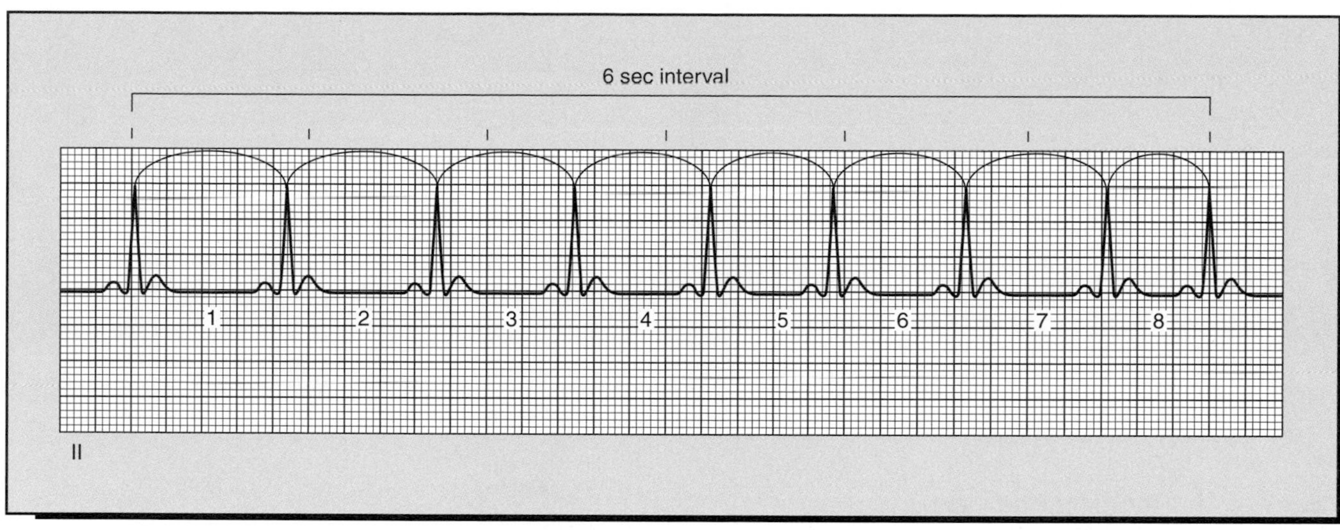

Figure 9-10 Determination of heart rate.

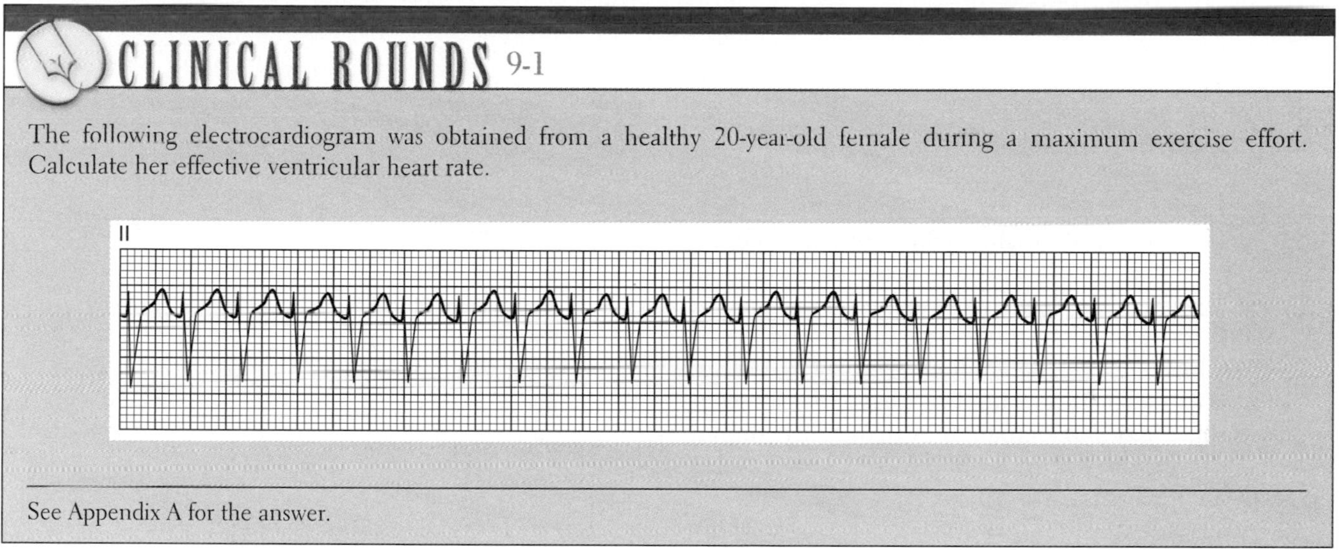

CLINICAL ROUNDS 9-1

The following electrocardiogram was obtained from a healthy 20-year-old female during a maximum exercise effort. Calculate her effective ventricular heart rate.

See Appendix A for the answer.

The amplitude and duration of U waves are considerably less than those of the T wave; however, the polarity of the U wave is normally in the same direction as the preceding T wave. When present, U-wave amplitude is made more prominent by hypokalemia and bradycardia.[7]

Interpretation of Electrocardiograms

Alterations in the initiation and the conduction of electrical impulses through the heart can result in abnormal cardiac rhythms or arrhythmias (also called dysrhythmias). A typical interpretation of an ECG contains information about the effective atrial and ventricular rates, an estimation of the mean ventricular electrical axis, and the presence of arrhythmias. The following sections of this chapter provide basic techniques for interpreting ECGs.

Determination of Rate

Figure 9-10 shows a practical method to determine the heart rate from an ECG. To calculate the heart rate, count the number of cardiac cycles during a 6-second period interval and multiply this number by 10. This can be easily accomplished because most ECG paper has vertical markings on the top of the paper corresponding to 3-second intervals when the paper speed is 25 mm per second. Alternatively, if the patient's heart rate is fairly constant, you can calculate the effective ventricular rate by counting the number of millimeters between two successive R waves (i.e., the R-R interval) and dividing this number into 1500 (25 mm per second equals 1500 mm per minute). The atrial rate can be calculated similarly by dividing the P-P interval or the number of millimeters between two successive P waves into 1500. Test your ability to calculate heart rate using the ECG shown in Clinical Rounds 9-1.

Mean Electrical Axis

As discussed previously, the mean ventricular axis of the heart represents the average direction and magnitude of the electrical activity of the heart. Figure 9-11 illustrates a method for determining the mean ventricular axis. Ordinarily, the frontal plane electrical axis is determined from the standard

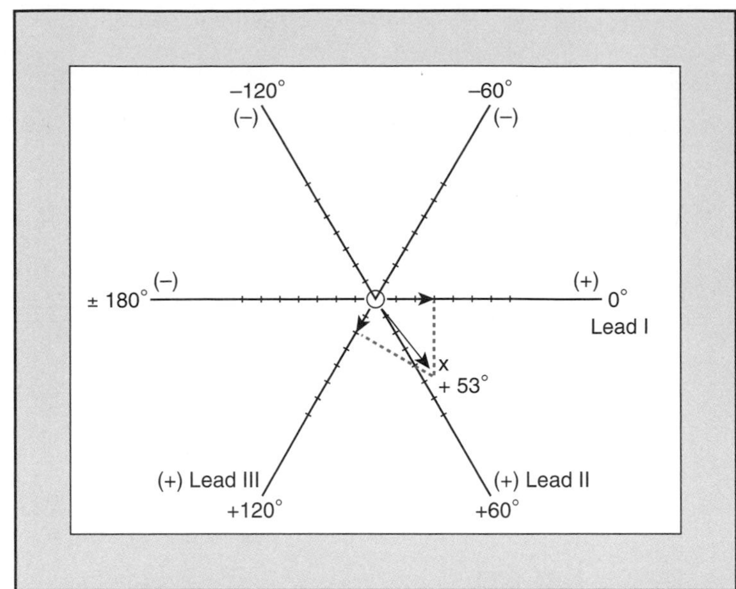

Figure 9-11 Simplified method for calculating mean ventricular axis. The amplitude of the QRS complexes is plotted on the lead I and lead III axes, respectively. The axis is established by determining the resolved vector for these two values.

limb leads. In healthy subjects, the mean ventricular axis is between −30 and +105 degrees because of the anatomic position of the heart within the thorax and because the muscle mass of the left ventricle is approximately three times greater than that of the right ventricle. The axis rotates more to the left in normal subjects during expiration and when a subject lies down because the diaphragm rises. Rotation to the right occurs during inspiration and when a subject assumes an upright position. Chronic changes in the mean ventricular axis of the heart occur in pathologic conditions, such as left or right ventricular hypertrophy, myocardial infarction, and during interventricular conduction delays or bundle branch blocks.

Pattern Regularity

To determine the presence of an abnormal rhythm, you should ask the following questions while observing the ECG. First, are P waves present? Is each QRS complex preceded by a P wave, that is, is there a 1:1 relationship between the number of P waves and the number of QRS complexes present? Does each of the P waves present have the same contour or do they vary from beat to beat? Is the time interval between the initiation of the P wave and the QRS complex less than 0.2 seconds? Furthermore, does the PR interval have a repeatable value or does it continually vary? Notice the contour of the QRS complexes. Is the QRS interval less than 0.1 seconds? If the QRS complexes are prolonged, do the QRS complexes show any abnormal notching? Next, look at the contour of the T wave. Is it peaked, depressed, or inverted? Finally, evaluate the position of the ST segment. Is it elevated or depressed below the isoelectric line by 2 mm for 0.08 seconds or greater? As you will see in the following section on identifying specific arrhythmias, using these criteria will lessen much of the difficulty associated with interpreting ECGs. Box 9-1 summarizes the various criteria that can be used to identify common arrhythmias encountered in clinical practice.

Box 9-1 Interpretation of Electrocardiograms

1. Rate
   a. Atrial rate
   b. Ventricular rate
2. Rhythm (Supraventricular versus Ventricular Rhythm)
   a. Presence of P waves
   b. Measure the PR interval
   c. QRS duration
   d. QT duration
   e. Presence of premature atrial or ventricular beats
3. Conduction Disturbances
   a. AV Blocks
   b. Intraventricular (bundle branch) blocks
4. Mean Ventricular Electrical Axis
   a. Chamber enlargement (hypertrophy)
5. Ischemia and Infarction
   a. ST segment displacement
   b. T wave changes
   c. Abnormal Q waves
6. Miscellaneous Findings
   a. Drug effects
   b. Electrolyte disturbances

Box 9-2 lists the most common rhythms and dysrhythmias encountered in clinical medicine. They are described briefly in the following sections; examples of each may be found in

Figures 9-12 through 9-20. Also note that unless stated otherwise, each of the arrhythmias shown is illustrated using lead II.

Box 9-2 Common Cardiac Rhythms and Arrhythmia Encountered in Clinical Practice

Supraventricular Rhythms

Sinus Rhythms
- Normal sinus rhythm
- Sinus tachycardia
- Sinus bradycardia
- Respiratory sinus arrhythmia

Atrial Tachycardia

Atrial Flutter

Atrial Fibrillation

Junctional (Nodal) rhythms

Ventricular Rhythms

Ventricular tachycardia

Ventricular fibrillation

Wolff-Parkinson-White syndrome

Heart Blocks

Intraventricular (bundle branch) blocks

Atrioventricular Blocks
- First degree
- Second degree (Mobitz I and Mobitz II)
- Third degree (complete)

Abnormal Beats

Premature atrial beat

Premature junctional beats

Premature ventricular beats

Sinus Rhythms (Figure 9-12)

Remember that under normal circumstances, the heart rate is determined by the number of times that the SA node depolarizes per minute. In healthy subjects, if the resting heart rate is 60 to 100 beats per minute and each QRS complex is preceded by a normally appearing P wave, then the rhythm is referred to as a **normal sinus rhythm.**

In **sinus tachycardia,** the SA node remains the source of cardiac excitation; but the ventricular rate exceeds 100 beats per minute. Stimulation of the autonomic nervous system, as occurs with the administration of sympathomimetic amines (e.g., isoproterenol or epinephrine) or drugs that block parasympathetic impulses to the heart (e.g., atropine) cause considerable increases in heart rate. Sinus tachycardia can also result from exertion, ingestion of large quantities of caffeine or nicotine, fever, anemia, hypoxemia, hypotension, myocardial ischemia, thyrotoxicosis, pulmonary emboli, and congestive heart failure.

Sinus bradycardia refers to heart rates that are less than 60 beats per minute. Again, each QRS complex is preceded by a P wave. This rhythm is caused by increased vagal tone, as occurs during carotid sinus massage and after the administration of β-adrenergic blocking agents (e.g., propranolol). Clinically, sinus bradycardia is most often associated with hypothermia, eye surgery, increased intracranial pressure, cervical and mediastinal tumors, vomiting, myxedema, and vasovagal syncope. (Note that well-trained athletes may demonstrate sinus bradycardia because of an improved ventricular stroke volume. It is not uncommon for these individuals to have resting heart rates as low as 40 beats per minute.)

The term **sinus arrhythmia** is used to describe a regular acceleration of the heart rate during inspiration followed by a slowing of the heart rate during expiration. It should be noted that although these variations in heart rate may be quite exaggerated, all QRS complexes have a normal duration and they are all preceded by P waves. Additionally, the PR

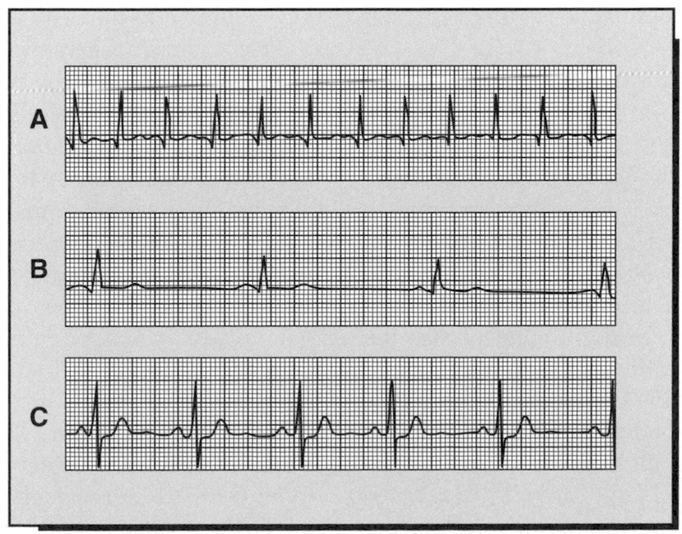

Figure 9-12 Sinus rhythms. **A,** Sinus tachycardia; **B,** sinus bradycardia; **C,** respiratory sinus arrhythmia.

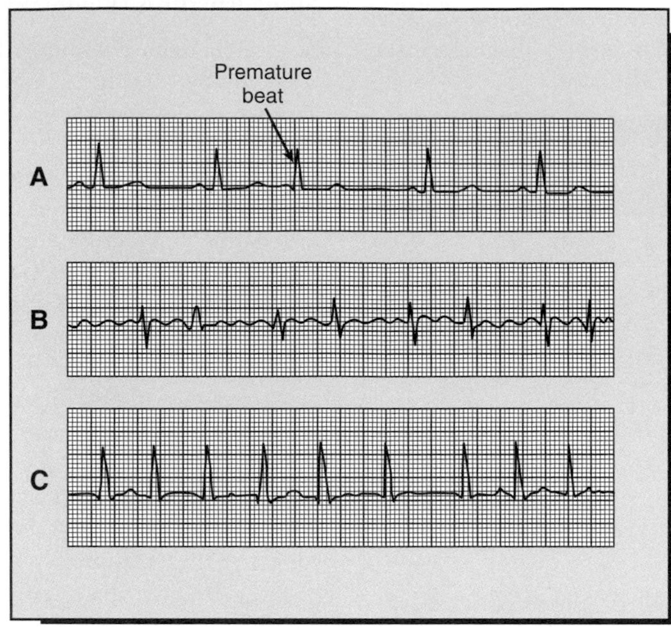

Figure 9-13 Supraventricular arrhythmias. **A,** Atrial premature depolarizations; **B,** atrial flutter; **C,** atrial fibrillation.

interval has a normal duration. Sinus arrhythmias are common findings in children and young adults. (It has been suggested that sinus arrhythmias result from the lung inflation reflex or from activation of the Bainbridge reflex-inspiration causes a reduction in intrathoracic pressure, an increase in venous return, and a consequent stretching of the atria, which ultimately leads to an increase in heart rate. Conversely, during expiration, intrathoracic pressure rises, atria filling declines, and heart rate slows.)

Supraventricular Arrhythmias

Included within this class of arrhythmias are atrial premature contractions, atrial flutter, atrial fibrillation (Figure 9-13), and junctional rhythms (Figure 9-14).

Atrial premature depolarizations are ectopic beats that can originate in any part of the atria. Atrial premature contractions, premature atrial beats, and atrial extrasystole are used synonymously when discussing these arrhythmias. These beats are characterized by P waves that come before the next expected sinus depolarization. Because the atrial premature beat may cause depolarization of the SA node, the interval between the premature P wave and the next normal sinus P wave is equal to or slightly longer than the usual P-P interval. The configuration of the atrial premature beat's P wave will vary, depending on the site of the ectopy and upon the lead being examined. For example, using lead II, if the impulse is generated high in the atria, then the P wave will have a normal upright appearance. If, however, the focus is low in the atria, then the P wave will appear inverted because the P wave axis is directed superiorly.

Atrial tachycardia usually involves atrial rates of 150 to 250 beats per minute. It can be caused by a number of agents, including stimulants such as caffeine, tobacco, and alcohol; sympathomimetic drugs; hypoxia; elevation of atrial pressure; and digitalis intoxication.

Paroxysmal atrial tachycardia (PAT) is a distinct clinical syndrome characterized by repeated episodes of atrial tachycardia with an abrupt onset lasting from a few seconds to many hours. The genesis of this type of arrhythmia is a premature atrial depolarization with a prolonged AV conduction time.[1] The prolonged AV conduction time permits the impulse to be reflected back into the atrium (i.e., reentry), resulting in the production of this type of supraventricular tachycardia. Vagal stimulation, caused by gagging, carotid sinus massage, face immersion, or the Valsalva maneuver, is often helpful in determining the underlying rhythm because these maneuvers will generally convert PAT to a normal sinus rhythm. Although PAT can be well-tolerated in healthy young adults, it can cause serious problems in elderly patients with other forms of heart disease, such as coronary atherosclerosis and valvular stenosis. In this latter group of patients, PAT can lead to myocardial ischemia, infarction, or pulmonary edema.

In **atrial flutter,** the atrial rate is regular and ranges from 250 to 350 beats per minute. The ventricular rate typically is about 125 to 150 beats per minute and it is regular if a constant degree of AV block is present. Atrial flutter waves (*F waves*) replace the normal P waves to give the ECG a characteristic: "sawtooth" or "picket fence" appearance.

As with atrial flutter, **atrial fibrillation** is characterized by gross irregularities in both atrial and ventricular depolarization. The atrial rate is usually 400 to 700 per minute, but generally cannot be quantified. P waves are replaced with fibrillatory waves. As shown in Figure 9-13, these fibrillatory waves vary in size and shape and they are irregular in rhythm, causing an undulation of the baseline on the ECG. The ventricular rate is between 120 and 200 beats per minute. Note that this ventricular rate occurs because not every atrial depolarization that reaches the AV node will be transmitted because of the inherent refractoriness of the AV node. Thus only depolarization that arrive at a period when the AV node is not refractory, as well as have sufficient strength will be transmitted into the ventricles.

Atrial fibrillation may occur intermittently or as a chronic arrhythmia, in which case it is the result of some underlying form of heart disease, such as mitral stenosis, thyrotoxicosis, chronic pericarditis, and congestive heart failure. It is also a common finding in patients recovering from a myocardial infarction, particularly during exercise. It may, however, occur paroxysmally in individuals with no apparent heart disease.

Junctional rhythms (Figure 9-14) are impulses that originate in or near the AV node. The P wave may precede, coincide with, or follow the QRS depending on the relative conduction times from the site of origin of the impulse in the AV node to the atria and ventricles. Thus impulses generated high in the AV node will likely be associated with a P wave occurring before the QRS complex, whereas impulses generated low in the AV node will result in a P wave that will follow the QRS complex. Note that because of the retrograde transmission of the impulse into the atria that the P wave will appear inverted in those ECG leads that face the left side of the heart (e.g., leads II, III, aVF), whereas it will appear upright in those leads that face the right side of the heart (e.g., leads aVR, V_1).

Junctional rates may vary from 40 to 60 beats per minute to well over 100 beats per minute. In the case of slower heart rates, the junctional rhythm may serve as an escape mechanism to protect ventricular function. This phenomenon occurs when the SA node either fails to depolarize or impulses generated by the SA node or atria fail to be conducted to the AV node. If the AV node is not depolarized within 1 to 1.5 seconds, it will initiate an impulse called an escape beat. A series of these beats is therefore called a **junctional escape rhythm.** Junctional rates greater than 100 beats per minute can occur because of an inherent instability in the AV node caused by ischemia or by some toxin. This latter type of junctional rhythm is referred to as junctional tachycardia.

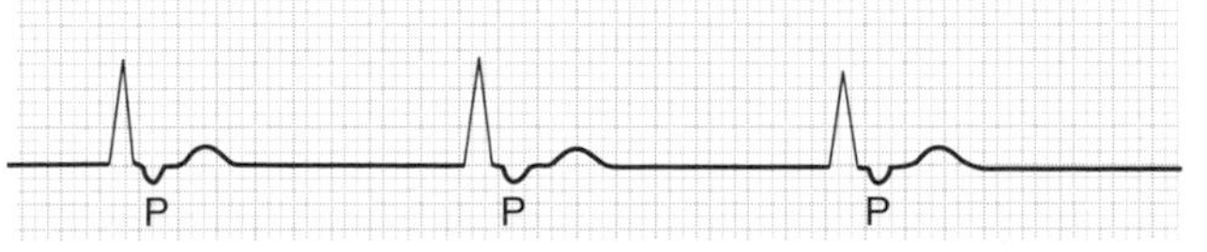

Figure 9-14 Junctional rhythm.

Ventricular Rhythms

Ventricular arrhythmias include **premature ventricular beats, ventricular tachycardia,** and **ventricular fibrillation** (Figure 9-15). Premature ventricular beats (PVBs), which are often called premature ventricular contractions (PVCs), occur when ectopic impulses originate in the ventricles before the normal sequence of depolarization beginning at the SA node. PVBs are characterized by the absence of P waves and the presence of wide QRS complexes (duration >0.12 seconds) that result from sequential activation of the two ventricles rather than the usual simultaneous activation. (Also, remember that the QRS duration will be prolonged resulting from cell-to-cell conduction rather than through the normal high-speed conduction pathways in the His-Purkinje system.) Because this type of abnormal depolarization affects repolarization, T waves will also be affected (i.e., inverted T waves).

In some instances, ectopic beats originating in the ventricles are conducted to the AV node and into the atria, resulting in inverted P waves. However, in most cases, this does not occur, and the impulses generated in the ventricles are blocked from entering the atria; consequently, the SA node is unaffected by the abnormal impulse. Thus the SA node will continue to fire at its own inherent rate. Because the ventricles will be refractory to any stimuli after activation, the ventricles will typically show a "compensatory pause" between the generation of the PVB and the next normally conducted depolarization. You can see this on an ECG by noting that the duration of two cardiac cycles (including the PVB) is the same as the duration of two normal cycles.

Premature ventricular depolarizations may occur alone or as multiples. Ventricular bigeminy refers to a rhythm in which every other beat is a premature ventricular beat. Ventricular trigeminy is used to describe the presence of a PVB on every third beat. **Ventricular tachycardia** exists when three or more PVBs occur in succession at a rate in excess of 100 beats per minute. Usually during ventricular tachycardia there is atrioventricular dissociation, meaning simply that the atria are depolarizing at a rate that is independent of the ventricular rate. P waves may be discernible between successive QRS complexes in ventricular tachycardia, but generally they are hard to find. Occasionally, an impulse originating in the SA node reaches the AV node and ventricles during a period when the ventricles are not in a refractory period. The SA node depolarization will therefore be conducted into the ventricles resulting in the production of a normal QRS complex or a "captured" beat.

PVBs can occur in normal healthy subjects who ingest large quantities of caffeine, alcohol, or tobacco, or who are experiencing abnormally high levels of physical or mental stress. Ventricular tachycardia is usually associated with myocardial ischemia and infarction, excessive adrenergic

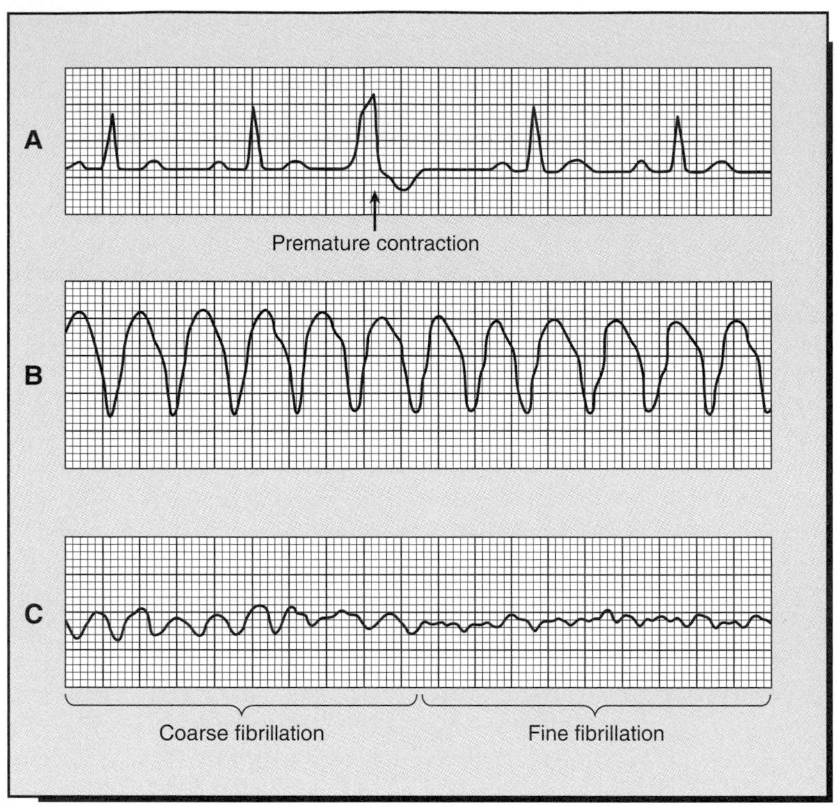

Figure 9-15 Ventricular arrhythmias. **A,** Premature ventricular beats; **B,** ventricular tachycardia; **C,** ventricular fibrillation.

stimulation, and digitalis toxicity. Premature ventricular depolarization that occurs during the T wave (i.e., during the ventricle's vulnerable period or supernormal period that occurs in the period immediately after the relative refractory period) may cause ventricular tachycardia and possibly even ventricular fibrillation.

In ventricular fibrillation, there are no effective ventricular contractions occurring, with the result that there is no cardiac output. The ECG can show "coarse" or "fine" fibrillatory waves that have replaced the normal PQRST waves. The terms coarse and *fine* refer to the amplitude of the fibrillatory waves. Ventricular fibrillation should be treated immediately with cardiopulmonary resuscitation (CPR), including the establishment of a patent airway so that the patient can be ventilated either by mouth-to-mouth or with a self-inflating (bag-valve-mask) resuscitator, external chest wall compressions; pharmacologic agents to maintain circulation; and the employment of electrical defibrillation. Coarse fibrillatory waves usually indicate that cardiovascular collapse has occurred recently and thus may respond to prompt defibrillation. Fine fibrillatory waves usually indicate that some time has elapsed since the onset of fibrillation and that the success rate for resuscitation may be significantly reduced.

Wolff-Parkinson-White (WPW) syndrome is an unusual rhythm that results from the presence of an abnormal route of conduction that bypasses the AV nodes as the impulse travels from the atria to the ventricles.[6,8] For most cases, this abnormal route is attributed to a group of muscle fibers called the Bundle of Kent. (It should be noted that other bypass tracts between the atria and the ventricles could also cause the WPW pre-excitation syndrome.) WPW syndrome is characterized by the presence of a P wave; however, the PR interval is abnormally short. Probably the most ominous sign of WPW is the presence of an early slurred upstroke of the QRS wave, often referred to as a delta wave. Thus there is a prolongation of the QRS complex, not because of a delay as the impulse travels through the ventricles, but because it started earlier than usual (pre-excitation). Figure 9-16 illustrates a typical tracing from a patient with WPW syndrome.

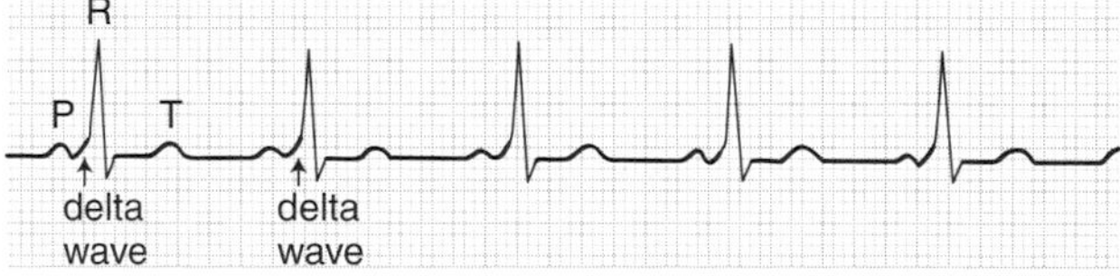

Figure 9-16 Wolff-Parkinson-White syndrome.

Ventricular asystole is the complete absence of any ventricular electrical activity and thus the absence of ventricular contractions. Ventricular asystole typically occurs after ventricular fibrillation; however, it may occur as a primary event during cardiac arrest.

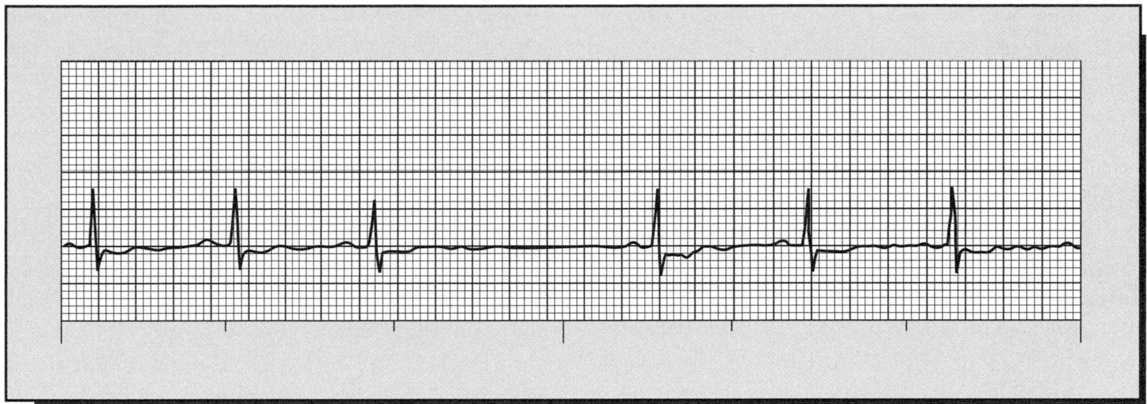

Figure 9-17 Sinoatrial conduction block.

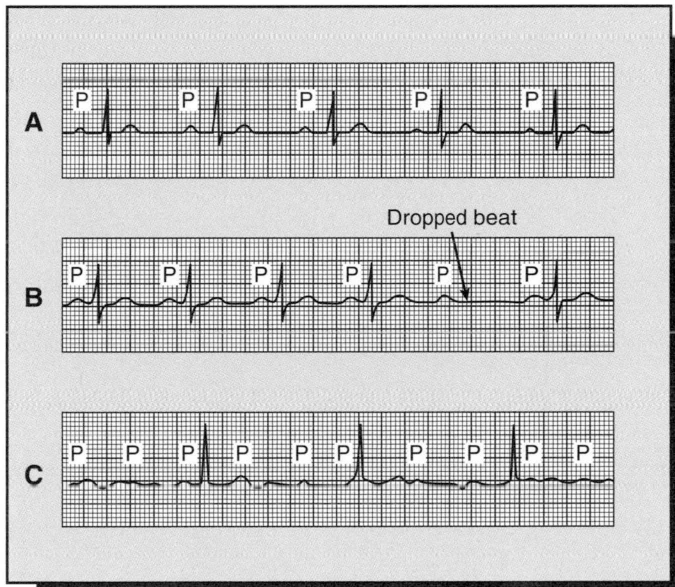

Figure 9-18 Atrioventricular blocks. **A,** First-degree block; **B,** second-degree (Mobitz II) block; **C,** third-degree block.

Heart Blocks

Heart blocks or abnormal conduction delays may occur anywhere in the heart when the refractory period at a certain point in the conduction path is prolonged. Generally, heart blocks are divided into three categories: (1) SA, (2) AV, and (3) intraventricular (bundle branch) blocks.

Sinoatrial blocks. SA blocks (Figure 9-17) occur when the impulse generated at the SA node is blocked before it can enter the atrial muscle. Typically, the ECG shows a sudden loss of P waves resulting from the absence of atrial depolarization. The contour of the QRS complex is normal but the R-R intervals are usually prolonged, indicating the presence of a junctional escape rhythm. Transient sinoatrial blocks usually do not produce symptoms; prolonged SA blocks can cause dizziness and syncope, particularly if the escape rhythm is slow.

Atrioventricular blocks. AV blocks occur when impulses generated at the SA node are abnormally prolonged or blocked in or near the AV node. Clinically, AV blocks are classified as first-degree, second-degree, or third-degree blocks. Figure 9-18 illustrates ECGs from patients demonstrating each of these conduction delays.

First-degree (1°) AV blocks are characterized by a prolongation of the PR interval (i.e., longer than 0.2 seconds), although every impulse does result in ventricular depolarization. Patients with first-degree AV blocks are generally asymptomatic if they do not demonstrate any other cardiovascular problems.

Second-degree (2°) AV blocks occur when some of the impulses generated at the SA node fail to pass through the AV node into the ventricles. The ECG shows characteristic "dropped" beats (i.e., P wave not followed by a QRS complex), resulting from a failure to conduct every impulse from the atria to the ventricles. Second-degree AV blocks may be further described as Mobitz type I (*Wenckebach*) blocks and Mobitz type II (*non-Wenckebach*) blocks. In the Mobitz type I block there is a progressive prolongation of the PR interval until at some point a QRS complex does not follow the P wave. In the Mobitz type II AV block, the PR interval does not show the progressive lengthening prior to the dropped beat.

Mobitz type I blocks are usually associated with blocking of the atrial impulses at the level of the atrial-AV node junction and they are often the result of increased parasympathetic tone or to the effects of drugs, such as digitalis or propranolol. Mobitz type II blocks typically occur below the level of the AV node, at the junction of the AV node and the bundle of His. Mobitz type II blocks are most often associated with an organic lesion in the conduction pathway. Mobitz I blocks usually do not require treatment, whereas Mobitz II blocks typically require the insertion of a permanent artificial pacemaker.

Third degree (3°) AV blocks are often referred to as complete AV blocks because there is a complete dissociation of atrial and ventricular conduction. The SA node continues to depolarize at a normal or elevated rate, but the ventricles "escape" to a slower rate. The ECG shows an atrial rate that is completely dissociated from the ventricular rate. Treatment of third-degree AV blocks usually necessitates the insertion of an artificial pacemaker if the ventricular rate is too low to permit normal activity.

Intraventricular blocks. Intraventricular blocks are also referred as *bundle branch blocks* occur when impulses are delayed or blocked in either the right or left branches of the Purkinje fiber system. The hallmark of this type of conduction delay is a prolongation of the QRS complex because, distal to the block, ventricular excitation must occur by cell-to-cell conduction.

In **right bundle branch blocks** (Figure 9-19, A), the QRS complex shows a characteristic rSR' pattern in the right precordial leads (i.e., leads V_1, V_2, and V_3) and a prolonged deep S wave in the left precordial leads (leads V_4, V_5, and V_6). Vector analysis of ECGs from patients with right bundle branch blocks demonstrate that the mean ventricular axis is shifted to the right (>90 degrees) resulting from the delayed cell-to-cell conduction through the right ventricle. Right bundle branch blocks are associated with hypertensive cardiac disease, cardiac tumors, rheumatic heart disease, pulmonary emboli, and congenital cardiac defects.

Left bundle branch blocks (Figure 9-19, *B*) are characterized by the absence of Q waves in the left limb leads (i.e., leads I and aVL) and in the left precordial leads (i.e., leads V_4, V_5, and V_6). The QRS complexes in the left precordial leads show an rsR' configuration. The mean ventricular axis is shifted to the left in this type of block (<30 degrees). Although left bundle branch blocks are less common than right bundle branch blocks, they are almost always indicative of coronary artery disease or systemic hypertension. (Other possible etiologies include aortic stenosis, myocarditis, and congenital cardiac diseases.)

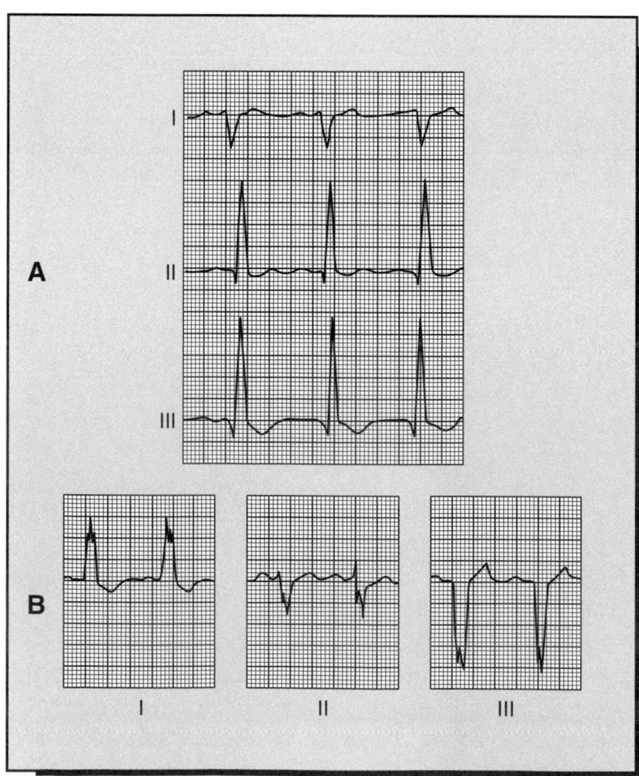

Figure 9-19 Intraventricular (bundle branch) blocks. **A,** Right bundle branch block; **B,** left bundle branch block.

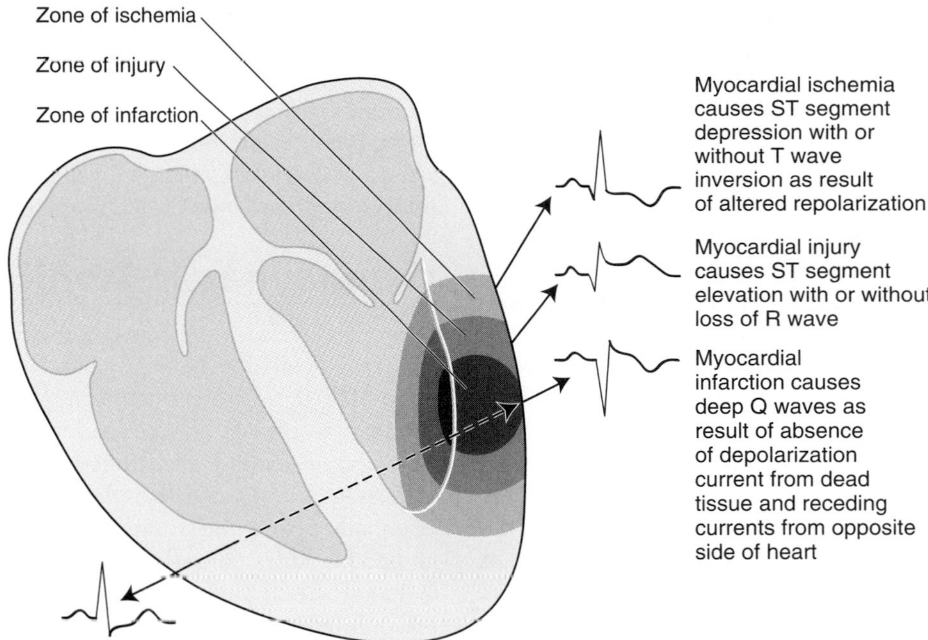
Zone of ischemia
Zone of injury
Zone of infarction
Myocardial ischemia causes ST segment depression with or without T wave inversion as result of altered repolarization
Myocardial injury causes ST segment elevation with or without loss of R wave
Myocardial infarction causes deep Q waves as result of absence of depolarization current from dead tissue and receding currents from opposite side of heart

Figure 9-20 Electrocardiogram changes associated with myocardial ischemia, injury, and infarction. (Courtesy Novartis, New York, NY.)

Table 9-2 Localization of acute myocardial infarction

ANTERIOR INFARCTS	
Anterolateral (occlusion of the anterior interventricular branch of the left coronary artery)	Deep Q waves in precordial leads V_3 to V_5 Loss of R waves in the left precordial leads (V_4 and V_5) ST segment elevation in lead I; ST segment depression in lead III
Anteroseptal (occlusion of the right division of the interventricular branch of the coronary artery)	Deep Q wave in precordial leads V_2 and V_3 Normal QRS complexes in limb leads I, II, and III S-T segment depression in limb lead II
Apical (occlusion of the terminal portions of the anterior interventricular branch of the left coronary artery)	Loss of R waves with deep Q waves in limb lead I and in precordial leads V_3 and V_4 ST segment elevation in lead I; S-T segment depression in lead III
Anterobasal (occlusion of a branch of the circumflex artery)	Small Q wave in limb lead I; large Q waves in precordial lead V_6 S-T segment elevation in leads I and V_6 T wave inversion in leads I and V_6
POSTERIOR INFARCTS	
Posteroseptal (occlusion of the right coronary artery)	S-T segment depression in precordial leads V_3 and V_4
Posteroinferior (occlusion of the posterior interventricular branch of the right coronary artery)	Large Q waves in limb leads II and III and aVF S-T segment depression in leads I, V_3, and V_4; S-T segment elevation in lead aVF
Posterolateral (occlusion of the circumflex artery)	Q waves in leads aVL and V_6 S-T segment elevation and T wave inversion in limb leads II, III, and aVL

Myocardial Ischemia and Infarction

If coronary blood flow is severely limited, as occurs with atherosclerosis or as a result of obstruction secondary to thromboembolism, the heart's oxygen demand exceeds its oxygen delivery and myocardial ischemia results. The inability of the coronary circulation to provide blood flow sufficient to meet the increased metabolic demands of the myocardium is manifest in the electrocardiogram.

As illustrated in Figure 9-20, three types of ECG changes are associated with myocardial ischemia, injury, and infarction. They are: T-wave inversion, ST segment elevation and depression, and abnormal Q waves. T-wave inversion occurs during periods of transient ischemia. Transient ischemia will affect repolarization waves before any other on ECG because this period represents the most energy sensitive activity of the heart.

ST segment alterations occur if ischemia progresses to injury. During myocardial injury, the cardiac cell membrane or sarcolemma is not able to maintain its integrity, and ions continue to stream into and out of the myocardial cells. These so-called currents of injury are responsible for depression or elevation of the ST segment.

If cardiac tissue is deprived of blood for a prolonged amount of time, the tissue will die, leading to a myocardial infarction or MI. The most characteristic finding in myocardial infarction is the presence of abnormal Q waves. These abnormal Q waves are most notable on the left precordial leads in those myocardial infarctions that involve the left anterior descending and circumflex branches of the left coronary artery. These Q waves occur because there is a lack of counterbalancing electrical forces on the affected side, thus resulting in the unaffected side demonstrating the predominant electrical forces. As a consequence, downward deflection (Q wave) rather than an upright (R) wave appears on the ECG.

Both clinical and basic research has provided valuable information about localizing myocardial infarctions by electrocardiography. Table 9-2 lists the common electrocardiographic changes associated with inadequate blood flow to various arteries supplying the heart.[6] A note of caution should be mentioned concerning ECG findings associated with myocardial infarction. Abnormal T waves, ST segment amplitude, and Q waves can occur with other serious cardiac disorders. For example, T-wave changes and ST-segment displacements (elevation or depression) are associated with pericarditis, as well as myocardial ischemia, injury, and infarction (Clinical Rounds 9-2).

Hemodynamic Monitoring

Hemodynamic measurements provide valuable information about the mechanical function of the cardiovascular system as compared with the electrocardiogram, which provides information about the electrical activity of the heart. To fully appreciate the significance of these measurements, you should recognize that the cardiovascular system is essentially a hydraulic system, which consists of a pump that propels liquid (i.e., blood) through a series of branched tubes or blood vessels (i.e., arteries, capillaries, veins) to supply the various organ systems of the body.

A functional description of any hydraulic system requires simultaneous evaluation of a variety of parameters to provide a reasonable estimate of its performance characteristics.[9,10] Thus the amount of force that the heart must generate to

CLINICAL ROUNDS 9-2

A 45-year-old male is admitted to the emergency department complaining of shortness of breath and angina. The patient appears diaphoretic and cyanotic. The following 12-lead electrocardiogram was obtained on admission. What are the most significant electrocardiographic findings?

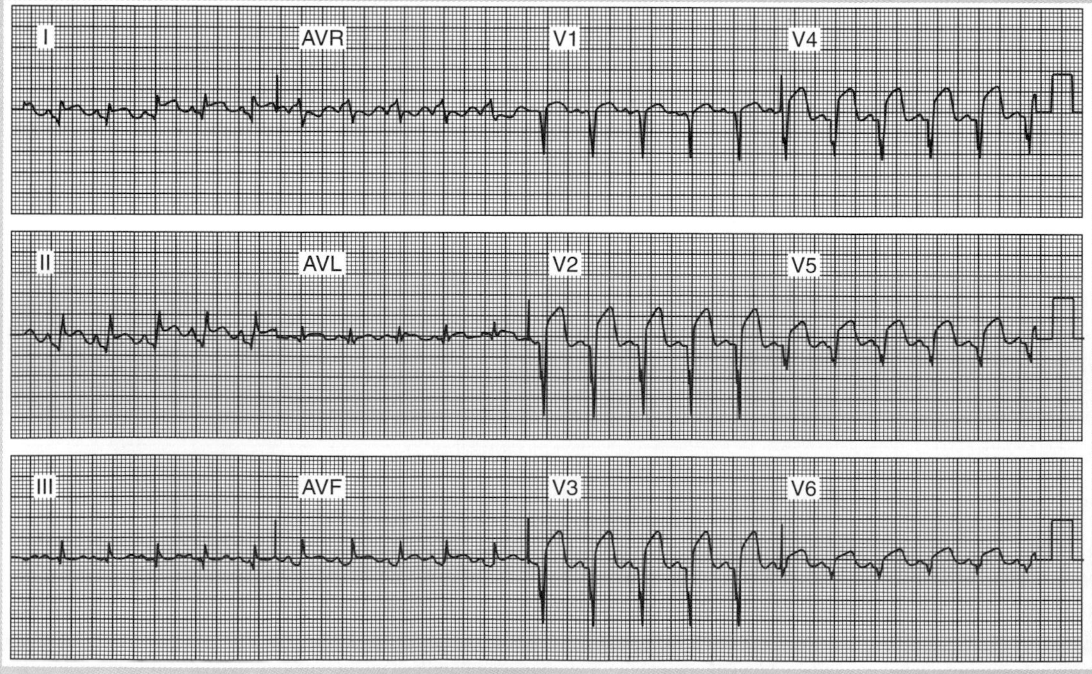

See Appendix A for the answer.

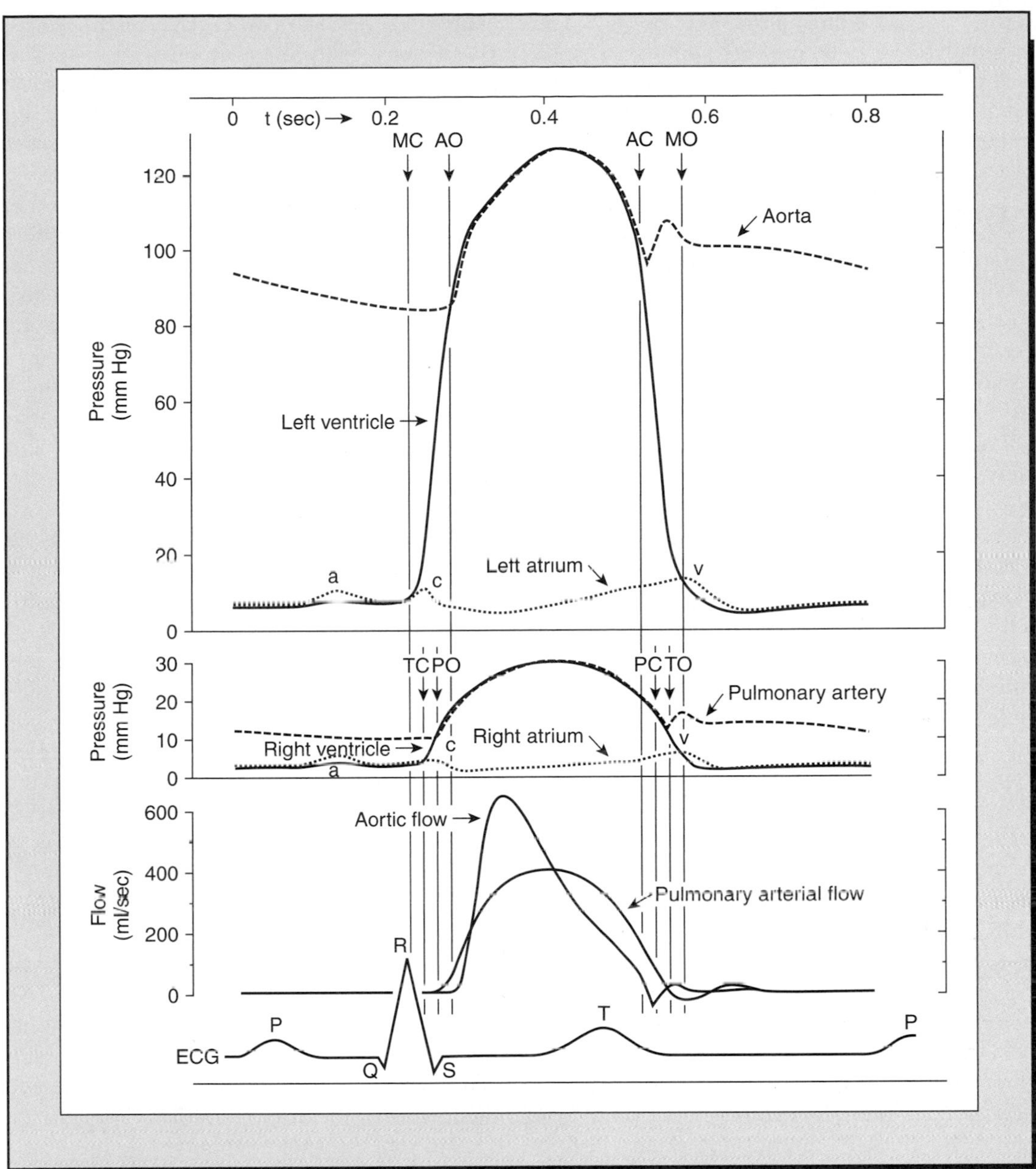

Figure 9-21 Pressure, volume, and flow changes that occur in the ventricles and great vessels during a typical cardiac cycle for a normal healthy individual. (Redrawn from Milnor WR: *Hemodynamics*, ed 2, Baltimore, 1989, Williams & Wilkins.)

propel the blood through the circulation depends on the impedance offered by these blood vessels. As such, measurements of intracardiac and intravascular pressures and cardiac output, along with computation of vascular resistance can provide fundamental information about the mechanical properties of the cardiovascular system and its ability to perform under varying conditions.

Technologic advances in the design of sensors, recording devices, and data analysis systems have greatly improved our ability to obtain accurate and reliable data that can be used in the diagnosis and treatment of patients with various types of cardiopulmonary dysfunction. Indeed, advances in solid-state electronics made during the past decade will present possibilities for the future that were previously unimaginable.

Before describing the various devices that are routinely used to obtain hemodynamic measurements, it is worthwhile to review some basic physical principles as they apply to the heart and circulation.

Cardiac Cycle

An appropriate place to begin our discussion of hemodynamics is to describe the pressure, volume, and flow events that occur in the heart and great vessels during a single heartbeat or **cardiac cycle.** Figure 9-21 shows these events as they occur in the left and right heart chambers and the great vessels (i.e., the aorta and the pulmonary artery).[10] The cardiac cycle is typically divided into two periods: a systolic period when the heart muscle is contracting and ejecting blood and a diastolic period when the heart is relaxing and filling with blood. As illustrated in Figure 9-21, the cardiac cycle can be further divided into ventricular and atrial events.

Ventricular Events

Ventricular systole begins with a period of **isovolumetric contraction,** which follows the peak of the R wave on the ECG. During this period of contraction, ventricular muscle fibers shorten but the volume of blood in the ventricle remains constant. The volume remains constant because the atrioventricular valves (i.e., mitral and tricuspid valves) and the semilunar valves (aortic and pulmonary valves) are closed. (Although the term isometric contraction is often used to describe this period, it is not a true isometric contraction because some of the fibers are shortening, whereas others increase in length.[2]) During this period the left ventricular pressure increases from 0 to about 80 mm Hg, whereas the right ventricular pressure increases from 0 to about 12 mm Hg.

As the ventricular muscle fibers continue to shorten and the left ventricle pressure exceeds the aortic diastolic pressure (i.e., ~80 mm Hg) and the right ventricle pressure exceeds the pulmonary artery diastolic pressure (i.e., ~12 mm Hg), a period of ejection occurs and blood flows rapidly out of the ventricles as the semilunar valves open. At this point in the cycle, the pressures in the aorta and pulmonary artery increase from their diastolic values toward their peak systolic pressures (~120 mm Hg and ~25 mm Hg, respectively). A longer phase in which the ejection of blood is considerably reduced immediately follows this period of rapid ejection and lasts until the pressures in the aorta and pulmonary artery decrease to ~80 mm Hg and ~15 mm Hg, respectively. The rapid ejection period can be distinguished from the reduced ejection period by examining the contour of the aortic and pulmonary artery flow curves. During the rapid ejection period the volume flow from the ventricle decreases sharply after the first third of the ejection. During the final two-thirds of ejection corresponding to the period of reduced ejection the flow curve tapers. Thus blood flow into the aortic and pulmonary artery increase dramatically during the early period of ejection and gradually decrease during the latter stage of ejection. Notice that the pressures in the ventricles are higher than the pressures in the great vessels during the first third of ejection whereas the reverse is true during the latter two-thirds of ventricular systole. Although it may not be apparent, the point of peak ejection occurs when the ventricular and aortic or pulmonary artery pressure tracings intersect.[1]

A period of **ventricular diastole** begins with closure of the aortic and pulmonary valve and can be identified by the presence of an **incisura** on the descending limb of the aortic or pulmonary artery pressure tracings. (It is thought that this incisura, which is a small negative deflection on the aortic and pulmonary artery tracing is associated with a transient reversal of flow that results from elastic recoil of these vessels following ventricular systole, thus forcing the blood to push against the respective semilunar valve.) The period of time between the closure of the semilunar valves and the opening of the atrioventricular valves is called **isovolumetric relaxation** because the pressure in the ventricle falls dramatically, whereas the volume of the ventricle remains constant. As was described for isovolumetric contraction, the atrioventricular and semilunar valves are closed during isovolumetric relaxation. The aortic pressure gradually returns to its resting or diastolic value. This gradual decrease in pressure results from the inertia of blood flowing from the heart and to the elastic recoil of the aorta, which serves to propel the blood through the systemic circulation even after ventricular systole, has concluded. Upon opening of the atrioventricular valves, which occurs as the ventricular pressure drops below the atrial pressure, rapid ventricular filling begins. This rapid filling period typically occurs during the first third of ventricular filling and it is followed by a longer period of reduced filling or **diastasis.** Figure 9-22 illustrates the pressure-volume changes that occur during each cardiac cycle. Although it may not be apparent, these changes are expressed independent of time and thus appear as a pressure-volume loop, with pressure expressed on the abscissa or x-axis and volume plotted on the ordinate or y-axis. As you will see later in this chapter, this approach to expressing hemodynamic data can be very useful when describing the consequences of pathologic changes in cardiac and circulatory function.

Atrial Events

Atrial systole begins immediately after the P wave, which, as mentioned previously, is associated with atrial depolarization on the ECG. Atrial systole is indicated on the atrial pressure tracing as an *"a" wave.* Under normal circumstances, ventricular filling occurs mainly during the period of atrial diastole when the atrioventricular valves are open between the atria and ventricles. Atrial systole (i.e., the "atrial kick" mentioned previously) occurs just before the beginning of ventricular systole. Contraction of the atria normally contributes only a small amount of blood to ventricular filling. It can, however, contribute a significant amount of blood to ventricular filling if the heart rate is increased and the period of diastasis is reduced. This occurs during ventricular tachycardia because the higher heart rate results in a reduction in the volume of blood that passively enters the ventricle during atrial diastole.

The next important wave to notice on the atrial pressure tracing is the *"c" wave,* which occurs at the beginning of *atrial diastole.* This wave coincides with the period of ventricular systole and it is associated with a transient increase in atrial pressure as the pressure in the ventricle increases and forces the closed AV valves backwards into the atrial chamber. It should be noted that the pressures in the two atria are normally only slightly higher than the ventricular pressures, indicating that there is minimal resistance between

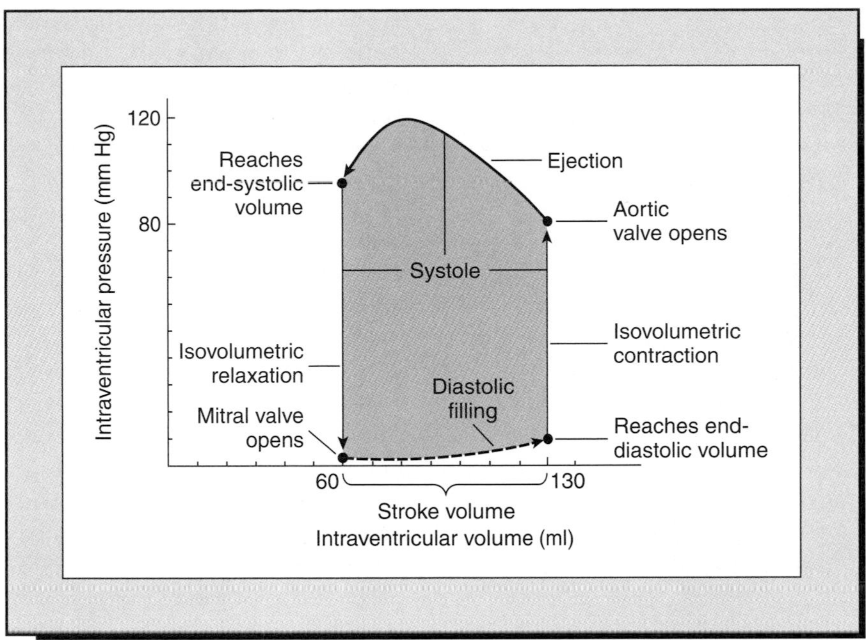

Figure 9-22 Pressure-volume graph illustrating changes during a normal cardiac cycle.

these two chambers when the valves are open. The atrial pressure wave does show a slight increase during atrial filling when the AV valves are closed and can be seen as a "*v*" *wave.* After the valves open, the pressure in the ventricle falls below the atrial pressure and the atrial pressure tracing drops sharply as blood flows from the atria into the ventricles, thus initiating the period of ventricular filling.

Heart Sounds

Four heart sounds are usually associated with the various ventricular and atrial events that occur during the cardiac cycle. These normal heart sounds are shown graphically in Figures 9-1, *A*, and 9-1, *B*. The first heart sound, typically designated as S_1, occurs at the onset of ventricular contraction and is associated with closure of the atrioventricular valves and opening of the semilunar valves. It is a relatively low-pitched, high-intensity sound that can be best heard over the apex of the heart. It has the longest duration of the four heart sounds. The second heart sound (S_2) occurs at the beginning of ventricular relaxation and is associated with closure of the semilunar valves and opening of the atrioventricular valves. It has a higher pitch and a lower intensity than the first heart sound. The duration of S_2 is shorter than S_1. The third heart sound (S_3) occurs during early ventricular filling and it is normally characterized as a low-intensity, low-frequency sound. The fourth heart sound (S_4) occurs during atrial contraction. It is also a low-intensity, low-pitched sound. Under normal circumstances, only the first two heart sounds are audible through a stethoscope. The third and fourth heart sounds are not typically heard with a stethoscope but can be amplified and recorded graphically as a **phonocardiogram.** The relationship between ventricular systole and diastole can be correlated with these various heart sounds by simply recognizing that ventricular systole occurs between S_1 and S_2 and ventricular diastole occurs during the period from S_2 to the next S_1. This division of the cardiac cycle based on heart sounds can be very useful when describing **murmurs** or abnormal heart sounds, which are associated with the generation of turbulent blood flow resulting from abnormal mechanical function of the heart, such as occurs when a valve fails to open or close properly. Thus clinicians typically describe a murmur as being a systolic murmur or a diastolic murmur depending on when it is heard relative to S_1 and S_2. Test yourself on this principle by determining whether a stiff, calcified aortic valve will cause a systolic or diastolic murmur.

Pressure Measurements

As stated in Chapter 1, pressure (P) may be defined as the force (F) exerted per unit area (A) or,

$$P = F/A$$

where pressure can be measured in pounds per square inch (lb/in^2), dynes per square centimeter (dynes/cm^2), millimeters of mercury (i.e., mm Hg), torr, centimeters of water (cm H_2O), or kilopascals (kPa). You might also remember that there are a variety of devices for measuring atmospheric pressures, most notably the mercury barometer and the aneroid barometer. In this chapter, we will focus our attention on pressure measuring devices that are routinely used to determine intracardiac and intravascular pressures. For the purposes of continuity, we will first describe those devices that are routinely used to perform noninvasive measurements of arterial pressure and then turn our attention to those devices that are used for invasive blood pressure measurements.

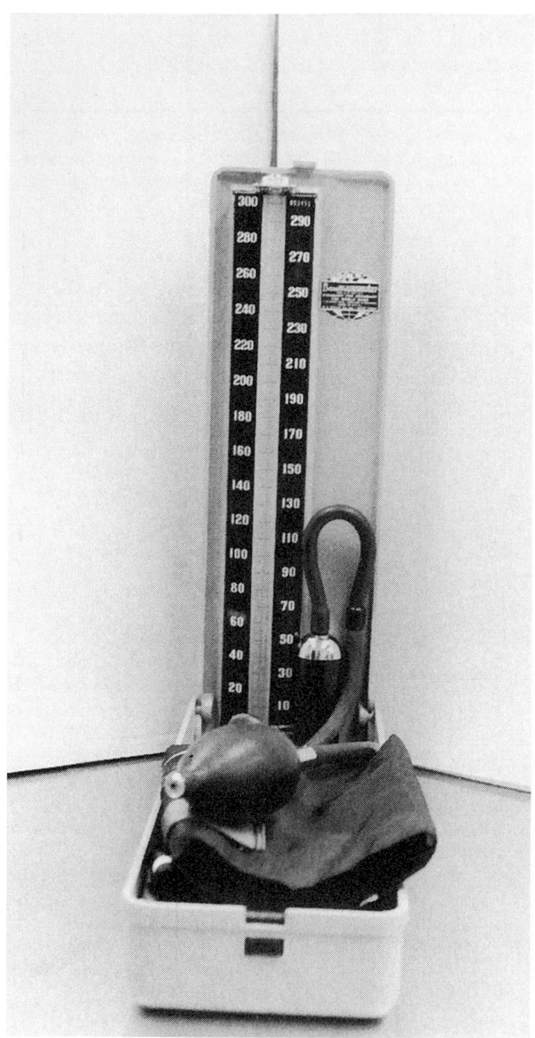

Figure 9-23 Sphygmomanometer. (Courtesy WA Braum, New York.)

Noninvasive Devices

The simplest and most widely used technique for measuring arterial blood pressure involves the **sphygmomanometer** (Figure 9-23). This device consists of an aneroid manometer connected via rubber tubing to an inflatable cuff, which can be inflated with a hand bulb. Deflation of the cuff is controlled by means of a pressure control valve that is attached to the tubing that connects the hand bulb to the inflatable cuff.

The technique is accomplished by placing the deflated cuff snugly around the patient's arm so that the bottom edge of the cuff is approximately 2 to 3 centimeters above the antecubital fossa. It is important to select the appropriately sized cuff when making these measurements because using a cuff that is too big or too small can seriously affect the accuracy of the measurement. The width of the cuff used should be approximately 40 to 50% of the circumference of the patient's arm. The length of the cuff should be approximately 80 to 100% of the patient's arm. For example, the standard blood pressure cuff used for adults is 5 inches wide and approximately 8 to 10 inches in length. Pediatric cuffs are also available for children younger than 5 years of age. These cuffs typically range from 1.5 to 3 inches in width and 3 to 6 inches in length.[11,12] It is suggested that the measurements are made on an arm that is not being used for the infusion of fluids or drugs because inflation of the cuff can obstruct the blood vessel and slow the infusion of the fluids.

While palpating the patient's radial artery in the arm being used for the measurement, the cuff is inflated to a pressure that is about 30 mm Hg above the pressure at which the radial pulse disappears. A stethoscope is placed over the brachial artery and the cuff is gradually deflated at a rate of about 5 mm Hg per second. The pressure at which a tapping sound is first heard as the cuff is deflated is the systolic pressure. The pressure at which these sounds become inaudible during cuff deflation is the diastolic pressure. The tapping sounds heard with the aid of the stethoscope are referred to as **Korotkoff sounds,** which are sounds that are attributed to turbulent blood flow that occurs when blood is forced through a partially occluded artery.[10] As the diameter of the vessel becomes larger with deflation of the compression cuff, blood flow becomes more laminar in character and the turbulence that caused the tapping sound essentially disappears.

Automated blood pressure measurement systems such as the one shown in Figure 9-24 operate on similar principles to a manual sphygmomanometer system. These systems are particularly convenient for situations when frequent determinations of blood pressure are required, such as during surgical procedures or in the intensive care unit.[11] Automated blood pressure measurement systems use electricity in the form of either a 110-V, 60-Hz alternating current or a battery as the power source. As with the manual systems, the automated devices can be attached to different size disposable cuffs. A microphone or ultrasound transducer attached to the cuff is used instead of the stethoscope to detect pressure pulsations that occur as the blood is forced through the partially occluded blood vessel during cuff deflation.

When the system is first activated, the cuff is inflated to a preset pressure and held constant for a period of pressure stabilization (e.g., 160 mm Hg). The system then determines if pressure oscillations are present and records the pressures as the cuff is deflated in a stepwise manner to atmospheric pressure. Figure 9-25 illustrates this sequence of events graphically. If oscillations are sensed during the period of pressure stabilization, indicating that the initial cuff pressure was less than the patient's peak systolic pressure, the system will increase the inflation pressure on the next cycle. Conversely, the system will decrease the inflation pressure on the next cycle if the inflation pressure was too high. Systolic and diastolic blood pressure along with mean arterial blood pressure can be recorded graphically on an oscilloscope or registered on an light-emitting diode (LED) display. The system automatically zeros itself periodically by opening the transducer to the atmosphere.

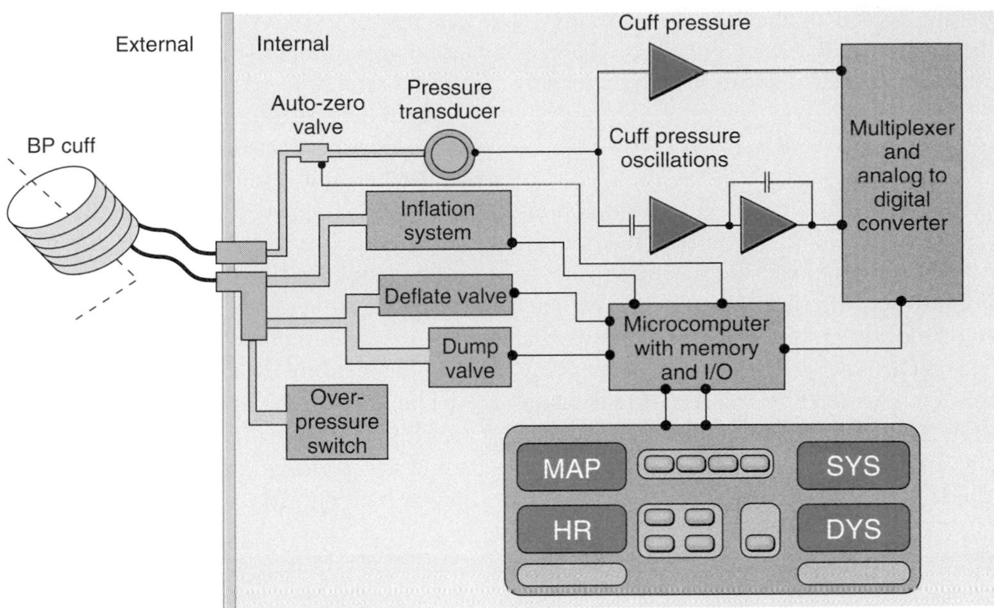

Figure 9-24 Automated blood pressure system. (Courtesy, Viasys, Puritan Bennett, Pleasanton, Calif.)

Automated systems can automatically determine the maximum inflation pressure in the cuff, cuff inflation time, and cuff deflation rate by relying on a specially designed control circuit. These circuits are also designed to automatically reject oscillation artifacts that can interfere with the accuracy of the measurements. Audible and visual alarm systems are available on all systems. In many systems, the alarms are set at default values but can be manually adjusted by the operator.[12] In several commercially available systems, the alarms are automatically set around the initial readings of the patient's peak systolic, diastolic, and mean arterial pressure.

The most common errors encountered when determining arterial blood pressure with both the manual sphygmomanometer and the automated blood pressure monitoring systems involve failure to use the proper cuff size, improper positioning of the cuff, improper deflation of the cuff, and motion artifacts. For example, blood pressure determinations made with an undersized cuff will cause falsely elevated readings, whereas using an oversized cuff will falsely underestimate the actual blood pressure.[13] Mechanical problems, such as a defective pressure control valve or old porous connecting tubing, can also lead to erroneous results. Improper cuff placement, such as moving it more peripherally away from the level of the heart, will typically result in an abnormally high reading for the systolic pressure and an erroneously low diastolic pressure. The most common problem encountered with deflation of the cuff occurs in automated systems that fail to deflate because of obstruction of the cuff vent. This latter problem may also cause an erroneous zero setting, resulting in lower than actual pressure readings. Motion artifacts caused by patient shivering, tremors, convulsions, or simply by restless movements can affect the measurement. Although most

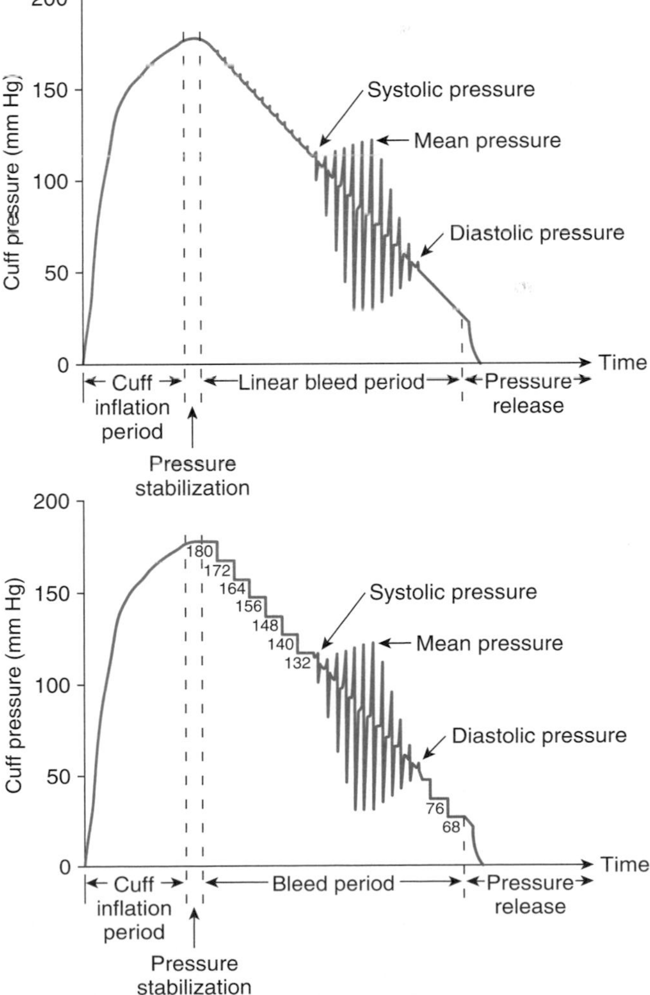

Figure 9-25 Pressure oscillation method for automated blood pressure. (Courtesy Tyco Healthcare, Pleasanton, Calif.)

automated systems are capable of rejecting these extraneous signals, it should be mentioned that these systems occasionally fail to reject an extraneous signal and thus lead to misleading information.

Invasive Devices

Invasive measurements, which allow for the determination of intravascular and intracardiac pressures, require the insertion of fluid filled catheters into the vascular space. In the case of arterial blood pressure measurements, a catheter made of polyvinyl chloride is inserted into a peripheral artery, such as the radial, brachial, or dorsalis pedis artery. The choice of the site for catheter insertion should be based on assessment of integrity of the vessel and the presence of adequate collateral circulation. This can be accomplished using the modified Allen's test, which is described in Chapter 10. Box 9-3 contains a summary of the technique for the insertion and maintenance of an indwelling arterial line catheter.[13]

Right heart pressure measurements are accomplished by inserting a catheter into a peripheral vein and slowly guiding it into the right atrium, right ventricle, and ultimately the pulmonary artery with the aid of fluoroscopy or real-time pressure measurements. A significant improvement in right heart catheterization, including fewer complications and the ability to perform this procedure at the bedside came with the introduction of the balloon-tipped, flow-directed pulmonary artery catheter by Swan and Ganz in 1970.[14]

The standard balloon flotation catheter (Figure 9-26) is a multiple lumen catheter constructed of polyvinyl chloride. Adult and pediatric catheters are available. The standard adult catheter is 110 cm in length and comes in 5 or 7 French

Box 9-3 Technique for the Insertion and Maintenance of an Indwelling Arterial Line Catheter

1. Perform Allen test before radial artery cannulation. Ischemic complications will be lowest if ulnar artery refill time is <5 seconds.
2. Use sterile technique for insertion (antiseptic preparation, gloves, drapes).
3. Choose percutaneous insertion over surgical cutdown when possible.
4. Use 20-gauge catheter if patient's wrist circumference is small.
5. Use continuous flush system with a nondextrose solution (normal saline) containing heparin.
6. Use transducer with disposable dome.
7. Assess daily:
   a. Catheter site for evidence of inflammation
   b. Distal extremity for evidence of ischemia
8. Limit cannulation to 4 to 5 days at one site.
9. Remove catheter for:
   a. Distal ischemia
   b. Local infection
   c. Persistently damped pressure tracing
   d. Difficulty with blood withdrawal

From Matthay RA, Wiedemann HP, Matthay MA: Cardiovascular function in the intensive care unit: invasive and noninvasive monitoring, *Respir Care* 30:432-449, 1985.

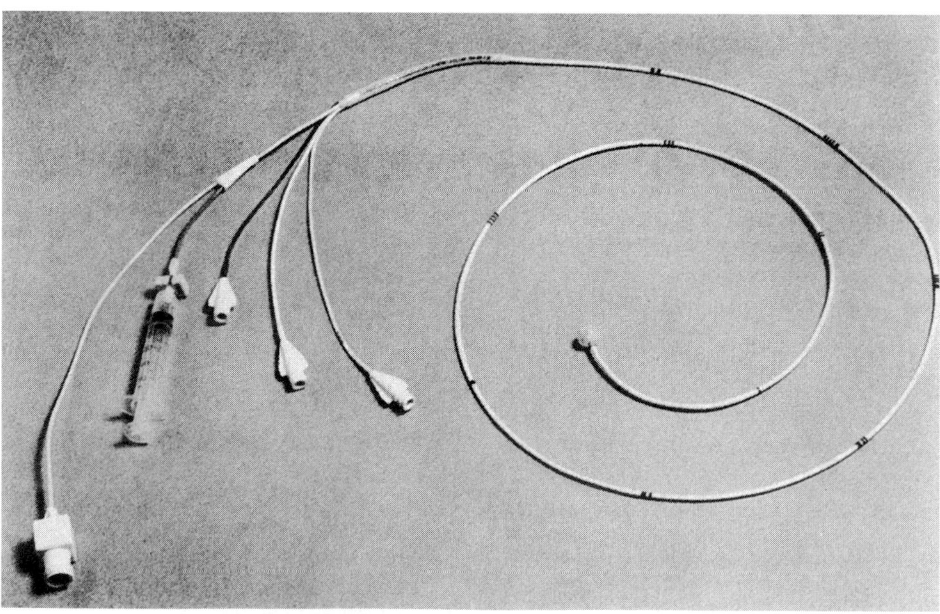

Figure 9-26 Balloon-tipped, flow-directed (Swan-Ganz) right heart catheter. (Courtesy Edwards-American Hospital Supply, Santa Ana, Calif.)

external diameter (the French number divided by 3.14 or π is the external diameter of the catheter in millimeters).[2] Pediatric catheters are 60 cm in length and available in either 4 or 5 French external diameter sizes. All catheters are marked at 10-cm increments. The Swan-Ganz catheter, as it is commonly identified, has an inflatable balloon attached to the tip of the catheter with multiple lumens that can be attached to pressure manometers or used for the injection of fluids.

Dual-lumen catheters have one lumen that connects to a balloon that is located at the tip of the catheter. A second lumen that runs the length of the catheter terminating at a port that is located at the distal end of the catheter. The second lumen's distal port can be used to monitor right ventricular and pulmonary artery (PA) pressures or it can be used to obtain mixed venous blood samples when the catheter's distal end is positioned in the pulmonary artery. Triple-lumen catheters have an additional lumen that is connected to a proximal port located 30 cm from the tip of the catheter. When the catheter is placed properly, the proximal port is located in the area of the right atrium and thus can be used to monitor central venous pressures (CVP). Specially designed thermodilution catheters have a fourth lumen, which contains electrical wires that connect a thermistor located approximately 2 cm from the tip of the catheter to a cardiac output computer like the one shown in Figure 9-27. We will discuss thermodilution cardiac output measurements in the following section on cardiac output measurements.

The catheter is introduced percutaneously into a peripheral vein, such as the antecubital, subclavian, internal or external jugular, or femoral veins. Surgical cut-down may be necessary if the antecubital route is used. It is advanced using fluoroscopy or with the aid of continuous pressure monitoring and electrocardiography until the tip of the catheter enters the intrathoracic vessels. Alternatively, the distance required to enter the intrathoracic vessels can be ascertained by noting the 10 cm marks on the catheter. If the catheter is introduced through the antecubital route, this distance is approximately 40 to 50 cm. The femoral route distance is approximately 30 to 40 cm and 10 to 15 cm if the internal jugular route is chosen.

After the catheter is positioned in the intrathoracic vessels, the balloon is inflated with a small volume of air (~0.8 mL). (Carbon dioxide [CO_2] is sometimes used to inflate the balloon so that in the event that the balloon should rupture, the CO_2 is absorbed by the tissues rather than cause an air embolism.) The balloon on the tip of the catheter is carried by the blood (like a sail being pushed by the wind) into the ventricle and then to the pulmonary artery. It can be further advanced and wedged into a small pulmonary artery for measurement of the pulmonary artery occlusion pressure (PAOP). The PAOP (which is often used interchangeably with the term *pulmonary artery wedge pressure or PAWP*) can be used as an estimate of the left atrial pressure and thus preload of the left ventricle (i.e., the left ventricular end diastolic pressure [LVEDP], which is not easily measured in the critical care setting). Deflation of the balloon after it is wedged in a small pulmonary artery will typically cause the catheter to drift backward into the main pulmonary artery. Figure 9-28 illustrates a typical pressure tracing for a healthy adult subject during a right heart catheterization using a Swan-Ganz catheter.

Box 9-4 provides a summary of the most common problems encountered during right heart catheterization. (See Clinical Rounds 9-3 for an exercise involving right heart catheterization.) It has generally been accepted that the number of critical incidences and problems associated with the use of balloon flotation catheters in critical care medicine have been relatively low if one considers the number of catheterizations that have been performed during the past 30 years. However, recent editorials and articles appearing in the medical literature have raised questions regarding the risk-benefit ratio when this procedure is used

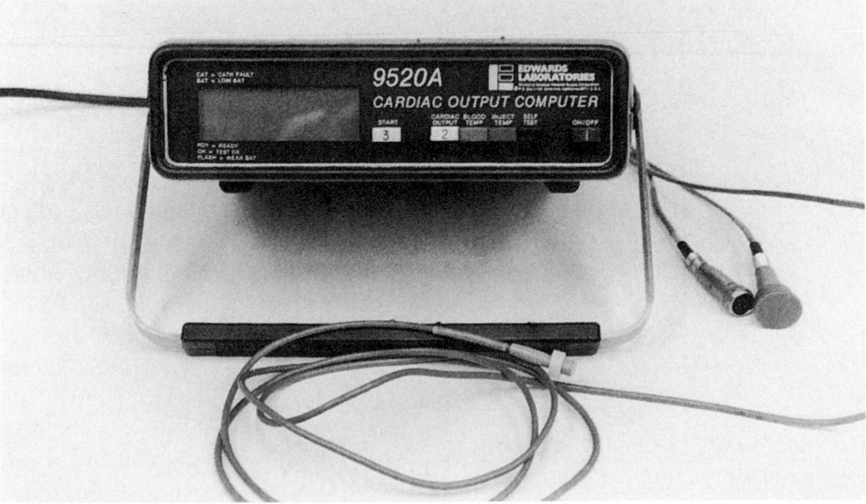

Figure 9-27 Cardiac output computer. (Courtesy Edwards-American Hospital Supply, Santa Ana, Calif.)

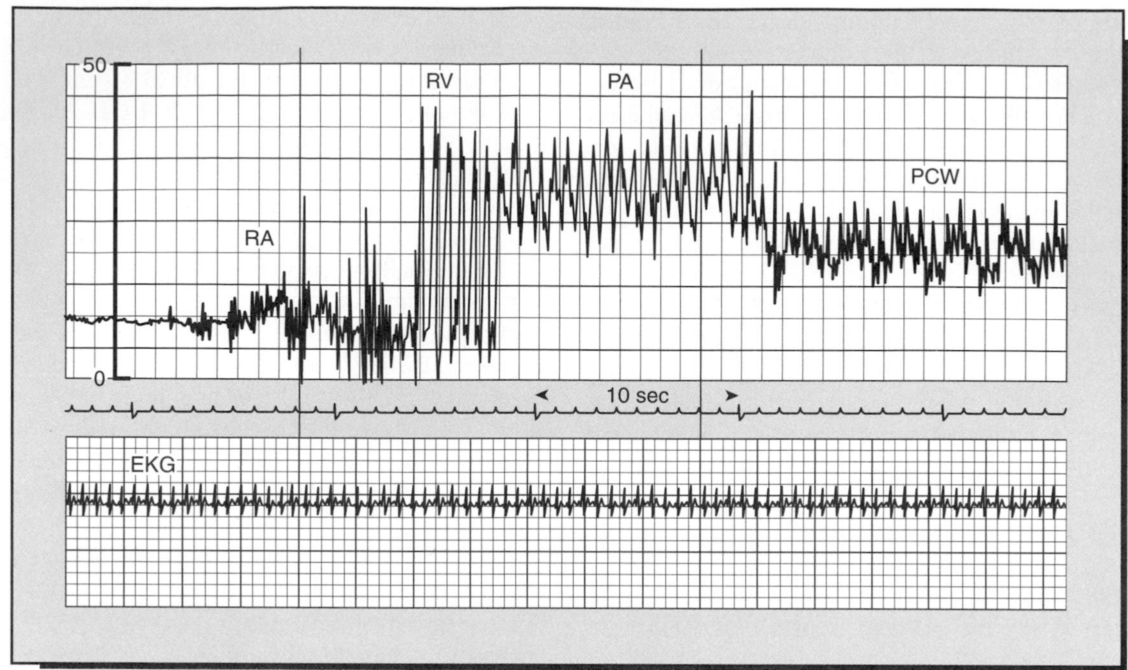

Figure 9-28 Pressure tracing obtained during a typical right heart catheterization. (Redrawn from Grossman W: *Cardiac catheterization and angiography,* ed 3, Philadelphia, 1986, Lea & Febiger.)

Box 9-4 Common Problems Encountered During Right Heart Catheterization

1. Arrhythmias
   a. Transient premature ventricular contractions (PVCs)
   b. Sustained ventricular tachycardia
   c. Ventricular fibrillation
   d. Atrial fibrillation
   e. Atrial flutter
2. Right bundle branch block
3. Pulmonary infarction
4. Pulmonary artery rupture
5. Catheter-related infections
6. Balloon rupture
7. Catheter knotting
8. Endocardial damage to:
   a. Valve cusps
   b. Chordae tendineae
   c. Papillary muscles
9. Complications at insertion site
   a. Pneumothorax
   b. Arterial puncture
   c. Venous thrombosis or phlebitis
   d. Air embolism

From Wiedermann HP, Matthay MA, Matthay RA: Cardiovascular-pulmonary monitoring in the intensive care unit, *Chest* 85:537-549, 656-658.

CLINICAL ROUNDS 9-3

A number of factors can lead to inaccurate pressure measurements during right heart catheterization with a balloon flotation catheter. Briefly describe how each of the following conditions would adversely affect these measurements:

1. Hypovolemic patient ventilated with PEEP
2. Therapist is unable to obtain a PAOP measurement
3. Attending physician notes that the pressure tracings are erratic and difficult to decipher

See Appendix A for the answer.

in critically ill patients. A special commission established by the American College of Chest Physicians, the American Society of Anesthesiologist, and the American Thoracic Society was formed in 2001 to address these issues. A final report from the commission proposed and ultimately succeeded in implementing an educational program to better prepare clinicians using this technology. The program is administered through online education and can be easily accessed through the American College of Chest Physicians' website.

Left heart catheterization, which involves placement of a catheter into the aorta, left ventricle, and left atrium, requires a retrograde approach in which the catheter is inserted into a peripheral artery (usually the brachial or femoral artery) using fluoroscopy to guide catheter placement.[15] A transseptal approach for left heart catheterization can also be used. In the transseptal technique, a specially designed catheter containing a retractable needle is introduced into a peripheral vein and positioned in the right atrium.[15] The clinician then extends the needle and punctures the interatrial septum thus establishing a communication between the distal tip of the catheter or needle, which lies within the left atrium and the proximal opening of the catheter, which can be attached to a pressure transducer. As you might have surmised, left heart catheterizations are performed in specially designed cardiac catheterization laboratories unlike right heart catheterization, which can be performed either in a cardiac catheterization laboratory or at the bedside in the intensive care unit. Specific information on the procedures for left heart catheterization can be found in the references at the end of this chapter.

Pressure Transducers

A transducer may be defined simply as a sensor that converts one form of energy into another form. A pressure transducer is an electromechanical device that converts a pressure signal into an electrical signal, which can be recorded or displayed on some type of output device. The number and variety of pressure transducers that are available for clinical practice has increased during recent years. The principles upon which these devices are based are the electrical properties, resistance, capacitance, and inductance.

Figure 9-29 illustrates these three types of electromechanical transducers.[16] A resistance type transducer (Figure 9-29, A) consists of a thin metal diaphragm attached to fours wires forming a Wheatstone bridge. Remember from Chapter 1 that a Wheatstone bridge is an electronic circuit consisting of four resistors connected in parallel. One branch of the circuit contains two resistors (R1 + R2) that form a fixed resistance whereas a second branch of the circuit is made up of two resistors (R3 + R4) that form a variable resistance. As pressure is applied to the metal diaphragm, the attached wires are stretched, thus changing their length and diameter and their electrical resistance. This change in electrical resistance changes the output voltage by an amount that is proportional to the applied pressure.

The variable capacitance transducer (Figure 9-29, *B*) also uses a flexible diaphragm to sense pressure changes. In this type of device, linking a thin metal diaphragm to an electrode forms a capacitor. Notice that when the diaphragm is not flexed, there is a small gap of air between the diaphragm and the electrode. As pressure is applied to the diaphragm, the gap narrows and ultimately causes the capacitor to discharge. As with the resistance type transducer, the output voltage is directly proportional to the movement of the diaphragm and thus the pressure applied to it.

Variable inductance transducers (Figure 9-29, *C*) consist of a stainless steel diaphragm attached to a soft iron core positioned between two coils. Applying pressure to the diaphragm results in a downward displacement of the iron core ultimately causing a change in the inductance of the two coils. The change in inductance caused by the movement of the iron core between the two coils is proportional to the applied pressure.

Strain gauge and variable inductance pressure transducers are the most frequently used devices because of their abilities to respond quickly to pressure changes. They both have good frequency response characteristics over a wide range of pressures. These devices are also quite stable and relatively insensitive to vibration and shock.[17] Variable capacitance transducers are usually large, bulky, and very sensitive to vibrations. They also have poor frequency response characteristics compared with strain gauge and variable inductance types of transducers.

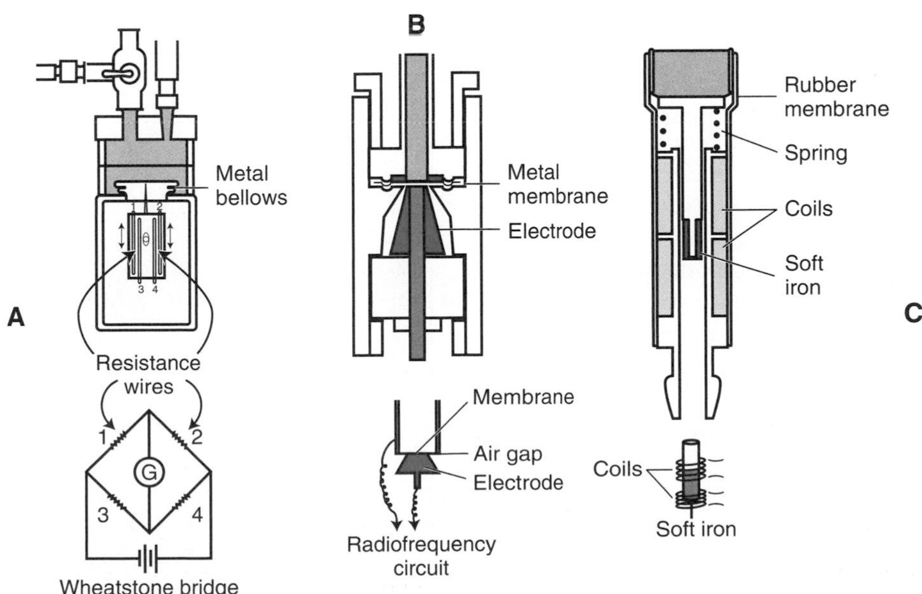

Figure 9-29 Electromechanical pressure transducers. **A,** Resistive; **B,** variable capacitance; **C,** variable inductance.

Cardiac Output Measurements

Historically, invasive techniques involving right heart catheterization have been the preferred method of determining cardiac output in clinical medicine. The direct Fick method, which is based on a principle that was formulated by Adolph Fick, has served as the gold standard for cardiac output measurements for more than a century. Development of thermistors and the thermodilution technique for measuring cardiac output have largely supplanted the use of the Fick method in clinical medicine during the past 20 years. More recent advances in the development of noninvasive technologies, which are based on impedance plethysmography and the Doppler effect, may very well prove to be the methods of choice for measuring cardiac output in critically ill patients because of their accuracy and safety.

Noninvasive methods of measuring cardiac output, such as impedance plethysmography and the indirect Fick method, are currently available but are not routinely used by most critical care clinicians for cardiac output determinations. It is reasonable to assume, however, that clinician will gain more confidence in these techniques and recognize their value in critical care medicine because they can provide another means of assessing the cardiopulmonary status of patients with minimal risk.[17]

Invasive Techniques

Direct Fick Method

The Fick principle states that the total uptake of a substance by an organ ($\dot{V}_x$) is directly related to the blood flow through the organ (Q) and the arteriovenous concentration or content difference of the substance across the organ ($Ca_x - Cv_x$), or

Equation 9-1

$$\dot{V}O_2 = Q \times (CaO_2 - C\dot{v}O_2)$$

We can determine the output of the right ventricle (i.e., pulmonary blood flow) by simultaneously measuring the total uptake of oxygen by the lungs or oxygen consumption ($\dot{V}O_2$) and the arteriovenous oxygen content difference between an arterial blood (CaO_2) and mixed venous blood ($C\bar{v}O_2$). The $\dot{V}O_2$ is determined from measurements of the volumes and oxygen concentrations in a subject's inspired and expired gases, whereas the arteriovenous oxygen difference is determining by measuring the oxygen content of arterial blood obtained from a peripheral artery and from a mixed venous sample of blood obtained from the pulmonary artery ($C\bar{v}O_2$). The cardiac output can by derived by simply applying equation 9-1.

Equation 9-2

$$\dot{Q} = \dot{V}O_2 \div (CaO_2 - C\bar{v}O_2)$$

Clinical Rounds 9-4 contains a clinical scenario to test yourself on calculation of cardiac output determination using the Fick method.

Indicator Dilution Methods

The indicator dilution method of determining cardiac output, which is also known as the *Stewart-Hamilton* dye dilution technique is commonly used to measure cardiac output during cardiac catheterization because of its accuracy and simplicity.[15] The technique is accomplished by injecting a known amount of dye, such as indocyanine green or Evan's blue, into a peripheral vein. The passage of dye through the pulmonary artery and its appearance and changing concentration in the arterial blood are recorded by continuously passing samples of arterial blood obtained from an indwelling radial, brachial, or femoral arterial line through a densitometer, which determined the concentrations of the dye in the blood. The results are recorded as time-concentration curves, which can then be displayed on an oscilloscope and digitally processed to determine the cardiac output, using the following relationship,

Equation 9-3

$$\dot{Q} = I/C_o,$$

where, $\dot{Q}$ is the cardiac output, I equals the total amount of dye injected in mg/min, and C_o is the average concentration of dye in the first pass through the circulation, which is measured in mg/L. As shown in Figure 9-30, if the first-pass curve is extrapolated with regard to time (as shown by a dashed line), the effects of recirculation can be eliminated and thus the cardiac output can be calculated by integrating the area under the curve.

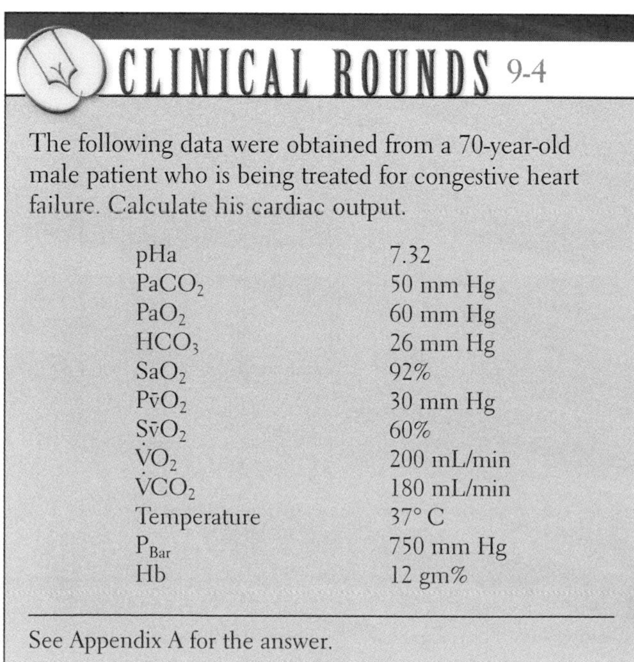

CLINICAL ROUNDS 9-4

The following data were obtained from a 70-year-old male patient who is being treated for congestive heart failure. Calculate his cardiac output.

pHa	7.32
$PaCO_2$	50 mm Hg
PaO_2	60 mm Hg
HCO_3	26 mm Hg
SaO_2	92%
$P\bar{v}O_2$	30 mm Hg
$S\bar{v}O_2$	60%
$\dot{V}O_2$	200 mL/min
$\dot{V}CO_2$	180 mL/min
Temperature	37° C
P_{Bar}	750 mm Hg
Hb	12 gm%

See Appendix A for the answer.

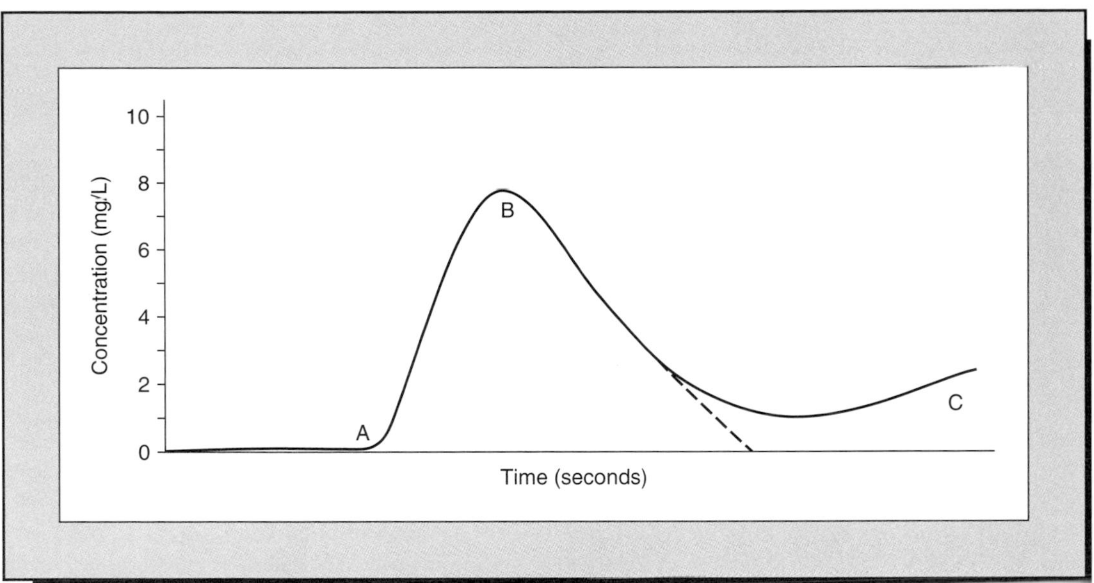

Figure 9-30 Indicator dilution curve.

Several factors must be considered when using this technique. Cardiac output determinations will be adversely affected in patients with intracardiac shunts and also in those patients with low cardiac outputs. In low cardiac output states, the downslope of the time-concentration curve may be prolonged because of the slower movement of dye pass the detector, thus making it difficult to differentiate recirculated dye from that of the dye that appears in the first-pass sample.

The thermodilution technique of determining cardiac output is another variation of the indicator dilution method. For the thermodilution technique, approximately 10 mL of cold (or room temperature) sterile 0.9% saline or 5% dextrose is injected through the proximal port of an indwelling balloon-tipped, flow-directed catheter, and a small thermistor located at the tip of the catheter senses changes in the temperature of the blood. In this technique, a cardiac output computer, which is connected to the catheter through electrical contacts, calculates the cardiac output by relying on temperature relationships (similar to the time-concentration relationships mentioned with the dye dilution technique) that occur as the injected fluid changes the temperature of the blood sensed by the catheter's thermistor.

The thermodilution technique for determining cardiac output is widely used in the critical care setting. The advantage of this technique is that it does not require monitoring arterial blood samples; measurements only require small volumes of injectate (i.e., cold normal saline), thus making multiple determinations possible, and there is essentially no problem with recirculation. Inaccuracies can occur in patients with tricuspid valve insufficiency and intracardiac shunts. Measurements are also affected by the presence of a low cardiac output. When making measurements of cardiac output on patients being mechanical ventilated, injection of the normal saline should occur during the end-expiration portion of the ventilatory cycle to insure that consistent measurements are obtained.

Noninvasive Techniques

Impedance Plethysmography

Impedance plethysmography as it is used in cardiac output measurements is based on the principle that changes in blood volume associated with pulsations of blood as it passes through a blood vessel will cause changes in the electrical impedance or resistance of the tissue surrounding the blood vessel.[17] This electrical impedance can be measured by passing a small amount of alternating current through the body segment in question. The amount of alternating electrical current is small enough that the patient does not feel any sensation from the electrical current flow. An important application of this principle is for the diagnosis of deep venous thrombosis.

Impedance cardiography, which is a variation of this technique, can be used to measure cardiac output by placing a series of two pairs of electrodes on the thorax, as shown in Figure 9-31. The assumption is that changes in bioimpedance that occur with changes in the thoracic blood volume during ventricular systole and diastole can be used to calculate beat to beat changes in stroke volume and thus cardiac output. Electrical voltage signals sensed by the measuring electrodes are then processed along with a simultaneous recording of the person's ECG and an impedance cardiograph curve is derived. Different points on the impedance cardiograph curve can then be labeled and used to calculate variables, such as stroke volume and systolic time intervals.

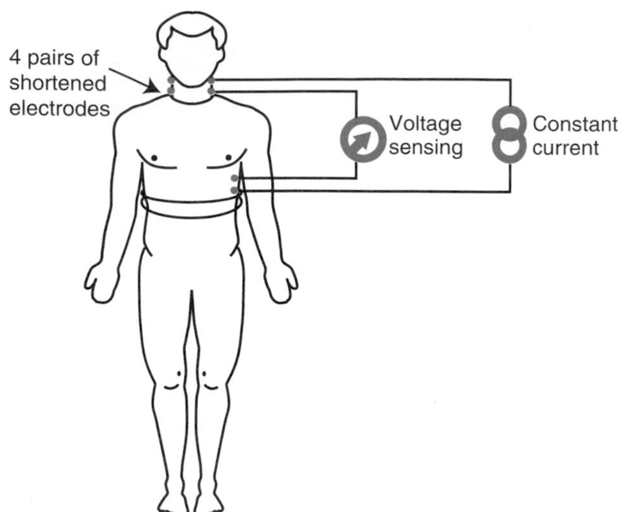

Figure 9-31 Impedance cardiograph.

Studies have demonstrated that cardiac output measurements made with thoracic electrical bioimpedance correlate with those obtained by thermodilution and the direct Fick method.[17] The potential uses for impedance cardiography include screening for the possible presence of cardiac disease, pacemaker adjustments, long-term continuous monitoring of cardiac output during surgery and in the intensive care unit, noninvasive hemodynamic measurements during cardiopulmonary stress testing, and as a means of monitoring the effects of pharmacological interventions.

Indirect Fick Method

As you might have surmised from the name of this technique, the indirect Fick method is based on the Fick principle, which was described previously. In the indirect technique, however, the cardiac output is determined by relying on continuous measurements of CO_2 production rather than oxygen consumption. Arterial and mixed venous oxygen differences are replaced with noninvasive measurements of arterial CO_2 content and mixed venous CO_2 content, respectively.[18] CO_2 production is obtained from continuous measurements of F_ECO_2 and V_E. F_ECO_2 is mixed expired CO_2 and V_E is expired minute ventilation. Arterial CO_2 content is calculated from partial pressure of end-tidal CO_2 ($P_{ET}CO_2$) measurements (to approximate partial pressure of CO_2 in the arteries [$PaCO_2$]) and mixed venous CO_2 is derived from measurements of partial pressure of mixed expired CO_2 when the patient intermittently rebreathes a 10% CO_2 mixture (using 10- to 15-second intervals). The cardiac output is therefore calculated as

Equation 9-4

$$\dot{Q} = \dot{V}CO_2/(P_{\bar{v}}CO_2 - P_{ET}CO_2)$$

Results indicate that the indirect Fick technique may prove to be useful in measuring cardiac output in most patients; however, more studies are required to determine the accuracy of this technique in critically ill patients.

Interpretation of Hemodynamic Profiles

Interpreting hemodynamic data is a fairly straightforward task. Using this information in the management of patients can be considerably more challenging for even the most skilled clinician. It is reasonable to state that the hemodynamic profile will ultimately focus on those factors that influence cardiac output, namely heart rate, preload, contractility, and afterload. Preload, which is typically defined as the filling pressure of the ventricle at the end of ventricular diastole is estimated by measuring the end-diastolic pressures. As such, the RVEDP is used as an indicator of the right ventricular preload and the LVEDP is used to estimate the left ventricular preload. Because both of these intracardiac pressures are difficult to measure in the critical care setting, clinicians rely on measurements of the CVP and PAWP to estimate the RVEDP and LVEDP, respectively.

Contractility, which is related to the force that the ventricle generates during each cardiac cycle, can be estimated using the ejection fraction or the ratio of the stroke volume to the ventricular end-diastolic volume. The ventricular afterload is the resistance the ventricle must overcome to eject blood and is estimated from calculations of the systemic and pulmonary vascular resistance.

The information that follows in this section is meant to provide an overview of basic measurements obtained in a standard hemodynamic profile. It is not our purpose to provide an extensive analysis of the various factors and conditions that can influence a patient's hemodynamic status. A number of excellent references related to hemodynamic monitoring in clinical practice are listed at the end of this chapter for those readers interested in obtaining more detailed information about this area of clinical physiology.

Cardiac Output

Cardiac output is defined as the volume of blood that is pumped by the heart per minute and is usually expressed in L/min or mL/min. It can be calculated by multiplying the heart rate times the stroke volume, which is the volume of blood pumped by the heart per beat and measured in mL/beat or L/beat. Alternatively, it can be measured using one of the techniques described in the previous section of this chapter on cardiac output determinations.

In many cases, the cardiac output and the stroke volume may be expressed relative to the person's body surface area, which can be easily obtained using a *Dubois* chart such as the one found in Appendix C. This indexing technique allows the clinician to compare an individual's cardiac output or stroke output to normal healthy individuals of the same weight and height (i.e., body surface area is calculated using these two anthropometric values). Cardiac index is calculated by dividing the cardiac output by the body surface area or

Equation 9-4

$$\text{Cardiac Index} = \dot{Q}/\text{BSA}$$

Similarly, stroke index is calculated by dividing stroke volume by body surface area, or

Equation 9-5

$$\text{Stroke Index} = \text{SV/BSA}$$

The normal cardiac index for an adult is approximately 3.5 L/min/m^2. The stroke index normally ranges from 40-50 ml/beat/m^2. Cardiac output can be reduced by decreases in either heart rate or stroke volume. Decreases in the effective ventricular rate are usually associated with an increase in parasympathetic tone or with the presence of various types of bradyarrhythmias. Decreases in stroke volume are typically associated with reductions in the preload or contractility of the heart or with an abnormally high afterload. Increases in cardiac output are associated with increases in heart rate or stroke volume. Tachycardia associated with an increase in sympathetic tone or a decrease in parasympathetic tone will increase cardiac output. Increases in stroke volume are associated with increases in preload and contractility, and with reductions in afterload. Note that profound increases in heart rate can actually decrease cardiac output by reducing the ventricular filling time and the resultant ventricular preload.

Vascular Resistance

The vascular resistance represents the impedance or opposition to blood flow offered by the systemic or pulmonary vascular beds and it influences the force that the ventricular muscle must generate during cardiac contractions (remember that $\Delta P = Q \times R$). It has been reported historically as dyne sec cm^{-5}; however, more recent publications have used the units of mm Hg/L/min. In this text, we will use the units of dyne sec cm^{-5}.

Vascular resistance is usually described as **systemic vascular resistance (SVR)** or **pulmonary vascular resistance (PVR).** A simple way to think of these calculations is to understand that ΔP represents the pressure gradient across the vascular bed and Q is the blood flow through the vascular bed. Thus systemic vascular resistance can be calculated as follows

Equation 9-6

$$\text{SVR} = (\text{MAP} - \text{MRAP/SBF})\ 80$$

where MAP is the mean arterial blood pressure, expressed in mm Hg; MRAP is the mean right atrial pressure, also expressed in mm Hg; and SBF is the systemic blood flow or cardiac output. Multiplying the equation by 80 is routinely used by clinicians to convert the units of mm Hg/L/min to dyne sec cm^{-5}. Similarly, pulmonary vascular resistance is calculated as

Equation 9-7

$$\text{PVR} = (\text{MPAP} - \text{MLAP/PBF})\ 80$$

where MPAP is the mean pulmonary artery pressure, MLAP is the mean left atrial pressure, both measured in mm Hg, and PBF is the pulmonary blood flow or cardiac output, expressed in L/min. Note that PAWP can be used in place of MLAP.

The normal SVR ranges from 900 to 1500 dyne sec cm^{-5} and the PVR ranges from 100 to 250 dyne sec cm^{-5}. A variety of factors can influence vascular resistance, most importantly, the caliber of the blood vessels and the viscosity of the blood. Remember that $R = 8\eta l/\pi r^4$, where in this case η is the viscosity of the blood, l is length, and r represents the radius of the vessel. Thus SVR can be increased in left ventricular failure and hypovolemia because of the vasoconstriction that results from stimulation of the baroreceptor reflex. SVR may also be increased by an increase in blood viscosity as occurs in polycythemia. SVR is reduced by systemic vasodilation, such as occurs with moderate hypoxemia or following the administration of pharmacologic agents like nitroglycerin or hydralazine.

PVR can increase significantly during periods of alveolar hypoxia or in cases where high intraalveolar pressures are generated, such as during positive pressure ventilation. Low cardiac outputs can increase PVR by causing derecruitment of pulmonary vessels. PVR is reduced by the administration of pulmonary vasodilator drugs such as tolazoline and prostacyclin.

Cardiac Work

In Chapter 1, we defined work as the product of a force acting on an object to move it a certain distance. In calculations of **cardiac work,** the pressure generated by the heart during a ventricular contraction is used quantify the amount of force developed and the distance traveled is replaced with the volume of blood pumped by the heart either as cardiac output or more often as stroke volume. We can actually quantify the amount of work performed by each ventricle during the cardiac cycle by applying the following formulae,

Equation 9-8

$$\text{LSW} = \text{MAP} \times \text{SV} \times 0.00136$$

Equation 9-9

$$\text{RSW} = \text{MPAP} \times \text{SV} \times 0.00136$$

where LSW and RSW are left ventricular stroke work and right ventricular stroke work, respectively, MAP is the mean arterial pressure, MPAP is the mean pulmonary artery pressure, SV represents stroke volume, and 0.00136 is a factor to convert mL-mm Hg to gram-meters. In most clinical situations, stroke work measurements are indexed to body surface area by dividing LSW or RSW by the patient's body surface area. Thus, left ventricular stroke work index (LSWI) and right ventricular stroke work index (RSWI) is calculated as

Equation 9-10

$$LSWI = LSW / BSA$$

Equation 9-11

$$RSWI = RSW / BSA$$

LSWI normally ranges from 0.50 to 0.60 kg-m/m^2 and RSWI ranges are normally between 0.07 and 0.10 kg-m/m^2. It should be apparent from these equations that conditions which increase the stroke volume or mean pressure generated by the ventricles will increase the amount of work that the ventricle must perform.

Summary

Assessment of cardiovascular function is an integral part of the management of patients with cardiopulmonary dysfunctions. Conventional electrocardiography provides valuable information about the electrophysiologic properties of the heart. In this chapter, we have reviewed the basic principles of electrocardiography and related ECG findings associated with major pathophysiologic processes. It should be stated that although an abnormal ECG should alert the clinician to alterations in the excitability, rhythmicity, and conductivity of the heart, the absence of abnormal findings does not rule out the possibility of a mechanical dysfunction of cardiac tissue.

Hemodynamic monitoring can provide information on the pressure, volume, flow, and resistance characteristics of the cardiovascular system. The introduction of the balloon-tipped, flow-directed pulmonary artery catheter in the early 1970s significantly extended the application of hemodynamic measurements in the diagnosis and treatment of patients with various types of cardiovascular problems. When used appropriately, these devices can provide valuable information that can be used for the successful management of critically ill patients.

Review Questions

1. Which of the following correctly describe the permeability characteristics of the resting membrane potential for a ventricular myocyte?
   a. $K^+ > Na^+$
   b. $Ca^{++} > Na^+$
   c. $Ca^{++} > K^+$
   d. $Na^+ = K^+$

2. Which of the following statements is true concerning nodal tissue action potentials?
   a. The action potential demonstrates five phases like ventricular myocytes
   b. The amplitude of this type of action potential is the same as an action potential for a ventricular myocyte
   c. The threshold potential for this type of tissue is more negative than the threshold potentials for a ventricular myocyte
   d. The slope of the phase 4 of the SA node is greater than that of the ventricular myocyte

3. For the lead aVF configuration, the positive electrode is placed on the:
   a. right arm
   b. left arm
   c. right leg
   d. left leg

4. A patient's ECG tracing shows an R-R interval of 15 millimeters. What is this patient's effective heart rate?
   a. 50 bpm
   b. 75 bpm
   c. 100 bpm
   d. 150 bpm

5. Which of the following electrocardiographic leads provides information related to the horizontal plane of the heart?
   a. I
   b. III
   c. V_4
   d. aVR

6. The last structure of the heart to depolarize is the:
   a. left bundle branch
   b. apex
   c. endocardial surface of the right ventricle
   d. epicardial surface of the base of the left ventricle

7. Which of the following is NOT characteristic of a respiratory sinus arrhythmia?
   a. The SA node is the pacemaker of the heart.
   b. The R-R interval is constant.
   c. A P wave precedes every QRS.
   d. The heart rate varies throughout the respiratory cycle.

8. The heart rate of an individual who demonstrates sinus tachycardia typically shows a ventricular rate of:
   a. less than 60 beats per minute
   b. 40-60 beats per minute
   c. 60-100 beats per minute
   d. greater than 100 beats per minute

9. For a person with a mean ventricular axis of 90 degrees, the amplitude of the QRS is typically greatest (upstroke) in which of the following leads?
   a. Lead I
   b. Lead III
   c. Lead aVF
   d. Lead V_3

10. Which of the following rhythms is characterized by the presence of delta waves on their ECG?
    a. First-degree AV block
    b. Bundle branch block
    c. Wolff-Parkinson-White syndrome
    d. Atrial fibrillation

11. Which of the following rhythms is characterized by a constant PR interval with intermittent loss of a QRS complex?
    a. Intraventricular conduction delay
    b. Second-degree (Mobitz I) AV block
    c. Second-degree (Mobitz II) AV block
    d. Respiratory sinus arrhythmia

12. Which of the following statements is true concerning ventricular action potentials?
    a. The action potential demonstrates three phases (phases 0, 3, and 4)
    b. The amplitude of this type of action potential is typically about 60 mV
    c. The threshold potential for this type of tissue is more negative that the threshold potentials for a nodal myocyte
    d. The slope of the phase 4 of the SA node is greater than that of the SA node myocyte

13. During a normal cardiac cycle:
    I. the first heart sound is associated with atrial contraction
    II. the period of isovolumetric contraction follows closure of the semilunar valves
    III. the dicrotic notch of the aortic pressure tracing is associated with closure of the aortic and pulmonary valves
    IV. the pressure in the left ventricle is higher than aortic pressure during the period of maximum ejection
    a. I and II only
    b. III and IV only
    c. I, III, and IV only
    d. I, II, III, and IV

14. An increase in right ventricular preload can be estimated clinically by measuring:
    a. LVEDP
    b. RVEDP
    c. PAWP (PCWP)
    d. MPAP

15. A 30-year-old female has a stroke index of 50 ml/beat/m^2. If her body surface area is 2.0 m^2 and her heart rate is 60, what is her cardiac output in liters per minute?
    a. 3.4 L/min
    b. 4.0 L/min
    c. 5.6 L/min
    d. 6.0 L/min

References

1. Berne RM, Levy MN: *Cardiovascular physiology*, ed 6, St Louis, 2001, Mosby.
2. Levitzky MG, Cairo JM, Hall SM: *Introduction to respiratory care*, Philadelphia, 1990, WB Saunders.
3. Scheidt S: *Basic electrocardiography*, West Caldwell, NJ, 1989, CIBA-GEIGY.
4. Cromwell L, Weibell FJ, Pfeiffer EA: *Biomedical instrumentation and measurements*, ed 2, Englewood Cliffs, NJ, 1980, Prentice-Hall.
5. Lipman BC, Cascio T: *ECG assessment and interpretation*, Philadelphia, 1994, FA Davis.
6. Scheidt S: *Interactive electrocardiography*, New York, 2000, NOVARTIS.
7. Guyton AC, Hall JE: *Textbook of medical physiology*, ed 10, Philadelphia, 2000, WB Saunders.
8. Katz AM: Physiology of the heart, Philadelphia, 2001, Lippincott Williams & Wilkins.
9. Fishman AP, Richards DW: *Circulation of the blood*, Bethesda, Md, 1982, American Physiological Society.
10. Levine RL, Fromm RE: *Critical care monitoring*, St Louis, 1995, Mosby.
11. Parbrook GD, Kenny GNC, Davis PD: *Basic physics and measurement in anaesthesia*, New York, 1999, Butterworth-Heinnemann.
12. Perloff D, Grim C, Flack J, et al: Human blood pressure determination by sphygmomanometry, *Circulation* 88(5):2460-2470, 1993.
13. Kascmarek RM, Hess D, Stoller JM: Monitoring in respiratory care, St Louis, 1993, Mosby.
14. Swan HJC, Ganz W, Forrester J, et al: Catheterization of the heart in man with the use of a flow-directed balloon tipped catheter, *N Engl J Med* 75:83-89, 1975.
15. Baim DS, Grossman W: *Grossman's cardiac catheterization, angiography, and intervention*, ed 6, Philadelphia, 2000, Lippincott Williams & Wilkins.
16. Rushmer RF: Structure and function of the cardiovascular system, ed 2, Philadelphia, 1976, WB Saunders.
17. Weiss S, Calloway E, Cairo J, et al: Comparison of cardiac output measurements by thermodilution and thoracic electrical impedance in critically ill versus non-critically ill patients, *Am J Emerg Med* 13:626-631, 1995.
18. Durbin CG: Noninvasive hemodynamic measurements, *Resp Care* 35(7):709-718, 1990.

Internet Resources

American Association for Respiratory Care Clinical Practice Guidelines: http://www.aarc.org

American College of Chest Physicians: http://www.chestnet.org

The Heart: An Online Exploration: http://sln2.fi.edu/biosci/heart.html

Heart Disease: http://www.pathguy.com/lectures/heart.htm

Introduction to Cardiothoracic Imaging: http://www.info.med.yale.edu/intmed/cardio/imaging/

MD Consult: http://www.lsuhsc.edu/mdconsult

The Merck Manual Online Resources: http://www.merckmedicus.com

The Virtual Human Gallery: http://www.vhgallery.gsm.com

WWW Virtual Library-Biosciences: http://www.ohsu.edu/cliniweb/wwwvl

Chapter 10

Blood Gas Monitoring

J.M. Cairo

Chapter Outline

Chapter Learning Objectives

Upon completion of this chapter, the reader should be able to:

1. Describe how to perform and evaluate the modified Allen test.
2. Identify various sites used to obtain samples for blood gas analysis.
3. Label the components of a modern, in vitro blood gas analyzer.
4. Compare the operational principles of the pH, partial pressure of carbon dioxide (PCO_2), and partial pressure of oxygen (PO_2) electrodes.
5. Apply values for PO_2 at which 50% saturation of hemoglobin occurs (P_{50}), bicarbonate, buffer base, and base excess in the interpretation of arterial blood gases (ABGs).
6. Explain the operational principle of CO-oximetry.
7. Name the components of a quality assurance program for blood gas analysis.
8. Compare the effect of hyper- and hypothermia on ABGs.
9. Describe physiological and technical factors that can affect pulse oximeter readings.
10. Identify various factors that can influence transcutaneous PO_2 and PCO_2 measurements.
11. State criteria for identifying four types of acid-base disorders.

Key Terms

Absorbance Sensors
Actual Bicarbonate
Allen Test
Amperometric
Base Excess/Deficit
Buffer Base
Capillary Blood Gas (CBG)
Central Processing Unit (CPU)
Clark Electrode
Clinical Laboratory Improvement Amendments of 1988 (CLIA-88)
Electrochemical Sensors
Electrodes
Fetal Hemoglobin (HbF)
Fluorescent Sensors
Fractional Hemoglobin Saturation
Functional Hemoglobin Saturation
Glucose Oxidase
Half-Cells
Henderson-Hasselbalch Equation
Hyperbilirubinemia
In Vitro
In Vivo
Invasive
Levy-Jennings Charts
Light-Emitting Diodes (LEDs)
Microcuvette
Nernst Equation
Noninvasive
One-Point Calibration
Optical Plethysmography
Optical Shunting
Oxygen Content (O_2ct)
$PaCO_2$
PaO_2
pH
Photoplethysmography
Point of Care Testing
Potentiometric
Quality Assurance (QA)
Quality Control (QC)
Sanz Electrode
Servo-Controlled
Siggaard-Andersen Alignment Nomogram
Standard Bicarbonate
Sulfhemoglobin (HbS)
Superior Palpebral Conjunctiva
Temperature Correction
Three-Point Calibration
Total Hemoglobin (THb)
Two-Point Calibration

Measurements of arterial blood gases (ABGs) and pH are used extensively in the diagnosis and treatment of patients with acute and chronic illnesses. This is most evident in the management of critically ill patients, for whom ABG analysis can provide valuable information, such as acid-base status, ventilatory function, and oxygenation status.

Blood gas techniques are generally classified as either **invasive** or **noninvasive.** Invasive blood gas analysis, which involves the direct exposure of a sample of blood to a series of electrochemical sensors or electrodes, is considered the gold standard for measuring the pH, partial pressure of carbon dioxide (PCO_2) and partial pressure of oxygen (PO_2) of arterial blood. Until recently, invasive blood gas analysis could only provide intermittent in vitro measurements of a patient's blood gas and acid-base status; but the development of fiberoptic catheters has extended the possibilities of in vivo blood gas monitoring by allowing for real-time determinations of pHa, partial pressure of carbon dioxide in the arteries (**$PaCO_2$**), and partial pressure of oxygen in the arteries (**PaO_2**).

Noninvasive techniques, which include pulse oximetry and transcutaneous monitoring, do not require blood samples and can be performed by sensors placed on the surface of the body. Both pulse oximetry and transcutaneous monitoring can provide continuous estimates of blood gases with minimal risk to the patient, so they are indispensable tools for managing patients with unstable ventilatory and oxygenation status. Appropriate use of noninvasive monitoring can significantly reduce the need for more expensive invasive blood gas analysis.

In this chapter, the various devices and techniques commonly used to determine ABGs and pH will be described. Some basic principles to ensure an understanding of how blood gas measurements can be used to assess a patient's acid-base and respiratory status will be presented. You should remember, however, that ABGs must be interpreted relative to other clinical indices, including other laboratory tests (e.g., hematology and electrolytes), chest radiographs, patient history, and physical examination findings. Interpretation of blood gases without consideration of other clinical findings can lead to serious mistakes and, ultimately, patient harm.

Invasive Blood Gas Analysis

Invasive blood gas analysis can be performed in a variety of settings, including hospitals, clinics, physician offices, and extended care facilities. The primary indications for invasive blood gas analysis are to quantify a patient's response to a diagnostic or therapeutic intervention and to monitor the severity and progression of a documented disease process.[1]

The American Association for Respiratory Care (AARC) has published a series of Clinical Practice Guidelines for ABG analysis to help ensure that these tests are performed in a safe and standardized manner.[1-3] Besides providing information on the equipment required to obtain blood samples, the guidelines also list the indications, contraindications, hazards, and complications of ABG analysis. The AARC Clinical Practice Guideline for blood gas analysis and hemoximetry[2] is summarized in Clinical Practice Guideline 10-1.

Health care professionals performing blood gas analysis should understand patient assessment techniques and the relationship of patient history, physical findings, and various cardiopulmonary dysfunctions. Therefore individuals involved in the performance of blood gas analysis should be formally trained in respiratory care, cardiovascular technology, clinical laboratory sciences, nursing, medicine, or osteopathy.[1,2] Periodic reevaluation of these individuals should focus on all aspects of blood gas analysis, including the proper technique for obtaining blood samples, postsampling care of the puncture site, and safe handling of blood, needles, and syringes.[1,2]

Collection Devices and Sampling Techniques

Specimens for ABG analysis can be drawn from a peripheral artery via a percutaneous needle puncture or from an indwelling intravascular cannula. Mixed venous blood samples can be obtained with a flow-directed (Swan-Ganz) intracardiac catheter. For percutaneous sampling, blood is most often drawn from the radial, brachial, or femoral arteries or the dorsalis pedis artery of the foot.[3-5] Capillary blood samples from an earlobe or a side of the heel may be substituted when arterial blood cannot be obtained. As will be discussed later, **capillary blood gas (CBG)** values may vary considerably from ABG values.

In the case of percutaneous puncture of the radial artery, a modified **Allen test** should always be performed before obtaining the sample (Figure 10-1).[4,5] For the Allen test, patients clench their fist to force blood from their hand. While the fist is formed, pressure is applied to the radial and ulnar arteries. The patient is then instructed to release the fist, and the hand should appear blanched. When pressure on the ulnar artery is released, blood should return to the hand, causing the palm to blush and indicating that the ulnar artery is patent. If the palm does not blush, the ulnar artery is either absent or partially or totally occluded. Another sampling site, such as the brachial artery, should be chosen if the modified Allen test is negative. Note that a similar test can be performed when obtaining blood from the dorsal artery of the foot. The artery is occluded by applying pressure directly over it, and then pressure is applied to the nail of the big toe, causing it to blanch. When pressure on the big toe is released, color will return to the toe if there is sufficient collateral circulation from the posterior tibial and lateral plantar arteries.[6]

After it has been determined that sufficient collateral circulation is present, the site should be prepared for puncture by being cleaned with 70% isopropyl alcohol or another suitable antiseptic solution.[7] In some cases, it may be necessary to anesthetize the puncture site by injecting a local anesthetic such as 1% lidocaine HCl.[1,4,5] Proper administration of the anesthetic can alleviate some of the pain associated with the procedure and reduce some patient anxiety.

Samples to be analyzed should be obtained with a small-gauge needle (23 to 25 gauge) attached to a glass or plastic syringe of low diffusibility containing an anticoagulant (sodium or lithium heparin, 1000 units/mL) (Figure 10-2).[1,2] For infants, 25- to 26-gauge scalp vein needles can be used to collect arterial samples. The blood should be drawn anaerobically to prevent contamination by room air. Room air that is inadvertently drawn into the syringe should be removed before analysis because contamination with room air can lead to erroneous results and ultimately compromise patient care. Clinical Rounds 10-1 gives an example of this type of problem in the clinical setting.

After blood is withdrawn and the needle removed, direct pressure should be applied to the puncture site to prevent formation of a hematoma. For adult patients with indwelling cannulas, 1 to 2 mL of blood should be removed and discarded before blood is removed for analysis. For infants, the discarded volume is typically only about 0.2 to 0.5 mL.*

**Remember that the volume of blood removed and discarded should be minimal; this is particularly important in neonates.*

Clinical Practice Guidelines 10-1

Blood Gas Analysis and Hemoximetry

Setting

1. Hospital laboratories
2. Hospital emergency areas
3. Patient-care areas
4. Clinical laboratories
5. Physician offices

Indications

1. Evaluate the adequacy of a patient's ventilatory, acid-base, or oxygenation status, oxygen-carrying capacity, and intrapulmonary shunt.
2. Quantify a patient's response to therapeutic intervention and/or diagnostic evaluation.
3. Monitor the severity and progression of documented disease processes.

Contraindications

1. Improperly functioning analyzer or an analyzer that has not had its functional status validated by analysis of commercially prepared quality control products or tonometered whole blood, or participation in a proficiency testing program.
2. A specimen that has not been properly anticoagulated.
3. A sample that contains visible air bubbles.
4. A sample that has been stored in a plastic syringe at room temperature for longer than 30 minutes, stored at room temperature for longer than 5 minutes for a shunt study, or stored at room temperature in the presence of an elevated leukocyte or platelet count.
5. Sample is submitted without adequate background information, including patient's name or other unique identifier (e.g., medical record number, birth date or age, date and time of sampling), location of the patient, name and signature of the requesting physician or authorized individual, clinical indication and tests to be performed, sample source (arterial line, central venous catheter, peripheral artery), respiratory rate, F_IO_2, ventilator settings (tidal volume, respiratory rate, mode, F_IO_2), body temperature, activity level, and working diagnosis. It is also imperative to have the signature of the person who obtained the sample.

Hazards/Complications

1. Infection of the specimen handler from blood containing HIV, hepatitis B, or other blood-borne pathogens.
2. Inappropriate patent medical management treatment based on improperly analyzed blood sample or from analysis of an unacceptable specimen, or from incorrect reporting of results.

Limitations of Procedure

1. Sample clotting due to improper anticoagulation or improper mixing.
2. Sample contaminated air, improper anticoagulant or anticoagulant concentration, saline or other fluids, inadvertent sampling of systemic venous blood.
3. Delay in sample analysis.
4. Incomplete clearance of analyzer calibration gases and previous waste or flushing solution(s)
5. Hyperlipidemia (interference with electrode membranes).
6. Failure to obtain an adequate sample size.
7. Calculation of derived variables may be in error (e.g., SaO_2 may underestimate O_2Hb resulting from the presence of carbon monoxide or methemoglobin).
8. Errors in measurement of the patient's temperature may cause erroneous temperature corrected results.

Validation of Results

1. Analytic procedure conforms to recommended, established guidelines, and follows manufacturer's recommendations.
2. Results of pH-blood gas analysis fall within the calibration range of the analyzer and quality control product range.
3. Laboratory procedures and personnel are in compliance with quality control and recognized proficiency testing programs.
4. Questionable results should be reanalyzed (preferably on a separate analyzer) and an additional sample should be obtained if the discrepancy cannot be resolved. Note results of analysis of discarded sample should be documented with reason for discarding.

Assessment of Need

1. The presence of a valid indication in the subject to be tested supports the need for sampling and analysis.

Infection Control

1. Staff, supervisors, and physician-directors associated with the pulmonary laboratory should be knowledgeable of Centers for Disease Control and Prevention (CDC) and Hospital Infection Control Practices Advisory Committee (HICPAC) "Guidelines for Isolation Precautions in Hospitals."
2. Laboratory manager and its medical director should maintain communication and cooperation with the institution's infection control service and the personnel health service to help assure consistency and thoroughness in complying with the institutions policies related to immunization, post-exposure prophylaxis, and community related-illnesses and exposures.

For a copy of the complete text, see AARC Clinical practice guideline: Blood gas analysis and hemoximetry: 2001 Revision and Update, *Respir Care* 46:498-505, 2001.

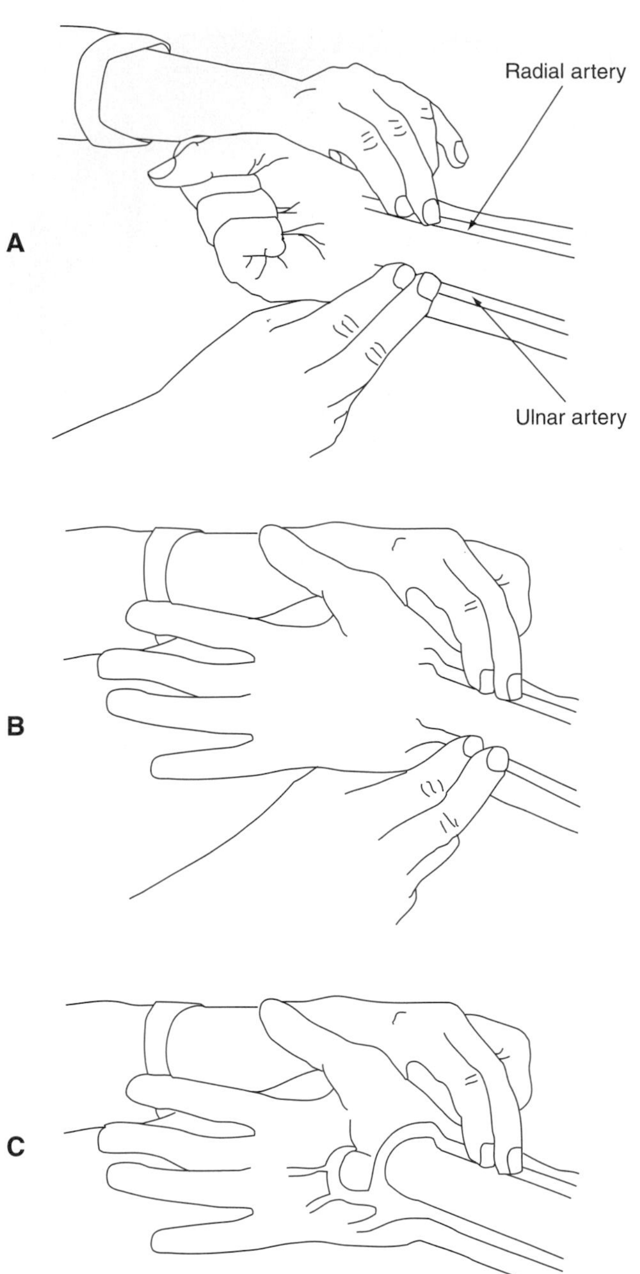

Figure 10-1 Modified Allen Test. **A,** The hand is clenched into a tight fist and pressure is applied to the radial and ulnar arteries; **B,** the hand is opened (but not fully extended), and the palm and fingers are blanched; **C,** pressure on the ulnar artery is removed, which should result in flushing of the entire hand. (From Shapiro BA Peruzzi WT, Templin R: *Clinical application of blood gases*, St Louis, 1994, Mosby.)

After removing the blood sample to be analyzed, the cannula should be flushed with several milliliters of normal saline to prevent blood coagulation within the cannula and avoid loss of a functioning indwelling line.

As mentioned previously, CBG samples obtained from an earlobe or the side of the heel may be substituted for arterial blood samples in certain situations.[8] CBGs are most often used in pediatrics, especially in the neonatal intensive care unit, to avoid multiple arterial sticks.[9-11] The site should be warmed before the sample is obtained to increase perfusion to the area (i.e., "arterializing"). "Arterialized" capillary samples actually contain a combination of arterial and venous blood and may therefore not be equivalent to an arterial blood sample.[11,12] The correlation between capillary and arterial pH and PCO_2 measurements is better than the correlation of capillary and arterial PO_2 measurements. Consequently, CBGs are used more often to discern acid-base status rather than to assess a patient's oxygenation status. Table 10-1 contains accepted normal ABG values. Clinical Rounds 10-2 shows how CBGs can be used in clinical decision making.

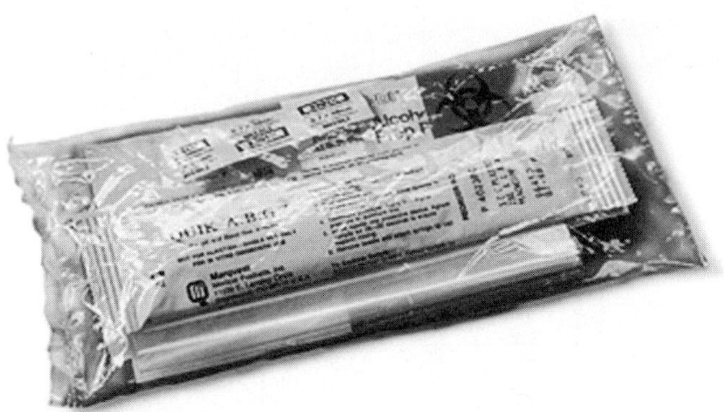

Figure 10-2 A commercially available blood gas kit. (Courtesy Marquest Medical Products, Vital Signs, Newark, NJ.)

CLINICAL ROUNDS 10-1

How would a large air bubble affect the PCO_2 and PO_2 of an arterial blood sample taken from a normal person breathing room air?

See Appendix A for the answer.

Personnel responsible for performing blood gas analysis should understand that they are dealing with a potential biohazard and take appropriate precautions when performing these tests.[13,14] Such precautions include wearing gloves, protective eyewear (goggles), and other barriers deemed necessary for preventing exposure. Needles used for blood sampling should be recapped with the one-hand, "scoop" technique, or they can be removed after being inserted into a cork or similar device to shield the sharp end. Unused blood samples, needles, and other "sharps" should be discarded in appropriately marked containers. (See Chapter 5 for a full discussion of infection control principles in respiratory care.)

Specimens should be transported to the blood gas laboratory and analyzed as soon as possible after drawing because blood cells remain metabolically active in vitro, so a prolonged time delay (>5 minutes) between obtaining and analyzing a specimen can lead to erroneous results (i.e., a reduction in PO_2 and a rise in PCO_2). This problem is particularly evident for patients with high leukocyte counts.[4,5] Chilling the specimen to <5° C by placing the syringe in ice water can reduce the metabolic rate of the white blood cells, thus minimizing this problematic effect.

Modern in Vitro Blood Gas Analyzers

Modern in vitro blood gas analyzers (Figure 10-3) contain three electrodes for determining the pH, PCO_2, and PO_2 of a blood sample. They also contain a **central processing unit (CPU)** for data management and outputs for displaying measured and derived variables. Many of these systems may also contain sensors for providing hemoglobin, oxyhemoglobin, carboxyhemoglobin, and methemoglobin measurements, along with serum electrolyte and blood glucose measurements. Table 10-2 lists the normal values for derived variables that are commonly recorded during blood gas analysis. Unlike early blood gas analyzers, which were cumbersome to operate and required large quantities of blood to make accurate measurements, modern analyzers are fully automated, self-calibrating devices that can analyze blood samples as small as 50 to 100 μL.

Table 10-1 Normal blood values*

pH	7.40 ± 0.05
$PaCO_2$	40 ± 5 mm Hg
PaO_2	80-100 mm Hg
HCO_3^-	24 ± 2 mEq/L
Base excess	± 2 mEq/L
O_2Hb	95%-100%
COHb	<1.5%
MetHb	<1.5%
THb	12-18 gm/dL
NA^+	140 ± 5 mWq/L
K^+	4 ± 0.5 mEq/L
CL^-	101 ± 4 mEq/L
Ca^{++}	5 ± 0.5 mEq/L
Glucose	70-105 mg/dL
P_{50}	27 ± 2 mm Hg

*Values are expressed for a healthy adult.

pH and Hydrogen Ion Concentration

S.P.L. Sorenson introduced the term ***pH*** as a shorthand way to express the hydrogen ion activity of solutions.[15,16] It is defined as the negative logarithm (base 10) of the hydrogen ion concentration, or

$$pH = -\log_{10}[H^+].$$

For example, a hydrogen ion concentration of 0.0000007 mol/L, or 1×10^{-7} mol/L, can be expressed as a pH of 7.0. Although there has been an increased scientific effort to express hydrogen ion concentrations in Système International (SI) units (i.e., nanomoles per liter [nmol/L]), the concept of pH is still recognized as a convenient and useful way of discussing a patient's clinical acid base status.[16,17] Table 10-3 shows the relationship between hydrogen ion concentration and pH. Note that pH decreases as hydrogen ion

CLINICAL ROUNDS 10-2

A CBG sample is obtained from a 2-day-old infant in apparent respiratory distress. The results indicate respiratory alkalosis (high pH, low PCO_2) and apparent hypoxemia (low PO_2). How would you interpret these findings?

See Appendix A for the answer.

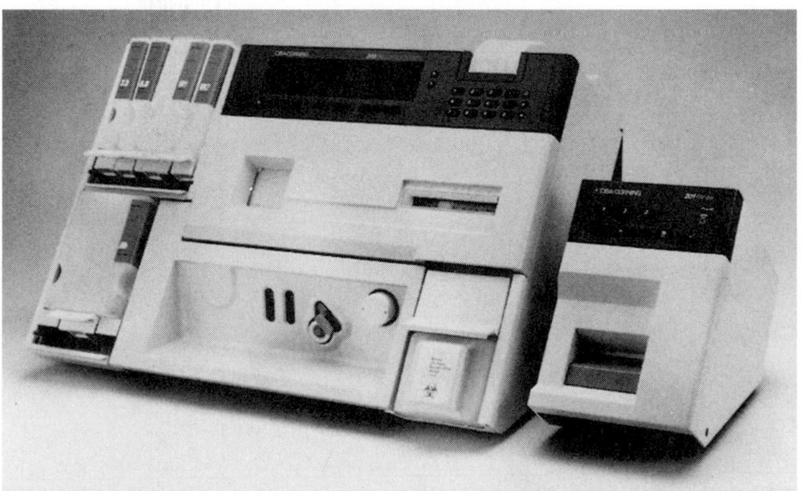

Figure 10-3 A modern in vitro blood gas analyzer. (Courtesy Corning Instruments, Chiron Diagnostics, Norwood, Mass.)

concentration increases and increases as hydrogen ion concentration decreases. Despite the fact that hydrogen ion activity is not exactly equal to hydrogen ion concentration, these two terms are interchangeable for practical purposes in clinical situations.

In general chemistry textbooks, the pH scale is described as ranging from 1 to 14, with a pH of 7.0 representing universal neutrality. (Neutrality is defined as the pH of pure water, which contains 1×10^{-7} mol/L of hydrogen ions and 1×10^{-7} mol/L of hydroxyl ions.) A solution with a pH less than 7.0 is acidic, and a solution with a pH higher than 7.0 is alkaline. Although the pH of arterial blood can vary from 6.90 to 7.80, it normally ranges (± 2 SD) from 7.35 to 7.45, with a mean pH of 7.40. For interpretative purposes, a blood pH less than 7.4 is considered acidic, and a blood pH higher than 7.4 is alkaline.

pH Electrode

The standard pH electrode, which is sometimes called the **Sanz electrode,** is composed of two **half-cells** that are connected by a potassium chloride (KCl) bridge (Figure 10-4).[18] One of the cells, which is the measurement half-cell, has a special glass membrane permeable to hydrogen ions (H^+); the measuring electrode is made of silver-silver chloride (Ag/AgCl) and immersed in a phosphate buffer solution with a pH of 6.840. The second cell, which is called the reference half-cell, is composed of mercury-mercurous chloride (Hg/HgO_2) (calomel) and is immersed in a solution of saturated KCl.

According to the Nernst equation, the electrical potential generated as H^+ ions pass through the glass membrane

Table 10-2 Normal values for derived blood gases

Parameter	Symbol	Normal Values
Oxyhemoglobin	O_2Hb	≥95%
Carboxyhemoglobin	COHb	<1.5%
Methemoglobin	MetHb	<1.5%
Deoxygenated hemoglobin	HHb	<2.0%
Sulfhemoglobin	SulfHb	<1.0%
Total hemoglobin	THb	Males: 15.8 ± 2.3 gm/dL Females: 14.0 ± 2.0 gm/dL
Partial pressure of oxygen at 50% saturation	P_{50}	27.0 ± 2.0 mm Hg

Table 10-3 Hydrogen ion-pH relationships

pH	$[H^+]$*
7.80	16
7.70	20
7.60	26
7.50	32
7.40	40
7.30	50
7.20	63
7.10	80
7.00	100
6.90	125
6.80	160

*Reported in nanomols per liter.

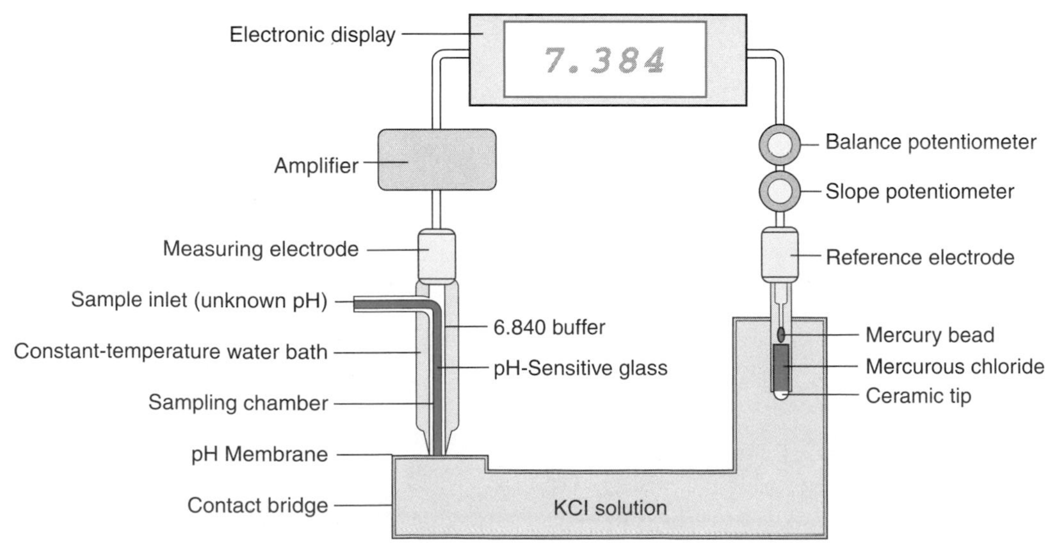

Figure 10-4 A schematic of the pH electrode. (From Hess et al: *Respiratory care: principles and practice,* St Louis, 2002, WB Saunders. Modified from Shapiro, et al: *Clinical application of blood gases,* ed 4, St Louis, 1989, Mosby.)

(EH^+) is a logarithmic function of the ratio of hydrogen ion concentration across the membrane, or

$$EH^+ = (RT/F) + \ln[(H_o^+)/(H_i^+)],$$

where R is the gas constant, F is Faraday's constant, T is the absolute temperature in Kelvin, H_o^+ is the hydrogen ion concentration outside the membrane, and H_i^+ is the hydrogen ion concentration inside the membrane. If you consider that at body temperature (37° C, or 310 K) the quantity (RT/F) is 61.5 mV, then the equation becomes,

$$EH^+ = 0.0615 \times \log_{10}[H^+], \text{ or}$$
$$EH^+ = 0.0615 \times pH.$$

Thus a voltage of 61.5 mV will be developed for every pH unit difference between the sample and the measuring electrode, which is constant (6.840). Consider the following example. A voltage difference of 30.75 mV is measured when a sample is analyzed. This voltage difference equals 0.500 pH units (30.750 ÷ 61.500 = 0.500). The resultant pH can be calculated as 6.840 + 0.500 − 7.34.

It should be apparent that these devices are quite sensitive, and therefore are adversely affected by changes in the permeability of the glass membrane as can occur when the electrode is damaged or coated with protein. As will be discussed later in this chapter, maintaining an effective quality assurance program can prevent these types of problems.

Partial Pressures of Carbon Dioxide (PCO_2) and Oxygen (PO_2)

In Chapter 1, it was stated that the partial pressure that a gas exerts in a gas mixture is calculated by multiplying the fractional concentration of the gas by the total pressure of the gas mixture. For example, if oxygen makes up about 21% of the atmosphere, and the barometric pressure is 760 mm Hg, then the partial pressure of oxygen in room air is approximately 159 mm Hg (0.21 × 760 mm Hg).

The **partial pressure of carbon dioxide in arterial blood ($PaCO_2$)**, which is primarily regulated by the respiratory system, can vary from 10 to 100 mm Hg. Subjects breathing room air at sea level typically have a $PaCO_2$ in the range of 35 to 45 mm Hg (the mean is 40 mm Hg; the range represents ±2 SD). The **partial pressure of oxygen in arterial blood (PaO_2)** can range from 30 mm Hg to 600 mm Hg, depending on the fractional concentration of inspired oxygen. For healthy people breathing room air at sea level, the PaO_2 is usually from 80 to 100 mm Hg.

PCO_2 Electrode

The PCO_2 electrode was first described by Stowe in 1957, but later refined by Severinghaus and associates,[41] so the standard PCO_2 electrode is commonly called the Stowe-Severinghaus electrode (Figure 10-5). It is basically a pH electrode covered with a carbon dioxide-permeable Teflon or silicon elastic (Silastic) membrane. A bicarbonate buffered solution is held between the Teflon (or Silastic) membrane and the pH glass electrode by a nylon spacer. Carbon dioxide from the blood diffuses across the semipermeable Teflon (or Silastic) membrane and reacts with the water to form carbonic acid, which dissociates into hydrogen ions and bicarbonate. The reaction can be written as:

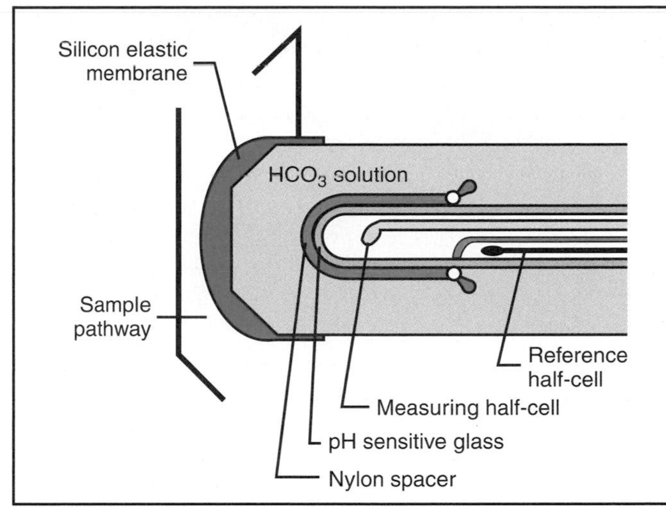

Figure 10-5 A Stowe-Severinghaus PCO_2 electrode. (Redrawn from Shapiro BA, Peruzzi WT, Templin R: *Clinical application of blood gases*, ed 5, St Louis, 1994, Mosby.)

$$CO_2 + H_2O \rightarrow H_2CO_3 \rightarrow H^+ + HCO_3^-$$

H^+ ions from the bicarbonate buffered solution then diffuse across the glass electrode, and the pH of the solution is measured as described earlier. The pH is related to the PCO_2 by using the following modification of the **Henderson-Hasselbalch equation,**

$$pH = pK + \log(HCO_3^-/PCO_2)$$

Thus the PCO_2 is determined as a function of the change in pH of the bicarbonate solution (i.e., the pH changes by 0.1 unit for every 10 mm Hg increase in PCO_2).

The most common problems encountered with PCO_2 electrodes involve interference with the diffusion of CO_2 across the Teflon (Silastic) membrane and the H^+ ions across the glass membrane (e.g., worn or cracked electrodes, protein deposits, etc.). If the bicarbonate solution dehydrates between the Teflon (Silastic) membrane and the pH glass electrode, erroneous data can result. As with the pH electrode, these problems can be minimized by using an effective quality assurance program.

PO_2 Electrode

The partial pressure of oxygen in blood is most commonly measured using the Clark electrode.[18] As Figure 10-6 shows, the **Clark electrode** consists of a negatively charged platinum electrode (cathode) and a positively charged Ag/AgCl reference electrode (anode) immersed in a phosphate/potassium chloride buffer, the pH of which can range from 7.0 to 10, depending on the manufacturer. The cathode and anode are connected together by a KCl bridge. An external voltage is applied to the platinum electrode, creating a small potential

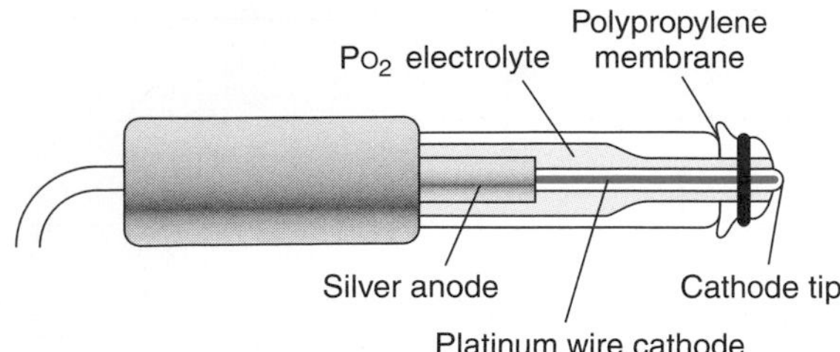

Figure 10-6 A Clark PO_2 electrode. (From Hess et al: *Respiratory care: principles and practice*, St Louis, 2002, WB Saunders. From Shapiro BA, Peruzzi WT, Templin R: *Clinical application of blood gases*, ed 5, St Louis, 1994, Mosby.)

difference of about 0.5 to 0.6 mV between it and the anode.* The active surface of the electrode is separated from the blood to be analyzed by a polyethylene or polypropylene membrane that is permeable to oxygen.

Figure 10-7 illustrates the principle of PO_2 measurement. Oxygen from the blood sample diffuses across the semipermeable plastic membrane into the KCl solution and reacts with the platinum cathode, altering the conductivity of the electrolyte solution. Specifically, the platinum cathode donates electrons, which reduce oxygen to produce hydroxyl ions,

$$O_2 + 2H_2O + 4e^- \rightarrow 4OH^-$$

The electrons donated by the cathode are derived from oxidation of Ag at the anode,

$$4Ag \rightarrow 4Ag^+ + 4e^-$$
$$Ag^+ + Cl^- \rightarrow AgCl$$

The volume of oxygen reduced at the cathode is directly proportional to the number of electrons used in the reaction. Therefore the amount of oxygen diffusing across the membrane into the electrolyte solution can be determined by measuring the current change that occurs between the anode and the cathode when the electrode is exposed to a blood sample containing oxygen. Because PO_2 is determined by measuring current changes that occur as oxygen is reduced, this technique is an example of an **amperometric** measurement; determinations of pH and PCO_2 as described above are examples of **potentiometric** measurements (i.e., they are based on voltage changes).

The electrical output of the Clark electrode, and thus its sensitivity for measuring PO_2, can be altered by several factors, including protein buildup, cracked electrodes, and loss of electrolyte. When analyzing blood samples, the consumption of oxygen by the electrode leads to an underestimation of the partial pressure of oxygen in a blood sample by 2% to 6%. This phenomenon, which has been called the blood gas factor, is due to the slow rate of oxygen diffusion in fluids (i.e., oxygen consumed by the electrode is not replaced by oxygen from the blood).[19] The magnitude of the blood gas factor depends on the diameter of the cathode and the thickness of the membrane between the sample and the cathode. Exposure of the PO_2 electrode to nitrous oxide and halothane (gaseous anesthetic agents) may also alter its electronic output by increasing the production of peroxide ions.[17]

Because an external polarizing voltage is applied to create this potential difference, the Clark electrode is called a polarographic electrode.

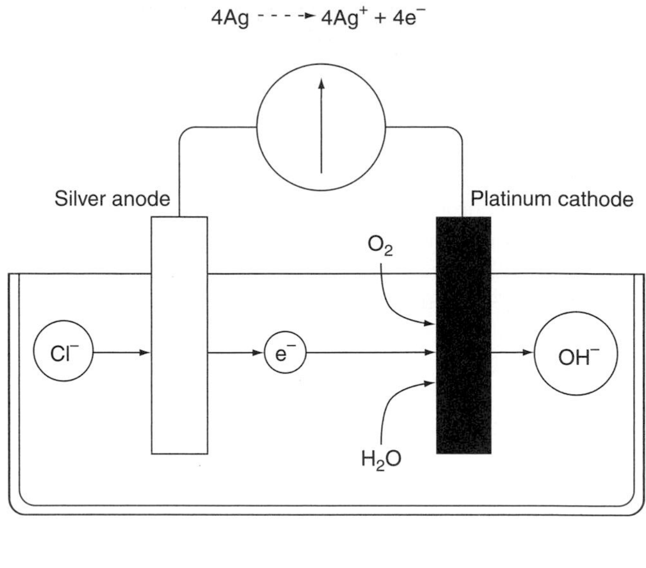

Figure 10-7 Principles of PO_2 measurements; see text for discussion. (From Shapiro BA, Peruzzi WT, Templin R: *Clinical application of blood gases*, ed 5, St Louis, 1994, Mosby.)

Derived Variables

Several variables can be calculated from the measurements of pH, $PaCO_2$, and PaO_2. Oxygen saturation of hemoglobin, P_{50}, bicarbonate, **buffer base,** and **base excess/deficit** are examples of derived variables. Although most modern blood gas analyzers have computer software that automatically calculates these variables, they can also be determined using formulae or nomograms that incorporate accepted constants. Note, however, that these derived variables are calculated and not measured. As such, they may be inaccurate when compared with actual measurements because they may not necessarily account for all confounding factors. For example, calculations of oxygen saturation of hemoglobin do not account for the presence of dyshemoglobins, such as carboxyhemoglobin and methemoglobin.

Oxygen Saturation of Hemoglobin (SO_2)

The percentage of available hemoglobin that is saturated with oxygen can be calculated by using an equation empirically derived from the oxyhemoglobin saturation curve. These calculations do not account for all of the variables (e.g., the actual $PaCO_2$ or the presence of dyshemoglobins) that can affect this value, and therefore can lead to erroneous conclusions about the level of oxyhemoglobin saturation. Direct measurement of oxyhemoglobin saturation will be discussed along with oximetry later in this chapter. Directly measured values are more reliable and should be used

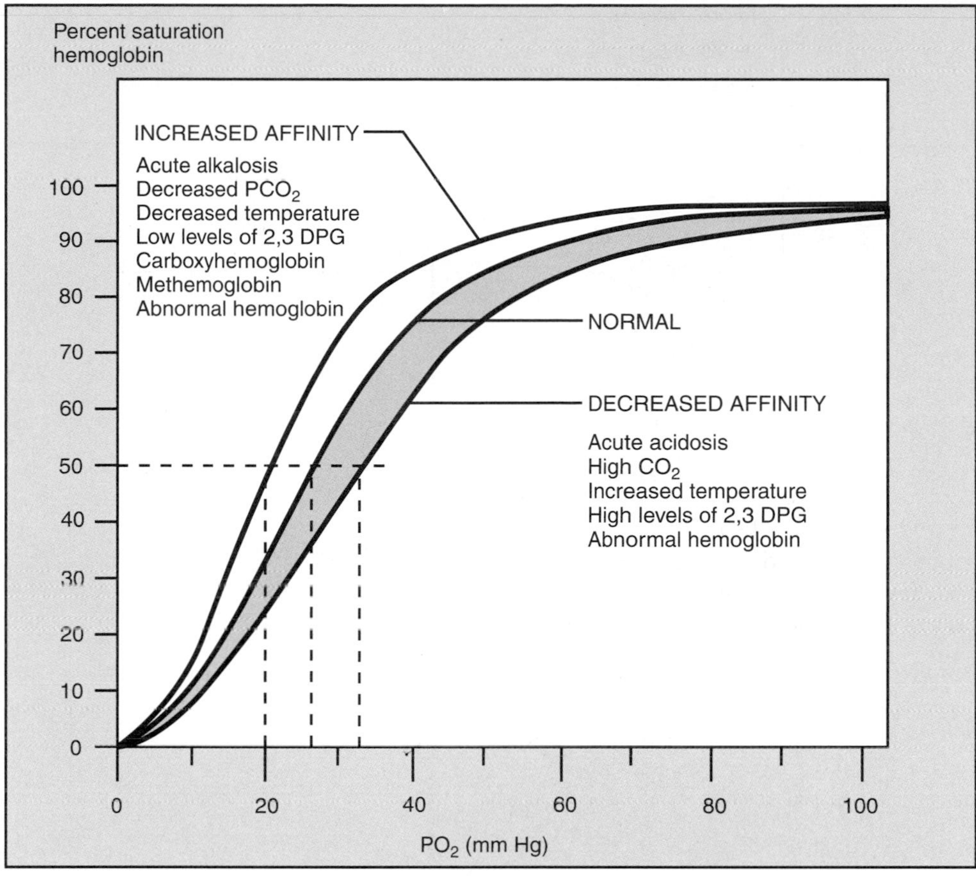

Figure 10-8 Effects of changes in pH, PCO_2, and 2,3 DPG on the oxyhemoglobin dissociation curve. (Redrawn from Lane EE, Walker JF: *Clinical arterial blood gas analysis*, St Louis, 1987, Mosby.)

instead of a derived oxygen saturation value when making decisions about a patient's oxygenation status. Notice that although both calculated and measured SO_2 are identical in many cases, this is not always true.

P_{50} Determinations

P_{50} is a convenient way of describing hemoglobin affinity for oxygen because it identifies the PO_2 in mm Hg when hemoglobin is 50% saturated with oxygen. It is determined by equilibrating a blood sample with various oxygen concentrations at 37° C, which can be accomplished with a tonometer connected to a series of certified gas mixtures.* As Figure 10-8 illustrates, alterations in hemoglobin affinity for oxygen are associated with shifting of the oxyhemoglobin dissociation curve. It is well established that the affinity of hemoglobin A (HbA, or normal adult hemoglobin) for oxygen, and thus the P_{50}, can be altered by changes in the pH, PCO_2, temperature, and 2,3 diphosphoglycerate concentration of arterial blood. The presence of **fetal hemoglobin (HbF)** and carboxyhemoglobin (COHb) can also alter the oxyhemoglobin curve. P_{50} determinations are not routinely performed, but they can be helpful in diagnosing and managing hypoxemia associated with various types of hemoglobinopathies.

**The P_{50} measurements are standardized for a pH of 7.40, $PaCO_2$ of 40 mm Hg, and a temperature of 37° C.*[18,19]

Bicarbonate, Buffer Base, and Base Excess

The actual bicarbonate is the concentration of HCO_3^- in the plasma of anaerobically drawn blood.[16] It is derived from measurements of pH and $PaCO_2$ using the Henderson-Hasselbalch equation. (Note that the standard bicarbonate is also derived from the Henderson-Hasselbalch equation, but it represents the bicarbonate concentration in a fully oxygenated plasma sample measured at a temperature of 37° C and a $PaCO_2$ of 40 mm Hg.) Plasma bicarbonate levels are normally from 22 to 26 mmol/L. The HCO_3^- becomes elevated in metabolic alkalosis and chronic respiratory acidosis and reduced in metabolic acidosis and chronic respiratory alkalosis.

The buffer base represents the sum of all the anion buffers in blood, including bicarbonate, hemoglobin, inorganic phosphate, and negatively charged proteins.[18] The buffer base usually ranges from 44 to 48 mmol/L. The base excess/deficit is the number of millimoles of strong acid required to titrate a blood sample to a pH of 7.4 at a PCO_2 of 40 mm Hg. Theoretically, the buffer base and the base excess are not affected by changes in respiratory function, so they can be used to identify nonrespiratory disturbances in acid-base status. Figure 10-9 is a **Siggaard-Andersen alignment nomogram** for calculating actual and standard bicarbonate, buffer base, and base excess concentrations.

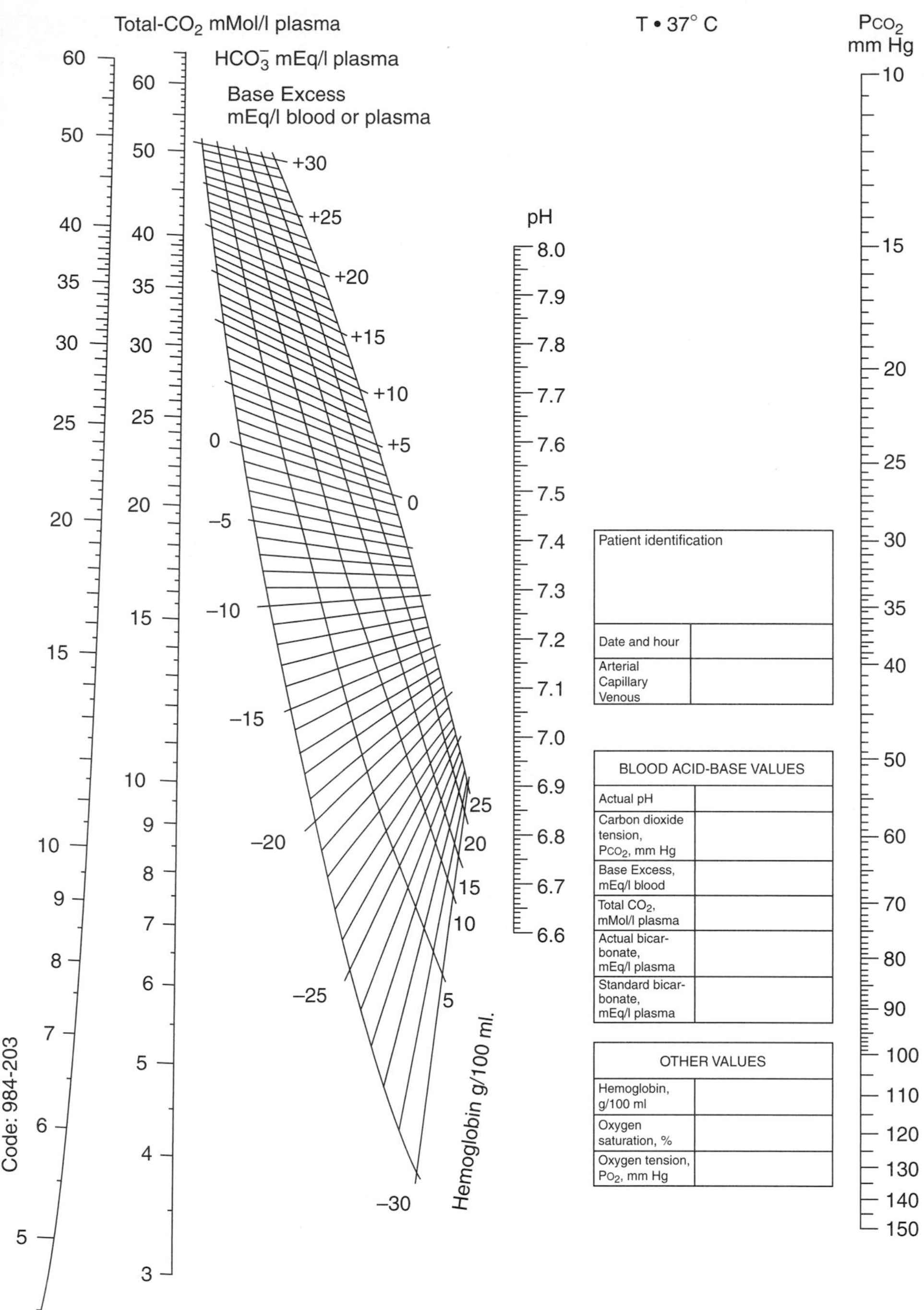

Figure 10-9 Siggaard-Andersen alignment nomogram: a line is drawn between pH and PCO_2, and actual bicarbonate is read directly at the intersection of this line. BE_b is hemoglobin dependent and can be read at the intersection of the constructed line and the patient's Hb value. Standard bicarbonate can be determined by constructing another line through the BE-Hb point and the Pco_2 of 40 mm Hg, and by reading the HCO_3^- scale. Buffer base can be computed from the equation BB = 41.7 + (0.42 × Hb) + BE. BE_{ECF} is calculated similarly to BE_b, but the BE_{ECF} is read off at the intersection of the constructed line and one-third of the patient's Hb value. (Modified from Siggaard-Andersen O, Radiometer A/S: Arterial blood gas analyzers. In Burton G, Hodgkin JE, Ward JJ: *Respiratory care: a guide to clinical practice*, ed 4, Philadelphia, 1997, JB Lippincott.)

Whole Blood Analysis: Electrolytes and Glucose

Many blood gas analyzers incorporate sensors for measuring electrolytes (e.g., Na^+, K^+, Cl^-, Ca^{++}) and metabolites (e.g., glucose). Table 10-4 contains the normal values for plasma electrolytes. The sensors used for electrolyte measurements are ion-selective electrodes, but those used to measure glucose are coated with an enzyme called glucose oxidase. Electrolytes are determined by potentiometric measurements, but metabolites are determined by amperometric measurements.

Table 10-4 Normal values for plasma electrolytes

Parameter	Symbol	Normal Values
Sodium	Na^+	136-145 mEq/L
Potassium	K^+	3.5-5.0 mEq/L
Total calcium	Ca^{++}	9.9-11.0 mEq/L
Magnesium	Mg^{++}	1.5-2.5 mEq/L
Chloride	Cl^-	98-106 mEq/L
Glucose*	–	100 ± 20 mg/dL

*Although glucose is not classified as an electrolyte, it is included in this table for reference because many blood gas analyzers can now provide determinations of serum glucose concentrations.

The typical electrolyte sensor is composed of a measuring half-cell and an external reference half-cell, which form a complete electrochemical cell. The measuring half-cell is made of a silver/silver chloride wire that is surrounded by an electrolyte-specific solution. For example, the electrolyte solution used in the sodium and chloride sensors contains a fixed concentration of sodium and chloride; the potassium sensor electrolyte contains a fixed concentration of potassium; and the calcium electrolyte contains a fixed concentration of calcium. The electrolyte solution is separated from the sample solution by an ion-selective membrane, and as the sample comes in contact with the membrane, a transmembrane potential develops across the membrane because of the exchange of ions across it. The potential developed across the membrane is compared with the constant potential of the external reference sensor, and the magnitude of the potential difference is proportional to the ion activity of the sample.

A glucose type of sensor consists of four electrodes:

1. The measuring electrode, which is made of platinum and glucose oxidase, is enclosed in a binder.
2. A second reference electrode, which is composed of silver/silver chloride.
3. A "counter" electrode, which is composed of platinum, ensures that a constant polarizing voltage is applied to the sensor.
4. A second "counter" electrode, which does not contain the enzyme glucose oxidase, is used to quantify interfering substances in the sample.

As the sample contacts the measuring electrode, glucose oxidase on the surface of the electrode converts the glucose in the sample to hydrogen peroxide and gluconic acid. The polarizing voltage applied to the electrode causes the hydrogen peroxide to oxidize, resulting in the loss of electrons. The loss of electrons causes current flow to be directly proportional to the glucose concentration of the sample.

Quality Assurance of Blood Gas Analyzers

The Joint Commission on Accreditation of Healthcare Organizations (JCAHO), the Centers for Medicare & Medicaid Services (formerly Health Care Financing Administration), and The College of American Pathologists (CAP) have published standards that clinical blood gas laboratories must follow to ensure the accuracy and reliability of blood gas measurements. These standards, which are based on recommendations from the **Clinical Laboratory Improvement Amendments of 1988 (CLIA-88)**, require routine calibrations of instruments, and programs for assessing **quality control (QC)** and **quality assurance (QA)**.[2,20,21]

Calibration standards for most blood gas analyzers are buffers for pH electrodes and specially prepared gases for the PCO_2 and PO_2 electrodes.[22] (Note that buffers and calibration gases must be clearly labeled with reference values and defined confidence limits.) Verification of the instrument's calibration may vary according to the regulatory agency under which the laboratory is accredited or licensed (e.g., CAP, JCAHO).[2] Generally, every instrument in operation must undergo routine one- and two-point calibrations, which should include high and low pH, PCO_2, and PO_2 values. The **one-point calibration** involves adjusting the electronic output to a single, known standard. With two-point calibrations, the electrode's electronic output is adjusted to two known standards. A one-point calibration should be performed before an unknown sample is analyzed, unless the analyzer is programmed to automatically perform a one-point calibration at regular intervals (e.g., every 20 to 30 minutes). **Two-point calibrations** are usually performed at least three times daily, usually every 8 hours. In many cases, analyzers can be programmed to perform a two-point calibration at predetermined intervals. A **three-point calibration** should be performed every 6 months, or whenever an electrode is replaced. Three-point calibrations involve adding a third standard that is intermediate to the other standards to ensure linearity of the electrode response. A fourth level may be required if samples containing high O_2 levels are analyzed with the instrument.[2]

The National Institute of Standards and Technology (NIST) and the International Federation of Clinical Chemistry (IFCC) have established standards for the calibration of blood gas electrodes. A nearly normal pH buffer (pH = 7.384) is used for one-point calibrations; a second, lower pH buffer (pH = 6.840) is analyzed in the two-point calibration to ensure that the electronic output of the electrode is linear over a wide range of pHs. The PCO_2 electrode is calibrated with two gas concentrations: a 5% CO_2 mixture for establishing the lower end of CO_2s encountered and a 10% CO_2 mixture for the high end of the range. The 5% mixture is used for one-point calibrations, but both mixtures are used in the two-point calibration to establish a linear slope for the electrode's electronic output. The PO_2 electrode is also calibrated with two gas mixtures: usually a gas mixture with 0% O_2 and another with 12% or 20% O_2.[18] The accuracy of oxygen electrodes may vary by as much as 20% for high PO_2s because of the lack of linearity between electronic output and oxygen tensions above 150 mm Hg. It has been suggested that the latter problem can be minimized by using additional calibration gases with higher concentrations of oxygen (i.e., >20% O_2).

Quality control may be defined as a system that includes analyzing control samples (with known pH, PCO_2, and PO_2), assessing the measurements against defined limits, identifying problems, and specifying corrective actions. Internal quality control can be accomplished by periodically analyzing commercial products with known pH, PCO_2, and PO_2 values. Quality control materials include human or bovine whole blood samples that have been tonometered to exact gas tensions or commercially prepared aqueous buffers and perfluorocarbon emulsions that have been equilibrated with a series of known PCO_2 and PO_2 values by the manufacturer. Although tonometry remains the gold standard method for quality control of PCO_2 and PO_2 electrodes, most laboratories use commercially prepared quality control systems for biosafety and convenience. It should be mentioned, however, that commercially prepared controls provide information on the instrument's precision—not the accuracy of the data. (Remember that precision refers to the reproducibility of repeat measurements, and accuracy relates to how close the measurement is to the correct value.) Additionally, commercial controls are susceptible to variations in room storage temperature and do not reflect temperature and protein errors in blood gas analyzers.[18]

Regardless of the type of quality control material used to assess an instrument's performance, results should be recorded in a manner that allows the operator to detect changes in the operation of the blood gas analyzer. The most common method of recording quality control data involves the use of **Levy-Jennings charts** (Figure 10-10). These charts allow the operator to detect trends and shifts in electrode performance, thus helping to avoid problems associated with reporting inaccurate data due to analyzer malfunction. For example, a trend (Figure 10-10, *A*) is typically associated with protein buildup on an electrode membrane or an electrode nearing the end of its life expectancy. A shift (Figure 10-10, *B*) can be due to a tear in the electrode membrane or loss of the electrolyte that bathes the electrode.

Quality assurance involves testing the proficiency of both personnel and equipment, providing a dynamic process of identification, evaluation, and resolution of problems that affect blood gas measurements.[22] CAP and the American Thoracic Society (ATS) currently offer two proficiency testing programs that provide a means of assessing blind samples (periodically) and the technical competence of laboratory personnel, and a means of reporting the variability of individual blood gas analyzers.

Proficiency testing materials usually include a series of unknown samples with target values that have been established by previously identified reference laboratories. At regular intervals throughout the year (i.e., a minimum of three times per year), all participating laboratories analyze unknown samples (typically three to five samples are used) and forward their results to the sponsoring organization collating the results from all laboratories. The criteria for acceptable results are defined, and the laboratory personnel are notified of their laboratory's performance. (Generally, an acceptable pH is within ±0.04 of the target value; PCO_2 values must be ±3 mm Hg or ±8% of the target value, whichever is greater; and PO_2 values must be within ±3 standard deviations.)[18,19] An unsatisfactory performance, which is a failure to achieve any of the target values at a single event, necessitates that remedial action is taken and documented. Unsuccessful performance, which is associated with a failure to achieve the target values for an analyte in two consecutive events or in two out of three consecutive events, can result in sanctions placed on the laboratory.[10-20] These sanctions can lose revenue for the laboratory because of suspension of Medicare and Medicaid reimbursement. The laboratory can only be reinstated by additional staff training, increased quality control procedures, and reapplication with evidence that the problems have been corrected.

Temperature Correction of Blood Gases

With most modern blood gas analyzers, the blood sample is heated and maintained at a constant temperature of 37° C during analysis. The term ***temperature correction*** refers to the application of mathematical formulae to adjust blood gas tensions to more accurately reflect the patient's core temperature (i.e., the temperature in the artery from which

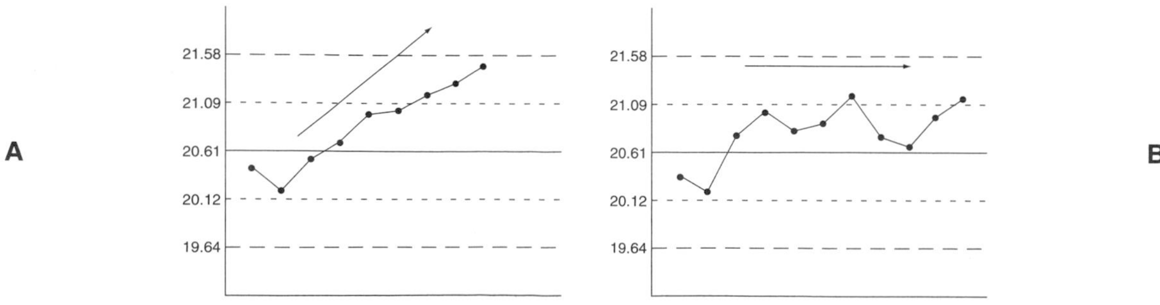

Figure 10-10 Levy-Jennings charts demonstrating two types of trend **(A)** and shift **(B)**.

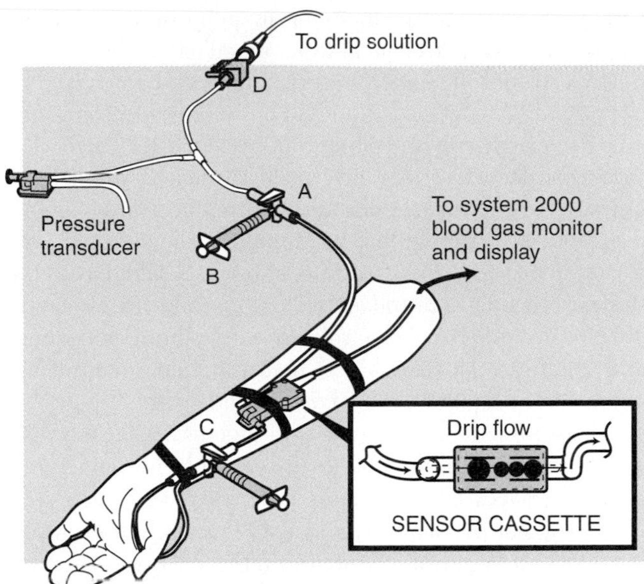

Figure 10-11 A fiberoptic blood-gas monitor. (Redrawn from Shapiro BA, et al: Clinical performance of a blood gas monitor: a prospective, multicenter trial, *Crit Care Med* 21:487, 1993.)

the blood sample was obtained). There is considerable debate as to whether it is necessary or even desirable to make these temperature corrections. Those favoring temperature corrections for blood gas analysis point out that corrected results are a true reflection of the oxygenation and acid-base status of an individual. According to Mohler and associates,[23] the PaO_2 changes approximately 7% for each degree Celsius; the $PaCO_2$ changes about 4% per degree Celsius; and the pH changes by 0.0146 per degree Celsius. Proponents of reporting blood gases at 37° C believe that pH and $PaCO_2$ values standardized to a body temperature of 37° C reliably reflect the in vivo acid-base status of the patient and that correction of pH and $PaCO_2$ do not affect the calculated HCO_3.[18] Furthermore, most acid-base nomograms are calculated for 37° C, and considerable errors occur if temperature-corrected blood gas data are used with these nomograms. Although all commercial blood gas analyzers contain solid-state circuitry that can easily perform temperature corrections, most laboratories still report blood gases at 37° C because of the lack of consensus on the topic.

In Vivo Blood Gas Monitors

As previously mentioned, recent advances in fiberoptics technology have made it possible to obtain continuous, in vivo ABG and pH measurements. A typical in vivo blood gas monitor contains one or more optical sensors that are imbedded in a gas or ion-permeable polymer matrix. The sensors are connected to a central processing unit via a fiberoptic cable. The fiberoptic sensor is inserted into the intravascular space through an indwelling 20-gauge cannula. Light of a specific wavelength and intensity from the central processing unit is transmitted along the fiber to a microcuvette containing a fluorescent dye. The incident light striking the microcuvette is modified in proportion to the PO_2, PCO_2, or pH levels of the blood, which is in contact with the microcuvette. The modified light is then transmitted back to the monitor, through either the same optical path or a second fiber parallel to the fiber carrying the incident light.[24] Figure 10-11 shows an alternative extra-arterial blood gas monitor. In this case, the blood gas sensor is located in series with the arterial catheter.

Optical blood gas sensors are generally categorized by how they modify the initial optical signal; they are classified as either **absorbance** or **fluorescent sensors.**[18] For absorbance sensors, when light of a known wavelength and intensity is transmitted down the fiber and through the microcuvette, a fraction of the incident light is absorbed, and the remaining light is transmitted. The concentration of the analyte can be determined by measuring the intensity of the light striking the photodetector because the amount of light transmitted is proportional to the concentration of the analyte in question (i.e., the pH, PCO_2, or PO_2)

Fluorescent sensors use dyes that fluoresce when they are struck by light in the ultraviolet or nearly ultraviolet visible range. Light from the monitor is transmitted to the microcuvette containing the dye. The dye absorbs the light energy of the optical excitation signal and emits a fluorescent signal that is returned to the monitor along the fiberoptic cable. The concentration of the analyte in question can be measured by determining the ratio of fluorescent light emitted to the original excitation light signal. The pH, PCO_2, or PO_2 of arterial blood can be determined by using sensing fibers containing dye systems that are analyte-specific (i.e., most commercially available systems contain three analyte-specific sensing fibers).

Fluorescent sensors currently in use can measure pH values from 6.8 to 7.8, PCO_2 values from 10 to 100 mm Hg, and PO_2 values from 20 to 600 mm Hg. When compared with in vitro blood gas analysis, intraarterial blood gas monitoring systems are comparable for pH, however, the correlation may not be as good for PCO_2 and PO_2 measurements.[24]

Calibration of Intraarterial Blood Gas Monitors

Intraarterial blood gas monitoring systems must be calibrated before being inserted into a patient by immersing the sensor in a buffer containing known pH, PCO_2, and PO_2 values. In vivo calibrations are complicated and subject to error because adjustment must be made using single-point measurements from laboratory (in vitro) ABG analysis.

In many cases, temperature corrections may be required because the sensor may be in a peripheral artery where the measured temperature may not equal the patient's core temperature. Temperature corrections are usually accomplished by combining a temperature measuring thermocouple with the analyte-specific sensor. By measuring the sensor's temperature, the pH or blood gas value may then be displayed as measured, or corrected to 37° C (or some other user-entered patient temperature).

Point-of-Care (POC) Testing

Point-of-care testing involves testing outside of the main hospital laboratory. POC testing typically involves using portable devices that can be located at or near the point of patient care. As such, these are lightweight, portable devices (total weight is approximately 1 lb) that allow in vitro ABG and pH measurements in the emergency room, intensive care unit, physician's office, or in a transport vehicle.[25] Figure 10-12 shows a typical POC blood gas analyzer. POC devices are usually battery-powered but can be powered by a standard AC electrical outlet. The system uses solid-state sensors, which rely on either fluorescence technology or thin-film electrodes that have been fabricated onto silicon chips. The microelectrodes are incorporated into a single-use disposable cartridge that also contains calibration reagents, a sampling stylus, and a waste container. In addition to the standard blood gas cartridges, several modules are also available for the analysis of electrolytes (e.g., sodium, potassium, and chloride), lactates, blood urea nitrogen, glucose, and hematocrit. Results are shown on a liquid crystal display.

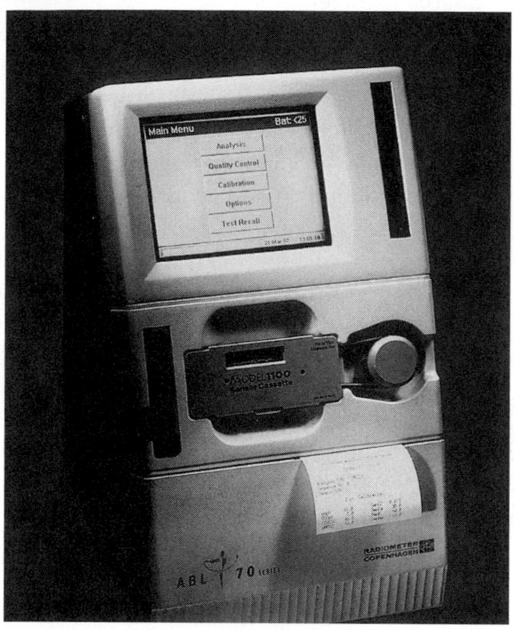

Figure 10-12 A point of care blood gas analyzer. (Courtesy Radiometer America, Cleveland).

Measurements can be made on blood samples less than a milliliter in volume in 60 to 120 seconds. Manufacturers of POC devices state that these devices are accurate over a wide range of pH, $PaCO_2$, and PaO_2 values. For example, iSTAT (East Windsor, NJ) states that its device has a range of 6.8 to 8.0 for pH, 10 to 100 torr for $PaCO_2$, and 5 torr to 800 torr for PaO_2. The use of these devices is growing, especially as a replacement for "stat" laboratory services. Table 10-5 compares four commercial POC blood gas analyzers currently available.[25] Box 10-1 summarizes the potential advantages and disadvantages of using POC testing.

CO-Oximetry

An oximeter is a device that can measure the oxyhemoglobin saturation of arterial, venous, mixed venous, or intracardiac blood. Two types of oximeters are routinely used in respiratory

Table 10-5 Comparison of four point-of-care blood gas analyzers

	StatsPal II	Gem 6	Gem Stat	Gem Premier
Measured values	pH	pH	pH	pH
	PCO_2	PCO_2	PCO_2	PCO_2
	PO_2	PO_2	PO_2	PO_2
		Hct	Hct	Hct
		Ca^{++}	Ca^{++}	Ca^{++}
		K^+	K^+	K^+
			Na^+	Na^+
Calculated values	6	5	4	4
Sample volume	0.2 mL	2 mL	0.5 mL	0.2 mL
Analysis time	60 sec	130 sec	109 sec	92 sec
Samples/module	25	50 in 72 hr	50 in 72 hr	150 or 300 in 7 d
Interface	–	RS 232		
Data management	–	Hard copy of module in use	Hard copy of module in use	Hard copy or floppy disk storage of module in use

From Levine RL, Fromm Jr RE: Critical care monitoring: from pre-hospital to the ICU, St Louis, 1995, Mosby.
StatPal II (PPG Industries, Inc), Gem 6, Gem Stat, and Gem Premier (Mallinckrodt Sensor Systems).
PCO_2, Partial pressure of carbon dioxide; *PO_2*, partial pressure of oxygen; *Hct*, hematocrit; *Ca*, calcium.

Box 10-1 Advantage and Disadvantages of Point-of Care Testing

Potential Advantages	Potential Disadvantages
Decreased therapeutic turnaround time	Lack of adequate documentation
Rapid data availability	QC and proficiency testing issues
Augmented clinical decision making	Unauthorized testing
Increased real-time patient management	Poor analytic performance
Shortened length of stay	Problems with training and competency
Decreased preanalytic error	Increased preanalytic error
Decreased patient cost per episode	Data not recorded
Test clustering	Sample handling error
Decreased iatrogenic blood loss	Limited test menu
Increased patient throughput	Decreased entry of results in patient record
Fewer redundant blood tests	Postanalytic error (e.g., transcription error or communication failure)
Convenient for the clinician	Need for separate license(s)
Improved clinician-patient interface	Failure to comply with regulations
Customized instrumentation	Increased costs
Convenient when laboratory is inaccessible	Duplication of instruments and methods
Rapid response to critical results	No critical values notification system and/or documentation
Integration with performance maps, algorithms, and care paths	

From Kost GJ, Ehrmeyer SS, Chernow B: The laboratory-clinical interface, point of care testing, *Chest* 115(4):1142, 1999.

care: CO-oximeters and pulse oximeters. A CO-oximeter can provide simultaneous in vitro measurements of various hemoglobin gases, including oxyhemoglobin (HbO_2), carboxyhemoglobin (HbCO), methemoglobin (HbMet), **Sulfhemoglobin (HbS),** and fetal hemoglobin (HbF) using whole blood samples. Pulse oximeters are noninvasive devices that can only provide measurements of arterial oxyhemoglobin saturation. Pulse oximeters will be discussed in detail in the section on noninvasive assessment of ABGs.

Oximeters operate on the principle of spectrophotometry, which is based on the relative transmission or absorption of portions of the light spectrum.[26] The various forms of hemoglobin mentioned previously can be identified because each form has its own absorption spectrum. (Figure 10-13 illustrates the light spectra for each hemoglobin.) The concentration of a certain hemoglobin type can be determined using the Lambert-Beer law, which states that the transmission of a specific wavelength of light through a solution is a logarithmic function of the concentration of the absorbing species in the solution.[18,27]

The principle of operation of a typical CO-oximeter is fairly straightforward. A blood sample is heated to 37° C and hemolyzed (either chemically or by high-frequency vibrations), creating a translucent solution. The solution is placed in a cuvette, which is positioned between a light source and a condenser and two photodetectors. A series of monochromatic light beams are simultaneously directed through the cuvette containing the sample of blood and through a blank solution (containing no hemoglobin).[18] The condenser lens system focuses the light passing through the sample cuvette onto a photodetector, which generates an electric current that is proportional to the intensity of the transmitted light and inversely proportional to the amount of light absorbed by the sample. The light passing through the blank solution is simultaneously focused onto a reference photodetector, which generates an electric current proportional to the light transmitted through the blank solution. The absorbance of the blank solution is then subtracted from the absorbances of the blood sample, and the resultant values are used to calculate the concentration of each type of hemoglobin in the blood sample. The normal concentrations of the various hemoglobin types are shown in Table 10-1.

Although blood can contain six different types of hemoglobin, most commercially available CO-oximeters provide measurements of only four types: HbO_2, deoxyhemoglobin (Hb), HbMet, and HbCO. Sulfhemoglobin and fetal hemoglobin are not usually determined by CO-oximetry, although Radiometer (Radiometer America, Westlake, Oh) has introduced a CO-oximetry procedure to determine fetal hemoglobin. Although these results are different from reference methods such as radioimmunoassay and chromatographic procedures, CO-oximeter analysis of fetal hemoglobin has been clinically acceptable. Other reported values may include **total hemoglobin (THb)** and **oxygen content (O_2ct).**

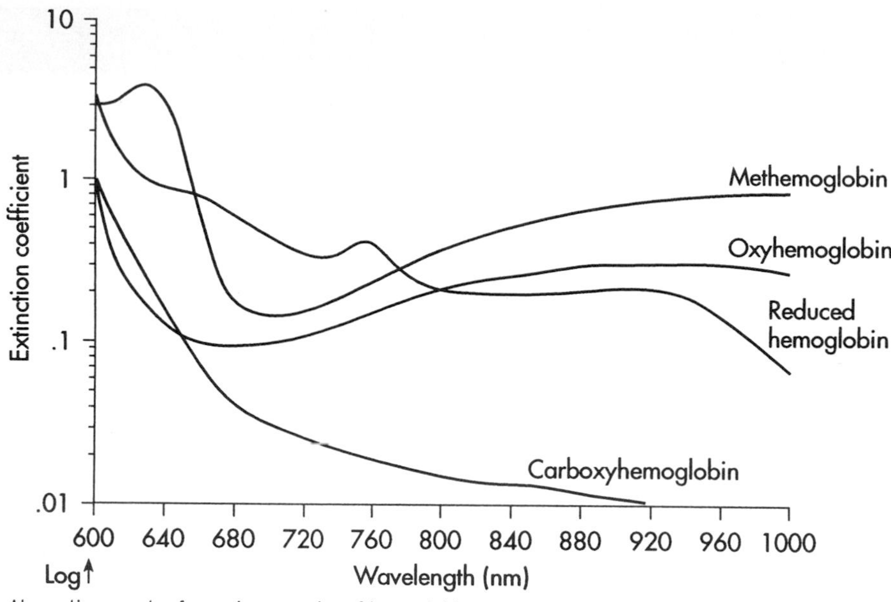

Figure 10-13 Absorption spectra for various species of hemoglobin. (From Pilbeam S: *Mechanical ventilation: physiological and clinical applications*, ed 3, St Louis, 1998, Mosby.)

A number of factors can interfere with CO-oximetry measurements. Incompletely hemolyzed red blood cells, lipids or air bubbles in the sample can scatter some of the incident light, thus producing erroneous measurements.[28,29] The presence of bilirubin (>20 mg/dL of whole blood) or intravenous dyes (particularly methylene blue and indocyanine green) can also alter measurements because they absorb near-infrared (IR) and IR light. Absorbance of light by these substances lowers the actual oxyhemoglobin measured. The presence of fetal hemoglobin can also lead to false HbCO readings. Oxygenated fetal hemoglobin produces a 4% to 7% false carboxyhemoglobin level; reduced fetal hemoglobin yields a 0.2% to 1.5% false carboxyhemoglobin level.[18]

Calibration of CO-Oximeters

CO-oximeters should be routinely calibrated with solutions supplied by the manufacturer. These solutions are typically dye-based propylene glycol solutions that only allow for the calibration of total hemoglobin. Determination of the various forms of hemoglobin is accomplished by relating the relative absorbances recorded at the wavelengths tested. That is, the percentage of a particular hemoglobin type reported is derived from absorbance ratios at predetermined wavelengths.

Noninvasive Assessment of ABGs

Noninvasive blood gas monitoring has become a standard practice in respiratory care and anesthesiology. The importance of these devices in the management of patients with cardiopulmonary dysfunctions cannot be overstated. In just 30 years, pulse oximeters and transcutaneous pH, PCO_2, and PO_2 monitors have gone from expensive, bulky units to compact, affordable devices that can provide both continuous and intermittent pH, PCO_2, and PO_2 measurements that are reliable and accurate.

Pulse Oximetry

Pulse oximetry provides continuous, noninvasive measurements of arterial oxygen saturation and pulse rate via a sensor placed over a digit, an earlobe, or the bridge of the nose that measures the absorption of selected wavelengths of light beamed through the tissue. Advances in microprocessor technology, coupled with improvements in the quality of **light-emitting diodes (LEDs)** and photoelectric sensors have greatly improved the accuracy and reliability of these devices. Pulse oximetry is now considered by most clinicians as an indispensable tool for monitoring the oxygenation status of patients at risk of hypoxemia.

Theory of Operation

Pulse oximetry is based on the principles of spectrophotometry and **photoplethysmography.**[30-32] As with CO-oximeters, pulse oximeters use spectrophotometry to determine the amount of hemoglobin (and deoxyhemoglobin) in a blood sample. Oxyhemoglobin and deoxygenated hemoglobin are differentiated by shining two wavelengths of light (660 and 940 nm) through the sampling site. As Figure 10-13 shows, at a wavelength of 660 nm (red light), deoxygenated hemoglobin absorbs more light than oxyhemoglobin. Conversely, oxyhemoglobin absorbs more light at 940 nm (IR light) than deoxygenated hemoglobin.

Photoplethysmography, or **optical plethysmography,** estimates heart rate by measuring cyclic changes in light

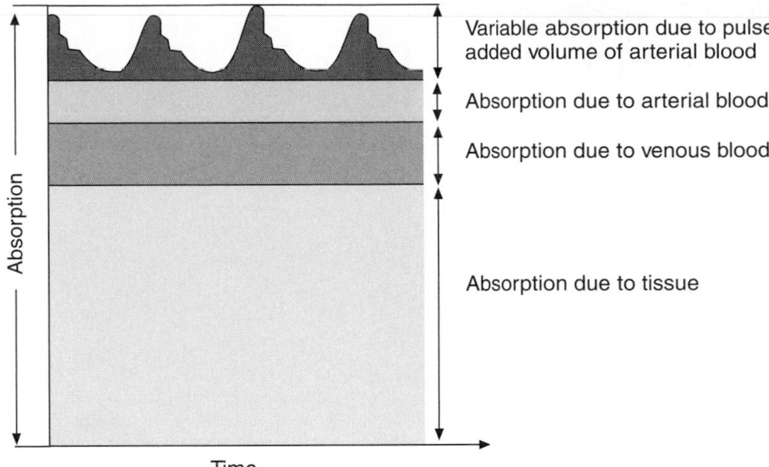

Figure 10-14 Pulsatile and nonpulsatile components of a typical pulse oximetry signal. (From McGough EK, Boysen PG: Benefits and limits of pulse oximetry in the ICU, *J Crit Ill* 4(2):23, 1989.)

transmission through the sampling site during each cardiac cycle. That is, as the blood volume in the finger, toe, or ear lobe increases during ventricular systole, light absorption increases and transmitted light decreases. Conversely, as blood volume decreases during diastole, absorbency decreases and transmitted light increases. The pulsatile and non-pulsatile components of a typical pulse oximetry signal are shown in Figure 10-14.

The percentage of oxyhemoglobin in a sample can be determined by first calculating the ratio of absorbencies for pulsatile and non-pulsatile flow at the two specified wavelengths, or

$$\text{Red/Infrared} = \frac{\text{Pulsatile}_{660\text{ nm}}/\text{Non-pulsatile}_{660\text{ nm}}}{\text{Pulsatile}_{940\text{ nm}}/\text{Non-pulsatile}_{940\text{ nm}}}$$

This ratio is then applied to an algorithm that relates the ratios of these two absorbencies to oxyhemoglobin saturation.[32]

As mentioned previously, four types of hemoglobin can be measured by oximetry: reduced or deoxygenated hemoglobin (HHb), oxyhemoglobin (O_2Hb), COHb, and methemoglobin (MetHb). Two terms that are often used when describing oxyhemoglobin saturation determinations are fractional and functional saturations. **Fractional hemoglobin saturation** is calculated by dividing the amount of oxyhemoglobin by the amount of all four types of hemoglobin present, or

$$\text{Fractional } O_2Hb = O_2Hb \div [HHb + O_2Hb + COHb + MetHb]$$

Functional hemoglobin saturation is calculated by dividing the oxyhemoglobin concentration by the concentration of hemoglobin capable of carrying oxygen. It may be written as,

$$\text{Functional } O_2Hb = O_2Hb \div [HHb\ O_2Hb]$$

Although laboratory CO-oximeters measure all four types of hemoglobin by using a series of wavelengths of light to identify each species, pulse oximeters use only two wavelengths to quantify the amount of O_2Hb and HHb present. Thus laboratory CO-oximeters can report fractional oxyhemoglobin saturation, and pulse oximeters can estimate functional oxyhemoglobin saturation.

Physiological and Technical Considerations

It is important to recognize that both physiological and technical factors can influence the accuracy of pulse oximetry measurements. A brief discussion of how each factor can affect pulse oximeter accuracy follows.[33]

Low Perfusion States

The accuracy of a pulse oximeter reading depends on the identification of an arterial pulse, therefore many conditions can interfere with proper pulse oximeter function. Hypovolemia, peripheral vasoconstriction from drugs or hypothermia, and heart-lung bypass (i.e., extracorporeal membrane oxygenation [ECMO]) are associated with a diminished pulsatile signal resulting in either an intermittent or absent oxygen saturation measured by pulse oximeter (SpO_2) reading.[30] Some oximeters compensate for the weak signal associated with low perfusion states by increasing the signal output. The problem with this approach is that augmenting the signal also causes an increase in the signal-to-noise ratio, which can result in high levels of background noise that can contribute to erroneous results. A simpler approach is to reposition the oximeter sensor in an area of higher perfusion. For example, placement of the oximeter probe on the ear instead of the finger may alleviate some of the problems associated with reductions in peripheral perfusion.

Dysfunctional Hemoglobins

It is well-established that high levels of dysfunctional hemoglobins (i.e., COHb and MetHb) can adversely affect oxyhemoglobin measurements by pulse oximeter.[30] High COHb levels can alter SpO_2 measurements because O_2Hb and COHb have similar absorption coefficients for red light

CLINICAL ROUNDS 10-3

Assessment of a patient admitted to the emergency department after exposure to an enclosed fire included evaluation of SpO_2 and ABGs. Results were obtained while the patient was breathing room air: SpO_2 = 98%, pH = 7.38, $PaCO_2$ = 35 mm Hg, PaO_2 = 95 mm Hg, and SaO_2 = 97%. What is your interpretation of these findings?

See Appendix A for the answer.

(660 nm), but COHb is relatively transparent to IR light (940 nm). Accordingly, significant levels of HbCO, as occur in carbon monoxide poisoning, lead to an overestimation of SpO_2.[30] (See Clinical Rounds 10-3 for a decision-making problem involving pulse oximetry.)

Methemoglobinemia, a complication associated with administering certain types of drugs (e.g., nitrites, benzocaine [a local anesthetic], dapsone [an antibiotic used to treat malaria and *Pneumocystis carinii*]), can lead to erroneous SpO_2 values because MetHb absorbs both red and IR light.[30] Methemoglobinemia is also associated with nitrate poisoning. If enough MetHb is present to dominate all pulsatile absorption, the pulse oximeter will measure a red to IR ratio of 1:1, corresponding to a SpO_2 of about 85%. Consequently, the pulse oximeter reading will over- or underestimate the true oxyhemoglobin saturation.[30]

Dyes

Intravascular dyes can adversely affect SpO_2 values by absorbing a portion of the incident light emitted by the pulse oximeter diodes. Injection of methylene blue and indigo carmine during cardiac catheterization causes a false drop in SpO_2; indocyanine green has been shown to have little effect on pulse oximeter readings.[33]

Dark nail polishes (particularly blue and black nail polish) can severely affect SpO_2 readings. It has been suggested that nail polish may affect pulse oximetry values by causing the shunting of light around the finger periphery.[34,35] In **optical shunting,** transmitted light never comes in contact with the vascular bed, so SpO_2 values can be erroneously high or low, depending on whether this light is pulsatile. This problem can be alleviated to a large extent by placing the device over the lateral aspects of the digit instead of over the nail. Theoretically, skin pigmentation should not affect pulse oximeter readings; but in practice, SpO_2 readings are inconsistent for patients with dark pigmentation possibly because of optical shunting.[36] **Hyperbilirubinemia,** which is a yellow discoloration of the skin associated with hepatic dysfunction, does not seem to affect pulse oximetry readings.[18]

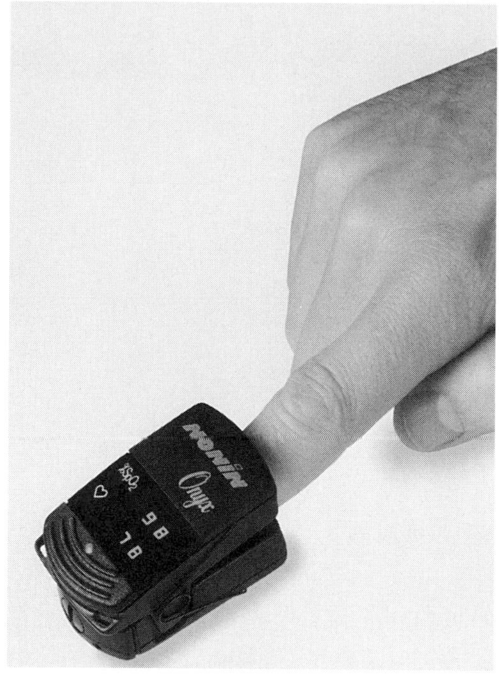

Figure 10-15 A hand-held pulse oximeter. (Courtesy Nonin Medical, Inc, Plymouth, Minn.)

Ambient Light

Fluorescent lights and other external light sources (e.g., heat lamps, fiberoptic light sources, and surgical lamps) have been shown to adversely affect heart rate and SpO_2 readings.[37] Most commercially available pulse oximeters attempt to compensate for this interference by continually cycling the transmitted red and infrared light on and off at a rate of about 480 cycles per second. In this process, the pulse oximeter cycles in three modes:

1. Red light on, IR off.
2. IR on, red light off.
3. Red light and IR off.

By using this sequence, ambient light interference can be determined when both red and IR light sources are off. Subtracting any light measured during Phase 3 from that measured during Phases 1 and 2 provides a means of minimizing ambient light interference.

Calibration of Pulse Oximeters

Pulse oximeters are calibrated by manufacturers with data obtained from studies of healthy humans. Specifically, SpO_2s are compared with invasive hemoximetry oxygen saturations (SaO_2) measured simultaneously while each subject breathes several gas mixtures of different fractional inspired oxygen (F_IO_2). Therefore the accuracy and reliability of a pulse oximeter is ultimately dependent on the initial calibration algorithm that is programmed into the device by the manufacturer. Generally, pulse oximeters are accurate for oxygen saturations higher than 80%. Pulse oximeter saturations lower than 80% are questionable and should be confirmed with ABG analysis and hemoximetry.

Clinical Practice Guidelines 10-2

Pulse Oximetry

Indications

Based on current evidence, pulse oximetry is useful for:

1. Monitoring arterial oxyhemoglobin saturation
2. Quantifying the arterial oxyhemoglobin saturation response to therapeutic intervention
3. Monitoring arterial oxyhemoglobin saturation during bronchoscopy

Contraindications

Pulse oximetry may not be appropriate in situations in which ongoing measurements of pH, $PaCO_2$, and total hemoglobin are required. The presence of abnormal hemoglobins may be a relative contraindication

Limitations

A number of factors, agents, and situations may affect readings, limit precision, and performance of pulse oximetry, including:

1. Motion artifacts
2. Abnormal hemoglobins (especially COHb and MetHB)
3. Intravascular dyes
4. Exposure of the measuring sensor to ambient light sources
5. Low perfusion states
6. Skin pigmentation
7. Nail polish
8. Low oxyhemoglobin saturations (i.e., below 83%)

Monitoring

The following information should be recorded during pulse oximetry:

1. Probe type, and measurement site, date and time of measurement, and patient position and activity level
2. F_IO_2 and mode of supplemental oxygen delivery
3. ABG measurements and CO-oximetry results that may have been made simultaneously
4. Clinical appearance of the patient (e.g., cyanotic, skin temperature)
5. Agreement between pulse oximeter heart rate and heart rate determined by palpation or ECG recordings.

For a copy of the complete text, see AARC clinical practice guideline: pulse oximetry, *Respir Care* 36:1406, 1991.

Clinical Applications of Pulse Oximetry

Pulse oximetry probes are available in neonatal, pediatric, and adult sizes. Advances in LED and solid-state technology have led to the miniaturization of pulse oximeters and the manufacture of hand-held devices (Figure 10-15). The response time of a pulse oximeter (i.e., how long it takes for a change in central [left heart PO_2] to be detected by the pulse oximeter) depends on the location of the probe. Probes placed on fingers show a delay of 12 seconds or more than when the probe is placed on the ear lobe. Probes placed on the toe show an even greater lag time for detecting PO_2 changes.

Pulse oximetry is well-recognized as an early warning system for detecting hypoxemia of patients with unstable oxygenation status. It can provide a continuous display of oxygen saturation, which can be used to monitor the oxygenation status of patients during surgery, mechanical ventilation, or bronchoscopy. It can also provide intermittent measurements of SpO_2, which can be useful, for example, in the management of home-care patients.

Although pulse oximetry can be quite effective when adjusting oxygen therapy in hospitalized patients, its use in prescribing oxygen therapy for home-care patients is questionable. Therefore caution should be exercised when using pulse oximeter readings to prescribe oxygen therapy. Carlin and associates[38] demonstrated that using only pulse oximetry measurements could disqualify a significant number of patients applying for reimbursement for oxygen therapy. The Centers for Medicare and Medicaid Services (formerly HCFA) guidelines for qualifying for oxygen therapy require that the patient demonstrate a PaO_2 of ≤ 55 torr or a saturation of $\leq 85\%$ saturation.[39] Because any of the physiological or technical problems discussed previously can significantly affect pulse oximetry measurements, it is wise to use invasive ABG analysis to establish the need for oxygen therapy for chronically ill patients.

Clinical Practice Guideline 10-2 summarizes the AARC CPG for pulse oximetry, which provides valuable information to ensure that SpO_2 values are valid.

Transcutaneous Monitoring

Transcutaneous monitoring provides another method of indirect ABG assessment. Unlike pulse oximetry, which relies on spectrophotometric analysis, transcutaneous monitoring uses modified blood gas electrodes to measure the oxygen and carbon dioxide tension at the skin surface.[40-42] The conjunctival PO_2 electrode, which is a modification of the standard transcutaneous PO_2 electrode, measures the PO_2 of the palpebral conjunctiva surrounding the eyeball.

Transcutaneous PO_2

Figure 10-16, A is a schematic of a transcutaneous PO_2 ($PtcO_2$) electrode, which consists of a **servo-controlled** heated (Clark) polarographic electrode connected to a CPU.[40,42] The electrode is covered with a Teflon membrane, and the entire electrode assembly attaches to the skin surface with a double-sided adhesive ring. The electrode is heated to 42° to 45° C to produce capillary vasodilation below the surface of the electrode. Heating improves gas diffusion across the

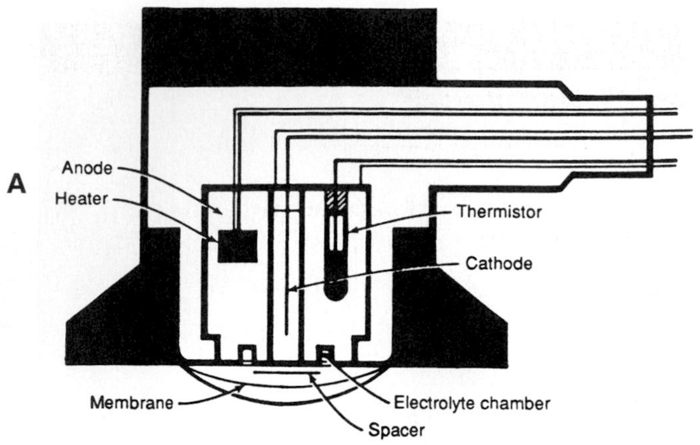

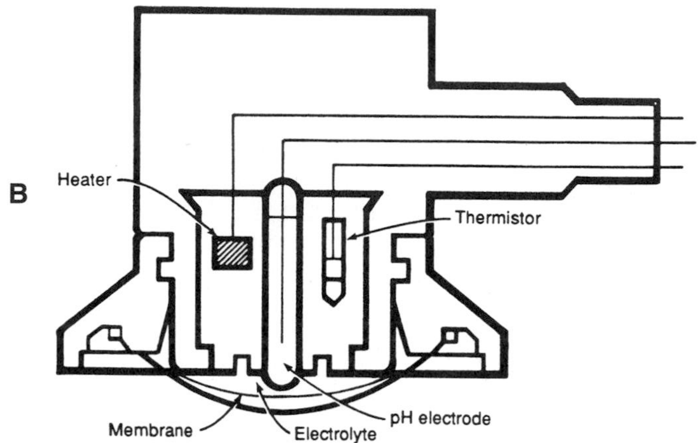

Figure 10-16 Transcutaneous electrodes: **A,** $PtcO_2$; **B,** $PtcCO_2$. (From Novametrix Medical Systems, Wallingford, Conn.)

skin because it increases local blood flow at the site of the electrode and alters the structure of the stratum corneum. The stratum corneum has been described as a mixture of fibrinous tissue within a lipid and protein matrix. It has been suggested that heating the skin to temperatures greater than 41° C melts the lipid layer, thus enhancing gas diffusion through the skin.[43]

The ratio of transcutaneous PO_2 to PaO_2 measured by hemoximetry (i.e., the $PtcO_2/PaO_2$ index) has been shown to be good for neonatal use, but it is often unreliable for critically ill adults.[44,45] Decreases in peripheral perfusion caused by reductions in cardiac output or increases in peripheral (cutaneous) resistance can significantly affect the accuracy of $PtcO_2$ measurements.[45,46] Current data indicate that when the cardiac index is >2.2 L/min/m^2, the $PtcO_2/PaO_2$ index is 0.5, but when the cardiac index is <1.5 L/min/m^2, it is only 0.1.[47] Thus hypoperfusion of the skin caused by pathologic states (e.g., septic shock, hemorrhage, or heart failure) or by increased vascular resistance (e.g., hypothermia or pharmacological intervention) can lead to erroneous data. Because $PtcO_2$ is influenced by blood flow to the tissues as well as by oxygen utilization by the tissues, changes in $PtcO_2$ may be an early indicator of vascular compromise or shock. In fact, many $PtcO_2$ monitors display the power supplied to the electrode heater as a way of identifying perfusion problems at the site.

Transcutaneous PCO_2

The standard transcutaneous carbon dioxide ($PtcCO_2$) electrode is a modified Stowe-Severinghaus blood gas electrode composed of pH-sensitive glass with a Ag/AgCl electrode (see Figure 10-16, *B*). As with the $PtcO_2$ electrode, the $PtcCO_2$ electrode is heated to 42° to 45° C. The $PtcCO_2$ values are slightly higher than the $PaCO_2$ value primarily because of the higher metabolic rate at the site of the electrode caused by heating the skin. Most commercial instruments incorporate correction factors into their system's software to remove the discrepancy between $PtcCO_2$ and $PaCO_2$.

Technical Considerations for Transcutaneous Monitoring

Clinical Practice Guideline 10-3 contains guidelines for transcutaneous monitoring of neonatal and pediatric patients that relate to care, placement, and calibration of the electrodes. Several points deserve special attention:

1. Transcutaneous signals are adversely affected by dirt and hair, so before an electrode is placed on the patient's skin, the site should be cleansed with an alcohol swab. In cases in which hair may be present, the site should be shaved to ensure good contact between the electrode and the skin. When attaching the electrode to the patient, placing a drop of electrolyte gel or deionized water on the electrode surface enhances gas diffusion between the skin and the electrode.
2. Transcutaneous PO_2 monitors are calibrated with two-point calibration in which room air ($PO_2 \sim 150$ torr) is the high PO_2 of the calibration and an electronic zeroing of the system is the low PO_2 of the calibration. The $PtcCO_2$ electrodes are also calibrated with a two-point calibration procedure. In this latter calibration, a 5% CO_2 calibration gas and a 10% CO_2 calibration gas are used for low and high calibration points, respectively. Electrodes should be calibrated before their initial use on a patient. Manufacturers typically suggest that an electrode should be calibrated each time it is repositioned.
3. Transcutaneous electrodes are bathed with a small volume of electrolyte solution that can easily evaporate because heat is applied to the electrode. Loss of electrolyte either through evaporation or leakage from a torn membrane can adversely affect electrode operation. The electrolyte and the sensor's membrane should be checked regularly and changed weekly or whenever a signal drift during calibration is noticed. Because silver can deposit on the cathode, the electrode should be periodically cleaned per manufacturer recommendations.

Clinical Practice Guidelines 10-3

Transcutaneous Blood Gas Monitoring for Neonatal and Pediatric Patients

Indications

1. Monitoring the adequacy of arterial oxygenation or ventilation.
2. Quantifying a patient's response to diagnostic and therapeutic interventions.

Contraindications

Transcutaneous monitoring may be a relative contraindication in patients with poor skin integrity or adhesive allergy.

Hazards/Complications

1. False-negative or false-positive results may lead to inappropriate treatment of patients.
2. Tissue injury at the measuring site (e.g., blisters, burns, skin tears).

Limitations

The following factors may increase the discrepancy between arterial and transcutaneous values:

1. Hyperoxemia (PaO_2 >100 mm Hg)
2. Hypoperfused state (e.g., shock)
3. Improper electrode placement
4. Vasoactive drugs
5. The nature of the patient's skin (skinfold thickness or presence of edema)

Validation

1. High and low limit alarms are set appropriately.
2. Appropriate electrode temperature is set.
3. Systematic electrode site change occurs.
4. Manufacturer recommendations for maintenance, operation, and safety are followed.

Monitoring

The following information should be recorded at regular intervals (e.g., 1 to 4 hours): date and time of measurement, patient position, respiratory rate, activity level, F_IO_2, mode of ventilatory support and settings, electrode placement site, electrode temperature, time of placement, results of simultaneously obtained in vitro ABG analysis, as well as the clinical appearance of the patient, including perfusion, pallor, and skin temperature.

For a copy of the complete text, see AARC clinical practice guideline: transcutaneous blood gas monitoring for neonatal and pediatric patients, *Respir Care* 39(12):1176, 1994.

4. When transcutaneous PO_2 and PCO_2 readings are reported, the date and time of the measurement, the patient's activity level and body position, the site of electrode placement, and the electrode temperature should be noted. The inspired oxygen concentration and the type of equipment used to deliver supplemental oxygen should always be included. The clinical appearance of the patient, including assessment of peripheral perfusion (i.e., pallor, skin temperature), is important data to note. When invasive ABG measurements are available, they are recorded for comparison with $PtcO_2$ and $PtcCO_2$ readings.[46]

Burns are probably the most common problem that clinicians encounter during transcutaneous monitoring because the site of measurement must be heated to 42° to 45° C. Repositioning the sensor every 4 to 6 hours can minimize this problem. For transcutaneous monitoring of neonates, the sensor should be repositioned more often.

Interpretation of Blood Gas Results

As stated previously, ABGs can provide valuable information about a patient's acid-base, ventilatory, and oxygenation status. Blood gas analysis is also an integral part of more sophisticated procedures, such as cardiopulmonary and hemodynamic monitoring. It is beyond the scope of this book to fully discuss the interpretive value of blood gas measurements. We will therefore only provide a framework for ABG interpretation, but the titles of several texts and monographs on blood gas analysis are listed at the end of the chapter.

Acid-Base Status

Acid-base disorders can be categorized as either acidosis or alkalosis. Acidosis is associated with an increase in the plasma hydrogen ion concentration and a fall in the pH. Alkalosis is associated with a decrease in plasma hydrogen ion concentration and a rise in pH. The Henderson-Hasselbalch equation can be used to describe how changes in HCO_3 and $PaCO_2$ can be used to determine if a metabolic, respiratory, or a combined acid-base disorder is present. Consider the following equations:

$$pH = pKa + \log (HCO_3^-) / (PaCO_2 \times 0.03),$$

or

$$pH \sim (HCO_3^-) / (PaCO_2)$$

Acute decreases in HCO_3^- and increases in $PaCO_2$ are associated with decreases in pH and metabolic and respiratory acidosis, respectively. Conversely, acute increases in HCO_3^- and decreases in $PaCO_2$ are associated with increases in pH and metabolic and respiratory alkalosis, respectively. If only one of the parameters changes and the other stays within normal limits, then the problem can be classified as an acute or uncompensated acid-base disorder.

Table 10-6 pH, $PaCO_2$, and HCO_3^- findings for various acid-base disturbances

	pH	PCO_2 (mm Hg)	HCO_3^-
RESPIRATORY ACIDOSIS			
Acute	<7.35	>45	Normal
Partly compensated	<7.35	>45	>26
Compensated	>7.35 <7.40	>45	>26
RESPIRATORY ALKALOSIS			
Acute	>7.45	<35	Normal
Partly compensated	>7.45	<35	<22
Compensated	<7.45 >7.40	<35	<22
METABOLIC ACIDOSIS			
Acute	<7.35	Normal	<22
Partly compensated	<7.35	<35	<22
Compensated	>7.35 <7.40	<35	<22
METABOLIC ALKALOSIS			
Acute	<7.35	Normal	>26
Partly compensated	>7.45	>45	>26
Compensated	<7.45 >7.40	>45	>26

From Harwood R: *Exam review and study guide for perinatal/pediatric respiratory care*, Philadelphia, 1999, FA Davis.

For example, a reduced pH with an increase in $PaCO_2$ and a normal HCO_3^- is indicative of an acute or uncompensated respiratory acidosis. If the reduced pH is associated with a decreased HCO_3^- and a normal $PaCO_2$, then an acute or uncompensated metabolic acidosis is suggested. Note that a mixed acidosis or mixed alkalosis is also an uncompensated event. In the case of a mixed acidosis, the pH is less than 7.35 with the $PaCO_2$ greater than 45 torr and the HCO_3^- less than 22 mEq/L. A mixed alkalosis is characterized by a pH greater than 7.45, a PCO_2 less than 35 torr and a HCO_3^- greater than 26 mEq/L. With compensated acid-base disorders, both $PaCO_2$ and HCO_3 are out of their normal range of values. Interpreting arterial blood gases can therefore be an arduous task particularly when trying to differentiate the source of the acid-base disturbance and the compensatory response. The following is offered as one method that can be used for interpreting ABG measurements where compensation occurs. First, look at the pH and determine if an acidosis or alkalosis is present. To determine the primary disorder, look at the $PaCO_2$ to decide if a respiratory problem could have caused the altered pH. Next, look at the HCO_3^- to determine if a metabolic disorder is responsible for the altered pH. After the origin of the acid-base disorder has been established, compensation can be discerned by examining if the other variable has also changed. Consider the following situation. If a patient's pH is below 7.40, then the original problem could be caused by an increase in $PaCO_2$ (i.e., respiratory acidosis) or a decrease in HCO_3^- (i.e., metabolic acidosis). The compensation for a respiratory acidosis would be a rise in the HCO_3^-, whereas the compensation for a metabolic

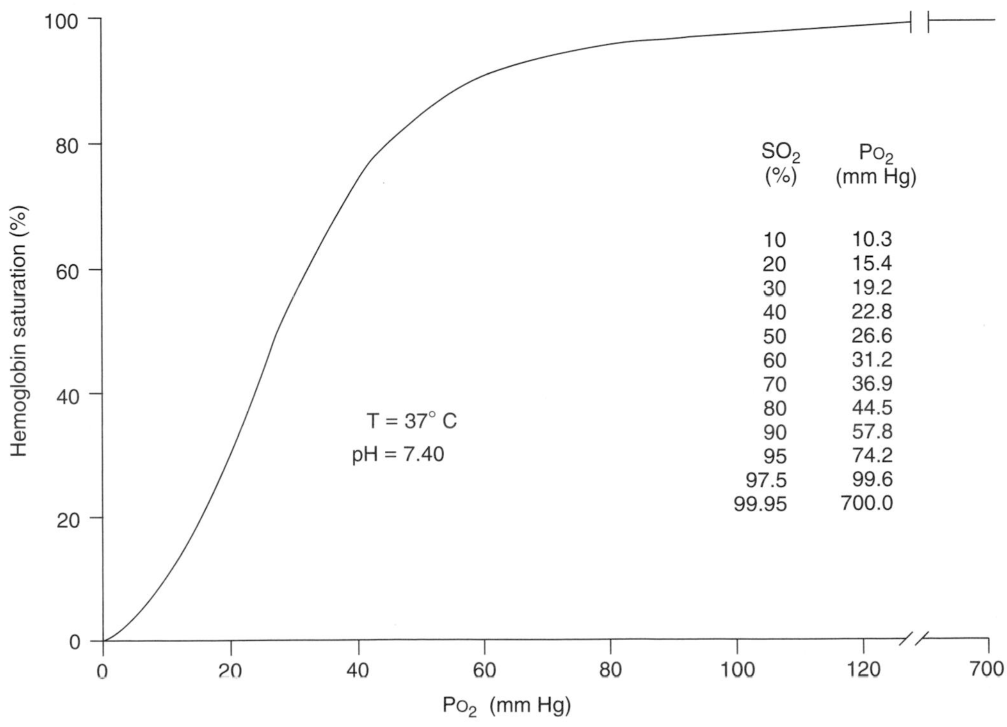

Figure 10-17 Oxyhemoglobin dissociation curve. (From Lane EE, Walker JF: *Clinical arterial blood gas analysis*, St Louis, 1987, Mosby.)

Table 10-7 Criteria for classifying hypoxemia using PaO_2 measurements

Hypoxemia	PaO_2
CONDITIONS: ROOM AIR IS INSPIRED; THE PATIENT IS <60 YR	
Mild*	<80 mm Hg
Moderate	<60 mm Hg
Severe*	<40 mm Hg
CONDITIONS: SUPPLEMENTAL OXYGEN IS INSPIRED; THE PATIENT IS <60 YR	
Uncorrected	Less than room air acceptable limit
Corrected	Within the room air acceptable limit; <100 mm Hg
Excessively corrected	>100 mm Hg

Adapted from Shapiro BA, et al: *Clinical application of blood gases*, ed 4, Chicago, 1989, Mosby.
*Subtract 1 mm Hg of oxygen to limits of mild and moderate hypoxemia for each year over 60. A PaO_2 <40 mm Hg indicates severe hypoxemia in any patient at any age.

acidosis would be a reduction in $PaCO_2$. The converse of this situation would follow the same line of logic. If the patient's pH is greater than 7.40, then the original problem could be caused by a reduction in $PaCO_2$ (i.e., respiratory alkalosis) or an increase in HCO_3^- (i.e., metabolic alkalosis). The compensation for a respiratory alkalosis is to lose HCO_3^-, whereas the compensation for a metabolic alkalosis is CO_2 retention.

The level of compensation is usually described as partially compensated or fully compensated. If the pH is within the range of normal limits, then the acid-base disorder is fully compensated. If not, then it is partially compensated. For example, a respiratory acidosis is associated with a decreased pH and an increased $PaCO_2$. If the HCO_3^- has also increased, then there is evidence of metabolic compensation. If the pH is between 7.35 and 7.40, then this is interpreted as a fully compensated respiratory acidosis. Table 10-6 summarizes the pH, $PaCO_2$, and HCO_3^- findings associated with various types of acid-base disturbances.

Ventilatory Status

A patient's ventilatory status can be assessed by looking at the $PaCO_2$. An increase in $PaCO_2$ is associated with hypoventilation and a respiratory acidosis. Conversely, a decrease in $PaCO_2$ is associated with hyperventilation and a respiratory alkalosis. As a general rule, a $PaCO_2$ greater than 50 mm Hg is classified as ventilatory failure and is often used as a criterion for initiating mechanical ventilatory support. Note that changes in $PaCO_2$ must be interpreted relative to the patient's clinical condition. For example,

Box 10-2 Examples of Disease States Associated with Various Types of Acid-Base Disorders

Metabolic Acidosis

- Diabetes mellitus
- Diarrhea
- Methanol ingestion
- Renal dysfunction
- Salicylate intoxication

Metabolic Alkalosis

- Administration of excessive amounts of bicarbonate
- Diuretic therapy
- Ingestion of excessive amounts of antacids
- Nasogastric suctioning
- Vomiting

Respiratory Alkalosis

- Acute airway obstruction
- Ingestion of excessive amounts of sedative, opiates, and other respiratory depressants
- Neuromuscular disorders
- Pneumothorax
- Restrictive pulmonary disease

Respiratory Alkalosis

- Anxiety
- Encephalitis
- Excessive mechanical ventilatory support
- Progesterone

patients with COPD often demonstrate chronic ventilatory failure (e.g., $PaCO_2$ higher than 50 mm Hg with pH within normal limits). Thus acute ventilatory failure is only said to exist in COPD patients if the $PaCO_2$ increases well above 50 mm Hg and the pH is below 7.30.

Oxygenation Status

A patient's oxygenation status can be evaluated by looking at the PaO_2 or the SaO_2. The relationship between these then can be illustrated graphically with an oxyhemoglobin dissociation curve, like the one shown in Figure 10-17. Note that a PaO_2 of 45 mm Hg is associated with an SaO_2 of approximately 80%; a PaO_2 of about 60 mm Hg corresponds to an SaO_2 of 90%; and a PaO_2 of 75 mm Hg is equivalent to an SaO_2 of 95%. For interpretative purposes, a PaO_2 from 60 to 80 mm Hg is classified as mild hypoxemia; a PaO_2 from 40 to 60 mm Hg is classified as moderate hypoxemia; and a PaO_2 less than 40 mm Hg is classified as severe hypoxemia. Table 10-7 provides PaO_2 and SaO_2 ranges for evaluating a patient's oxygenation status.

Box 10-2 lists examples of conditions and disease states associated with various acid-base disorders. As mentioned previously, blood gas measurements are only meaningful when they are interpreted relative to other clinical findings. Interpretation of ABGs without other supporting clinical data can be misleading and lead to potentially harmful decisions in patient management.

Summary

Blood gas analysis is an integral part of managing patients with cardiopulmonary dysfunctions. Modern in vitro blood gas analyzers are fully automated systems that only require small amounts of blood for analysis and can provide intermittent measurements of pH, $PaCO_2$, and PaO_2, which give valuable information about a patient's acid-base, ventilatory, and oxygenation status. Many blood gas analyzers also allow for determinations of plasma electrolytes and metabolites, such as sodium, potassium, calcium, and glucose. Noninvasive devices, including pulse oximetry and transcutaneous monitoring, provide an alternative to the standard in vitro blood gas analysis and allow for continuous blood gas surveillance. Two relatively new devices, the in vivo intraarterial catheter and the point-of-care blood gas analyzer, hold considerable promise for providing accurate and reliable blood gas analysis at the bedside.

The importance of blood gas analysis cannot be overstated. It is important to recognize that blood gas measurements should be interpreted relative to other clinical indices, including history and physical examination, chest radiographs, and other clinical laboratory tests.

Review Questions

See Appendix A for the answers.

1. Which of the following are current safety guidelines for the protection of the therapist drawing an ABG sample?
   I. Gloves
   II. Gown
   III. Protective eyewear (goggles)
   IV. Shoe covers
   a. I and III only
   b. II and III only
   c. II and IV only
   d. I, II, and III only

2. A positive Allen test indicates the presence of:
   a. an occluded radial artery
   b. a patent ulnar artery
   c. inadequate arterial oxygenation to the hand
   d. inadequate collateral circulation to the hand

3. The site most often used for sampling arterial blood in adults is which of the following arteries?
   a. Brachial
   b. Dorsal foot
   c. Radial
   d. Femoral

4. Interpret the following ABG findings:
   pH = 7.50; $PaCO_2$ = 30 mm Hg; PaO_2 = 60 mm Hg; HCO_3^- = 24 mEq/L.
   a. Acute metabolic alkalosis with mild hypoxemia
   b. Chronic metabolic acidosis with moderate hypoxemia
   c. Acute respiratory alkalosis with mild hypoxemia
   d. Chronic respiratory alkalosis with moderate hypoxemia

5. Which of the following conditions is associated with an acute respiratory acidosis?
   a. Barbiturate intoxication
   b. Excessive ingestion of antacids
   c. Emphysema
   d. Anxiety

6. A patient is admitted to the emergency department of the hospital after a motor vehicle accident. In your initial assessment of the patient, you find that he is pale and his pulse is weak. You are unable to obtain a steady pulse oximeter reading. Which of the following is the most probable cause of the erratic pulse oximetry readings?
   I. Poor perfusion state
   II. Increased levels of carboxyhemoglobin
   III. Low PaO_2
   IV. Anemia
   a. I only
   b. I and II only
   c. I, II, and III only
   d. I, II, III, and IV

7. Which of the following can alter pulse oximeter readings?
   I. Low perfusion states, such as hypovolemic shock
   II. Dark blue nail polish
   III. Methemoglobinemia
   IV. Hyperbilirubinemia
   a. I and III only
   b. II and III only
   c. II and IV only
   d. I, II, and III only

8. A patient's P_{50} is 37 mm Hg. Which of the following conditions could be responsible?
   I. Hypercarbia
   II. Decreased plasma levels of 2,3 diphosphoglycerate
   III. Acute acidosis
   IV. Carbon monoxide poisoning
   a. I and III only
   b. II and III only
   c. II and IV only
   d. I, II, and IV only

9. To function effectively, the reference pH electrode must be bathed in which of the following solutions?

a. 1% sodium bicarbonate
b. Saturated potassium chloride
c. 5% hydrochloric acid
d. 0.9% sodium chloride

10. While assessing the Levy-Jennings graphs for PCO_2 values, you notice that results for the last five quality assessment tests have increased progressively. Which of the following is the most likely cause of this finding?
a. A leak in the electrode membrane
b. Protein build-up on the electrode
c. A damaged wire
d. This is a normal membrane function

11. Which of the following is NOT an anion buffer?
a. Hemoglobin
b. Inorganic phosphate
c. Bicarbonate
d. Organic calcium

12. Based on CLIA standards, laboratory instruments used in the hospital for blood sample testing should have three-point calibrations performed at least:
a. Daily
b. Weekly
c. Monthly
d. Every 6 months

13. Compare the processes of quality control and quality assurance.

14. Arterial blood was obtained from a patient after open heart surgery. The patient's temperature is 35° C, and the measured PaO_2 is 80 mm Hg before temperature correction. The patient's actual PaO_2 is approximately:
a. 70 mm Hg
b. 80 mm Hg
c. 90 mm Hg
d. It cannot be determined from the information provided

15. What are the consequences of maintaining the temperature of the transcutaneous PO_2 probe at 48° C?
a. Thermal injury
b. Low $PtcO_2$ readings
c. Fire hazard
d. Malignant hyperthermia

16. Which of the following tests is indicated for determining the presence of carbon monoxide poisoning?
a. Pulse oximetry
b. ABGs
c. CO-oximetry
d. Transcutaneous $PtcO_2$

References

1. American Association of Respiratory Care: Clinical practice guideline: sampling for arterial blood gas analysis, *Respir Care* 37:913, 1992.
2. American Association of Respiratory Care: Clinical practice guideline: Blood gas analysis and hemoximetry: 2001 Revision and Update, *Respir Care* 46:498, 2001.
3. Browning JA, Kaiser DL, Durbin CG: The effect of guidelines on the appropriate use of arterial blood gas analysis in the intensive care unit, *Respir Care* 34:269, 1989.
4. Bruck E, et al: *Percutaneous collection of arterial blood for laboratory analysis*, National Committee for Clinical Laboratory Standards 1985, H11A, 5(3):39.
5. National Committee for Clinical Laboratory Standards: *Procedures for the collection of diagnostic blood specimens by skin puncture*, ed 3, Villanova, Penn, 1992, The Committee.
6. Koch G, Wendel H: Comparison of pH, carbon dioxide tension, standard bicarbonate and oxygen tension in capillary blood and in arterial blood during the neonatal period, *Acta Paediatr Scand* 56:10, 1967.
7. Burritt MF, Fallon KD: *Blood gas preanalytical considerations: specimen collection, calibration, and controls*, National Committee for Clinical Laboratory Standards 1989, C27-T 9(11):685.
8. Ehrmeyer S, Laessig RH: Measurement of the proficiency of pH and blood gas analyses by interlaboratory proficiency testing, *J Med Tech* 2:33, 1985.
9. Koch G, Wendel H: Comparison of pH, carbon dioxide tension, standard bicarbonate and oxygen tension in capillary blood and in arterial blood during the neonatal period, *Acta Paediatr Scand* 56:10, 1967.
10. Duc GV, Cumarasamy N: Digital arteriolar oxygen tension as a guide to oxygen therapy of the newborn, *Biol Neonate* 24:134, 1974.
11. McLain BI, Evans J, Dear PFR: Comparison of capillary and arterial blood gas measurements in neonates, *Arch Dis Child* 63:743, 1988.
12. Desai SD, et al: A comparison between arterial and arterialized capillary blood in infants, *S Afr Med J* 41:13, 1967.
13. Centers for Disease Control: Update: universal precautions for prevention of transmission of human immunodeficiency virus, hepatitis B virus, and other blood-borne pathogens in health care settings, *MMWR* 37:377, 1988.
14. Department of Labor, Occupational Safety and Health Administration: Occupational exposure to bloodborne pathogens, 29 CFRR Part 1910.1030, *Federal Register*, Dec 6, 1991.
15. Moran RF, et al: Oxygen content, hemoglobin oxygen, "saturation," and related quantities in blood: terminology, measurement, and reporting, National Committee for Clinical Laboratory Standards 1990, C25-P 10:1.
16. Davenport HW: *The ABC of acid-base chemistry*, ed 3, Chicago, 1975, University of Chicago Press.
17. Brensilver JM, Goldberger E: *A primer of water, and acid-base syndromes*, ed 8, Philadelphia, 1996, FA Davis.
18. Shapiro BA, et al: *Clinical application of blood gases*, ed 5, St Louis, 1994, Mosby.
19. National Committee for Clinical Laboratory Standards: *Clinical laboratory technical procedure manual*, ed 2, Pub GP2-A2, Illinois, 1992, Villanova.
20. Clinical Laboratory Improvement Amendments of 1988: Final rule, subpart H, *Federal Register*, Feb 1992.

21. Medicare, Medicaid and CLIA Programs: CLIA-88 continuance of approval of the Joint Commission on Accreditation of Healthcare Organizations (JCAHO) as an accrediting organization. *Federal Register* 67(207):65585, 2002.

22. Hansen JE, et al: Assessing precision and accuracy in blood gas proficiency testing, *Am Rev Respir Dis* 141:1190, 1990.

23. Mohler JG, et al: Blood gases. In Clausen JL, editor: *Pulmonary function testing: guidelines and controversies*, New York, 1982, Academic Press.

24. Barker SJ, Hyatt J: Continuous measurement of intraarterial pH, $PaCO_2$, and PaO_2 in the operating room, *Anesthesia Analg* 73: 43, 1991.

25. MacIntyre NR, et al: Accuracy and precision of a point-of-care blood gas analyzer incorporating optode, *Respir Care* 41(9):800, 1996.

26. Brown LJ: A new instrument for the simultaneous measurement of total hemoglobin, % oxyhemoglobin, % carboxyhemoglobin, % methemoglobin, and oxygen content in whole blood, *IEEE Trans Biomed Engineering* 27:132, 1980.

27. Falholt W: Blood oxygen saturation determinations by spectrophotometry, *Scan J Clin Lab Invest* 15:67, 1963.

28. Severinghaus JW, Astrup PB: History of blood gas analysis, VI oximetry, *J Clin Monitoring* 2:270, 1986.

29. Nillson NJ: Oximetry, *Physiol Rev* 40:1, 1960.

30. Tremper KK, Barker SJ: Pulse oximetry, *Anesthesiol* 70:98, 1989.

31. Yang K, Brown SD, Gutierrez G: Noninvasive assessment of blood gases. In Levine RL, Fromm RE, editors: *Critical care monitoring, from pre-hospital to ICU*, St Louis, 1995, Mosby.

32. Pilbeam S: *Mechanical ventilation*, ed 3, St Louis, 1998, Mosby.

33. Scheller MS, Unger RJ, Kelner MJ: Effects of intravenously administered dyes on pulse oximetry readings, *Anesthesiol* 65:550, 1986.

34. Cote CJ, et al: The effect of nail polish on pulse oximetry, *Anesth Analg* 67:685, 1988.

35. Rubin AS: Nail polish color can affect pulse oximeter saturation, *Anesthesiol* 68:825, 1988.

36. Emery JR: Skin pigmentation as an influence on the accuracy of pulse oximetry, *J Perinatol* 7:329, 1987.

37. Amar D, et al: Fluorescent light interferes with pulse oximetry, *J Clin Monit* 5:135, 1989.

38. Carlin BW, Claussen JL, Ries AL: The use of cutaneous oximetry in the prescription of long-term oxygen therapy, *Chest* 94:239, 1988.

39. Kacmarek RM, Hess D, Stoller JK: *Monitoring in respiratory care*, St Louis, 1993, Mosby.

40. Lubbers DW: Theory and development of transcutaneous oxygen pressure measurement, *Int Anesthesiol Clin* 25:31, 1987.

41. Severinghaus JS, Bradley FA: Electrodes for blood PO_2 and PCO_2 determination, *J Appl Physiol* 13:515, 1958.

42. Severinghaus JS, Stafford M, Bradley FA: Transcutaneous PO_2 electrode design, calibration, and temperature gradient problems, *Acta Anesthesiology Scan* (suppl) 68:118, 1978.

43. Baecjert P, et al: Is pulse oximetry reliable in detecting hypoxemia in the neonate, *Adv Exp Med Biol* 220:165, 1987.

44. Reed RL, et al: Correlation of hemodynamic variables with transcutaneous PO_2 measurements in critically ill patients, *J Trauma* 25:1045, 1985.

45. Lubbers DW: Theoretical basis of transcutaneous blood gas measurements, *Crit Care Med* 9:721, 1981.

46. American Association of Respiratory Care: Clinical practice guideline: transcutaneous blood gas monitoring for neonatal and pediatric patients, *Respir Care* 39(12):1176, 1994.

47. Wahr JA, Tremper KK: Non-invasive oxygen monitoring techniques, *Crit Care Clin* 11(1):199, 1995.

Internet Resources

AARC Clinical Practice Guidelines: http://www.aarc.org

Acid-Base Balance (Alan W. Grogono, MD): http://www.tmc.tulane.edu/anes/acidbase/ practical.html

American College of Physicians—Annals of Internal Medicine: http://www.acponline.org/journals/annals/ annaltoc.htm

American Lung Association: http://www.lungusa.org

Anesthesia for Elephants: http://www.csen.com/anesthesia/elephants.htm

Carbon Monoxide Headquarters (David G. Penney, PhD): http://www.phymac.med.wayne.edu/facultyprofile/ penney/COHQ/col.htm

Clinical Laboratory Improvement Act (CLIA-88 and Updates): http://www.phppo.cdc.gov/clia/default.asp

College of American Pathologists: http://wwww.cap.org

Joint Commission on Accreditation of Healthcare Organizations: http://www.jcaho.org

Medical Vendors with Internet Addresses: http://www.med.utah.edu/usrc/national.htm

New England Journal of Medicine: http://www.nejm.org

NIH Clinical Center Nursing Department—procedure for obtaining blood samples from pediatric patient with arterial lines: http://cc.nih.gov/nursing/obsppar1.html

The Virtual Hospital: http://www.vh.org

Chapter 11

Introduction to Ventilators

Susan P. Pilbeam

Chapter Outline

CHAPTER OUTLINE continued

Chapter Learning Objectives

Upon completion of this chapter, the reader will be able to:

1. List the two primary power sources used in mechanical ventilators.
2. Compare and contrast negative- and positive-pressure ventilation.
3. Explain how a closed-loop ventilator system can perform self-adjustment.
4. Define volume and pressure ventilation.
5. Provide three additional names for pressure and volume ventilation.

6. Name three volume-displacement designs and three flow-control valves.
7. Compare the location of expiratory valves on current ICU ventilators with that on older model ventilators.
8. Draw the flow and pressure curves produced by linear drive and rotary drive piston ventilators.
9. Explain the two fundamental principles of fluidics.
10. Evaluate available PEEP valves to determine if a flow-resistor or a threshold resistor is being used.
11. Evaluate patient information to determine which expiratory maneuver is indicated: negative end expiratory pressure (NEEP), CPAP, PEEP, expiratory pause, or expiratory retard.
12. Troubleshoot IMV and freestanding CPAP systems.
13. Describe the four phases of a breath.
14. Explain how pressure, flow, and volume triggering mechanisms work to begin the inspiratory phase of a breath.
15. Identify the graph of the flow-time, volume-time, and pressure-time curves for time-triggered, volume- or pressure-limited, time-cycled breaths.
16. Identify a pressure-time curve showing patient triggering.
17. Compare the feature of sloping or ramping the beginning part of a pressure-targeted breath with a nonsloping breath.
18. Explain the concept of having an adjustable flow drop-off feature for ending inspiration in pressure support ventilation.
19. Name at least one current use of NEEP.
20. Define the modes of ventilation by their triggering, limiting (controlling), and cycling mechanisms.
21. Compare the two types of dual -control modes of ventilation.
22. Contrast the three methods of achieving minimum minute ventilation as used by current generation ventilators.
23. Define each of the following modes of ventilation: APRV, PAV, and ASV.
24. List the five common methods of delivering high-frequency ventilation.
25. Identify the most common causes of high- and low-pressure alarm activations.
26. From a clinical situation with a ventilated patient, differentiate between problems associated with the ventilator and those caused by a patient problem.
27. Analyze ventilator graphics to determine modes of ventilation and common problems occurring during ventilation.

Key Terms

Part I: Physical Characteristics of Ventilators

Beam Deflection
Blowers
Chest Cuirass
Closed-Loop System
Coanda Effect
Combined-Powered Ventilators
Combined Pressure Devices
Compressors
Continuous-Flow IMV and CPAP Systems
Control Panel
Demand Flow IMV and CPAP Systems
Direct Drive Pistons
Drive Mechanisms
Electrically Powered
External Circuit
Flip-Flop Valves
Flow-Control Valves
Flow Resistors
Fluidics
Fluid Logic
Gas Streaming
Internal Circuit
Iron Lung
Linear Drive Piston
Loop
Microprocessor Controlled
Negative Pressure Ventilators
Open-Loop System
Patient Circuit
Pneumatic
Pneumatic Circuit
Pneumatically Powered
Positive-Pressure Ventilators
Power Source
Power Transmission Systems
Proportional Amplifier
Rotary Drive Pistons
Rotary Compressors
Separation Bubble
Sinusoidal
Spring-Loaded Bellows
Threshold Resistors
User Interface
Ventilator Circuit
Volume-Displacement Devices
Y Connector

Part II: Basic Components of Breath Delivery

Baseline Pressure
Control Variables
Cycle Variable
Expiratory Hold (End-Expiratory Pause)
Expiratory Positive Airway Pressure (EPAP)
Expiratory Retard
Flow Triggering
Inspiratory Pause
Inspiratory Positive Airway Pressure (IPAP)
Inspiratory Hold
Intensive Care Unit (ICU)
Mandatory Breath
Negative End-Expiratory Pressure (NEEP)
Patient Triggering
Peak Inspiratory Pressure (PIP)
Pendelluft
Phase Variables
Plateau Pressure ($P_{plateau}$)
Pressure Triggering
Positive End-Expiratory Pressure (PEEP)
Pressure Triggering
Rise Time
Sloping

Spontaneous Breaths
Static Compliance
Taylor Dispersion
Total Cycle Time (TCT)
Trigger Sensitivity
Trigger Variable
Work of Breathing (WOB)

Part III: Basic Modes of Ventilation

Adaptive Support Ventilation (ASV)
Airway Pressure-Release Ventilation (APRV)
Assist/Control Mode
Assisted Breaths
Autoflow
Auto-PEEP
Bi-level Positive Airway Pressure (BiPAP, Bi-level Pressure-Assist, Bi-Level Pressure-Support)
Continuous Positive Airway Pressure (CPAP)
Control Mode
Control Ventilation
Dual Modes of Ventilation
High-Frequency Flow Interruption (HFFI)
High-Frequency Jet Ventilation (HFJV)
High-Frequency Oscillatory Ventilation (HFOV)
High-Frequency Percussive Ventilation (HFPV)
High-Frequency Positive-Pressure Ventilation (HFPPV)
High-Frequency Ventilation (HFV)
Intermittent Mandatory Ventilation (IMV)
Mandatory Minute Ventilation (MMV)
Pressure-Controlled Ventilation (PCV)
Pressure-Controlled, Inverse Ratio Ventilation (PCIRV)
Pressure-Regulated Volume Control (PRVC)
Pressure-Support Ventilation (PSV)
Pressure Ventilation (PV) (Pressure-Limited Ventilation, Pressure-Controlled Ventilation, Pressure-Targeted Ventilation)
Proportional Assist Ventilation (PAV)
Synchronized Intermittent Mandatory Ventilation (SIMV)
Variable Pressure Control
Variable Pressure Support
Volume-Controlled Inverse Ratio Ventilation (VCIRV)
Volume Support
Volume Ventilation

Part IV: Troubleshooting During Mechanical Ventilation

Scalars

Part I: Physical Characteristics of Ventilators

Computer technology has advanced rapidly in the past 5 years. Nowhere is the impact of computer advancement more noticeable than in medical devices, particularly mechanical ventilators. A wide variety of mechanical ventilators are available for managing patients of different ages and in various settings. Although a large number of ventilators are available, all share certain characteristics, as well as important functional properties. This information will be discussed in this chapter. In addition, an explanation of expiratory valves and spontaneous breathing systems is included. Another important aspect of mechanical ventilation presented is the use of specific ventilator modes. The discussion of modes in this chapter includes not only those most commonly used, but also servo-controlled and high-frequency ventilation methods. Managing the patient-ventilator system is less difficult with an understanding of ventilator alarms, an ability to identify problems using ventilator graphics, and a knowledge of some of the fundamentals of troubleshooting. These concepts will also be described in this chapter.

Perspectives on Ventilator Classification

The use of ventilators in patient management is relatively young. In the United States, the earliest ventilators appeared in the 1950s and 1960s and were originally classified by a system used by Mushin and associates,[1] the purpose of which was to try to describe ventilator function. The technology of mechanical ventilation has expanded so rapidly that the original classification system needed modification. Practitioners were becoming confused about terms used to describe ventilators and modes. In the late 1980s and early 1990s Chatburn and Branson[2-4] tried to solve this problem by establishing a newer classification system. Although a welcome change, this system was difficult for some practitioners to adopt.[5]

Historically, classification systems tried to describe the physical function of the ventilator. Chatburn and Branson's method was different and attempted to do two things. First, it described certain characteristics of the ventilator, for example, that which powers the ventilator—electricity or compressed gases. Second, it provided a description of the breath or breathing pattern delivered to the patient.[3] For example, does the therapist seek to target a specific volume to deliver to a patient, or was he more concerned about pressure? Was the gas flow started when the patient takes in a breath or did the machine determine when flow started?

Although this classification system seemed appropriate, some respiratory therapists and physicians remained confused by the names applied to different modes and breath types. Part of this confusion exists because of what manufacturers use to name a "new" mode. They give it a different name from anyone else's ventilator. They will do this even though the mode is the same as that on another machine. For example, Autoflow on the Dräger Evita-4 ventilator is similar in function to pressure-regulated volume control (PRVC) on the Servo 300, but one is called Autoflow and the other is called PRVC.

Chatburn and Branson made every effort to eliminate this naming problem, but many students found the classification cumbersome.[5] In 2001, Chatburn and Primiano modified the ventilator classification to provide a better description of newer ventilators and their modes. The reader is referred to their reference for a complete description of this system.[6]

An Introduction to Ventilators

A ventilator is basically a box that is connected to a **power source** and provides a breath or gas flow to a patient. The operator sets certain controls on the **control panel**, sometimes called the **user interface.** What is set with the controls determines the pattern of gas delivery the patient receives.

The classification of a ventilator begins with a description of the physical characteristics of the ventilator itself as shown in Box 11-1. It then proceeds to describe the type of breaths and combinations of breaths, also referred to as modes.

Power Source

Power sources, which provide the energy to perform the work required to ventilate a patient, fall into three categories: **pneumatically powered, electrically powered,** or **combined-powered ventilators.**

Pneumatically Powered Ventilators

Pneumatically powered ventilators connect to high-pressure gas sources, and use the high pressure to power gas flow to the patient. In general, pneumatically powered ventilators used in an intensive care unit (ICU) operate using two 50 psi gas sources (oxygen and air) and have built-in reducing valves so that the operating pressure is lower than the source pressure. Two basic types of pneumatic ventilators are used: **pneumatic** and **fluidic.** Pneumatic ventilators may incorporate components such as venturi devices or air entrainers, needle valves, flexible diaphragms, and spring-loaded valves to perform certain functions. For example, venturi devices may be used to control an expiratory valve (see the section on resistive expiratory valves under Additional Devices Used During Patient Ventilation in this chapter). A needle valve may control the rate of gas flow during inspiration. On the other hand, fluidic ventilators use fluidic components that are based on special pneumatic principles. The section on fluidics later in this chapter provides a description of fluidic function.

Box 11-1 Physical Characteristics of Ventilators[7]

Ventilator power source or input power (electric or gas source)
- Electrically powered ventilators
- Pneumatically powered ventilators
- Combined-power ventilators

Positive- or negative-pressure ventilators

Control systems and circuits
- Open- and closed-loop systems to control ventilator function
- Control panel (user interface)
- Pneumatic circuit

Power transmission and conversion system
- Volume-displacement, pneumatic designs
- Flow-control valves

From Pilbeam SP: *Mechanical ventilation: physiological and clinical applications*, St Louis, 1998, Mosby.

Electrically Powered Ventilators

Electrically powered ventilators most often use standard electrical outlets to power the internal components. They may also contain internal direct-current (DC) batteries, which can provide electrical power during patient transport or in the event of a power failure. Some ventilators can also be connected to external DC batteries. Electrically powered ventilators may use the electricity to power internal motors for operating air compressors, pistons, electrical solenoids, transducers, and microprocessors, all of which either provide gas flow to the patient or help control gas flow to the patient.

Combined Power Ventilators: Pneumatically Powered and Electronically or Microprocessor-Controlled

One of the most common types of ventilators used in the ICU today is pneumatically powered and **microprocessor-controlled.** Two 50 psi gas sources provide the pressure to deliver inspiratory gas flow. This gas flow is usually the same gas the patient receives during inspiration. Control of the inspiratory flow waveform is governed by a microprocessor. For example, the waveform or pattern of gas flow may be constant, producing a constant flow waveform, or it may be rapid at the beginning of inspiration and gradually taper down, producing a descending ramp waveform (see the section on inspiratory waveform and ventilator graphics later in this chapter). Programming of the microprocessor and its interaction with electrically operated flow valves or mechanical devices control this function. These ventilators require both electric and pneumatic power sources.

Pressure Delivery

A ventilator does all or part of the **work of breathing (WOB)** for the patient. A ventilator can increase lung volume during inspiration either by creating negative- or positive-pressure gradients. The pressure gradient that is applied to the body results in gas flow to produce ventilation (Box 11-2).

Box 11-2 Types and Examples of Pressure Ventilators

Negative-Pressure Ventilators
- Iron lung
- Chest cuirass

Positive-Pressure Ventilators
- Most ventilators in use today are this type, such as the Puritan-Bennett 7200, the Servo 300, and the Hamilton Galileo

Positive/Negative Pressure Ventilators
- High-frequency oscillators

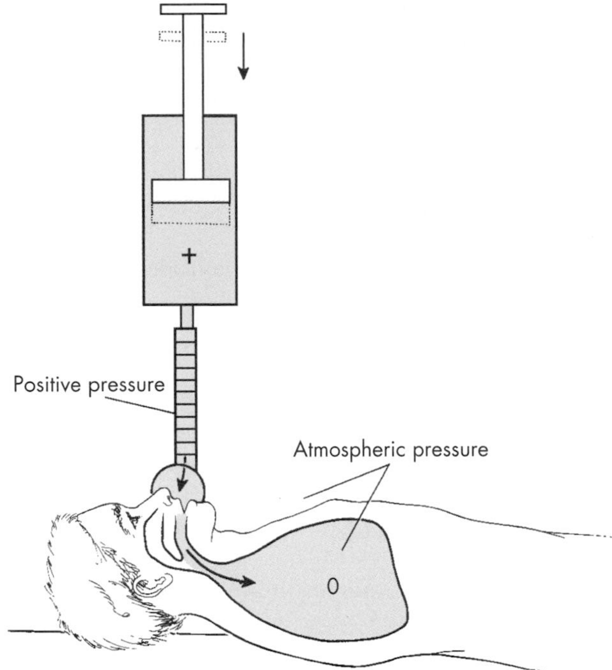

Figure 11-1 Application of positive pressure at the airway provides a pressure gradient between the mouth and the alveoli; therefore, gas flows into the lungs.

Positive-Pressure Ventilators

A pressure gradient must exist for gas flow to occur. During normal spontaneous breathing, contraction of the inspiratory muscles initiates inspiration. During inspiration, the diaphragm contracts and descends and the external intercostal muscles contract. The action of these muscles, especially the diaphragm, results in an increase in the intrathoracic volume. Intrapleural and intraalveolar pressures becomes subambient. This produces a pressure gradient from the mouth, which is at ambient pressure, to the alveoli, which are below ambient pressure. Consequently, air flows into the lungs. Expiration follows because passive relaxation of the respiratory muscles reduces the intrathoracic volume. Intraalveolar pressure become slightly positive (above ambient), and air flows out of the lungs.[7]

During positive-pressure ventilation, a supra-atmospheric pressure is created at the mouth while intraalveolar pressure is ambient. As a result, air flows into the lungs, expanding them and the chest wall (Figure 11-1). **Positive-pressure ventilators** are by far the most common method of ventilation used today.

Negative-Pressure Ventilators

Negative-pressure ventilators generally enclose the thoracic area and create a subatmospheric pressure around the chest wall (Figure 11-2). This negative pressure is transmitted across the chest wall, resulting in reduced intrapleural and intraalveolar pressures. The pressure at the mouth is atmospheric pressure, creating a pressure gradient between the mouth and alveoli similar to the normal spontaneous pressure gradient. Air flows into the lungs. During exhalation, the negative pressure around the chest is returned to ambient, the intraalveolar pressure becomes slightly positive, and air flows out of the lungs. Examples of these types of devices are the **iron lung** and the **chest cuirass.** Chapter 14 describes and illustrates these devices in more detail. Presently these ventilators are not widely used, but are occasionally used in the home.

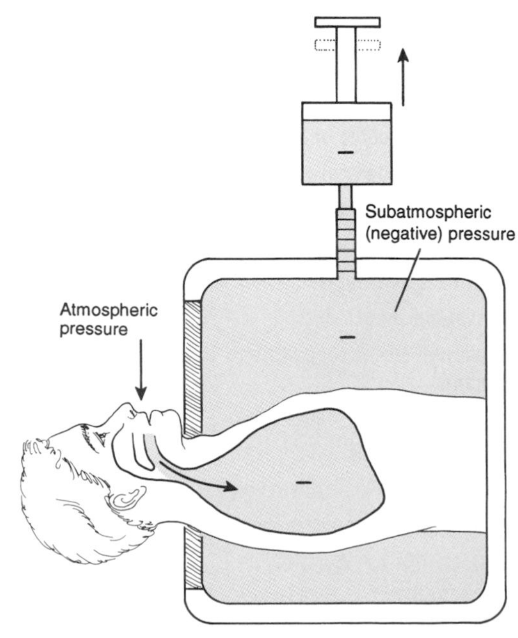

Figure 11-2 By applying subatmospheric pressure around the chest wall, a pressure drop in the alveoli occurs and air flows into the lungs.

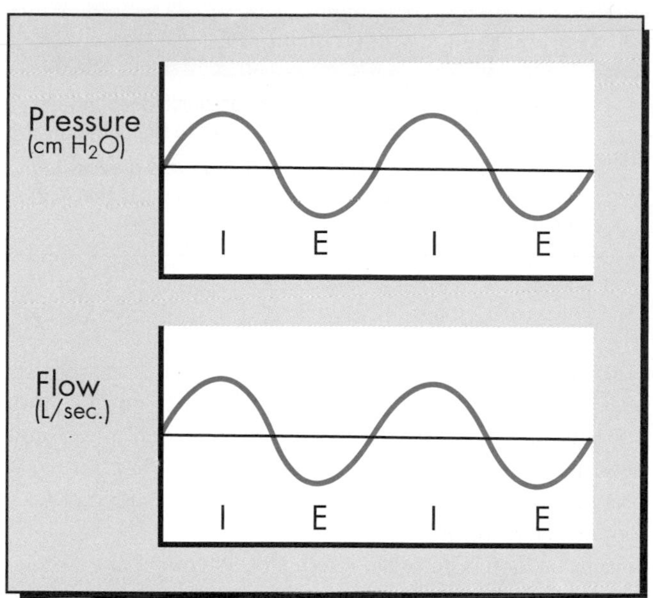

Figure 11-3 The sinusoidal waveform produced by an oscillator. *I*, Inspiration, *E*, expiration.

Combined-Pressure Devices

The most common example of a combined-pressure device is a **high-frequency oscillator.** This is a form of **high-frequency ventilation (HFV)** that produces oscillating gas pressure waveforms at the upper airway. The waveform is a **sinusoidal** pattern with positive- and negative-pressure oscillations produced at the upper airway by an oscillating device (Figure 11-3). The section in this chapter on high-frequency ventilation explains oscillator function. Oscillators are being used with neonatal patients and occasionally in adults. The chapter on infant and pediatric ventilation provides an example of this type of device.

Control Systems and Circuits

A combination of mechanical, pneumatic, or electronic devices within the ventilator represent the control or decision-making functions of the unit. These control systems and circuits govern ventilator operation and can either be an **open-loop** or a **closed-loop** system.

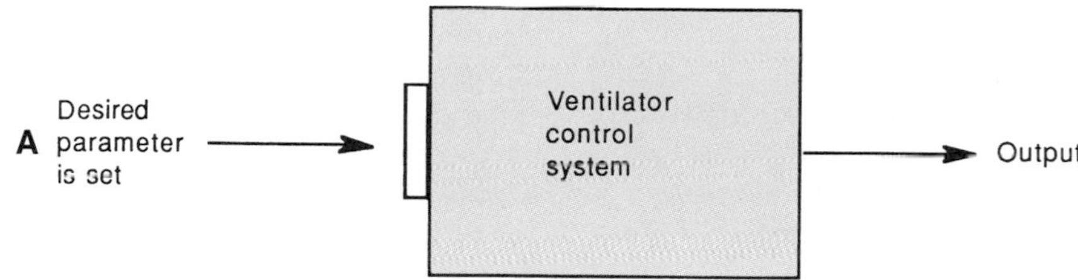

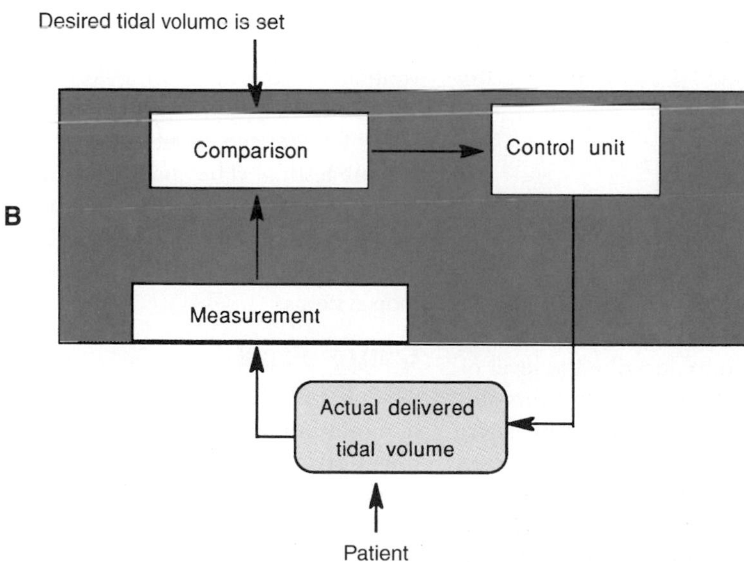

Figure 11-4 A, Open-loop system. The path through the device is straight from the control panel, to the internal device and out to the patient. No feedback is provided to the ventilator about the output. In **B** the ventilator "closes the loop" by measuring gas exhaled from the patient, comparing it to the set value and feeding this information back to the machine. (See text for further explanation.) (From Pilbeam SP: *Mechanical ventilation: physiological and clinical applications*, ed 3, St Louis, 1998, Mosby.)

Box 11-3 Hierarchical Control

With hierarchical control the output is forced to follow or match an operator preset input based on several layers of conditional logic. For example, in the pressure augmentation mode of the Bear 1000, inspiration starts out delivering a constant pressure. This action is modified by a series of "if-then" statements. **If** the set volume has not been met by the time flow decreases to the set value, **then** switch to volume ventilation, and maintain the flow at the set value.

Box 11-4 Smart Modes, Handguns and Tequila[9]

Rob Chatburn reminds us of a very appropriate quotation about the use of closed-loop ventilation. "A computer lets you make more mistakes faster than any invention in human history . . . with the possible exception of handguns and tequila."

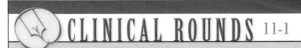

Open-Loop and Closed-Loop Systems

Part I

A respiratory therapist sets a ventilator tidal volume at 650 mL and the peak inspiratory pressure is 8 cm H_2O. Volume measured at the exhalation valve is 500 mL. These measurements occur over the next several breaths with no changes. Is this open-loop or closed-loop logic?

Part II

A respiratory therapist sets the tidal volume at 650 mL. After one breath, the exhaled volume measures 500 mL and the peak pressure is 8 cm H_2O. After a second breath, the exhaled volume is 600 mL and the pressure is 14 cm H_2O. After a third breath, the exhaled volume is 649 mL and the peak pressure is 16 cm H_2O. What type of system is this?

See Appendix A for the answer.

Open- and Closed-Loop Systems

The terms open-loop and closed-loop describe the level of control within a ventilator. Unintelligent ventilators are called open-loop systems. When the operator establishes a setting, such as tidal volume (V_T), the unit delivers the set amount of volume. In reality, this volume might leak into the room and never reach the patient. Unfortunately, an open-loop system cannot discern a difference between the volume actually delivered and the set volume and respond to this difference (Figure 11-4, A).[2] For example, suppose a robot is pouring water from a 1 L beaker of water into a 0.75 L container. If not programmed otherwise, the robot will pour the liter of water filling the container, but spill the excess (0.25 L) on the ground. On the other hand, an intelligent robot that can see the container and determine when it is full has the ability to stop pouring, if programmed to do so. This example demonstrates a closed-loop programming.

Closed-loop systems are intelligent systems.[8] For example, the manufacturer programs a responsive system into the computer to deliver a specific quantity (e.g., V_T). This system measures the volume delivered by the ventilator and exhaled by the patient, makes a comparison, and adjusts the volume delivery based on this comparison to deliver the amount of volume set on the control panel. Figure 11-4, *B*, shows an algorithm for a closed-loop system.[2] This system is similar to cruise control on a car. You set the cruise control at the speed you want the car to go. The car then compares what the speed actually is with how fast you want to go. If the car is going too slowly, the cruise control accelerates the car. You do not have to make any adjustments; the cruise control does it for you. This is a closed-loop system. It is closed because it compares the input to the output and "closes the loop" as illustrated in Figure 11-4, *B*. These systems are also called feedback systems and servo-control systems. Another term for closed-loop or intelligent systems is hierarchical control (Box 11-3).[6] All new commercially available ventilators now have some form of hierarchical control. They are not, however, without problems. New hierarchical control modes can be introduced on the market without any patient testing. The manufacturer only has to prove the mode does the intended function and that the software is validated (Box 11-4).[9] Clinical Rounds 11-1 provides an exercise to test your understanding of closed- and open-loop systems.

Box 11-5 Types of Internal Circuits

- A single circuit is one in which the gas supply that powers the ventilator is the same gas that goes to the patient.
- A double circuit has a source gas that powers the unit by compressing a bag or bellows containing the gas that will go to the patient.

Control Panel

The control panel or user interface is located on the front of most ventilators and contains the controls for the operator to adjust such as respiratory rate (f), tidal volume (V_T), set pressure (P_{set}), and inspiratory time (T_I).

Pneumatic Circuit

The **pneumatic circuit** consists of a series of tubing that directs gas flow both within the ventilator (the **internal circuit**) and from the ventilator to the patient (the external or **patient circuit**).

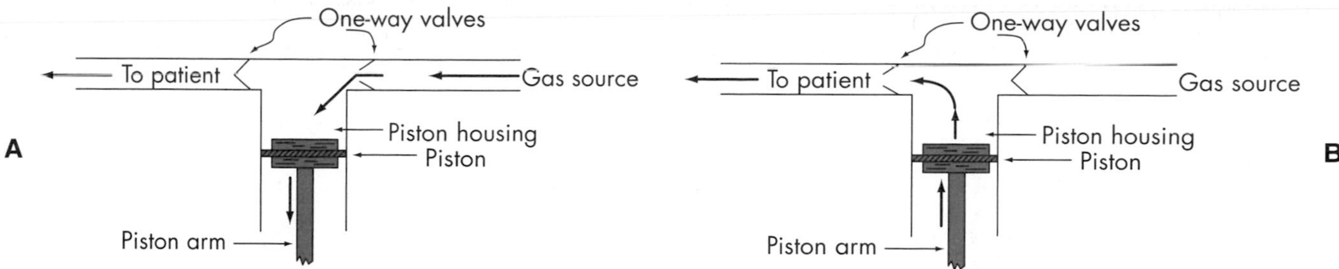

Figure 11-5 A ventilator using a single-circuit design. Gases are drawn into the cylinder during the expiratory phase **(A).** During inspiration, the piston moves upward into the cylinder sending gas directly toward the patient circuit **(B).** (From Pilbeam SP: *Mechanical ventilation: physiological and clinical applications*, ed 3, St Louis, 1998, Mosby.)

Internal Circuit

The internal circuit conducts gas generated by the power source, passes it through various mechanical or pneumatic mechanisms, and finally directs it to the **external circuit.** Internal circuits are either single or double circuits (Box 11-5).

In a single-circuit ventilator, the gas enters the ventilator goes directly to the patient (Figure 11-5). A double-circuit ventilator consists of two gas sources. One gas source goes to the patient from a bag or bellows; the other actively compresses the bag or bellows. Double circuits are also called "bag-in-a-box" designs. Figure 11-6 shows an example of a compressor blowing gas into a chamber. This gas lifts the bellows. Gas in the bellows goes to the patient. This design was originally used in Puritan-Bennett's MA-1 ventilator. The figure is not drawn to scale.

External Circuit

The external circuit conducts the gas from the ventilator to the patient and from the patient through an expiratory valve to the room. The external circuit is commonly called the **ventilator circuit,** or the patient circuit. The components of the patient circuit are illustrated in Figure 11-7. Part *A* shows a ventilator circuit with an externally mounted expiratory valve, and *B* shows a ventilator circuit with an internally mounted exhalation valve.

With an external circuit, gas flows both through the main inspiratory line to the patient and to the expiratory valve line during inspiration. This line inflates a balloon or puts pressure on a diaphragm that closes a hole. The hole in the exhalation valve is where the patient's exhaled gases normally vents into the room. During inspiration the hole is covered by the balloon or diaphragm. During exhalation, no gas goes through the main inspiratory line or the expiratory valve line. The balloon deflates and the patient's exhaled volume passes through the open hole (Figure 11-7, A, enlarged portion.)

Almost all new ventilator circuits use a patient circuit with the exhalation valve mounted inside the machine. These internal valves are usually low-resistance, large diameter, flexible plastic diaphragms. They operate in a similar fashion as the externally mounted expiratory valve. During inspiration either gas pressure or a mechanical

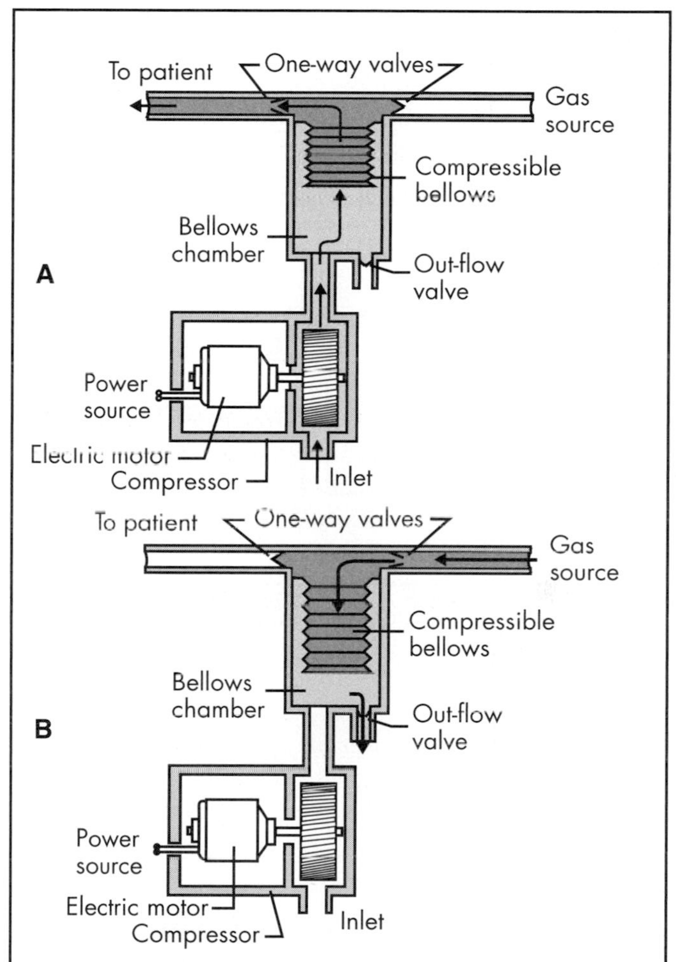

Figure 11-6 A ventilator using a double-circuit design. The compressor produces a high-pressure gas source, which is directed to a chamber that holds a collapsible bellows. The bellows contains the desired gas mixture that will go to the patient. The pressure from the compressor forces the bellows upward, resulting in a positive-pressure breath **(A).** After the inspiratory breath is delivered, the compressor no longer directs pressure to the bellows chamber and exhalation occurs. The bellows drops to its original position and fills with the desired gas in preparation of the next breath **(B).** (From Pilbeam SP: *Mechanical ventilation: physiological and clinical applications*, ed 3, St Louis, 1998, Mosby.)

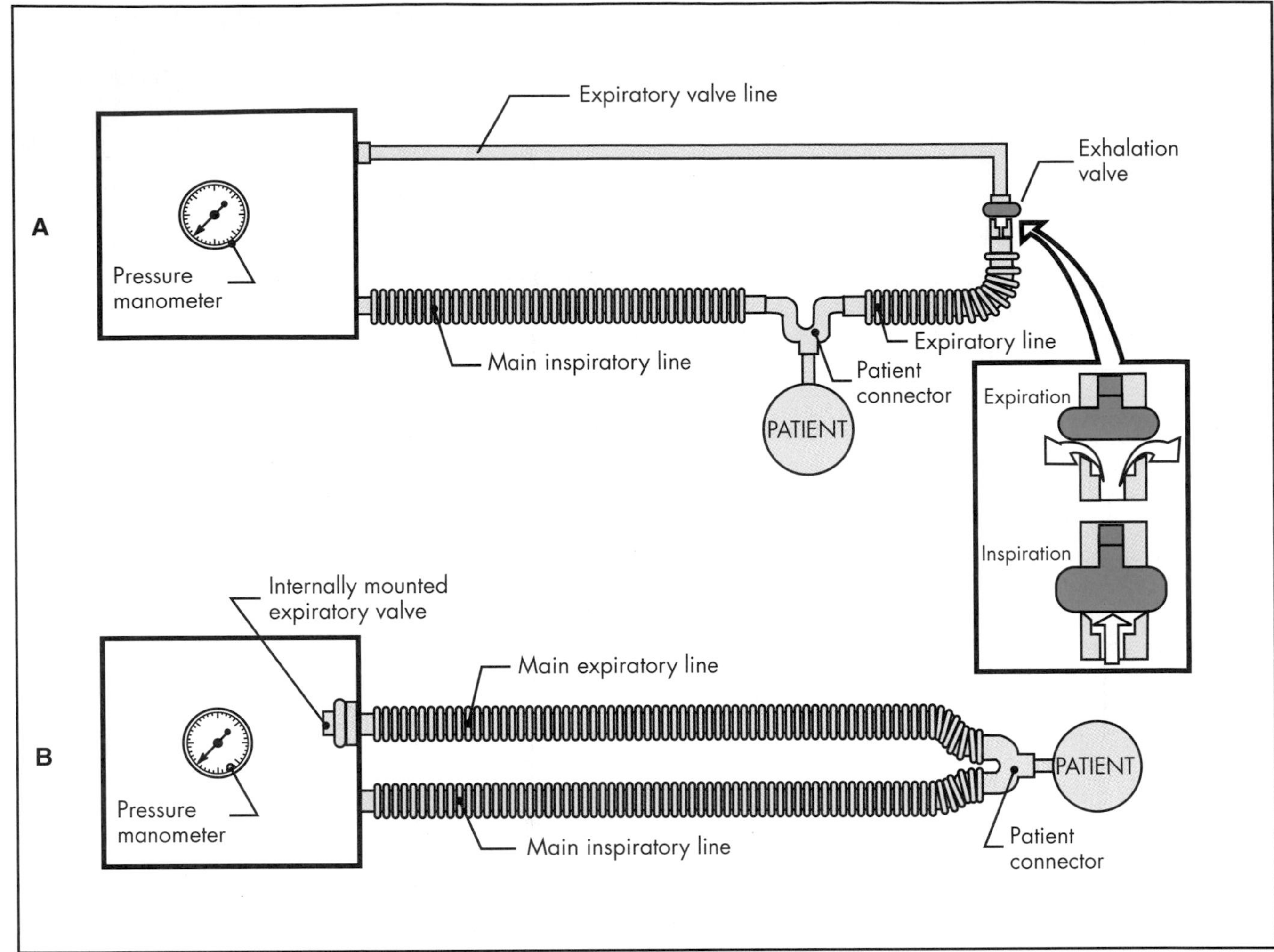

Figure 11-7 **A,** Ventilator circuit with an externally mounted expiratory valve; **B,** Ventilator circuit with an internally mounted exhalation valve. (See text for further explanation.)

device pushes the valve over the exhalation hole. Exhaled gas normally passes through this hole. During exhalation the valve is opened and the patient's exhaled volume can pass through the hole.

Drive Mechanisms (Power Transmission Systems)

The power sources, gas or electricity, provide the energy to power mechanical devices. This energy and the devices they control ultimately generate a pressure gradient. The pressure gradient, negative or positive, provides all or part of the patient's work of breathing. These internal drive mechanisms are also called the **power transmission systems.** They transmit the original energy source—gas or electricity or both—to direct gas flow to the patient.

From an engineering point of view, two basic categories describe the power transmission systems in most conventional ventilators: those controlling volume delivery, and those controlling flow delivery.[10-12] For electrically powered ventilators that control volume delivery, these systems might be compressors or blowers, and volume-displacement devices. For pneumatically powered systems, the power transmission unit may consist of venturi entrainers, flexible diaphragms, or specially designed pneumatic or fluidic elements. For pneumatically powered, microprocessor-controlled units the power transmission devices might be flow-control valves.

In the past respiratory therapy students spent a great deal of time studying ventilator systems because respiratory therapists were often called upon to repair the systems or, at least, to be able to answer questions about them. Now, less emphasis is being placed on this information. Respiratory therapists no longer repair these devices. That function has been given to bioengineering departments. The following section will briefly review examples of these ventilator drive mechanisms. Some of these mechanisms are still in use. Knowing about ventilator systems helps the reader acquire a better understanding of situations in which internal mechanisms alter ventilator functions.

Compressors or Blowers

Compressors can be driven by pistons, rotating blades (vanes), moving diaphragms, or bellows. Large, piston-type, water-cooled compressors are used by hospitals to supply high-pressure air for wall air outlets (see Chapter 2, section on Medical Gases). Small portable compressors are used for powering small-volume nebulizers and similar devices. The most common type of compressor used for ventilators is the rotary compressor. The rotor acts as a fan, drawing air from the room, compressing it, and directing it through the ventilator's internal circuit. Figure 2-16 shows an example of a rotary compressor. External compressors not built into the ventilator can provide a 50-psi gas source to power the unit when a wall outlet is not available. Historical Note 11-1 and Figure 11-6 provide a historical perspective on ventilators that used compressors as power sources.

HISTORICAL NOTE 11-1
Use of the Rotary Compressor

Some of the older ventilators developed in the 1950s and 1960s were never connected to wall air sources because at that time wall outlets for air were scarce. An internal compressor was sometimes used within the ventilator as the power source itself. For example, the rotating vane compressor in the MA-1 provided the driving pressure to power the drive mechanism. In this case, an electric motor powered a blower that held a series of blades, similar to a fan. The rotary blower caused gas to flow to a canister containing a bellows, which forced air into the canister. The bellows emptied, sending the gas inside it to the patient (see Figure 11-6).

Volume-Displacement Designs

Some ventilators use volume-displacement devices, including pistons, bellows, concertina bags, or similar "bag-in-a-chamber" mechanisms to deliver a positive-pressure breath.[10] Many of the older ventilators, such as the MA-l and the Emerson Post-Op, used the bag-in-a-chamber and the piston design. Figure 11-5 is an example of a single-circuit piston design used in the Emerson Post-Op ventilator during the 1960s and 1970s. During the downward stroke of the piston, gas

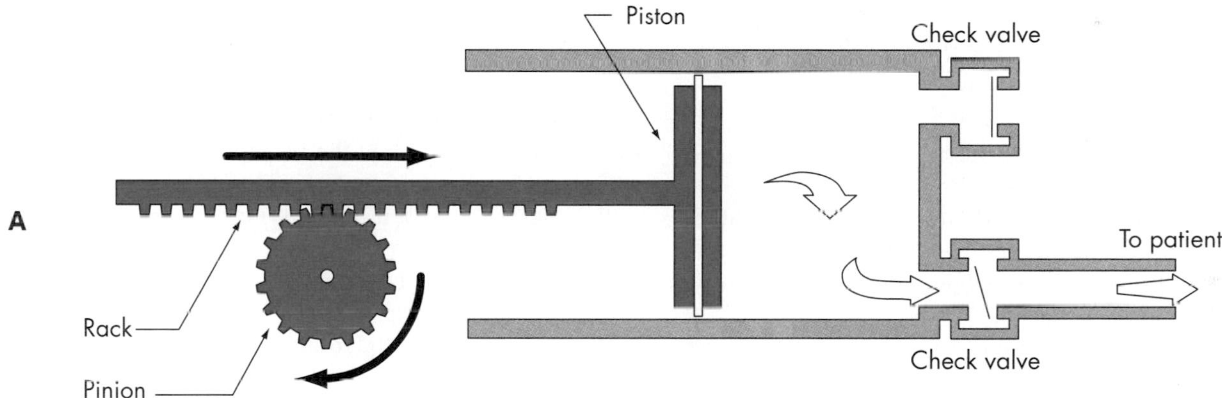

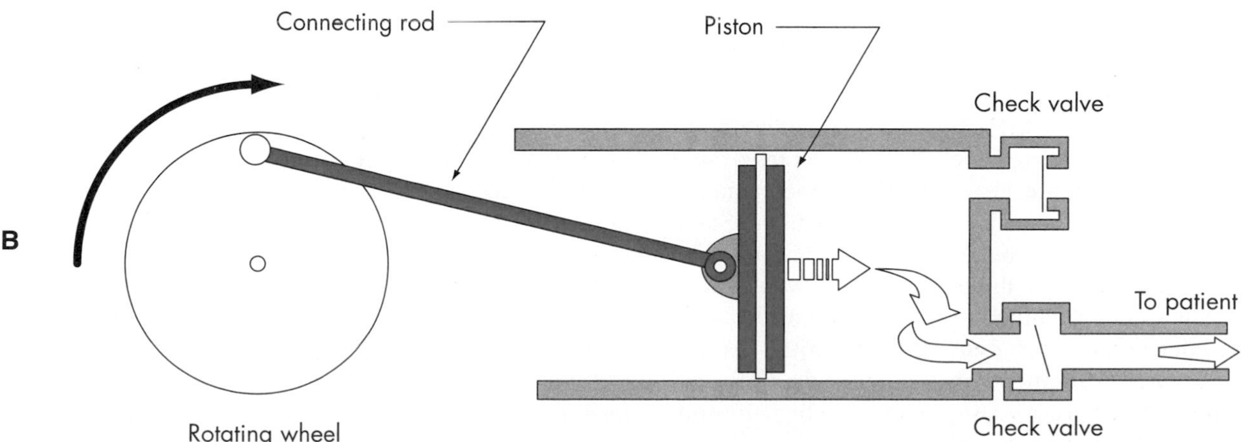

Figure 11-8 **A,** Linear, and **B,** rotary, piston-driven mechanisms for ventilators. (Redrawn from Dupuis Y: *Ventilators*, ed 2, St Louis, 1992, Mosby.)

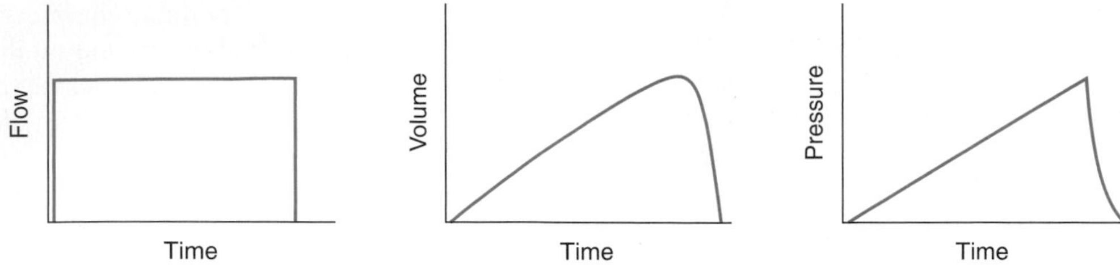

Figure 11-9 The flow-time, volume-time, and pressure-time curves generated by a linear drive piston.

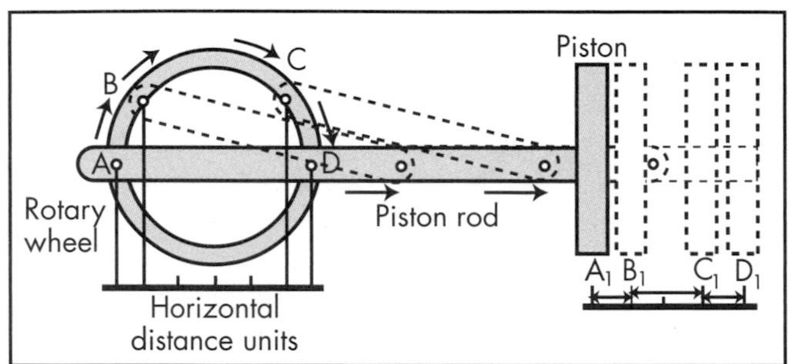

Figure 11-10 A diagram of the rotary-driven piston's movement. The times between points *A* and *B*, *B* and *C*, and *C* and *D* are equal. The piston travels different distances in the same amount of time and therefore moves at different speeds from A_1 to B_1, from B_1 to C_1, and from C_1 to D_1.

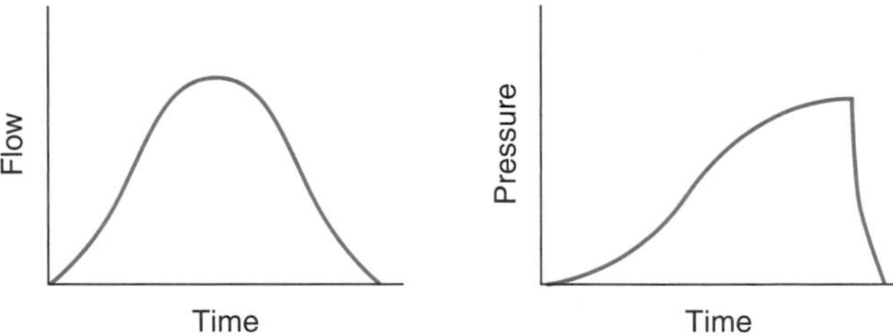

Figure 11-11 Flow-time and pressure-time curves created by a rotary-driven piston, positive-pressure ventilator during volume delivery.

was drawn into the piston's cylinder (see Figure 11-5, A). On the upward stroke of the piston, gas flowed out of the cylinder, through the ventilator circuit, and to the patient (see Figure 11-5, B). Some home-care ventilators also use pistons. The Puritan-Bennett 740 and 760 ventilators use a piston design (see Chapter 12). Another ICU ventilator, the Venturi, uses a bag-in-a-chamber circuit (see the EVOLVE website for this text.)

Pistons

Two piston designs are commonly used: the direct drive and the indirect drive. In a direct, or **linear drive piston**, special gearing connects an electrical motor to a piston rod or arm (see Figure 11-8, A). The rod moves the piston forward linearly inside the cylinder housing at a constant rate. This movement normally produces a constant or rectangular waveform of gas flow to the patient, an ascending ramp volume waveform, and a relatively linear ascending ramp pressure waveform (Figure 11-9). Ventilators incorporating linear drive pistons are usually single-circuit units. Some high-frequency ventilators use **direct drive pistons.** The recently incorporated use of the rolling-seal or low-resistance materials have helped eliminate the friction of the early piston-cylinder designs. For example, the Puritan-Bennett 740 uses a very low-resistance piston that provides all the gas flow to patient and does not require an external high-pressure gas source to function (electrically powered).[10] It also has the ability to produce not only a constant flow, but also a descending flow waveform.

Rotary or nonlinear drive pistons are sometimes called eccentric drive pistons (Figure 11-8, *B*). Figure 11-10 shows a complete forward cycle of such a unit. The piston is connected to the outer edge of the rotary wheel. The piston's forward motion is short at the beginning of inspiration (A1 to B1), rapid at mid-inspiration (B1 to C1), and slow again at the end of inspiration (C1 to D1). This change in speed produces the sine-wavelike flow curve (Figure 11-11). Gas flow is slowest at the beginning and end of inspiration and the fastest at mid-inspiration, producing a sine-wavelike flow pattern. Note that the **rotary drive piston** produces half of the sinusoidal wave during the inspiratory phase, but it is commonly referred to as a sine wave or a pattern similar to a sine wave.

Bag in a Chamber

Piston-driven ventilators can be double- or single-circuit ventilators. A double-circuit, piston-driven ventilator is shown in Figure 11-12. A piston drives air into a chamber, which compresses a bag containing the gas for the patient. Although not a common design for most ICU ventilators, the Venturi ventilator uses this concept in its patient circuit. In the Venturi, pressured gas from a wall source (oxygen) is the power source that compresses the bag (see the Evolve website for this text).

Spring-Loaded Bellows

Another volume design unit uses a **spring-loaded bellows** to act as the force delivering the breath (Figure 11-13). A mixture of oxygen and air at the desired fractional inspired oxygen (F_IO_2) flows into a bellows, which is spring-loaded. The operator can tighten the tension on the spring to increase the force exerted against the bellows and the pressure

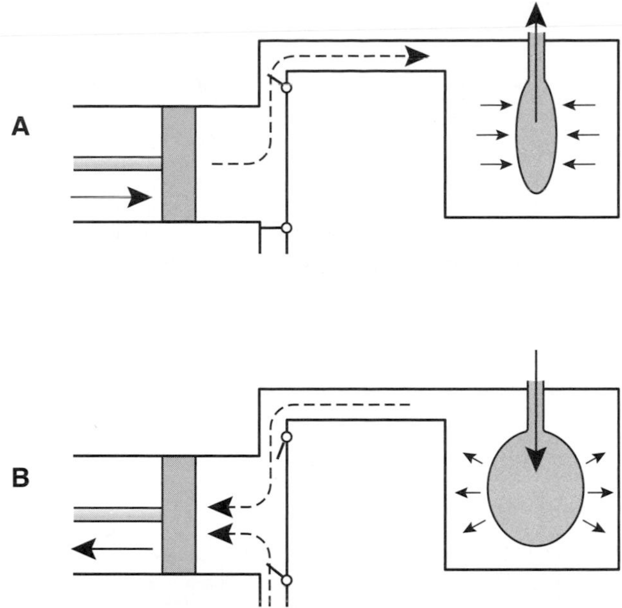

Figure 11-12 A simple diagram of a piston-driven, double-circuit system (i.e., bag-in-a-chamber). **A** shows the forward stroke of the piston which causes gas to flow to the chamber containing the bag. The bag collapses sending gas to the patient (inspiration). **B** shows the backward stroke of the piston with gas entering the piston cylinder. Gas also enters the bag filling it for the next patient inspiration. (See text for description.)

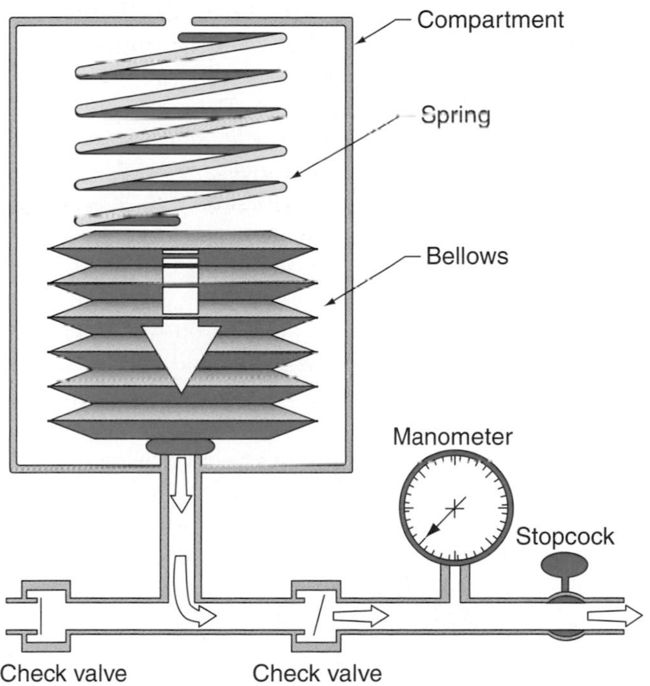

Figure 11-13 A spring-loaded bellows unit. (See text for description.) (Redrawn from Dupuis Y: *Ventilators*, ed 2, St Louis, 1992, Mosby.)

delivered to the patient. The Servo 900C ventilator uses this type of power transmission system, which can be adjusted up to 120 cm H_2O.

The flow and pressure curves produced by this system will be like those of a linear drive piston when the working

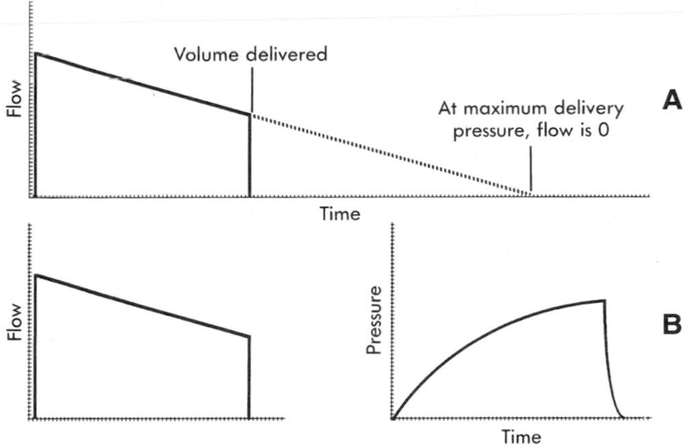

Figure 11-14 **A,** The primary flow-time curve from a spring-loaded bellows with a low working pressure and a high system resistance (i.e., high patient airway resistance and low lung compliance). **B,** Flow-time and pressure-time curves for this system when the breath is time-cycled.

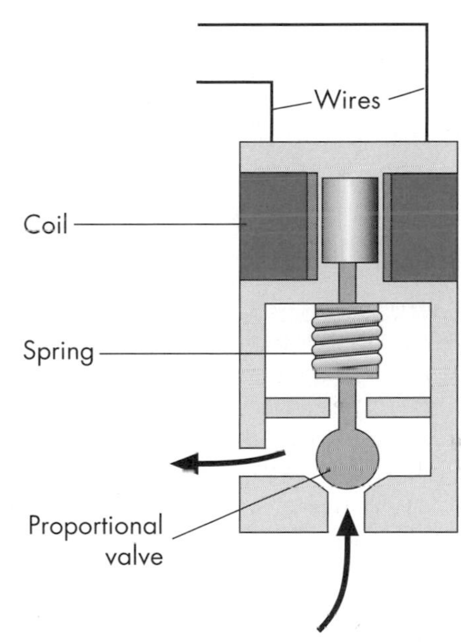

Figure 11-15 A proportional solenoid valve. (See text for description.) (Redrawn from Sanborn WG: *Respir Care* 38:72, 1993.)

pressure is high and the system resistance (patient lung condition and patient circuit) is low (see Figure 11-9). When the working pressure is low, especially when the system resistance is high, the flow curve descends during inspiration (Figure 11-14).

Flow-Control Valves

Most of the current ICU ventilators use valves that precisely control flow to the patient. In general, high-pressure sources of air and oxygen are mixed and delivered at the desired F_IO_2 to accumulator chambers. These chambers are often of similar shape to medical gas cylinders. They hold about 2 to 3 L of gas under pressure and act as reservoirs from which inspired gas for the patient can be withdrawn.

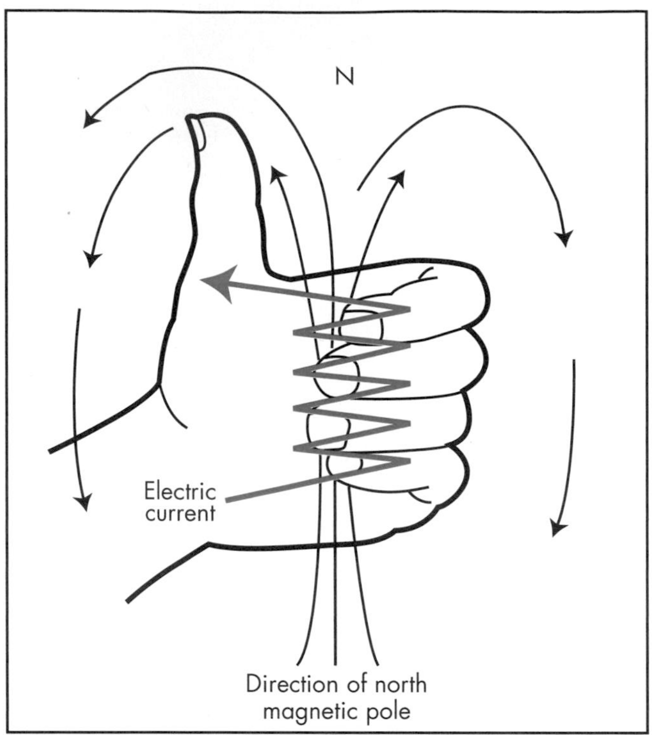

Figure 11-16 A solenoid uses a coil of wire. An electrical current is passed through the coil, generating a magnetic field. The direction of the magnetic field is indicated by the arrows. If you hold your left hand with your thumb pointed up and your fingers slightly curved, the curve of your fingers is the direction of the electric current through the coil, and your thumb is in the direction of magnetic north. (See text for further explanation.)

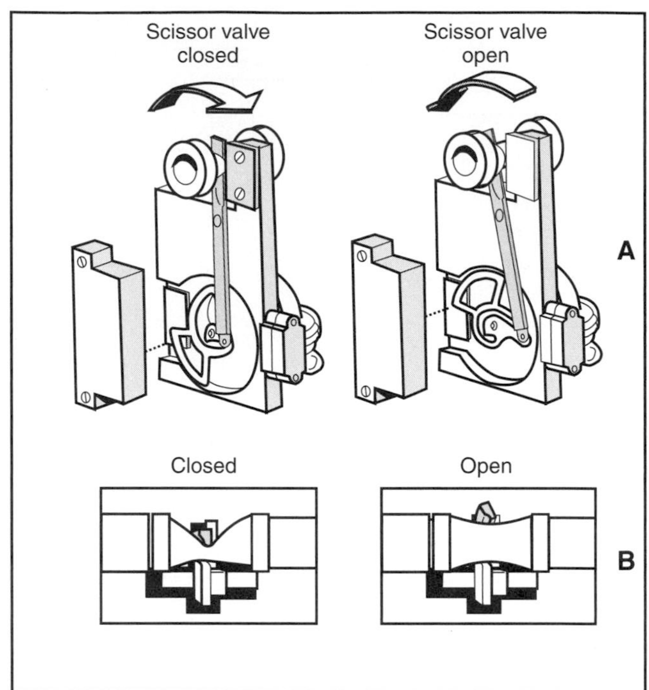

Figure 11-17 A stepper motor with a scissor valve in the Siemens Servo 900C ventilator. **A,** A cam on the motor controls the moving arm. On the left, the valve is shown in the closed position, and on the right, it is completely open. **B,** The closing and opening of the internal circuit by the scissor valve. (**A,** Courtesy Siemens Life Support Systems, Danvers, Mass.)

From these chambers, gas is sent through a valve that controls the inspiratory gas flow. These valves can be moved in small precise increments and at varying rates because their activity is governed by a microprocessor. Flow-control valve response is so rapid that it has precise control over the exact pattern of gas and pressure. The more advanced technology has become, the more rapid and dependable flow valves have become. Three common flow-controlling valves are worth further discussion: proportional solenoids, stepper motors with valves, and digital valves with on/off configurations.

Proportional Solenoid Valves

Proportional solenoid valves control flow by using an on/off switch (Figure 11-15). Commonly, this valve contains a gate or plunger, a valve seat, an electromagnet, a diaphragm, a spring, two electrical contacts, and an adjustable electric current.

The operation of this device is based on a basic principle of physics concerning electricity and magnetism. When a current flows through a wire, it creates a magnetic field. Winding a wire into a coil increases the strength of the magnetic field around the wire. Adding an iron rod within the coiled wire further increases the magnetism and produces an electromagnet.

The polarity of an electromagnet can be determined using the left-hand rule shown in Figure 11-16. The curved fingers indicate the electric current and the upward pointing thumb points to the north magnetic pole. With the rod connected in line within the center of the coiled wire, the rod will move up and down depending on the strength of the electric current and the magnetic field it creates. The action of this electromagnet describes basically how solenoid valves operate.

The variation in the amount of current flowing through the coiled wire results in movement of the rod or plunger and causes the plunger to assume a specific position. Some solenoids are called proportional solenoid valves because the valves move in proportion to the current applied and open a hole or gate a proportional amount.

Besides using an electrical current, which is often microprocessor-controlled or controlled by an electric timer, solenoids can also be controlled by manual operation and by pressure. Manual operation closes a switch, which sends a current to the electromagnet and alters the valve position. Air pressure changes often caused by an actively breathing patient can cause a diaphragm to descend, closing an electric contact and altering valve position. Examples of ventilators with proportional solenoid valves are the Puritan Bennett 7200, the Hamilton

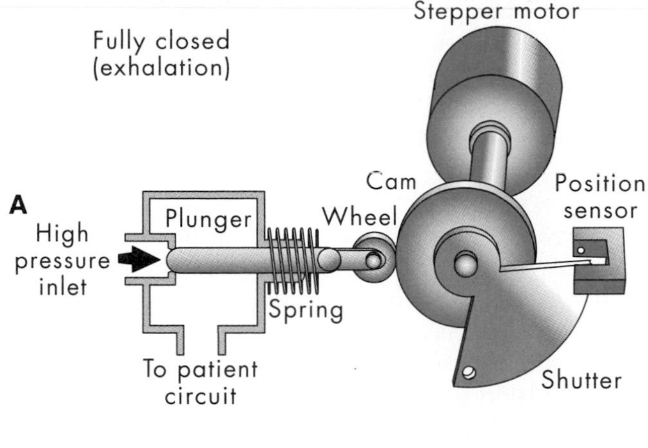

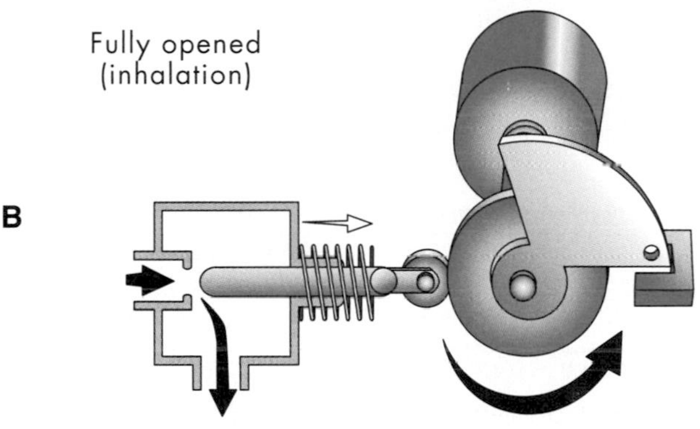

Figure 11-18 A schematic of a microprocessor-operated flow valve. (See text for description.) (Redrawn from Dupuis Y: *Ventilators*, ed 2, St Louis, 1992, Mosby.)

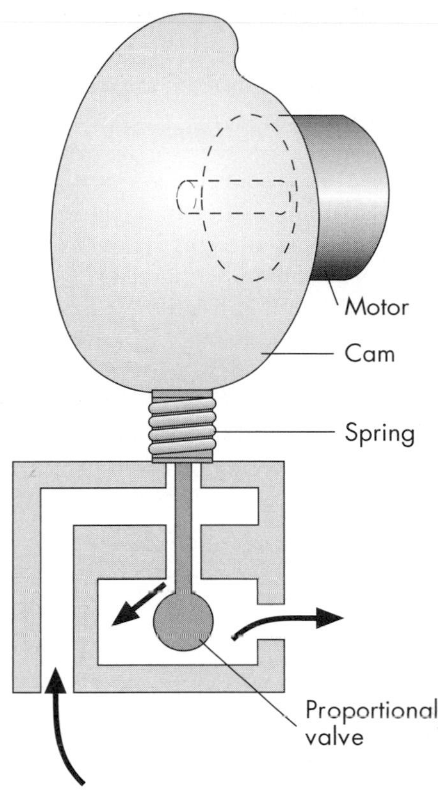

Figure 11-19 Example of an externally actuated proportional valve. (See text for description.) (Redrawn from Sanborn WG: *Respir Care* 38:72, 1993.)

VEOLAR and GALILEO, the Dräger Evita, and the Siemens Servo 300.

Figure 11-15 illustrates a proportional solenoid valve used to govern gas flow. Gas enters the bottom of the valve when the metal rod with the ball at the base moves upward. This movement opens a hole into the valve. The flow can then be directed out another hole and to the patient.

Stepper Motor with Valve

Stepper motors can move in very rapid, discreet steps to open or close a valve. Figure 11-17, A, shows an example of a stepper motor. Notice the lever arm colored in light green. It is connected at its base to a rotating metal "wheel." The wheel moves in very fixed steps, almost like the teeth on a gear. This movement is very rapid. As the wheel moves, the arm moves forward and back. The arm moves toward a fixed metal post located to the right of the moving arm. The movement is like closing a pair of scissors. It closes a plastic tube *(B)* as shown on the lower left. When the arm moves away from the metal post, the tube reopens and gas can now flow through it (right side of figure). Electricity is used to power the motor that controls the movement of a lever arm.

Stepper motors are considered digital valves as opposed to analog valves, which do not move in discreet steps. A stepper motor is used in the Siemens Servo 900C ventilator. Precisely controlled gas flow to the patient is accomplished by the stepper-motor—driven scissors-like valve that pinches a silicon tube (see Figure 11-17).

Figure 11-18 shows a microprocessor-controlled stepper motor, which consists of a cam connected to a stepper motor and a spring-loaded plunger attached to a wheel. The tension of the spring pushes the wheel against the perimeter of the cam. During exhalation, the plunger occludes the gas outlet and stops flow to the patient (Figure 11-18, A). During inspiration, the motor turns the cam, and the spring tension relaxes, although contact is still maintained. Because of this action, the plunger moves to the right (Figure 11-18, *B*), and gas flows to the patient. An optical sensor and a shutter, which sends information to the microprocessor about the position of the cam are not shown, but are also present. Through microprocessor control, the motor can rotate the cam in many specific steps and at different speeds, allowing the microprocessor to deliver gas flow in the pattern and amount the operator selects.[13]

Although several ventilators incorporate stepper motors as flow-control valves, several different motor and cam designs for controlling valve or poppet positions are used in each. For example, Puritan Bennett Adult Star Ventilator uses a flow-metering orifice directly coupled to a stepper motor. The Bear 1000 and the Bird 8400 ventilators incorporate stepper-motor—driven cam devices that actuate flow-control valves. Figure 11-19 shows one example of an externally actuated proportional valve. Several different motor and cam designs are available for controlling valve or poppet position.

Digital Valve On/Off Configuration

With a digital valve on/off configuration, several valves operate simultaneously, assuming either an open or closed position (Figure 11-20). A given valve produces a specific flow by opening or closing a certain size orifice. Depending on which valves are open, the amount of flow can be varied. The Infant Star ventilator uses this type of valve configuration.

Fluidic Elements in Power Transmission Design

Units using **fluidics** or **fluid logic** to deliver gas flow to the patient do not require moving parts or electrical circuits to function. Control is provided solely through fluid dynamics. Fluidic units use air and oxygen as the operating medium and employ all of the same basic functional controls as electrically operated ventilators.[13] The Sechrist IV-100B, the Bio-Med MVP 100, and the Monaghan 225 are examples of fluidic ventilators.

Because some are immune to failure from electromagnetic interference, as encountered near magnetic resonance imaging (MRI) equipment, fluidic ventilators can be used in this environment. They must, of course, be constructed of non-ferrous metals, such as aluminum. The Monaghan 225 has such a design. Modifications can also be made to other ventilators to make them MRI-compatible.[14]

Fluidic devices use two basic physical principles: wall attachment and beam deflection. The principle of wall attachment is commonly called the Coanda effect (Historical Note 11-2 and Figure 11-21), a phenomenon that occurs when an air stream (jet stream) is forced through an opening. The jet exits the opening, creating a localized

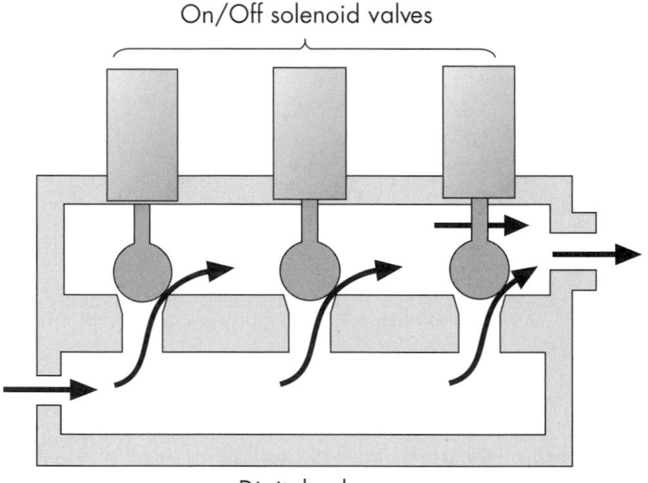

Figure 11-20 On/off digital-valve design for flow control. Each valve controls a critical orifice and thus a specified flow. The number of discreet flow steps (from zero upward) becomes 2^n, where n is the number of valves. (Redrawn from Sanborn WG: *Respir Care* 38:72, 1993.)

HISTORICAL NOTE 11-2
The Coanda Effect

In 1932, Dr. Henri Coanda, a Romanian aeronautical engineer, first described the "wall attachment" phenomenon. Consequently, this effect now carries his name.[13]

As gas travels faster over a pocket of turbulent air, the increased forward molecular velocity of the gas causes a decreased lateral pressure by the pocket as adjacent molecules are sheared away by the jet stream. The surrounding gas molecules (i.e., those not in the stream) then possess a higher pressure, thus holding the stream against the wall (see Figure 11-21, *B*).

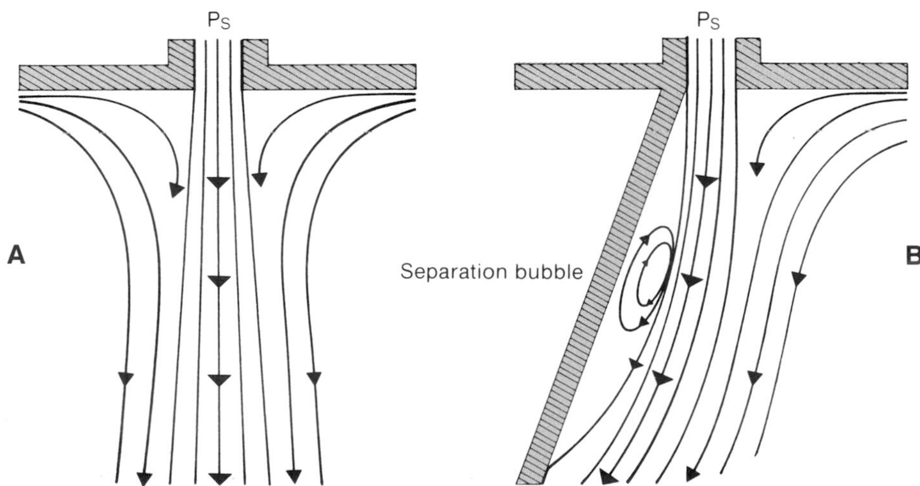

Figure 11-21 The Coanda effect, or the wall attachment phenomenon: **A,** Turbulent jet flow causes a local drop in lateral pressure and draws air inward. **B,** A wall placed adjacent to the jet stream creates a low-pressure vortex or separation bubble. The gas stream tends to bend toward that wall. (From Dupuis Y: *Ventilators*, ed 2, St Louis, 1992, Mosby.)

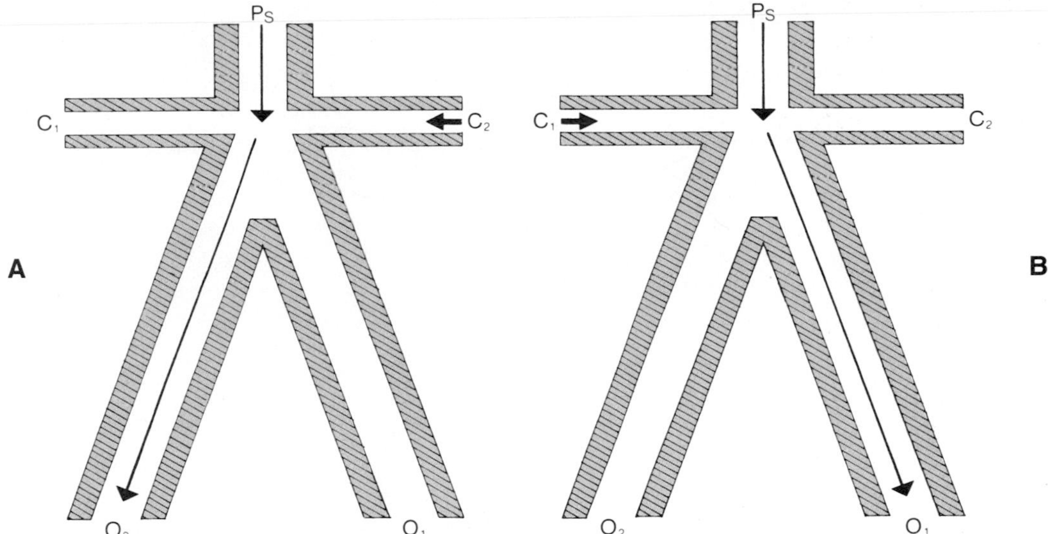

Figure 11-22 A diagrammatic representation of a flip-flop valve showing the principle of beam deflection. (See text for explanation.) (From Dupuis Y: *Ventilators*, ed 2, St Louis, 1992, Mosby.)

drop in pressure adjacent to itself. Ambient air is drawn toward the jet stream on all sides as a result of the localized low pressure associated with the rapid movement of the jet through the air (Figure 11-21, A). When a wall is added to one side of the jet stream, as seen in Figure 11-21, *B*, the entrained gas can only enter from the opposite side. However, a separation bubble (a low-pressure vortex) develops between the wall and the jet stream. The bubble attracts or bends the jet stream toward the wall. The pocket of turbulence forms an air foil, similar to that seen with an airplane wing.[13] When the gas entrained into the bubble from the jet stream equals the amount of air moving from the vortex flow of the bubble back to the jet stream, the attachment is stable.

The second important phenomenon of fluid logic is beam deflection. When a beam or jet of gas is moving through a fluidic device (Figure 11-22, A, Ps to O_2), the direction of the beam can be changed by hitting the beam with another jet of gas (Figure 11-22, *B*, C_1). The second gas jet usually comes from the side, at a right angle to the main jet stream (Figure 11-22, *B*, C_1 to C_2).

These two principles can be applied to design a host of other devices. These, in turn, are used in the construction of fluidic ventilators. The nomenclature used in fluidics has its origin in digital electronics, which is why many of the terms seem unusual in relation to those for medical terminology. Terms include names such as Flip-Flop component and the OR/NOR gate. More details about fluidics are beyond the scope of this text. (Additional information on fluidic devices can be found on the Evolve website for this text.)

Additional Devices Used During Patient Ventilation

Expiratory Valves for Providing Positive End Expiratory Pressure (PEEP)

Expiratory valves in a ventilator normally close during inspiration, directing gas flow into the patient's lungs, and open during exhalation, allowing the patient to exhale through a valve. Optimally designed expiratory valves allow unrestricted flow from the patient. Older valves often increased resistance to gas flow when expiratory flow was high or when the patient coughed into the ventilator circuit.[15] Newer ventilator systems try to avoid this problem by using very low resistance, large diameter valves.

Besides allowing exhalation to occur naturally with pressures returning to atmospheric, ventilator can also apply positive pressure during exhalation to increase the patient's functional residual capacity. In certain types of patients, this application of positive pressures helps improve oxygenation. This technique is referred to as positive end expiratory pressure or PEEP.

When PEEP is selected, it is the threshold-resistive characteristics of the expiratory valve that provide PEEP. PEEP valves can also be used in the freestanding PEEP/continuous positive airway pressure (CPAP) systems described later in this section. In newer ventilators, the PEEP valve is often located inside the ventilator housing. Older ventilators, such as the Bear 3 and the MA-1, had expiratory valves both external to the ventilator and integrated into the patient circuit (see Figure 11-7, A). Pressure on exhalation is accomplished in one of two ways: **flow resistance** or **threshold resistance.**

Flow resistors direct expiratory flow through an orifice or resistor, such as a screw clamp, and act as expiratory retard

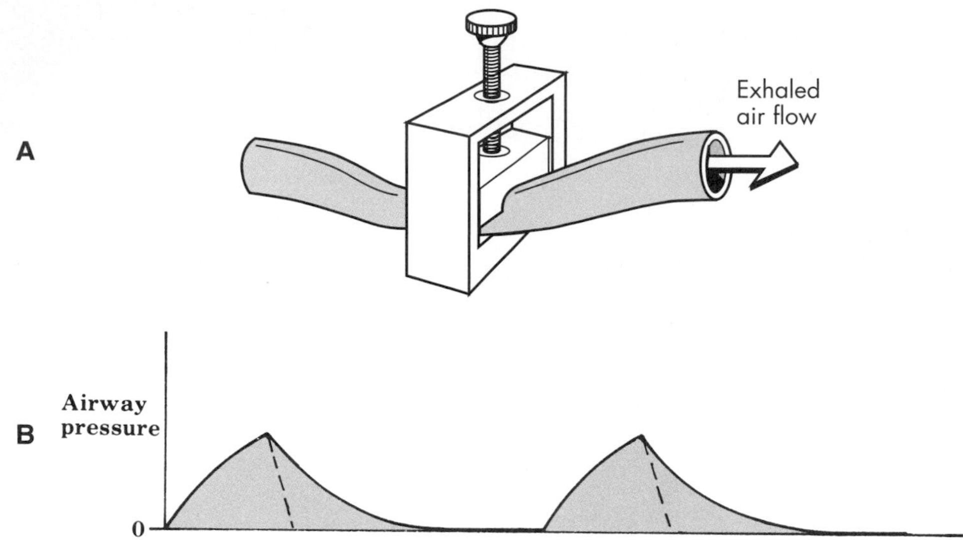

Figure 11-23 **A,** Screw clamp as an example of a flow resistor. **B,** Pressure-time curve for a normal breath with normal exhalation (dashed line) and with expiratory retard (solid line). (From Pilbeam SP: *Mechanical ventilation: physiological and clinical applications*, ed 3, St Louis, 1998, Mosby.)

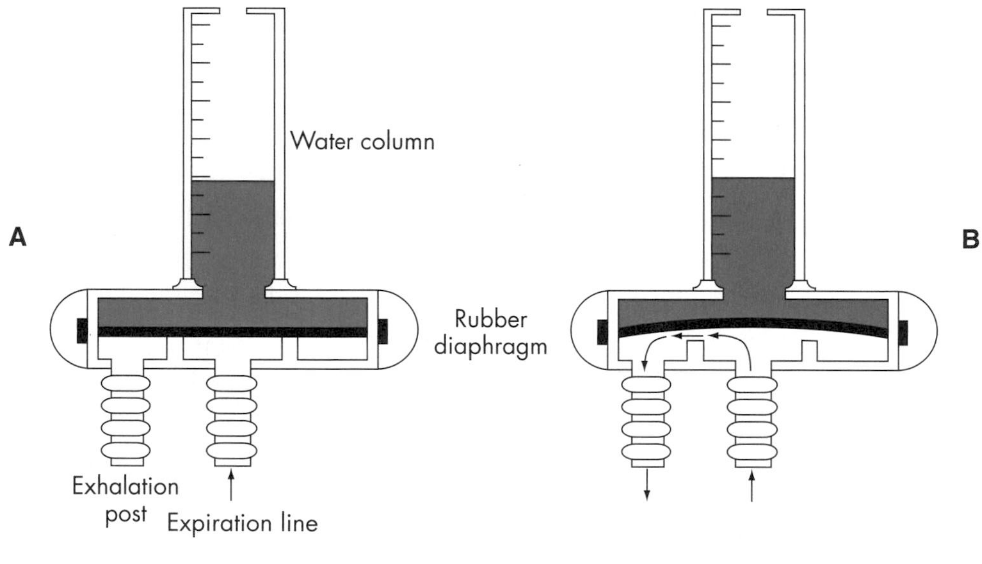

Figure 11-24 A water-weighted diaphragm PEEP valve is an example of a threshold resistor. The exhalation valve has a large diaphragm to reduce any resistance when flow is high. The diaphragm is weighted with water that determines the amount of pressure during exhalation. Although almost a pure threshold resistor, this Emerson water column PEEP valve has slight flow resistance as well. (From Pilbeam SP: *Mechanical ventilation: physiological and clinical applications*, ed 2, St Louis, 1992, Mosby.)

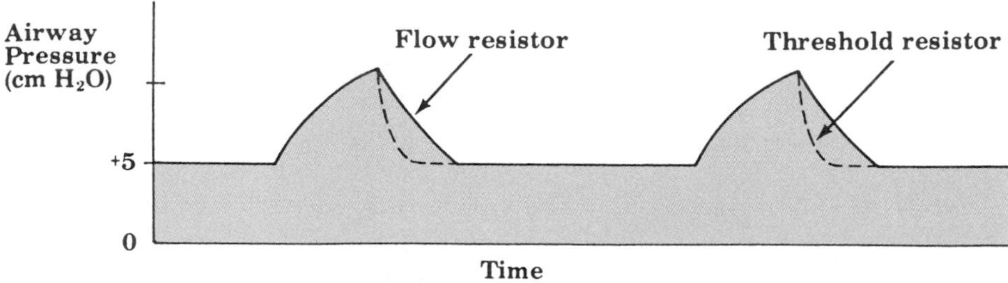

Figure 11-25 This airway pressure curve shows a mandatory breath plus PEEP with two different expiratory flow curves. The solid line illustrates pressure with a flow resistor. Pressure can vary with flow. The dashed line represents a threshold resistor. Flow leaves the lungs rapidly until the set baseline is reached. (From Pilbeam SP: *Mechanical ventilation: physiological and clinical applications*, ed 3, St Louis, 1998, Mosby.)

HISTORICAL NOTE 11-3
Underwater Column PEEP Valves

The underwater column was used during the early development of PEEP. All one had to do was to connect a line to the exhalation valve of a ventilator. By submerging one end of the line into a bucket of water, PEEP would be created. The depth of the line below the water level in centimeters would be the amount of PEEP in cm H_2O (Figure 11-26). The line had to be the same diameter as the main exhalation valve line or increased flow resistance resulted. The problem with this arrangement is that water would often splash onto the floor when the exhaled gas bubbled through the water. Housekeeping was not too happy.

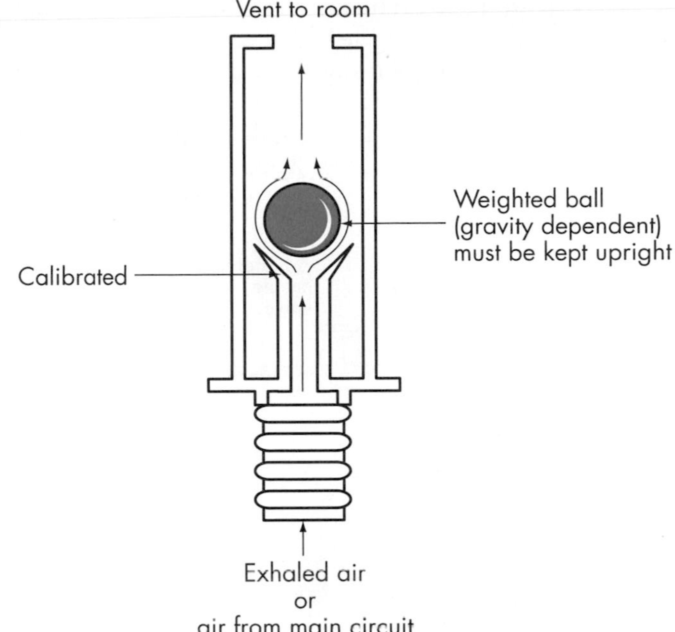

Figure 11-27 A weighted-ball PEEP valve. (From Pilbeam SP: *Mechanical ventilation: physiological and clinical applications*, ed 2, St Louis, 1992, Mosby.)

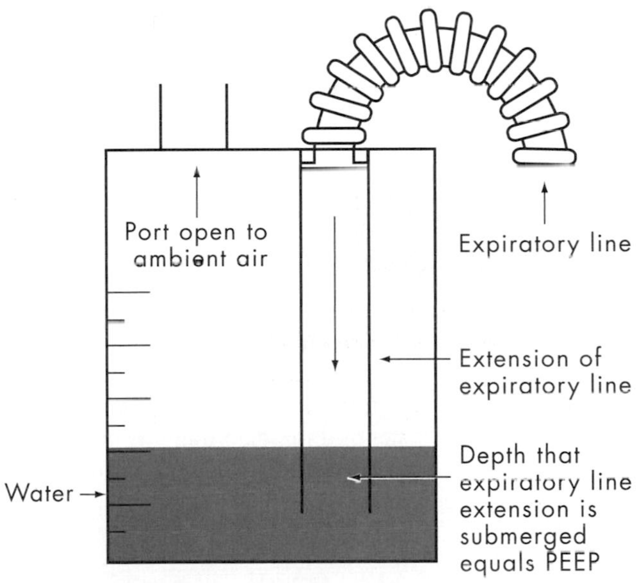

Figure 11-26 An underwater-column PEEP valve. See Historical Note 11-3 for a historic note and explanation on underwater-columns. (From Pilbeam SP: *Mechanical ventilation: physiological and clinical applications*, ed 2, St Louis, 1992, Mosby.)

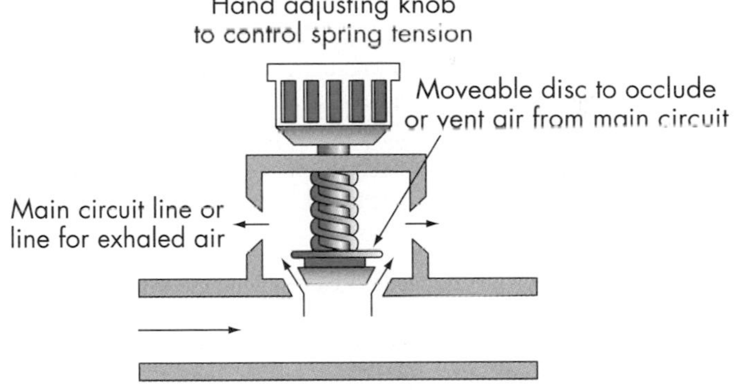

Figure 11-28 A spring-loaded PEEP valve. (From Pilbeam SP: *Mechanical ventilation: physiological and clinical applications*, ed 2, St Louis, 1992, Mosby.)

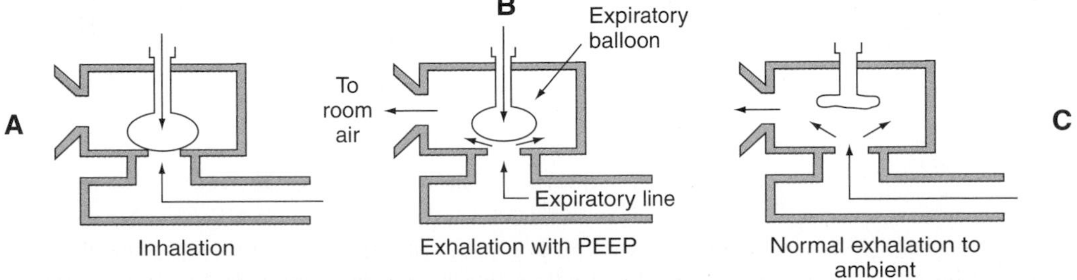

Figure 11-29 Balloon or diaphragm type of expiratory valves for applying PEEP. (See text for description.) (From Pilbeam SP: *Mechanical ventilation: physiological and clinical applications*, ed 2, St Louis, 1992, Mosby.)

devices (Figure 11-23). The higher the rate of gas flow, the higher the pressure generated. If the expiratory period is extended, the baseline pressure can return to zero. One example of the use of flow resistors is a positive expiratory pressure (PEP) mask used for combating atelectasis and aiding secretion removal (see Chapter 7). It is used less commonly in ventilator circuits because the rapid flow from a patient's cough can cause pressure to be very high.

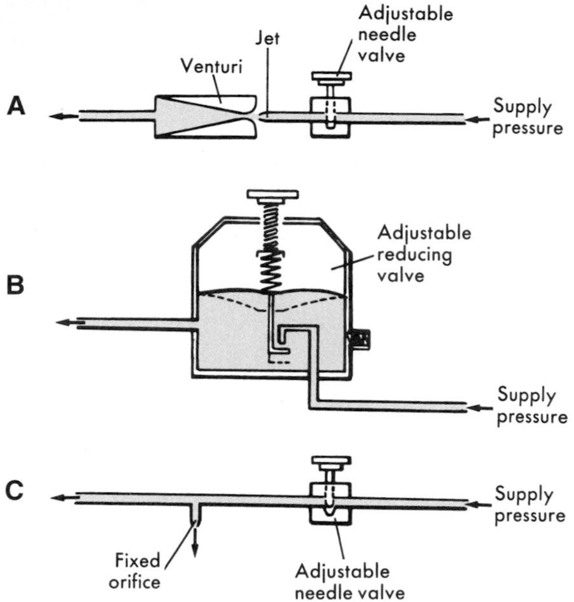

Figure 11-30 Three methods for pressurizing the expiratory line to provide PEEP with balloon or diaphragm expiratory valve devices: **A,** Using a Venturi device to control pressure in the balloon. Opening the needle valve increases pressure. **B,** Using a reducing valve to provide pressure to the balloon. Tightening the spring increases the pressure. **C,** Using a fixed orifice and an adjustable needle valve. As the needle valve is opened, more gas flows from the supply pressure, increasing pressure against the leak of the fixed orifice. This increased pressure is applied to the expiratory line for the balloon and increases PEEP.

Threshold resistors allow expiratory flow to continue unimpeded until the pressure in the circuit equals the threshold value set—that is, the desired PEEP level. A true threshold resistor is unaffected by rate of flow (Figures 11-24 and 11-25). This action is further described below under water-weighted diaphragm. Most newer generation ventilators have PEEP capabilities built into their design and operate through the expiratory valves that are generally located internally. Ventilators such as the MA-1 and the IMV Emerson had PEEP valves located near or built into the expiratory valve, which was located outside the ventilator in the patient circuit.

Threshold expiratory resistor valves are placed into two categories: gravity-dependent and non-gravity-dependent.[16,17] Gravity-dependent resistors include underwater columns (Historical Note 11-3 and Figure 11-26), water-weighted diaphragms (see Figure 11-24), and weighted balls (Figure 11-27). Non-gravity—dependent devices include spring-loaded valves (Figure 11-28), balloon or diaphragm type of expiratory valves (Figure 11-29), opposing gas flow systems (Figure 11-30), and magnetic and electromagnetic PEEP valves (Figures 11-31 and 11-32).[17]

The following two devices (water-weighted diaphragm and weighted ball) are added here as a historical note because they are seldom—if ever—used these days.

Water-Weighted Diaphragm

The J.H. Emerson Co. produces a water-column PEEP device that uses the weight of the water to push on an expiratory diaphragm (see Figure 11-24). During active expiration the pressure in the patient circuit is greater than that exerted by the water and the diaphragm is pushed up, opening the outflow port. When the pressure in the tubing circuit equals the pressure exerted by the water, the diaphragm

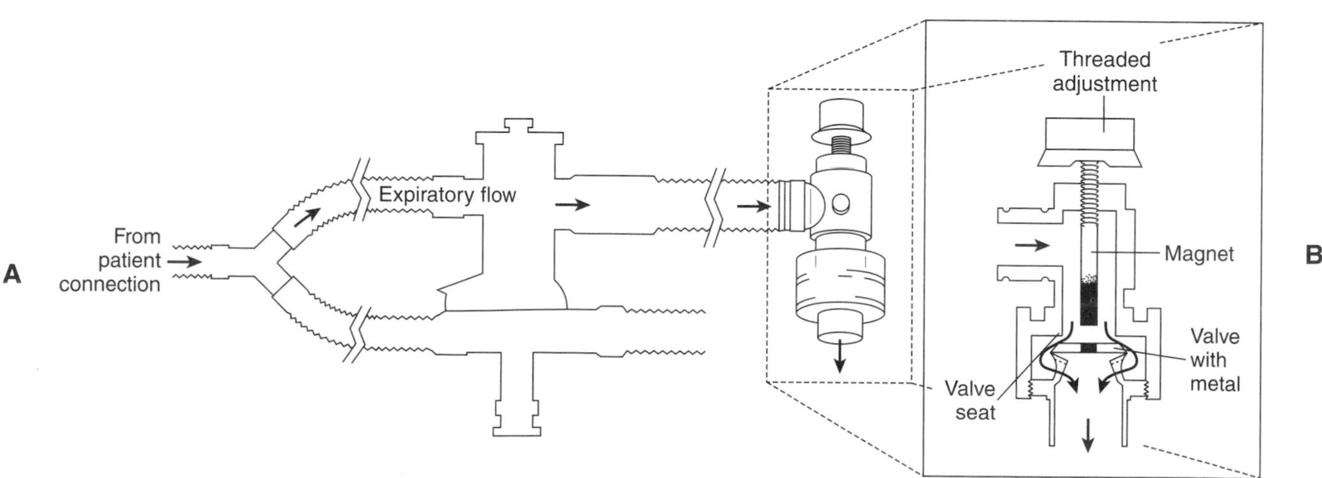

Figure 11-31 A magnetic PEEP valve. **A,** The valve is connected to a typical ventilator circuit with the expiratory valve mounted in-line. Arrows show the direction of expiratory flow. **B,** Detail of the magnetic valve. The threaded adjustment moves the magnet closer to or farther from the metal valve, which increases or decreases, respectively, the magnetic attraction. The greater the attraction, the greater the pressure needed to lift the valve from its seat.

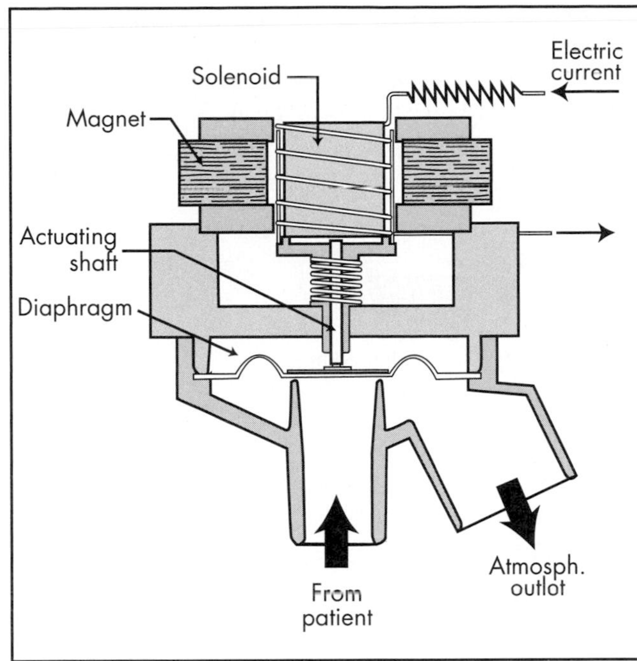

Figure 11-32 The electromagnetic threshold resistor of the Hamilton VEOLAR. (Redrawn from Hamilton Medical Corp, Reno, Nev.)

closes, keeping pressure within the circuit and the patient's airway. The weight of the water above the diaphragm and the surface area of the diaphragm determine the PEEP level (Box 11-6). This device is a true threshold resistor that is not significantly affected by changes in expiratory gas flow until flows exceed approximately 200 L/min.[13]

The Weighted Ball

Figure 11-27 illustrates a weighted-ball threshold resistor. A device containing a weighted valve is connected vertically to the main expiratory line of a patient circuit. The pressure generated varies directly with the weight of the ball. The diameter of the expiratory line and the opening connected to this valve must be equal to or greater than the valve connector to prevent flow resistance, which would affect the PEEP level. An example of this threshold resistor is the Boehringer valve.

Spring-Loaded Valves

A spring-loaded valve may also be used to create PEEP (see Figure 11-28). Changing the spring tension adjusts the amount of pressure needed to move the valve off its seat and allows expiration to occur. When the circuit pressure equals the force applied on the valve by the spring, the valve closes. Some of these devices may have flow-resistor characteristics when expiratory flows are high. Examples include Vital Signs (multiple springs against a disc) and the LTV ventilator.

Box 11-6 Water-Weighted Diaphragm for PEEP Administration

In this device (see Figure 11-24), the calibrations on the column for centimeters of water pressure are not the actual centimeter distance because of the relationship between the surface areas on the water side of the diaphragm and on the diaphragm's seat.

Balloon Valve or Diaphram Type of Expiratory Valves

Balloon valve or diaphragm type expiratory valves commonly incorporate a balloon or diaphragm and are a part of the patient-circuit expiratory valve assembly (see Figures 11-7 and 11-29). During inspiration (see Figure 11-29, A), the expiratory valve line pressurizes the balloon (or diaphragm) and closes the expiratory orifice. During normal expiration (see Figure 11-29, *C*), pressure in the line is released and the patient's expiratory gas flow occurs unimpeded. When PEEP is applied (see Figure 11-29, *B*), a proportional pressure is held within the expiratory tubing, partially inflating the balloon, which provides resistance to expiratory gas flow. When expiratory flow varies, PEEP also varies (flow resistance). Thus these valves have both flow- and threshold-resistor properties. Figure 11-30 illustrates three methods of pressurizing the expiratory line.

Opposing Gas Flow Systems

The output pressure from a venturi can be used to oppose gas flow to a one-way valve. Figure 11-30, A, shows a system in which a venturi applies pressure against a one-way valve (expiratory diaphragm). The valve normally opens, allowing a patient's expiratory gas to flow out. Gas flow from the venturi creates a pressure that opposes opening of the valve resulting in PEEP in the patient circuit. When pressure on the patient circuit side of the valve is greater than the venturi pressure, gases flow through the one-way valve and out the open ports near the venturi jet. When pressure on the patient circuit side is less, the valve closes. Examples of this include the Bourns BP 200 and the Puritan Bennett 7200a.

Magnetic PEEP Valves

Some PEEP valves use magnetic forces to oppose gas pressure (see Figure 11-31). A metallic valve is held on its seat by magnetic attraction supplied by an adjustable magnet. The threaded adjustment moves the magnet closer to or farther from the metal valve, causing an increase or decrease, respectively, in magnetic attraction. The greater the attraction, the greater the pressure needed to push the valve off its seat and allow gas flow from the circuit. If the cross-sectional area of the device is small or restricted, a magnetic PEEP valve can act as a flow resistor.

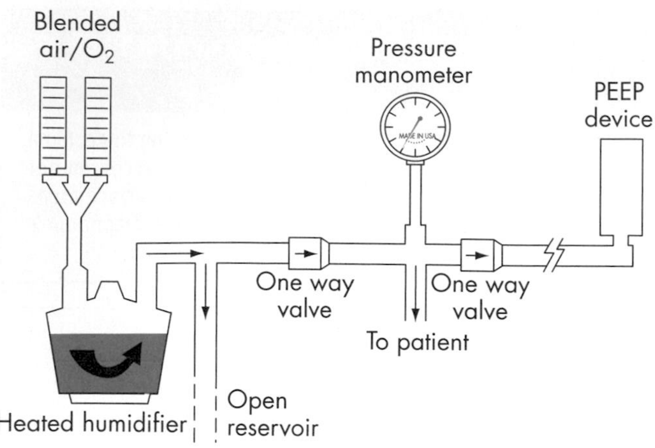

Figure 11-33 Freestanding demand-flow sPEEP (CPAP) circuit (open system). (See text for description.) (From Pilbeam SP: *Mechanical ventilation: physiological and clinical applications*, ed 2, St Louis, 1992, Mosby.)

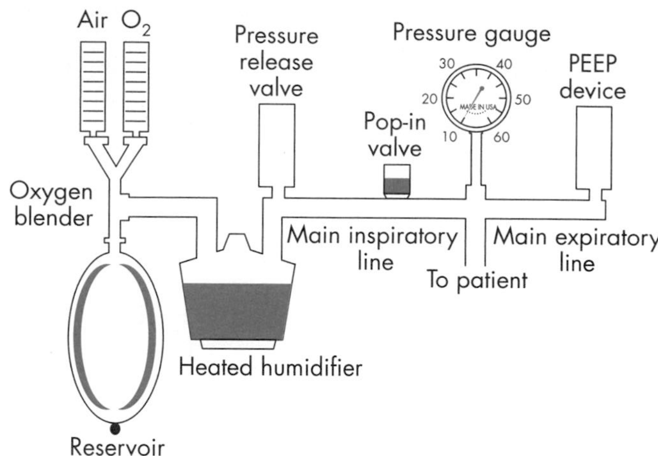

Figure 11-34 Freestanding, continuous-flow CPAP system. (See text for description.) (From Pilbeam SP: *Mechanical ventilation: physiological and clinical applications*, ed 2, St Louis, 1992, Mosby.)

Electromagnetic Valves

Electromagnetic valves often use solenoids in their construction. The operation of solenoids was described earlier (see Figures 11-15 and 11-16). Figure 11-32 shows the electromagnetically activated piston used in the Hamilton VEOLAR, which uses a solenoid. The amount of electric current that flows to a solenoid is regulated by a rheostat. The solenoid creates a downward force through an actuating shaft. The actuating shaft pushes against a diaphragm that opposes expiratory gas flow. The stronger the current, the stronger the downward force and the higher the PEEP level.

Low-resistance threshold resistors are the expiratory valve of choice when ventilating patients. These valves can help reduce expiratory resistance (expiratory work) and reduce the potential for barotrauma.

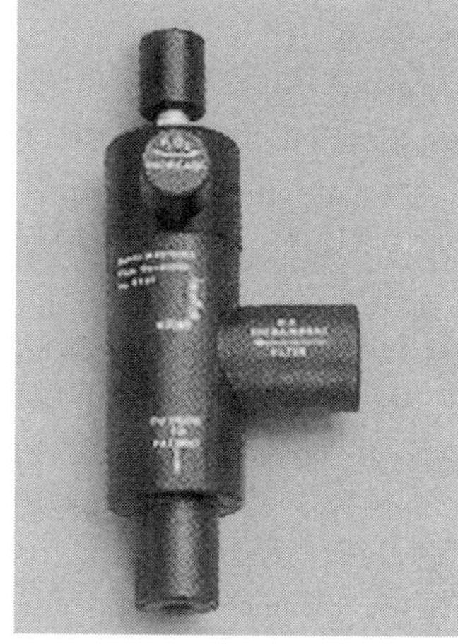

Figure 11-35 Downs CPAP generator. (Courtesy Vital Signs Corp, Totowa, NJ.)

Continuous Positive Airway Pressure (CPAP) Devices

CPAP is very similar to PEEP. CPAP provides positive airway pressure, but it is restricted to spontaneously breathing patients. CPAP devices designed for use in patients' homes for the treatment of sleep apnea are discussed in Chapter 14. Some are used for neonates and are covered in the chapter on infant and pediatric ventilators (Chapter 13). CPAP can also be used for certain types of hospitalized patients who are able to spontaneously breath, but who need help with oxygenation. Examples of illnesses for which CPAP is often indicated include cardiogenic pulmonary edema and hypoxemic respiratory failure. CPAP in this environment can be provided by a ventilator or on its own in a freestanding system.

Freestanding CPAP Systems

Presently, hospitals often use ventilators for this function, but some occasionally use a freestanding CPAP systems. These systems can be constructed to provide CPAP and avoid the use of an expensive ventilator to perform the same task. The disadvantage of using a freestanding system is having to add monitoring and safety systems, which are incorporated in a ventilator. For example, it would be wise to monitor the patient with a pulse oximeter for heart rate and oxygen saturation.

Freestanding CPAP systems can be either demand- or continuous-flow devices. Figure 11-33 provides an example of a demand-flow CPAP (spontaneous PEEP [sPEEP]) system. It is called *sPEEP* in this situation because positive pressure is only applied during exhalation—not during inhalation. The patient must open a one-way valve to receive gas flow from a warmed, humidified, blended gas (air/oxygen) source. The patient must drop circuit pressures from the set CPAP level to ambient to open the valve and receive flow.

In a continuous-flow CPAP system, blended gas passes into a reservoir that can be pressurized to equal the desired positive pressure. The blended gas can come from air and

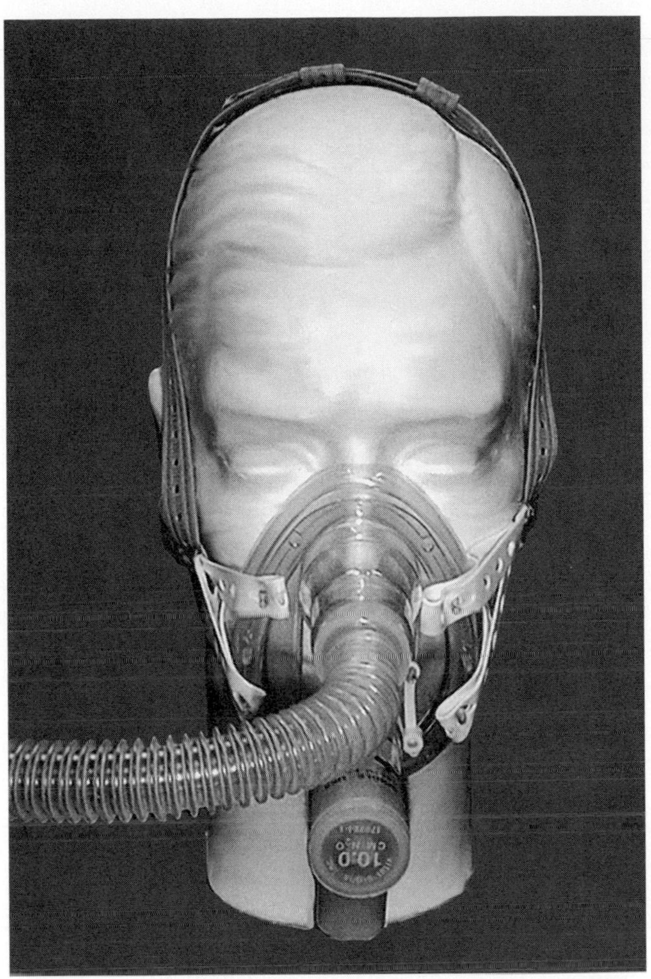

Figure 11-36 Patient with a CPAP mask connected to the Downs CPAP generator. (Courtesy Vital Signs Corp, Totowa, NJ.)

CLINICAL ROUNDS 11-2

Troubleshooting Freestanding CPAP Systems

Problem 1

A patient attached to a freestanding, continuous-flow CPAP system set at 10 cm H_2O appears to be in distress (e.g., supraclavicular retractions, accessory muscle use, pale and diaphoretic). The operator notices that the manometer drops to –1 cm H_2O during inspiration and rises to 10 cm H_2O during expiration. What do you think is the problem?

Problem 2

The low oxygen saturation alarm is sounding on a patient connected to a freestanding, continuous-flow CPAP system. The operator notices that the manometer fluctuates around the zero point during both inspiration and expiration. What is the problem?

See Appendix A for the answer.

oxygen flowmeters, from a blender, or from a CPAP generator. The gas is then warmed and humidified. A threshold resistor is attached to the expiratory end of the system (Figure 11-34), and a manometer is used to monitor circuit pressure. A safety pressure-release valve is incorporated into a CPAP system. Its threshold resistance equals the desired CPAP level plus 5 cm H_2O. For example, if the CPAP is 10 cm H_2O, the safety pressure release is 15 cm H_2O. If the normal threshold resistor jams, preventing gas flow from exiting the system, the valve can act as a pop-off valve. Adding a safety pop-in valve is also important in case the source gas is accidentally turned off so that a source of ambient air for the patient is available. Some institutions add a one-way valve in the main expiratory line to keep gas flowing in one direction, which can be important in patients with high-flow demands who may begin to rebreathe some of their own exhaled air.

As mentioned previously, one possible gas source for a freestanding CPAP system is a CPAP generator. Figure 11-35 shows an example of a Downs CPAP generator that connects to a high-pressure gas source and then attaches via large-bore tubing to a CPAP mask. The mask has a CPAP valve attached to its face. Most valves are spring-loaded with fixed pressures (e.g., 5 cm H_2O, 7.5 cm H_2O), but others can be adjusted by tightening the spring (Figure 11-36).

A variety of problems can occur with a freestanding CPAP system, so the operator must be sure that the safety systems (i.e., pop-off and pop-in valves) are in place and the patient is monitored. Some examples of problems follow: (1) inadequate flow to the patient; (2) leaks in the system; (3) loss of source gas flow; and (4) jamming or obstruction of the expiratory threshold resistor (Clinical Rounds 11-2).

Part II: Basic Components of Breath Delivery

For a ventilator to accomplish breath delivery, it must be able to provide the four basic phases of a breath and assume all or part of the patient's work of breathing. The four phases, which are controlled by **phase variables,** are listed in Box 11-7. The following sections discuss these concepts in more detail.

Model Description of Shared Work of Breathing

Two forces are available to perform work of breathing: the patient's muscles and the ventilator. The ventilator must also be adjustable so the operator can balance the work between these two components. This balance is best described by the equation of motion (Box 11-8) and is shown in Figure 11-37. For a single breath, the compliance and resistance of the respiratory system do not change significantly, but the volume, pressure, flow, and time can vary and are regulated by the ventilator.[2,18]

Box 11-7 The Four Phases of a Breath During Mechanical Ventilation and Their Phase Variables

Breath Phases

1. End of expiration and beginning of inspiration
2. Delivery of inspiration
3. End of inspiration and beginning of expiration
4. Expiratory phase

The Phase Variables

Phase variables are controlled by the ventilator and are responsible for each of the four parts of a breath.

Triggering: begins inspiratory gas flow

Limiting: places a maximum value on a control variable (pressure, volume, flow, or time) during delivery of a breath

Cycling: ends inspiratory gas flow

Box 11-8 Equation of Motion

There are two pressures to move gas into the lung, the pressure needed to move gas through the airway (flow resistance pressure) and the pressure to expand the lung (elastic recoil pressure). These two pressures are provided by the respiratory muscles (muscle pressure) or by a ventilator (ventilator pressure).

Equation 1:

Muscle Pressure + Ventilator Pressure = Elastic Recoil Pressure + Flow Resistance Pressure

Or, using an abbreviated form,

Equation 2:

$Pmus + P_{TR} = V/C + (Raw \times flow)$

Where:

Pmus is the pressure generated by the muscles of ventilation (i.e., muscle pressure).

If these muscles are not active, Pmus equals zero.

P_{TR} is the transrespiratory pressure (Pawo − Pbs)

In other words, the airway opening pressure, Pawo, minus the body surface pressure, Pbs. Basically P_{TR} is the pressure read on the ventilator gauge during inspiration with intermittent positive-pressure ventilation (ventilator pressure).

V is volume delivered.

C is respiratory system compliance.

V/C is elastic recoil pressure.

Raw is respiratory system resistance.

Flow is the gas flow during inspiration (i.e., Raw × flow, flow resistance).

Because P_{TA} = Raw × flow, and alveolar pressure (P_A) = V/C,

the following substitutions can be made in the equation above:

$Pmus + P_{TR} = P_A + P_{TA}$

From Pilbeam SP: *Mechanical ventilation: physiological and clinical applications,* St Louis, ed 3, 1998, Mosby.

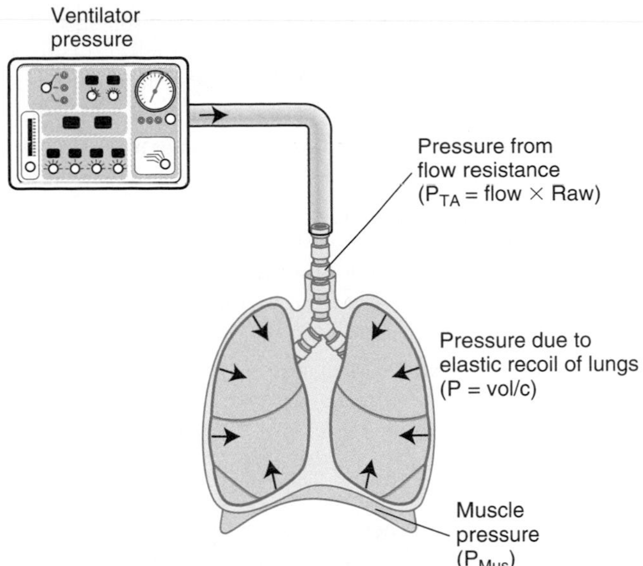

Figure 11-37 Model of the equation of motion: Muscle Pressure + Ventilator Pressure = Elastic Recoil Pressure + Flow Resistance Pressure. (See text for description.)

Box 11-9 Chatburn and Primiano–A New Classification System: Assisted Breath[6]

An assisted breath, that is a mechanically assisted breath is a breath "during which all or part of inspiratory or expiratory flow is generated by a change in transrespiratory pressure (i.e., airway pressure [Paw] minus body surface pressure [Pbs]; Paw–Pbs) due to an external agent (e.g., manual or mechanical ventilator)."

Type of Breath Delivery

As mentioned previously, work of breathing can be provided by the ventilator and by the patient, so more than one type of breath delivery is possible. If the ventilator does all the work of breathing (i.e., starts the breath, controls inspiratory gas delivery, and ends inspiration), the breath is called a **mandatory breath. Assisted breaths,** on the other hand, are those in which inspiration is begun by the patient, but the ventilator controls the inspiratory phase and ends inspiration and may assist exhalation as well. Box 11-9 provides Chatburn and Primiano's new definition of an assisted breath.[6] **Spontaneous breaths** are those which the patient controls transition from inspiration to exhalation.

Another important aspect of breath delivery is whether the operator wishes to control the volume or the pressure delivered to the patient. **Volume-targeted ventilation** is also called volume ventilation and volume-limited ventilation. It involves setting a desired tidal volume. **Pressure-targeted ventilation** is sometimes called *pressure ventilation (PV)* or *pressure-limited ventilation* and refers to setting a desired pressure (Box 11-10). Confusion results from many names having the same meaning.

Box 11-10 Other Names for Volume and Pressure Ventilation

Volume Ventilation
Volume-limited ventilation
Volume-controlled ventilation
Volume-targeted ventilation

Pressure Ventilation
Pressure-limited ventilation
Pressure-controlled ventilation
Pressure-targeted ventilation

Phases of a Breath

When the term *breath* is used, it is usually used for inspiration, but a breath really consists of a total respiratory cycle; that is, the time required for both inspiration (T_I) and expiration (T_E) and the events that occur during that time. This time frame is also called the total cycle time (TCT). A ventilator must be capable of separating a breath into the following four parts (see Box 11-9):

1. The **trigger variable** begins inspiration.
2. Breath delivery (inspiration) is accomplished when the settings on the ventilator front panel establishes what will be controlled: pressure, flow, volume, or time. These four are also called **control variables.**
3. The **cycle variable** ends the inspiratory phase and begins exhalation.
4. Pressures and flows can be controlled during exhalation, thus the ventilator can be involved in the expiratory phase.

Beginning of Inspiration: The Triggering Variable

The trigger variable begins the inspiratory phase. Ventilator breaths can be time-, pressure-, flow-, or volume-triggered. For example, when the trigger variable is time, the ventilator controls the beginning of inspiration based on the set rate. For example, if you set a rate of 12 breaths/min, a breath will occur every 5 seconds. Inspiratory flow starts 5 seconds after the last inspiration, thus providing **time triggering.** When pressure, flow, or volume begins the breath, the patient controls the beginning of inspiration. This is called **patient triggering.**

The triggering variable must not be confused with the cycling variable. Triggering begins inspiration; cycling, discussed later, ends inspiration. The purpose for mentioning this difference is that the term cycle previously meant the variable that began the breath, although some journal articles and technical manuals still occasionally use this terminology.

Time Triggering

As noted, with time triggering, the ventilator controls the beginning of inspiration based on the set rate. Time-triggered breathing is sometimes called **control ventilation.** The breath is mandatory.

Patient Triggering

Ventilators can be adjusted to sense patient inspiratory effort. The control set by the operator is commonly called the sensitivity setting, or **trigger sensitivity.** Pressure and flow are the most common variables used for patient triggering. **Pressure triggering** occurs when the ventilator senses a drop in pressure below baseline in the circuit. Pressure triggering is usually set from –0.5 to –2.0 cm H_2O. In other words, the pressure must drop by this amount below baseline to begin inspiration (Figure 11-38). **Baseline pressure** is the pressure maintained at the airway during exhalation and the pressure from which inspiration begins. (See the discussion of the expiratory phase later in this section.)

Pressure is generally measured in three different locations on ventilators because pressure transducers or sensors can be placed at three common locations:

1. within the internal ventilator circuit near the point where the main gas flow leaves the unit,
2. where expired gas enters the unit, or
3. at the proximal airway (near the **Y connector**).

In the latter case, a small-bore plastic tubing extends from the front of the ventilator to the patient's **Y** connector (Clinical Rounds 11-3). (See Chapter 8 for further information on pressure monitoring devices.)

Flow triggering occurs when a drop in flow is detected. In some ventilators a pneumotachograph (Chapter 8) is situation between the ventilator circuit and the patient to measure flow. In others, a background flow, also called a **base** or **bias** flow, is set by the operator. This flow is present during the expiratory phase. It is normally set from approximately 5 to 10 L/min. A flow trigger is also set and can range from about 1 to 5 L/min, although this value varies with the type of ventilator used, the patient's size (baby vs. adult), and inspiratory effort. Most ventilator manufacturers recommend a value.

The ventilator measures the base flow during exhalation. When the flow drops by the amount set on the flow trigger, inspiration begins. For example, if the base flow is set at 7 L/min and the trigger is set at 3 L/min, the ventilator will begin inspiration when the expiratory flow is measured at 4 L/min (7 L/min – 3 L/min = 4 L/min). Figures 11-39 and 11-40 show flow trigger graphics and a flow-triggering device. Clinical Rounds 11-4 presents a practice problem on flow triggering.

Volume triggering occurs after a specific volume has been inhaled by the patient from the circuit. This type of triggering is currently used on the Venturi ventilator. By adjusting the trigger sensitivity from 1 mL to 250 mL, the operator can change the effort required by the patient to begin inspiration. Just to give an example of how sensitive this can be, a tuberculin syringe has a volume of 1 mL. The operator can adjust the Venturi's sensitivity so that only 1 mL must be inhaled from the circuit to start inspiration. Volume triggering is also used in some infant ventilators (see Chapter 13).

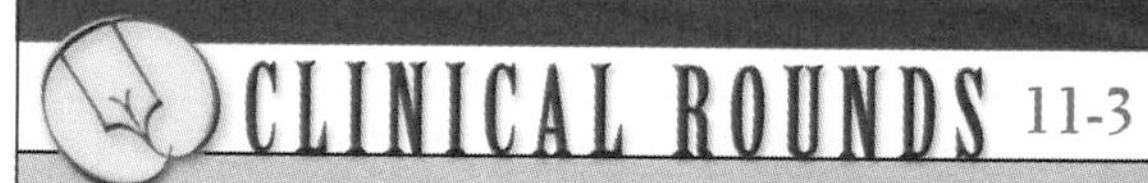

A patient has a baseline pressure of 10 cm H_2O during mechanical ventilation. The trigger sensitivity is set at –1 cm H_2O. At what pressure will the ventilator sense a patient effort and start inspiration?

See Appendix A for the answer.

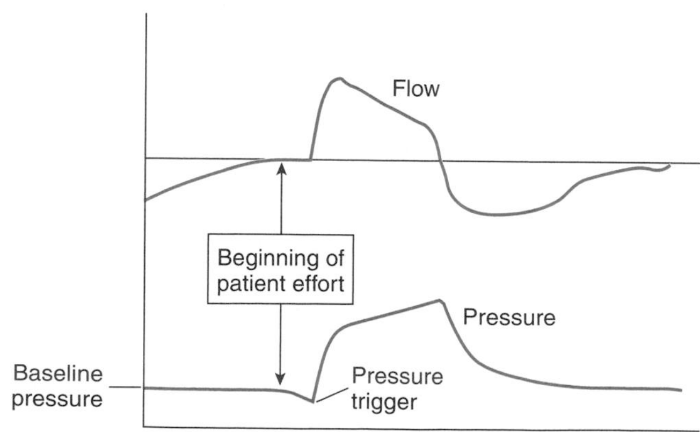

Figure 11-38 A pressure triggered breath. When the pressure drops to the trigger level, the inspiratory flow begins. (From Hess DR, MacIntyre NR: *Respiratory care: principles and practices*, Philadelphia, 2002, WB Saunders.)

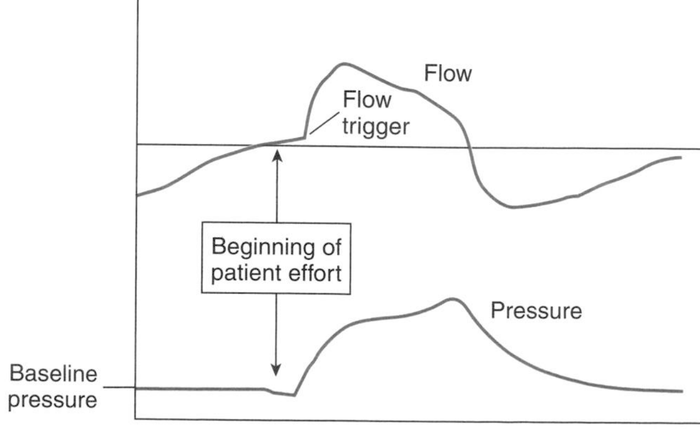

Figure 11-39 Flow triggered breath. When the flow reaches the set flow-trigger level, inspiratory flow begins. (From Hess DR, MacIntyre NR: *Respiratory care: principles and practices*, Philadelphia, 2002, WB Saunders.)

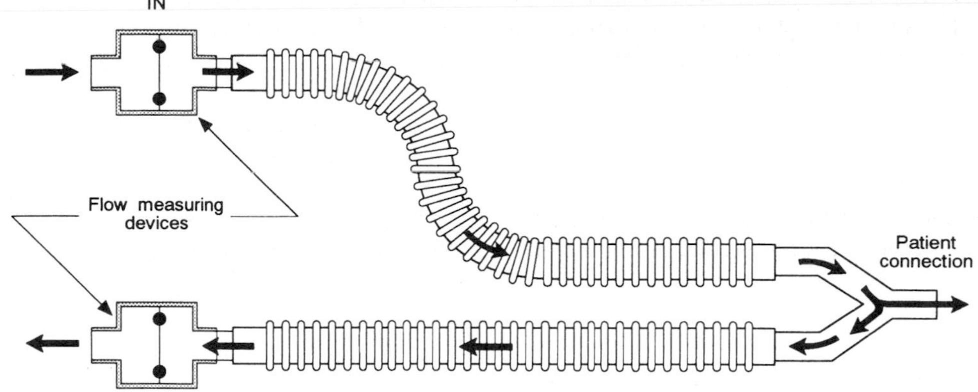

Figure 11-40 Schematic representation of flow triggering, which occurs when the patient makes an inspiratory effort and drops the flow through the patient circuit to the trigger level. (From Dupuis Y: *Ventilators*, ed 2, St Louis, 1992, Mosby.)

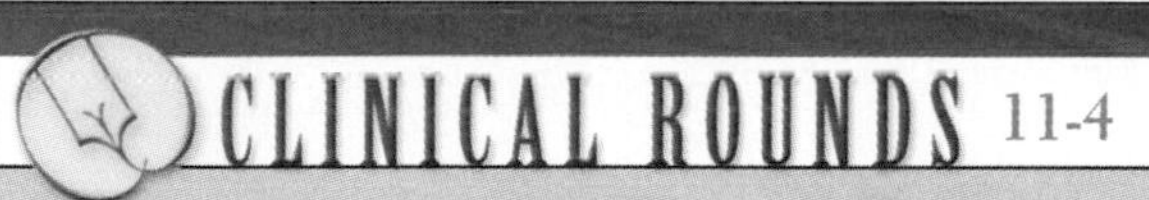

The operator decides to use flow triggering for a patient and sets the base flow at 6 L/min and the trigger flow at 2 L/min. The base flow measurement must drop to what value before the ventilator will begin the inspiratory phase?

See Appendix A for the answer.

HISTORICAL NOTE 11-4
Classification[1,7]

Classification was Previously Based on the Power Source

For example, the IMV Emerson ventilator was described as a high-pressure drive ventilator. A powerful electric motor was used to drive its rotary piston. Regardless of changes in patient lung characteristics, the ventilator could deliver the set volume, although pressure would increase as the work load increased.

Classification was also Based on the Flow Waveform Produced

For example, the IMV Emerson was also referred to as a non—constant-flow generator because the flow produced was not constant (in this case, it was sine-wavelike) and produced the same sine pattern breath after breath, regardless of changes in patient lung characteristics.

Other methods of triggering include the following.

1. Manual triggering in which the operator activates the "manual breath" control and delivers a mandatory breath based on the set variables.
2. Triggering from chest wall movement as is available in the Star Sync module on the Infant Star ventilator (see Chapter 13).

The Inspiratory Phase

One of the most important ventilator functions is delivery of inspiratory gas flow. The first positive-pressure volume ventilators were often classified by how strong the force was behind inspiratory delivery and by the evaluation of the pressure, flow, and volume curves produced during inspiration (Historical Note 11-4). Many current ICU ventilators, such as the Viasys Avea, the Bear 1000, and the Newport e500, can actually alter their function enabling different inspiratory flow patterns to be selected by the operator. A ventilator can now be instructed to produce specific waveform patterns for pressure, volume, flow, or time.

The two most commonly controlled variables during inspiration are volume and pressure, as mentioned previously. The type of breath being delivered is defined or identified by the waveforms produced for pressure, volume, flow, and time.

A Volume-Targeted Breath (Volume-Controlled, Volume-Limited)

When the volume waveform is maintained in a specific pattern, the delivered breath is a volume breath. The volume waveform remains constant, but the pressure waveform varies with changes in the patient lung characteristics (i.e., lung compliance and airway resistance). Ventilators capable of measuring flow and time during inspiration can use these variables to calculate volume.

Note that any ventilator with a set volume waveform has a set flow waveform (flow = volume/time). So, a volume

> **Box 11-11 A Flow-Controlled Breath**
>
> Any breath having a set flow waveform that does not change from one breath to the next—regardless of changes in lung characteristics—is a flow-controlled breath. If flow is controlled, the volume is also controlled. Thus the breath is also a volume-controlled breath.

breath is one in which flow is also controlled (i.e., a flow-controlled breath) (Box 11-11).*

A Pressure-Targeted Breath (Pressure-Controlled, Pressure-Limited)

When the pressure waveform has a specific pattern that is not affected by changes in lung characteristics, but where volume and flow vary, then the breath is a pressure-targeted breath or a pressure-controlled breath.[19,20]

A Time-Controlled Breath

When a ventilator delivers a time-controlled breath, pressure, volume, and flow may vary with changes in lung characteristics. Time is constant. Examples of timed breaths are those produced during **high-frequency jet ventilation** and **high-frequency oscillation.** Time-controlled ventilation is less commonly used than pressure or volume ventilation.

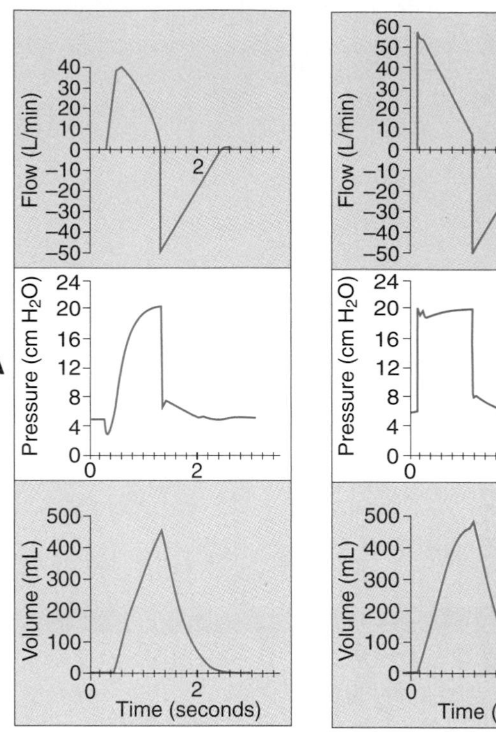

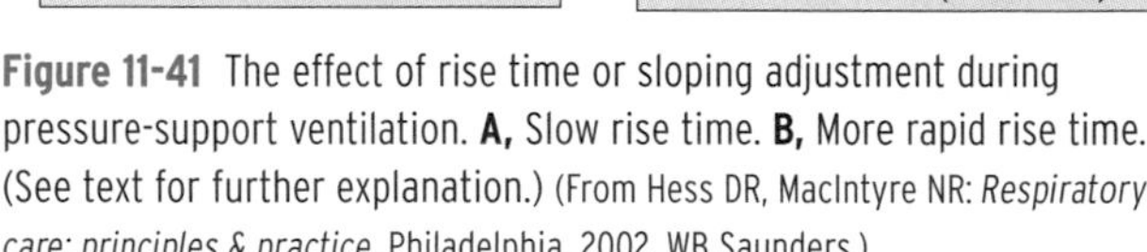

Figure 11-41 The effect of rise time or sloping adjustment during pressure-support ventilation. **A,** Slow rise time. **B,** More rapid rise time. (See text for further explanation.) (From Hess DR, MacIntyre NR: *Respiratory care: principles & practice,* Philadelphia, 2002, WB Saunders.)

Initial Operator Selection of Ventilator Parameters

The operator may consider the following selections when choosing a ventilator for patient use:

1. The type of pressure delivery (positive- or negative-pressure ventilation).
2. The type of control variable (pressure-, volume-, flow-, or time-controlled).
3. The type of triggering (time or patient), which determines if the breath is mandatory, assisted, or spontaneous.
4. The type of flow or pressure waveform. The two most common flow waveforms used for volume ventilation are the constant (rectangular) and the descending ramp (decelerating ramp) waveforms. The two most commonly occurring pressure waveforms are the constant and the ascending exponential waveform.[19,20]

NOTE: During volume-targeted ventilation, some ventilators will not respond to a patient's inspiratory demand and flow waveforms remain constant regardless of the flow the patient desires. A few ventilators are changing. For example, the Servo 300 will give the patient more flow during volume ventilation if the patient's effort is adequate (Chapter 12, Servo 300).

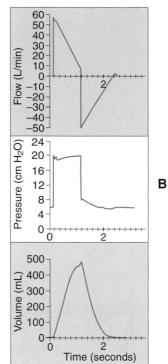

5. The type of interface with the patient, a mask for noninvasive ventilator or an endotracheal tube for invasive ventilation. (Noninvasive ventilation of adults is reviewed in Chapter 14; for children, see Chapter 13.
6. In newer ventilators the operator can select a parameter called **sloping** or **rise time.** This setting is most commonly available in pressure-targeted ventilation. Historically, in pressure ventilation the ventilator was designed to begin inspiration and achieve the set pressure as quickly as possible. Thus the gas flow rapidly rose and hit against the airway. This situation can actually cause an abrupt rise in the pressure, creating discomfort for the patient. By setting a slope or rise time adjustment, the clinician prevents the patient from receiving the set pressure immediately. Instead, the pressure gradually rises to the set level (Figure 11-41).[20]

Waveforms and Graphics

Monitoring and evaluating graphic waveforms produced during ventilation has become a popular method to determine how patients are being ventilated and whether or

**In this text, the terms volume-targeted or volume-controlled also mean flow-controlled or flow-limited.*

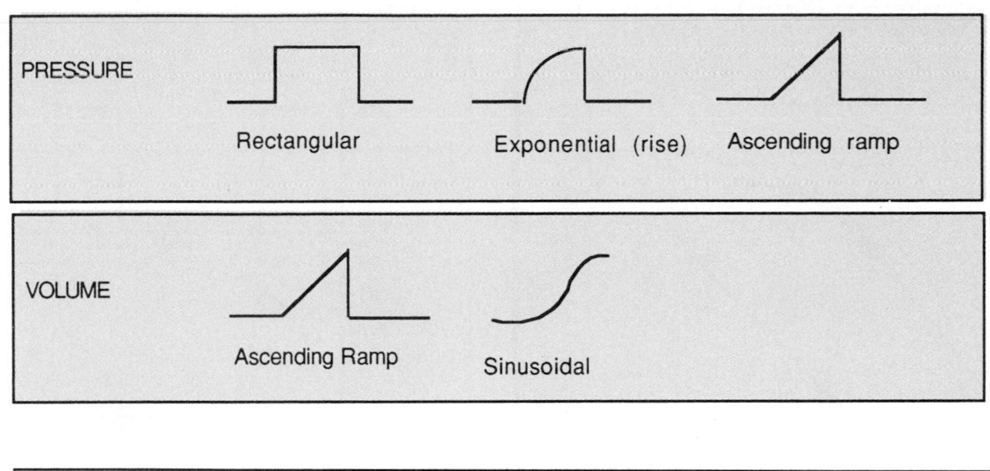

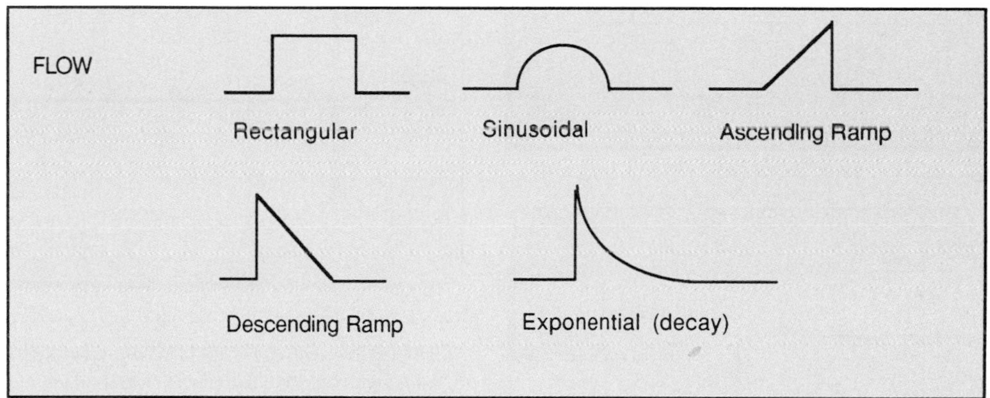

Figure 11-42 Examples of curves for pressure, volume, and flow. Pressure curves are usually constant, rising exponential, or ascending ramps. Volume curves are usually ascending ramp or sinusoidal (sine-wave-like). Flow curves are commonly rectangular (constant), sine, ramp (ascending or descending), and decaying exponential. (From Pilbeam SP: *Mechanical ventilation: physiological and clinical applications*, ed 3, St Louis, 1998, Mosby.)

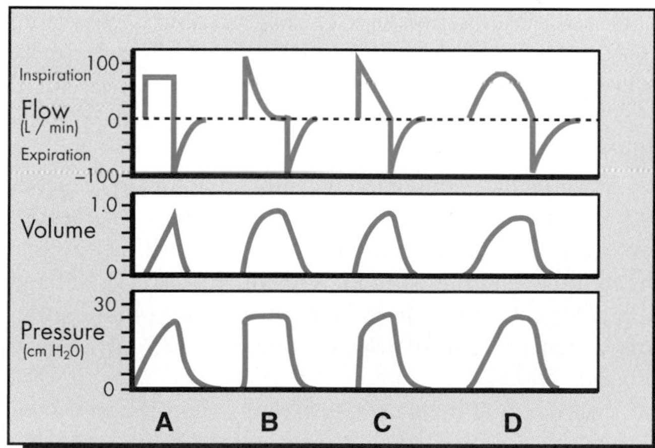

Figure 11-43 Characteristic waveforms for pressure, volume, and flow in the following forms of ventilation: **A,** volume breath with constant flow; **B,** pressure breath (pressure-controlled) with a constant pressure delivery, a long T_I time (flow returns to zero), and time-cycling; **C,** volume breath with a descending ramp flow pattern; and **D,** volume breath using a sine-like flow pattern. (From Pilbeam SP: *Mechanical ventilation: physiological and clinical applications*, ed 3, St Louis, 1998, Mosby.)

not problems are occurring during ventilation. Although more detailed descriptions of waveform use are available elsewhere,[7] a summary of the more common waveforms produced during ventilation is provided here.

Pressure, volume, and flow graphed over time are also called **scalars** (i.e., pressure-time, volume-time, and flow-time).[21] Six basic waveforms are produced for pressure, volume, and flow over time during ventilation (Figure 11-42). Figure 11-43 shows examples of the pressure, volume, and flow waveforms produced with several methods of pressure and volume ventilation. Another type of graphic is called a **loop.** A loop is a display of two variables plotted on the x (horizontal) and y (vertical) axes. Pressure-volume (Figure 11-44, *A*) and flow-volume loops (*B*) are the two most frequently used.

Remember that during pressure ventilation the delivered set pressure pattern stays the same, regardless of changes in the patient's lung condition, but volume and flow delivery vary (Figure 11-45). During volume ventilation, the selected volume and flow wave patterns stay the same, but the pressure varies (Figure 11-46).

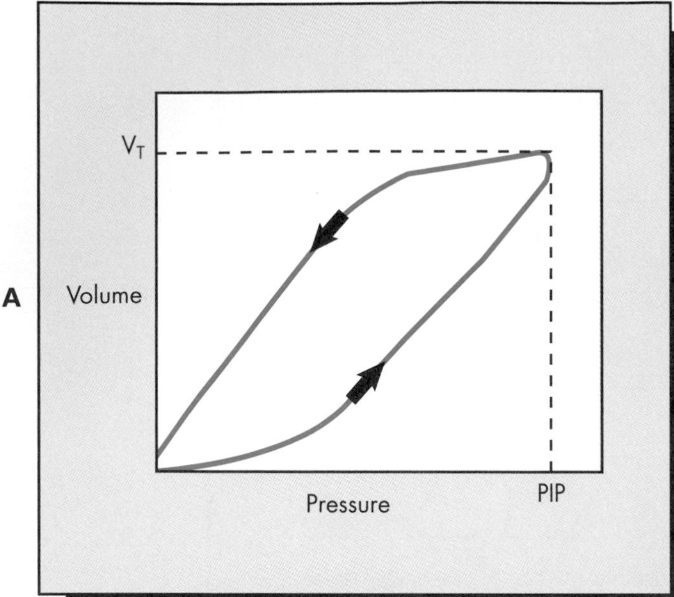

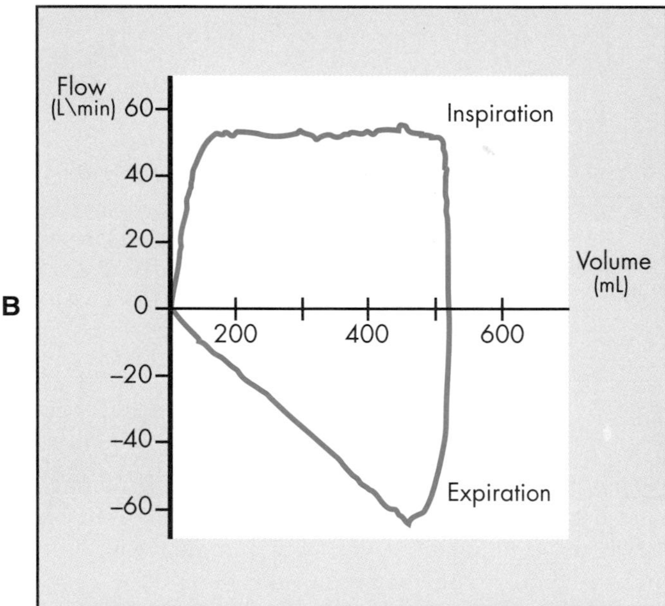

Figure 11-44 **A,** Typical pressure-volume curve for a positive-pressure breath. The highest points for tidal volume (V_T, vertical axis) and peak inspiratory pressure (PIP, horizontal axis) represent the dynamic compliance for the pressure-volume relationship. **B,** Normal flow-volume loop during volume ventilation. The inspiratory curve is on the top; the expiratory curve is on the bottom. Note the linear change in expiratory flow from peak to end-expiration. Note also that end-expiratory flow is zero. (From Pilbeam SP: *Mechanical ventilation: physiological and clinical applications*, ed 3, St Louis, 1998, Mosby.)

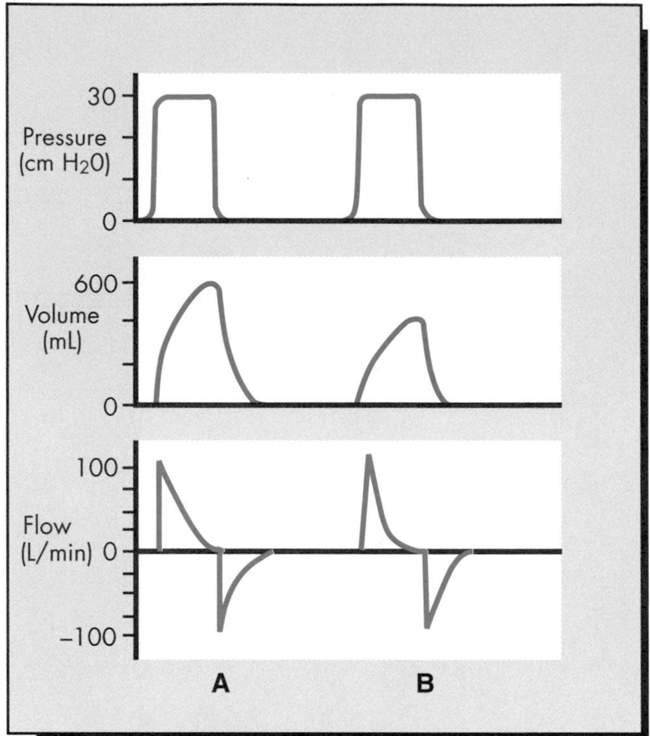

Figure 11-45 An example of patient's lungs getting worse with pressure targeted ventilation: **A,** normal pressure, volume, and flow curves; **B,** curves with reduced lung compliance, showing reduced volume delivery.

Limiting Factors During Inspiration

As reviewed previously, the ventilator controls one of the four control variables during inspiration and can also limit the remaining variables. A limiting variable has a maximum value that cannot be exceeded during inspiration because the ventilator will not allow it; however, reaching its limit does not end inspiratory flow. For example, in a bag-in-a-box ventilator, the volume is limited to the gas volume within the bag. It cannot exceed that volume; however, delivering the volume does not necessarily end the breath. The ventilator may continue to hold the bag in a collapsed state for a brief period after the bag is empty. This would add a brief period of time following breath delivery in which the ventilator pauses before beginning exhalation. In this example, inspiration is time-cycling and volume-limited.

A ventilator is considered flow-limited if the flow reaches a maximum value before the end of inspiration but does not exceed that value. For example, if the forward motion of a linear drive piston is constant, then the flow is constant and limited to the rate of forward motion and the volume within the piston housing (flow = volume ÷ time; see Clinical Rounds 11-5).

Pressure limiting sets a maximum value for pressure, which is not exceeded during inspiration. After the pressure is reached, inspiration may continue, but no more pressure (and thus no more volume) is delivered to the patient (Figure 11-47). Excess pressure is vented through a pressure-release mechanism. Some ventilators have pressure-limited capabilities and use a mode called time-cycled pressure limited ventilation (see Chapter 12, Viasys Avea ventilator).

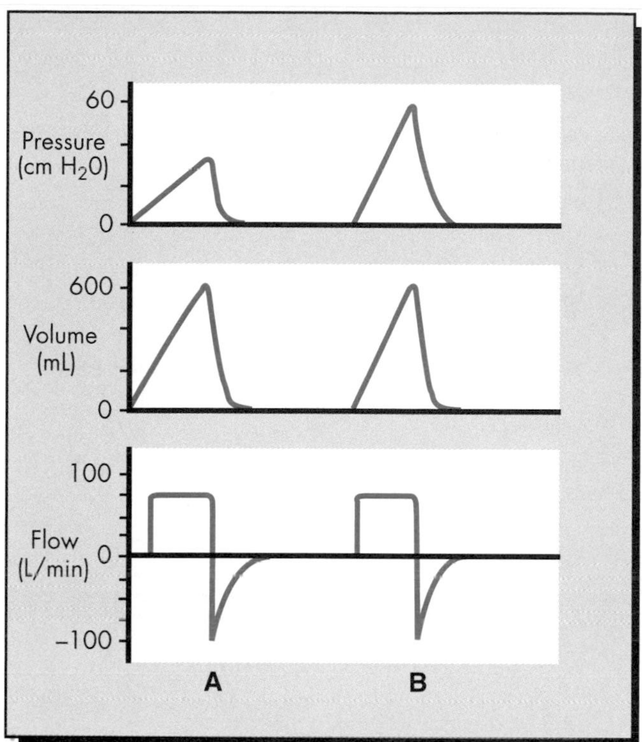

Figure 11-46 An example of patient's lung getting worse with volume targeted ventilation: **A,** normal pressure, volume, and flow curves; **B,** curves with reduced lung compliance, showing increased pressure delivery. Volume and flow waveforms remain constant.

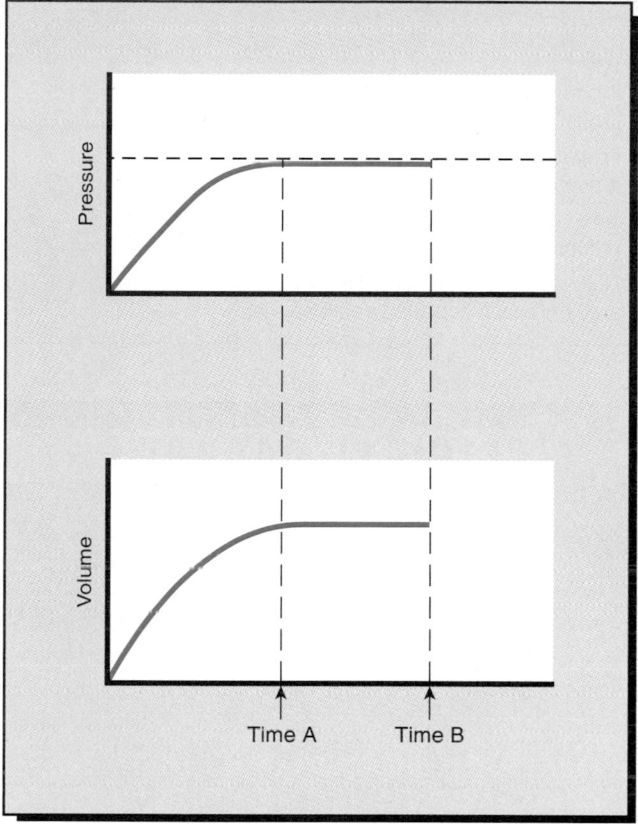

Figure 11-47 The pressure-time and volume-time waveforms illustrate a time-cycled, pressure-limited breath. The pressure peaks and the volume is delivered by time *A*. The pressure reaches the set limit and stays constant. No more volume enters the patient's lungs after time *A*. Between *A* and *B* excess pressure is vented. Inspiration ends at time *B* (time-cycled).

CLINICAL ROUNDS 11-5

Before inspiration the pressure drops to −1 cm H_2O on the pressure manometer and then inspiratory flow begins. During inspiration the pressure rises to 20 cm H_2O in 0.5 second and then stays at 20 cm H_2O for 0.5 more second. Then, expiration begins. What are the trigger, limit, and cycle variables?

See Appendix A for the answer.

Box 11-12 Common Names for Maximum Safety Pressure Control

- Pressure limit
- Upper pressure limit
- Normal pressure limit
- High pressure limit
- Peak/maximum pressure

Maximum Safety Pressure

All ventilators come with some type of feature that allows inspiratory pressure to reach—but not exceed—a maximum value during inspiration. This pressure is usually set by the operator at 10 cm H_2O above the peak pressure reached during inspiration. This particular setting on the control panel can have a variety of names (Box 11-12); the purpose of this feature is to prevent excessive pressure from damaging lung tissue. In most adult ventilators, reaching this pressure ends inspiratory gas flow; thus the ventilator pressure cycles out of inspiration. Unfortunately, the labeling used on the control panel of most ventilators includes the term pressure limit, which leads to a lot of confusion because this feature usually cycles the ventilator out of inspiration and does not just limit the pressure.

Termination of the Inspiratory Phase: Cycling Mechanism

The phase variable measured and used to end inspiration is called the *cycle variable.* A breath can be volume-cycled, pressure-cycled, time-cycled, or flow-cycled (Boxes 11-13 and Clinical Rounds 11-6). Even though the ventilator may measure a specific volume output during volume-

Box 11-13 Cycling Variables

Volume-cycled: The ventilator ends inspiration after a predetermined volume has been reached.

Pressure-cycled: The ventilator ends inspiration after a predetermined pressure has been reached.

Time-cycled: The ventilator ends inspiration after a predetermined time has been elapsed.

Flow-cycled: The ventilator ends inspiration after a predetermined flow has been achieved.

CLINICAL ROUNDS 11-6

During volume ventilation in current ICU ventilators, the operator sets a volume, flow, and respiratory rate. The ventilators do not measure volume. They calculate and set the inspiratory time needed to achieve the set volume based on the set variables (volume, flow, and time [rate]). This technically makes them time-cycled.

However, clinicians commonly consider them volume-cycled because they do achieve volume delivery by the time inspiratory flow ends, but technically do not "measure" the volume using a volume-measuring device like a bellows or bag.

Defend the argument that these ventilators are volume-cycled instead of time-cycled.

See Appendix A for a discussion.

cycled ventilation, the amount delivered to the patient may be less. This discrepancy can be due to leaks in the system or compression of some of the volume in the patient circuit (tubing compressibility).

Tubing Compliance or Compressibility

Tubing expansion can easily be seen when high pressure is generated in a patient circuit. The circuit can be seen to expand during inspiration and return to normal volume during exhalation. Part of the tidal volume delivered from the ventilator contributes to the expansion of the circuit and never reaches the patient. This volume is important in infants and small children. For this reason, infant patient circuits are made from a lower compliance plastic and thus expand less.

Some ventilators automatically measure and calculate the loss of volume from tubing compliance and compensate by increasing actual volume delivery. An example is the Puritan Bennett 7200. Others, such as the Bear 1000, will allow you to measure the tubing compliance (compressibility) and enter this number into the ventilator. After completing these two steps, the ventilator can then compensate for volume compressed in the tubing during inspiration. Box 11-14 gives an example of how to calculate tubing compliance. Most adult ventilator patient circuits have a tubing compliance factor from 1 to 3 mL/cm H_2O. In other words, for every centimeter of water pressure generated during ventilation of a patient, 1 to 3 mL is lost (compressed) to tubing compliance. For example, if peak inspiratory pressure (PIP) = 10 cm H_2O, and tubing compliance (C_T) = 2 mL/cm H_2O, the volume lost to the circuit will be 10 cm $H_2O \times 2$ mL/cm H_2O = 20 mL. If the tidal volume leaving the ventilator is 500 mL, only 480 mL will reach the patient. Clinical Rounds 11-7 provides problems as exercises.

Box 11-14 Tubing Compliance or Compressibility Calculation

To calculate tubing compliance, perform the following procedure before connecting the ventilator to a patient:

1. Set ventilator volume to 100 or 200 mL.
2. Select a low flow setting (e.g., 40 L/min).
3. Set the upper pressure limit to the maximum and the PEEP to zero.
4. Occlude the patient Y connector.
5. Manually cycle the ventilator, record the measured peak inspiratory pressure (PIP), and measure the exhaled volume (V).

Tubing compliance (C_T) equals measured volume divided by measured pressure (C_T = V/PIP).

CLINICAL ROUNDS 11-7

Calculating Tubing Compliance

Part I

Calculate the tubing compliance of a circuit. The volume was measured as 90 mL during the test and peak inspiratory pressure (PIP) was 45 cm H_2O. What is the tubing compliance?

If this circuit is used to ventilate a child with a set tidal volume of 300 mL and a PIP of 20 cm H_2O, how much volume is lost to the circuit? How much of the volume will go to the patient?

Part II

An adult patient circuit has a compliance of 3 mL/cm H_2O. During inspiration the peak inspiratory pressure reaches 28 cm H_2O. The tidal volume is set at 640 mL on the ventilator. How much volume is lost to the circuit and how much will reach the patient?

See Appendix A for the answers.

Flow Termination

A recent addition to inspiration termination criteria is adjustable flow-cycling. This option resulted from the problem of dyssynchronous patient breathing during pressure support ventilation (PSV). PSV is a patient-triggered, pressure-targeted breath. Historically, PSV was the only mode that was flow-cycled out of inspiration. That is, inspiration ended when the ventilator detected that flow had dropped by some percentage of the peak flow measured during inspiration. Originally, pressure support breaths ended when gas flow dropped to about 25% to 30% of peak inspiratory flow (e.g., Bear 1000) or when a specific flow was measured. For example, in the Puritan-Bennett 7200, when the inspiratory gas flow drops off at the end of inspiration to 5 L/min, inspiratory flow delivery ends.

Because not all patients have similar breathing patterns, fixed ending points did not always synchronize with the patient's breathing pattern. Newer ventilators, such as the Puritan Bennett 840 and the Hamilton Galileo, allow the operator to adjust the flow termination point. In some units this feature can be adjusted from 5% to 80% of the peak flow measured during inspiration. Careful adjustment by the clinician is required. Eventually, the next generation of ventilators will be able to assess patient synchrony during pressure ventilation and adjust inspiratory termination on a breath-by-breath basis.[20,22] Figure 11-48 illustrates two different PS breaths. In part A pressure is set at about 13 cm H_2O, peak flow is about 30 L/min and inspiration ends when the flow drops to about 5 L/min (about 17% of peak flow). The breath is long enough to reach its set value and produce a pressure plateau. In part *B* pressure is set at about 20 cm H_2O, peak flow is about 35 L/min and inspiration ends when flow drops to about 20 L/min (about 57% of peak flow). Inspiration is short, and a visible pressure plateau does not occur.

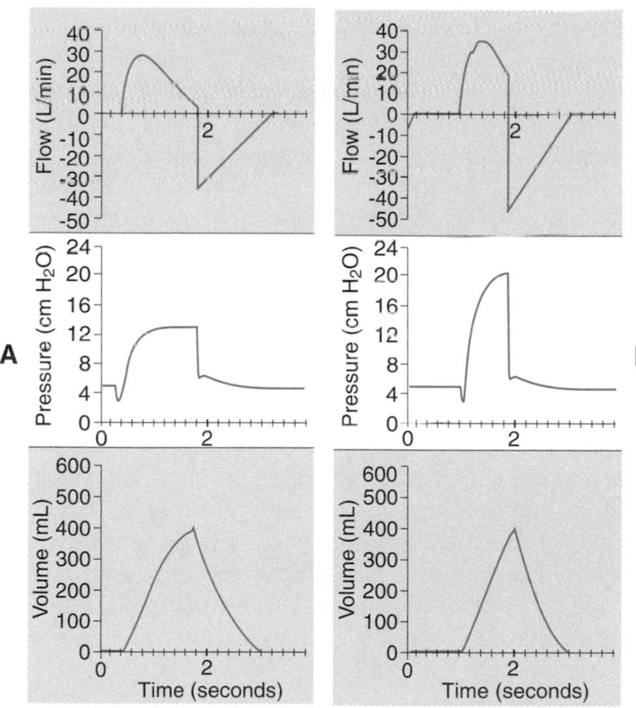

Figure 11-48 The effect of changes in termination flow (flow drop-off) during pressure support ventilation. Termination flow is set as a small percentage of peak inspiratory flow **(A)** and as a greater percentage of peak inspiratory flow **(B).** (See text for further explanation.) (From Hess DR, MacIntyre NR: *Respiratory care: principles & practice*, Philadelphia, 2002, WB Saunders.)

The Expiratory Phase

Normally, when inspiratory flow ceases during ventilation, the expiratory valve opens, allowing expiratory flow to begin. The expiratory phase is the time between inspiratory phases. Expiratory flow can be delayed by keeping the expiratory valve momentarily closed, thus preventing gas flow from leaving the circuit. This maneuver is referred to as an **inspiratory pause,** or inflation hold, and extends inspiratory time.

Inspiratory Pause

Inspiratory pause is also called *inspiratory plateau* and *inflation hold.* An inspiratory pause is not a part of the expiratory phase. It normally extends inspiratory time (T_I). Inspiratory pause can occur in either pressure or volume ventilation. In volume ventilation, it is commonly used to obtain a reading of **plateau pressure ($P_{plateau}$)** for estimating alveolar pressure and calculating **static compliance** ($C_s = V \div [P_{plateau} - PEEP]$) (Box 11-15 and Figure 11-49). It can also be used to extend inspiratory time and increase mean airway pressure for mandatory breaths. A control for this function is located on the operating panel. The inspiratory pause control enables the operator to select a time from fractions of a second up to about 2 seconds.

Box 11-15 Peak, Plateau, and Transairway Pressure

As volume is delivered, pressure rises to a peak (peak inspiratory pressure [PIP]) at the end of inspiration. PIP represents the pressure needed to overcome both airflow resistance and compliance.

When an inspiratory pause is selected, the volume is briefly held in the lungs at the end of inspiration, and the pressure reading drops to a plateau. The plateau or static reading indicates the pressure needed to overcome the static (lung) compliance alone. $C_S = Vol \div (P_{plateau} - PEEP)$.

The difference ($PIP - P_{plateau}$) is the transairway pressure (P_{TA}) and represents pressure associated with airflow resistance and is used to calculate airway resistance: $Raw = P_{TA} \div flow$.

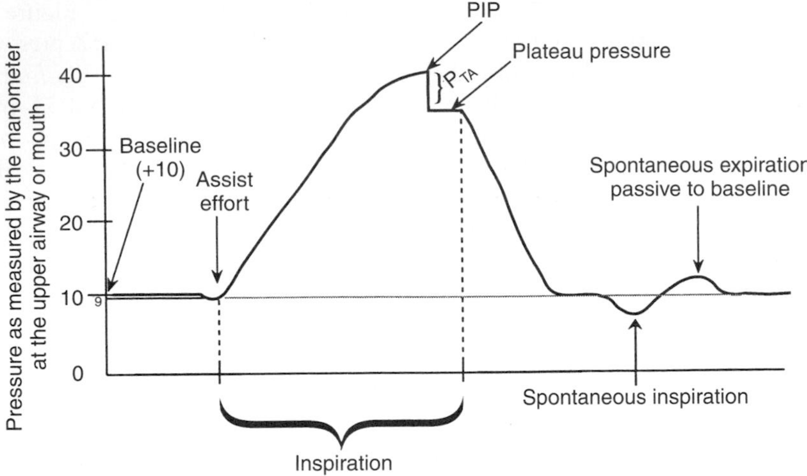

Figure 11-49 A volume breath with an inspiratory hold providing a pause before expiratory flow begins, allowing plateau (alveolar) pressure to be estimated. To be performed accurately, the patient cannot be making spontaneous breathing efforts. Also shown is baseline pressure, at a PEEP of 10 cm H_2O, transairway pressure (P_{TA} = PIP - $P_{plateau}$), and pressure changes during a spontaneous breath. (From Pilbeam SP: *Mechanical ventilation: physiological and clinical applications*, ed 3, St Louis, 1998, Mosby.)

Box 11-16 PEEP and CPAP

PEEP **is the term most commonly used when mandatory ventilator breaths are being delivered with a positive baseline pressure.**

CPAP **is the term most commonly used to describe the positive baseline pressure continuously applied to the airway of a spontaneously breathing patient. Patients doing well on CPAP alone do not require mandatory breaths from a ventilator.**

During pressure ventilation, an **inspiratory hold** pressure can also be observed when T_I is sufficient to allow the selected pressure to equilibrate with the patient's lungs. In this situation, inflation hold is not actually selected as a parameter on the control panel. Flow reads zero during this time, before expiratory flow is allowed to begin (see Figure 11-43, *B*). This phenomenon can be observed with pediatric ventilators when a pressure-relief valve is used. In this situation, the pressure-relief valve opens during the inspiratory phase and allows the pressure to be maintained at a constant level within the circuit until the ventilator cycles into expiration (pressure-limited, time-cycled ventilation) (see Figure 11-47).

Baseline Pressure

Baseline pressure is the pressure level at which inspiration begins and exhalation ends. It is a variable controlled by the ventilator during the expiratory phase. Baseline pressures above zero are commonly called **PEEP (positive end-expiratory pressure)** or **CPAP (continuous positive airway pressure)** (Box 11-16 and Figures 11-49 and 11-50). Exhalation valves designed to provide PEEP were described earlier in this chapter, as were freestanding CPAP devices.

Expiratory Retard

Expiratory retard is a technique that offers resistance to expiratory gas flow by incorporating a variable orifice in the expiratory outflow tract (see Figure 11-23). Its purpose is to maintain pressure in the circuit and the airway during expiration to help prevent flaccid airways from collapsing in patients with chronic obstructive pulmonary disorders. This maneuver is thought to mimic pursed-lip breathing, which is not effective when an endotracheal or tracheostomy tube is in place.[16] It may increase mean intrathoracic pressure, potentially increase expiratory time (especially during spontaneous breathing), and alter inspiratory to expiratory (I:E) ratios. An expiratory retard control, although present on older ventilators, is rarely seen as a control in newer ventilators.

Positive End-Expiratory Pressure (PEEP)

PEEP occurs because a resistance, applied during exhalation, limits lung emptying and increases functional residual capacity (FRC) to increase mean airway pressure and to improve lung recruitment. The use of PEEP is described elsewhere and is beyond the scope of this text.[7,20] Increased pressure is accomplished by using a resistance device, which can be either a flow or threshold resistor, as described earlier in this chapter.

Continuous Positive Airway Pressure (CPAP)

CPAP, also described previously, refers to a technique in which a patient breathes spontaneously at an elevated baseline pressure (see Figure 11-50). As with PEEP, the increased pressure is accomplished with the use of some type of expiratory resistance device. CPAP can be achieved

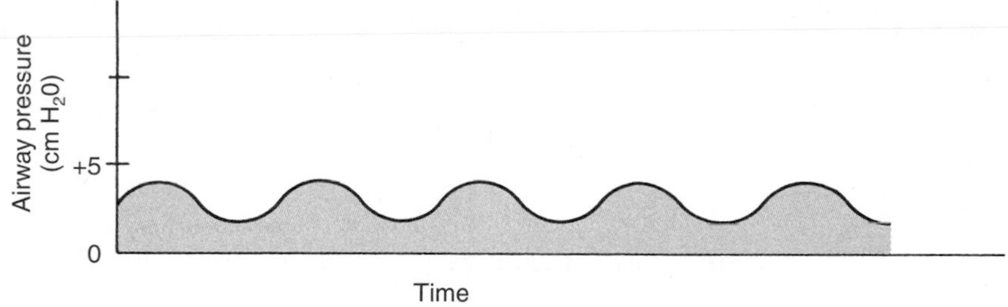

Figure 11-50 Curve of pressure and time for CPAP. (From Pilbeam SP: *Mechanical ventilation: physiological and clinical applications*, ed 3, St Louis, 1998, Mosby.)

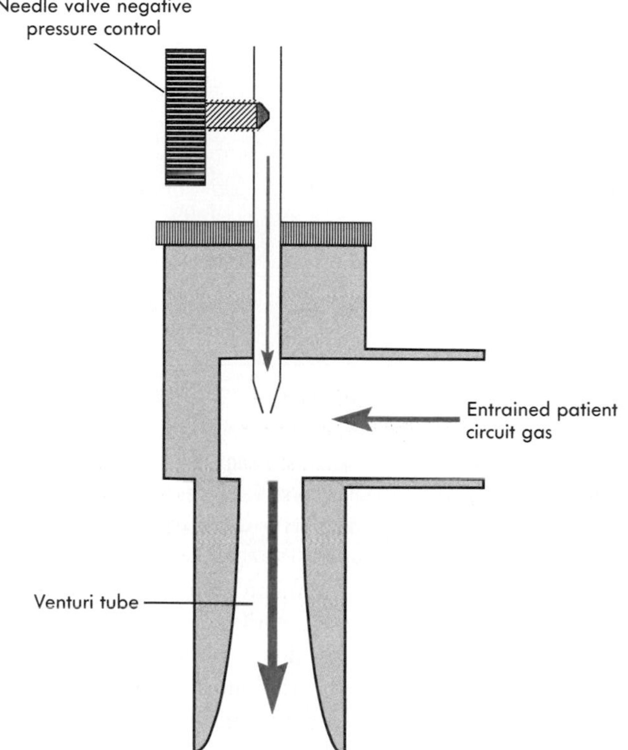

Figure 11-51 Example of a NEEP mechanism. (See text for description.)

through a mechanical ventilator or via a free-standing spontaneous breathing system. (See the section in this chapter on additional devices used during patient ventilation.)

As with PEEP, CPAP can be used to increase FRC to increase mean airway pressure (MAP) and to improve lung recruitment. It is also used for the treatment of sleep apnea (see Chapter 15).

Continuous Gas Flow During Exhalation

Ventilators that provide flow-triggering frequently have a flow of gas passing through the circuit throughout expiration called base flow or bias flow. Normally, this flow does not begin until about one-third of the expiratory time has occurred; thus helping prevent resistance to exhalation. But, because this bias flow is present in the patient circuit during the remainder of expiration, it provides immediate flow to a patient at the beginning of the next inspiratory effort.

Subambient Pressure, or Negative End-Expiratory Pressure

Historically, negative pressure during expiration was called **negative end-expiratory pressure (NEEP).** One of the designs for NEEP used a venturi at the upper airway to actively draw air from the airway (Figures 11-51 and 11-52). This older technique was intended to counterbalance the increase in mean intrathoracic pressures caused by positive-pressure ventilation and permit more rapid respiratory rates in infants.

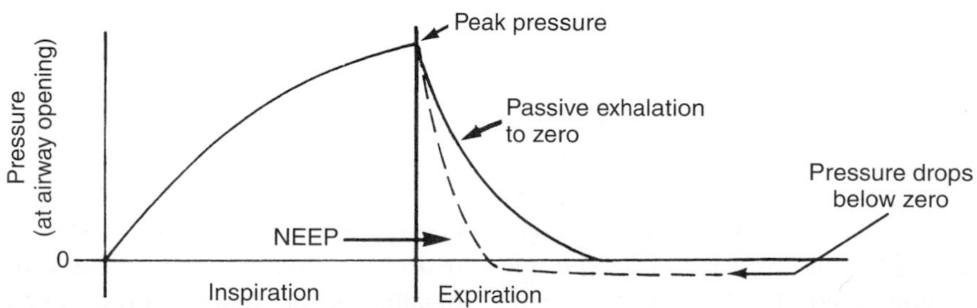

Figure 11-52 Pressure-time curve for a mandatory breath, showing normal passive exhalation to zero baseline *(solid line)* and exhalation using NEEP *(dashed line)*. (From Pilbeam SP: *Mechanical ventilation: physiological and clinical applications*, ed 3, St Louis, 1998, Mosby.)

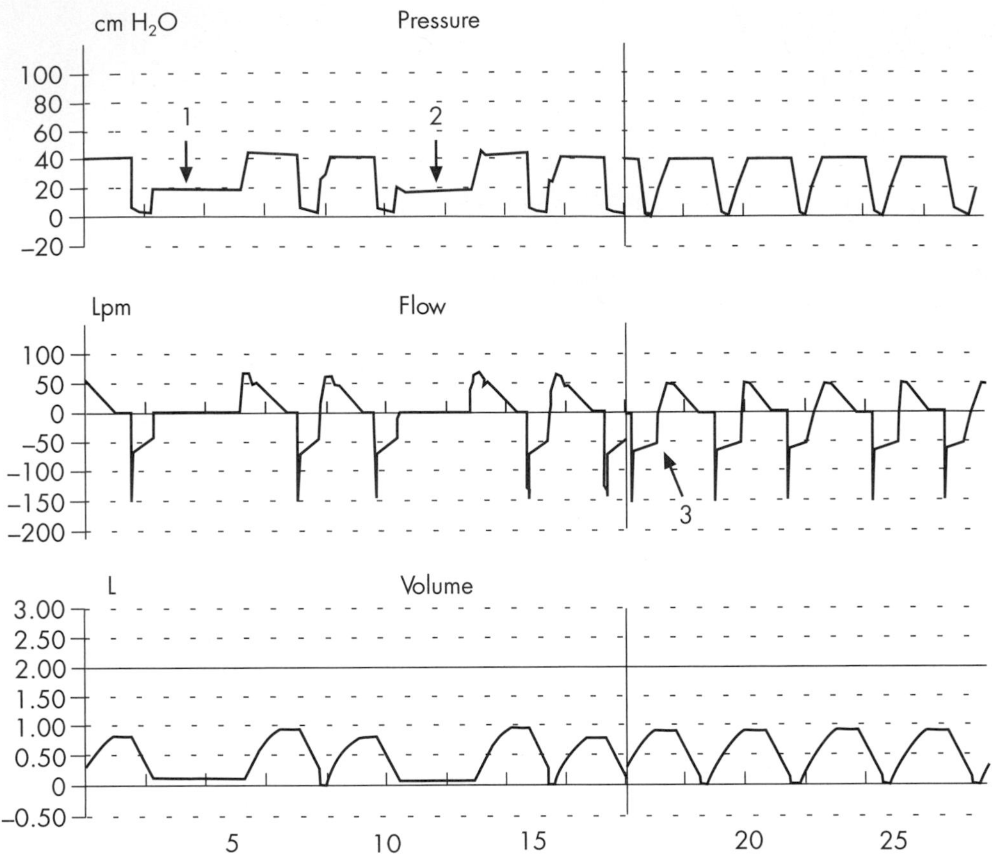

Figure 11-53 Pressure-time, flow-time, and volume-time curves showing the use of end-expiratory pause, allowing the estimation of auto-PEEP (*1* and *2*). Without using a pause, the presence of auto-PEEP can be detected from the flow curve. Flow does not return to zero before the next mandatory breath *(3)*. (See text for complete description.) (Redrawn from Nilsestuen JO, Hargett K: Managing the patient-ventilator system using graphic analysis: an overview and introduction to Graphics Corner, *Respir Care* 41:1105, 1996.)

Current use of negative pressure during expiration occurs during high-frequency oscillation (see Figure 11-3). The ventilator actually creates a wave of negative pressure, drawing air out of the airway. Another use for it is to facilitate expiration on patients being ventilated with the Venturi ventilator (Cardiopulmonary Corp, see the Evolve website for this text). The Venturi provides a slight negative pressure at the very beginning of exhalation. This low negative pressure is believed to facilitate removal of air from the circuit and to reduce the patient's expiratory resistance.

Expiratory Hold: End-Expiratory Pause

Expiratory hold or **end-expiratory pause** is performed to estimate pressure in the patient's lung and ventilator circuit due to trapped air. Air trapping or auto-PEEP can occur when high minute ventilation is used (> 10 L/min). It can also occur in patients with obstructive airway disease in which airway resistance is high and exhalation takes longer than normal. In both of these instances, there is not enough time for the patient to completely exhale.

Normally, expiratory flow is finished about half way through the expiratory phase. The second half of expiration is a pause with no flow. The expiratory portion of a flow-time curve normally shows flow returning to zero during exhalation. When a patient has air-trapping and auto-PEEP is present, the expiratory flow does not return to zero. A new inspiration begins before the patient has had time to completely exhale. As a result air remains trapped in the lungs. To be watchful of air-trapping, the operator must be sure that the flow curve returns to zero before the next breath. If it does not, as illustrated by arrow 3 in Figure 11-53, then auto-PEEP is present. The operator can then perform an expiratory pause to determine how much pressure is being trapped.

The expiratory pause maneuver is performed at the end of exhalation after a mandatory breath. For this measurement to be accurate the patient must not make any spontaneous breathing efforts or a stable end expiratory pressure reading cannot be obtained. Activating the expiratory pause control closes both the inspiratory and expiratory valves at the end of expiration and delays delivery of the next mandatory breath. This delay allows time for equilibration of pressures in the circuit and for the operator to obtain a reading of end-expiratory pressure. Figure 11-53 illustrates this procedure.

In the pressure-time curve at the top, arrow number *1* shows the first use of the expiratory pause control. Just before this plateau, a mandatory breath was given and the patient appeared to exhale to baseline pressure. What is actually occurring is the manometer measuring pressure is exposed to atmospheric pressure when the expiratory valve opens to allow exhalation to begin. Thus the pressure reading is false and is reflecting atmospheric pressures and not pressures in the patient's lungs.

When the operator enables the expiratory pause control, the resulting rise in pressure shows about 20 cm H_2O is still present in the patient's lung and the ventilator circuit. Note in the corresponding flow curve that the flow is at zero. All valves are closed and the delivery of the next timed breath is delayed.

Arrow number 2 shows another activation of the expiratory pause control and the resulting end expiratory pressure reading. The valves reopen when the control is released or after a set time period, usually a maximum of 20 seconds.

To help eliminate auto-PEEP, the operator should try to use a lower minute ventilation if possible. Also, increasing inspiratory flow can shorten inspiratory time and allow more time for exhalation. The use of bronchodilators may help patients with bronchoconstriction by reducing their airway resistance.

Time-Limited Exhalation

Time limiting of exhalation is also used as a safety feature during ventilation, especially in infants when rapid respiratory rates dictate a short TCT. Breath stacking can occur and become a hazard. Time-limiting can also be used as a safety feature to end inspiratory flow if inspiration is prolonged.

Part III: Basic Modes of Ventilation

Modes of ventilation describe the pattern of breath delivery to a patient. The use of the terms associated with ventilator modes indicates the type of breath being delivered and how the breaths are triggered, controlled, and cycled. Most ventilator control panels have a mode-selection switch. Unfortunately, naming of modes varies among manufacturers and causes confusion.

For a discussion of the purpose of different ventilator modes and how they are set, the reader is referred elsewhere.[7,12,20] The following discussion will focus on definitions of the modes and technical aspects of their functions.

Controlled Mechanical Ventilation, or Control Mode

The **control mode** is the delivery of a preset volume (volume-targeted) or pressure (pressure-targeted) breath at set intervals (time-triggered breaths). Breaths are time- or volume-cycled and pressure- or volume-limited, and each breath is mandatory. Controlled ventilation is generally used when patients make no inspiratory effort, as with drug overdoses, neurological or neuromuscular disorders, or seizure activities that require sedation and sometimes induced paralysis. Historical Note 11-5 provides a historic note about the control mode. Figure 11-54 shows the pressure, flow, and volume scalars for controlled ventilation, *A*, volume-targeted and *B*, pressure-targeted.

Note that controlled ventilation should never be deliberately selected on the operating panel. That is, the ventilator should never be insensitive to the patient's inspiratory effort. Generally, if a practitioner wants to control breathing, he or she must sedate and paralyze the patient. Control of breathing can be provided by any mode of ventilation except spontaneous mode settings (i.e., CPAP

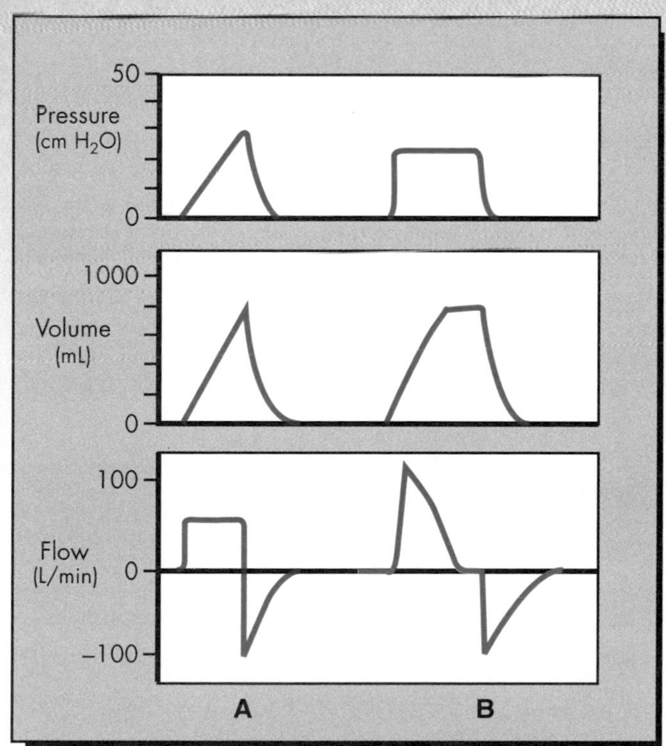

Figure 11-54 Pressure, volume, and flow scalars for volume targeted ventilation with constant flow **(A)** and pressure targeted ventilation **(B)**, both in the control mode.

HISTORICAL NOTE 11-5
The Control Mode

Early volume ventilators had no sensitivity control to monitor and respond to patient efforts during inspiration. If patients tried to breathe on their own, they simply ended up "fighting the ventilator." Sensitivity controls were soon added to allow patient triggering. When this control was first added, clinicians would sometimes turn the sensitivity off so that patients could be controlled. When patients did make efforts at inspiration under these conditions, their "fighting the ventilator" was sometimes treated with sedation and/or paralytics.

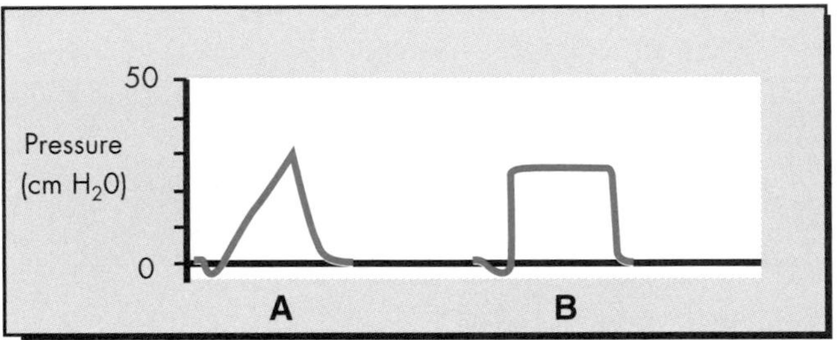

Figure 11-55 Pressure-time curves for volume **(A)** and pressure **(B)** ventilation in the assist/control mode. Note the deflection of the pressure below baseline before breath delivery.

and pressure support). Newer ventilators do not have pure "control mode" options (i.e., a knob that says "control mode").

Note also that when practitioners in the clinical setting hear the term *control mode* or **assist/control mode,** described in the following section, they assume that volume ventilation is being used. This assumption has come about through the historical development of this mode. On the other hand, the phrase **pressure-controlled ventilation (PCV)** is assumed to mean controlled ventilation that is pressure targeted (pressure-limited). Being specific about the meanings of terms is important so that misunderstandings do not occur.

Assist, Assist/Control Ventilation

Sensing mechanisms are designed to detect a drop of pressure, flow or volume in the circuit when a patient makes an inspiratory effort (patient triggering). When all breaths are patient-triggered, the mode is referred to as the **assist** mode. When a backup rate is set and some breaths are time- and patient-triggered, the mode is called the assist/control mode. Operators set a back-up rate when using assist/control to ensure patient safety, should the patient become apneic.

The pressure-time waveform reflects the downward deflection of a patient-assisted breath when breaths are

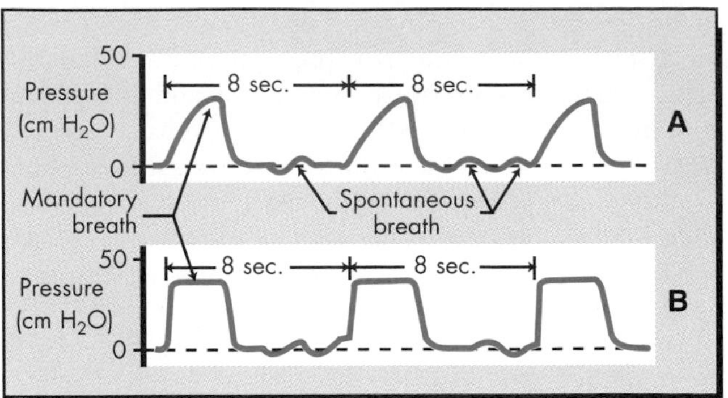

Figure 11-56 Pressure-time curves for volume ventilation **(A)** and pressure ventilation **(B)** with IMV.

patient-triggered (Figure 11-55). Breath intervals may be irregular, but each breath will deliver the set volume or pressure, regardless of how it was triggered. If the patient's rate drops below the set rate (i.e., if the time between patient-initiated breaths is longer than the ventilator cycle time [60 seconds/set rate]), timed breaths occur. Mandatory breaths continue at the set rate until the patient's rate increases again or patient effort occurs before the timed ventilator interval. Control and assist/control modes are commonly labeled continuous mandatory ventilation (CMV) on newer generation ventilators.

In summary, assist and assist/control (CMV) are patient-triggered or time-triggered, volume- or pressure-targeted, and usually volume- or time-cycled. In volume ventilation, breaths are volume- or flow-limited. In pressure ventilation, breaths are pressure-limited.

Intermittent Mandatory Ventilation

Intermittent mandatory ventilation (IMV) is designed to deliver volume- or pressure-targeted breaths at a set minimum frequency (time-triggered). Between mandatory breaths, the patient can breathe spontaneously from the ventilator circuit without getting the set volume or pressure from the ventilator itself. During this spontaneous breathing period, the patient breathes from the set baseline pressure, which may be ambient pressure or a positive baseline pressure (PEEP/CPAP). Spontaneous breaths can also be aided by the use of pressure support (see the section on pressure support later in this chapter). Because patients have an opportunity to spontaneously breathe, they must assume part of the work of breathing. For this reason, IMV and SIMV (described later) are commonly used for patients who can provide part of the ventilatory work.

Figure 11-56 illustrates the pressure-time graph for IMV with volume and pressure ventilation. During IMV with volume ventilation (IMV vol.), mandatory breaths are time-triggered, volume-targeted, and volume-cycled. During IMV with pressure ventilation (IMV press.), mandatory

HISTORICAL NOTE 11-6
Demand-Flow IMV Systems

In the 1970s demand-flow IMV represented the earliest type of IMV design. Demand-flow IMV required the patient to open a one-way valve that needed an effort of –0.5 to –2 cm H_2O. In the demand-flow system pictured (see Figure 11-57), a one-way valve is positioned near the patient's Y-connector. When the ventilator provided a mandatory breath, the expiratory valve closed and the pressure from the breath also closed a one-way valve, which connected the demand system with the patient circuit. Gas was forced from the ventilator to the patient.

During spontaneous inspiration between mandatory breaths, the patient opened the one-way valve connecting the patient circuit to the IMV demand system. The patient received gas from a separate heated, humidified source consisting of two flowmeters (air and oxygen) or a blender. This gas passed from the added humidifier through a large bore tube to the T-piece that housed the one-way valve. An additional piece of tubing connected to the T-piece opened into room air. Gas was continuously flowing through this tube.

Figure 11-57 is a schematic of a volume ventilator with a demand-flow IMV circuit added. The enlarged portion of the demand IMV circuit shows the one-way valve that connects the two circuits, the demand circuit, and the patient ventilator circuit.

breaths are time-triggered, pressure-targeted, and time-cycled.

Historically, IMV circuits had to be added to the patient circuit to provide for IMV ventilation. Newer ventilators have this system built-in and provide SIMV rather than IMV, but IMV circuits are still added to home-care ventilators. For this reason, add-on IMV system will be included.

When IMV or SIMV is used for weaning, the mandatory breath rate can be progressively decreased, allowing for more spontaneous breaths from the patient.

Setting up a Ventilator with IMV

Add-on IMV circuits are also used with some home ventilators. Two basic types of designs for an IMV system are used: demand flow and continuous flow. Demand-flow systems, also called parallel flow or open-circuit IMV, were the earliest type of design. Historical Note 11-6 provides a historical note on this system. Figure 11-57 shows a diagram of a demand flow system.

The problem with the original demand-flow design was that much of the system's tubing was close to the patient's airway, added weight, and caused pulling on the artificial airway. Additionally, the patient was required to perform the work of opening the valve. When PEEP was applied, the patient had to reduce patient-circuit pressure to below ambient to receive airflow from the IMV circuit. The patient was required to generate such large negative pressures because the IMV circuit and the patient-circuit pressure was at the set PEEP level (Figure 11-58).

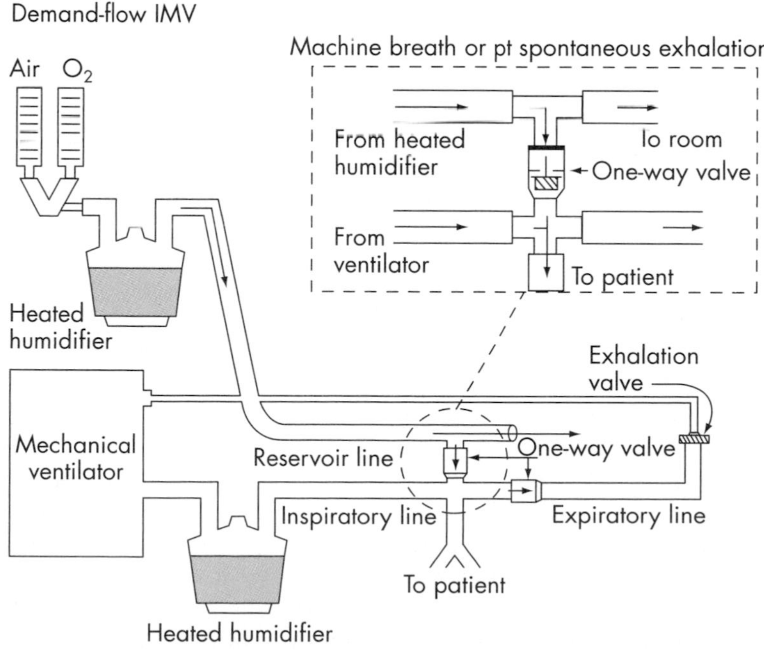

Figure 11-57 Demand-flow IMV. (See text for further explanation.) (From Pilbeam SP: *Mechanical ventilation: physiological and clinical applications*, ed 2, St Louis, 1992, Mosby.)

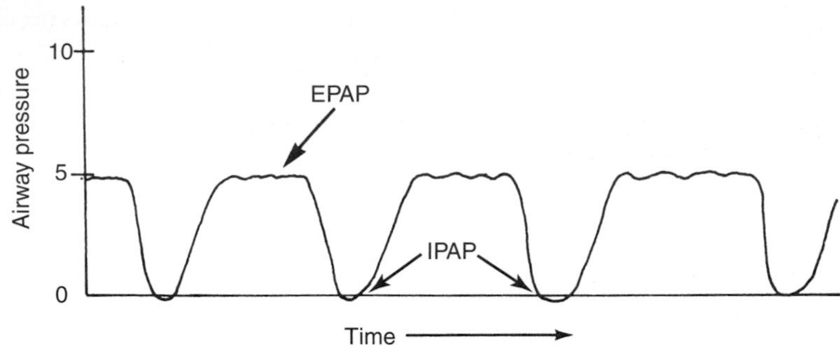

Figure 11-58 Spontaneous breathing with a demand-flow IMV system with PEEP. During inspiration, the pressure drops to slightly below ambient, which is required to open the one-way valve. Inspiratory positive airway pressure (IPAP) is at or below zero, and expiratory positive airway pressure (EPAP) is at the set-PEEP level. (From Pilbeam SP: *Mechanical ventilation: physiological and clinical applications*, ed 3, St Louis, 1998, Mosby.)

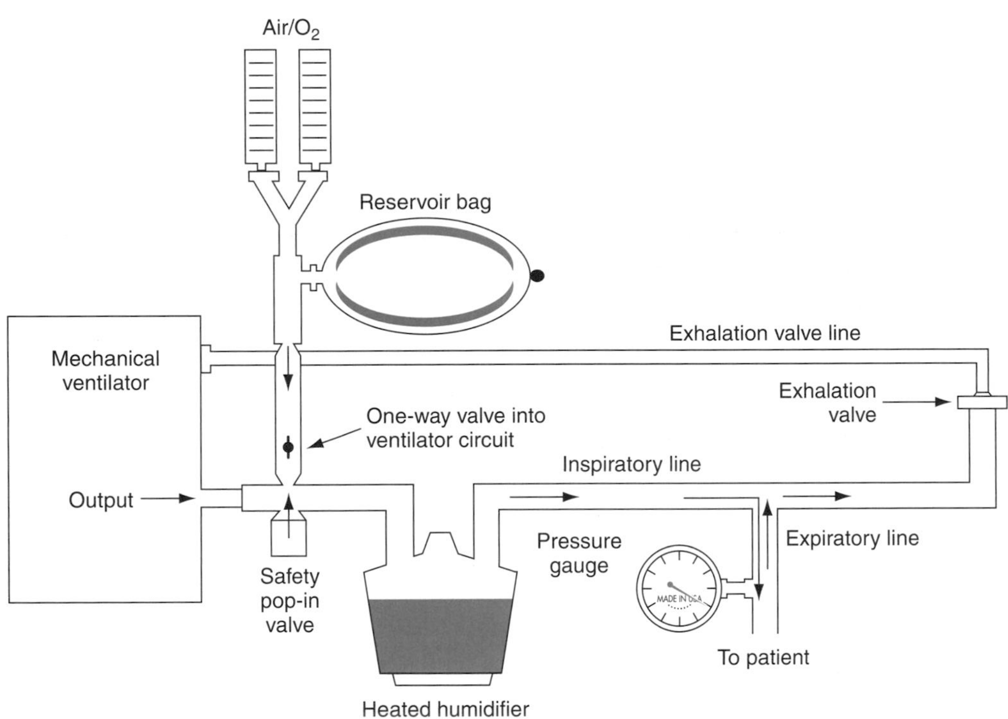

Figure 11-59 Continuous-flow IMV system added to a volume ventilator. (See text for explanation.) (From Pilbeam SP: *Mechanical ventilation: physiological and clinical applications*, ed 2, St Louis, 1992, Mosby.)

The design of continuous-flow or closed-circuit IMV systems takes advantage of the heated humidifier on the ventilator. It incorporates a reservoir, along with a continuous flow of gas, so that the one-way valve opening toward the patient circuit remains open by the continuous flow and does not have to be opened by the patient. Figure 11-59 shows an example of a continuous-flow IMV system. A blended gas source (i.e., air and oxygen flowmeters or a blender) provides gas flow to a reservoir bag. The gas reservoir is attached to the ventilator circuit by a one-way valve on the proximal side of the humidifier (the side closest to the main outlet of the ventilator). This valve remains open during the spontaneous breathing period, so that the patient can receive a continuous flow of gas past his or her airway. The pressure generated by a mandatory breath closes the one-way valve so that the mandatory breath is delivered to the patient and not to the reservoir. Adding a safety pop-in valve, as shown in Figure 11-59 is imperative. If gas flow from the outside source is accidentally shut off, patients can open the one-way valve and receive ambient air.

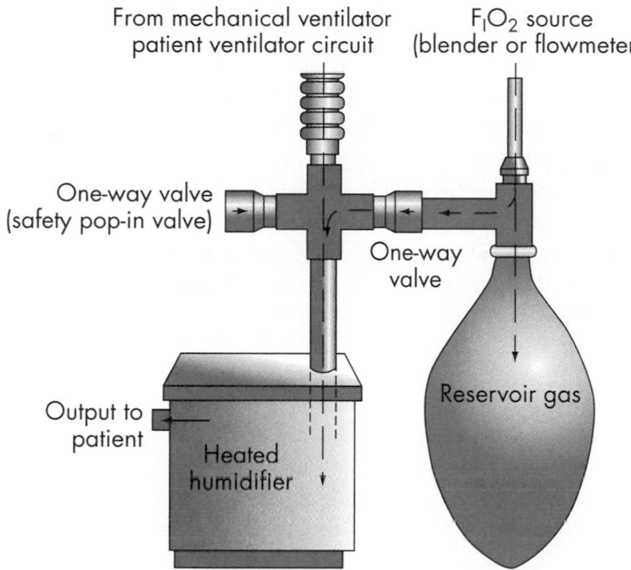

Figure 11-60 Schematic of a continuous-flow IMV circuit. (From Pilbeam SP: *Mechanical ventilation: physiological and clinical applications*, ed 2, St Louis, 1992, Mosby.)

Box 11-17 Disadvantages and Safety Considerations with IMV Circuits

Continuous-flow systems have certain disadvantages. First, the continuous flow often causes inadvertent PEEP at the patient's airway. Second, the constant flow of gas through the expiratory valve during the spontaneous period prevents the use of an inspiratory plateau to measure plateau pressure. Closing the expiratory valve for any reason with this type of assembly results in continuous flow of gas into the circuit and the patient's lungs, increasing system pressure. Third, measurement of V_T at the exhalation valve is impossible because of the constant gas flow, so it must be measured at the endotracheal tube. An accurate measurement of exhaled V_T can be obtained by placing a respirometer directly between the endotracheal tube and the ventilator Y connector.

Figure 11-60 shows another example of a continuous-flow IMV assembly. Blended gas fills the reservoir and flows through the one-way valve into the patient circuit. Because of their shape, add-on systems are sometimes called H-valve assemblies. If PEEP is used, the reservoir can be pressurized to keep its pressure at or near the set PEEP level. Box 11-17 describes some disadvantages and safety concerns with IMV add-on systems.

Adjusting the Ventilator with Add-on IMV Circuits

When an IMV system is added, the ventilator sensitivity is either turned off (as long as a safety pop-in valve allowing access to room air is added) or reduced so it does not normally respond to patient effort. The pressure limit must be set at about 10 cm H_2O above peak inspiratory pressure for a mandatory breath. This adjustment is important because a mandatory breath may occur immediately after a spontaneous inspiration, resulting in a very high-volume delivery. When adjustments are made to the F_IO_2 control on the ventilator front panel, the F_IO_2 must also be changed at the source providing flow to the IMV system.

Synchronized Intermittent Mandatory Ventilation (SIMV)

Unlike IMV, **synchronized intermittent mandatory ventilation (SIMV)** is built into the ventilator. SIMV delivers a set volume or pressure breath to the patient in response to the patient's effort. Similar to IMV, a minimum respiratory rate is set by the operator with SIMV. SIMV breaths can be volume- or pressure-targeted. Between these assisted breaths, the patient can breathe spontaneously and will not receive the set mandatory volume or pressure.

During the spontaneous period, the patient breathes from the baseline pressure, which may be ambient or positive (PEEP/CPAP). Spontaneous breaths can also be aided by the use of pressure support (see the section later in this chapter on pressure support). The main difference between IMV and SIMV is that SIMV tries to synchronize delivery of the mandatory breath with patient effort (patient triggering). When the time for a mandatory breath occurs, the unit waits briefly for a patient effort. If the patient triggers the breath, then the ventilator automatically delivers the mandatory breath.

The use of the terms mandatory and assist in relation to IMV/SIMV should be noted. Recall that a mandatory breath is completely machine-controlled, and an assisted breath is patient-triggered with the ventilator determining how inspiration is delivered and when it ends (cycles). If a patient fails to trigger a breath during SIMV, the machine will time-trigger the breath, which makes it a mandatory breath. If the patient triggers the breath, it is technically an assisted breath. However, when referring to the IMV/SIMV mode, labeling breaths "mandatory" breaths is easier when they are volume- or pressure-targeted breaths, regardless of how the breaths are triggered. This concept will become clearer as the function of SIMV, PCV, and PSV are reviewed.

In SIMV, as in IMV, the operator sets a minimum respiratory rate and a desired volume (volume-targeted, SIMV-vol.) or pressure (pressure-targeted, SIMV-press). Between mandatory breaths, the patient breathes spontaneously.

If the pressure waveform has a downward deflection before the delivery of a mandatory breath, the breath is patient-triggered (Figure 11-61). If no downward deflection of the pressure waveform occurs before a mandatory breath, the breath is time-triggered.

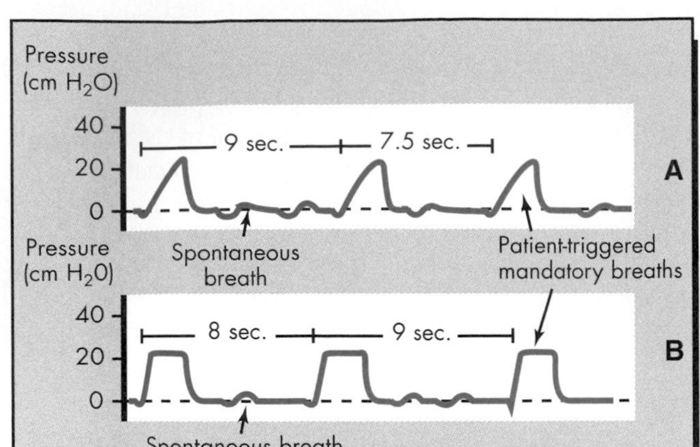

Figure 11-61 Pressure-time curves for volume ventilation **(A)** and pressure ventilation **(B)** with SIMV. (See text for explanation.)

Current ICU ventilators have controls on the front panel labeled SIMV. These controls can actually deliver IMV or SIMV (IMV/SIMV). Sometimes these controls are labeled "SIMV(vol.)" and "SIMV(press.)" on the control panel to distinguish between volume- and pressure-targeted SIMV.

In summary, SIMV incorporates both mandatory and spontaneous breaths. Mandatory breaths are patient- or time-triggered, pressure- or volume-targeted, and usually time- or volume-cycled. Spontaneous breaths are from the set baseline and can be assisted with pressure support. Box 11-18 outlines how the controls are set for volume and pressure targeted breaths in either assist/control or IMV/SIMV ventilation.

Box 11-18 Operator-Selected Controls for Volume- and Pressure-Targeted Breaths in Assist/Control and IMV/SIMV

For volume-targeted breaths in assist/control and IMV/SIMV, the operator normally selects from two options:

1. With volume-cycled (or flow/time*) ventilators, volume, flow, and rate are set.
2. With time-cycled ventilators, volume, rate and inspiratory time are set.

For pressure-targeted breaths in assist/control and IMV/SIMV modes, the operator normally selects the following:

1. Pressure
2. Respiratory rate
3. Inspiratory time

*Flow and time are measured, and the ventilator cycles when it estimates that set volume has been delivered.

Pressure-Controlled Ventilation

PCV is the common name applied to pressure-targeted (pressure-limited) ventilation in the assist/control mode. It is also called pressure assist/control.[23] The operator sets a target pressure. Sensitivity is also set to allow for patient triggering. A rate and an inspiratory time are set to establish the total cycle time. The rate guarantees a minimum respiratory rate.

When the breath is triggered, the ventilator produces a rapid inspiratory flow to achieve the set pressure. When the pressure is reached as the lungs fill, the flow decreases (descending ramp). The breath ends when the inspiratory time has passed. Volume delivery varies with the set inspiratory time and the patient's lung characteristics and whether or not the patient is actively inspiring. For example, when the patient's lungs are stiff, less volume is delivered for the same amount of pressure. As the lungs improve, less pressure is required to deliver the same volume. If the patient actively inspires, the ventilator will increase flow delivery to maintain the set pressure, which can increase volume delivery. If inspiratory time is too short, the ventilator will not have sufficient time to deliver all the pressure to the lungs, and the volume may be lower than desired.

Recently, new ICU ventilators offer the feature of sloping or tapering the inspiratory pressure curve, described previously in this chapter. Many of them also offer flow-cycling for PC ventilation. Rather than waiting for a certain time to pass, the ventilator ends the breath as flow begins to drop off signaling the end of inspiration. This flow drop-off can be set on new ventilators including the **Servo i** ventilator (Siemens Servo Corp.) and the **Venturi** ventilator (Cardiopulmonary Corp.).

In its early development, PCV was used with inverse I:E ratios and was termed **pressure-controlled inverse ratio ventilation (PCIRV).** Inverse ratios were used to increase the mean airway pressure, with the intent of improving oxygenation of the patient.

Pressure-Support Ventilation

Pressure-support ventilation (PSV) is a spontaneous mode that allows the operator to select a pressure to support the patient's work of breathing. It is patient-triggered, pressure-limited, and flow-cycled.[24] PSV can also be used to support the work of breathing for spontaneous breaths during IMV/SIMV ventilation. Figure 11-62 shows the waveforms for SIMV + PSV for both volume- and pressure-targeted mandatory breaths.

As with pressure-controlled ventilation, the ventilator delivers a high flow of gas to the patient when a breath is triggered during pressure-support ventilation. As the lungs fill, the flow and the pressure gradient between the machine and the patient decrease. The flow curve appears as a descending waveform, but never falls all the way to zero during inspiration because ventilators are programmed to sense the drop in flow until it reaches a predetermined amount. Some ventilators end inspiration when flow drops to 25% of peak flow during inspiration. Others end inspiration

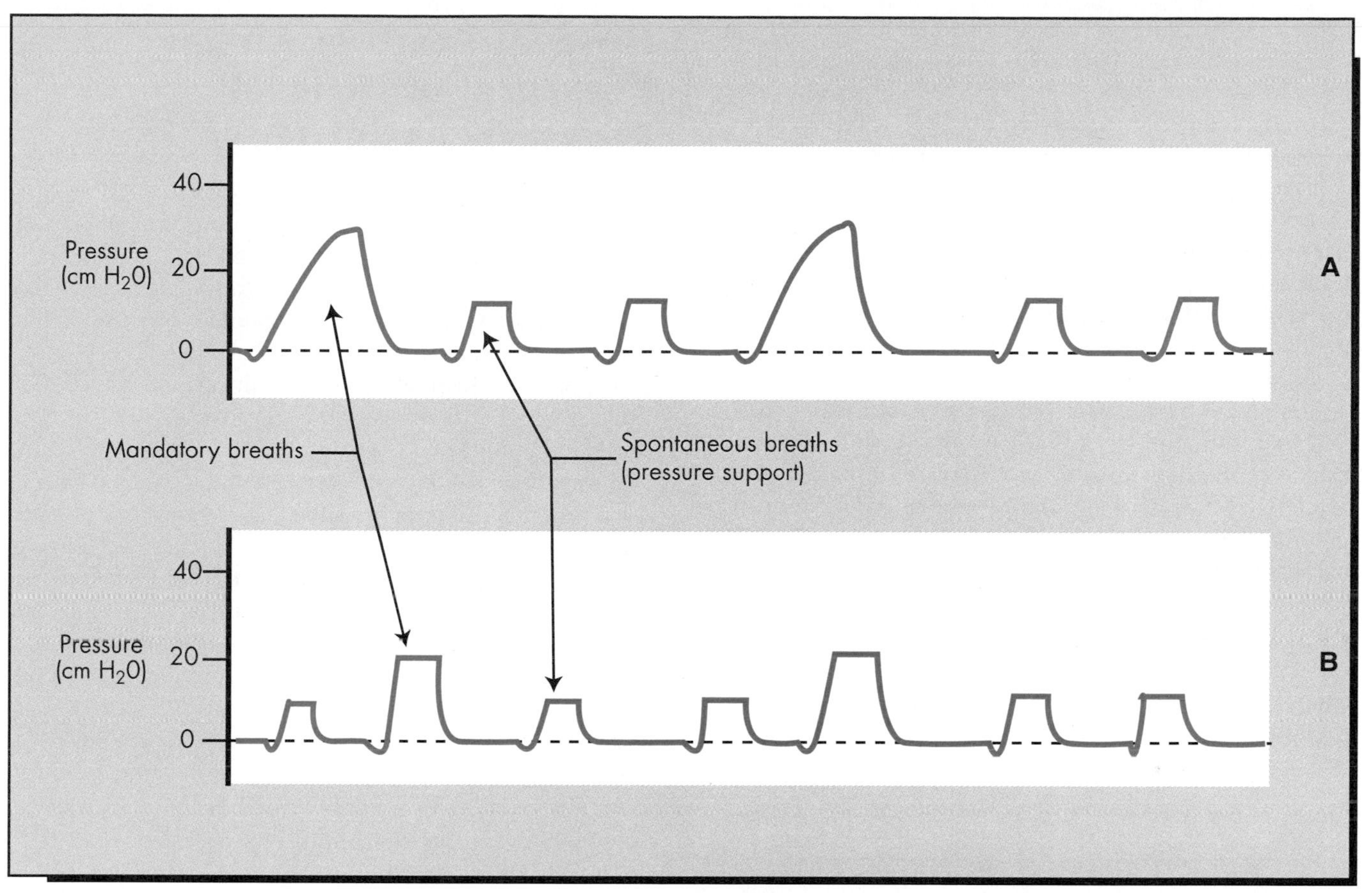

Figure 11-62 Pressure waveforms of SIMV(vol) + PSV **(A)** and SIMV(press) + PSV **(B).** (See text for explanation.)

at fixed rates (e.g., the 7200ae cycles when flow drops to 5 L/min). Still newer ventilators, as mentioned previously, provide flow cycling as an adjustable parameter, allowing the operator to change the cycle level (% flow) based on the type of patient being ventilated. Examples of these ventilators include the Hamilton Galileo, the Servo i, and the Newport e500. In the future new software may automatically adjust the flow-cycling threshold by monitoring such factors as the pulmonary time constant at the end exhalation and the slope of the pressure waveform at the end-inspiration. This monitoring may allow adjustment of the flow cycling threshold by the ventilator.[25]

If the flow does not decrease (e.g., with a leak in the system), inspiration will be time-cycled (1 to 5 seconds) out of inspiration. The breath can also be pressure-cycled (set pressure + 2 to + 3 cm H_2O), if the pressure begins to rise higher than the set pressure level, which might occur if the patient begins to actively exhale. These safety back-up systems are available with any ventilator providing PSV.

The volume delivery in PSV is determined by three factors: the set pressure, the patient's lung characteristics (resistance and compliance), and the patient's inspiratory effort.

PSV has two common uses. The first is to reduce the patient's work of breathing when resistance to breathing is increased because of an artificial airway and the ventilatory circuit. The work of breathing imposed by small endotracheal tubes can be a major contributor to fatigue. A review of Poiseuille's law illustrates the basic theory of pressure support when airway resistance (Raw) is increased (see Chapter 1). Decreasing the diameter of the airway significantly increases the resistance to gas flow, which can be a contributing factor to the difficulty of weaning some patients (Box 11-19).

Box 11-19 Use of PSV with Increased Raw

Pressure support increases the pressure gradient for gas flow across a tube. Theoretically, if the pressure gradient across the tube is high enough, the effect of the increased resistance due to the tube is negated.

Where the increased work of breathing is associated with the artificial airway or the ventilator system, the initial pressure-support level set does not have to be very high. Commonly 5 to 10 cm H_2O are used. Another way to estimate the starting pressure level in this case is to calculate the patient's transairway pressure ($P_{TA} = P_{peak} - P_{plateau}$), which is the difference between peak and plateau pressure. P_{TA} reflects pressure generated to overcome the resistance caused by the ventilator circuit, the endotracheal tube, and the patient airways.[7] The P_{TA} value is a safe starting point for PS. The pressure support levels can then be readjusted after it is activated to fit the patient's needs.

Newer ventilators, like the Dräger E-4, actually have an artificial airway compensation feature, called tube compensation. When the type of artificial airway the patient has—endotracheal or tracheostomy—and the size of the tube are programmed into the ventilator, the ventilator calculates and delivers the amount of pressure support needed to compensate for the airway.

A second use for PSV is for spontaneously breathing patients who have intact respiratory centers. PSV can be adjusted so that much of the work of breathing is provided by the ventilator with a simple increase of the set pressure level. This result can be accomplished by measuring volume delivery while adjusting pressure. A desired V_T is based on the patient's ideal body weight (IBW) and lung condition. For example, 5 to 6 mL/kg may be appropriate for a patient, but tidal volume needs vary with different lung conditions.[7,20] Box 11-20 lists patients who might benefit from PSV; Clinical Rounds 11-8 provides an exercise about PSV.

Box 11-20 Candidates for Pressure-Support Ventilation

Patients with an artificial airway in place and any of the following conditions:

- Airways smaller than optimal size.
- Spontaneous respiratory rates >20 breaths/min (adults).
- Minute ventilation >10 L/min.

Patients being supported with IMV/SIMV or CPAP (with spontaneous breaths) and any of the following conditions:

- A history of chronic obstructive pulmonary disorder (COPD)
- Evidence of ventilatory muscle weakness requiring ventilatory support.

Bi-level Positive Airway Pressure, or Bi-level Pressure-Assist (BiPAP)

Bi-level positive airway pressure is similar to CPAP in that they both provide positive pressure during inspiration and expiration. With CPAP, the pressure tends to stay at a fairly constant baseline with a slightly negative pressure as the patient breathes in and a slightly positive pressure as the patient breathes out (see Figure 11-49). With bi-level positive airway pressure, **inspiratory positive airway pressure (IPAP)** is usually higher than **expiratory positive airway pressure (EPAP)** (Figure 11-63).

This form of patient ventilatory assistance is called several names including bi-level positive airway pressure, **bi-level pressure-assist,** bi-level PEEP, bi-level CPAP, bi-level positive pressure, and **bi-level pressure-support.** One of the original units manufactured is the Respironics BiPAP S/T. The term **BiPAP,** although a brand name for this unit, has become the popular term used by clinicians to describe this method of ventilation.

BiPAP via a nasal or a face mask is most commonly used to treat obstructive sleep apnea. Units that provide BiPAP generate a high gas flow through a microprocessor-controlled valve. Operator controls for both IPAP and EPAP are present. Inspiration is normally patient-triggered, but it can be time-triggered when a rate control is provided.

CLINICAL ROUNDS 11-8

If the algorithm (computer program) that controls the ventilator's function determines the cycling time in PSV, then how would you argue that this breath is classified as a spontaneous breath? Isn't the ventilator determining cycling time and not the patient?

See Appendix A for the answer

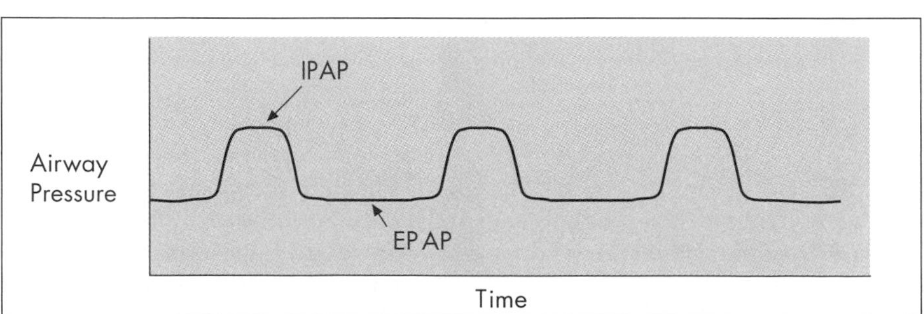

Figure 11-63 Bi-level positive airway pressure (BiPAP) showing inspiratory positive airway pressure (IPAP) and expiratory positive airway pressure (EPAP). Note that both pressures are higher than a zero baseline pressure. (From Pilbeam SP: *Mechanical ventilation: physiological and clinical applications*, ed 3, St Louis, 1998, Mosby.)

BiPAP units can be flow- or time-cycled. Hospitals also use these units for noninvasive positive-pressure ventilation (NIPPV) for patients who do not necessarily require intubation. Chapter 14 provides more detail about the BiPAP S/T and other devices that can provide bi-level pressure support and noninvasive ventilation.

Most BiPAP units also provide leak compensation. The normal interface between the unit and the patient is a mask, and because masks commonly have leaks around them, these units can measure flow to the patient and flow from the patient. If a discrepancy exists between these flows (i.e., a leak), the unit can determine the amount of leak and increase its output to compensate. It can continue its normal triggering and cycling, even with a small leak.

Inverse Ratio Ventilation

In the early 1970s, Reynolds reported success using mechanical ventilation in infants when the inspiratory phase exceeded the expiratory phase, using an inspiratory hold.[26,27] Since then, much more extensive use of inverse ratios has occurred both in infants and adults. The primary purpose of this technique was for treatment of acute respiratory distress syndrome (ARDS). By extending inspiratory time, mean airway pressure is increased and oxygenation can be improved. Sometimes air-trapping (auto-PEEP) occurs, which increases the functional residual capacity of the lung. The occurrence of auto-PEEP in this instance can keep alveoli open that would otherwise collapse on exhalation.

Box 11-21 Interrelation Among Tidal Volume, Flow Rate, Inspiratory Time, Expiratory Time, Total Cycle Time, and Respiratory Rate

Calculating total cycle time (TCT)

Total cycle time equals inspiratory time (T_I) plus expiratory time (T_E)

$$TCT = T_I + T_E$$

Example: If T_I = 1 second and T_E = 2 seconds, TCT = 3 seconds

Calculating respiratory rate

Respiratory rate (f) equals 1 min (60 sec) divided by total cycle time (TCT)

$$f = \frac{(1\ \text{min})}{TCT} = \frac{60\ \text{seconds}}{TCT\ (\text{seconds})} = \text{breaths/min}$$

Example: If TCT = 3 seconds, $f = \frac{60\ \text{seconds}}{3\ \text{seconds}} = 20$ breaths/min

Calculate TCT from f.

$$TCT = \frac{(60\ \text{sec})}{f}$$

Example: If rate = 20 breaths/min, $TCT = \frac{60\ \text{sec}}{(20\ \text{breaths/min})}$,

$$TCT = \frac{60\ \text{sec}}{(20\ \text{breaths}/60\ \text{sec})} \text{ and } TCT = 3 \text{ seconds}$$

Calculate T_E from TCT and T_I. Because TCT = T_I + T_E, then T_E = TCT - T_I

Example: if T_I = 1 second and TCT = 3 seconds, T_E = 3 sec - 1 sec

And, T_E = 2 sec.

Calculate T_I from TCT and T_E. Because TCT = T_I + T_E, then T_I = TCT - T_E

Example: if T_E = 2 second and TCT = 3 seconds, T_I = 3 sec - 2 sec

And, T_I = 2 sec.

Calculate T_E from f and T_I.

$$T_E = \left[\frac{60\ \text{sec}}{f}\right] - T_I$$

Which is the same as T_E = TCT - T_I, because $TCT = \frac{60\ \text{sec}}{f}$

Example: If rate is 10 breaths/min and T_I is 1.5 seconds, T_E will be

$$T_E = \left[\frac{60\ \text{sec}}{f}\right] - T_I, \text{ and } T_E = \left[\frac{60\ \text{sec}}{10}\right] - 1.5\ \text{sec} = 6\ \text{sec} - 1.5\ \text{sec}$$

And, T_E = 4.5 sec.

Reducing the I:E ratio to its simplest form, divide the numerators by T_I.

$$\text{I:E ratio} = \frac{T_I}{T_I} : \frac{T_E}{T_I}$$

Example: T_I = 2 seconds and T_E = 4 seconds

$$\text{I:E ratio} = \frac{T_I}{T_I} : \frac{T_E}{T_I} = \frac{2\ \text{seconds}}{2\ \text{seconds}} : \frac{4\ \text{seconds}}{2\ \text{seconds}} = 1:2$$

Inverse ratio ventilation equals the division of both the numerators by T_E.

$$\text{I:E ratio} = \frac{T_I}{T_E} : \frac{T_E}{T_E}$$

Example: T_I = 4 seconds and T_E = 2 seconds

$$\text{I:E ratio} = \frac{T_I}{T_I} : \frac{T_E}{T_I} = \frac{4\ \text{seconds}}{2\ \text{seconds}} : \frac{2\ \text{seconds}}{2\ \text{seconds}} = 2:1$$

Calculate T_I from V_T and flow rate ($\dot{V}$)

$$T_I = V_T/\dot{V}$$

Example: V_T = 500 mL (0.5 L) and flow = 60 L/min = 60 L/60 sec = 1 L/sec

T_I = 0.5 L/(1 L/sec) and T_I = 0.5 sec

Calculate V_T from T_I and $\dot{V}$

$$V_T = \dot{V} \times T_I$$

Example: $\dot{V}$ = 60 L/min = 1 L/sec and T_I = 0.5 sec

V_T = (1 L/sec) $\times$ 0.5 sec, V_T = 0.5 L or 500 mL

Calculate $\dot{V}$ from V_T and T_I.

$$\dot{V} = V_T/T_I$$

Example: If V_T = 500 mL (0.5 L) and T_I = 0.5 sec

Then $\dot{V}$ = 0.5 L/0.5 sec = 1 L/sec

Or 60 L/min

From Pilbeam SP: *Mechanical ventilation: physiological and clinical applications*, ed 3, St Louis, 1998, Mosby.

Auto-PEEP should be monitored and measured along with the PEEP levels selected by the operator so that alveolar pressures do not exceed 30 cm H_2O. Levels above this value are known to be damaging to the lungs of a variety of experimental animals. Even though the clinical studies on humans are limited, the recommendation is that pulmonary pressures be kept lower than 30 cm H_2O rather than risk potential lung injury.[28-29]

PCIRV and VCIRV

Inverse ratio ventilation can be performed using either pressure ventilation (**pressure-controlled inverse ratio ventilation [PCIRV]**) or **volume ventilation (volume-controlled inverse ratio ventilation [VCIRV])**. When inspiration is time-cycled, inspiratory time is extended and expiratory time shortened, assuming the ventilator can accommodate these settings. ICU ventilators are normally time-cycled when pressure-controlled ventilation is used. However, not all units have controls for inspiratory time during volume ventilation. To extend the inspiratory time, the operator can reduce flow rates, use a descending ramp waveform, which extends T_I in non-time—cycled volume ventilation, or use an inspiratory pause. Box 11-21 provides a list of equations describing the relationship among inspiratory time, expiratory time, I:E ratio, flow, respiratory rate, and volume. For a more detailed explanation of the relationship between these parameters, the reader is referred elsewhere.[7,12,20]

Currently, rather than trying to improve oxygenation with inverse ratio ventilation, the emphasis is on ventilating patient's with low lung volumes ($V_T \leq 6$ mL/kg of ideal body weight),[28,29] finding an optimum PEEP level, and preventing alveoli from collapsing and reexpanding.[30] These strategies are designed to reduce lung injury and improve oxygenation.

Airway Pressure-Release Ventilation

Airway pressure-release ventilation (APRV) provides two levels of CPAP and allows for spontaneous breathing at both levels. This mode was originally invented by Drs. Christine Stock and Jay Block in the late 1980s.[31] APRV is available on such ventilators as the Dräger E 4. The Viasys Avea, and the Puritan-Bennett 840. On these other ventilators APRV may be referred by another name. For example, in the Puritan Bennett 840, it is currently called **Bilevel** ventilation.

This mode works even for apneic patients. It is time-triggered, pressure-limited, and time-cycled. Some ventilators even allow patient triggering and cycling. APRV was first introduced as a way of controlling mean airway pressure and improving oxygenation in patients with severe lung injuries, and often employs inverse I:E ratios.[31] Patients are given an elevated baseline pressure that approximates their optimum CPAP level. The baseline pressure is periodically released to a lower level (usually above zero) for a very brief period (about 0.2 to 1.5 sec).[32,33] The high CPAP level increases mean airway pressure to improve oxygenation. The intervals during which pressure briefly drops to a lower CPAP level reduces the patient's functional residual capacity and allows for ventilation (i.e., exhalation of carbon dioxide). As soon as this expiratory period is complete, pressures return to the higher CPAP level (Figure 11-64).

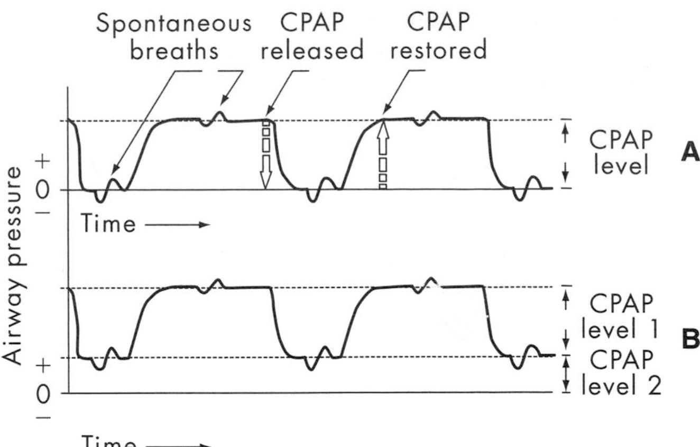

Figure 11-64 Pressure-time curve for airway pressure release ventilation (APRV). **A,** APRV when pressure is released to atmospheric pressure, and **B,** APRV when pressure is released to above atmospheric pressure (CPAP level 2). (Redrawn from Dupuis Y: *Ventilators*, ed 2, St Louis, 1992, Mosby.)

APRV is available on the Dräger Evita, E-4, **Savina**, the Viasys Avea, and the Puritan Bennett 840, but other current and newly developed ICU ventilators will undoubtedly be reprogrammed to make this mode available, if further clinical research supports its benefits.

Servo-Controlled Modes of Ventilation

Intelligent, closed-loop ventilator systems have been available for several decades. The advent of faster computer systems, more sophisticated programming, and higher levels of technology in monitoring have provided for a variety of intelligent systems. Now several forms of closed-loop or servo-controlled modes are available. One such system that has been available since the 1970s is **mandatory minute ventilation (MMV)**, which guarantees delivery of a set minimum minute ventilation ($\dot{V}_E$) and has been used as a method of weaning as well as a method of backing-up ventilation.

Other forms of servo-controlled ventilation sprang from a solution to a problem that clinicians had with pressure-controlled ventilation (PCV). When lung characteristics change during PCV, the volume delivery changes and can affect overall $\dot{V}_E$, acid-base status, and oxygenation. Two closed-loop modes of ventilation were developed and became available in the 1990s to overcome this problem (Historical Note 11-7).

These modes guaranteed volume delivery using pressure target ventilation. One such method guarantees the volume for each breath delivered, and the other guarantees the volume over a several breaths. Thus the benefits of pressure ventilation (i.e., limiting maximum pressure and allowing a more compatible flow pattern and better gas distribution) can still be incorporated while volume is guaranteed. Both methods have also been referred to as **dual control modes of ventilation.**[34] These and other more recently developed modes are described in the following section (Box 11-22). The dual mode available with new generation ventilators is described in Chapter 12 in detail for each ventilator that has this feature.

Mandatory Minute Ventilation

Mandatory (or minimum) minute ventilation (MMV) is a closed loop form of volume or pressure-targeted ventilation used in patients who can perform part of the work of breathing and are progressing toward weaning from mechanical ventilation.[35] MMV guarantees a minimum $\dot{V}_E$, even though the patient's spontaneous ventilation may change. The minimum $\dot{V}_E$ set by the operator in MMV is usually less than the patient's projected spontaneous. When the measured $\dot{V}_E$ falls below a minimum level, the ventilator increases either pressure, rate, or volume to return the ventilator to the minimum $\dot{V}_E$. The Hamilton Veolar is an example of a unit that increases pressure using pressure-support breaths for MMV. The Bear 1000 is an example of a unit that uses rate to adjust MMV during volume ventilation. The Servo 300 has volume support that functions like MMV and increases tidal volume to maintain minute volume. The operator must set high rate and low tidal volume alarms in most units to indicate when the patient's rate rises too high and tidal volume falls too low (Clinical Rounds 11-9), which indicates an increased work of breathing—even if the patient could maintain the desired $\dot{V}_E$ (Table 11-1).

HISTORICAL NOTE 11-7
Volume Ventilation

Historically, in the United States, respiratory therapists and physicians had been trained to set a desired tidal volume and rate for a patient. Consequently, when PCV was first used, clinicians were reluctant to use PCV as a common ventilator mode because they could not guarantee a volume delivery. As a result, researchers and manufacturers struggled to develop ways to use pressure ventilation, which had certain advantages, but to guarantee volume delivery. Thus these "volume-targeted" pressure modes became popular.

Box 11-22 Servo-Controlled Modes of Ventilation

1. Mandatory minute ventilation, as in the Bear 1000, the Hamilton VEOLAR, the Ohmeda Advent, and several others.
2. Pressure-targeted ventilation with volume guaranteed every breath: as in pressure augmentation (Paug) in the Bear 1000 ventilator and volume-assured pressure support (VAPS) in the Bird T-Bird and the Bird 8400STi.
3. Pressure-targeted ventilation with volume guaranteed over several breaths as in pressure-regulated volume control (PRVC) and volume support (VS) in the Servo 300, and Autoflow in the Dräger E-4.
4. Proportional Assist Ventilation (PAV) as a prototype in development (possibly available in the Dräger E-4 upgrade and with other ventilators when upgrades are available).
5. Adaptive Support Ventilation (ASV) in the Hamilton Galileo.

Table 11-1 Constant Minute Ventilation with Changing Alveolar Ventilation

Tidal Volume (mL)	Dead Space (mL)	Respiratory Rate (breaths/min)	Alveolar Ventilation (L/min)	Minute Ventilation (L/min)
800	150	10	6.50	8.0
667	150	12	6.20	8.0
533	150	15	5.75	8.0
400	150	20	5.00	8.0
250	150	32	3.20	8.0

From Pilbeam SP: *Mechanical ventilation: physiological and clinical applications*, ed 3, St Louis, 1998, Mosby.

Assuming a constant anatomic dead space volume of 150 mL, minute ventilation can stay constant while alveolar ventilation decreases, rate increases, and tidal volume falls.

Pressure-Targeted Ventilation with Volume Guaranteed for Every Breath

Pressure augmentation (Paug; Bear 1000 ventilator) and volume-assured pressure-support (VAPS; T-Bird and Bird 8400st) are examples of dual modes that provide **pressure-limited ventilation** with volume guaranteed for every breath. In Paug and VAPS, the patient initiates a breath (patient-triggering), and pressure climbs to a set level. During inspiration, the ventilator monitors V_T delivery. If volume is delivered before flow drops to its set value (value on flow control), then inspiration flow-cycles. If volume is not delivered by the time flow drops to its set value, then flow continues at the amount set on the flow control until the set V_T is delivered. Inspiration then becomes volume-cycled (based on measured flow and time elapsed). Figure 11-65 provides examples of these types of breaths.

> **CLINICAL ROUNDS 11-9**
>
> A patient on MMV has a set minute ventilation of 4 L/min and a measured minute ventilation of 6 L/min (spontaneous V_T = 600 mL; spontaneous rate = 10 breaths/min). Over several hours, the patient's tidal volume drops to 300 mL, and the rate increases to 25 breaths/min. Will the ventilator increase its ventilation delivery to reduce the patient's work of breathing?
>
> See Appendix A for the answer

Pressure-Targeted Ventilation with Volume Guaranteed over Several Breaths

Another dual control mode of ventilation uses patient-triggered (or time-triggered), pressure-limited ventilation and adjusts the pressure level to achieve the volume delivery selected. Examples of ventilators that provide this form of ventilation are the Servo 300, the Servo i, and the Dräger E-4.

In **pressure-regulated volume control (PRVC)** on the Servo 300, and the Viasys Avea breaths are patient- or time-triggered, pressure-limited and time-cycled. The operator sets a maximum safety pressure, a desired V_T and a desired $\dot{V}_E$. The ventilator gives a test breath and calculates system compliance and resistance. The ventilator determines the pressure needed to deliver the set volume. As it ventilates the patient, the ventilator monitors pressure, volume, rate, and minute ventilation. The ventilator adjusts pressure delivery to accomplish volume delivery in increments of 1 to 3 cm H_2O at a time—up to the maximum pressure which equals the set upper pressure limit minus 5 cm H_2O (Servo 300) or to a maximum pressure limit (Viasys Avea). It will go as low as the set baseline (PEEP level). If the volume cannot be delivered within these parameters, the ventilator alarms alert the clinician.

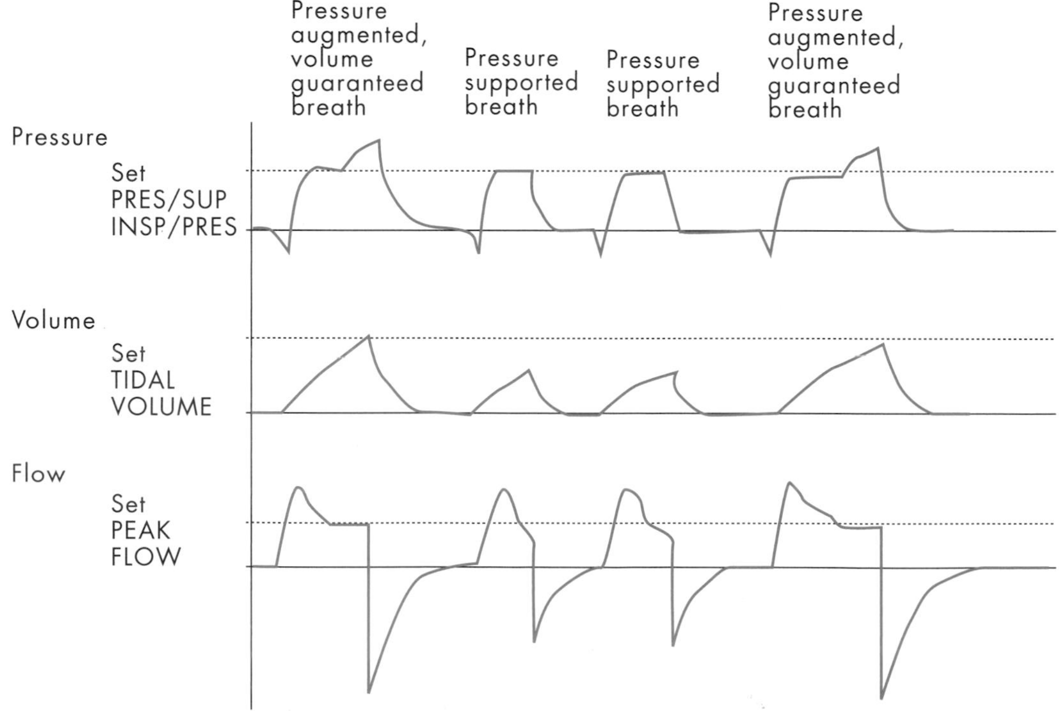

Figure 11-65 Examples of breath delivery in Paug with SIMV plus PSV. Note that the flow curve for a mandatory breath rises rapidly, descends to the set flow value, and remains constant at the set flow until the volume is delivered. For PSV breaths, flow is a descending-ramplike curve and ends when it is about 30% of the peak inspiratory flow rate. (Courtesy Viasys Corp, Yorba Linda, Calif.)

If the patient's respiratory rate declines, a set back-up rate is available. The **autoflow** mode on the Dräger E-4 and the **variable-pressure control (VPC)** mode on Cardiopulmonary Corporation's Venturi ventilator are similar to PRVC on the Servo 300.

Volume support (VS) on the Servo 300 is similar to PRVC, except that there is no back-up rate with volume support. VS is a purely assist mode. VS is patient-triggered, pressure-limited, and flow-cycled, which basically makes it a form of PSV except that volume delivery is guaranteed over a time frame of several breaths. As with PRVC, pressure increases and decreases within the same limits described to maintain V_T. If the patient's respiratory rate drops and the set $\dot{V}_E$ is not being maintained, the Servo 300 increases V_T delivery (up to 150%) in an attempt to achieve the set $\dot{V}_E$. Again, this aspect is similar to MMV. If the patient becomes apneic, the ventilator automatically switches to PRVC, delivers whatever respiratory rate is set, and sounds an alarm to alert the practitioner. The patient may experience difficulty with breath synchrony with VS ventilation.[36,37] The **variable pressure support (VPS)** mode available on Cardiopulmonary Corporation's Venturi ventilator is similar to VS on the Servo 300.

Switching Modes During Ventilation

Closed-loop ventilation has gone a step further. Ventilators can now switch modes based on monitored information. For example, the Servo 300 has a control called **Automode.** When this feature is turned on, the ventilator can switch from a control mode to a support mode and back again based on how the patient is breathing. Suppose the patient is in PRVC with the Automode on. When the ventilator detects two consecutive patient efforts, it determines the patient is able to spontaneously ventilate. It then switches to volume support. If the patient is in the pressure control mode with Automode on, the ventilator can switch to pressure support. In volume control it switches to volume support. In other words, the ventilator is switching from a more supportive breath to a more spontaneous breath, thus allowing the patient to have more control over his or her breathing. This feature is now available on other ventilators although it has a different name. For example, in the Venturi, the ventilator switches from VPC to VPS if the minute ventilation falls too low or, from SIMVpc to CPAP when spontaneous breathing improves. Each of these mode switches is described in more detail in the section on the ventilator in question (Chapter 12).

Proportional Assist Ventilation

Proportional assist ventilation (PAV) is a method of assisting spontaneous ventilation in which the practitioner adjusts the amount of the work of breathing assumed by the ventilator. PAV is an approach to ventilatory support in which pressure, flow, and volume delivery at the airway increase in proportion to the patient's inspiratory effort. PAV augments the underlying breathing pattern of a patient who experiences increased work of breathing associated with worsening lung characteristics (increasing airway resistance [Raw] or decreasing compliance [C]). The more effort the patient exerts during inspiration, the more pressure and flow the machine provides. PAV allows patients to comfortably reach whatever ventilatory pattern suits their needs.[38-40] The operation of PAV is based on the

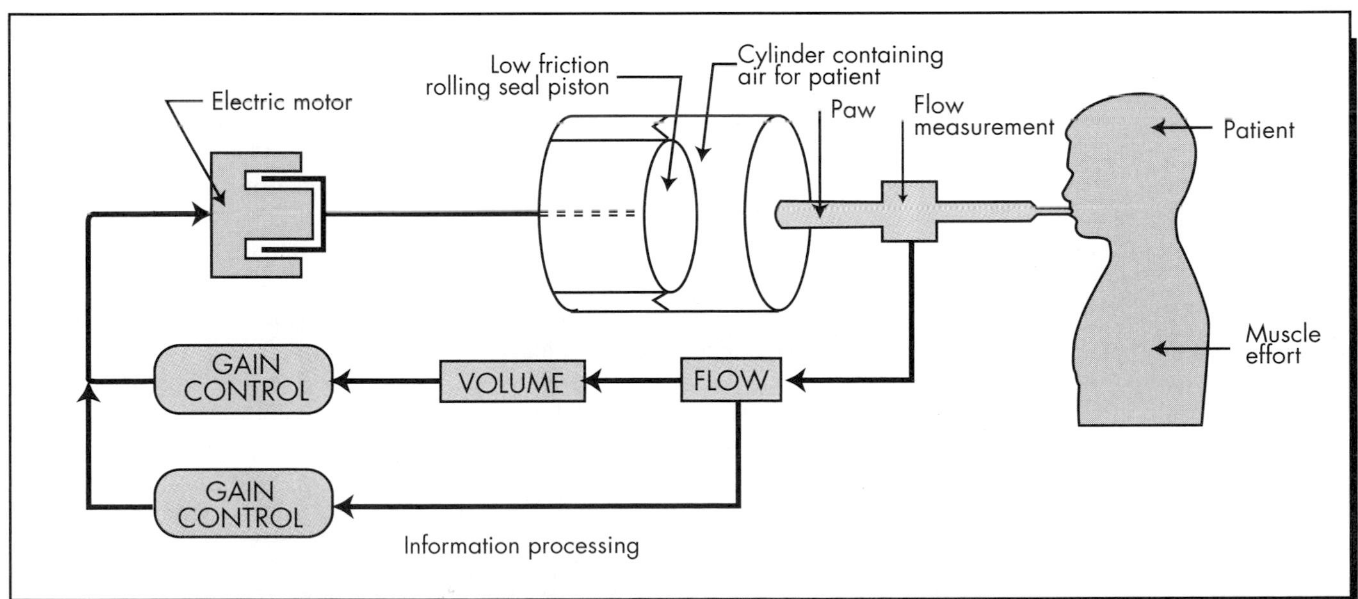

Figure 11-66 Simplified diagram of a PAV-delivery system. A piston is coupled to an electric motor that generates force in proportion to the supplied current. The current is determined by the measured rate of volume delivery and gas flow to the patient. The gain controls are set by the operator and determine what proportion of patient effort will be assisted.

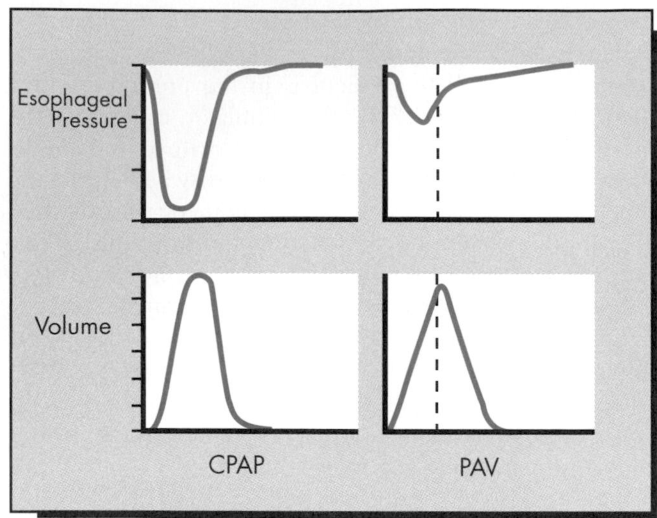

Figure 11-67 Volume and esophageal pressure curves for a CPAP breath and a volume proportional assist breath. (Redrawn from Schulze A, et al: *Am J Respir Crit Care Med* 153:671, 1996.)

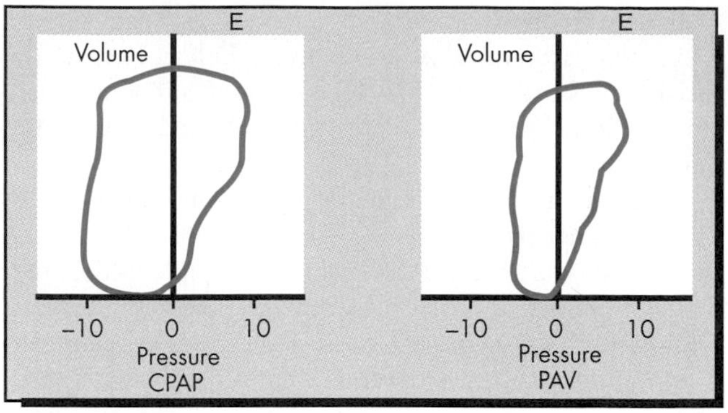

Figure 11-68 Pressure-volume loop changes comparing CPAP with PAV showing inspiration (I) and expiration (E). PAV reduces work of breathing (WOB). Inspiratory WOB is the area within the loop to the left of the vertical axis. Expiratory WOB is the area within the loop to the right of the vertical axis. (Redrawn from Schulze A, et al: *Am J Respir Crit Care Med* 153:671, 1996.)

equation of motion previously described (see Box 11-8). The amount of pressure generated by the patient's own respiratory muscles is used as an index of inspiration effort:

Pmus = (V × e) + (flow × R) − Paw, where Pmus is pressure generated by the respiratory muscles, V is volume, e is elastance (1/compliance), R is resistance, and Paw is airway pressure. Pmus can be calculated when e and R are known. The signal obtained from these variables can be used as a reference for the amount of pressure the ventilator needs to produce.[39]

Figure 11-66 shows an example of a device for delivering proportional assist ventilation. A cylinder, within which a rolling-seal piston moves, is filled with air intended for a patient. The cylinder is connected to the patient by way of an artificial airway. The piston operates on a very low resistance arm connected to an electrically powered motor. When the patient inhales, air moves from the cylinder toward the patient. The piston moves forward to assist the patient's inspiration. The air movement is sensed by a flow-measuring device, which creates flow and volume signals that are sent to a microprocessor. The microprocessor then signals the piston in a positive feedback manner. The greater the patient effort, the greater the piston force. The electric motor supplies current to the piston in proportion to the flow and volume signals. The sum of these two signals determines the amount of electric current going to the motor. A gain control determines how much pressure will be exerted based on where the gain is set. The gain set for the flow determines how much pressure is generated for each unit of flow (cm H_2O/L/sec [i.e., resistance units]). The gain set on the volume signal establishes how much pressure will result for each unit of the volume signal (cm H_2O/L [i.e., elastance units]).[39]

For a better understanding of the concept behind this technique, consider the following example. Suppose a patient is connected by endotracheal tube to a sealed rigid box. When the patient spontaneously inhales, the pressure inside the box decreases in proportion to the volume of air the patient inspires. The pressure drop inside the box represents an increased workload. If the box is replaced with a ventilator that provides instantaneous pressure delivery as soon as the patient breathes in, and does so in proportion to the amount of air inspired, then the ventilator basically "unloads" the amount of work. This response represents "volume" proportional assist. Figure 11-67 compares a patient on CPAP with a patient on volume proportional assist ventilation.[41,42]

Here is another example. A patient is connected by endotracheal tube to a narrow tube. When the patient inspires, pressure in the tube drops. In flow-proportional assist ventilation (flow-PAV) the ventilator increases pressure during inspiration in proportion to the rate of inspiratory flow generated by the patient. The increased pressure delivered by the ventilator has the affect of unloading the work (Figure 11-68).[41,42]

When volume- and flow-proportional assist ventilation are used together, they respond to both the elastance (1/C) and resistance (R) components of breathing and help to unload the work of breathing in proportion to patient effort. The greater the volume and flow demand of the patient, the higher the force (pressure) provided by the ventilator.

For PAV the following settings are established by the operator:

1. Baseline pressure
2. Gain for volume (elastance component)
3. Gain for flow (resistance component)

For example, if gain is set at 50% of the patient's elastance and 50% of the resistance, the ventilator will provide half

Box 11-23 Determining Proportional Assist

Paw = (f1 × volume) + (f2 × flow)

Where

f1 = ventilator supported load of elastance or the amount of volume assist

volume = ventilating volume

f2 = the ventilator support for resistance load or the amount of flow assist

flow = flow during ventilation

Table 11-2 Adaptive-Support Ventilation in the Hamilton Galileo

Parameter	Range
Respiratory rate range	5 to 60 breaths/min
Tidal volume range	4.4 to 22.0 mL/kg
Inspiratory time	0.5 sec (or expiratory time constant [RCe]) to 2 × RCe or 3 seconds

the work performed by the patient required to overcome the forces of elastance and resistance (Box 11-23). If the patient makes no effort, the ventilator does no work. Thus PAV is better suited for patients with abnormalities in resistance and compliance and less so for those with neuromuscular weakness with an inability to generate a strong inspiratory effort.

An example of a ventilator with PAV is the Stephan Medizintechnik's Stephanie Infant Ventilator. This mode may soon be available on ventilators in the United States, such as the Puritan Bennett 840.

Adaptive Support Ventilation in the Hamilton Galileo

Adaptive support ventilation (ASV) is a closed-loop mode of ventilation in which the ventilator determines dynamic compliance ($C_D = V_T/[PIP - PEEP]$) and expiratory time constant (exhaled V_T/peak expiratory flow rate) for the patient and establishes a respiratory rate and V_T delivery based on monitored and set parameters. Its purpose is to target respiratory rate and V_T to establish the least amount of work possible for the patient based on lung characteristics.[43] The clinician sets the following parameters:

1. Patient's IBW and percentage of $\dot{V}_E$ that the operator wants the ventilator to supply
2. Maximum pressure limit and baseline pressure (PEEP)
3. Pressure or flow trigger
4. Rise time (pressure ramp)

When the patient is apneic, breaths are time-triggered, pressure-targeted, and time-cycled. Both respiratory rate and V_T are calculated to establish the optimum $\dot{V}_E$ based on the patient's IBW and lung mechanics. The maximum pressure limit determines the upper limit of pressure delivery.

When the patient can perform some spontaneous breaths, patient-triggered breaths are supported at a calculated pressure using PSV (minimum P = PEEP +5 cm H_2O). The difference between the actual number of spontaneous breaths and the calculated number established by the ventilator equals the number of mandatory breaths delivered.

In spontaneously breathing patients with an adequate spontaneous rate, the ventilator adjusts pressure delivery to keep patients in the optimal calculated range for rate and V_T. The ranges for respiratory variables in ASV are presented in Table 11-2. Chapter 12 provides a more in-depth discussion of ASV and the Hamilton Galileo ventilator.

Similar modes are being rapidly designed with the development of each new ventilator. Readers are advised to read about the specific ventilator they plan on using in Chapter 12 to learn more details about the newer closed-loop modes in use with each unit.

High-Frequency Ventilation[44-47]

HFV is a technique of ventilation rather than a mode. It uses respiratory rates higher than normal and tidal volumes lower than normal. The Food and Drug Administration defines high-frequency ventilation as any form of mechanical ventilation in which respiratory rates are greater than 150 breaths/min. Five basic types of HFV are available:

1. High-frequency positive-pressure ventilation (HFPPV)
2. High-frequency jet ventilation (HFJV)
3. High-frequency oscillatory ventilation (HFOV)
4. High-frequency flow interruption (HFFI)
5. High-frequency percussive ventilation (HFPV)

For particularly high rates, frequencies are usually given in Hertz (Hz) or cycles per second, with 1 Hz equaling 60 cycles (breaths)/min

High-Frequency Positive-Pressure Ventilation

HFPPV uses a conventional volume- or pressure-limited ventilator with a low compliance patient circuit. With HFPPV, the airway is intermittently pressurized with gas with no air entrainment. Respiratory rates are about 60 to 110 breaths/min. Breath rates are sometimes given in Hertz (1 Hz = 1 cycle/sec). In this case 60 to 100 breaths/min would be 1.0 to 1.8 Hz, respectively. HFPPV was developed by Sjöstrand and associates in the late 1960s to minimize the cardiovascular side effects of positive-pressure ventilation.[45]

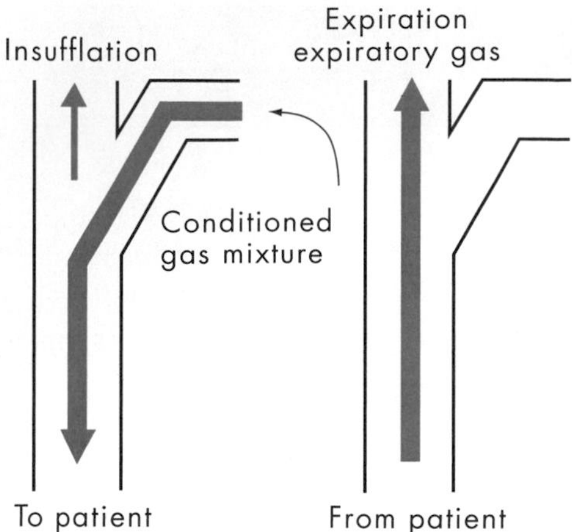

Figure 11-69 This pneumatic valve assembly used with HFPPV introduces a gas mixture during inspiration. Because of the Coanda effect, the gas stream hugs the channel. No air entrainment occurs, and only a small amount of gas leaks from the expiratory limb. (From Pilbeam SP: *Mechanical ventilation: physiological and clinical applications*, ed 1, St Louis, 1986, Mosby.)

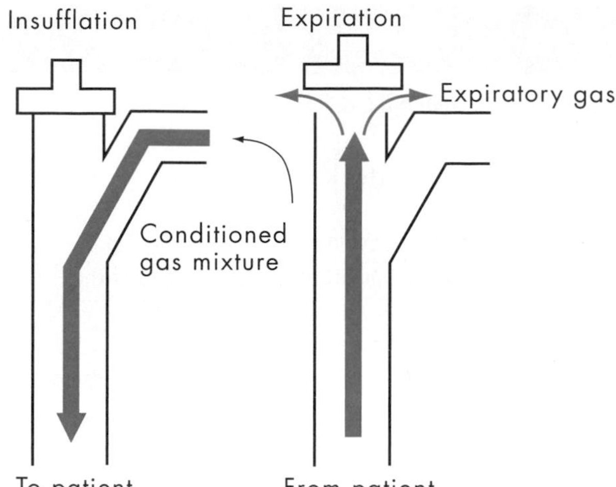

Figure 11-70 A modification of the H-valve for HFPPV uses an expiratory valve that closes during inspiration to prevent gas leaking. (From Pilbeam SP: *Mechanical ventilation: physiological and clinical applications*, ed 1, St Louis, 1986, Mosby.)

Animal studies also showed its effectiveness in eliminating intracranial pressure variations normally associated with breathing, thus providing a better surgical field for microneurosurgical procedures.

Early prototypes used an H-valve assembly in which the circuit was connected to an insufflation catheter attached to the endotracheal tube. The catheter was fitted with either a pneumatic (fluidic) valve (Figure 11-69) or a rapidly responding exhalation valve (Figure 11-70).

Two possible problems could occur with the use of HFPPV. One, the short inspiratory times and high rates could prevent adequate V_T delivery. Breath stacking could occur with these rates as only passive exhalation occurred.[48-49] That is, when respiratory rates are this rapid, sometimes the air has enough time to enter the lungs but not enough to leave. Breaths begin to "stack up" in the lungs, resulting in trapped air, which creates pressure called auto-PEEP. With other modes of HFV now becoming more popular and the use of other techniques for the management of acute lung injury (e.g., permissive hypercapnia and open lung ventilation),[20] HFPPV is not often used clinically.

High-Frequency Jet Ventilation

In 1977 Klain and Smith developed a method of HFJV that used a percutaneous transtracheal catheter. The catheter was connected to an air source that provided a jet injection of air controlled by a fluidic logic ventilator. Rates up to 600 breaths/min (10 Hz) were employed. Later this technique used a catheter that allowed for air entrainment.[47]

This technique offers rates of about 100 to 600 breaths/min (1.7 to 10 Hz, respectively) with V_T smaller than anatomic dead space volume. Historical Note 11-8 lists some of the earlier uses of HFJV. In general, HFJV operates by passing gas from a high pressure source through a variable regulator that reduces the pressure to the desired working level. The gas then passes through a device, usually a solenoid or a fluidic valve, which governs the amount and duration of flow. The gas jet is then delivered through a specially made triple-lumen endotracheal tube (Figure 11-71, *A*), which is similar to conventional endotracheal tubes except that two additional small lines are added. One is for delivering jet ventilation and the other is for monitoring distal airway pressures. The jet stream exits the tube at about one third of the tube's length from the distal end. The pressure tube is located at the distal tip of the tube. If a jet tube is not used, a special jet adapter can be attached to the endotracheal tube (Figure 11-71, *B*). Another technique to use when a special jet tube is not in place is to use a small catheter inserted either through a conventional endotracheal or tracheostomy tube. Studies have shown that the best position for the jet is close to the proximal end of the trachea near the vocal cords.[48]

HISTORICAL NOTE 11-8
Early Uses of HFJV

1. To provide surgical fields undisturbed by ventilatory movement.
2. For use with bronchoscopy and laryngoscopy to provide better surgical field access while maintaining ventilation.
3. To reduce cardiovascular side effects associated with IPPV.
4. To reduce the risk of barotrauma.
5. To maintain ventilation when large air leaks are present (e.g., bronchopleural fistula).

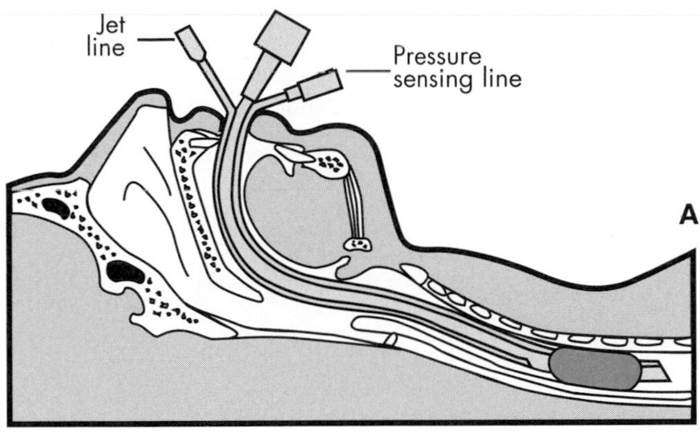

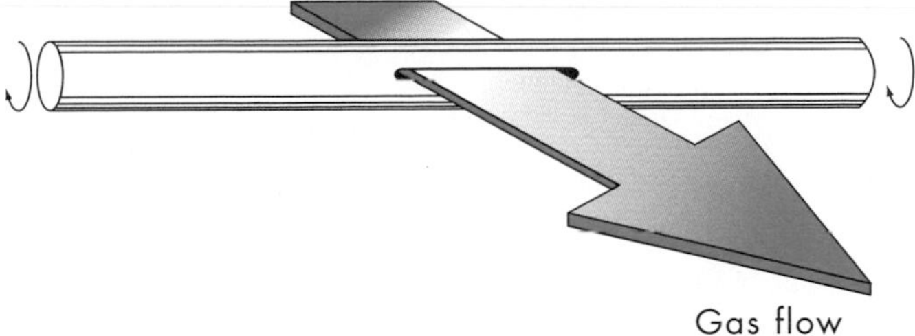

Figure 11-72 A flow interrupter. Flow is interrupted at high frequencies as a rotating metal bar allows flow to pass through during some portions of the breath and blocks it at others. (From Pilbeam SP: *Mechanical ventilation: physiological and clinical applications*, ed 1, St Louis, 1986, Mosby.)

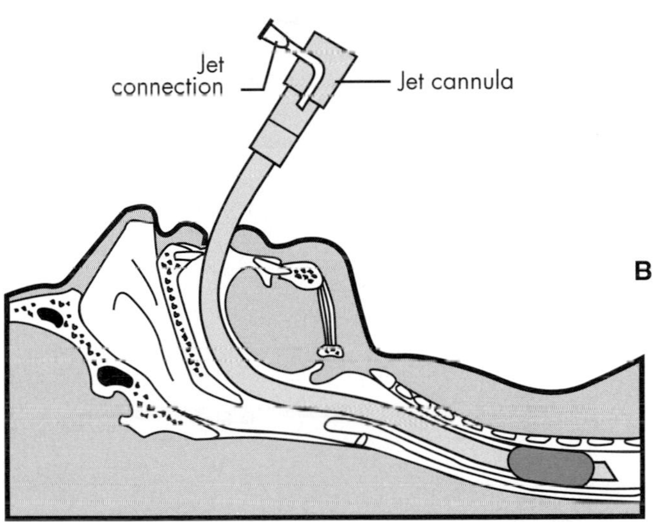

Figure 11-71 Diagram of an endotracheal tube used in high frequency jet ventilation **(A)** and a jet connection with a jet cannula attached to a standard endotracheal tube **(B).**

The operational principle of HFJV involves the delivery of short breaths or pulsations (20 to 34 ms) under pressure through a small lumen at high rates (4 to 11 Hz).[48] The tidal volume of the breath depends on the following four basic factors:

1. Length of the pulsation
2. Amplitude or driving pressure of the jet
3. Jet orifice size
4. Patient lung characteristics

Under certain conditions, gas can be entrained around the jet through the physical process of jet mixing. It results from the viscous shearing of the jet gas layer with stagnant gas in the airway. This gas is dragged downstream in an entrainment-like effect. The volume of entrained gas can alter V_T delivery depending on patient lung characteristics.[44] Examples of jet ventilators include the Bunnell's Life Pulse and the Adult Star 1010.

High-Frequency Oscillatory Ventilation

HFOV uses some type of reciprocating pump to generate an approximation of a sine wave (Figures 11-3 and 13-37). Examples of devices that provide this function are reciprocating pumps (usually pistons), diaphragms, and loudspeakers. Although not true oscillators, high-frequency flow interrupters (HFFIs), discussed in the following section, can be used in ventilators to provide a similar effect. These ventilators are called "pseudo-oscillators."

With HFOV pressure is positive in the airway during the inspiratory phase (forward stroke) and negative during the expiratory phase (return stroke). Thus both inspiration and expiration are active, and bulk flow rather than jet pulsations is produced. HFOV uses frequencies in the range of 1 to 50 Hz (60 to 3000 cycles/min), and V_T is less the anatomic dead space volume. Some ventilators have a fixed I:E ratio, and others allow the I:E ratio to be adjusted.

HFOV is one of the most widely used forms of HFV in infants and pediatric patients. One example of an oscillator is the Sensormedics 3100A from Viasys Critical Care (Yorba Linda, Calif) (Chapter 13). The 3100A uses a diaphragm-shaped piston that is driven magnetically, much like a stereo speaker (see Figure 13-38). The mean airway pressure control sets the tension on the diaphragm. Gas is oscillated back and forth by the action of the diaphragm. The amplitude of the wave set by the power control determines the forward and backward excursion of the piston, which helps determine V_T. In the 3100A, rigid plastic circuits provide the bias flow of warmed and humidified air that is delivered to the patient.

High-Frequency Flow Interruption

HFFI is similar to HFJV, but differs in its technical design. In HFFI a control mechanism interrupts a high-pressure gas source. One common mechanism is a rotating ball with a flow port in the center. Another example is a rotating bar with a slit through its center (Figure 11-72). Frequencies with HFFI are as high as 15 Hz. As in HFJV, the high pressure bursts of gas can entrain static gas supplied by the

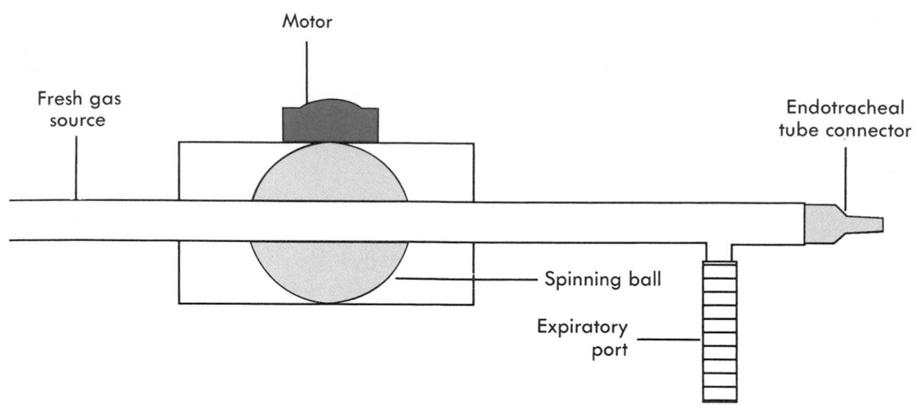

Figure 11-73 Example of a high-frequency oscillatory device, the spinning ball.

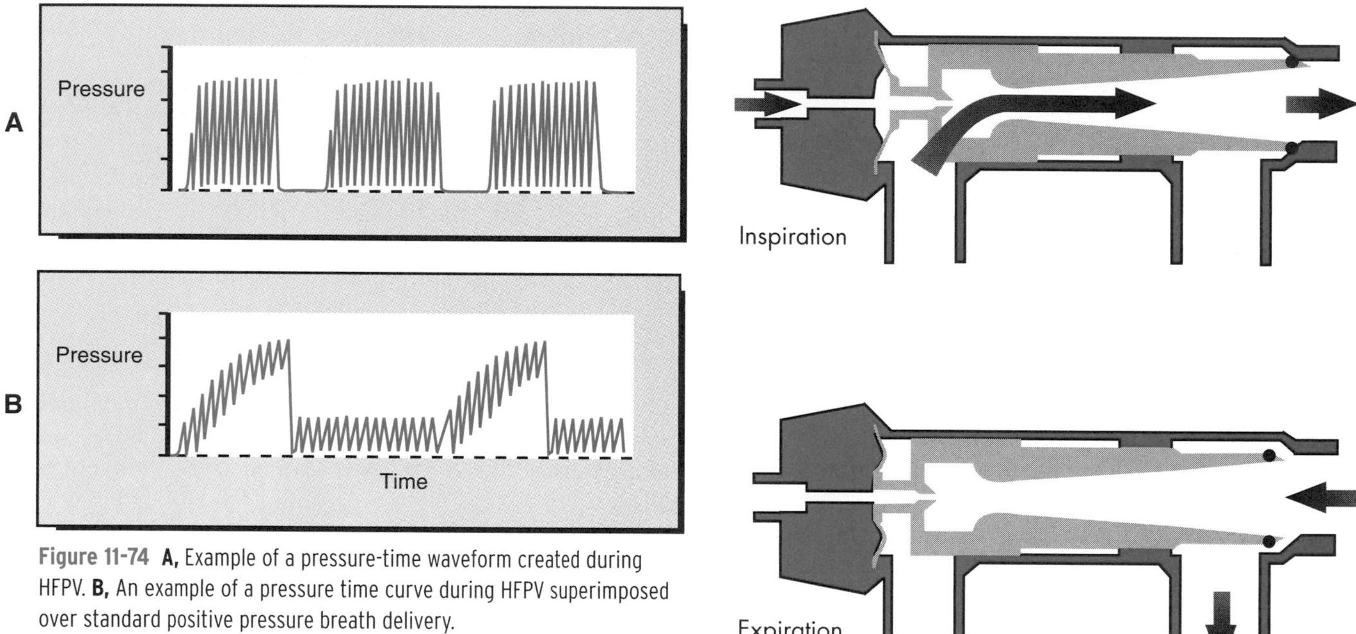

Figure 11-74 **A,** Example of a pressure-time waveform created during HFPV. **B,** An example of a pressure time curve during HFPV superimposed over standard positive pressure breath delivery.

Figure 11-75 Design of the sliding venturi for a high-frequency percussive generator used to provide HFPV. (See text for explanation.) (From Pilbeam SP: *Mechanical ventilation: physiological and clinical applications,* ed 3, St Louis, 1998, Mosby.)

addition of a bias flow circuit, which enhances volume delivery. An example of this device was invented by Emerson, whose HFFI uses a spinning ball and consists of a conduit that conducts a gas flow. Inside the conduit is a ball with a flow port in its center. The ball is moved back and forth in the conduit by an electric motor at rates up to 200 cycles/min. As it moves, the ball interrupts the outflow of gas (Figure 11-73).[44] An example of a HFFI (a pseudo-oscillator) is the Infant Star ventilator (see Chapter 13).

High-Frequency Percussive Ventilation

Dr. Forrest M. Bird, a pioneer in ventilatory devices, designed a high-frequency percussive ventilation device in which he incorporated the beneficial characteristics of both a conventional positive-pressure ventilator and a jet ventilator. It operates in such a way that high-frequency breaths can be provided at ambient pressures. Figure 11-74, *A*, shows the rapid pressure waves representing high frequency pulses with pauses following where these pulses are interrupted. High-frequency pulses can also be superimposed onto conventional positive pressure breaths. In this case the pulses would still occur but the baseline would rise as a positive pressure breath was delivered (Figure 11-74, *B*). These can be compared with time-cycled, pressure-limited ventilation when high-frequency pulsations (up to 100 to 225 cycles/min, or 1.7 to 5.0 Hz) are injected throughout the inspiratory phase. The resulting unit is called a high-frequency percussive ventilator.

A ventilator that incorporates this principle is the Bird VDR-4, which operates using a sliding venturi (Figure 11-75).

At the mouth of the venturi is a jet orifice. Around the jet is a continuous bias flow of warm, humidified air. During inspiration, a diaphragm connected to the venturi fills with gas. This action slides the venturi forward, toward the patient's airway, simultaneously blocking the expiratory port. During this time, the jet is activated and begins delivering short pulses of gas. At the same time, a large amount of air is entrained through the now open inspiratory ports, so that flow to the patient is high. The large gas flow is due to the pressure gradient between the jet and the patient connector. As inspiration progresses and pressure builds in the patient's airway, this gradient is reduced. Therefore, flow is reduced. However, the jet pulsations continue throughout inspiration. When the set inspiratory time is reached, inspiration ends. The diaphragm is no longer pressurized, and the venturi slides back away from the patient, opening the expiratory port. During exhalation, a counterflow of gas is directed at the airway to maintain the set PEEP level.[44]

Ventilation is controlled by respiratory rate and peak airway pressure. Oxygenation is determined by PEEP level, inspiratory time, I:E ratio, and peak airway pressure. The high-frequency pressure oscillations also affect gas exchange, which makes clinical monitoring of these variables an important part of frequency adjustments.

Clinical benefits of HFPV may include facilitation of secretion removal, as well as provision of a mode of continuous ventilation. HFPV has been used prophylactically in patients with thermal airway injury to help prevent pneumonia and atelectasis.[48]

Mechanisms of Action of HFV

The mechanisms of action of the various forms of HFV are not clearly understood; however, ventilation successfully occurs even when V_T is less than a patient's anatomic dead space volume (V_D). Alveoli located close to the airways are thought to be ventilated by convection, just as in conventional ventilation.* The following additional mechanisms may be responsible:

1. Pendelluft
2. Gas streaming or helical diffusion
3. Taylor dispersion
4. Molecular diffusion
5. Spike formation

Pendelluft is the movement of gases from one area of the lungs to another resulting from differences in the compliance and resistance of various lung regions. It is also called out-of-phase ventilation. This movement occurs through normal anatomic channels (e.g., alveolar ducts, the pores of Kohn, the canals of Lambert). When lung tissue is oscillated, as occurs with HFV, this phenomenon may be enhanced.

Convection is the movement of air molecules associated with the pressures of ventilation.

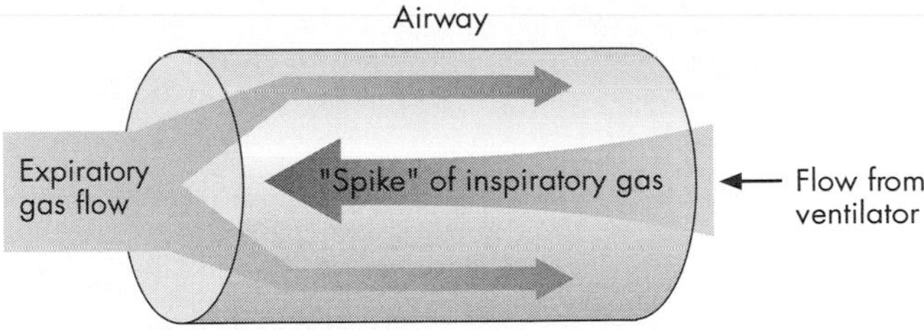

Figure 11-76 Effects of streaming in HFJV: forward movement of the gas in the center produced by pulsations from the jet causes gas along the airway walls to be pushed backward. (From Pilbeam SP: *Mechanical ventilation: physiological and clinical applications*, ed 3, St Louis, 1998, Mosby.)

Streaming or asymmetric velocity profiles occur when gas flows in both directions at once through a conductive airway. Inspired gas is believed to move into the lungs down the center of the airways in a parabolic fashion, while exhaled gas tends to move near the walls and out of the lungs (Figure 11-76). This wall air movement may occur in a helical fashion and has been called helical diffusion.

Taylor dispersion is thought to occur in HFOV. It is the enhanced mixing of gases associated with the turbulent flow of high velocity gases moving through small airways and their bifurcations. Taylor dispersion can occur where two gas streams meet. The erratic pattern of eddies and streams created is thought to enhance gas mixing and diffusion.

Simple molecular diffusion also occurs, at least at the terminal air spaces and is another mechanism that adds to gas mixing. It is the result of the random thermal oscillation of molecules.

One theory is that a spike (parabolic shaped front) of high energy wave impulse of gas travels rapidly through the center of the airway like a bullet. This gas movement may provide a larger area of gas mixing in the distal portions of the lungs.[49]

Because HFV is used infrequently in many institutions, and because it has not demonstrated improved outcomes in comparison with conventional ventilation, HFV has not been a dominant technique of ventilatory support of patients. It has, however, gained popularity in some hospitals, especially in the management of infants and children. How important its position will be is still uncertain and depends on not only further clinical research but also increased popularity with a larger group of clinicians.

Part IV: Troubleshooting During Mechanical Ventilation

Ventilator-patient interaction can result in a variety of problems. Some problems are related to equipment malfunction and others to operator error.[50] Some problems develop in the patient or from inadequate adjustment of the ventilator to make it more responsive to patient needs. This section will review alarm situations and solving ventilator problems using graphics.

Ventilator Alarms

A variety of alarms are available with all mechanical ventilators. These alarms can be audible, visible, displayed on screens, or a combination of these. Some can be inactivated by the operator; others cannot. Alarms critical to unit function, such as loss of power (electric or pneumatic) or detection of an internal operational error (technical error), cannot be silenced and require immediate attention. The American Association for Respiratory Care (AARC) has suggested a classification system for the levels of priorities of alarms (Table 11-3). Box 11-24 lists the most common types of alarms available. Appendix 11-1, at the end of this chapter, provides algorithms to help solve common alarm situations.

Identifying and Solving Alarm Situations

Alarms sometimes inform the operator of a potential problem, but the problem still must be solved. Most of the time the solution is easy because the alarm provides a light or message telling the operator the problem that has occurred is currently present. For example, when a ventilator reaches its high pressure limit, it normally provides an audible high-pressure alarm. This alarm sounds only once to signal the event. Most ventilators have a small light that remains lit

Table 11-3 Events and Monitoring Sites for Ventilator Alarms

Event	Possible Monitoring Site
LEVEL 1	
Power failure (including when battery in use)	Electrical control system*
Absence of gas delivery	Circuit pressure,* circuit flows, timing monitor, CO_2 analysis
Loss of gas source	Pneumatic control system*
Excessive gas delivery	Circuit pressures,* circuit flows, timing monitor
Exhalation valve failure	Circuit pressure, circuit flows, timing monitor
Timing failure	Circuit pressures, circuit flows, timing monitor
LEVEL 2	
Battery power loss (not in use)	Electrical control system*
Circuit leak*	Circuit pressure,* circuit flows
Blender failure	F_IO_2 sensor
Circuit partially occluded	Circuit pressures, circuit flows
Heater/humidifier failure	Temperature probe in circuit
Loss of/or excessive PEEP	Circuit pressures
Autocycling	Circuit pressures, circuit flows
Other electrical or preventive subsystem out of limits without immediate overt gas delivery effects	Electrical and pneumatic systems monitor
LEVEL 3	
Change in central nervous system drive	Circuit pressures, circuit flows, timing monitor
Change in impedances	Circuit pressures, circuit flows, timing monitor
Intrinsic PEEP (auto) >5 cm H_2O	Circuit pressures, circuit flows

From AARC consensus statement on the essentials of mechanical ventilation, *Respir Care* 37:1007, 1992.
*Alarms currently defined in the ISO and ASTM standards.

Box 11-24 Common Alarms for Mechanical Ventilators

1. Loss of power (electric or pneumatic)
2. Apnea
3. Pressure alarms: low and high circuit pressure, low and high baseline pressures (PEEP/CPAP), and failure of pressure to return to baseline
4. High and low expired V_T or $\dot{V}_E$
5. Low and high respiratory rate
6. Inappropriate T_I or T_E
7. Inspired temperature alarm
8. High and low F_IO_2 alarms

Box 11-25 Common Causes of Low-Pressure Alarm Situations

Patient disconnect

Circuit leaks
- Mainline connections to humidifiers, filters, or water traps
- In-line metered dose inhalers
- In-line nebulizers
- Proximal pressure monitors
- Flow monitoring lines
- Exhaled gas monitoring devices
- In-line closed suction catheters
- Temperature monitors
- Exhalations valve leaks: cracked or leaking valves, unseated valves, or improperly connected valves

Airway leaks
- Use of minimum leak technique
- Inadequate cuff inflation
- Leak in pilot balloon
- Rupture of tube cuff
- Chest tube leaks

From Pilbeam SP: Mechanical ventilation. In Burton GG, Hodgkin JE, Ward JJ, editors: *Respiratory care: a guide to clinical practice*, ed 4, Philadelphia, 1997, JB Lippincott.

until a manual reset button is activated by the operator. In this way, the ventilator keeps a visual record of the alarm event that the operator can observe even after the alarm has ceased.

Some of the common causes of low- and high-pressure alarms are provided in Boxes 11-25 and 11-26, respectively. Whenever an alarm is activated, the clinician's primary responsibility is to ensure that the patient is being adequately ventilated. Sometimes the solution is immediately obvious. For example, a patient may be disconnected from the ventilator at the Y connector. If this situation is readily seen, it is easily solved by reconnecting the patient. Other times the problem is less obvious. When the problem is not apparent, the most immediate and important solution is to disconnect the patient from the ventilator and perform manual ventilation with a resuscitation bag. If the patient improves, the problem resides with the ventilator. Examples of mechanical problems include leaks, expiratory valve failures, power source failures, inappropriately assembled circuits, I:E ratio problems, and incompatible settings. If the patient does not improve, the problem is with the patient. Patient problems can include airway obstructions, pneumothorax, pulmonary thromboembolism, cardiac problems, and air trapping.

Box 11-26 Common Causes of High-Pressure Alarm Situations

Common causes
- Patient coughing
- Secretions or mucus in the airway
- Patient biting oral endotracheal tube

Airway problems
- Kinking of tube inside the mouth or in the back of the throat
- Impinging of the tube on the carina
- Change in the tube position
- Cuff herniated over the end of the tube

Patient-related conditions
- Reduced compliance (e.g., pneumothorax or pleural effusion)
- Increased airway resistance (e.g., secretions, mucosal edema, or bronchospasm)
- Patient "fighting the ventilator" (e.g., dyssynchrony with ventilator settings)

Ventilator circuit
- Accumulation of water in the patient circuit
- Kinking in the circuit
- Ventilator's inspiratory or expiratory valves malfunctioning

From Pilbeam SP: Mechanical ventilation. In Burton GG, Hodgkin JE, Ward JJ, editors: *Respiratory care: a guide to clinical practice*, ed 4, Philadelphia, 1997, JB Lippincott.

Troubleshooting Problems Using Ventilator Graphics

Clinicians can rely on ventilator alarms, changes in patients' signs and symptoms, and changes in ventilator data to help solve problems and alarm situations. In the last few years, ventilator graphic display screens have become more widely available and are another tool for evaluating and determining problems. Although it is beyond the scope of this text to cover all the possible graphic changes that can help determine problems, the most common methods of identifying these problems will be reviewed.[7]

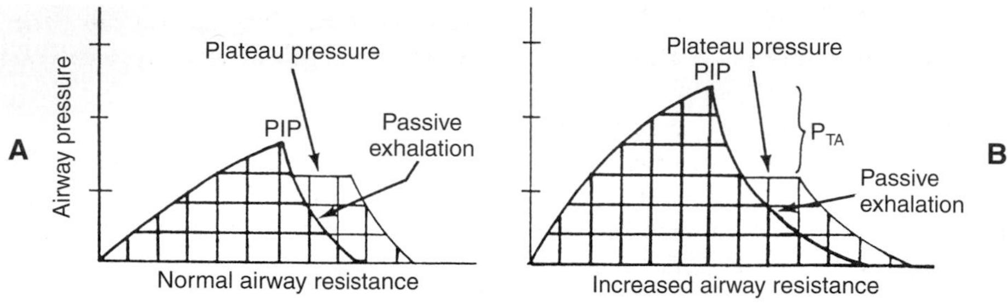

Figure 11-77 **A,** Normal pressure difference between peak inspiratory pressure (PIP) and plateau pressure when airway resistance is normal during volume ventilation. When airway resistance is increased, the difference between PIP and plateau pressure is increased (i.e., more pressure is lost to the airways [P_{TA}]). **B,** Note that peak inspiratory pressure is also increased. (From Pilbeam SP: *Mechanical ventilation: physiological and clinical applications*, ed 3, St Louis, 1998, Mosby.)

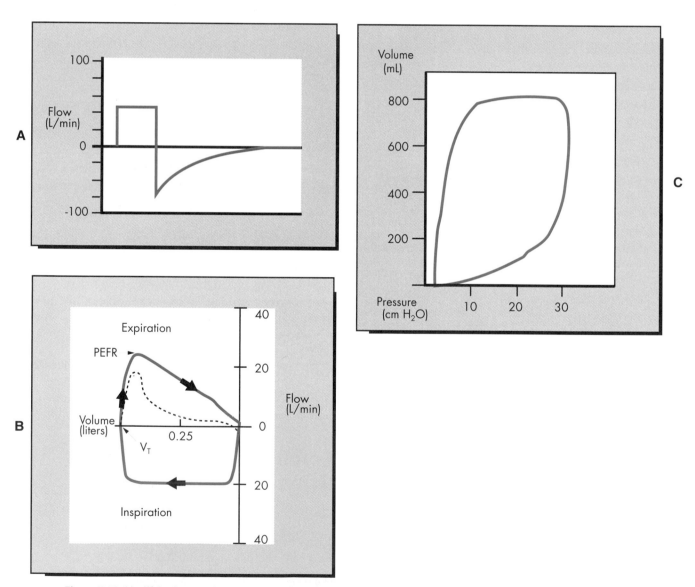

Figure 11-78 Identifying increased Raw with ventilator graphics: **A,** Flow-time curve showing increased length of expiratory flow from the patient. **B,** Flow-volume loop showing normal expiratory flow (solid line) and reduced expiratory flow (dashed line). **C,** Pressure-volume loop showing increased airway resistance with an increase in the hysteresis of the loop (i.e., the loop is has a larger area than normal). (From Pilbeam SP: *Mechanical ventilation: physiological and clinical applications*, ed 3, St Louis, 1998, Mosby.)

Increased Airway Resistance

Figure 11-77 shows the difference between PIP and $P_{plateau}$ increases (increased P_{TA}) as one method of identifying an increase in airway resistance (Raw). In addition, prolonged expiratory flows in a flow-time curve (Figure 11-78, *A*), reduced flows in flow-volume loops (*B*), and an increase in the hysteresis of a pressure-volume loop (*C*) can all help establish the presence of increased airway resistance.

Decreased Compliance

When both PIP and $P_{plateau}$ increase proportionally during volume ventilation, lung compliance is decreased. In this example, P_{TA} will remain the same, indicating that the problem is in the lungs and not the airways. Another way of identifying a reduced compliance is to observe the shift of a pressure-volume loop to the right, (i.e., more pressure is required for a similar volume delivery) (Figure 11-79).

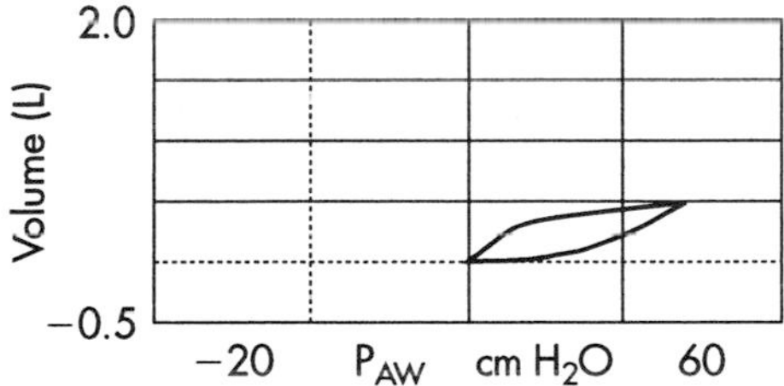

Figure 11-79 Airway pressure-volume loop recorded on a patient with reduced lung compliance. Note the decrease in area (i.e., the loop is narrower), representing nonelastic inspiratory and expiratory work. The curve is "shifted" (i.e., leans) to the right. (Redrawn from Kacmarek RM, Hess D, Stoller JK: *Monitoring in respiratory care*, St Louis, 1993, Mosby.)

Auto-PEEP

Air-trapping or auto-PEEP can be identified when the expiratory flow curve does not return to zero (baseline) before the next breath triggers into inspiration. This event can be seen in the flow-time and the flow-volume loops (Figures 11-53 and 11-80).

Inadequate Flow

When a fixed flow is delivered during volume ventilation, sometimes the amount of flow is inadequate for the patient.

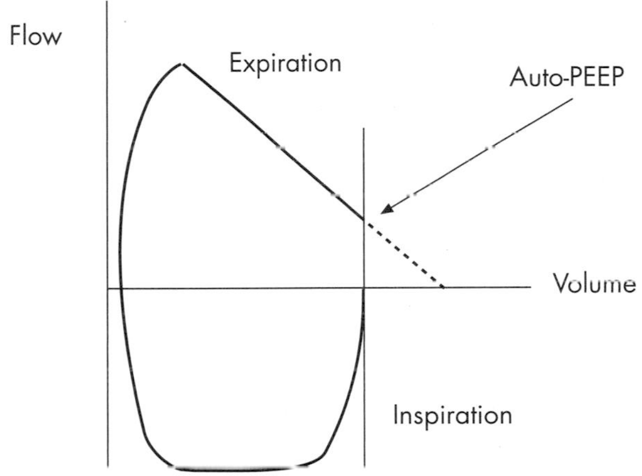

Figure 11-80 Flow-volume loop showing the presence of auto-PEEP. Flow does not return to zero during exhalation.

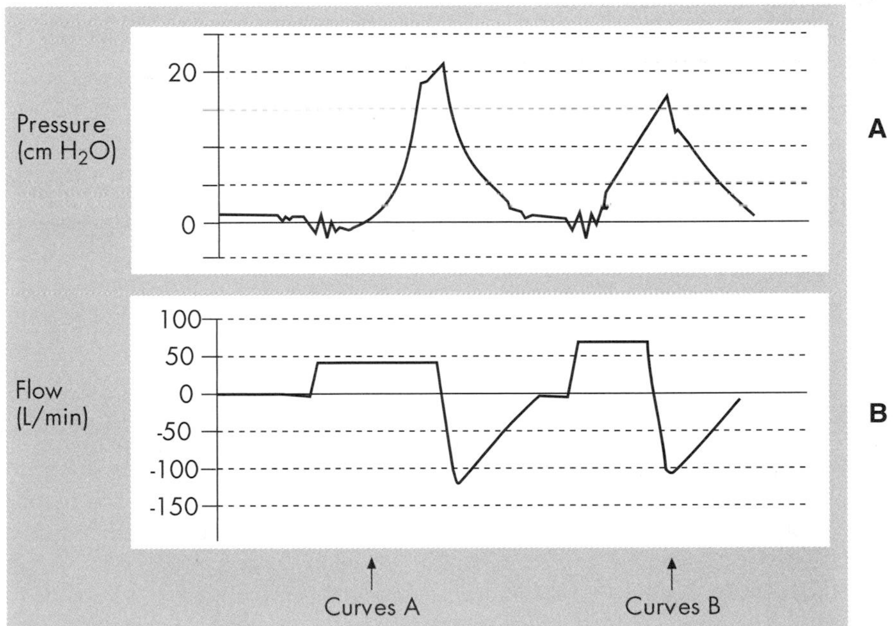

Figure 11-81 These are examples of volume breaths with constant flow delivery. **A,** The flow, which is set at approximately 50 L/min, is too low for patient demand. Note the concave appearance of the pressure curve. **B,** In this curve, flow has been increased to about 75 L/min, and the pressure rise is normal. The erratic pattern of pressure just before the mandatory breath suggests that sensitivity may not be set appropriately. (From Pilbeam SP: *Mechanical ventilation: physiological and clinical applications*, ed 3, St Louis, 1998, Mosby.)

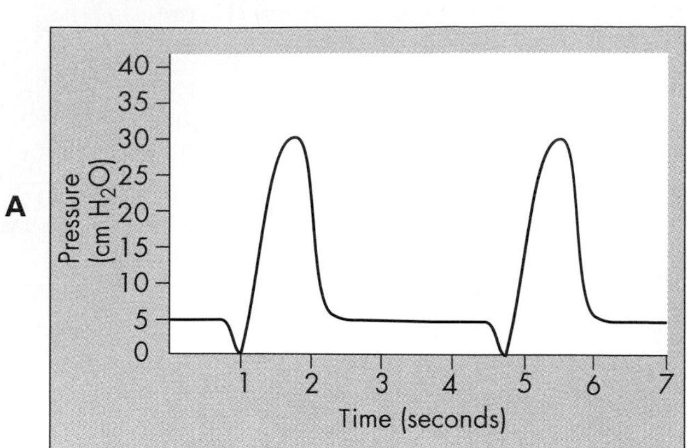

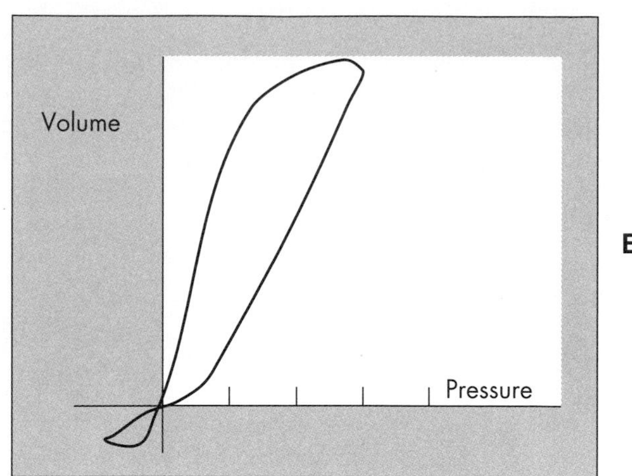

Figure 11-82 Inadequate sensitivity: **A,** pressure drops well below baseline before a breath delivery. In this case, baseline is 5 cm H_2O of PEEP. **B,** Pressure-volume loop showing a deflection to the left on inspiration much higher than normal. (From Pilbeam SP: *Mechanical ventilation: physiological and clinical applications*, ed 3, St Louis, 1998, Mosby.)

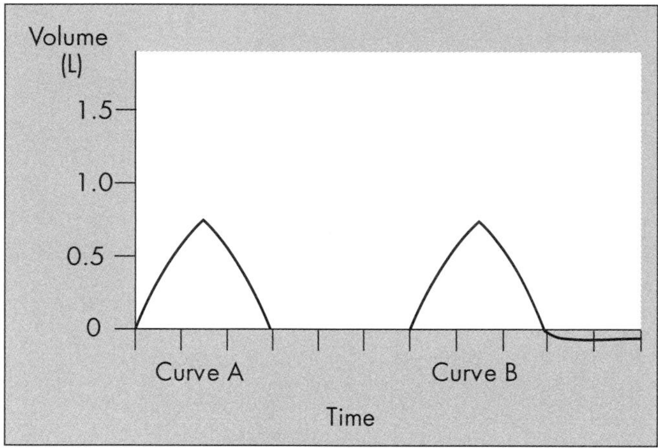

Figure 11-83 Curve *A* is a normal volume-time curve. Curve *B* shows the expiratory portion of the volume below the zero baseline (see text for explanation). (From Pilbeam SP: *Mechanical ventilation: physiological and clinical applications*, ed 3, St Louis, 1998, Mosby.)

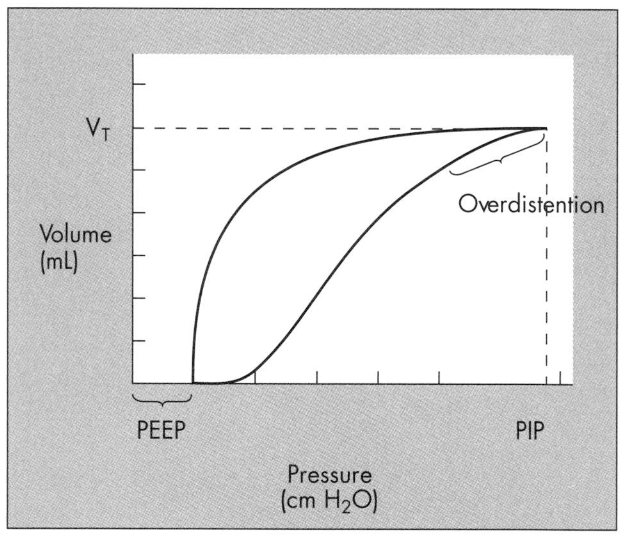

Figure 11-84 Pressure-volume loop in a patient with acute over-distention of the lung during positive-pressure ventilation. Notice the duck-billed appearance of the top, right-hand portion of the curve. This feature signifies over-distention. (From Pilbeam SP: *Mechanical ventilation: physiological and clinical applications*, ed 3, St Louis, 1998, Mosby.)

An inadequate inspiratory flow produces a concave pressure-time curve (Figure 11-81).

Inadequate Sensitivity Setting

If the patient appears to be struggling for a breath and inspiratory pressures are deflecting too far below baseline, then the ventilator is not sensitive enough to patient effort (Figure 11-82). Sometimes sensitivity is set appropriately, but the patient still cannot trigger a breath. This can occur if auto-PEEP is present, making it more difficult for the patient to reduce upper airway pressures low enough to trigger inspiration.

Active Exhalation or Out of Calibration

When a volume-time curve shows expiratory volume going below baseline, two possible problems are suggested. The patient is air trapping and is forcibly exhaling, or the expiratory flow transducer is out of calibration and is recording expiratory flow below the baseline (Figure 11-83).

Overinflation

When a pressure-volume loop shows a sharp, beak-shaped spike to the right (i.e., pressure increases without much or any volume change during volume ventilation), then the patient's lungs are overinflated, or overdistended (Figure 11-84).

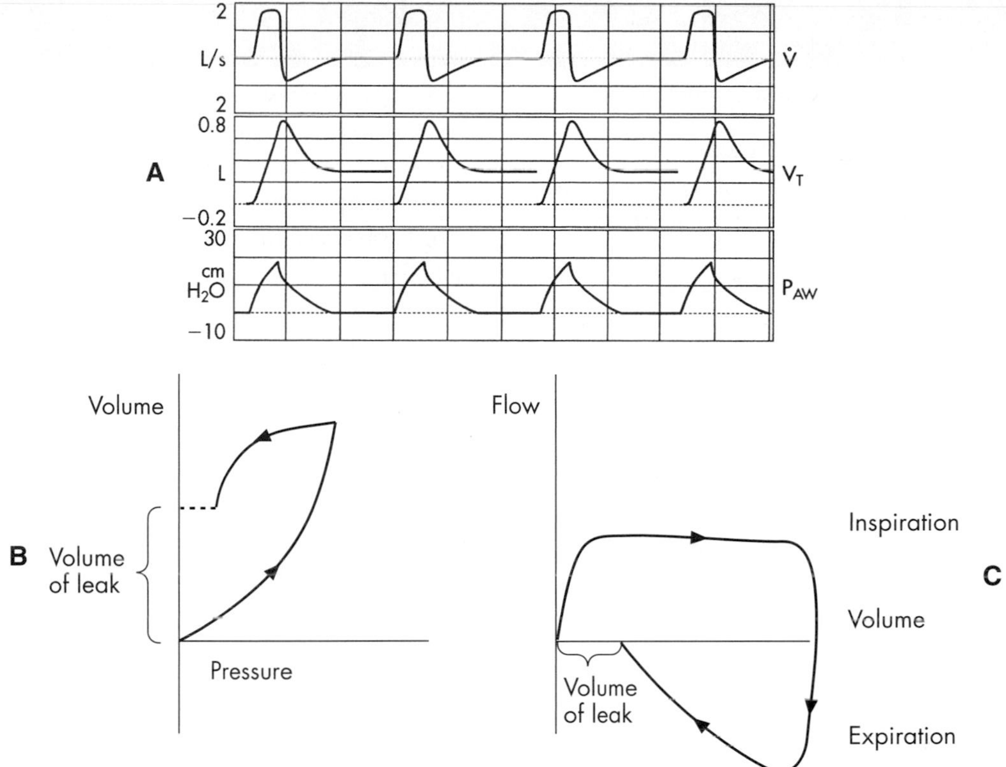

Figure 11-85 **A,** Airway pressure *(Paw)*, tidal volume (V_T), and flow $(\dot{V})$ curves during volume ventilation. Note that the exhaled volume curve does not return to zero. The ventilator's computer returns the volume curve to the baseline at the beginning of the next breath. By measuring the difference between inspired and expired volume, the leak can be quantified. **B,** A pressure-volume loop showing an air leak. **C,** A flow-volume loop showing an air leak. (From Pilbeam SP: *Mechanical ventilation: physiological and clinical applications*, ed 3, St Louis, 1998, Mosby; **A,** Redrawn from Kacmarek RM, Hess D, Stoller JK: *Monitoring in respiratory care*, St Louis, 1993, Mosby.)

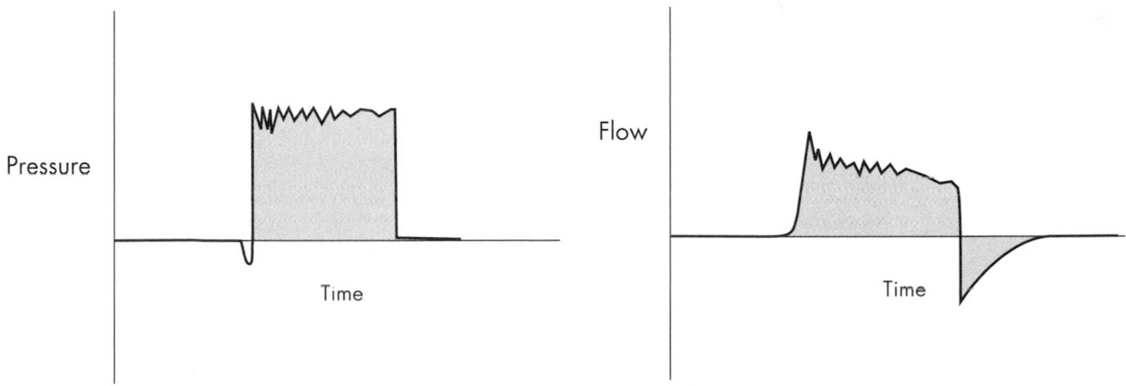

Figure 11-86 Ringing or oscillation in the circuit, occurring when working pressure and airway resistance are high. (See text for further explanation.) (From Pilbeam SP: *Mechanical ventilation: physiological and clinical applications*, ed 3, St Louis, 1998, Mosby.)

Leaks

Leaks in the circuit can be quickly identified when the expiratory volume curve does not return to baseline or zero. This event is true for volume-time curves (Figure 11-85, A), volume-pressure loops *(B)*, and flow-volume loops *(C)*.

Ringing or Oscillation in the Circuit

The initial flow of gas in pressure ventilation may be the maximum flow for the ventilator. If this flow is too rapid, it can cause a spike in the pressure curve. When this flow is extremely high, "ringing" occurs. For example, if the working pressure is set too high on the Servo 900, "ringing" or an oscillation in pressure delivery results. This condition can create patient discomfort, end a breath prematurely, and reduce volume delivery (Figure 11-86).[51] This is most likely to occur in patients with small endotracheal tubes, such as infants. Oscillations can also occur when there is water in the circuit.

Box 11-27 Ventilator Troubleshooting: Responding to Alarms and Abnormal Waveforms

Alarm Situation, or Abnormal Waveform Present, in All Situations Do the Following:

1. Look at the patient to evaluate distress.
2. Assess patient to be sure of ventilation and oxygenation.
3. If necessary, disconnect patient from ventilator and manually ventilate, increasing F_IO_2.
4. Check that alarms are set appropriately.
5. Once the cause of problem has been determined, resolve the cause.
6. If the problem cannot be resolved, change the ventilator.

Common Alarm Situations

Low-Pressure Alarm

1. Check for patient disconnection.
2. Check for leaks in the patient circuit, related to the artificial airway, and through chest tubes.
3. Check the proximal Paw line to be sure that it is connected and not obstructed.
4. This alarm may be accompanied by a low $\dot{V}_E$ or low V_T alarm.

High-Pressure Alarm

1. If patient is coughing, be sure that secretions have not built up in the airway and that patient is not biting the tube.
2. Check for kinking of the endotracheal tube, displacement of the tube balloon, and position of the tube.
3. Check to see if the patient's Raw has increased or if C_L has decreased.
4. Be sure that the main inspiratory or expiratory lines are not kinked or obstructed.
5. Check that patient is breathing synchronously with ventilator.
6. Determine if auto-PEEP has developed.
7. Be sure the expiratory valve is functioning properly.

Low PEEP/CPAP Alarms

1. Check the low PEEP alarm setting to be sure it is below the PEEP level.
2. See if the patient is actively inspiring below baseline.
3. Determine if a leak is present.
4. Check to be sure that the patient is not disconnected.
5. Assess the proximal Paw line to be sure it is not occluded.

Apnea Alarm

1. Determine if the patient is apneic.
2. Check for the presence of leaks.
3. Check the sensitivity setting to be sure the ventilator can detect patient effort.
4. Check the alarm-time interval and the volume setting, when appropriate.

Low Source-Gas Pressure or Power Input Alarm

1. Check 50 psi gas source (e.g., wall connection or air compressor).
2. Check high-pressure hose connections to the ventilator.
3. Check electrical power supply, and reconnect if necessary.
4. Check line fuse or circuit breaker.
5. Try using the reset button.
6. If alarms continue, replace the ventilator.

Ventilator Inoperative Alarm or Technical Error Message

1. Internal malfunction present; try turning ventilator off and restarting it.
2. If alarm continues, replace the ventilator.

Operator Settings are Incompatible with Machine Parameters

1. Error message usually indicates that a parameter must be reset (e.g., flow is not high enough to deliver V_T within an acceptable T_I to keep I:E ratio below 1:1 [based on f, V_T, and flow]).
2. Readjust the appropriate controls.

I:E Ratio Indicator and Alarm Activated

1. Usually indicates an I:E ratio of greater than 1:1.
2. If inverse I:E ratio is a goal, disable the I:E ratio limit.
3. If normal I:E ratios are a goal, check alarm causes:
   - Has increased Raw or decreased CL resulted in a lower flow? Treat the cause.
   - Is the flow setting too low for the desired V_T delivery? Increase flow or change flow waveform.

Other Possible Alarms

1. High PEEP/CPAP alarms
   - Similar to causes of high-pressure alarms.
   - In flow-cycled modes, check for system leaks.
2. Low V_T, low $\dot{V}_E$, or low f alarms
   - Similar to situations that cause low-pressure alarms.
   - The patient's spontaneous ventilation has decreased for some reason.
   - The alarms may be set inappropriately.
   - Flow sensor disconnection or malfunction.
3. High V_T, high $\dot{V}_E$, or high respiratory rate (f) alarms
   - Check machine sensitivity for auto-triggering.
   - Check for possible cause of increased patient $\dot{V}_E$.
   - Be sure alarms are set appropriately.
   - If external nebulizer is in use, reset the alarm setting until the treatment is finished.
   - Check flow sensors for miscalibration, contamination, or malfunction.
4. Low F_IO_2 and high F_IO_2 alarms
   - Check gas source.
   - Check built-in oxygen analyzer for proper functioning.

From Pilbeam SP: *Mechanical ventilation: physiological and clinical applications*, ed 3 St Louis, 1998, Mosby.

Solving Problems During Alarm Situations

Box 11-27 and Appendix 11-1 at the end of this chapter provide some solutions to problems encountered during ventilation by identifying alarm situations, establishing the cause of the alarm, and finding some potential solutions. For more in-depth coverage of ventilator graphics and management of patient-ventilator problems, readers are referred elsewhere.[7,20,52-55]

Summary

Many important aspects of mechanical ventilation must be understood before a practitioner begins managing a patient-ventilator system. Most common aspects of mechanical ventilation related to the physical characteristics and technical operation of ventilators have been reviewed here. The main focus has been on physical function and terms and explanations of fundamental concepts related to mechanical ventilation. Chapters 12, 13, and 14 review the use and operation of a variety of mechanical ventilators.

Review Questions

See Appendix A for the answers.

1. Name the two common power sources for mechanical ventilators.

2. What type of system is described in this example? A ventilator measures a drop in tidal volume during pressure ventilation and automatically increases the pressure to return the volume to its original value.

3. During operation of a ventilator, the respiratory therapist sets the tidal volume, respiratory rate, and flow all of which are appropriate settings for what type of ventilation?
   a. Pressure-targeted ventilation
   b. Volume-targeted ventilation

4. List three additional names for pressure ventilation.

5. Which of the following devices represent flow-control valves?
   I. Rotary drive piston
   II. Proportional solenoid
   III. Bag-in-a-chamber
   IV. Stepper motor with valve
      a. I only
      b. II only
      c. II and IV only
      d. I, III, and IV only

6. When a jet stream passes through an opening and with a wall adjacent to its left side, the jet will deflect away from the wall because of the formation of a separation bubble—true or false?

7. Classify and describe controlled volume ventilation with a constant flow waveform.

8. What are the trigger mechanisms in assisted ventilation?

9. During volume ventilation, the volume-time curve shows that inspired volume is greater than expired volume. The expired volume curve does not return to zero during exhalation. What is the most likely problem?

10. Graphic findings on a patient indicate an increase in the difference between the peak inspiratory pressure and the plateau pressure and a prolonged expiratory flow on a flow-time curve. What do you think is the problem?

11. An apneic patient is severely hypoxemic. The physician wishes to use an elevated baseline pressure. Which would you recommend: PEEP or CPAP?

12. The flow-time curve for a paralyzed and sedated patient receiving PCIRV reveals that a mandatory breath occurs before flow returns to zero at the end of exhalation. Which of the following maneuvers would you perform?
    a. Inflation hold
    b. Cuff pressure measurement
    c. Maximum inspiratory pressure measurement
    d. End-expiratory pause

13. A physician wants to use pressure ventilation that guarantees volume delivery of every breath. Which of the following modes of ventilation would you recommend?
    a. Pressure-regulated volume control
    b. Pressure augmentation
    c. Proportional-assist ventilation
    d. Airway pressure-release ventilation

14. What HFV technique provides an active inspiratory and expiratory phase?

15. Which of the following conditions is NOT a cause of a high-pressure alarm?
    a. Patient coughing
    b. Increased airway resistance
    c. A ruptured endotracheal tube cuff
    d. Water in the patient circuit

16. Which of the following devices is an example of a PEEP valve that primarily has threshold resistor quality and is gravity-dependent?
    a. Balloon type of expiratory valve
    b. Underwater column
    c. Spring-loaded diaphragm
    d. Restrictive orifice

17. A patient is being ventilated via a continuous-flow IMV system. The respiratory care practitioner notices that during spontaneous inspiration the reservoir bag completely collapses and fills slowly during expiration.

To solve this problem what should the practitioner consider doing?
   a. Check the function of the one-way valve between the reservoir bag and the ventilator circuit
   b. Increase the flow to the reservoir bag
   c. Increase the sensitivity setting on the ventilator
   d. Check the expiratory valve line connection

18. Describe the four phases of a breath and the phase variables.

19. A patient on flow-triggering has a base flow of 10 L/min and a flow trigger of 3 L/min. At what measured flow will the ventilator begin inspiration? If you wanted to make the ventilator more sensitive to the patient, how would you adjust the flow trigger.

20. While viewing the ventilator graphics, the respiratory therapist notices no downward deflection of the pressure curve before inspiratory flow begins. The inspiratory flow curve is constant and repeatedly has a fixed inspiratory flow time of 1.0 second. The peak inspiratory pressure has increased over the past 24 hours. What are the trigger and cycle mechanisms and is this breath volume or pressure-targeted? Locate the graph of the flow-time, volume-time, and pressure-time curves for time-triggered, volume- or pressure-limited, time-cycled breaths.

21. During PCV the flow rises sharply to its peak of 100 L/min and progressively decreases. The pressure-time curve shows such a sharp rise to peak that a small spike appears at the beginning of the curve before the pressure-time curve settles into a normal plateau. What adjustment could the therapist make to eliminate this sharp rise in pressure and maintain current status?
   a. Switch to volume-targeted ventilation
   b. Adjust the flow drop-off for flow cycling
   c. Adjust the sloping or rise time control
   d. Switch to APRV ventilation

22. During PSV the therapist notices that inspiration seems to end quickly without adequate time for the patient to benefit from the breath. The flow only rises to 30 L/min. What adjustment might increase the inspiratory time?
   a. Inspiratory time control
   b. Flow drop-off or flow termination adjustment
   c. Sensitivity control
   d. Peak inspiratory flow control

23. The Venturi ventilator uses what feature to reduce the resistance to exhalation at the beginning of the expiratory phase?
   a. It has a control that applies a negative pressure to the patient circuit during this time
   b. The Venturi has a control that adjusts NEEP
   c. No such feature is present on the Venturi
   d. It uses high frequency oscillation to achieve negative pressure during exhalation

24. Which of the following modes is commonly defined as patient- or time-triggered, pressure-targeted, and time-cycled?
   I. Pressure assist/control
   II. Pressure limited ventilation
   III. Pressure ventilation
   IV. Pressure control ventilation
      a. I and III only
      b. II and IV only
      c. I, II, and III only
      d. I, II, III, and IV

25. PRVC is different from Paug in terms of what primary characteristic?
   a. PRVC is pressure targeted
   b. PRVC guarantees volume over several breaths
   c. PRVC guarantees volume for every breath.
   d. PRVC is not a servo controlled mode.

26. Which of the following ventilators will increase tidal volume in to maintain a mandatory minute ventilation?
   a. Cardiopulmonary Venturi
   b. Hamilton Veolar
   c. Siemen's Servo 300
   d. Bear 1000

27. Which of the following modes responds by giving more flow and pressure when a patient demands more? In this mode the operator sets the amount needed to unload the work imposed by elastance and resistance?
   a. APRV
   b. PAV
   c. ASV
   d. PRVC

28. List the five common methods of delivering high-frequency ventilation.

29. What is the most common condition likely to cause a high pressure alarm?
   a. Deflated endotracheal tube cuff
   b. Disconnection of the patient at the Y connector
   c. Leak around a face mask
   d. Patient coughing

30. During mechanical ventilation of a patient, the therapist notes that the volume-time curve rises normally during inspiration, but fails to return to zero during the expiratory phase. What is the most likely cause of this problem, the patient or the ventilator system?

References

1. Mushin WW, et al: *Automatic ventilation of the lungs*, Philadelphia, 1980, FA Davis.
2. Chatburn RL: *Classification of mechanical ventilation*, Dallas, 1988, American Association for Respiratory Care.
3. Chatburn RL: A new system for understanding mechanical ventilators, *Respir Care* 36:1123, 1991.
4. Branson RD, Hess DR, Chatburn RL: *Respiratory care equipment*, Philadelphia, 1995, JB Lippincott.

5. Blanch PB, Desautels DA: Chatburn's ventilator classification scheme—a poor substitute for the classic approach, *Respir Care* 39:762, 1994.

6. Chatburn RL, Primiano FP: A new system of understanding modes of mechanical ventilation, *Respir Care* 46:604-621, 2001.

7. Pilbeam SP: *Mechanical ventilation: physiological and clinical applications*, ed 3, St Louis, 1998, Mosby.

8. Raniere VM: Optimization of patient-ventilator interactions: closed loop technology to turn the century (editorial), *Intensive Care Med* 23:936-939, 1997.

9. Branson RD: Dual control modes, closed loop ventilation, handguns and tequila (editorial), *Respir Care* 46:232, 2001.

10. Sanborn WG: Microprocessor-based mechanical ventilation, *Respir Care* 38(1):72, 1993.

11. Desautels D: Ventilator classification: a new look at an old subject, *Current Rev Respir Ther* (lesson 11) 1:81, 1979.

12. Scanlan CL, Wilkins RL, Stoller JK: *Egan's fundamentals of respiratory therapy*, ed 7, St Louis, 1999, Mosby.

13. Dupuis Y: *Ventilators: theory and clinical application*, ed 2, St Louis, 1992, Mosby.

14. Morgan SE, Kestner JJ: Modification of a critical care ventilator for use during magnetic resonance imaging, *Respir Care* 47:61, 2002.

15. Banner MJ: Expiratory positive pressure valves and work of breathing, *Respir Care* 32:431, 1987.

16. Kacmarek RM, et al: Technical aspects of positive end-expiratory pressure (PEEP) (I, II, and III), *Respir Care* 27:1478, 1490, 1505, 1982.

17. Spearman CB. Positive end-expiratory pressure: terminology and technical aspects of PEEP devices and systems, *Respir Care* 33:434, 1988.

18. Chatburn RL: Dynamic respiratory mechanics, *Respir Care* 31:703, 1986.

19. MacIntyre N, Nishimura M: The Nagoyo conference on system design and patient-ventilator interactions during pressure support ventilation, *Chest* 97:1463, 1990.

20. Hess DR, MacIntyre NR, *Respiratory care: principles and practice*, Philadelphia, 2002, WB Saunders.

21. Nilsestuen JO, Hargett K: Managing the patient-ventilator system using graphic analysis: an overview and introduction to Graphics Corner, *Respir Care* 41:1105, 1996.

22. Chatmongkolchart S, Williams P: Evaluation of inspiratory rise time and inspiratory termination criteria in new-generation mechanical ventilators: A lung model study, *Respir Care* 46:666, 2001.

23. Williams P, Mueluer M: Pressure support and pressure assist/control: are there differences? An evaluation of the newest intensive care unit ventilators, *Respir Care* 45:1169, 2000.

24. Campbell RS, Branson RD: Ventilatory support for the '90s: pressure support ventilation, *Respir Care* 38:526, 1993.

25. Miller Cyndy: Director of Clinical Education, Personal Communication, Newport Medical Instruments, Costa Mesa, Calif, May 2002.

26. Reynolds EOR: Effect of alterations in mechanical ventilator settings on pulmonary gas exchange in hyaline membrane disease, *Arch Dis Child* 46:152, 1971.

27. Reynolds EOR, Taghipadeh A: Improved prognosis of infants mechanically ventilated for hyaline membrane disease, *Arch Dis Child* 49:405, 1974.

28. Kallet RH, Corral W: Implementation of a low tidal volume ventilation protocol for patients with acute lung injury or acute respiratory distress syndrome, *Respir Care* 46:1024, 2001.

29. Brochard L, Roudot-Thoraval F: Tidal volume reduction for prevention of ventilator-induced lung injury in acute respiratory distress syndrome. The multicenter trail group on tidal volume reduction in ARDS, *Amer J Respir Crit Care Med* 158:1831, 1998.

30. Amato MBP, Barbas CSV: Effect of a protective-ventilation strategy on mortality in the acute respiratory failure syndrome, *N Engl J Med* 338:347, 1998.

31. Stock MC, Downs JB: Airway pressure release ventilation: a new approach to ventilatory support during acute lung injury, *Respir Care* 32:517, 1987.

32. Martin LD, Wetzel RC: Optimal release time during airway pressure release ventilation in neonatal sheep, *Crit Care Med* 22:486, 1994.

33. Foland JA, Martin J: Airway pressure release ventilation with a short release time in a child with acute respiratory distress syndrome, *Respir Care* 46:1019, 2001.

34. Branson RD, MacIntyre NR: Dual-control modes of mechanical ventilation, *Respir Care* 41:294, 1996.

35. Hewlett AM, Platt AS: Mandatory minute volume: a new concept in weaning from mechanical ventilation, *Anaesthesia* 32:163, 1977.

36. Sottiaux TM: Patient-ventilator interactions during volume-support ventilation: asynchrony and tidal volume instability—a report of three cases, *Respir Care* 46:255, 2001.

37. Keenan HT, Martin LD: Volume support ventilation in infants and children: analysis of a case series, *Respir Care* 42:281, 1997.

38. Younes M: Proportional assist ventilation. In Tobin MJ, editor: *Principles and practice of mechanical ventilation*, New York, 1994, McGraw-Hill

39. Younes M: Proportional assist ventilation: a new approach to ventilatory support. Part I: Theory, *Am Rev Respir Dis* 145:114, 1992.

40. Younes M, et al: Proportional assist ventilation: results of an initial clinical trial, *Am Rev Respir Dis* 145:121, 1992.

41. Schulze A, Schaller P: Proportional assist ventilation: a new strategy for infant ventilation? *Neonatal Respir Dis* 6:1, 1996.

42. Schulze A, et al: Effects of ventilator resistance and compliance on phrenic nerve activity in spontaneously breathing cats, *Am J Respir Crit Care Med* 153:671, 1996.

43. Otis AB, Fenn WO, Rahn H: Mechanics of breathing in man, *J Appl Physiol* 2:592, 1950.

44. Watson K: Ventilatory support in newborn and pediatric patients. In Pilbeam SP: *Mechanical ventilation: physiological and clinical applications*, ed 3, St Louis, 1998, Mosby.

45. Sjöstrand U: High-frequency positive pressure ventilation (HFPPV): a review, *Crit Care Med* 8:345, 1980.

46. Boros SJ, et al: Using conventional infant ventilators at unconventional rates, *Pediatrics* 74:487, 1984.

47. Klain M, Smith RB: High-frequency percutaneous transtracheal jet ventilation, *Crit Care Med* 5:280, 1977.

48. Calkins JM: High-frequency jet ventilation: experimental evaluation. In Carlon CG, Howlan WS, editors: *High-frequency ventilation in intensive care and during surgery*, New York, 1985, Marcel Dekker.

49. English P, Mason SC: Neonatal mechanical ventilation. In Hess DR, MacIntyre NR: *Respiratory care: principles & practice*, Philadelphia, 2002, WB Saunders.

50. Blanch PB: Mechanical ventilation malfunctions: a description and comparative study of six common ventilator brands, *Respir Care* 44:1183, 1999.

51. Cohen IL, Bilen Z, Krishnamurthy S: The effects of ventilator working pressure during pressure support ventilation, *Chest* 103:588, 1993.

52. Pilbeam SP: Mechanical ventilation. In Burton GG, Hodgkin JE, Ward JJ: *Respiratory care: a guide to clinical practice*, Philadelphia, 1997, JB Lippincott.

53. Kacmarek RM, Hess D, Stoller JK: *Monitoring in respiratory care*, St Louis, 1993, Mosby.

54. Meliones JN, Cheifetz IM, Wilson BG: *Use of airway graphic analysis to optimize mechanical ventilation strategies*, L1312, Palm Springs, Calif, 1995, Bird Products Corporation.

55. Wilson BG, Cheifetz IM, Meliones JN: *Optimizing mechanical ventilation in infants and children with the use of airway graphics*, L1326 Rev B, Palm Springs, Calif, 1995, Bird Products Corporation.

Internet Resources

American Association for Respiratory Care: www.aarc.org.

Check "Resources," Clinical Practice Guidelines, and look for the following:
a. Patient-Ventilator System Check
b. Ventilator Circuit Changes

American Journal of Respiratory and Critical Care Medicine: http://ajrccm.atsjournals.org

Bird and Bear Ventilators and the Avea: www.viasyscriticalcare.com

Cardiopulmonary venturi ventilator: www.venturi.com

Drager ventilators: www.draegermedical.com

Hamilton Medical: www.hamilton-medical.com

Medscape: www.medscape.com

National Board for Respiratory Care: www.nbrc.org

National Library of Medicine: http://text.nlm.nih.gov

Percussionaire: www.percussionaire.com

Puritan Bennett: www.PuritanBennett.com

Respironics: www.respironics.com

Sechrist Industries: www.sechristind.com

Siemens Medical: www.siemensmedical.com

Society of Critical Care Medicine: www.sccm.org

Ventilator information: www.ventworld.com

Virtual Hospital at www.vh.org

Look into Adult Critical Care Core Curriculum—Auto-PEEP

Look into Radiology

Appendix 11-1

Algorithms for Alarm Situations

In any alarm situation, it is imperative that patients be assessed to determine if they are in distress. If so, they should be disconnected from the ventilator and manually ventilated with 100% oxygen. If the patient improves, the problem is most likely in the ventilator system. If the patient does not improve, the problem is with the patient or the artificial airway. The following algorithms review common alarm situations when the problem is with the ventilator or the artificial airways. Patient problems, such as pneumothorax and pulmonary embolism, are beyond the scope of this text.

Because some alarms often occur at about the same time, the situations are grouped together and include the following:

1. Increased V_T, $\dot{V}_E$, or rate alarms (Figure A11-1)
2. Low pressure, low PEEP/CPAP, low $\dot{V}_E$, low V_T, or low rate alarms (Figure A11-2)
3. High pressure or high PEEP/CPAP alarms (Figure A11-3)

Additional alarms to be reviewed are as follows:

1. Inverse I:E ratio indication activated (Figure A11-4)
2. Apnea alarm (Figure A11-5)
3. Loss of power alarm (Figure A11-6)

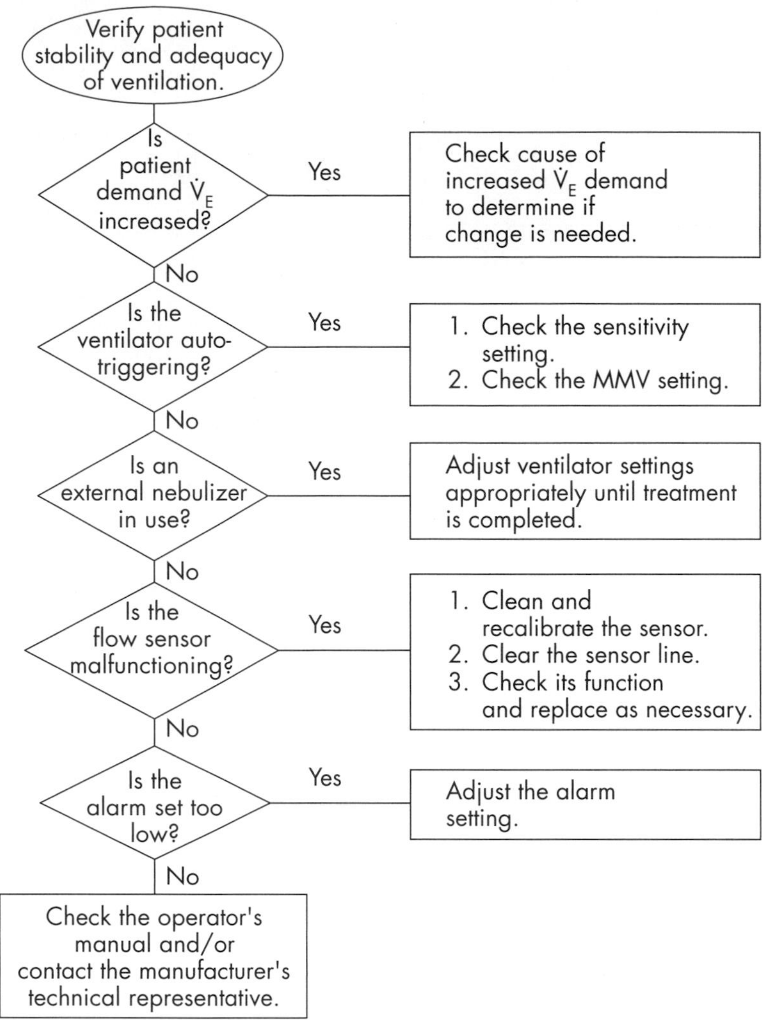

Figure A11-1 Increased V_T, $\dot{V}_E$, or rate alarm.

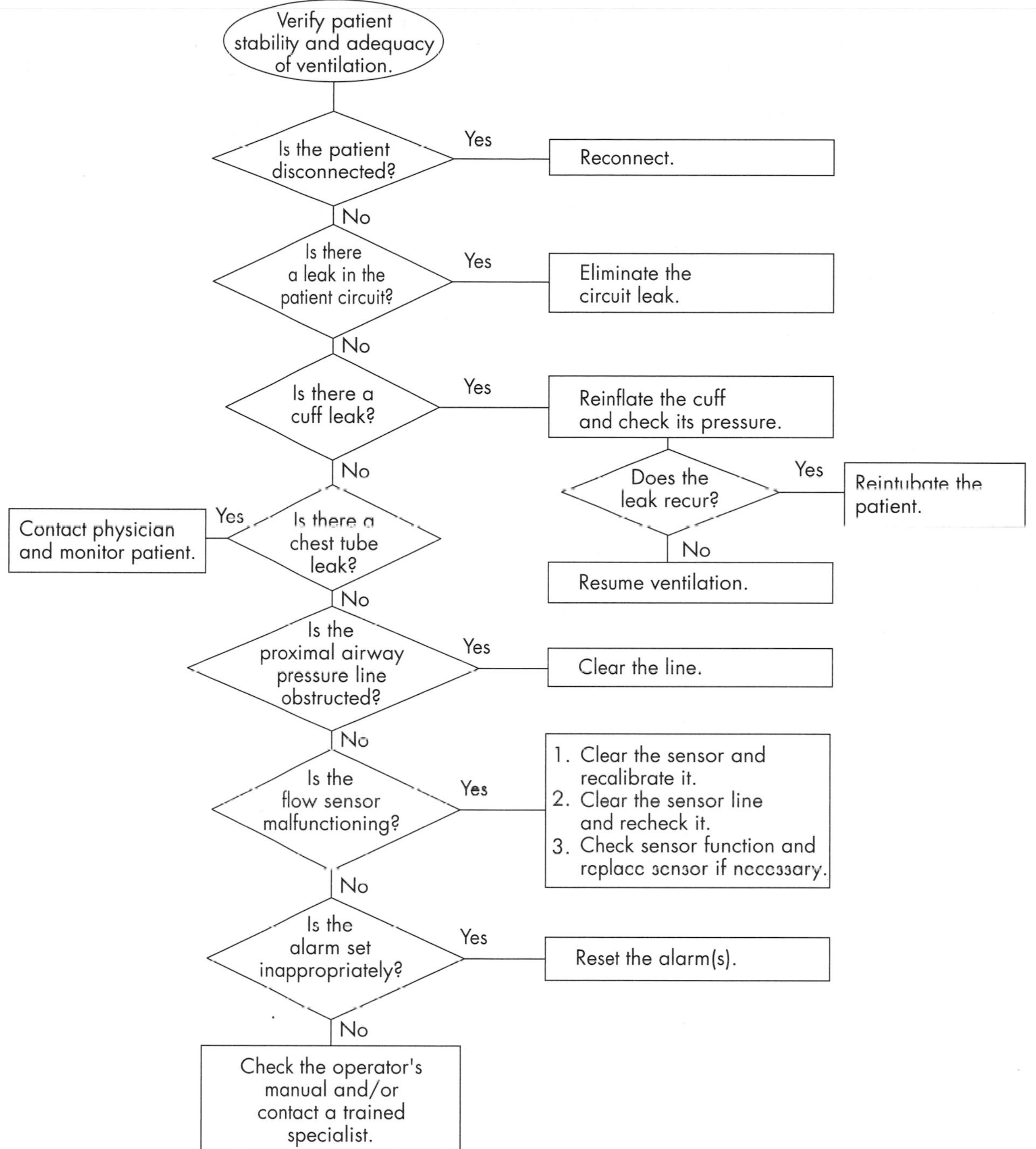

Figure A11-2 Low pressure, low PEEP/CPAP, low $\dot{V}_E$, low V_T, or low rate alarms.

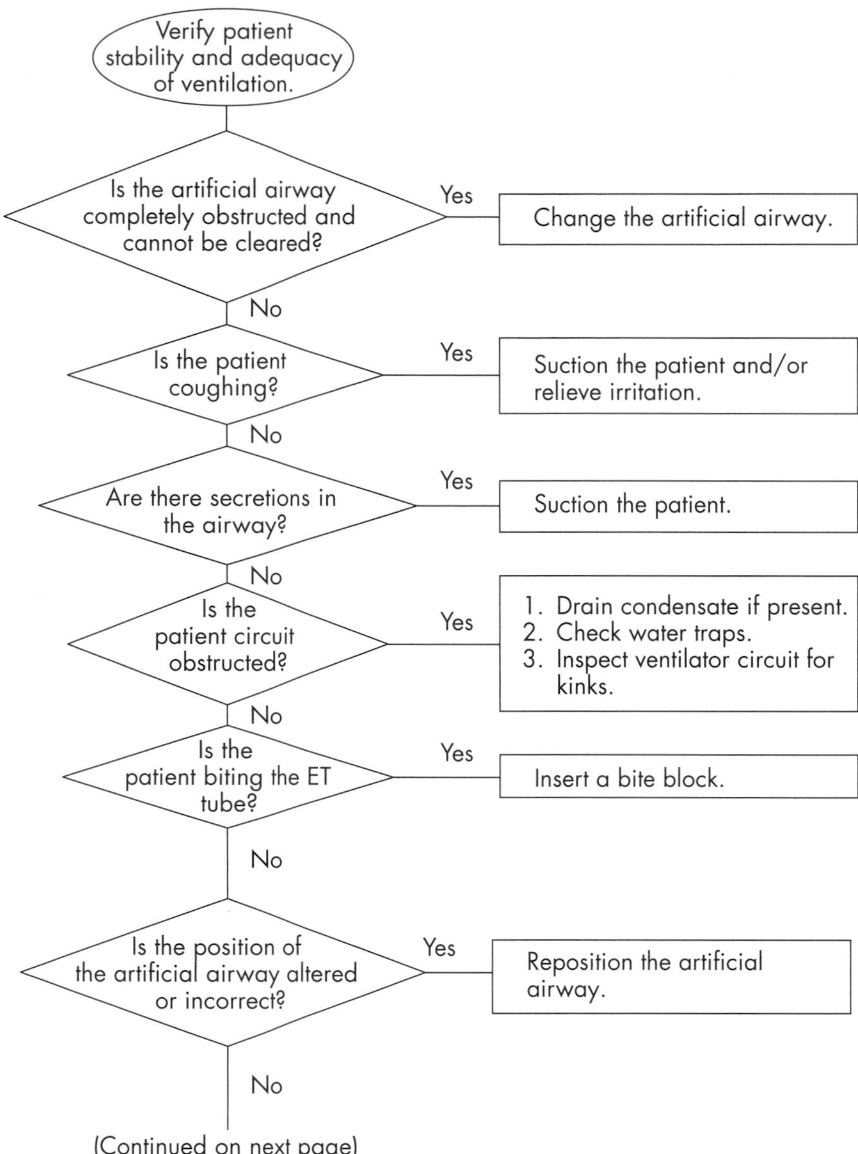

Figure A11-3 High-pressure or high-PEEP alarms.

(Continued from previous page)

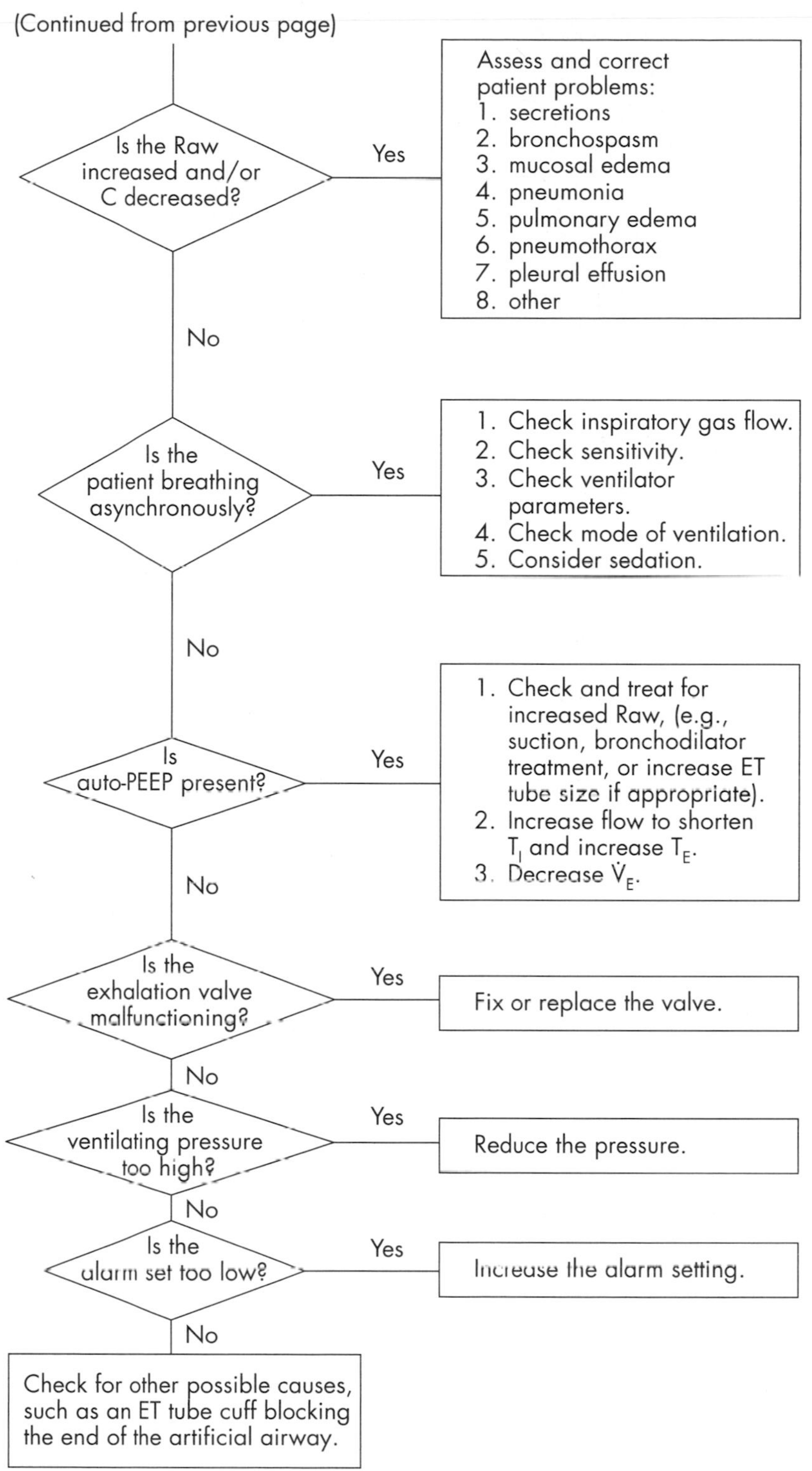

Figure A11-3, cont'd

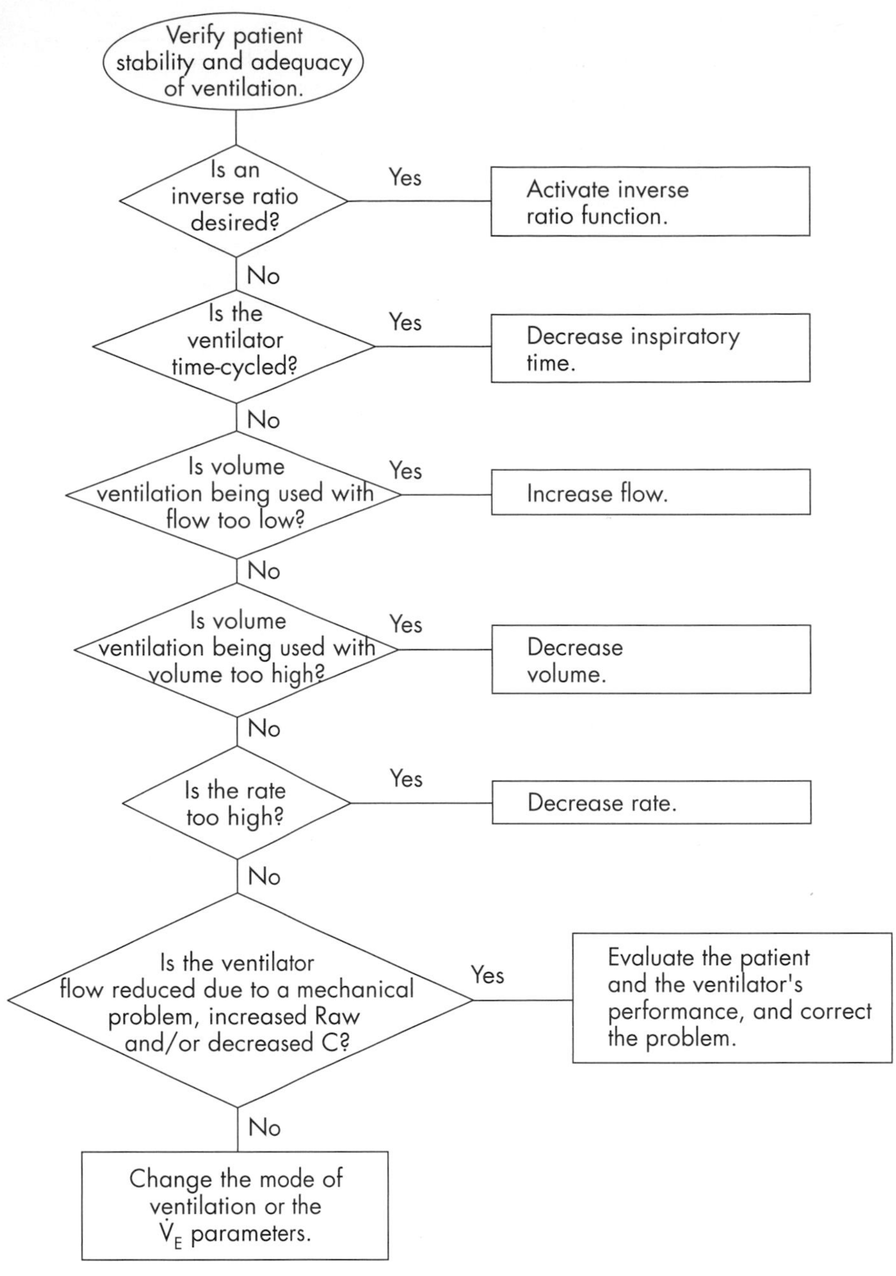

Figure A11-4 Inverse I: E ratio indicator activated.

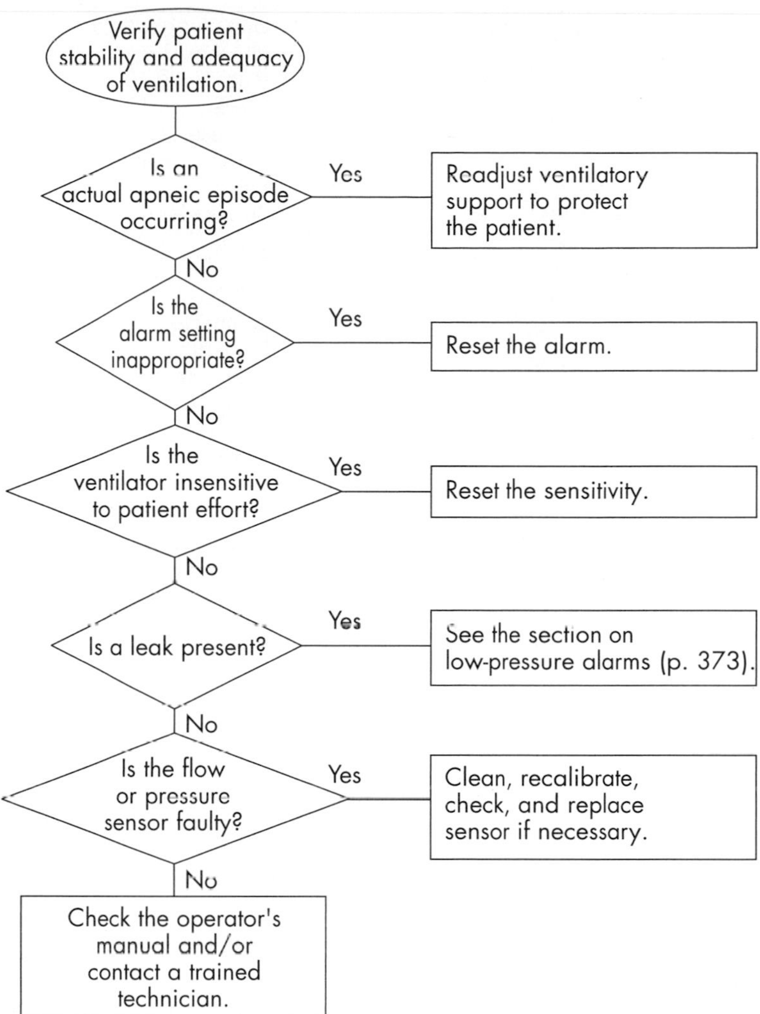

Figure A11-5 Apnea alarm.

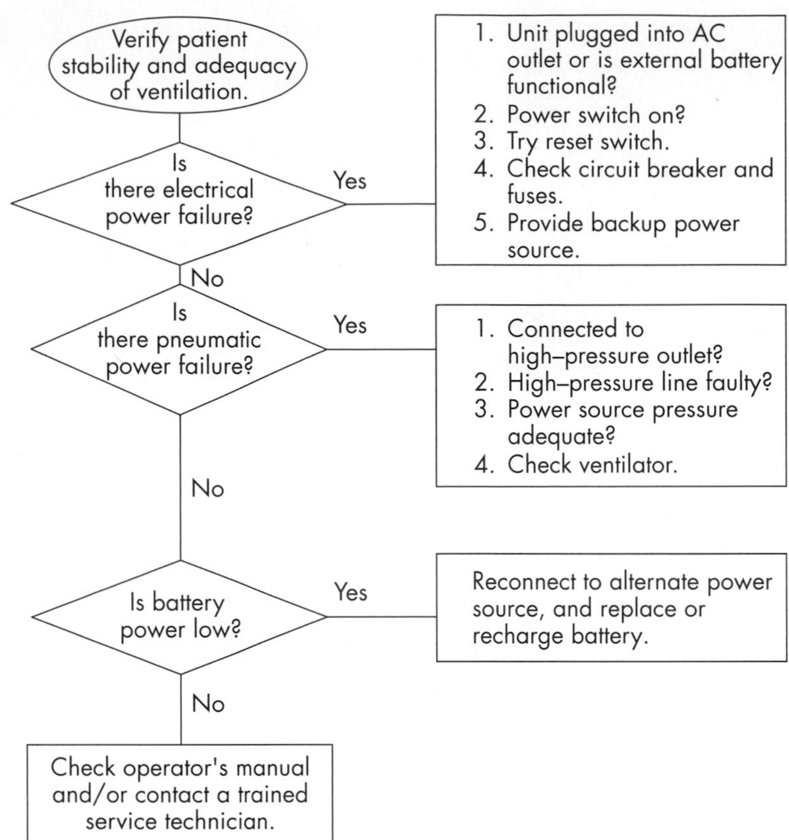

Figure A11-6 Loss of power alarm.

Chapter 12

Mechanical Ventilators: General-Use Devices

Susan P. Pilbeam

Chapter Outline

CHAPTER OUTLINE continued

CHAPTER OUTLINE continued

CHAPTER OUTLINE continued

CHAPTER OUTLINE continued

CHAPTER OUTLINE continued

Chapter Learning Objectives

Bear 1000

Upon completion of this section, the reader should be able to:

1. Describe the major components of the internal mechanisms of the Bear 1000.
2. Identify the controls and discuss the function of each.
3. Explain how the controls are set.
4. Discuss how the alarms are set.
5. Assess what alarm-activated LEDs and alarm messages indicate, and state possible causes.
6. Compare each of the modes of ventilation on the Bear 1000, including the trigger and cycle mechanisms and the target variable (pressure or volume).
7. Evaluate a graph or a description of a graphic display that shows pressure sloping or pressure augmentation (Paug) to determine if the ventilator is set appropriately.

8. Explain the function of the compliance comp. control.
9. Identify a resource that can help determine the causes of a functional problem of the Bear 1000.

Bird 8400STi

Upon completion of this section, the reader should be able to:

1. Describe the internal mechanism.
2. Explain the location and function of the controls on the front panel.
3. From a description, establish which alarm is active and state a possible cause for the alarm.
4. Recommend a solution to an alarm situation.
5. Compare the pressure-targeted breath setting to the volume-targeted breath setting.
6. Determine what parameter is cycling the breaths in VAPS based on the description of a pressure/time graph.

T-Bird

Upon completion of this section, the reader should be able to:

1. Describe the power source, patient circuit, and internal mechanism of the T Bird.
2. Explain how the control parameters and adjustable alarms are set.
3. Assess an alarm situation and name possible causes and solutions.
4. Compare VAPS on the T-Bird with PAug on the Bear 1000.
5. Recommend an information source for reviewing user verification tests.
6. Explain the operation of the special functions.

Dräger Evita

Upon completion of this section, the reader should be able to:

1. Describe and label the components of the front panel on the Dräger Evita.
2. Discuss the function of each control on the front panel.
3. Explain the CMV mode, including the associated features of pressure limiting and PCV.
4. Given appropriate ventilatory parameters, determine the spontaneous breathing window during SIMV ventilation.
5. Identify and correct an alarm situation.
6. Draw or describe a pressure/time graph for a patient breathing spontaneously during APRV.
7. Describe the method for setting APRV ventilation.
8. Explain the set-up and measurement of intrinsic PEEP and occlusion pressure (P0.1) on the Dräger Evita.

Dräger E-4 (Evita-4)

Upon completion of this section, the reader should be able to:

1. Describe the front panel on the Dräger E-4.
2. Discuss the function of each control on the E-4 front panel.
3. Compare the set-up of a ventilator mode on the E-4 with that on another microprocessor-controlled ICU ventilator.
4. Assess an alarm situation, describe its priority level, and suggest a possible cause and solution.
5. Identify a pressure/time graph for a patient breathing spontaneously during PCV ventilation.
6. Compare upper Paw alarm limit to the Pmax pressure limit.
7. Describe the method for setting PCV and APRV and compare it with the two modes of ventilation.
8. Discuss the similarities and differences between AutoFlow and PRVC on the Servo 300 (see Chapter 11).
9. List the features available when Neoflow is added as an upgrade to the Dräger E-4.
10. Explain the set-up and function of proportional pressure support.

Dräger Evita 2 Dura

Upon completion of this section, the reader should be able to:

1. Discuss the function of each control on the front panel of the Dräger Evita 2 Dura.
2. Compare the set-up of a ventilator mode on the Dräger Evita 2 Dura to that on the E-4.
3. Assess an alarm situation, describe its priority level, and suggest a possible cause and solution.
4. Describe the special functions available on the Dura.
5. Compare and contrast the modes on the Dräger Evita 2 Dura.

Hamilton VEOLAR^{FT}

Upon completion of this section, the reader should be able to:

1. Describe the function of each control, alarm, and monitor parameter on the Hamilton VEOLAR^{FT}.
2. Calculate peak inspiratory flow from ventilator settings.
3. Explain the set up of both the MMV and the PCV modes of ventilation.
4. Describe the set-up of PCV on the VEOLAR^{FT}.
5. Discuss the function of the hold control.

Hamilton Galileo

Upon completion of this section, the reader should be able to:

1. Describe the function of the two knobs on the front of the GALILEO ventilator.
2. Explain how to select a ventilator mode and the parameters for that mode.
3. Explain how to select the alarm screen and set the alarms.
4. Compare the addition of APV to standard PCV.
5. Discuss how the microprocessor selects V_T, $\dot{V}E$, and rate values for a patient receiving ASV.
6. Describe the method the ventilator uses when starting ASV.
7. Assess a patient case representing one of the three common scenarios that describes the function of ASV to determine how the ventilator will function.
8. Troubleshoot a problem when an alarm indicator is activated.
9. Describe back-up ventilation in the GALILEO.

Puritan Bennett 740

Upon completion of this section, the reader should be able to:

1. Name the power source requirements.
2. Describe the internal mechanisms involved in breath delivery.
3. Explain how ventilator and alarm settings are made.
4. Assess an alarm situation and identify the probable cause.
5. Identify messages that appear in the message window.
6. Compare POST with SST.

7. Define the function of the various keys in the ventilator settings and patient status sections.
8. Interpret flashing vs. constantly lit indicators in the ventilator status section.
9. Explain the function of all modes of ventilation available on the 740, including apnea ventilation.
10. Identify functions that can be accessed through the menu key.
11. Describe the appropriate corrective action when the Vent.Inop. alarm is activated.

Puritan Bennett 760

Upon completion of this section, the reader should be able to:

1. List the options and breath types available on the 760 that are not on the 740.
2. Calculate T_I, T_E and I:E when these variables are selected in PCV
3. Explain the setting and function of exhalation sensitivity, rise time factor, and inspiratory and expiratory pause.
4. Identify the presence of auto-PEEP using the end expiratory flow value in the message window.

Puritan Bennett 840

Upon completion of this section, the reader should be able to:

1. Explain the three primary functions of the expiratory filter.
2. Identify a situation where the battery has become operational in the back-up power source.
3. Describe how an SST is run by the operator.
4. List the tests performed during SST.
5. Analyze a problem in ventilator cycling during PSV.
6. Provide a definition of the parameter settings in the lower screen.
7. List the information contained in the upper screen.
8. Describe the indicator lights on the Status Indicator Panel and the Breath Delivery Unit.
9. Compare the vertical and horizontal adjustments on the available waveforms and loops.
10. Identify the potential causes of problems during measurement of respiratory mechanics.
11. Explain the function of rise time percent and expiratory sensitivity.
12. Define the modes of ventilation available including trigger, limit and cycle parameters.
13. Contrast the function of the expiratory valve during PC and VC ventilation.

Newport Breeze E150

Upon completion of this section, the reader should be able to:

1. Describe the internal mechanisms of the ventilator.
2. Explain the setting of controls and alarms.
3. Assess a problem associated with trigger sensitivity and recommend a solution.
4. Solve a problem related to the use of the low CPAP alarm.
5. Describe the available modes of ventilation.
6. Discuss the timing of mandatory and spontaneous breaths during SIMV.
7. Compare a manual breath (inflation) delivered in volume control with one delivered in pressure control.
8. Describe the effects of using the nebulizer function on normal volume delivery.
9. Identify a situation in which the pressure-relief valve is in operation.
10. List and discuss the various alarms violations.

Newport Wave E200

Upon completion of this section, the reader should be able to:

1. Name the power sources required to operate the ventilator.
2. Describe the internal components.
3. Explain the function of the controls on the front panel.
4. Identify an alarm situation and suggest a possible cause and solution.
5. Assess a problem associated with using bias flow and trigger sensitivity during spontaneous ventilation and recommend a solution.
6. Solve a problem related to use of the low-pressure alarm.
7. Describe the available modes of ventilation.
8. Explain the function of the nebulizer control.
9. Compare the setting of pressure-targeted modes with that of volume-targeted modes.
10. Identify a situation when the pressure-relief valve is operating.

Pulmonetics LTV Ventilator

Upon completion of this section, the reader should be able to:

1. List the features that distinguish the LTV 800, 900, 950, and 1000.
2. Explain the attachment points on the LTV for the patient circuit, power cord, oxygen source, and remote cable connector.
3. Name the power sources that can be used with the LTV ventilator.
4. Describe the function of the panel controls and alarm settings.
5. Explain the setting and reading of PEEP values.
6. Review the procedures for turning on and off the ventilator, including the ventilator checkout tests.
7. Discuss the function of the Extended Feature menu items.
8. Identify the normal and alarm condition illumination of the screen displays and indicators.
9. Troubleshoot a clinical situation regarding sensitivity settings.
10. Identify alarm messages and their meaning.

Respironics Esprit Ventilator

Upon completion of this section, the reader should be able to:

1. List the power sources available.
2. Identify controls and indicators
3. Describe alarm function.
4. Verify ventilator preparedness with SST and EST.
5. Set apnea ventilation parameters
6. Set and adjust breath types and modes of ventilation.
7. Compare the functions of I-trigger and E-trigger.
8. Describe the optional functions of O_2 monitoring and graphics.

Siemens Servo 900C

Upon completion of this section, the reader should be able to:

1. Label the internal components on a diagram of the Servo 900C.

2. Explain the operation of each of the controls and alarms on the Servo 900C.
3. Given the ventilator control settings, calculate V_T, T_I, T_E, and I:E ratio during volume ventilation on the Servo 900C.
4. Estimate inspiratory flow during volume ventilation and SIMV when constant flow is selected and control settings are given.
5. Describe each of the modes of ventilation for the Servo 900C.
6. Indicate which control must be set for each mode.
7. Solve an alarm situation.

Siemens Servo 300

Upon completion of this section, the reader should be able to:

1. Label a diagram of the internal components of the Servo 300.
2. Explain the function of the controls on the operating panel of the Servo 300 and compare measured with set digital display values.
3. Recommend a safe method for changing rate and VT settings on the Servo 300.
4. Assess an alarm situation and recommend an action to correct the problem.
5. Compare each of the modes of ventilation on the Servo 300, including a review of triggering and cycling mechanisms and breath delivery (volume vs. pressure).
6. Explain the use of the select parameter guide (SPG) for setting up controls when switching to a new mode of ventilation.
7. Describe the function of volume support, PRVC, and Automode.

Dräger Savina

Upon completion of this section, the reader should be able to:

1. List the available power sources of the Dräger Savina.
2. Describe the procedure for setting ventilator parameters including those listed in the "Settings" screen and the "Configuration" screen.
3. Explain the function of the nebulizer key, the "O_2 ↑suction" key, and the manual inspiration key.
4. Compare AutoFlow to CMV A/C ventilation with the upper pressure limit (Pmax) set.
5. Name the feature used to adjust the rate of pressure and flow delivery at the beginning of inspiration.
6. Describe the function of the sigh feature on the Savina.
7. Discuss the modes of ventilation available with the Savina and the modifications that can be used with each.

Siemens Servo^i Ventilator

Upon completion of this section, the reader will be able to:

1. Describe the available power sources for the Servo^i and their function.
2. Compare the use of the front panel, the quick access knobs, and the main rotary dial during parameter and mode setting.
3. Describe parameter adjustment on the Servo^i ventilator.
4. Explain the function of the following: Servo^i Ultra Nebulizer, inspiratory rise time, inspiratory cycle off, breath cycle time, and trigger time-out.
5. Discuss setting the alarm limits on the Servo^i.

Viasys AVEA

Upon completion of this section, the reader should be able to:

1. Explain the power sources of the AVEA.
2. Describe the function of each of the membrane buttons.
3. Identify indicators located on the ventilator front.
4. Determine the current power source and battery status.
5. Outline the parameter set up when "New Patient" is selected.
6. Name the limit for the I:E ratio variable.
7. Compare the trigger, target (limit), and cycle variables for the available modes of ventilation.
8. Identify the icons and waveforms on the main screen.
9. Recognize visual and audio alarm signals for level of priority.
10. Explain how to access the following: ventilator set up, screen menu, main screen, advanced settings, alarm limits, and mode menu.
11. Describe the purpose of each of the advanced settings.

Newport e500

Upon completion of this section, the reader should be able to:

1. Describe the available power sources and indicators for their use.
2. Explain the function of the front panel controls, indicators and alarms.
3. Compare flow delivery during volume-targeted and pressure-targeted ventilation.
4. State what ventilator parameters become active when the ventilator is turned on.
5. Discuss the sloping feature of the e500 in terms of how it is set.
6. Identify the meaning of information provided in the monitor data section and the alarm section.
7. Describe how the Preset Vent Settings are used.
8. Recommend an appropriate response by a respiratory therapist to the message "Vol Target Not Met" when VTPC assist/control ventilation is active.
9. Determine the possible cause of an Insp Time Too Short alarm.
10. Name the common causes of the problems that might occur with the e500 ventilator.

Key Terms

Accumulator
Airway Pressure-Release Ventilation (APRV)
Alternating Current (AC)
Analog Pressure Manometer
Antisuffocation Valve
Apnea Ventilation
Apneic Period
Assist/Control (A/C)
Autoflow
Base Flow
Baseline Pressure
Bias Alert

Bias Flow
Continuous Mandatory Ventilation (CMV)
Continuous Positive Airway Pressure (CPAP)
Control Panel
Cyber Knobs
Cyber Pads
Default
Diffuser
Direct Current (DC)
Display Window
Drag Turbine
Electrically Powered
Electromagnetic Frequency Interference (EFI)
Electronic Logic
Expiratory Hold
Expiratory Pause
Expiratory Time (T_E)
External Battery
Flow Trigger
Flow Waveforms
High-Pressure Servo Valves
Inspiratory Hold
Inspiratory Pause
Inspiratory Time (T_I)
Internal Battery
Internal Demand Valve
Internal Mechanisms
Intrinsic Positive End-Expiratory Pressure (PEEP)
Inverse Ratio Ventilation (IRV)
Light-Emitting Diodes (LEDs)
Mandatory Breaths
Mandatory Minute Volume Ventilation (MMV)
Manual Trigger
Maximum Pressure Limit (Pmax)
Message Window
Microprocessor
Monitor
Nebulizer Control
Occlusion Pressure (P0.1)
Optical Encoder
Over Pressure-Relief Valve
Oxygen Sensor
Pneumatically Powered
Pneumotachograph
Power Indicators
Pressure Augmentation (Paug)
Pressure-Control Ventilation (PCV)
Pressure Slope
Pressure Support (PS)
Pressure-Support Ventilation (PSV)
Pressure-Targeted Ventilation
Pressure Trigger
Proximal Pressure Line
Radio Frequency Interference (RFI)
Sensitivity
Service Verification Test (SVT)
Slope
Sloping
Software
SmartTrigger
Smart Window
Subambient Overpressure-Relief (SOPR) Valve
Subambient Pressure Valve
Subambient Relief Valve
Synchronized Intermittent Mandatory Ventilation (SIMV)
Total Cycle Time (TCT)
Turbine
User Verification Testing (UVT)
Ventilator Inoperative Alarm (vent. inop.)
Volume-Assured Pressure Support (VAPS)
Volume-Targeted Ventilation

This chapter provides detailed information about a number of multipurpose mechanical ventilators that can be used for both pediatric and adult patients. Emphasis is placed on ventilators used primarily in the intensive care unit. Each ventilator presented includes a concise description so that the reader could literally work through how to operate the device using the information provided. It is not the author's intention that this chapter be read from beginning to end, but rather that it is used to gain knowledge about a specific ventilator or ventilators.

Every effort has been made to ensure that the information provided in this chapter is accurate. However, readers should always use the operating manuals and instructions from the manufacturer whenever using medical devices for patient care. Readers also need to be aware of what software changes may have been made to equipment they are using and to familiarize themselves with the changes.

Since the last edition of this text, an Evolve website has been added as a feature. The reader will be referred to that site for gaining information about some of the older model ventilators and newer ventilators. Specifically, the Bear 3, Hamilton Amadeus, and Puritan Bennett Adult Star ventilators, which were presented in the sixth edition, have been moved from the text to the website. In addition, the Cardiopulmonary Venturi ventilator has been added to the website. These changes have been introduced because of space constraints and also because, although these ventilators are still in use in some facilities, their use has declined significantly or they are no longer being produced and supported by the manufacturer.

The incorporation of microprocessors into mechanical ventilators in the 1980s forever changed their design. Ventilators with microprocessing features can rapidly monitor, manage, and store information, and even change machine function. Manufacturers can change or add new modes or features by simply adding new software, a circuit board, or maybe even a new face to the device.

Buy-outs are another phenomenon that has affected the character of ventilator purchases and use. For example, Bear Medical Corporation merged with Allied Health Corporation, which was then purchased by Thermo Electron Corporation, which also owns Bird Ventilator Products.

The original Bird Company was owned by Dr. Forrest Bird, who sold it to the 3M Corporation. In 2001, the company changed the name of the Bear and Bird Ventilator division to Viasys Healthcare, Critical Care Division. Likewise, Nellcor purchased the Puritan-Bennett Corporation as well as Infrasonics. In turn, Nellcor Puritan Bennett was bought out by Mallinckrodt, which was then purchased by Tyco. And so goes the buy-out phenomenon, which ultimately affects the availability of ventilators.

Both the economic situation and technological advances have resulted in a rapidly changing environment for mechanical ventilators. It is important for consumers to keep these factors in mind and to be aware that units used or purchased may not have the appropriate manufacturer support.

Common Features of Ventilators

Fierce competition among manufacturers has created an advantageous situation for consumers. Because ventilators can be reprogrammed, whenever a manufacturer advertises a new feature, it's usually not long until other manufacturers offer a similar option. For example, the Puritan-Bennett 7200 ventilator was one of the first to offer a back-up mode of ventilation. This "back-up" ventilation has preprogrammed parameters, such as tidal volume (V_T), rate, fractional inspired oxygen (F_IO_2), and flow, which would be activated if the ventilator detected the presence of apnea. Most ventilators now used in acute care have a back-up ventilation feature.

Distinguishing Different Models

Because programmable features can be added, clinical facilities can purchase a unit and then add new features as they are developed. This add-on concept has resulted in much confusion about the names and numbers given to various machines. For example, a hospital initially purchases a unit called the Magnolia 500; but, after developing several new alarm or monitoring capabilities, the manufacturer now calls it the Magnolia 500a or maybe the Magnolia 500 version 2.0. Keeping track of all of the new features added after the initial purchase is truly an art for both the purchaser and the sales representative, not to mention authors of ventilator texts. This places an important responsibility on the clinicians to learn about updates and to understand how they affect the functions of a particular ventilator.

Common Internal Mechanisms

The internal mechanisms of many microprocessor-controlled machines have several similarities. For example, they usually require high-pressure air and oxygen gas sources for pneumatic power, as well as electricity to power the internal microprocessors and various electronically operated components. Gas entering the ventilator's internal circuit is filtered before its temperature and pressure is measured. The gas pressure is then regulated, and both gases are mixed. The mixture is sometimes fed into a holding tank or pressurized cylinder that acts as a reservoir for gas under pressure. The gas is then routed to a microprocessor-controlled flow valve. Although these valves vary by manufacturer, they all provide rapid response for a variety of gas delivery methods. For example, they can give a constant flow and preset volume, or they can give a constant pressure while volume delivery varies. They can change the shape of the inspiratory flow waveform during volume ventilation and respond rapidly to a patient's spontaneous demand for gas flow. Chapter 11 provides additional information on the internal drive mechanisms of ventilators.

Historically, respiratory therapists (RTs) were required to learn the specific details about the internal parts of such ventilators as the Bird Mark 7 and the Emerson Post-Op ventilator. It was important for RTs to know this information so that they could disassemble and repair these devices. This is no longer the case. Trained specialists now repair the internal mechanism. Because of this, much of the discussion of the internal function of ventilators in this chapter will be presented in an abbreviated fashion. A majority of the schematic diagrams of the internal pneumatic and electric circuits which appeared in the sixth edition will be placed on the text's Evolve website for readers interested in this detail.

Patient Monitoring

Sophisticated new technology enables flow and pressure delivery to be monitored rapidly and accurately and allows a variety of monitors and alarms to be used. Pressure and flow are often measured internally, near the main ventilator outlet and return line (i.e., expiratory valve area), but some ventilators monitor flow, pressure or both, at the patient's upper airway. Although types of monitors vary, their function is usually the same. For example, ventilators incorporate flow-measuring devices, which may be variable-orifice **pneumotachographs** or heated thermistor beads, depending on manufacturer preference. Chapter 8 reviews the function of several of these devices.

Ventilators usually have digital displays of the following: V_T, rate (spontaneous and total), peak inspiratory pressure (PIP), plateau pressure ($P_{plateau}$), positive end expiratory pressure (PEEP), continuous positive airway pressure (CPAP), peak flow, oxygen percentage, and inspiratory:expiratory (I:E) ratio. Many also offer a graphic display screen as an add-on feature.

Parameters and Displays

Most ventilators now have **light-emitting diodes (LEDs)** on their control panels to show the operator the mode and parameters currently active. These **control panels** usually include a **display window** that can provide the operator with a written message.

The range of available volume, pressure, and flow also tends to be very similar in current ventilators. For example, the tidal volume range for units used for pediatric and adult patients tends to be from 50 to 2000 mL, although the range may be lower than 50 mL in units that can volume ventilate infants. The typical range of inspiratory pressure limits is from 0 to 120 cm H_2O, PEEP/CPAP values are usually from 0 to 50 cm H_2O, and pressure-support pressure levels generally range from 0 to 100 cm H_2O. Most units provide three **flow waveforms** in volume ventilation: constant, descending ramp, and sine waveforms.

Nearly every ventilator for use in acute care provides the following ventilatory modes: **assist/control (A/C)** and synchronized intermittent mandatory ventilation (SIMV) (either volume- or pressure-targeted), and spontaneous, which includes PEEP/CPAP and **pressure support (PS)**.

Alarms

Common alarms include high/low pressure, high/low oxygen percentage, high/low minute volume, high rate, and low PEEP/CPAP. Ventilators also have alarm-silencing buttons that usually silence audible alarms for 1 to 2 minutes. Sometimes the type of alarm that is active is shown in a display window. In their memory, microprocessors can save information about which alarms have occurred and can report these back to the operator in some form. Some ventilators illuminate the LEDs next to the violated alarms to indicate which alarms are being or have been activated. Some units scroll through the chronological order of the alarm events as the operator reads the display screen. Some do both.

Low gas supply and **ventilator inoperative alarms** (i.e., internal error detected by the microprocessor) are available and cannot be silenced.

Understanding Individual Ventilators

After clinicians have mastered the use of a newer, more sophisticated ventilator, it is usually not difficult for them to understand another brand. Manufacturers have tried to make their equipment user-friendly and provide a wide variety of materials and services to explain their operation: training videotapes, instruction and operation manuals, and trained technicians and representatives, CD-ROM interactive programs, and product specialists via telephone or Internet. And, as always, users are encouraged to read the directions.

Presentation of Specific Ventilators

It is assumed that readers have a basic understanding of the physical properties of ventilators as outlined in Chapter 11. The machines are presented in such a way as to help prepare readers to use them in a clinical setting, so the discussions do not focus too much detail on internal function or classification.

Bear 3 Ventilator

In 1988, the Bear 3 ventilator was introduced by Bear Medical Systems, Inc., a subsidiary of Thermo Electron Corporation, now called Viasys Healthcare. The Bear 3 is the third model of its kind. The Bear 1 and Bear 2 preceded the Bear 3, all three models being similar. Although the Bear 3 is currently the most common of these ventilators used in the United States, its use has declined as older generation models have been replaced by newer model ventilators, such as the Bear 1000. The material on the Bear 3 can be viewed by going to the EVOLVE website for this text.

Bear 1000 Ventilator

The Bear 1000 and the 1000T/ES ventilators[1,2] are manufactured by Viasys Healthcare, Critical Care Division, (Palm Springs, CA), formerly the Bear Medical Systems, Inc., a subsidiary of Thermo Electron Corporation. The Bear 1000 model will be the primary focus of this section (Figure 12-1). Special features added with the Bear 1000T/ES model are presented in the appropriate sections. The Bear 1000 can be programmed to provide ventilation for children and adults.

Power Source

The Bear 1000 is pneumatically powered and microprocessor-controlled. It is normally connected to external high-pressure sources of air and oxygen (30 to 80 psig). An air compressor can be added to the unit so that the ventilator can operate from a high-pressure air source without external gas connections; however, this eliminates the ability to increase F_IO_2. The power switch for the unit is on the back of the ventilator.

The patient circuit has a proximal pressure line to monitor airway pressure at the Y connector. The exhalation valve is mounted internally. Gas from the patient exits through the exhalation diaphragm and the external flow sensor, which is a hot wire anemometer (Box 12-1).

Internal Mechanisms

Compressed oxygen and air enter the Bear 1000 through filters and check valves to regulators that reduce the pressures to an internal driving pressure of 18.0 psig. Gas passes to a blender and is then directed to an **accumulator.** The accumulator holds 3.5 L of gas under driving pressure (18.0 psig) and acts both as a mixing chamber to blend gases and as a source of high flow (≥ 200 L/min). Gas exits the accumulator and passes to a flow-control valve that is

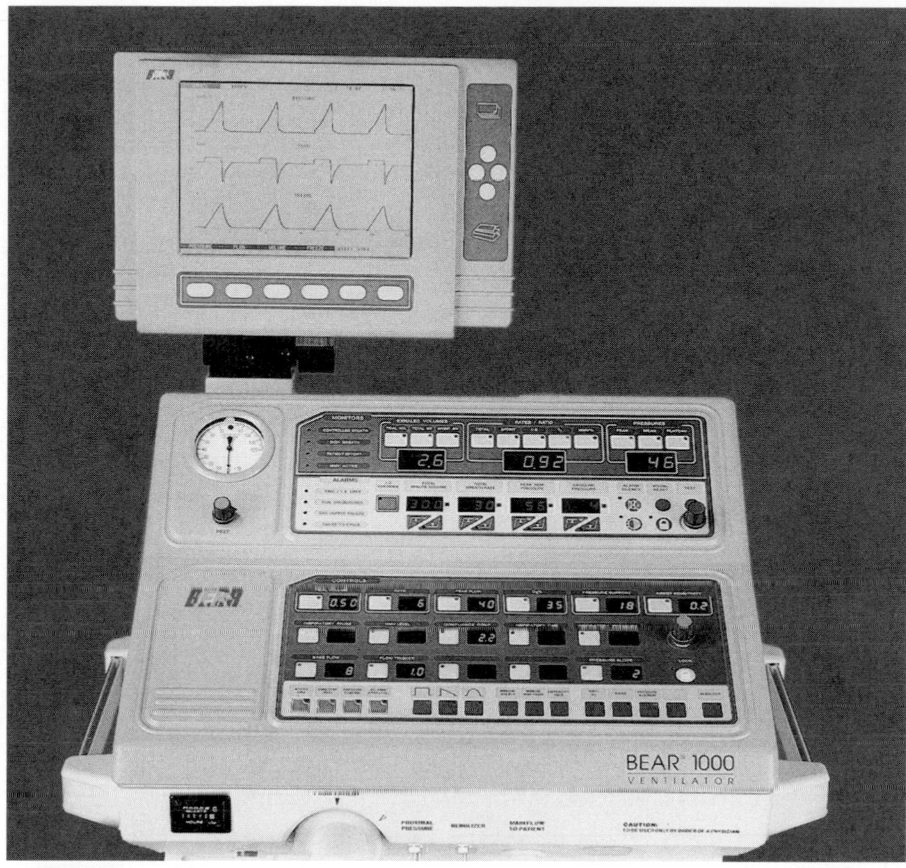

Figure 12-1 The Bear 1000 ventilator. (Courtesy Viasys Healthcare, Critical Care Division, Palm Springs, Calif.)

Box 12-1 Bear 1000 Exhalation Flow Sensor

Remember from Chapter 8 that a hot wire anemometer measures gas flow as the rate of heat loss from the hot wire. Therefore the greater the flow, the greater the current needed to maintain a high constant temperature.

positioned by a stepper motor, so that rapid changes in flow are possible (see Chapter 11). The flow delivery logic of the microprocessor uses information from the monitors and the control panel to determine outflow from the valve.

There are six pressure transducers that provide information to the microprocessor: (1) a proximal pressure transducer, (2) a differential pressure transducer, (3) a flow valve pressure transducer, (4) a machine pressure transducer, (5) air, and (6) oxygen source pressure transducers.

Both control panel settings and patient flow demand determine the output from the flow-control valve. The flow-control valve allows for delivery of flows from 10 to 150 L/min for volume breaths and in excess of 200 L/min for pressure breaths or on patient demand. From the flow-control valve, gas travels through the **subambient overpressure-relief valve (SOPR)** and out of the ventilator through the outlet check valve. A diagram of the internal circuitry is available on the EVOLVE site for this text.

Controls and Alarms

The operating panel of the Bears 1000 is separated into two sections (Figures 12-2 and 12-3). The lower section contains the control functions, and the upper section contains the alarms and monitors. Both panels contain a key that must be unlocked before any settings can be changed. Once unlocked, both panels also contain a CONTROL knob that adjusts the numerical value of any parameter selected. To select a parameter, the operator simply presses the touch pad for the parameter, and an LED illuminates and flashes to show that it has been selected.

Control Panel

The control panel is organized into four rows of controls (see Figure 12-3). With the exception of the CONTROL knob, each control variable (e.g., volume and rate) has a touch pad, a small LED to show when it is active, and a digital window to give the operator the selected value. A control can only be selected and changed if the LED for the variable is illuminated, and only those controls available in the current mode of ventilation illuminate. For example, to

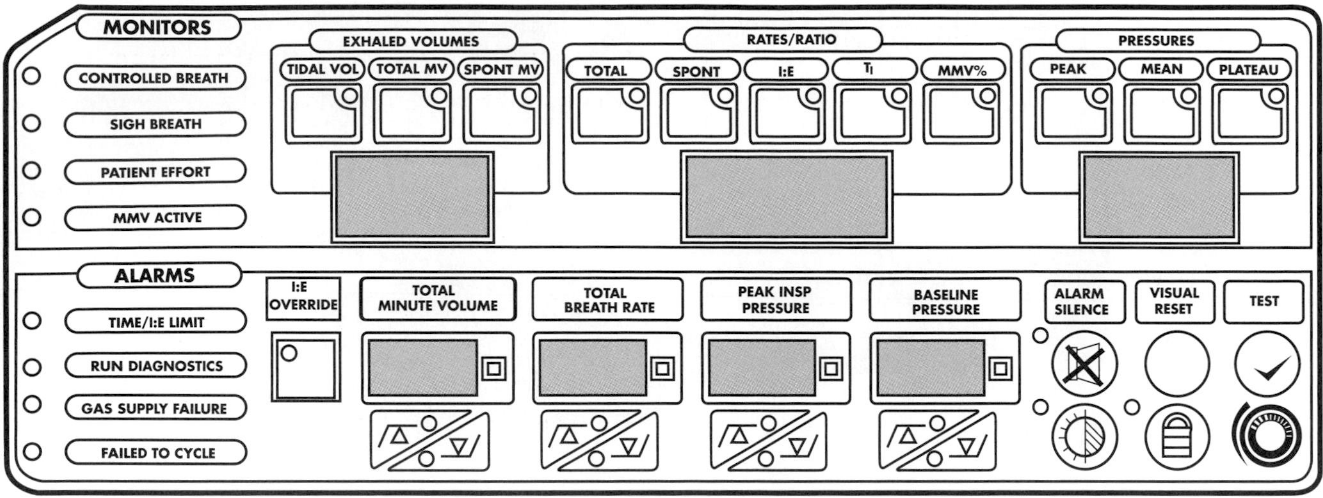

Figure 12-2 Monitor and alarm panel of the Bear 1000.

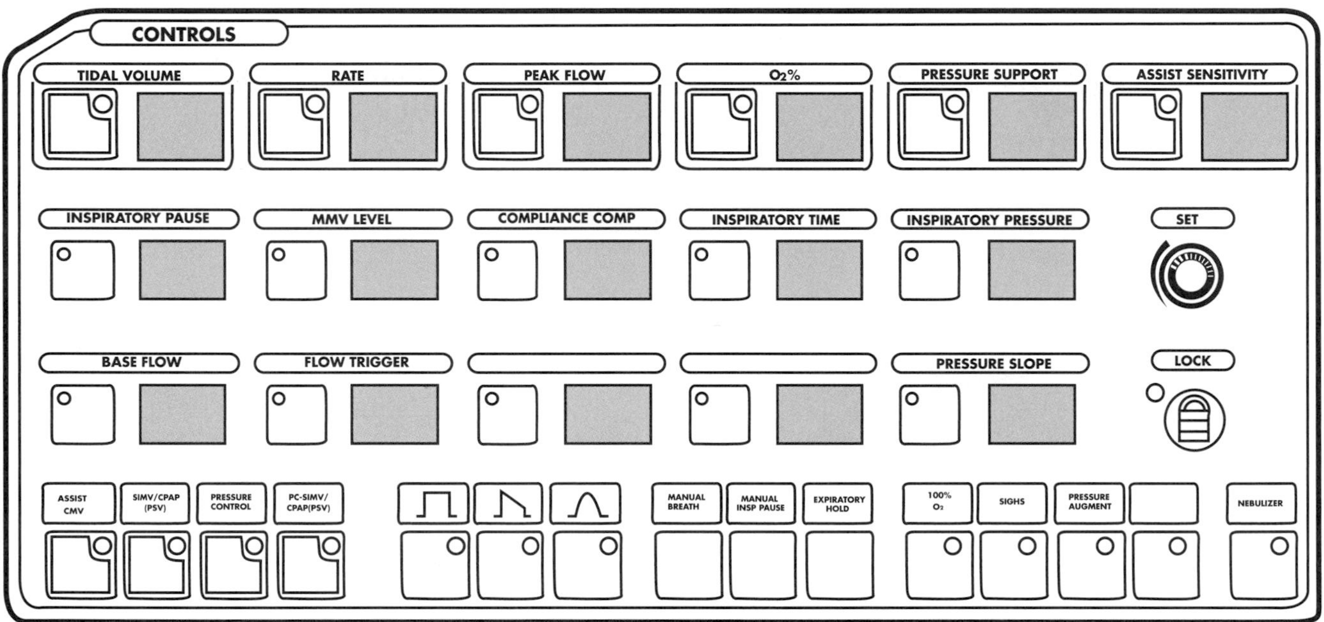

Figure 12-3 Control panel of the Bear 1000.

change V_T during volume ventilation, the touch pad next to the parameter is pushed, and then the control knob at the far right on the second row of controls is turned until the desired value for V_T appears. The change in the parameter's actual value occurs immediately.

The top row of controls on the control panel includes (from left to right) tidal volume (100 to 2000 mL), rate (0, or 0.5 to 120 breaths/min), flow (10 to 150 L/min), O_2% (21% to 100%), pressure support (0 to 80 cm H_2O), and assist sensitivity (0.2 to 5.0 cm H_2O). Units programmed for lower volumes can provide lower tidal volumes (30 to 99 mL) and flows (5 to 150 L/min). To obtain these lower variables, the operator must press and hold the touch pad for V_T or flow while turning the control knob. When a "P" is displayed in the adjacent digital window, the lower volume range has been obtained. When a pediatric circuit is used, it is recommended that the **pressure slope** control (in the third row) be turned to 0 or P0. This control can be readjusted using the ventilator's graphic display after it is attached to the patient (see the discussion of pressure sloping).

The second row of controls includes inspiratory pause (0.0 to 2.0 seconds), mandatory minute volume (MMV) level (0 to 50 L/min), COMPLIANCE COMPENSATION (0.0 to 7.5 mL/cm H_2O), **inspiratory time** (0.1 to 5.0 sec), inspiratory pressure (0 to 80 cm H_2O), and the CONTROL knob. With inspiratory pause, both the inspiratory and expiratory valves close and hold the delivered breath in the patient and the patient circuit after inspiration. Inspiratory pause is commonly used to measure plateau pressure for the calculation of static compliance. The MMV control sets the minimum minute ventilation ($\dot{V}_E$) that the operator wants the ventilator to provide for the patient (see the discussion on modes later in this chapter). The COMPLIANCE COMP. control compensates for the volume lost resulting from tubing compressibility (tubing compliance). The operator enters the numerical value of tubing compliance for the patient circuit being used. He or she obtains this value by performing a tubing test and calculation (see Chapter 11 for explanation). The ventilator adds volume to the set V_T (Equation 1) to establish volume output (Equation 2), so the desired V_T is delivered to the patient. The monitor display of V_T (monitor and alarm panel) shows the measured exhaled V_T minus the additional volume (Equation 3).

Equation 1:

volume added = (COMPLIANCE COMP. setting) × (PIP* − PEEP)

* PIP is the peak pressure from the previous breath

Equation 2:

volume output from ventilator = volume added (for tubing compliance) + set V_T

Equation 3:

volume displayed = measured exhaled V_T − volume added

When the INSPIRATORY TIME control is used with **pressure-control ventilation** (pressure control and PC-SIMV/CPAP[PS]), the breath is time-cycled out of inspiration. The INSPIRATORY PRESSURE CONTROL sets the level of pressure that the ventilator will maintain during inspiration for pressure control ventilation (PCV). (These modes will be reviewed in the discussion of modes later in this section.) In the original panel of the Bear 1000, the inspiratory pressure control was called "PRES SUP/INSP PRES" and controlled the pressure for pressure-support breaths, pressure-targeted breaths in PCV, and pressure augmentation. It was changed in the updated version so that SIMV could provide mandatory PCV and spontaneous PSV with different pressure levels for each. The CONTROL knob allows the operator to adjust the value of the selected parameter.

The third row of controls includes the **base flow** control (0, or 2 to 20 L/min), **flow trigger** control (from 1 to 10 L/min), two blank controls for future updates, pressure slope control (from -9 to 9 for adult settings and P-9 to P9 for pediatric settings), and the lock control. Base flow is the flow added to the circuit during exhalation in order to provide flow triggering. Flow trigger is the amount the flow must drop from the base flow value to trigger a patient-(flow)-triggered breath (see Chapter 11). The FLOW TRIGGER control can only be set if base flow is active. (*Note:* The unit can be set so that pressure and flow transducers for triggering a breath are active. The ventilator selects the signal that is most sensitive to patient effort and has the fastest response. The manufacturer calls this the "**SmartTrigger**" option.)

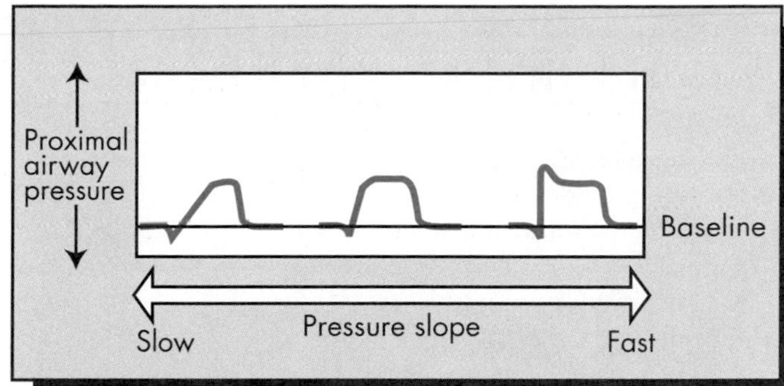

Figure 12-4 Pressure sloping function shown during pressure-support breaths on the Bear 1000; slow (-9) to fast (+9). See text for further explanation. (Courtesy of Viasys Healthcare, Critical Care Division, Palm Springs, Calif.)

Box 12-2 The Fourth Row of Controls on the Bear 1000 Operating Panel

Mode Controls

Assist CMV, SIMV/CPAP (PSV), Pressure Control, PC-SIMV/CPAP (PSV)

Flow Waveform Controls

Constant (rectangular), descending ramp, sinelike wave

Miscellaneous Controls

Manual breath, manual inspiratory pause, expiratory hold, 100% O_2, sighs, pressure augment, blank control (for future option), nebulizer

PRESSURE SLOPE provides control over the speed at which the inspiratory pressure level is achieved. The amount of slope can be monitored by observing how the pressure curve tapers at the beginning of a pressure breath (pressure control, pressure support, pressure augmentation). Significant tapering or sloping reduces pressure delivery at the beginning of the breath (negative values). Positive values for pressure slope provide rapid delivery of pressure at the beginning of the breath (Figure 12-4). The lock function locks and unlocks the control panel. When controls are locked, they cannot be changed.

The fourth row of controls is listed in Box 12-2. The mode controls are explained in the discussion of modes later in this section. The original version of the Bear 1000 did not provide a mode for SIMV with pressure-targeted breaths, but the newer version does. This control is called "PC-SIMV/CPAP(PSV)," with PSV indicating pressure

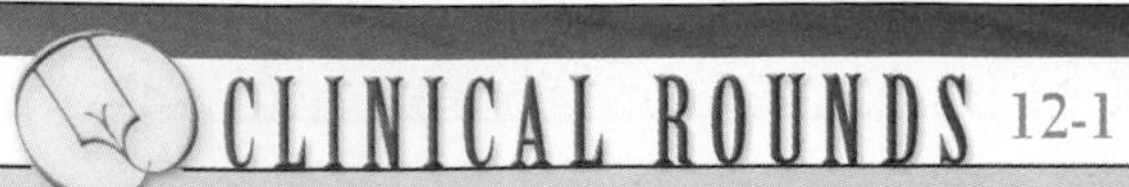

12-1

During volume ventilation with the Bear 1000, the length of inspiration depends on the flow, volume, and rate. For example, the following parameters are set:

- Peak flow = 60 L/min (1 L/second)
- Flow waveform = constant
- Volume = 0.5 L (500 mL)
- Rate = 12 breaths/min (TCT = 5 seconds)

Calculate the inspiratory time (T_I). What happens to T_I when the flow curve is changed to a descending ramp?

See Appendix A for the answer.

support ventilation. The FLOW WAVEFORM controls only operate during volume-targeted breaths. The constant flow waveform delivers flow at the peak flow setting. The descending ramp rapidly rises to the peak flow setting, then descends linearly until flow decreases to about 50% of peak. The sine flow progressively rises to peak flow and gradually falls to zero in a sinusoidal pattern (Clinical Rounds 12-1).

When activated during expiration, the MANUAL BREATH control delivers one mandatory breath in any mode based on the set values. (*Note*: The unit will not allow a manual breath to be delivered during inspiratory flow of another breath.) MANUAL INSPIRATORY PAUSE triggers a pause at the end of inspiration of the next volume breath and operates for as long as it is depressed—up to a maximum of 2 seconds. It can be used to obtain a plateau pressure reading when the patient is not actively breathing.

EXPIRATORY HOLD delays breath delivery when pressed during the end of exhalation. It closes the expiratory and inspiratory valves at the moment the next mandatory breath would have been delivered and stops breath delivery for as long as it is pressed (maximum time is 9 seconds). It is used for measuring auto-PEEP.

The 100% O_2 knob delivers 100% oxygen through the patient circuit until it is pressed a second time or 3 minutes have passed, whichever comes first.

Selecting the sigh control provides a sigh breath every 100th breath. The conditions of delivery vary with the mode. Sigh is not available with pressure control in either A/C or SIMV modes. With CPAP, only mandatory breaths are counted until the 100 mandatory breath, so sigh delivery is unlikely. The volume delivery is 150% of the set V_T. The pressure limit for sigh is 150% of the set pressure limit. When it is time for delivery, the sigh breath replaces the next volume breath. With A/C, total cycle time (TCT) is doubled. With SIMV, TCT does not change.

PRESSURE AUGMENTATION is another control in this row; it is reviewed in the discussion of modes of ventilation later in this section.

When **NEBULIZER control** is selected, a 10 psig gas source is available to the nebulizer port, which can be connected to a small-volume nebulizer for delivery of medication. Approximately 6 L/min of flow comes from this port. The ventilator automatically subtracts 6 L/min from the flow that would be delivered during inspiration so that V_T delivery does not change significantly. In addition, the nebulizer only operates when the flow from the main inspiratory line exceeds 20 L/min—regardless of the mode, pressure slope, or waveform selected. The nebulizer port operates for 30 minutes unless the control is turned off first.

The only control not part of the control panel is the PEEP control, which is a knob located below the analog manometer. The PEEP control has no numerical values next to it, so adjustment is determined by the PEEP value indicated on the analog manometer. PEEP ranges from 0 to 50 cm H_2O and is available with all modes. If a leak occurs in the patient circuit when baseline is above zero, the ventilator increases flow through the circuit to try to maintain the selected PEEP level.

The **analog pressure manometer** reads from -10 to 120 cm H_2O and provides monitoring in all modes. It is a back-up method of verifying digitally displayed pressure values (peak, mean, and plateau pressure).

Monitors and Alarms

The top panel of the Bear 1000 contains the alarms and monitors (see Figure 12-2). The first row of this section contains monitored information, and the second row contains alarm information. On the left of the panel is a list of four possible breath functions: controlled breath, sigh breath, patient effort, and MMV active. An LED adjacent to each of these illuminates to indicate the type of breath that has just been initiated. For example, the CONTROLLED-BREATH LED lights up if a set volume or pressure breath is either patient- or time-triggered. It also lights up for a sigh breath or a manually triggered breath. The SIGH BREATH LED lights during the inspiratory phase of a sigh breath. The PATIENT EFFORT LED indicates that patient effort was equal to or greater than the set assist sensitivity or flow trigger. The MMV ACTIVE LED indicates that the ventilator is giving back-up breaths to maintain a minimum level of ventilation (see MMV in the section under modes) and remains lit as long as the MMV backup is active.

The next section of the monitor panel is the exhaled volume section. There is one digital readout window and three potential volume readings: V_T, total $\dot{V}_E$, and spontaneous $\dot{V}_E$. The operator selects the desired displayed volume by pressing the touch pad below the volume. Volumes are measured by the flow sensor located near the main expiratory line. The expiratory flow sensor reads flow and converts it to volume readings at STPD (standard temperature [77° F, or 25° C], ambient pressure, dry gas). The microprocessor subtracts the volume attributed to humidity from the exhaled volumes to help correct readings.

Box 12-3 Calculating I:E Ratios on the Bear 1000

A patient on A/C volume ventilation on the Bear 1000 has the following settings: V_T = 1.0 L; rate = 10/min; flow = constant; peak flow = 60 L/min. Calculate the I:E ratio.

TCT = 60/10 breaths/min = 6 seconds

$T_I = V_T$/flow

Change flow to liters/second.

60 L/min = 1 L/sec

$T_I = V_T$/flow = 1 L/(1 L/sec) = 1 second

T_E = TCT - T_I = 6 seconds −1 second = 5 seconds

I:E = 1:5

(If you had trouble with this calculation, refer to Chapter 11.)

Box 12-4 Measuring Plateau Pressure

Plateau pressure measurement is an attempt to estimate the pressure in the patient's lungs at the end of inspiration; but it really measures pressure in both the lungs and the patient circuit.

When plateau pressure is measured, a patient cannot be actively breathing. If the patient tries to breathe in or out against the closed valves, which is only natural, the plateau reading will be inaccurate.

V_T represents the most recent breath of any type. $\dot{V}_E$, total or spontaneous, is the average of the most recent breaths. Any changes represent the actual exhaled volumes accumulated over a 1 minute. The V_Ts range from 0.00 to 9.99 L and the $\dot{V}_E$ (total and spontaneous) range from 0 to 99.9 L.

The next panel displays either respiratory rate (total or spontaneous), I:E ratio, inspiratory time or % MMV. Likewise, there is one digital display window, so the operator selects which parameter is to be displayed. Rate is an average of the most recent breaths and reflects a 60-second accumulated value. Available readings are from 0 to 155 breaths/min. The total represents all breaths, and the spontaneous rate only represents patient spontaneous breaths for CPAP or pressure-support breaths.

The I:E ratio ranges from 1:0.1 to 1:99.9 and can be calculated with the following ratio: 1:(T_E/T_I). The reading is based on the last breath and updates at the beginning of the next inspiration. It does not measure spontaneous or pressure-support breaths (Box 12-3).

T_I displays the inspiratory time for the previous breath. Similar to the I:E ratio, it does not work for spontaneous or pressure-supported breaths. Its values range from 0 to 9.99 seconds.

The MMV % monitor (0% to 100%) displays the average percentage of time in the last 30 minutes that the MMV backup rate has been used instead of the normal breath rate control.

The pressure monitors include peak, mean, and plateau. As with the other monitors, the operator must select which of the three is to be displayed. Peak pressure (0 to 140 cm H_2O) shows PIP for the most recent breath, but does not read spontaneous peak pressure. Mean (0 to 140 cm H_2O) shows the average mean pressure at the Y connector for the last breath. Plateau (0 to 140 cm H_2O) requires that an inspiratory pause of at least 0.1 seconds be provided. This can be done using the inspiratory pause control on the second row of controls or the manual inspiratory pause on the fourth row of controls. The window displays the plateau pressure of the previous breath. If no measurable plateau was present on the previous breath, it reads zero (Box 12-4).

Alarms

The alarms being monitored appear in the second row on the monitor and alarm panel. The left column of alarms represents built-in alarms. The TIME/I:E limit alarm is activated under two circumstances: when T_I is ≥ 5 sec + inspiratory pause time and T_I exceeds T_E, and when the I:E ratio exceeds 1:1 for mandatory breaths. For example, if an attempt is made to alter the ratio to 2:1, the alarm will sound. If these limits are exceeded, the ventilator ends inspiration. The first alarm condition cannot be disabled. To disable the second alarm condition, the operator must select the I:E override key, which is to the right of the TIME/I:E limit alarm. When the LED for the I:E override key is on, the ventilator will allow inverse ratios up to 4:1.

The RUN DIAGNOSTICS indicator tells the operator that the microprocessor has detected a system or electronic problem during the self test or normal operation. A troubleshooting code can be viewed in the total minute volume digital display by pressing the test key. The gas supply failure alarm activates if either source gas pressure falls below 27.5 psig. The ventilator will continue to operate from the remaining gas source, but this can alter F_IO_2 delivery. The FAILED TO CYCLE alarm activates if the ventilator does not cycle because of an external or internal condition. The error code appears in the total minute volume digital display window. An internal safety valve opens, allowing the patient to breathe room air. These four built-in alarms are both visual (flashing light) and audible. If any of these LEDs are lit but not flashing, this indicates that the alarm condition occurred but was corrected. Pressing the visual reset near the right side of this row of alarms turns the light off.

There are also four sets of adjustable alarms in the second row. The alarm sequence from left to right is: TOTAL MINUTE VOLUME, TOTAL BREATH RATE, PEAK INSPIRATORY PRESSURE, and BASELINE PRESSURE. They can all be adjusted in the same way. For each alarm panel, there is one digital display window used for both the high and low settings of a particular alarm. To the right of the digital window is an

LED that lights up when the alarm is violated. There are two touch pads below the digital window: the left one has an upward-pointing triangle and sets the upper limit; the right one has a downward-pointing triangle and sets the lower limit. To adjust either, the alarm panel must be unlocked with the LOCK control. Either the upper or lower limit touch pad should be touched for the desired alarm parameter. For example, if the upper alarm key for total minute volume is touched, its current numerical value appears in the digital display window. At the same time, the touch pad light that was touched begins to flash and will do so for 15 seconds or as long as the control knob continues to be turned. While it is flashing, the touch pad light can be adjusted by turning the ALARM CONTROL knob on the far right side of the alarm panel. It is important to note that the alarm level changes as soon as the knob is turned, even while the alarm indicator is flashing. While the first selected alarm parameter is still flashing, the operator can select another alarm to adjust by repeating the same process. Even though the indicators may be flashing, only one parameter can be adjusted at a time.

When the alarm parameters set by the operator have been exceeded, the small light to the right of the digital display (the alarm trigger indicator for that control) flashes and an audible alarm sounds. After the alarm condition is corrected, the alarm trigger indicator stays lit until the visual reset pad is pressed.

The high and low $\dot{V}_E$ alarms range from 0 to 80 and 0 to 50 L, respectively. High and low V_T rate alarms range from 0 to 155 and 1 to 99 breaths/min, respectively. HIGH and LOW PIP alarms are slightly more involved. The high PIP range is from 0 to 120 cm H_2O, and reaching this alarm limit ends inspiration. For a sigh breath, the PIP is 150% of the set high PIP limit, or 120 cm H_2O, whichever occurs first. When a high PIP alarm occurs, the pressure in the proximal line must drop to within 5 cm H_2O of the PEEP level (baseline). If there is a kink in the main expiratory line, the line pressure may not be able to drop, and the delivery of the next breath is delayed until pressure in the proximal line decreases. The range for the low PIP alarm is from 3 to 99 cm H_2O and cannot be set below 3 cm H_2O. It is not active for spontaneous breaths and is also inactive in PSV and PCV under the following condition:

$$[\text{PEEP} + (\text{Pressure Support or Inspiratory Pressure})] \leq 3 \text{ cm } H_2O$$

If the abbreviation *Pro* appears in the PIP alarm display window, the machine pressure is greater than the sum of the high PIP alarm setting + 10 cm H_2O. The *Pro* alarm is most commonly caused by a disconnection of the proximal pressure line from the machine or the patient circuit, but large leaks can also be responsible.

HIGH and LOW BASELINE PRESSURE alarms (0 to 55 cm H_2O and 0 to 50 cm H_2O, respectively) occur when monitored pressure limits are exceeded. Box 12-5 gives some examples of when these events can occur.

Box 12-5 Situations Affecting Baseline Pressure

PEEP is set at 8 cm H_2O, and the high and low PEEP alarms are set at 13 and 3 cm H_2O, respectively. If a leak occurs and pressure during expiration falls to zero, the low baseline pressure alarm activates. If the patient actively exhales or coughs during expiration and prevents pressure from falling to at least 8 cm H_2O, the high baseline pressure alarm will sound.

Five touch pads and the control knob are to the right of the alarms in this row. The top three touch pads are as follows:

1. Alarm silence: silences audible alarms for 60 seconds or until pressed again; cannot silence the failed to cycle alarm
2. Visual reset: resets visual alarms after alarm conditions are corrected
3. Test: has three functions: (1) activates the visual and audible indicators for 4 seconds during normal operation in order to check function; (2) displays any troubleshooting codes that might have occurred with the ventilator in the total minute ventilation digital window; or (3) if pressed before the ventilator is turned on and held while the power is turned on, it causes the ventilator to enter Operator Diagnostics, and the operating manual should be consulted

The bottom two touch keys are the dimmer key and the LOCK key. The DIMMER key adjusts the brightness of the LEDs on the control panel, and the LOCK key locks the alarm control panel so values cannot be accidentally changed. The LED near this key is lit when the panel is locked. Changes to alarm controls cannot be made until this key is pressed to unlock it.

Modes of Ventilation

The mode controls on the Bear 1000 include the following: assist continuous mandatory ventilation (CMV), SIMV/CPAP(PSV), pressure control, PC-IMV/CPAP(PSV), pressure augment, and MMV. Each of these will be reviewed.

Changing Ventilator Modes

The first four mode keys are on the lower left row of the control panel. The last, PRESSURE AUGMENTATION, is the farthest right control in this row. Mode keys have three conditions: OFF, SETUP, and ON. When changing an operating mode on the Bear 1000, the following procedure is used. The operator first presses the mode key for the new mode desired: OFF TO SETUP. This causes the LED by that mode's touch pad to flash while the original mode key's LED stays lit. The control panel illuminates the controls available for the new mode. Then the operator adjusts each control variable for the new mode to the desired setting, along with all desired alarm settings. After everything is set, the operator presses the new mode touch pad a second time: SETUP TO ON. It stays illuminated and the old mode switches off.

Assist CMV

Assist CMV is **volume-targeted ventilation** that can be time- or patient- (pressure- or flow-) triggered. All of the controls are available except MMV, inspiratory time, pressure support, or inspiratory pressure.

SIMV/CPAP (PSV)

SIMV/CPAP (PSV) is volume-targeted SIMV. The operator can provide a positive baseline (PEEP/CPAP) in this mode by using the PEEP control. Pressure support is also available for spontaneous breaths. Volume breaths can be patient-triggered or, if that fails, time-triggered. Volume breaths are based on the V_T, rate, peak flow, and flow waveform selected. Spontaneous breaths begin from the set baseline pressure. In addition, PSV can be provided for spontaneous breaths based on the set pressure support level. The set PSV pressure is added to the PEEP level. For example, if the PEEP is 5 cm H_2O, and the PSV is set at 15 cm H_2O, PIP during a PSV breath will be 20 cm H_2O. The PSV breaths are patient-triggered, pressure-limited, and flow-cycled at about 30% of the initial peak flow reached at the beginning of the breath.

When this mode control is active and the rate is turned to zero, the ventilator can provide either CPAP alone or PSV. Baseline can also be zero with PSV added for spontaneous breath support.

Pressure Control

Pressure control is **pressure-targeted ventilation** in which each breath is time- or patient- (flow- or pressure-) triggered, and the ventilator provides the pressure set on the inspiratory pressure control for each breath. Pressure-delivered equals the inspiratory pressure plus PEEP. In addition to inspiratory pressure, the operator sets the rate, T_I, assist sensitivity and/or base flow and flow trigger, and pressure sloping. Most other controls, including the waveforms, sigh, and pressure augment, are not available. It is very important to set the upper pressure limit in this mode because pressure can go above the set inspiratory pressure level. For example, if the patient coughs, the pressure may exceed the set value. A reasonable setting would be 10 to 15 cm H_2O above the peak inspiratory pressure.

PC-SIMV with CPAP and PSV

PC-SIMV/CPAP(PSV) is ventilation in which mandatory or assisted breaths are pressure-targeted and time-cycled. Remember the definitions of mandatory and assisted (Box 12-6; see Chapter 11). Baseline can be positive. Spontaneous breaths can occur with pressure support or simply from the set baseline. As in pressure control, the operator sets the rate, inspiratory pressure, triggering mechanisms, and T_I. PEEP and pressure support can also be set. Both the inspiratory pressure setting and the pressure support setting are added to the PEEP level. If the inspiratory pressure is 20 cm H_2O, the pressure support is 10 cm H_2O, and the baseline 10 cm H_2O, PIP for mandatory will be 30 cm H_2O, and all spontaneous breaths will be at 20 cm H_2O.

If rate is turned to zero, the ventilator allows the patient to spontaneously breathe at the set baseline (zero or PEEP/CPAP). If the sensitivity is appropriately set, the ventilator can monitor spontaneous breaths, which occurs when the patient's inspiratory effort meets or exceeds the set trigger value. These spontaneous breaths can also be pressure-supported.

Pressure slope can also be used in this mode and can affect the rate of flow during pressure-targeted mandatory, pressure-support breaths, or spontaneous breaths.

Box 12-6 Reviewing Definitions of Breath Types

Mandatory breath delivery is completely determined by the ventilator (i.e., triggering, delivery of inspiration, and cycling are ventilator-controlled). Breaths are commonly volume- or pressure-targeted.

An assisted breath is patient-triggered. The delivery of inspiration and the ending of inspiration (cycling) is determined by the ventilator.

With spontaneous breaths, the patient controls all phases of the breath.

Pressure Augment

Pressure augment, or pressure augmentation (PAug), is a servo-control (closed-loop) mode of ventilation that guarantees volume delivery for each breath. Because it is a fairly unusual form of ventilation, more time is spent reviewing its function.

PAug provides the benefits of pressure-targeted ventilation, such as high initial gas flows, a descending-ramp type of flow pattern, and a limited pressure, with the added feature that it can guarantee volume delivery. Key criteria for using pressure augmentation are that a patient must be able to initiate breaths and must have a consistent respiratory rate and a reasonable inspiratory effort. PAug is designed to work in any patient-triggered volume breath. For this reason, it only works in assist CMV and SIMV/CPAP(PSV). It is selected by pressing the pressure augment control so that it is illuminated. The operator also selects a V_T, a rate, an inspiratory pressure level above baseline, a peak flow, and a sensitivity setting. It is also important to set an appropriate pressure limit of about 10 cm H_2O above the inspiratory pressure plus PEEP. Regarding flow pattern, it is currently recommended that a constant flow pattern be selected to help keep T_I shorter.

PAug operates in the following manner. When the patient triggers a breath, the ventilator provides a high inspiratory gas flow to achieve the set pressure level. As it delivers this flow, it monitors flow and volume delivery. From this point, one of two possible scenarios unfolds. If patient inspiratory flow demand and the set pressure are high, the ventilator will see that the minimum volume is delivered quickly and it does not need to take any action. Inspiration ends when the flow drops to 30% of measured peak flow. If the patient demand is modest, however, the ventilator may find that the volume has not been delivered by the time the measured flow has dropped to a value equal to the flow set on the peak flow control. In this case, it will not allow the flow to drop further, but will maintain flow at the set peak flow and continue to provide this flow until it determines that the minimum volume has been delivered, at which point the breath ends.

Figure 12-5 illustrates some of the potential outcomes of PAug. Waveform A is an example of a typical pressure-support breath instead of a pressure-augmented breath, so that readers can make some comparisons with pressure augmentation. In **A**, the breath is patient-triggered, pressure-limited (25 cm H_2O), and flow-cycled at approximately 30% of the peak flow reached (100 L/min), and the patient achieved a V_T of about 1.0 L.

In Waveform **B**, the patient has a moderate inspiratory demand, and flow rises to reach and maintain the pressure (25 cm H_2O). Flow drops to the set value of 40 L/min and the ventilator determines that the set volume of 0.8 L has not been reached. It maintains the flow at 40 L/min. Because more flow is going into the patient's lungs, the pressure rises above the set value. When the ventilator determines that the volume was delivered, the breath ends. This is a classic pattern of a pressure-augmented breath.

In Waveform **C**, it appears that the set pressure of 25 cm H_2O is not adequate to quickly meet the volume setting for this particular patient. When the flow drops to the set value (40 L/min), it is maintained until the 0.8 L volume is delivered. Notice how long inspiration is compared with Waveforms **A** and **B**. To more appropriately provide pressure augmentation, the inspiratory pressure needs to be increased. The flow may need to be increased as well.

In Waveform **D**, the patient has a high inspiratory demand, flow rises rapidly to reach and maintain the set pressure, inspiratory pressure is set high, and minimum volume is surpassed. Volume delivery is high. In this situation, inspiration ends when the flow drops to about 30% of peak flow. PAug can provide whatever volume and flow the patient desires and still remain within a safe pressure limit.

In Waveform **E**, no patient effort is detected. The ventilator delivers a typical volume breath at a constant flow setting. Pressure rises to a peak, which depends on the volume delivered and the patient's lung characteristics.

When PAug is used in assist CMV, every breath is potentially augmented. With SIMV, only the patient-triggered mandatory breaths are augmented. It is strongly recommended that practitioners use the graphic waveforms for pressure, volume, and flow against time when adjusting PAug for a patient.

Because of its ability to perform pressure augmentation, the ventilator can also augment flow and volume. If patient inspiratory demand drops the measured airway pressure below the baseline pressure, the ventilator automatically

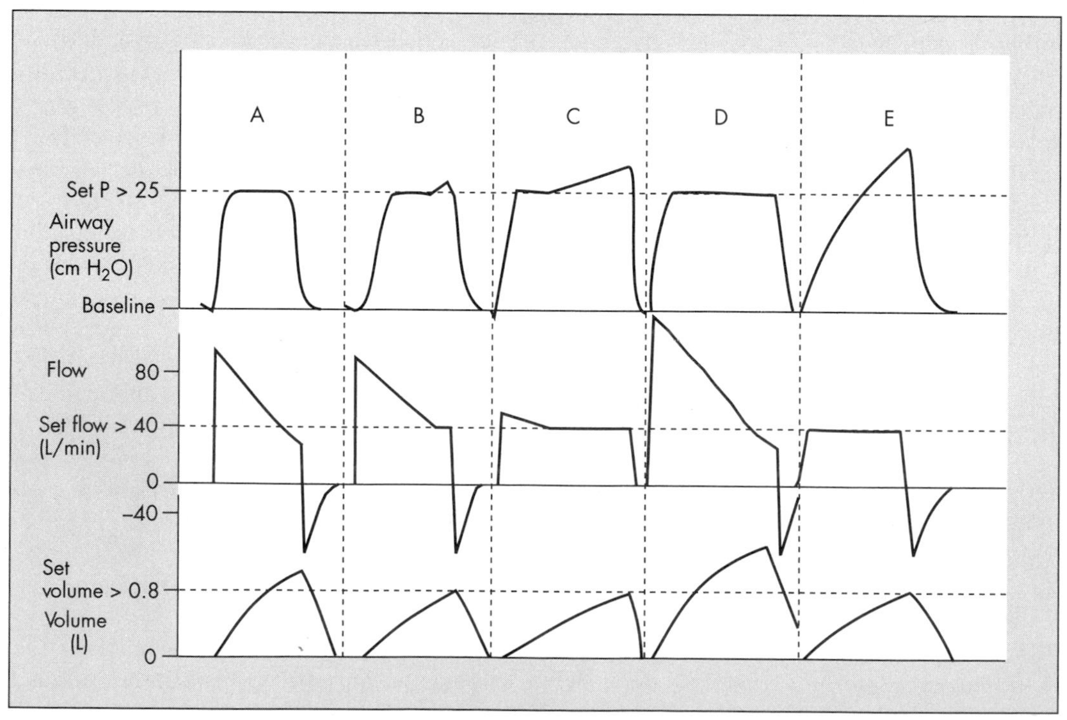

Figure 12-5 Various waveforms achievable with pressure augmentation. (From Pilbeam SP: *Mechanical ventilation: physiological and clinical applications*, ed 3, St Louis, 1998, Mosby.)

increases flow to maintain baseline. This augments flow to the patient and also increases volume delivery above the set value if the patient demands it. For example, in the CPAP mode or with SIMV + CPAP, if baseline pressure during spontaneous breathing drops below the set value due to patient demand, the ventilator increases flow to the patient to maintain the baseline and augment the patient's needs.

MMV Feature

MMV operates in the SIMV and CPAP modes to ensure that spontaneously breathing patient's minute volume does not drop below a set level. As long as the monitored total exhaled minute volume meets or exceeds the value set in the MMV setting, backup ventilator support is inactive. However, if the exhaled $\dot{V}_E$ falls below the set MMV, the breath rate automatically increases to ensure that the minimum $\dot{V}_E$ is delivered. The backup breath rate (breaths/min) is determined as follows.

$$\text{Backup Rate} = (\text{MMV Level})/V_T$$

The MMV ACTIVE indicator illuminates during inspiration and exhalation whenever the MMV mode is active. The MMV % indicator displays the percent of time during the last half-hour that the MMV backup rate has been in use instead of the clinician-set rate.

The ventilator returns to operation at the clinician-set rate when the monitored $\dot{V}_E$ exceeds the set MMV by 1 L/min or 10%, whichever is greater. (*Note*: MMV must be set to a value greater than the set $\dot{V}_E$ (rate × V_T). The Total Breath Rate alarm must be set appropriately to avoid high respiratory rates.)

Special Features

The BEAR 1000T/ES version of the Bear 1000 has some additional upgrades. Two more pressure transducer connectors have been added. One is intended for monitoring esophageal pressures (P_{ES}) and the second tracheal pressures (P_{TRACH}). The Balloon button on the control panel is used to initiate the filling of the esophageal balloon. When pressed once, the button results in a "negative leak test" being performed and then the balloon inflates to the proper fill volume (0.8 cc). When the button is pressed and held, the ventilator performs a "distension maneuver" causing the balloon to fill beyond its normal measuring volume (5 to 5.5 cc adults, 2 to 2.5 cc pediatric). It then returns to the proper fill volume.

The 1000T/ES also determines the inflection points on a pressure/volume loop using algorithms to identify the upper and lower inflection points. The 1000T/ES provides calculations of work of breathing and weaning data, which include the following:

- Ventilator, patient, and imposed work of breathing (Joules/L)
- AutoPEEPes (esophageal)
- AutoPEEPaw (airway),
- Maximum inspiratory pressure (MIP) (range 0 to –60 cm H_2O),
- P100, the pressure generated during the first 100 milliseconds of inspiration; range 0 to –20 cm H_2O,
- f/V_T ratio (rapid shallow breathing index; range 0 to 300),
- Change in esophageal pressure during inspiration (0 to –100 cm H_2O)

Graphics

The Bear 1000 has a graphics monitor and program that can easily be added to the ventilator unit. The graphics panel has a viewing screen (see Figure 12-1), below which are six operating keys. To the right of the screen are two icons and four operating keys that look like arrow heads. The power switch for the screen is on the back panel of the unit, and the screen is activated by touching the icon (that looks like pages of paper) on the upper right corner of the panel to the right of the screen. The icon at the bottom of the panel looks like a printer and allows the information on the screen to be printed when connected to a printer. The four directional arrows have two main functions: they can change the lighting on the screen; and when they are being used for functions, they can change the amplitude scale of the graphs. For example, if a pressure graph goes from 0 to 10 cm H_2O, the arrows can be used to change the range to 0 to 100 cm H_2O.

The operator's manual provides information about setting time and date and other start-up information. There are menus at the top and bottom of the basic waveform pages of the screen. The top menu provides access to waves, loops, set-up, and time and has several blank positions for future updates. The bottom menu provides information about what parameter is on the screen (e.g., flow or volume) and allows it to be selected and changed. The bottom menu also can freeze a screen, mark a particular graph for reference, and scale the x-axis of the graph.

Between one and three graphs can be displayed on the screen. For example, the operator may want to view pressure, volume, and flow scalars. These parameters can be selected by highlighting the desired parameter with the adjacent touch pads just below the screen and can be removed by simply unhighlighting the parameters. Loops or graphs can be provided by highlighting the options appearing at the top menu on the screen. The graphic display also has a mechanics page, which offers flow/volume and pressure/volume loops as well as compliance, resistance, and work of breathing calculations.

Troubleshooting

The variety of alarms and monitors and the availability of graphic monitoring make everyday troubleshooting fairly simple. In addition, the operator's manual contains a troubleshooting section with a table of symptoms, possible causes, and corrective actions. For example, suppose the low baseline pressure alarm activates. Possible causes might be the patient is disconnected from the ventilator, or there is a leak in the patient circuit, or there is a leak in the exhalation valve diaphragm. Solutions would include reconnecting the patient, checking the circuit for leaks, and, finally, checking the diaphragm for holes or tears. After correcting any problems it would then be appropriate to perform a leak test.

More than 20 possible problems are identified in the troubleshooting section of the operator's manual. It is beyond the scope of this text to cover all of them. Readers who intend to use this ventilator should consult that section for more information.

Radio frequency interference (RFI)/electromagnetic frequency interference (EFI) can affect the operation of the Bear 1000, just as it can with any medical device that uses a microprocessor. Walkie-talkies and cellular phones should not be used near these types of medical devices.

The manufacturer is continually updating the various programs and features that are available with the unit. It is important to be sure to check which system is in operation when troubleshooting a ventilator problem.

Bird 8400STi Ventilator

The Bird 8400STi ventilator[1-4] is a second-generation unit derived from the Bird 6400, and has largely replaced that unit. It was previously manufactured by Bird Medical Technologies, Inc., and is now a part of Viasys Healthcare, Critical Care Division (Figure 12-6, *A* and *B*). The Bird 8400Ti is designed for use with pediatric and adult patients.

The patient circuit has the usual main inspiratory and expiratory limb and an expiratory valve that is mounted within the unit.

Power Source

The Bird 8400STi is pneumatically powered and microprocessor-controlled. It requires a blender so that a blend of gases may enter the back panel and usually uses a Bird 3800 Microblender, which has two 50 psig (ranging from 30 to 70 psig) gas sources: air and oxygen. The blended and pressurized gas is used for pneumatic operation. A standard 120-volt AC outlet powers the microprocessor and the electrically operated components.

Internal Mechanism

The basic internal circuit of the Bird 8400STi ventilator is described here. The blended gases enter the unit where they are filtered and flow into a high-pressure, 1.1-liter reservoir. This large, pressurized reservoir allows for an augmented gas flow of up to 120 L/min to the patient. Gas passes from the reservoir to a pressure regulator, where the pressure is adjusted to 20 psig. From the regulator, gas passes to the pulsation dampener, a rigid chamber that dampens pressure pulses that may originate from the reservoir, thus minimizing pressure fluctuations.

Gas flow is then directed to the servo-control valve, which is an electromechanical stepper valve that works in the following way. Signals from the microprocessor cause an electric motor to rotate a shaft. These rotations occur in a series of precise steps, each of which opens or closes a poppet type of orifice inside the servo-control valve (see Chapter 11). The information about valve position, orifice size, and the relative flow output from the valve is programmed into the microprocessor, allowing it to precisely deliver the flow, flow pattern, volume, and/or pressure designated by the operator. The operator determines these by selecting the appropriate parameters and modes on the control panel. Flow from the inspiratory flow valve is then directed to the patient.

There is a flow transducer assembly used to monitor flow from the expiratory valve. It operates on the principle of a variable orifice transducer (see Chapter 8). The two small-bore connecting hoses from this unit send pressure information to an internal differential pressure transducer. This information is monitored and interpreted by the microprocessor and used to display information such as $\dot{V}_E$, V_T, respiratory rate, and I:E ratio. A diagram of the pneumatic diagram for the Bird 8400Sti can be found on the EVOLVE Website for this text

Controls and Alarms

The front panel of the Bird 8400STi has two rows of control knobs and a bottom row of touch pad controls (Figure 12-7). Display windows are above the knob controls, and the values displayed there are set, not measured, values.

Controls

The top row of controls has a mode and waveform selection switch on the far left (see Figure 12-7), which allows either A/C or SIMV to be selected. These modes can be either volume- or pressure-targeted. (*Note:* Pressure-targeted ventilation is an option available on the 8400STi ventilator, but is not a standard function.) In volume ventilation, the operator can choose either the constant flow or the descending ramp flow waveform. The next control knob determines either the target volume or pressure, but it normally regulates volume (ranges from 50 to 2000 mL). Pressure-targeted or PCV requires the use of the touch pad on the bottom row marked PRESS. CTRL. Pressing this pad activates the pressure-control mode. The desired pressure can then be selected with the TIDAL VOLUME/INSP.PRESS control. The letter *P*, followed by the amount of inspiratory pressure chosen by the operator (ranges from 5 to

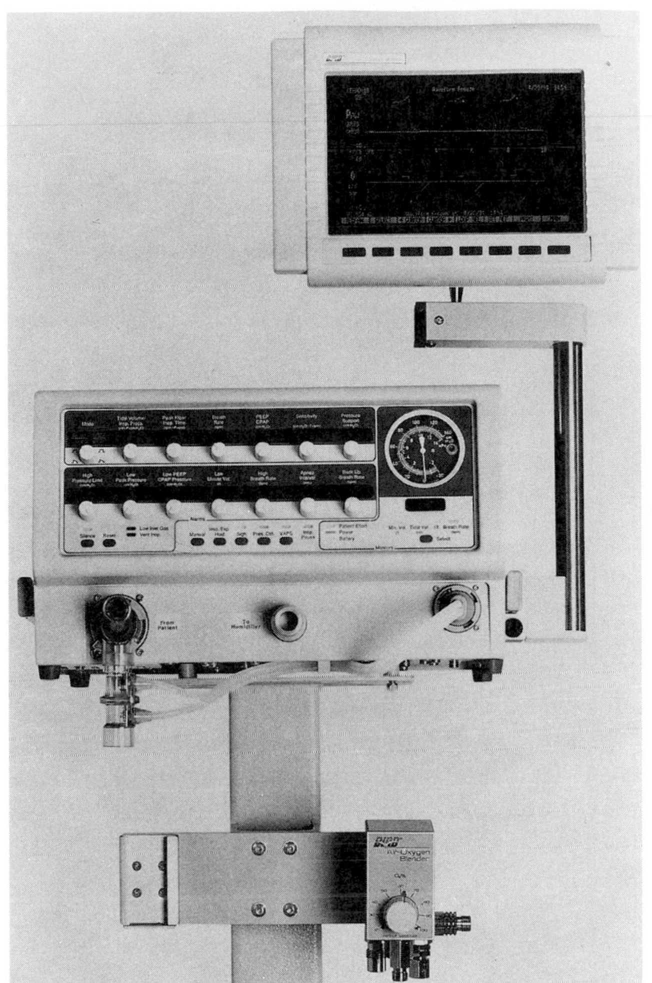

A

Figure 12-6 **A,** photo of the Bird 8400STi ventilator; **B,** the Bird 8400STi with a patient circuit attached. (Courtesy Viasys Healthcare, Critical Care Division, Palm Springs, Calif.)

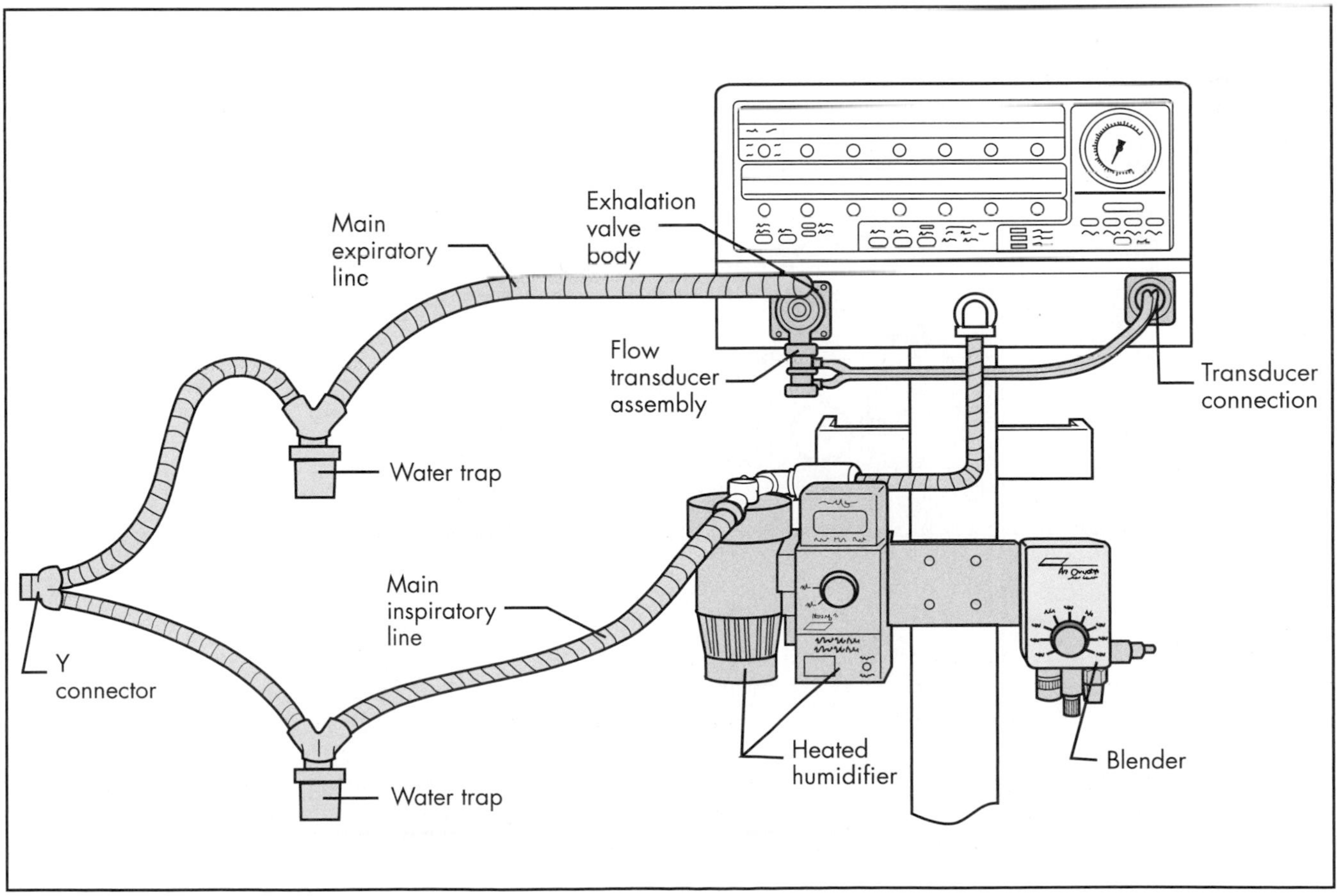

Main expiratory linc
Exhalation valve body
Flow transducer assembly
Transducer connection
Water trap
Y connector
Main inspiratory line
Water trap
Heated humidifier
Blender

B

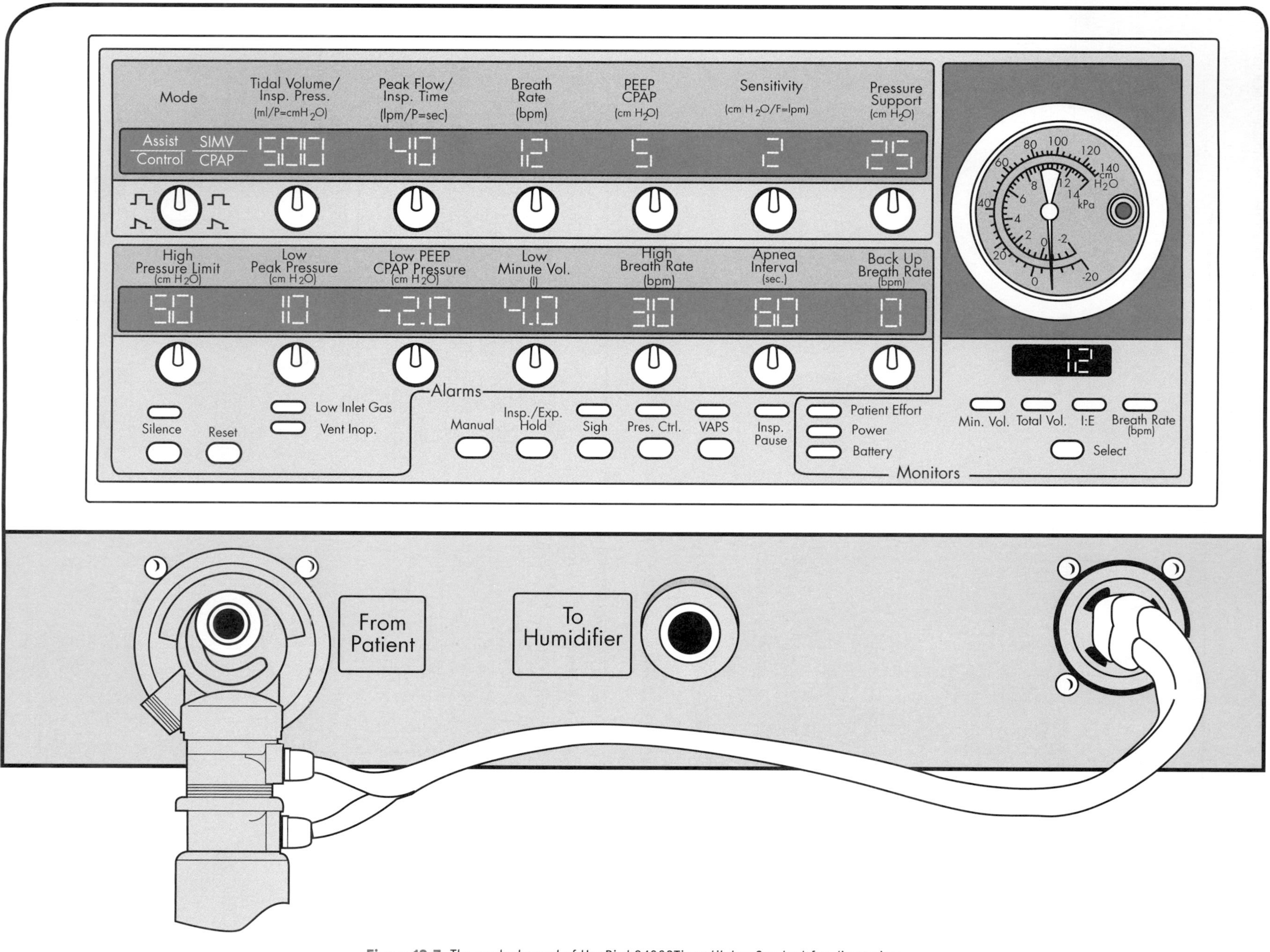

Figure 12-7 The control panel of the Bird 8400STi ventilator. See text for discussion.

100 cm H_2O) is displayed in the window above the knob. How to set up pressure control will be reviewed in the discussion of modes of ventilation in this section.

The next knob in the top row controls either peak flow (volume ventilation) or inspiratory time (PCV). When PCV is used, the numerical value is preceded by the letter *P*. For example, if the digital value is 50, the flow is 50 L/min (10 to 120 L/min). If it reads "P 0.5," the inspiratory time in PCV is 0.5 seconds (range, 0.1 to 9.8 sec).

The third knob on top regulates the respiratory rate (0 to 80 breaths/min), which determines the minimum mandatory rate in the A/C or SIMV mode. This is followed by the PEEP/CPAP control (0 to 30 cm H_2O) and the sensitivity knob. The unit can be pressure- or flow-triggered. Pressure-triggering ranges from –1 to –20 cm H_2O, or can be turned off. Flow-triggering uses a base flow of 10 L/min and a flow trigger range of 1 to 10 L/min (see Chapter 11). When flow-triggering is used, the letter *F* precedes the numerical value for the liters/minute trigger sensitivity. For example, if the number 2 appears in the window above the knob, the machine is pressure-triggering at –2 cm H_2O. If "F 2" is in the window, the flow-triggering sensitivity is set at 2 L/min. The last knob in this row controls pressure-support settings (1 to 50 cm H_2O, or is off). The pressure set by this control is above the set baseline or PEEP level. Pressure support is normally flow-cycled at 25% of measured peak flow, but it will time-cycle if inspiratory flow time exceeds 3 seconds. The second row of alarm controls is discussed in the section on monitors and alarms.

The final row of touch pads and indicators (the right portion after the alarm section) contains some additional controls. The first is the manual touch pad, which provides a manual breath at the set mandatory settings. The INSP/EXP HOLD control can provide either an inspiratory hold for measuring plateau pressure for a mandatory volume breath or an expiratory hold for measuring auto-PEEP when pressed. To obtain an **inspiratory hold,** the pad must be pressed, so the display window below the pressure manometer reads "I HLD." Pressing and holding the select key displays the inspiratory hold pressure. The pad must be pressed three times after this maneuver to return the display to its normal reading. To obtain an expiratory hold, the INSP/EXP HOLD pad must be pressed twice until "E HLD" is displayed in the monitor window. Next, the select key must be pressed and held to display the expiratory pressure (auto-PEEP). After this maneuver, the pad must be pressed twice to return the display to its normal reading. The maximum length for either inspiratory or expiratory hold is 6 seconds. (See Clinical Rounds 12-2 for an exercise in performing this function.)

Activation of the SIGH control provides a sigh breath every 100 breaths. The sigh breath is a mandatory breath equal to 150% of the set V_T (75 to 3000 mL). The upper pressure limit increases to 150% of the set value for this breath (maximum is 140 cm H_2O). The sigh function is available in all modes.

The PRES. CTRL. touch pad is used to set pressure control. The VAPS control is used to set volume-assured pressure support (VAPS) ventilation (see the discussion of modes of ventilation in this section).

At the end of the row of touch pads is an LED marked INSP. PAUSE. Inspiratory pause (0.1 to 3.0 seconds) can be selected for volume-targeted mandatory breaths in A/C or SIMV modes. To activate an inspiratory pause, the INSP./EXP HOLD key must be pressed three times until "IP 0.0" appears in the monitor window. Then the select key must be pressed as many times as necessary to obtain the desired value for pause time. Each time the pad is pressed, pause time increases by 0.1 seconds. After the desired value is obtained, the INSP./EXP HOLD touch pad must be pressed one more time. The INSP. PAUSE LED stays lit, and the display window returns to its original reading. To cancel inspiratory pause, the pad must be pressed four times until "IP X.X" appears in the display window. Pressing the RESET key returns the pause time to "IP 0.0." Pressing the INSP./EXP HOLD pad once more turns off the INSP. PAUSE LED.

Monitors and Alarms

To the right of the bottom row of controls is a section marked "Monitors." The first three monitors are LEDs for

> **CLINICAL ROUNDS 12-2**
>
> A respiratory therapist suspects that a ventilated patient has air trapping. How can she determine the end-expiratory pressure on the Bird 8400STi?
>
> See Appendix A for the answer.

Box 12-7 Parameters Shown in the Display Window Using the Select Touch Pad on the Bird 8400STi

Minute Volume (liters/minute)

Calculated from the last eight breaths (average volume per minute) and the rate for spontaneous and mandatory breaths, as follows:

$\dot{V}_E$ = Total breath rate $\times$

{[Sum of last 8 V_T (mL)] $\div$ 8} $\times$ (1 L/1000 mL)

Tidal Volume (milliliters)

Breath-by-breath

I:E Ratio

Calculated for mandatory breaths only; updated breath-by-breath; range of 1:1.0 to 1:99, or 1:0 to 99:1

Breath Rate (breaths/minute)

Based on an average of the last eight breaths (spontaneous or mandatory), calculated as follows:

Breath rate = 8 breaths divided by sum of the last 8 breath periods (minutes)

Box 12-8 Adjustable Alarm Controls for the Bird 8400STi

High-pressure limit (1 to 140 cm H_2O)
Low peak pressure (2 to 140 cm H_2O, or off)
Low PEEP/CPAP pressure (-20 to + 30 cm H_2O)
Low minute volume (0 to 99.9 L/min)
High breath rate (3 to 150 breaths/min)
Apnea interval (10 to 60 seconds)
Back-up breath rate (0 to 80 breaths/min)

Box 12-9 Low PEEP/CPAP Alarm in the Bird 8400STi

The low PEEP/CPAP alarm can be valuable in detecting the return of the inspiratory effort in patients who have been apneic. This alarm can be set below baseline. For example, if the alarm is set at −2 cm H_2O on a patient who is being heavily sedated, the clinician can be alerted to a change in the level of ventilatory effort. When the patient's inspiratory effort is sufficient to drop baseline pressure to −2 cm H_2O for just half a second, the low PEEP/CPAP alarm sounds. The clinician can then identify the circumstances and take appropriate actions.

PATIENT EFFORT, POWER, and BATTERY. The PATIENT EFFORT LED is lit whenever the ventilator detects a patient inspiratory effort sufficient to trigger a breath (spontaneous or mandatory). The POWER LED lights up when the unit is turned on and connected to an AC power source. The BATTERY LED is illuminated when an external battery is used. An external 12-volt (range 11.8 to 16 volts) direct-current battery can be connected to the unit, but the back panel switch must be changed to the ALT PWR SOURCE setting for the battery to become the source of power.

On the bottom right section of the control panel, there is a touch pad marked SELECT. Pressing this pad allows several parameters (listed in Box 12-7) to be displayed in the monitor window below the pressure manometer. The last front panel monitor is the pressure manometer, which displays airway pressure (ranges from −20 to 140 cm H_2O).

Alarms on the Bird 8400STi are both audio and visual. The second row of the front panel controls contains most of the available alarm settings. Box 12-8 lists the adjustable alarms, which function in the following fashion. Reaching the HIGH-PRESSURE LIMIT ends inspiration, so if the ventilator detects circuit pressures above the set HIGH-PRESSURE LIMIT for more than 0.3 seconds and/or above the baseline pressure 3 cm H_2O for more than 3 seconds, an internal safety valve opens that reduces the pressure. After pressure returns to baseline 3 cm H_2O, the ventilator attempts another mandatory breath. If the problem is not resolved, such as with a kinked expiratory line, the process repeats itself. After the problem is resolved, the ventilator resumes normal operation.

The LOW PEAK PRESSURE alarm is activated if the airway pressure does not exceed the set value during inspiration. The low PEEP/CPAP alarm is activated if the airway pressure drops below the set value at any time during a complete respiratory cycle (inspiration plus expiration) for more than 0.5 seconds (Box 12-9). The LOW MINUTE VOLUME alarm is activated whenever the minute ventilation drops below the value set on the alarm. The volume is measured by the flow transducer connected to the exhalation valve body outlet. (This applies to all types of breaths.) The HIGH BREATH RATE alarm is activated when the patient's total respiratory rate exceeds the set value on the alarm.

CLINICAL ROUNDS 12-3

A respiratory therapist is using a Bird 8400 STi to ventilate a patient. Suddenly a beep is heard, and the window above the apnea interval displays "AP" alternating with "20" seconds. The respiratory rate control is set at 6 breaths/min, and the mode was set on SIMV. However, the ventilator has switched to apnea back-up ventilation. The therapist presses the ALARM RESET button, but the ventilator remains in apnea back-up ventilation.

What mode will the ventilator switch to if apnea is detected? What will be the rate and V_T delivery? How can the ventilator be switched back to normal operation?

See Appendix A for the answer.

The APNEA INTERVAL determines the amount of time that must pass before an apneic condition is detected, based on all breaths—spontaneous and mandatory. When apnea is present, the ventilator will switch to apnea back-up ventilation. The apnea BACK-UP BREATH RATE is the final control knob in this row and can be set to zero or some value greater than the breath rate control. (*Note*: If the back-up ventilation breath rate is lower than the primary breath rate, the display value will be limited to the primary breath rate and will flash.) During back-up ventilation, the ventilator switches back to the A/C mode. The BACK-UP BREATH RATE becomes dominant, and the regular breath rate control is no longer functional. The settings for V_T (or inspiratory pressure), peak flow (or inspiratory time), PEEP/CPAP, and sensitivity remain active. Normal ventilation resumes if one of two conditions occur:

- Two consecutive spontaneous breaths occur and at least 50% of the set V_T is exhaled with each. (*Note:* In pressure ventilation mode, two consecutive spontaneous breaths will reset the unit.)
- The operator presses the reset button and activates the control setting for breath rate (Clinical Rounds 12-3).

Box 12-10 Nonadjustable Alarms Shown in the Display Window of the Bird 8400STi

"CIRC": Possible Circuit or Pressure Transducer Fault

How measured: compares measurements of the airway pressure transducer with those of the machine pressure transducer (both located internally).

Activates during inspiration if machine pressure is 29 cm H_2O greater than or 9 cm H_2O less than the airway pressure for >100 msec.

Activates during expiration if machine pressure is 29 cm H_2O greater than or 9 cm H_2O less than the airway pressure for >1.0 sec.

Results in opening of the expiratory valve and ending inspiratory flow. PEEP/CPAP is maintained. If prolonged (>12 seconds), the safety and expiratory valves open to allow spontaneous breathing of room air.

Common causes:

- Blocking of the airway pressure sensing port
- Occlusion or kinking of either the main inspiratory or the main expiratory line
- Transducer failure

"MODE/WAVEFORM" Discrepancy Display

A square appears in the display window, the corners of which flash sequentially. This indicates that the mode selection switch is not properly positioned and the ventilator is in operation. The 8400STi stays in the previous mode and settings. If this situation occurs when the ventilator is first turned on, the ventilator provides SIMV with a descending-flow waveform.

The next row contains several alarm indicators as well as several controls. The alarm indicators are on the left side of the panel. The first is the ALARM SILENCE control, which silences most audible alarms for 1 minute when touched. Three alarms cannot be silenced by a simple touch of this control. They are:

1. A loss of electrical power alarm
2. A VENT INOP. (ventilator inoperative) alarm
3. A LOW INLET GAS alarm, a circuit alarm, (Box 12-10 gives information on the circuit alarm)

During a loss of electrical power, the alarm can be silenced by pressing this button for 3 to 5 seconds.

The low inlet gas pressure (low inlet gas) alarm can be activated by insufficient gas supply pressure, a clogged inlet filter, malfunction of the internal regulator, or malfunction of the system pressure transducer. It cannot be silenced.

The ventilator inoperative alarm (VENT INOP.) will activate with one of the following three conditions:

1. Loss of electrical power
2. Detection of an internal system problem
3. Prolonged detection (>1 sec) of excessively high (>24 psig) or low (<16 psig) pressure at the blended gas inlet in an older ventilator version

Box 12-11 Control Settings During VAPS

Mode: A/C, SIMV, or SIMV. PS

Flow Waveform: constant (rectangular)

Pressure Support: at a pressure sufficient to provide the patient's current V_T; estimate using plateau pressure

Tidal Volume: set a minimum value

Flow: should be set high and readjusted after starting

Breath Rate: set a minimum guaranteed value

Back-up Breath Rate: below set rate

PEEP: appropriate for the patient

Trigger Sensitivity below PEEP: appropriate for the patient

Alarm Limits: appropriate for the patient

For example, the mode selected is SIMV with a constant flow waveform and a flow of 60 L/min. The breath rate is set at 10 breaths/min. The back-up rate is set at 8 breaths/min. V_T is 0.5 L. Pressure support is 20 cm H_2O, which is 2 cm H_2O above the patient's plateau pressure during volume ventilation at the same volume. PEEP is 3 cm H_2O, and trigger sensitivity is set so that a breath patient triggers at 2 cm H_2O (−1 cm H_2O below baseline).

(*Note*: Current unit production has changed this function because low inlet gas no longer produces a VENT INOP. condition.) If a VENT INOP. alarm situation occurs, a safety valve opens to provide the spontaneously breathing patient access to room air.

Although these alarm controls are easily seen on the control panel, there are two additional, nonprogrammable alarms (see Box 12-10). The cause of these alarms can be determined by viewing the monitor window on the right side of the front panel, between the pressure manometer and the row of LEDs.

Modes of Ventilation

The Bird 8400STi provides the usual modes of ventilation with volume- or pressure-targeting. In addition, it also has a servo-controlled, pressure-targeted mode that guarantees volume delivery, it is called volume-assured pressure support (VAPS).

Assist/Control

This mode is patient-triggered (pressure or flow) or time-triggered. Each breath can be either volume- or pressure-targeted. When volume-targeted, inspiration ends when the unit determines that the volume has been delivered (volume-cycled, based on flow and time calculations). When pressure-targeted, it is time cycled out of inspiration based on the set T_I.

Because pressure-targeted breaths for either A/C or SIMV are set slightly differently than on most ventilators, the setting of pressure-controlled (targeted) breaths is reviewed here. After selecting the desired mode, the operator presses the PRESSURE-CONTROL touch pad, and the LED above the touch pad flashes. The current settings are still operational, and a "P" flashes in the V_T control window. The operator selects the desired pressure delivery in this location by using the TIDAL VOLUME/INSP. PRESS control knob, and a flashing "P" appears in the PEAK FLOW/INSP. TIME window. The operator selects the desired T_I with this control. When these controls have been set and all other controls are at their desired settings, the operator presses the PRESSURE-CONTROL touch pad again to activate pressure-targeted mandatory breaths in the selected mode. The "P" stays continuously lit in the INSP. PRESS. and INSP. TIME display windows, and the PRES. CTRL. LED is also continuously illuminated.

When switching from pressure-controlled breaths back to volume ventilation, the inspiratory pressure must first be reduced to 5 cm H_2O to ensure that the V_T is not set too high and can be readjusted upward. Pressing the PRESSURE-CONTROL pad turns off pressure ventilation (the LED is no longer lit).

SIMV

The function of the SIMV mode of ventilation on the Bird 8400STi is similar to the SIMV mode on most ventilators. Mandatory breaths are patient- or time-triggered, but when they are volume-targeted, inspiration ends when the unit determines that the volume has been delivered. When mandatory breaths are pressure-targeted, they are time-cycled out of inspiration. Spontaneous breaths can occur at baseline pressure (zero or PEEP) and with pressure support.

Spontaneous Mode

To provide spontaneous ventilation, the breath rate control is set at zero, and the patient breathes spontaneously from the desired baseline pressure, allowing for CPAP. Spontaneous breaths can also be pressure-supported. For example, the clinician may select 5 cm H_2O of CPAP and PSV of 10 cm H_2O. The baseline pressure will be 5 cm H_2O, and the inspiratory pressure will reach 15 cm H_2O during a pressure-supported spontaneous breath.

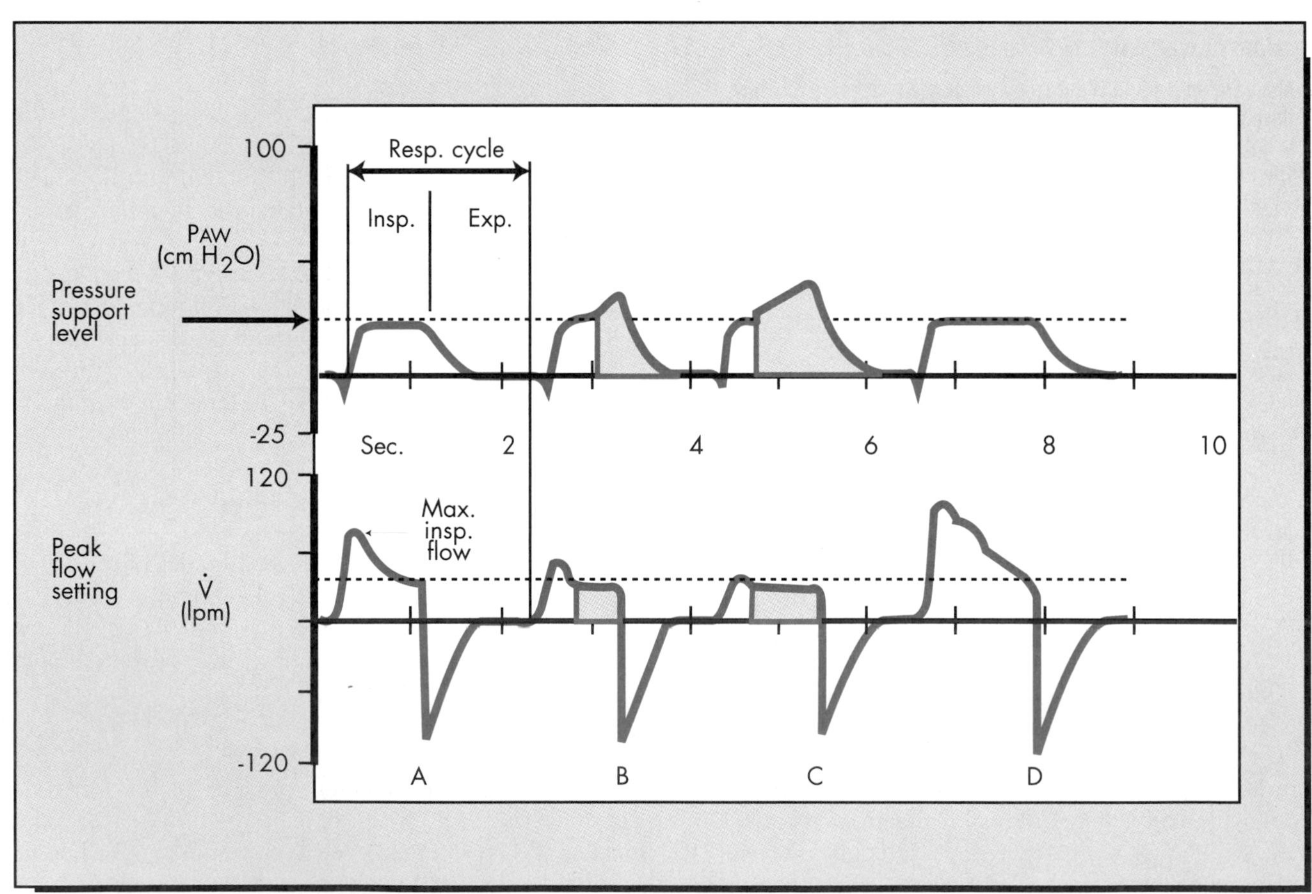

Figure 12-8 Examples of potential VAPS breath patterns: **A,** a pressure-generated breath with flow-cycling at the set flow value. The V_T was ≥ set V_T. **B,** an example where flow has dropped to the set value, but V_T has not been delivered, so flow is sustained until V_T is delivered. Note the rise in pressure as flow is continued. **C,** a breath where the set pressure is inadequate for the patient's lung conditions and inspiration is prolonged. **D,** an example of a breath in a patient with a high inspiratory flow demand. The ventilator responds by delivering an increased flow and V_T (not shown). (Courtesy Viasys Healthcare, Critical Care Division, Palm Springs, Calif.)

Volume-Assured Pressure Support

VAPS is a pressure-targeted mode of ventilation that guarantees volume delivery in each breath. It is a servo-control (closed-loop) mode (see Chapter 11). VAPS is similar in its function to the PAug mode discussed previously with the Bear 1000. Box 12-11 lists the control settings used in this mode.

VAPS is intended for use with spontaneously breathing patients. It functions as follows: when a patient triggers a breath, the ventilator pressure targets the breath and delivers the set PS level. Flow is rapid at the beginning of inspiration and gradually tapers down in a descending ramp pattern. As flow is delivered, the microprocessor monitors flow and volume delivery, and two common patterns emerge.

1. If the volume delivered is greater than or equal to the set minimum V_T, the ventilator ends the breath by flow cycling at the set flow value.
2. If volume delivered is less than the set volume, and the flow drops to the set flow value, the set flow is maintained until the volume is delivered. Figure 12-8 shows examples of different types of respiratory patterns that can occur during this mode of ventilation.

Graphic Display Screens

Figure 12-9 provides an overview of the basic controls on the Bird graphics monitor. The menu along the bottom provides a variety of functions. Waveforms of pressure, flow, and volume vs. time are available, in addition to a variety of loops including flow-volume and pressure-volume loops. The graphics package can also freeze screens, overlap graphs and loops, and indicate trending. Information on the screen can be printed out when a compatible printer is attached to

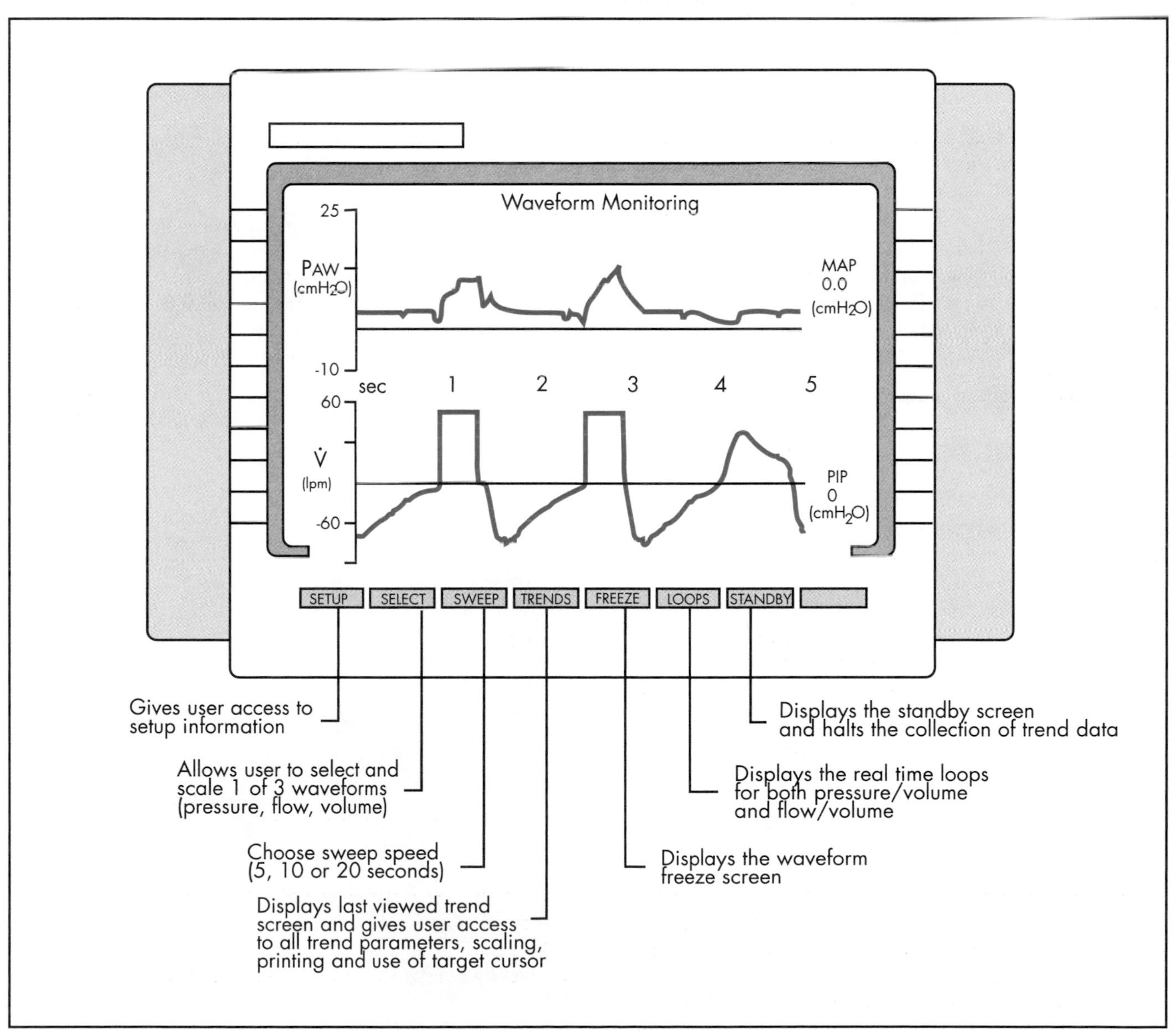

Figure 12-9 The Bird 8400STi waveform graphics monitor. (Courtesy Viasys Healthcare, Critical Care Division, Palm Springs, Calif.)

the unit. Complete instructions for operating the graphics package and troubleshooting guidelines are provided by the manufacturer's Instruction and Service Manual (PIN L 1282).

Special Features

Perhaps the most significant features of the Bird 8400 are its new mode of ventilation (VAPS) and its graphic monitor. An air compressor (Bird 6500) is also available and can be used to provide pneumatic power to the unit.

Troubleshooting

The monitors and alarms provide immediate information about the functioning of the unit. The manufacturer's instruction manual contains a table for troubleshooting clinical problems that includes symptoms, potential causes, and the corrective action to take. For example, one problem that is described is as follows:

- The VENT INOP. LED illuminates, an audible alarm sounds and all displays are disabled.
- Possible causes might be: (1) loss of electrical power, (2) extended low inlet gas pressure, or (3) a system failure.

Corrective actions might include restoring electrical power, restoring inlet gas pressure, or contacting the Viasys Healthcare Corporation in the case of a system failure.

A list of 19 potential clinical problems are outlined in the troubleshooting section of the operator's manual. The user is referred to that section for additional information.

As with other microprocessor-controlled medical equipment, it should be kept away from RFI and EFI equipment. In addition, Chapter 11 of this text reviews common problems encountered during mechanical ventilation.

Bird T-Bird

The T-Bird AVS is manufactured by Viasys Heathcare, Critical Care Division (Palm Springs, CA), formerly Bird Products Corp. (Figure 12-10). The T-Bird AVS comes in three configurations, depending on what options have been added. The AVS III comes with PCV and VAPS modes and also has the following options added: expiratory hold, inspiratory time, and MIP/negative inspiratory force (NIF) measurements. Of these features, the AVS II has expiratory hold and MIP/NIF measurements. The AVS I does not have these options.

Power Source

Similar to many of the newer generation ventilators, the T-Bird is also a microprocessor-controlled unit. It requires an electrical source to power the microprocessor and the electrical components of the internal circuits. Unlike some of the newer units, however, the T-Bird, does not require a high-pressure gas source to function because it possesses an electrically powered internal turbine. Silencers help to suppress the noise generated by turbine intake. Oxygen can be provided to the patient by using either or both of the two available high pressure oxygen connectors (range from 40 to 65 psig). Using two oxygen sources rather than one allows the transfer of sources without interruption.

The ON/STANDBY power switch, as well as the high-pressure oxygen connectors and the air inlet filter, is on the back panel of the ventilator. There is an internal battery (48 volts, direct current [DC]) that can provide a back-up power source. In addition, there is an external battery, which is manually loaded on the lower right side of the unit and provides another power source.

The patient circuit has an expiratory valve mounted inside the front of the unit and the standard main inspiratory and expiratory lines that connect to the patient Y adapter.

Internal Mechanism

Ambient air enters the unit through the air filter, and oxygen enters through one or both of the oxygen connections. The T-Bird is equipped with an internal blender that uses a series of electronically operated, microprocessor-controlled solenoids. The microprocessor evaluates the oxygen setting on the control panel and selects and mixes the appropriate blend of gases from the air inlet and the solenoids receiving

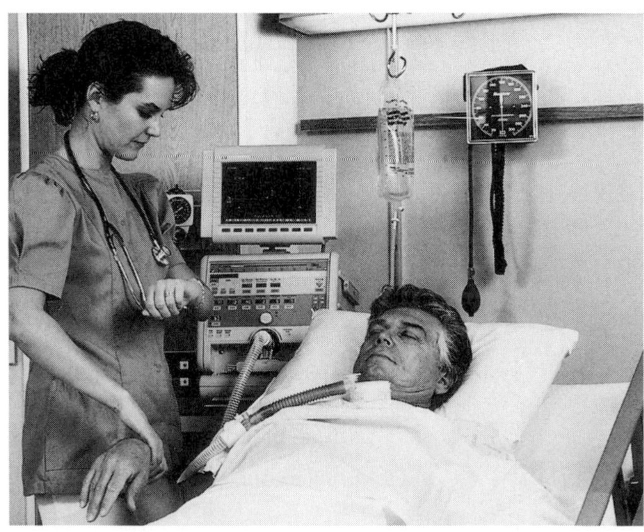

Figure 12-10 The Bird T-Bird AVS. (Courtesy Viasys Healthcare, Critical Care Division, Palm Springs, Calif.)

oxygen to provide the desired F_IO_2 for the patient. Blended gases are sent to an accumulator that also acts as a **diffuser** for initial mixing. The accumulator also helps silence the noise caused by the built-in turbine. (*Note*: See the EVOLVE website for this text to view a diagram of the internal circuit of the T-Bird AVS.)

The gas is then directed to the turbine inlet. The microprocessor monitors the speed and output pressure from the turbine and uses this information to establish breath delivery to the patient. The flow-control device in this unit is called a **drag turbine.** Inlet and outlet pressures for the turbine are monitored by a differential-pressure transducer. The microprocessor uses information about the pressure difference and the turbine speed (from the **optical encoder**) to control the precise flow delivered to the patient from the turbine. Volume delivery is the integration of flow for each unit of time (volume = flow × T_I).

An internal **subambient relief valve,** or **antisuffocation valve,** opens if the ventilator cannot provide an assisted breath to the patient. The patient can then inhale to open the valve and receive room air. This would occur, for example, during a ventilator inoperative condition (see the discussion of alarms in this section).

There are also internal transducers to measure expiratory and airway pressures. The expiratory flow transducer is a differential pressure transducer (see Chapter 8).

Controls and Alarms

The front panel of the T-Bird AVS provides a wide variety of controls, monitors, and alarms (Figure 12-11), some of which are touch pads that allow actions such as mode selection, mandatory breath delivery, or variable adjustment to be made.

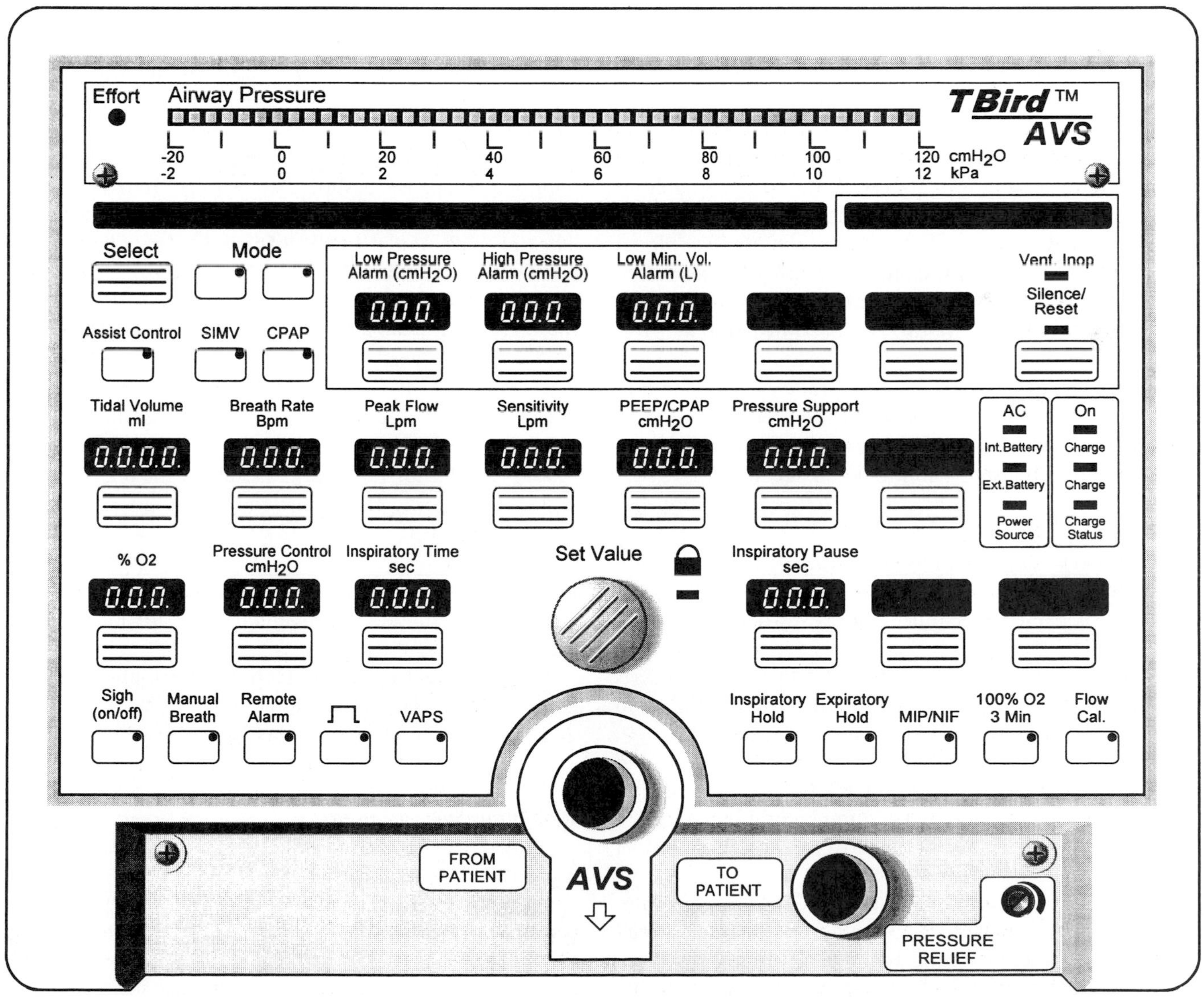

Figure 12-11 The front Panel of the T-Bird AVS. (See text for description of controls.) (Courtesy Yvon Dupuis.)

Box 12-12 Flashing Controls on the T-Bird

Flashing Occurs

When the following settings are used:

- $T_E < 250$ msec
- $T_I < 300$ msec
- High pressure alarm setting < 5 cm H_2O above set PEEP
- I:E > 4:1 (e.g., 5:1)
- Peak flow setting < bias flow setting
- Bias flow setting > peak flow

When a required control has not been set for the mode selected; for example, a low peak pressure alarm that has been turned off will flash until it is set.

When an alarm is active.

When the mode pad has been pressed once. It flashes for 15 seconds or until the mode is activated by pressing the pad a second time.

Box 12-13 Setting the Over Pressure-Relief Valve

1. Attach the patient circuit to a test lung.
2. Set the high-pressure limit to the maximum (120 cm H_2O).
3. Set high V_T and peak flow in order to achieve ≥100 cm H_2O (monitored display value).
4. During breath delivery, monitor PIP.
5. Adjust the pressure-relief valve until the desired maximum pressure is seen on the manometer.
6. Remember the high-pressure limit must be reset appropriately for the patient and the over pressure-relief valve must be 5 to 15 cm H_2O above this.

When a touch pad is active, the LED on its surface is lit. Above the touch pads controlling different variables (e.g., pressure and volume) are display windows that provide digital values of the set parameters. These windows may be bright or dim. A control is dim when it is not available in the currently active mode. For example, V_T is not available during pressure-controlled ventilation, so the V_T digital value is dim. Fortunately, the previous setting remains visible so that if the mode is changed, that setting is still available. In addition, a dimmed control can be adjusted so that it is at the desired setting before a ventilator mode is changed.

Sometimes the window for a control will be flashing to show that a parameter has been set incorrectly. Box 12-12 provides the usual reasons for these to be flashing.

In the center, there is a control knob, labeled SET VALUE, for adjusting all control and alarm levels. This knob has three basic functions:

1. To set variable controls (V_T, breath rate, pressure, etc.)
2. To select special functions
3. To activate tests during **user verification testing (UVT)**

To set a parameter (control variable), the operator presses the touch pad for the parameter and turns the control knob to change the numerical value of the parameter.

To select special functions, the control knob is pressed and held down until "VENT SETUP" appears in the monitor window (i.e., the window below the pressure manometer). The control knob is then released (see the discussion of special functions later in this section).

The UVT permits the operator to review several ventilator functions, such as a lamp test, a filter test, a leak test, etc. The operator's manual for the T-Bird covers this information, so it is not included here. These tests may be run during the set-up and check-out procedure before patient use.

A lock control allows the operator to lock the front panel and prevent accidental or unauthorized adjustments. Pressing the control knob locks it, preventing adjustable parameters from being changed. A green LED next to a lock icon lights when the control knob is locked. Pressing the knob again unlocks it. The only controls that do not lock are the monitor SELECT, MANUAL BREATH, and ALARM SILENCE/RESET.

There are also digital display windows above the alarm control touch pads that show their settings. Across the top of the front panel is a horizontally mounted pressure monitor. The main gas outlet to the patient is at the lower right corner of the front panel.

Connections for the main inspiratory and expiratory flow lines are below the operating controls of the front panel. In the lowest right corner is an adjustable control for the **over pressure-relief valve,** with which the maximum pressure allowed by the system can be set. Reaching this pressure does not end inspiration, but vents excess pressure to the room. It is set from 5 to 15 cm H_2O above the high-pressure limit. Box 12-13 describes this procedure.

Controls

Looking at the front of the control panel, the upper left area is where the mode control touch pads are located (see Figure 12-11).

The first touch pad in this section is the monitor SELECT control, which is used to do three things:

1. Select monitored parameters
2. Select special functions
3. Run UVTs

It is also used to clear some alarms.

Table 12-1 lists the monitored parameters visible in the top display window during normal operation. Their appearance is controlled by the SPECIAL FUNCTIONS control (explained in the later discussion of special functions) or by the monitor SELECT button. The parameters are displayed in sets of two or three and are automatically scanned (autoscanning) when either of these functions are turned on (i.e.,

Table 12-1 T-Bird monitored parameters

Parameter	Range
Total breath rate (f)	0 to 250 breaths/min
I:E ratio	99:1 to 1:99
$\dot{V}_E$	0 to 999 L/min
PIP	0 to 140 cm H_2O
Mean airway pressure (MAP)	0 to 99 cm H_2O
T_I	0.01 to 99.99 sec
PEEP	0 to 99 cm H_2O
Exhaled V_T (Vte)	0 to 4000 mL

enabled). Using the monitor SELECT control, the display can hold at a particular set of parameters or can be manually advanced through parameters.

To access special functions, press and hold the main control knob for about 2 seconds until "VENT SET-UP" appears in the monitor window. Then release the control knob. Turning the control knob now allows display of the special functions that can be selected (Table 12-2; see the later section on special functions).

The UVT can be accessed in the same way in which special functions are accessed. The UVT and the **service verification test (SVT)** appear after event codes, but cannot be accessed while the ventilator is in operation. The UVT and SVT are described in the operator's manual, so they are not covered here.

The next controls in this row are the mode touch pads, which are activated by pressing them. Modes include A/C, SIMV, and CPAP. When the selected mode is pressed twice, the LED on the corner of the pad is illuminated, and the mode becomes active. Set-up and operation of the modes will be covered in the discussion of modes of ventilation later in this section.

Alarm settings are to the right of the mode touch pads (see the discussion of alarms in this section).

The row of controls in the central part of the panel is as follows: tidal volume, breath rate, peak flow, sensitivity, PEEP/CPAP, and pressure support. There is a blank control at the end of this row to be used in future upgrades.

Tidal Volume

The V_T control (range 50 to 2000 mL) sets the V_T for volume ventilation and sets the volume goal for VAPS. The V_T is delivered in the selected flow waveform with the maximum flow as the peak flow setting. Even when a pressure-targeted mode or CPAP is selected, this control must be set at the appropriate level for back-up ventilation in case the patient becomes apneic. The value is dimmed in pressure ventilation (Box 12-14).

Table 12-2 Special functions and parameters

Special Function	Parameter Available
Vent set-up	Autoscan on/off
	Bias flow setting
	Enables/disables control lock function
	Bird graphic monitor (BGM) on/off
	Select display language
	Display software version
	Total hours of operation
	Display turbine serial no.
	Altitude compensation
Alarm set-up	Apnea interval
	Remote alarm status
Transducer data	Readings from various transducers*
Transducer test group	Autozero flow transducer
	Autozero expiratory flow transducer
	Autozero turbine pressure transducer
Events code group	Displays previous 256 event codes*

*See operator's manual for codes.

Box 12-14 Back-up Ventilation

When setting the controls for any mode of ventilation on the I-Bird, it is wise to set all settings. For example, even if you plan to use a pressure-targeting form of ventilation such as pressure control, you still need to set the V_T, f, peak flow, flow pattern, F_IO_2, and pressure limit. This way, if the apneic back-up mode of ventilation becomes active, its parameters will be appropriately set.

Breath Rate

The BREATH RATE control (2 to 80 breaths/min) sets the number of mandatory breaths. Breath rate is available in A/C, SIMV, and apnea back-up modes and should always be set in case the patient becomes apneic.

Peak Flow

The PEAK FLOW control (10 to 140 L/min) sets the maximum inspiratory flow during volume ventilation and interacts with the FLOW WAVEFORM control. When a constant waveform is selected, the peak flow is sustained during inspiration. When a descending ramp is selected, the set peak flow occurs at the beginning of inspiration, and flow gradually tapers toward the end of inspiration.

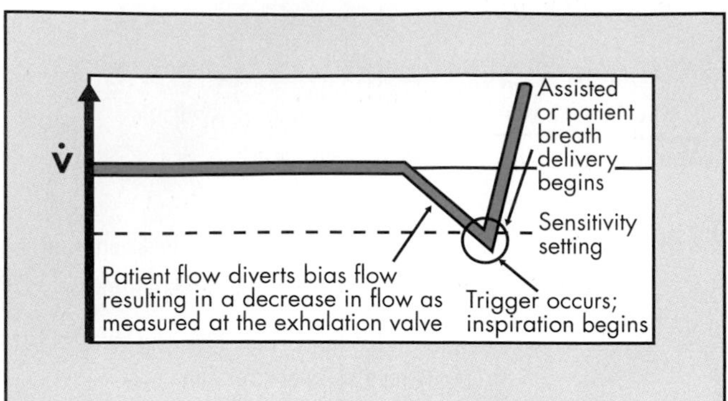

Figure 12-12 A graph showing the function of the flow trigger (sensitivity control). See text for further explanation. (Courtesy Viasys Healthcare, Critical Care Division, Palm Springs, Calif.)

With VAPS, the PEAK FLOW control sets the minimum flow generated, determines expiratory criteria, and establishes minimum flow for a guaranteed volume delivery (see the discussion of VAPS under the section on modes of ventilation).

Sensitivity

The SENSITIVITY control (1 to 8 L/min, or off) sets the threshold flow. During the latter part of exhalation, a constant flow of gas passes through the patient circuit. This flow is called bias or base flow. The expiratory flow sensor monitors the bias flow. When the bias flow drops by the amount set on the SENSITIVITY control, in any mode, inspiration is triggered (Figure 12-12). Chapter 11 provides additional information on flow triggering.

When SENSITIVITY is off, the unit can not be triggered by the patient, so it is recommended that the sensitivity never be turned off. (*Note:* The T-Bird does not use pressure-triggering.)

PEEP/CPAP

The PEEP/CPAP control (0 to 30 cm H_2O) sets the baseline pressure and maintains the airway pressure between breaths in all modes of ventilation. The high pressure alarm setting must be set at least 5 cm H_2O above the PEEP/CPAP setting.

Pressure Support

The pressure support control (1 to 60 cm H_2O, or off) sets the pressure level above PEEP for all pressure-support breaths. It is functional for spontaneous breaths in SIMV and CPAP modes.

Blank Control

The blank control is the last touch pad in this row and is for future upgrades.

Power Indicators

The section to the right of the row of controls described above contains battery and power source indicators.

The AC power source indicator activates when the unit is connected to a wall outlet (AC power). While the unit is connected, the optional external and internal battery are being charged. If power fails, the unit switches to the external battery source, if present. If no external battery is connected, it switches to the internal battery. An alarm occurs when the power source changes from AC to DC. To the right of this indicator is the ON indicator, which shows that the unit is turned on.

The internal battery has two light indicators, one to indicate battery use (INT. BAT.) and one to indicate battery charge status (CHARGE). Both lights change colors.

The INT. BAT. light comes on when it is in use. It is green when fully charged (about 7 to 24 minutes remain), yellow at medium charge (about 5 to 14 minutes remain), and red at low power (about 4 to 10 minutes remain). OFF indicates the unit is using either an AC wall outlet or the external battery for power. When the color changes (from green to yellow or yellow to red), an audible alarm is activated to alert the operator. The length of battery use depends on the amount of power being used by the unit.

The internal battery charge status indicators are as follows:

- Green = 90% to 100% charged
- Yellow = battery is being charged
- Red = low battery, needs to be charged*

When the external battery indicator is lit (EXT. BAT.), the unit is operating on external battery power. The available time from a fully charged battery depends on the power demand of the unit, but ranges from about 1.0 to 3.5 hours. Colors provide the following information about battery status:

- Green = sufficient power
- Yellow = charge is getting low (about 20 min to 1.5 hours remain)
- Off = not in use

When the battery is fully discharged, the ventilator switches to the internal battery and the EXT. BAT. alarm is activated.

The color of the external battery charge indicator (CHARGE) shows that the external battery is being charged and changes depending on the amount of charge present:

- Green = 90% to 100% charged
- Yellow = being charged (charge time about 7 to 11 hours)
- Red = low battery, needs to be charged
- Off = battery is not present or properly connected

Immediately below this row of controls are the following: % O_2, PRESSURE CONTROL, INSPIRATORY TIME, the SET VALUE (CONTROL KNOB), INSPIRATORY PAUSE, and two blank positions for use in future upgrades.

% O_2

The % O_2 control sets the delivered oxygen percentage from 21% to 100%.

**Charge time is about 6 to 7 hours.*

Pressure Control

The PRESSURE CONTROL position (AVS III only; ranges from 1 to 100 cm H_2O, or off) sets inspiratory pressure above baseline for pressure-targeted breaths in A/C, SIMV, and VAPS.

Inspiratory Time

The INSPIRATORY TIME control (AVS III only; TI in seconds, ranges from 0.3 to 10.0 seconds) sets the inspiratory time for pressure-control breaths. When selected, the new time begins with the next pressure-targeted mandatory breath.

Control Knob

The control knob is used to set each parameter as selected by the operator.

Lock Indicator

The indicator shows whether or not the control knob has been locked or unlocked.

Inspiratory Pause

The INSPIRATORY PAUSE control (0.1 to 2.0 seconds, or off) sets an inspiratory pause time for volume-targeted breaths in A/C and SIMV. An inspiratory pause occurs on the next and on all subsequent volume breaths.

The bottom row of controls consists of a series of touch pads as follows (left-to-right): SIGH, MANUAL BREATH, REMOTE ALARM, FLOW WAVEFORM CONTROL, VAPS (AVS III), INSPIRATORY HOLD, EXPIRATORY HOLD (AVS II or III), MIP/NIF (AVS II or III), 100% O_2 3 min, and FLOW CAL.

Sigh

When the sigh control (on/off) is activated, the ventilator delivers a sigh breath at the next mandatory breath and then at every 100th breath or 7th minute—whichever comes first. The sigh volume is 150% of the set V_T. Inspiratory time increases by 50% (to a maximum of 5.5 sec); and PIP increases by 50% (to a maximum of 120 cm H_2O). (*Note:* The over pressure-relief valve setting must be adjusted when sigh is selected.)

Manual Breath

Pressing the MANUAL BREATH touch pad delivers a mandatory breath based on set parameters. For example, during volume ventilation, the set V_T and the peak flow are delivered using the set flow waveform. During pressure ventilation, the set pressure and T_I are active. The MANUAL BREATH touch pad can only be activated after inspiration and the minimum T_E (250 msec) have occurred.

Remote Alarm

The REMOTE ALARM control turns the optical remote alarm transmitter on and off. The transmitter is a special feature that must be added to the unit (see the operating manual). When purchased, this feature provides a remote receiver that can be placed at an appropriate location and activated in case an alarm is triggered.

Square Waveform

The SQUARE WAVEFORM (on/off) button is located adjacent to the REMOTE ALARM control and provides a constant (rectangular) or descending (decelerating) ramp flow waveform during volume ventilation. The LED lights up when the square waveform is active. Pressing the button changes the waveform.

Volume Assured Pressure Support (VAPS)

The VAPS control turns the VAPS mode on and off (see the discussion of modes of ventilation).

Inspiratory Hold

The INSPIRATORY HOLD control is used to measure plateau pressure, which is used in calculating static compliance. Pressing and holding the button results in a message in the display window: "Paw xxx cm H_2O," where xxx is the real time value of airway pressure. At the end of inspiration, "Pplat xxx cm H_2O" appears, where xxx is the measured plateau pressure. The value is continually updated as it is displayed. Inspiratory pause ends when the button is released or 6 seconds has elapsed—whichever occurs first. After the maneuver, the window reads "Palvd xxx cm H_2O Cst xxx ml/cm H_2O," where Palvd xxx is the alveolar distending pressure, and Cst xxx is the static compliance. This maneuver fails if the inspiratory hold button is released too soon or a stable plateau cannot be obtained, which can occur if the patient is actively breathing against the closed valves.

Expiratory Hold

The EXPIRATORY HOLD control (AVS II and AVS III) is used to measure auto-PEEP during A/C and SIMV ventilation. When the button is pressed, the display window shows "Paw nn Pex mm AUTOPEEP pp cm H_2O," where nn is a display of actual airway pressure, mm is the end-expiratory pressure, and pp is the measured auto-PEEP.

First, the button is pressed. At the moment when the next mandatory breath would have been delivered, both the inspiratory and expiratory valves close. The value of Pex (total end expiratory pressure) is updated in the display window every 6 seconds or until the button is released. At the end of the maneuver, the auto-PEEP level is calculated by determining the difference between PEEP (regular baseline pressure) and Pex.

Maximum Inspiratory Pressure (MIP) or Negative Inspiratory Force (NIF)

The MIP/NIF control (AVS II and AVS III) allows the operator to perform an MIP (i.e., an NIF maneuver). The MIP/NIF control is pushed and held to initiate and perform an MIP maneuver. At the end of expiratory flow, the ventilator closes the inspiratory and expiratory valves, measures pressures in the patient circuit, and displays values in the display window as "Pstart ________," "Paw ________," and "MIP ________ cm H_2O." The value for MIP is updated each time a new maximum negative pressure is detected until the button is released or 30 seconds have passed—whichever occurs first.

100% O_2 3 min

Pushing this pad (LED illuminated) provides 100% oxygen through the patient circuit for 3 minutes. Touching it a second time turns the control off before the 3-minute limit.

Flow Calibration (Flow Cal.)

The FLOW CAL. control allows the operator to perform a manual flow calibration that measures the **bias flow** passing through the expiratory flow valve transducer. When the unit is first turned on, the display window gives the message "FLOW CAL." To clear the message, a flow calibration must be performed by pressing and holding down the FLOW CAL. pad down during the expiratory phase of a breath. The message "FC nn.n," where nn.n is the bias flow (L/min), appears. When "FC nn.n OK" appears, the FLOW CAL. touch pad can be released because calibration is complete. (*Note:* The ventilator will still operate with a "FLOW CAL" alert, but the accuracy of V_T and $\dot{V}_E$ measurements may be inaccurate.)

Monitors

Across the top of the control panel is the airway pressure manometer (–20 to 120 cm H_2O), which contains a series of LEDs, each equal to 2 cm H_2O when lit. LEDs to the right of zero represent positive pressure and to the left of zero represent negative pressure. The amber LEDs indicate the current high- and low-pressure alarm settings.

Just to the left of the pressure manometer is the effort LED, which (when lit) verifies that a patient's inspiratory effort has been detected after it reaches the sensitivity setting. Below the pressure manometer, there is a monitor window that displays ventilator parameters, messages, and other information.

Alarms

Most ventilator alarms are both audio and visual. In the top right section of the front panel is an alarm window. It displays messages for alarms and alerts (Box 12-15). Adjustable alarms and nonadjustable alarms are available with the T-Bird AVS.

Box 12-15 Inactivating T-Bird Alarms

1. After an alarm condition no longer exists, the audible alarm usually is silenced.
2. The visual alarms and messages usually clear after the alarm condition is resolved as well.
3. If the visual alarm remains on, press the alarm silence/reset button.
4. Some alarm conditions, such as the "BATTERY ON" alarm, require that the alarm silence/reset button be pressed twice for deactivation.

Adjustable Alarms

The adjustable alarm controls can be set using the control knob and the appropriate touch pad and digital display window. The adjustable alarm controls include the following: LOW PRESSURE, HIGH PRESSURE, LOW MINUTE VOLUME, and HIGH RATE.

The LOW PRESSURE ALARM control (2 to 60 cm H_2O) sets the lowest pressure that must be achieved in the patient circuit during a breath. If the unit fails to produce at least the set pressure, a low press alarm occurs.

The HIGH PRESSURE ALARM control (5 to 120 cm H_2O) sets the maximum amount of pressure in the patient circuit that the unit will allow, regardless of the type of breaths. Its lowest setting is 5 cm H_2O over the set PEEP. If a high press alarm is activated, inspiration ends (pressure-cycling). If circuit pressure does not drop to PEEP 5 cm H_2O within 3 seconds, all flow from the unit stops. When pressure falls below PEEP 5 cm H_2O, the alarm is automatically cleared, flow is restarted, and the next breath is delivered. During a sigh breath, the alarm is increased to 150% of the set high-pressure limit; but, this value does not appear in the display above the alarm control.

The LOW MINUTE VOLUME ALARM control (range 0.1 to 99.9 L) sets the minimum $\dot{V}_E$ level that must be exceeded to prevent an alarm. The expiratory flow transducer measures exhaled volume (average of last 8 breaths extrapolated to 1 minute) and compares measured values to the alarm settings. If exhaled $\dot{V}_E$ is below the set low $\dot{V}_E$ alarm setting, the low minute volume alarm is activated.

The HIGH BREATH RATE alarm (optional, range 3 to 150 breaths/min) counts both spontaneous and mandatory breaths before being activated and can be turned off. The display window gives the total respiratory rate (spontaneous mandatory) actually measured. If this equals or exceeds the alarm setting, the alarm is activated.

At the far right of the alarm control panel is the alarm SILENCE/RESET touch pad, which silences most audible alarms for 1 minute when pressed. Touching it again reactivates the controls. If a VENT. INOP. alarm occurs (indicator in same area), the manufacturer recommends that the unit be turned off before the alarm silence pad is touched. Of course, the patient should be disconnected from the machine and be ventilated manually. The VENT. INOP. indicator is activated whenever the ventilator detects a condition that could affect safe operation of the unit. The ventilator ceases to operate, opens the exhalation valve, and stops turbine flow so the patient can breathe spontaneously from room air. This requires that the operator immediately provide for patient ventilation and obtain another ventilator for the patient. The ventilator in question must be serviced by a certified technician.

Nonadjustable Alarms

The nonadjustable alarms for the T-Bird are listed in Box 12-16 and will be briefly reviewed here.

Box 12-16 Nonadjustable Alarms/Alerts on the T-Bird

AC power lost alarm
Apnea alarm
Bias alert
Check apnea back-up settings alert
Check filter alert
Circuit fault alarm
Control settings limit alert
Controls locked alert
Default setting alarm
EEPROM failure alert
Fan fault alarm
Flow calibration required alert
Flow sensor alert
Hardware fault alarm
High oxygen inlet pressure alarm
Internal operations check alarm
Invalid calibration values alert
Low external battery alarm
Low internal battery alarm
Low oxygen inlet alarm
New sensor alert
Remote alarm transmission fault alarm
Transducer fault alarm
Ventilator inoperative alarm

Apnea Alarm

The message window reads "xx sec APNEA." This alert occurs immediately after the power-on self-test (POST) and gives the operator the amount of seconds set on the apnea interval setting.

AC Power Lost Alarm

The message window reads "BATTERY ON." This alarm occurs if the ventilator has been operating from a standard AC electrical power source, and it has failed. The ventilator immediately switches to an external or internal battery power source.

Bias Alert

The message window reads "BIAS xx LPM." After the POST test, this informs the operator of the current bias flow setting.

Check Apnea Back-Up Settings Alert

The message window reads "CHECK BKUP," which reminds the operator to set the parameters needed for back-up ventilation. All parameters should be appropriate for the patient's size, age, and condition. This will ensure that the back-up ventilation parameters are also set. For example, in SIMV with pressure-targeted breaths, the following would be set: inspiratory pressure above PEEP, rate, and T_I.

Internal Operations Check Alarm

The message window reads "CHECK EVENTS," which occurs when the ventilator detects an unusual condition during one of its ongoing self-tests. The ventilator runs the POST test to recheck itself and records the type of error that occurred into memory (EEPROM). If the unit detects an error that compromises safe operation, it gives a VENT. INOP. alarm.

Circuit Fault Alarm

The message window reads "CIRC FAULT." This alarm occurs if the patient circuit becomes kinked, occluded, or disconnected, but also occurs if the internal transducer that measures patient circuit pressure has a problem that is detected by the ventilator.

Default Setting Alarm

The message window reads "DEFAULTS." The ventilator has a number of **default** settings that are set at the factory, but the operator actually overrides these default values when a new value is set. For example, the default value for V_T is 500 mL, but setting a different V_T overrides this value. The new setting is stored into memory (EEPROM) and replaces the set value. In this way, the ventilator can be turned off and it keeps the new settings when it is turned back on. If an error occurs that prevents retrieving the new value from memory, the factory-set values are always available.

EEPROM Failure Alert

The message window reads "EEPROM FAULT." This alert is caused when a hardware failure occurs, preventing the unit from retrieving ventilator settings from memory (EEPROM). If this fault occurs, a certified technician should be contacted.

Low External Battery Alarm

The message window reads "EXT BATTERY." This alarm occurs when the ventilator switches from external to internal battery power.

Fan Fault Alarm

The message window reads "FAN FAULT." When the speed of the cooling fan falls below its set acceptable low limit, this alarm is activated.

Check Filter Alert

The message window reads "FILTER." Every 500 hours, this alert will appear to remind the operator to check the air inlet filter because it may need cleaning or replacing.

Flow Calibration Required Alert

The message window reads "FLOW CAL" and occurs only when the unit is turned on. It requires that the operator perform a flow calibration.

Flow Sensor Alert

The message window reads "FLOW SENSOR." This alert occurs if the unit cannot detect that the expiratory valve body has been connected to the exhalation valve. The valve may need to be reseated or replaced.

High Oxygen Inlet Pressure Alarm

The message window reads "HIGH O_2." If the inlet pressure is >65 psi, and the oxygen percentage is set at >21%, the alarm will be activated.

Hardware Fault Alarm

The message window reads "HW FAULT." If a self-test detects a ventilator hardware problem, this alarm is activated. It also occurs if the internal temperature of the unit is too high for normal operation.

Control Settings Limit Alert

The message window reads "LIMITED" and appears if an incompatible setting is made. Clinical Rounds 12-4 gives an example. (*Note*: T_I must be at least 300 ms, T_E no less than 250 msec, I:E ≤ 4:1 [e.g., 1:1], and the high-pressure limit must be ≥ the set PEEP level + 5 cm H_2O.)

Controls Locked Alert

The message window reads "LOCKED." This alert appears if you try to change a control when the front panel is locked.

Low Internal Battery Alarm

The message window reads "LOW BATTERY." This alarm appears if the ventilator is operating from the internal battery and the charge in the battery drops to the medium level. The audible portion of this alarm is a chirping sound heard every 3 seconds, and the internal battery light indicator is yellow. If the alarm is continuous, the power level is low and the light indicator is red. The low power level alarm can be cleared by plugging the ventilator into an AC power source.

Low Oxygen Inlet Alarm

The message window reads "LOW O_2." If the oxygen inlet pressure is <35 psig, and the oxygen percentage is set at >21%, this message appears and an alarm activates.

New Sensor Alert

The message window reads "NEW SENSOR." The alert appears when a newly installed sensor is present in the exhalation valve body. Flow-sensor calibration is required when the valve body is replaced.

Invalid Calibration Values Alert

The message window reads "NO CAL DATA." During a POST, if the unit detects a problem with transducer calibration data that have been stored in memory (EEPROM), this alert will appear and cannot be cleared. Although the unit will still function, the accuracy of the volume and pressure measurements is reduced, so it is advisable to take the unit out of service and contact a Bird representative.

Remote Alarm Transmission Fault Alarm

The message window reads "REMOTE FAULT." This only occurs if a remote alarm transmitter has been installed, and the unit fails to transmit valid data to the remote receiver. The alarm remains active until the problem is corrected or the remote alarm button is turned off.

Transducer Fault Alarm

The message window reads "XDCR FAULT." This alarm occurs if the zero point of a transducer has drifted out of range. The unit will continue to operate, but volume and pressure measurements will be less accurate. Replacing the exhalation valve body and recalibrating the flow sensor usually clears the error.

Ventilator Inoperative Alarm

The message window reads "VENT.INOP." The ventilator has detected an unsafe operating condition and ceases to operate if this alarm occurs. The patient is able to breathe room air through the circuit, but the unit must be removed and replaced.

Modes of Ventilation

The modes of ventilation in the T-Bird AVS include A/C, SIMV, CPAP, and VAPS. A/C and SIMV can provide volume- or pressure-targeted breaths. CPAP provides spontaneous ventilation at the desired baseline and can also provide PSV, which is available whenever spontaneous breaths are provided (e.g., SIMV or CPAP). VAPS is a pressure-targeted breath with volume guarantee.

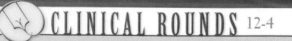

A respiratory therapist is changing a ventilator from pressure support of 18 cm H_2O to A/C using volume ventilation. The following parameters are set: Mode = A/C; V_T = 0.7 L (700 mL); f = 20 breaths/min; sensitivity = 2 L/min; peak flow = 20 L/min using a constant flow waveform; inspiratory pause = 1.2 seconds; and O_2% = 35%. An alarm sounds, and the message window reads "LIMITED." What does the alert indicate, and what should the therapist do to correct the situation?

See Appendix A for the answer.

CLINICAL ROUNDS 12-5

The following parameters are set for a patient being ventilated by the T-Bird: mode = assist/control/VAPS; V_T = 0.65 L (650 mL); f = 10 breaths/min; sensitivity = 3 L/min; flow pattern = constant; peak flow = 60 L/min; pressure control = 20 cm H_2O; O_2% = 30%.

While monitoring the patient, the respiratory therapist notices a breath that appears as shown in Figure 12-13. Was this breath flow- or volume-cycled out of inspiration? How can this be determined?

See Appendix A for the answer.

To select a mode, the operator presses the desired mode button. The LED flashes for 15 seconds, notifying the operator that the unit is ready to switch modes. The mode becomes operational at the selected parameters after the mode pad is pressed a second time, while the LED is still flashing. If the pad is not pressed a second time, the operation is canceled and the ventilator stays in the current mode.

Assist/Control (A/C)

The A/C mode provides a mandatory breath at the minimum set rate or whenever the patient triggers a breath. Volume ventilation is provided whenever PCV is off. When PCV is on, PRESSURE CONTROL and INSPIRATORY TIME are set by the operator, and any volume setting is ignored. The pressure delivered is in addition to any baseline (PEEP) set. (*Note:* PCV is available on the AVS III.)

Synchronized Intermittent Mandatory Ventilation (SIMV)

SIMV can provide volume ventilation for mandatory breaths (PCV off) or pressure ventilation for mandatory breaths (PCV on). PEEP can also be set. All volumes or pressures are delivered from the baseline pressure. Spontaneous breaths can occur at baseline pressures only or can be provided with pressure support (PS set where desired).

Pressure Support Ventilation (PSV)

PSV can be provided during SIMV or CPAP for the patient's spontaneous breaths. The operator sets the desired pressure-support level above the PEEP (baseline) setting. Sensitivity must be set appropriately. All PSV breaths are patient-triggered. Inspiration is flow-cycled at 25% of the measured peak inspiratory flow.

Continuous Positive Airway Pressure (CPAP)

CPAP is a purely spontaneous breathing mode setting. The patient can breathe from baseline pressure (CPAP level) and also receive pressure-support during inspiration if the pressure-support level is set above zero. During CPAP, certain parameters must be set on the control panel even though they are not operational. These parameters are the default settings if the ventilator switches to apnea back-up ventilation. In the display window, "CHECK BKUP" appears, telling the operator to verify that back-up rate, volume, flow, etc., have been set.

Volume Assured Pressure Support (VAPS)

The VAPS mode (AVS III only) is a servo-control mode of ventilation (see Chapter 11). The operator must select appropriate settings for the following based on the patient's size, age, and condition: V_T, peak flow, pressure control, PEEP/CPAP, sensitivity, pressure support (available with SIMV), inspiratory pause, and appropriate alarm settings. When VAPS is first turned on, the ventilator delivers a VAPS breath using whatever pressure-control level (plus baseline) is set. Two common events then result, as follows:

1. The ventilator ends inspiration if the V_T has been delivered by the time inspiratory flow decreases to the set value. That is, the ventilator flow cycles at the set peak flow value.
2. If V_T has not been delivered by the time flow has dropped to this value, the flow is maintained (constant waveform pattern) at the peak flow value until the V_T has been delivered. In this situation the unit volume cycles at the set V_T. Clinical Rounds 12-5 gives an example of delivery of a volume during VAPS (Figure 12-13).

(*Note*: If a VAPS breath meets the minimum V_T criteria and inspiratory pause is set at some value above zero, the inspiratory pause is active. However, if a VAPS breath does not meet the minimum V_T criteria and transitions to a volume-cycled breath, the ventilator will ignore inspiratory pause if it is set.[1]) Chapter 11 provides a more detailed explanation of this closed-loop form of ventilation that guarantees a volume for every breath.

Graphic Display Screens

The graphics monitor for the T-Bird is the same as the one adapted to use with the Bird 8400STi. Readers are referred to that section for more details.

Special Features

One of the advantages of the T-Bird is the availability of several unique features. For example, under the ventilator set-up options, it allows the operator to adjust for altitudes ranging from –1000 to 10,000 feet. Because of this, the unit can compensate for lower gas pressures and improve the

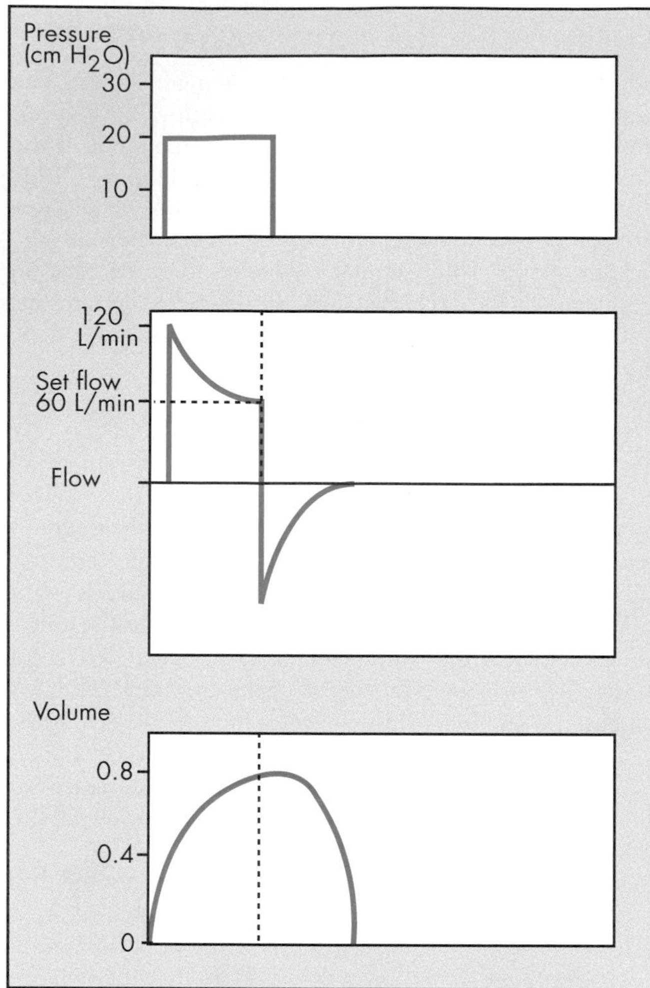

Figure 12-13 A graph of pressure, flow, and volume vs. time for a breath during VAPS on the T-Bird. The top curve shows constant pressure delivery at the set PC level. The baseline is 0 cm H_2O. The middle curve shows the flow rising rapidly at the beginning of inspiration and then descending to the set flow value, and at which point the breath ends. The V_T achieved is higher than the set value, so the patient must have been actively breathing.

accuracy of volume and flow delivery at varying elevations. The ventilator set-up options also contain the bias flow (10 to 20 L/min) control, which sets the level of continuous gas flow through the patient circuit.

The special functions alarm group allows for setting the apnea interval (ranges from 10 to 60 sec), which sets the time between breaths before the apnea alarm is activated. The ventilator then switches to apnea back-up and stays in this mode until the patient initiates two successive breaths or the operator hits the alarm silence/reset button twice.

The two groups of special controls that are most likely to be frequently used are the ventilator set-up group and the alarm set-up group (Table 12-3). The reader is directed to the operating manual for full descriptions of all the special function groups and tests.

Table 12-3 Ventilator and alarm set-up special function

Function	Description
VENTILATOR SET-UP GROUP	
Altitude	Altitude setting (-1000 to 10,000 ft)
Autoscan	Turns automatic scanning of monitored parameters on/off
BGM (MCH) interface	Switches ventilator interface with graphics monitor to activate or deactivate lung mechanics
Bias flow	Sets the bias flow from 10 to 20 L/min
Control lock enable	Turns on/off control lock function
Display language selector	Selects the display language preferred by the operator
Hour meter	Shows the total number of hours the unit has been in operation
Software versions	Displays the current software versions in use by the unit
Turbine	Shows the serial number of the internal turbine
ALARM SET-UP GROUP	
Apnea interval	Sets the apnea time interval from 10 to 60 seconds
Remote alarm status	Displays the remote alarm ID

Troubleshooting

The alarms and monitoring functions reviewed in this section provide the basic information needed to troubleshoot common problems. In addition, the operating manual contains a section on troubleshooting that describes potential problems, possible causes, and appropriate actions.

New Releases

In 2001-2002 the Viasys Healthcare, Critical Care Division, released a ventilator called the Vela Ventilator (Figure 12-14) that is alike in function to the T-Bird, and includes similar modes, parameters, and alarms. The computer interface provides a user-friendly screen that includes graphics monitoring. The flow-cycling criteria for pressure support in the Vela are adjustable from 5 to 30%. Pressure control can also be flow-cycled (Off to 30%), as well as time-cycled. Bias flow is adjustable from 10 to 20 L/min. The Vela also offers noninvasive positive pressure ventilation and measurement of MIP. For additional information the reader is directed to the company's website (www.ViasysCriticalCare.com).

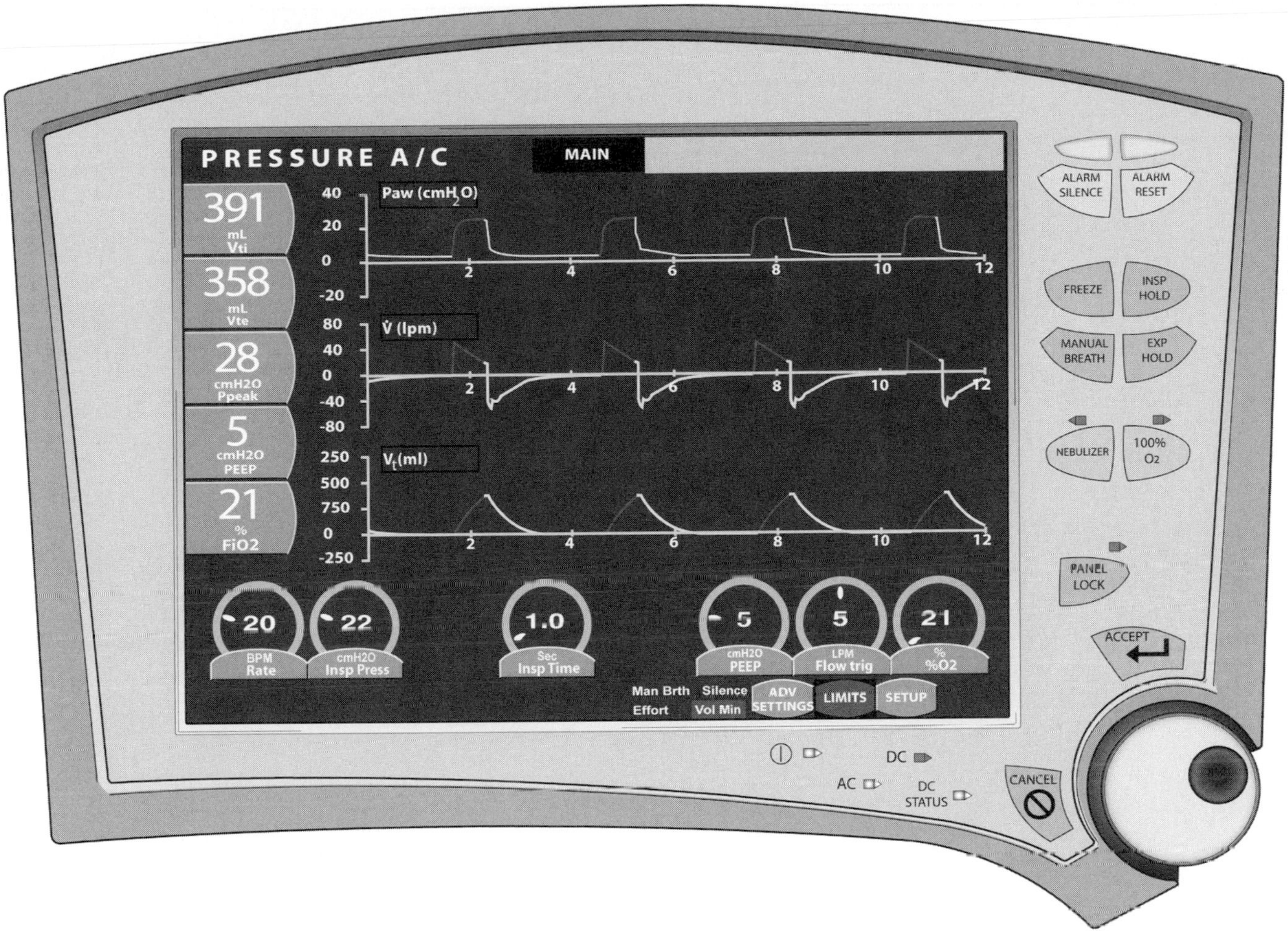

Figure 12-14 The Vela ventilator from Viasys Healthcare. (Courtesy Viasys Healthcare, Critical Care Division, Palm Springs, Calif.)

Dräger Evita

The Dräger Evita ventilator was the first in a series of ventilators manufactured by Drägerwerk in Lubeck, Germany and represented in the United States by the Dräger Corporation (Figure 12-15). The Evita 2 was a modified version of the Evita (Evita 1), but was never marketed in the United States. A second version, the E-2 Dura, replaced the Evita 2 and is sold internationally. And, finally, the Evita 4, or E-4, was the final version of that series. (*Note*: There was never an Evita 3.) All three of these units are presented here, starting with the Evita, which was designed primarily for adult use in the acute care setting.

Power Source

The Evita normally uses two high-pressure gas sources (40 to 87 psig) as its pneumatic power source, but it can also operate with a single-gas source, such as an air compressor with version 14.0 software or higher. Using a single-gas source, however, alters oxygen delivery capability. A standard AC 120-volt outlet is used to power the microprocessor and the electrical components. The on/off switch is located in the upper right corner of the unit's back panel.

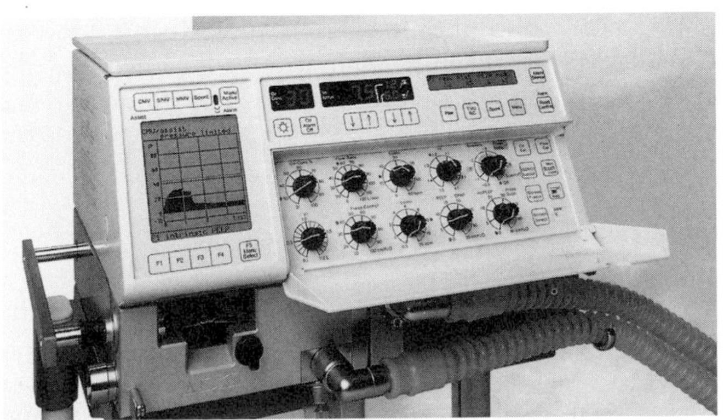

Figure 12-15 The Dräger Evita ventilator. (Courtesy Dräger Corp, Telford, Penn.)

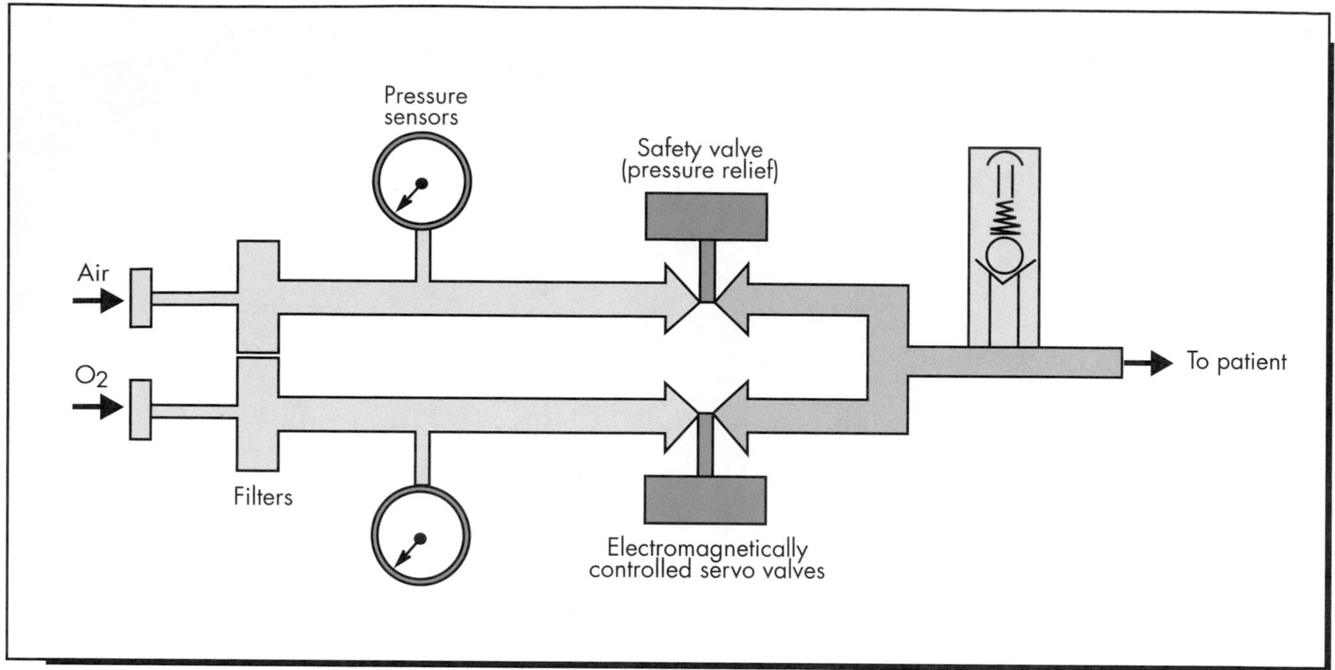

Figure 12-16 A simplified diagram of the internal mechanism of the Evita ventilator that shows the flow-control valves.

Internal Mechanism

In the Evita, the gas source enters the unit through high-pressure gas connections on the back panel (Figure 12-16). The gas is filtered, and the pressure is reduced to a lower working pressure. The incoming flow is then directed to two electromagnetically operated **high-pressure servo valves**. Gases are blended to match the F_IO_2 to be delivered, depending on the setting and assuming that oxygen and air are the source gases. Information from the settings on the front panel, the internal flow, the pressure transducers, and the position of the valves is sent to the microprocessor. The microprocessor uses this information to regulate the action of the servo valves and govern the amount and flow pattern of gas delivered to the patient.

A variety of multiple-pressure transducers monitor the internal gas flow, the output from the unit, and the return of expired gas from the patient through the expiratory valve.

Controls and Alarms

The Evita's front panel (Figure 12-17) is divided into the following three main sections:

1. A lower control panel covered by a protective cover
2. An upper section for displaying parameters and alarm settings
3. A main monitoring screen on the left

Control Parameters

The lower control panel consists of two rows of knobs and a section of touch pads (*right side*). The top row comprises the following (see Figure 12-17):

1. O_2 % control (range, 21% to 100%).
2. INSPIRATORY FLOW (6 to 120 L/min) sets the peak flow for all time-cycled breaths. In volume-targeted breaths, the flow waveform is constant. For pressure control ventilation and pressure-limiting, the ventilator sets the maximum flow at the beginning of the breath. Flow then decreases in a ramp-like fashion. (*Note*: For pressure support breaths, flow is governed by the rise time or slope control.)
3. CMV RATE control knob (5 to 60 breaths/min) sets the breath rate and the inspiratory time in SIMV and MMV.
4. I:E RATIO control (4:1 to 1:5).
5. Knob for SENSITIVITY in CMV and for SLOPE in pressure support.
   - For mandatory breaths in CMV, this knob controls the sensitivity (–0.5 to –5 cm H_2O). When the patient triggers a breath, the green assist LED at the top left corner of the main monitoring screen lights up. (*Note*: In SIMV and MMV, the pressure trigger is fixed at –0.7 cm H_2O, and in CPAP it is fixed at –0.2 cm H_2O.)

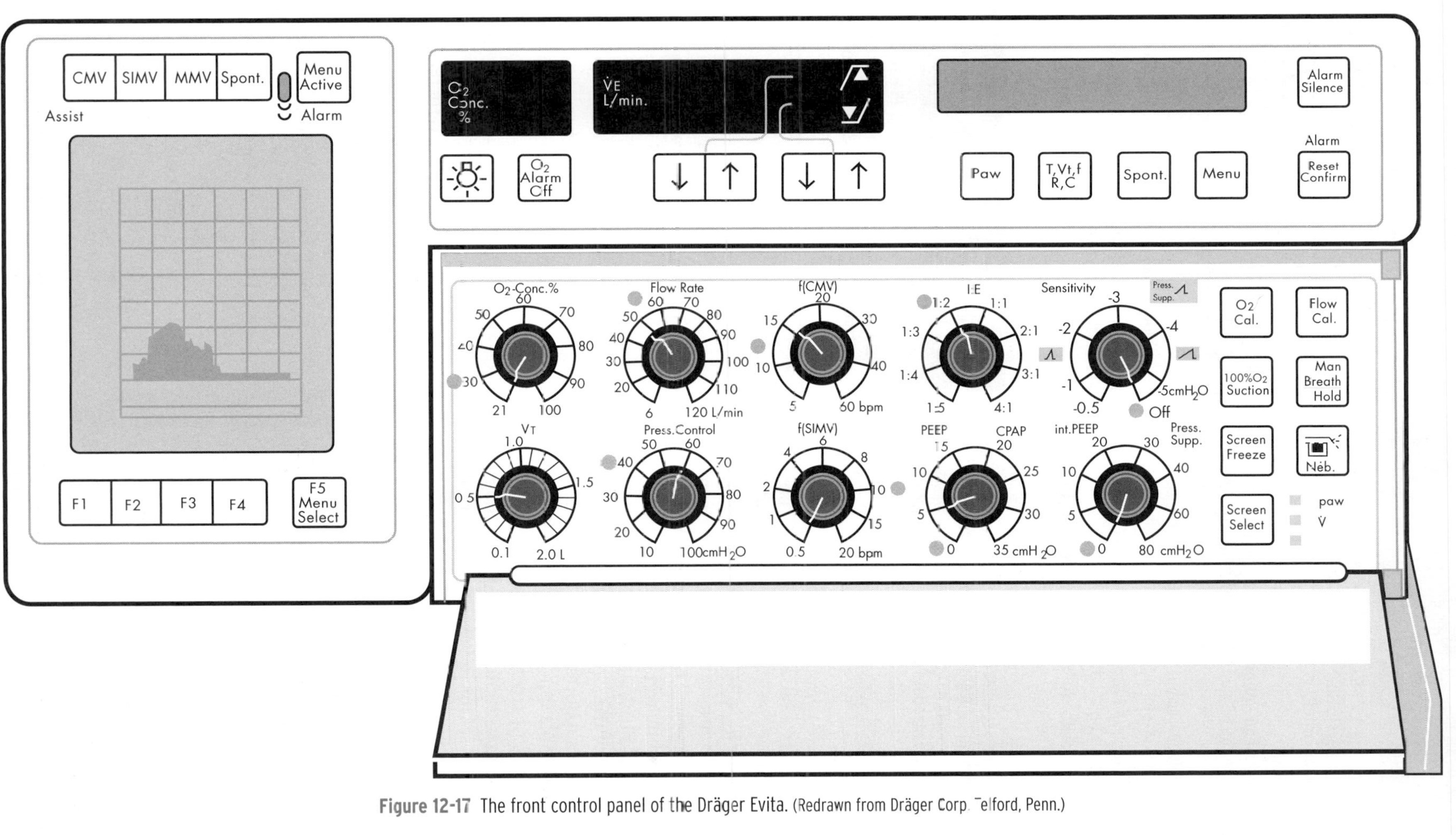

Figure 12-17 The front control panel of the Dräger Evita. (Redrawn from Dräger Corp. Telford, Penn.)

Box 12-17 Adjusting Sensitivity for Pressure-Support Breaths on the Dräger Evita

Setting the flow-triggering for PSV is performed by using the function touch pads or keys below the main monitor. They are selected in the following order:

1. Press menu select (F5)
2. From the displayed menu options appearing on the main monitor screen, use the F3 key to scroll through and select set value.
3. Activate the set value by using the F1 or F2 key. The set value appears on the screen against a dark background.
4. Confirm the set value using the F3 key. The value now appears dark against a light background.
5. To return the main monitor to its normal waveform display, press F5 or wait and the main screen will appear in 2 minutes.

Note that after the F5 key is activated and a menu appears, the menu provides enough information for you to proceed with the desired change. You do not need to memorize a list of steps or refer to the operator's manual to perform these exercises.

- When pressure support is active, this knob controls the rate of rise or slope in the pressure and flow curves for PS breaths in the SIMV, MMV, and PSV modes (range, 0 to 2 seconds). The knob determines how fast the high-pressure servo valves open. The time selected is the time it takes pressure to rise to the set value after the beginning of inspiratory flow. (For a further explanation of rise time, see the discussion of the pressure support mode in later section on modes of ventilation.)

Pressure support is flow-triggered (ranges from 1 to 15 L/min) instead of pressure-triggered. Box 12-17 shows how trigger sensitivity is set for pressure-support breaths.

The second row of controls includes the following:

1. TIDAL VOLUME (0.1 to 2.0 L) sets V_T delivery for volume-targeted breaths in CMV, SIMV, and MMV.
2. PRESS. CONTROL (range, 10 to 100 cm H_2O).
   - Sets the target pressure for mandatory breaths (pressure controlled breaths) in CMV, SIMV, and MMV.
   - Sets the pressure limit for all breaths in all modes. The microprocessor uses the set pressure control value plus 10 cm H_2O to establish the maximum pressure that may be reached in the patient circuit. For this reason, this control must be set at all times.
3. The SIMV rate control, "f(SIMV)," (range 0.5 to 20 breaths/min) sets the mandatory breath rate in the SIMV mode.
4. PEEP/CPAP (0 to 35 cm H_2O). To set the PEEP value, rotate the knob while observing the value for measured PEEP in the measured values window. To view the PEEP value, press the Paw touch pad below the measured values screen at the upper right of the top monitor panel (an LED appears) and rotate the PEEP/CPAP knob until the desired value appears in the measured values window.
5. Rotary knob for INT. PEEP and PRESS. SUPP.
   - The intermittent PEEP knob is turned to the desired pressure level. Intermittent PEEP acts as a sigh breath when it is selected. The baseline pressure is increased by the value set on the INT. PEEP knob (0 to 35 cm H_2O) for two consecutive breaths every 3 minutes during CMV only (Figure 12-18). The function becomes active as soon as it is set, and the top of the main monitoring screen reads "INT. PEEP ACTIVE" when it is selected.
   - The pressure support function of this control sets the PS level during SIMV, MMV, and PSV ventilation (3 to 80 cm H_2O). The value set on this control determines the maximum amount of pressure the ventilator will deliver with a pressure support breath (Box 12-18). When the pressure support function is active (SIMV, MMV, or SPONT. mode touch pad lit), the sigh (INT. PEEP) is not active. The green LEDs adjacent to and on either side of the knob appear to show which function is active.

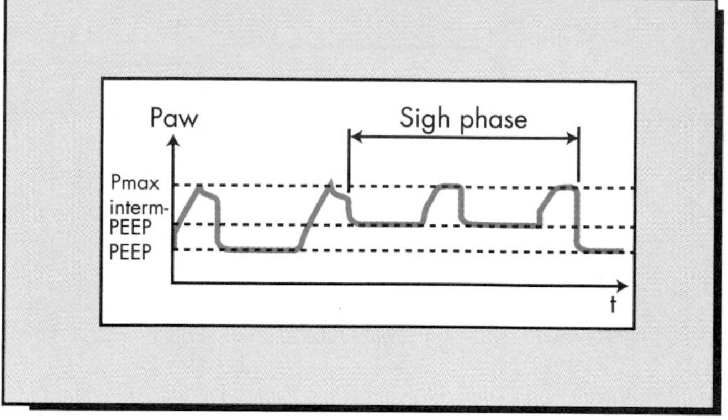

Figure 12-18 Intermittent PEEP for the delivery of sigh breaths. (Redrawn from Dräger Corp, Telford, Penn.)

Box 12-18 Setting the Pressure Level for Pressure Support on the Dräger Evita

If you want a pressure support of 15 cm H_2O, you must set the desired value above the baseline pressure (PEEP/CPAP). For example, if you want 15 cm H_2O of PS and the PEEP is set at 5 cm H_2O, set the PRESS. SUPPORT knob to 20 cm H_2O.

Each of these operating controls has a green LED indicator adjacent to it that illuminates when the knob needs adjustment or is operational. A flashing LED is warning of an extreme setting, such as an I:E ratio >1:1 or <1:3, and indicates that the knob is functional and the change has occurred, but is asking you to confirm that you do want this setting. Verify the setting by using the reset/confirm keypad. If multiple LEDs, such as V_T, flow, and I:E, are flashing, this is a warning that parameters are set incorrectly. For example, the V_T set may be too high to be achieved with the set flow and inspiratory time, so that the settings must be readjusted. The ventilator will stay at the original setting prior to the change until the error is corrected.

The touch pad controls on the right side of the panel serve the following functions:

1. Calibration of the built-in **oxygen sensor** (LED is yellow during calibration).
2. 100% O_2 suction that provides 100% oxygen during suctioning. When pressed, the ventilator delivers 100% oxygen through the circuit for 3 minutes. The main screen reads "O_2 enrichment 180 s," and the time remaining is displayed. A pressure of 4 cm H_2O is applied if a PEEP of <4 cm H_2O is set to help the ventilator identify when the circuit is disconnected and reconnected. All other parameters are unchanged. After disconnection has been identified, the unit provides 100% oxygen for 2 minutes after suctioning. During these 2 minutes, the audible alarm is silenced so that it is not a nuisance, and a flow of 4 L/min is provided through the circuit. This low flow is intended to reduce humidifier splash. After the patient is reconnected, ventilation is resumed, and an additional 2 minutes of 100% oxygen are provided to the patient. The alarms are reactivated, and the Evita returns to its normal operating mode. The main display screen reads "final O_2 enrich. 120 s." Pressing the RESET/CONFIRM key at any time stops the oxygenation procedure, which cannot be restarted for 15 seconds. (*Note*: The oxygenation procedure is interrupted if the Evita does not detect a disconnection within the first 3 minute period.)
3. SCREEN FREEZE freezes the waveform on the main monitor screen.
4. SCREEN SELECT allows selection of pressure-time or flow-time waveforms to appear on the main monitor screen. For example, the flow-time curve can be viewed by following the procedure in Box 12-19.
5. FLOW CAL cleans and calibrates the sensor (LED is yellow during calibration).
6. MANUAL BREATH HOLD either delivers a mandatory breath or performs an inspiratory breath hold. (LED is yellow when this key is pressed; maximum time is 15 seconds.)
7. NEBULIZER CONTROL; the nebulizer operates for 10 minutes and is synchronized with the inspiratory flow phase of a breath and provides 1.5 L/min (air or oxygen). (LED is green when the nebulizer is operating.) It is recommended that the Dräger reusable nebulizer provided be used for this function to maintain F_IO_2 and volume delivery as much as possible. Software upgrades (version 14.0) allow for flows of 6 to 9 L/min when other nebulizers are used. Cleaning and calibration of the flow sensor automatically occurs after the nebulizer function is used. (*Note*: The flow sensor is located on the expiratory end of the internal pneumatic circuit.)

Box 12-19 Viewing the Inspiratory Flow Curve on the Dräger Evita

1. **Press the screen select key (lower right panel) repeatedly until the LED for flow lights.**
2. **The waveform for flow-time appears on the left of the main monitoring screen.**

Monitors and Alarms

At the top of the display panel are three small LED screens or windows to provide digital information. The left screen displays the O_2 % being measured by the oxygen analyzer. The next screen shows the measured expired $\dot{V}_E$ with the set upper and lower $\dot{V}_E$ alarm limits. The right screen is the measured values display, which provides a digital display of selected measured values based on using the touch pads below the window.

To select alarm settings and measured values, the operator uses the touch pads adjacent to the LED windows. For example, below the O_2 % window is a key (touch pad) marked with a picture of a light bulb that is used to change the back lighting on the main viewing screen and the measured values screen. Next to it is the touch pad to turn the oxygen analyzer function on and off. When it is off, the yellow LED flashes. The displayed measured value may differ by ± 4% of the value set on the control knob. If it differs by more than this, an alarm is activated to indicate that the oxygen sensor needs to be calibrated or replaced (see the operator's manual).[1]

Below the $\dot{V}_E$ window there are four touch pads that contain arrows (up and down) for changing the upper alarm and lower alarm limits for $\dot{V}_E$.

There are four more touch pads below the measured values display screen. The first three allow the selection of the measured and calculated data listed in Box 12-20. When any of the three are activated, a green LED appears. When any of these pads are touched a second time, the dimensions (units) of the measurement are indicated. The fourth touch pad is the menu select button, which is used to adjust the contrast setting on the display and screen and to adjust the clock.

Box 12-20 Touch Pads on the Dräger Evita for Selecting Data Display

First Touch Pad (at Left) Provides the Following Values:

Peak pressure
Plateau pressure
PEEP
Mean airway pressure

Second Touch Pad Provides the Following Values:

Inspiratory gas temperature (T)
Exhaled tidal volume (V_{Te})
Frequency (f)
Resistance (R)
Compliance (C)

Third Touch Pad Provides the Following Data:

Spontaneously breathed exhaled $\dot{V}_E$
Spontaneously respiratory rate (f-spo)
Spontaneous respiration with positive airway pressure

Box 12-21 Alarm Messages for the Dräger Evita

Ventilation Alarms

- MV low or high
- Airway pressure low or high
- Oxygen concentration low or high
- Apnea
- High rate
- High temperature

Equipment Alarms

- Compressed air low
- Oxygen pressure low, or oxygen cal. Inactive
- Pressure measurement inoperative
- Mixer inoperative
- Malfunction fan
- Fan defect
- Flow measurement inoperative
- Suction inactive
- Expiratory valve inoperative
- Failure to cycle
- Oxygen measurement inoperative
- Service needed
- Pressure-relief opened
- RS 232 inoperative (defect in digital interface)

Main Monitoring Screen

The left side of the front panel contains a large LED screen, the main monitoring screen, which shows a constant display of the waveform pattern selected. At the top of this screen are the status and alarm displays. For example, the status display might indicate the mode of ventilation.

Above and below the monitoring screen are touch pads for selecting ventilator modes and specific functions. The top pads are used to select CMV, SIMV, MMV, and spontaneous modes of ventilation. (*Note*: When a mode is being set, these keys must be pressed and held until the LED lights.) In addition, there is a menu active key, which places the Evita in apnea ventilation or airway pressure-release ventilation (APRV), depending on which is selected from the menu. The touch pads below the screen give access to many additional menu functions. A few main functions are reviewed in the material here, but readers are advised to check the operator's manual for a complete review of the function keys.[1]

Alarm Conditions

When an alarm is activated, a red light flashes at the upper right corner of the main screen and an intermittent sound is emitted. An alarm message is displayed in the upper right corner of the main monitor screen. Box 12-21 lists the ventilation and equipment alarm messages that may occur. To silence the audible alarm for 2 minutes, the ALARM SILENCE key is pressed. When the problem is corrected, the alarm stops. Pressing the ALARM RESET key removes the alarm message from the main screen.

Airway Pressure Alarms

The alarm thresholds for pressure and PEEP are automatically set by the ventilator. The upper pressure limit is 10 cm H_2O above the setting on the PRESS. CONTROL knob, and is always active regardless of the mode. When this upper pressure limit is reached in the circuit, inspiratory gas flow stops and the expiratory valve opens. If the level reaches 15 cm H_2O above the setting, a second valve opens to vent the pressure more quickly.

The lower pressure limit is 5 cm H_2O below the PEEP/CPAP setting and is active in CMV, SIMV, MMV, and spontaneous.

Front Connections

There are several connectors below the front control panel (see Figure 12-15). There are large-bore connectors for the main inspiratory and expiratory lines of the patient circuit and a small connector for the nebulizer line. The expiratory flow transducer housing is below the main monitoring screen. To the right of the main inspiratory line connection is a screw adjustment for the protective cover over the oxygen analyzer and the room air intake filter (not shown in the figure).

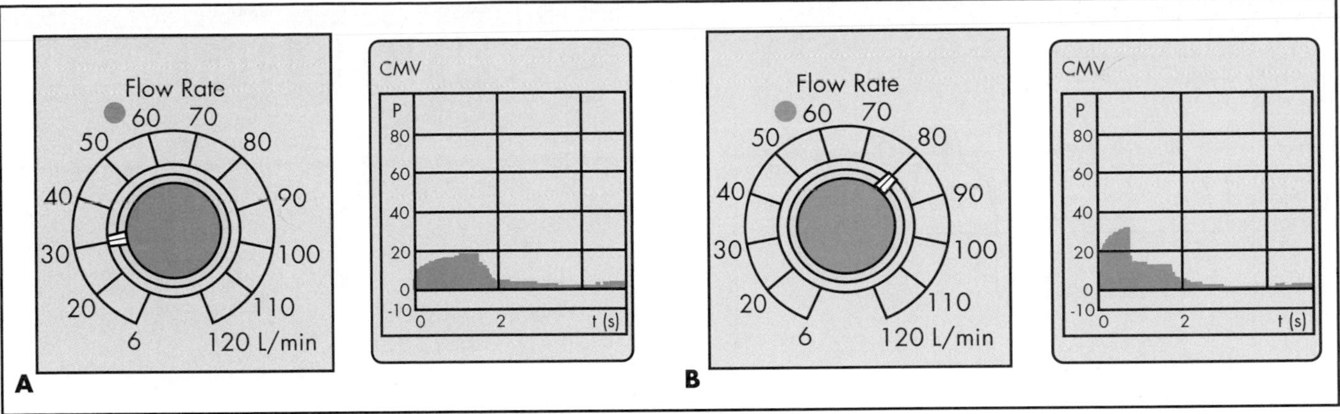

Figure 12-19 Comparison of high and low flow rates during CMV ventilation. Curve **A** shows a slow filling rate with a low peak pressure and a short pause. Curve **B** shows a rapid flow rate with a higher peak pressure and a longer pause time. (Redrawn from Dräger Corp, Telford, Penn.)

Modes of Ventilation

Modes of operation available on the Evita include CMV, SIMV, spontaneous (PSV and CPAP), MMV, apnea ventilation and APRV. (*Note*: APRV may also be referred to as BIPAP or biphasic positive airway pressure.) Before using the ventilator with a patient, a series of tests are performed as a part of standard maintenance. The operator's manual describes all of the essential steps for testing the unit's readiness.[1]

Continuous Mandatory Ventilation (CMV)

The CMV mode is an assist/control volume ventilation mode. The operator presses the CMV key until its LED remains continuously lit. The parameters that are set include V_T, flow, f (CMV), I:E, sensitivity, PEEP, F_IO_2, PRESS. CONTROL, and desired alarm settings. Breaths are patient- or time-triggered, volume-targeted, and time-cycled. (*Note*: If the sensitivity is turned all the way clockwise, the Evita is placed in controlled ventilation, i.e., time triggering and an "assist" message disappears from the top left portion of the main screen.) T_I is based on the rate and the I:E control settings. For example, if the rate is set at 10 breaths/min and the I:E at 1:2, the inspiratory time will be as follows:

1. Total cycle time (TCT) = 60 seconds/(10 breaths/min) = 6 seconds
2. I:E = 1:2, T_I = 2 seconds, and T_E = 4 seconds (see Chapter 11)
3. T_I = 2 seconds

All breaths deliver the set V_T. Flow to the patient is restricted to the flow setting value. The flow waveform is constant. If flow is high and V_T is delivered before T_I is achieved, the inspiratory valve closes (expiratory valve is already closed) and the breath is held. This event can be identified by an inspiratory pause pressure in the pressure-time curve and the flow curve returns to zero flow on the flow-time curve.

Box 12-22 Ventilating Infants with the Dräger Evita

Tidal volume may be reduced to approximately 50 mL by using the Pmax setting and inspiratory flow settings to limit pressure during inspiration during CMV.

Using high flow rates provides a longer pause time but also produces a higher peak pressure (Figure 12-19). (*Note*: When setting up volume-targeted breaths in CMV or any volume mode, the PRESSURE CONTROL knob must be set high enough so that a constant flow waveform is delivered. If there is a descending flow waveform, pressure and flow delivery will be limited.)

After the patient is connected, the measured values window can be accessed using the T, V_T, f, R, and C touch pads below the window. The values for each variable are then displayed in the window. Some adjustments can be made to accommodate pediatric patients (Box 12-22).

Pressure Limit Function

The high peak pressures that may occur with volume ventilation can be avoided by using a lower flow or by using the pressure limit function. The pressure limit is determined by the setting on the PRESS. CONTROL knob. The pressure limit function is also called "**Pmax**" and "pressure-limited ventilation (PLV)" by the manufacturer and is available on the E-4 and the Evita 2 Dura as well. Unlike other ventilators that end inspiration when the upper pressure limit is reached, in the Evita during volume ventilation, when the pressure set on the PRESS. CONTROL is reached, the pressure stays at that value. Inspiration is time-cycled, not pressure-cycled during volume ventilation.

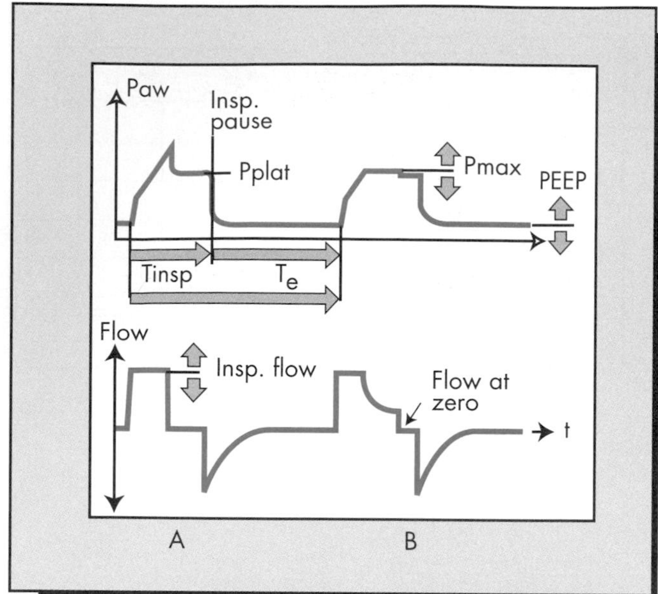

Figure 12-20 The pressure limit function operating during volume targeted mandatory breaths. The top curve is a pressure/time curve showing a typical volume delivered breath with a constant flow delivery **(A)** and a second breath delivery when pressure limit is selected **(B).** See text for further explanation. (Redrawn from Dräger Corp, Telford, Penn.)

CLINICAL ROUNDS 12-6

A patient being ventilated with the Dräger Evita is being switched from volume ventilation in the CMV mode to PCV. Current V_T is 0.65 L (650 mL), rate is 10 breaths/min, flow is 50 L/min, Ppeak is 20 cm H_2O, and $P_{plateau}$ is 16 cm H_2O. Answer the following questions:

1. How do you activate PCV?
2. Where would you set an initial pressure setting to deliver a similar V_T?
3. Where would you set the upper and lower $\dot{V}_E$ alarm values?
4. After PCV is activated, how do you check the delivered V_T?

See Appendix A for the answer.

The pressure limit function operates during volume ventilation in CMV, SIMV, and MMV modes in the following manner. When a breath begins, the pressure in the circuit rises rapidly. The speed at which the pressure is reached depends on how high the peak flow is set. After the set flow is reached, the ventilator maintains this value until:

- The tidal volume is delivered, at which time flow drops to zero and pressure is maintained in the circuit until T_I is reached (T_I is based on rate and I:E ratio settings), or
- The pressure limit is reached. This pressure will be maintained until T_I has elapsed. V_T will be delivered as long as the pressure limit is set appropriately. The pressure limit must be at least 3 cm H_2O above the plateau to ensure V_T delivery.

Figure 12-20 shows two examples of breath delivery during volume ventilation. In breath **A**, a typical volume-targeted breath is delivered. During inspiration the pressure rises rapidly to a peak value, then drops to the plateau after the set V_T is delivered. Flow delivery is at zero (i.e., no more volume is added, but pressure is maintained in the circuit. Inspiration continues until T_I has passed). In this situation the set pressure limit was not reached.

In Figure 12-20, breath **B**, the pressure limit has been set lower using the PRESS. CONTROL knob. The amount of pressure in the circuit cannot go above the set pressure value. The pressure curve shows a rise to the set value and the pressure curve then plateaus at that value. The flow rises rapidly, plateaus, and then tapers off as the difference between the pressure being delivered by the ventilator and the pressure in the lungs become closer in value. In breath **B**, the flow eventually falls to zero. At that point the pressure in the lungs and ventilator circuit are equal. This occurred before T_I had elapsed. In this case, the volume will be delivered. If T_I is too short, a plateau pressure will not appear, flow will not drop to zero and the V_T may be lower than the set value. (*Note:* The V_T remains constant at the set value *as long as the flow drops to zero before the end of inspiration* [i.e., an inspiratory hold]. If flow does not drop to zero for the pressure being provided by the unit, the volume cannot be delivered. This changes the breath delivery to a pressure-targeted breath.)

If the breath is now pressure-targeted, the volume delivery will also change as the condition of the patient's lung changes. For example, if the lungs become stiffer (less compliant), more pressure would be required to deliver the same volume. Pressure limit might need to be readjusted upward after an evaluation of the cause of the change.

Pressure Control Ventilation (PCV) and Inverse Ratio Ventilation (IRV)

In the CMV or SIMV modes, the Evita can provide PCV, which is activated by rotating the PRESS. CONTROL knob until the desired (target) pressure ("Ppeak") appears in the measured values window. It is recommended that V_T be set at 2.0 L, and it is important to turn off the volume not constant alarm in the function key pads, otherwise whenever a breath does not reach the set V_T (2.0 L), the alarm will activate.

Displays of pressure can be viewed on the digital monitoring screen by pressing the "Paw" key pad.

When a pressure value is set on the PRESS. CONTROL knob, pressure limit takes priority over volume delivery. For

Box 12-23 Setting Inverse Ratio Ventilation (IRV)

1. Select the flow-time curve on the main monitor to observe flow delivery while IRV is being adjusted. Avoid developing auto-PEEP during the procedure. The flow must return to zero before the next breath is delivered (see Chapter 11).
2. If PEEP is being used, it should be reduced for safety purposes. In other words, IRV increases mean Paw, as does PEEP, so you do not want the mean Paw too high to begin with.
3. Gradually increase the I:E ratio from 1:1 to 2:1, and so on while monitoring the patient.
4. The top of the main monitor screen reads "confirm I:E," and the green LED on the I:E knob flashes.
5. Confirm to the microprocessor that you want to go to IRV by pressing the reset confirm touch pad (at the top right of the front panel) until the change is confirmed; the LED stops flashing, and the message disappears.
6. Readjust the following control knobs: flow, pressure limit (press. control), PEEP, and I:E as necessary.
7. Be sure that $\dot{V}_E$ alarm limits are set appropriately.

example, if the volume is set at 2 L and the pressure is set at 20 cm H_2O, the Evita will go to the set pressure (20 cm H_2O) as soon as inspiration begins. It will stay there for the allotted T_I, based on rate and I:E ratio, and time-cycle out of inspiration. V_T delivery depends on the patient's lung compliance and the set pressure value (Clinical Rounds 12-6).

Flow waveforms during PCV resemble a descending ramp waveform. If flow reaches zero at the end of inspiration, the pressure generated by the ventilator is equivalent to the pressure in the lungs and circuit. Remember that changes in lung characteristics (resistance and compliance) will alter the volume delivered during pressure ventilation, so it is recommended that the high and low $\dot{V}_E$ alarms be set carefully so that they will be activated when a significant change in compliance or resistance has occurred (see Clinical Rounds 12-6).

Inverse ratio ventilation (IRV) can be provided in either volume- or pressure-targeted ventilation by using the I:E RATIO control knob, but is only available in the CMV mode. In Box 12-23, the procedure for setting and confirming the desired IRV is reviewed.

Synchronized Intermittent Mandatory Ventilation (SIMV)

SIMV provides a minimum number of mandatory breaths and allows the patient to breathe spontaneously between these breaths (see Chapter 11). Mandatory breaths can be patient- or time-triggered, volume- or pressure-targeted and time-cycled. In the SIMV mode, as in CMV mode, the volume breaths can be changed to pressure-targeted breaths by using the PRESS. CONTROL knob. They can also be set as pressure-targeted breaths by using the procedure for setting PCV described in the previous section on the CMV mode.

The operator selects the mandatory rate using the f(SIMV) control knob, which determines the time between mandatory breaths. This value is always set lower than the f(CMV) knob. The f(CMV) rate and the I:E ratio are also set and establish the inspiratory time of a mandatory breath. For example, suppose the following are set: f(CMV) = 10 breaths/min, I:E = 1:2, and f(SIMV) = 5 breaths/min. The T_I will be 2 seconds (Box 12-24). The patient can receive the set volume or pressure in 2 seconds (T_I), have the next 10 seconds to exhale, and breathe spontaneously during that time. The V_T and flow controls determine what part of T_I is spent delivering flow to the patient and what part provides a pause (Clinical Rounds 12-7).

All other adjustable parameters in SIMV are the same as those described in the previous section on CMV. Spontaneous breaths can be provided using pressure support. Pressure support breaths are patient-triggered, pressure-limited, and normally flow-cycled (see the following section on PSV).

Box 12-24 Calculations of T_I and SIMV Cycle Time in the Evita

Calculation:

60 seconds = 10 breaths/min = 6 seconds cycle time

Total Cycle Time (TCT)/(sum of I:E) = T_I

6/3 = 2 seconds

The mandatory breath is delivered in 2 seconds. Expiratory time is 4 seconds. The time between mandatory breaths is 60 seconds (divided by) 5 breaths/min, or 12 seconds.

CLINICAL ROUNDS 12-7

A respiratory therapist is ventilating a patient with the Dräger Evita in the SIMV mode. The ventilator parameters are as follows: V_T = 0.5 L (500 mL); f (CMV) = 15 breaths/min; I:E = 1:3; f (SIMV) = 4 breaths/min; flow = 60 L/min; PRESS. CONTROL is set at zero. Answer the following questions:

1. What will the flow waveform pattern look like?
2. What is the T_I of a mandatory breath?
3. What part of T_I is spent in flow delivery and what part in inspiratory pause?
4. What is the time interval between mandatory breaths?

See Appendix A for the answer.

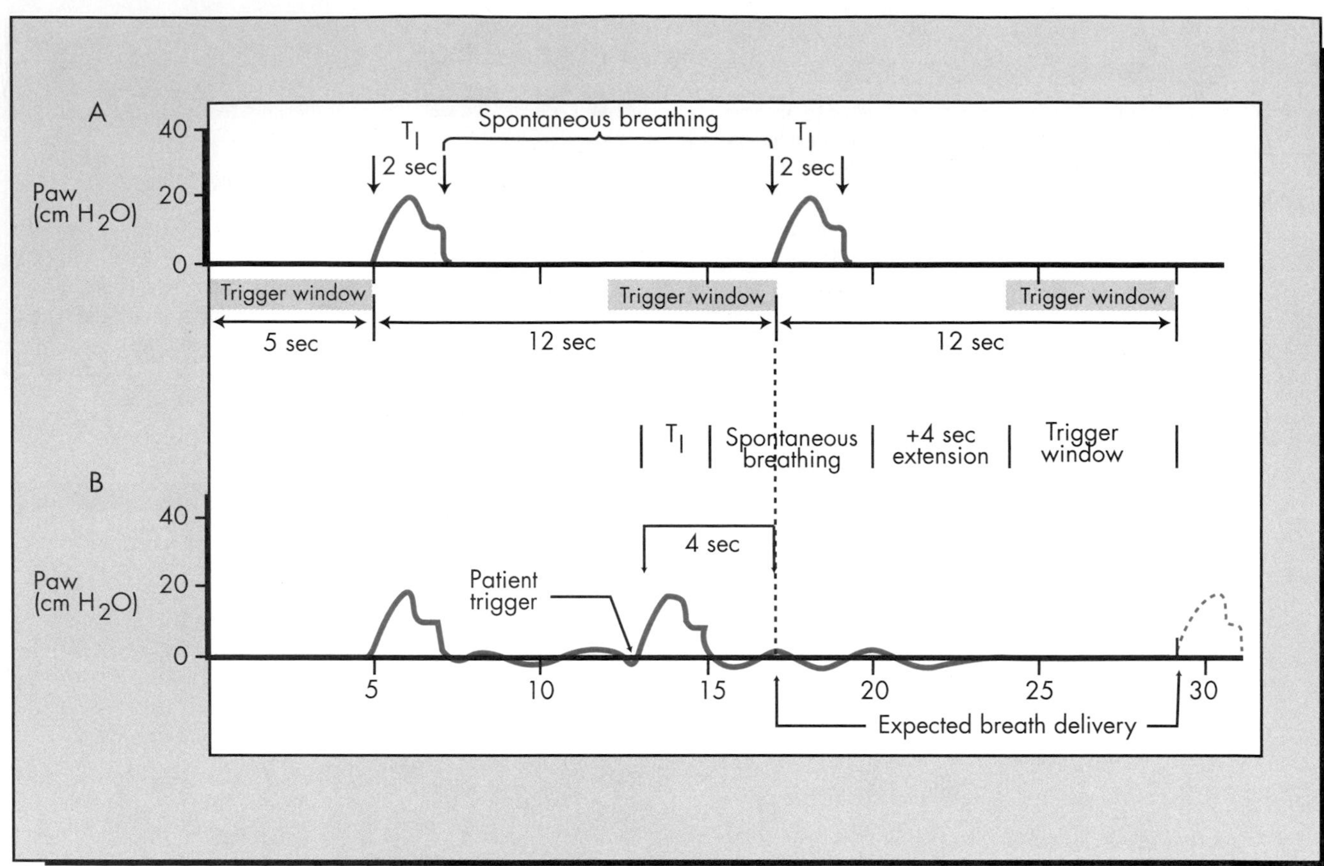

Figure 12-21 SIMV rate timing; see text for description.

When SIMV is first started, the patient has a 5-second window during which to make an inspiratory effort and trigger a mandatory breath. For example, suppose the following values are set:

- f(CMV) = 10 breaths/min
- f(SIMV) = 5 breaths/min
- T_I = 2 seconds, based on I:E and f(CMV)

The set SIMV time is 12 seconds (60 seconds/5 breaths/min). After a mandatory breath, the patient has 10 seconds during which to exhale and breathe spontaneously (12 seconds – 2 seconds = 10 seconds of spontaneous breathing time).

Suppose that the patient does not make a spontaneous effort and the ventilator time triggers the first mandatory breath at the end of the 5-second window (Figure 12-21, *A*). The next mandatory breath will occur 12 seconds after the beginning of this breath if the patient remains apneic.

Suppose that a patient breathes the first time-triggered mandatory breath spontaneously (see Figure 12-21, *B*). The patient has 5 seconds to do so before the next 5-second window appears. During the window, an adequate inspiratory effort triggers the next mandatory breath. Figure 12-21 shows the following example:

1. Mandatory inspiration (T_I) = 2 seconds
2. Spontaneous breathing time = 12 seconds – 2 seconds = 10 seconds
3. Mandatory window = 5 seconds
4. Spontaneous time without breath-triggering window = 10 seconds – 5 seconds

The patient breathes spontaneously for 5 seconds, and then the 5-second window begins. The next patient effort triggers a mandatory breath 1 second into the 5-second window. This is 4 seconds before the next mandatory breath (time-cycled) is due. If this early triggering continues, the actual mandatory breath rate will be higher than its set value. To compensate, the microprocessor calculates the difference between the actual breath delivery (see "patient trigger" in Figure 12-21, *B*) and the expected breath delivery (which is 4 seconds in this example). This amount of time is added to the next spontaneous window. The 4-second extension is added onto the spontaneous breathing time for the next mandatory breath delivery, preventing mandatory breaths from occurring too frequently and thus increasing the mandatory rate over the set SIMV rate.

In the Evita, the mandatory volume is also compensated in SIMV. Suppose that the patient spontaneously breathes in a large volume of air at the beginning of a mandatory breath. The ventilator takes this volume into account and reduces the inspiratory flow and time enough to keep the V_T constant at the set value, thus avoiding excessive volume delivery. The combination of adjustments to the SIMV rate and the V_T delivery helps to maintain a stable minimum $\dot{V}_E$.

Pressure Support Ventilation (PSV)

The Dräger Evita can provide PSV during SIMV, MMV, and spontaneous ventilation modes. To activate PSV in these modes, dial the desired PS level using the INT. PEEP/PRESS. SUPP knob. The main monitor will read "CPAP/PRESS. SUPP." PS breaths are patient-triggered, pressure-targeted, and usually flow-cycled (25% of the peak measured flow). Patient-triggering is based on the set flow-trigger value or when the inspired volume exceeds 25 mL (volume-triggering). The machine then provides the set pressure. Flow delivery is in a descending waveform pattern.

When PSV is active, the rate of rise in pressure and flow that occurs at the beginning of a PS breath can be adjusted using the SENSITIVITY/PRESS. SUPP control. When the left portion of the range is used, pressure and flow rise rapidly (range 0 to 1 seconds). When the right portion of the range is used, pressure and flow rise slowly (about 1 to 2 seconds) (Figure 12-22).

If the patient actively exhales or fights the ventilator during the start of a PS breath, inspiratory flow ends. This happens when either the flow goes to zero at the beginning of a breath or the patient is actively exhaling during the early portion of inspiration. Inspiratory flow during PSV will also time-cycle at 4 seconds. Prolonged T_I occurs most commonly if a leak is present. In this situation, an alarm (audio and visual) is activated.

When switching from spontaneous ventilation modes (PSV or CPAP) to CMV, the INT. PEEP/PRESS. SUPP knob must be readjusted. Remember that in switching back to CMV, the SENSITIVITY/PRESS. SUPP control now controls trigger sensitivity—not the rate of pressure and flow delivery, which must also be readjusted.

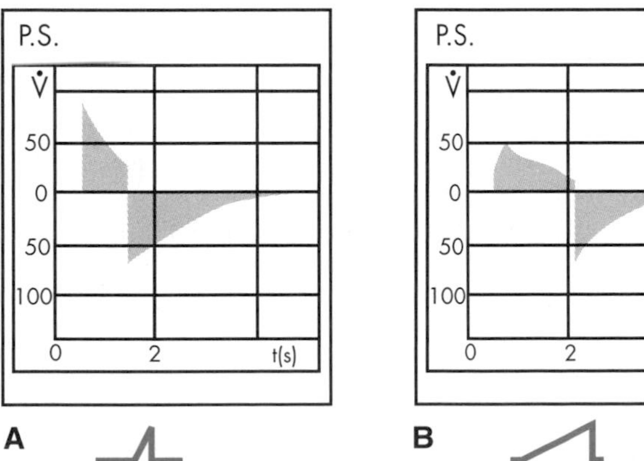

Figure 12-22 The sloping (adjustment of rise time) of the flow/time curve using the SENSITIVITY/PRESS. SUPP control with the Dräger Evita. Curve **A** shows a very rapid flow. Curve **B** shows a very slow flow. (Redrawn from Dräger Corp, Telford, Penn.)

Continuous Positive Airway Pressure (CPAP)

CPAP is available on the Evita by selecting the spontaneous mode touch pad. Set the desired CPAP level (cm H_2O) with the PEEP/CPAP knob. Set PS if spontaneous breaths are to be aided with PSV. The set PS level is the peak pressure for the breath (see Box 12-18). Be sure to set upper and lower $\dot{V}_E$ alarm limits, and remember that when switching from a spontaneous mode back to CMV, the INT. PEEP and SENSITIVITY/PRESS. SUPP controls must be readjusted.

Mandatory Minute Volume (MMV)

As described in Chapter 11, a patient can spontaneously breathe and contribute a portion or all of the overall $\dot{V}_E$ in the MMV mode. The difference between the spontaneous and the set $\dot{V}_E$ is provided by mandatory breaths at the set volume.

A desired minimum $\dot{V}_E$ is set using an appropriate rate and V_T to maintain the desired arterial blood gas values. A pressure support level should also be selected to help the patient's spontaneous breathing efforts between any mandatory set V_T breaths. Pressure support rise time can be used to slope the pressure-time curve during PSV. A HIGH RESPIRATORY RATE alarm is also set to monitor increased work of breathing.

The frequency of a mandatory breath is determined by the level of spontaneous breathing. If the patient is providing sufficient spontaneous $\dot{V}_E$, no mandatory breaths occur. However, if spontaneous $\dot{V}_E$ falls below what the ventilator anticipates to occur based on the set $\dot{V}_E$ ($V_T \times f$), mandatory breaths begin as soon as the balance between the set and the spontaneous $\dot{V}_E$ becomes negative. The software program for MMV ventilation is designed to allow for irregular patterns of spontaneous breathing with occasional short intervals of apnea. It permits these irregularities without allowing excessive time to pass with no spontaneous or mandatory breathing.

Apnea Ventilation

Apnea ventilation is an independent mode setup in the menu. It is not a backup for other modes and only supplies CPAP and PSV modes with backup. Apnea ventilation provides volume ventilation with a minimum breath rate if the patient becomes apneic. If the patient quits breathing for the length of time set on the apnea alarm control, the alarm is activated, the ventilator switches to CMV based on the control knob settings, and apnea ventilation begins.

Box 12-25 describes how to set apnea ventilation. If an apneic event occurs, the Evita will give an audio/visual alarm after 15 seconds. After the set apnea time has elapsed (15 to 60 seconds), ventilation with the CMV mode begins, using all rotary knobs that have green LEDs lit. The main screen shows a flashing "CMV" message, and the unit remains in apnea ventilation regardless of what the patient is doing. Pressing the reset/confirm key returns the ventilator to its previous function.

Box 12-25 Setting Apnea Ventilation on the Evita

1. Touch the F5 function key.
2. Select the APNEA VENT. menu using the F2 key.
3. Select apnea time using F2.
4. Set the desired apnea time using the F1 and F2 keys.
5. Confirm the new value by pressing the F3 key.
6. Return to the original screen using F5.
7. Press F1 to select apnea ventilation.
8. Press the menu active button until its LED is lit continuously; the new apnea time is set and apnea ventilation is now active.
9. Press the F5 key twice to return to the normal waveform screen.

Box 12-26 Performing an Intrinsic PEEP Maneuver with the Evita

1. Push the MENU SELECT (F5) key.
2. From the screen menu select F4, MEAS. MANEUVER.
3. With F1, select intrinsic PEEP.
4. Use F5 to select the waveform display (pressure-time curve).
5. The measurement is automatically performed when the F1 key is pressed; the measured values are displayed on the screen.
6. After the measurement, return to the pressure-time curve display (F5). (This screen automatically returns in 2 minutes.)

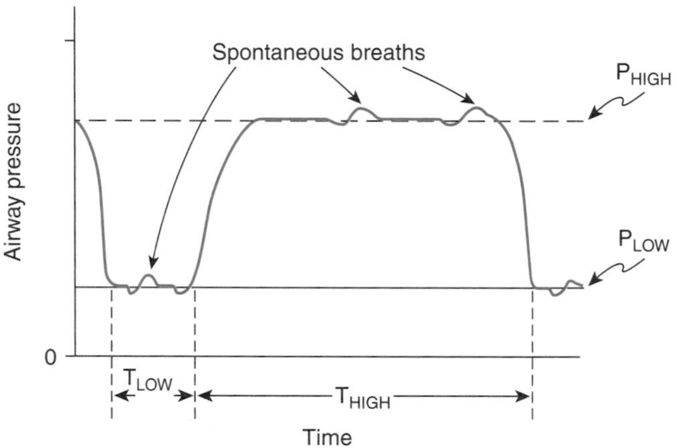

Figure 12-23 Pressure time curve for airway pressure-release ventilation; see text for further explanation.

Airway Pressure-Release Ventilation (APRV)

APRV is a mode of ventilation that can be selected from the extensions menu (F5). It provides two levels of CPAP (P_{high} and P_{low}) (Figure 12-23) and is intended for spontaneously breathing patients. Patients are able to breathe spontaneously at any time. P_{high} and P_{low} range from 0 to 35 cm H_2O. Changing from P_{high} to P_{low} or from P_{low} to P_{high} is synchronized with the set timed intervals. Chapter 11 provides additional information about this mode.

To set APRV, the operator selects the APRV mode from the ventilator modes menu. The upper and lower pressure levels are set using the F1 and F2 function keys and are confirmed with the F3 key. The unit times the length of both pressure levels. "T_{high}" is the length of time that high pressure is provided, and "T_{low}" is the length of time that low pressure is provided. APRV time levels range from 0.5 to 60 seconds. The duration of each is selected by first choosing F3 in the APRV menu. Then the settings are adjusted and confirmed using the F1, F2, and F3 keys. The menu prompts the operator through the steps. Function (F5) returns to the last menu.

To activate APRV, F1 is pressed and the MENU ACTIVE key is pressed until its green LED stays lit. (*Note*: To switch to another mode of ventilation, that specific mode key should be pressed and held until its LED remains lit. The menu from the mode that was previously active stays on the screen until it is changed with the function keys.)

Special Functions

Additional features on the Dräger Evita are the measurement of intrinsic PEEP and occlusion pressure.

Intrinsic Positive End-Expiratory Pressure (PEEPi)

An estimate of the amount of auto-PEEP present in the patient can be determined in addition to an estimate of the trapped volume (Vtrap) by using the intrinsic PEEP (PEEPi) function. These measurements can be performed only in the CMV mode and as long as no patient activity occurs during the measurement.

Box 12-26 describes the steps of performing this measurement. During the maneuver, the inspiratory and expiratory valves close, allowing for equilibration of pressure in the patient circuit during the expiratory phase. On the screen, values for PEEPINT and trapped volume (Vtrap) are shown. The auto-PEEP level can be viewed at any time on the pressure-time curve display.

Occlusion Pressure (P0.1)

Measurement of occlusion pressure (P0.1) is available as a special function in the Evita, but can only be performed during spontaneous breathing. Occlusion pressure is used to evaluate a patient's neuromuscular drive. At the beginning of inspiration, the ventilator occludes the inspiratory and expiratory valves 0.1 second after the beginning of

Box 12-27 Measurement of Occlusion Pressure in the Evita

1. Push the MENU SELECT (F5) key.
2. From the screen menu, select F4: MEAS. MANEUVER.
3. With F2, select OCCLUSION PRESSURE.
4. Use F5 to select the waveform display (pressure/time curve).
5. The measurement is automatically performed when the F1 key is pressed.
6. After the measurement is performed, return to the pressure-time curve display (F5). (This screen automatically returns in 2 minutes.)

Occlusion pressure can be set up in any mode, but can only be measured during the spontaneous mode.

inspiratory flow. The pressure measured at that time is displayed. The normal values range from –3 to –4 cm H_2O. Values below –6 cm H_2O may indicate impending exhaustion and respiratory muscle fatigue.

This procedure can be automatically performed using the steps outlined in Box 12-27. The value for occlusion pressure is shown on the screen; this measurement can only be carried out in the spontaneous breathing mode. Preparation for measurement, however, can be accomplished in any mode.

Ventilator Graphic Waveforms

The graphics monitor of the Dräger Evita is part of the main computer screen during standard operation. It can provide pressure-time or flow-time waveforms.

Troubleshooting

The alarms and monitored information provided by the Evita are a great help in solving most problems that might occur. In addition, the operator's manual contains a large troubleshooting section that lists ventilation and equipment alarm messages, common causes, and appropriate remedies. It is beyond the scope of this text to include this information. Users are advised to review the manual.

Dräger E-4 (Evita-4)

The Dräger E-4[1] and the Evita 2 Dura were developed after the original Evita ventilator. The Dräger E-4 ventilator was originally manufactured by Drägerwerk in Lubeck, Germany. Production of the E-4 and the E-2 Dura is now at Dräger, Inc., in Telford, PA. The E-4 and the E-2 Dura have many functional similarities. The E-4 is presented first (Figure 12-24). The manufacturer refers to the E-4 as the Dräger E-4 Pulmonary Work Station because it can monitor a variety of patient information.

The unit has a front panel that contains touch pads, a rotary (dial) knob, and a computer screen. The infrared touch screen uses light beam interruption technology. There are images or icons on the screen. Some of these are shaped like knobs (soft knobs, or **cyber knobs**), and some are shaped like touch pads (soft pads, or **cyber pads**). All of these dials and knobs are used to control the unit and are discussed later in this section.

Below the front operating panel are the connections for the main inspiratory and expiratory lines, the expiratory valve, and the nipple connector for the nebulizer line. The expiratory flow sensor is to the left of the expiratory valve. On the far right side below the unit's main control knob (rotary knob) is a protective cover that hides the oxygen sensor and the ambient air filter.

Power Source

The E-4 normally uses two 50 psig gas sources (air and oxygen, ranging from about 40 to 87 psig). The unit will operate on a single gas source if the second fails, but it will

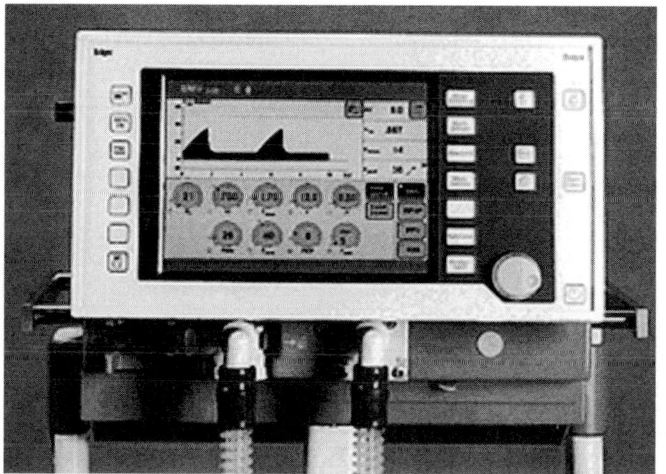

A

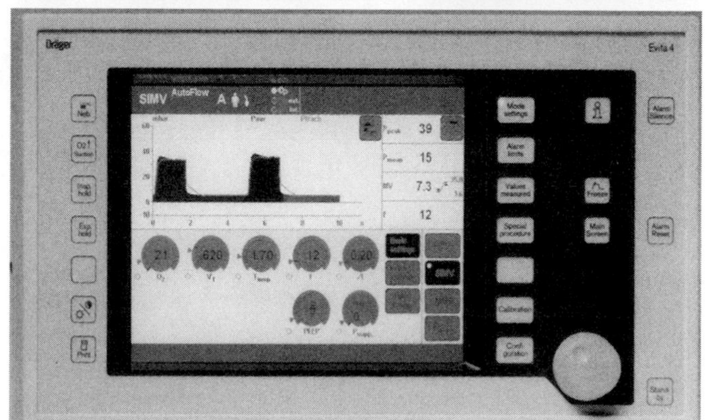

B

Figure 12-24 A, the Dräger E-4 ventilator; **B,** full screen with controls. (Courtesy of Dräger Corp, Telford, Penn.)

issue an alert when the other gas source runs low, altering oxygen-delivery capabilities. A standard AC 120-volt outlet is used to power the microprocessor and the electrical components. The on/off switch is located on the back panel of the unit.

Internal Mechanism

The internal mechanism is similar to those of many of the recently released ICU ventilators. The gas sources enter the unit through connections on the back panel. They are filtered, and their pressure is measured and reduced to a working pressure. The incoming flow is then directed to two flow-control valves. (*Note*: In the Dräger Dura and the E-4, these flow-control valves are high-pressure electromagnetic servo valves.) The function of these valves is controlled by the microprocessor, which uses information from the settings on the front panel, internal flow, pressure transducers, and the action of the valve itself to control the flow to the patient. These valves regulate the amount of pressure and flow and the flow waveform of the gas delivered depending on the selected modes and settings. The valves also control the F_IO_2 based on the set value, and the changes are instantaneous. From the flow-control valve, gas is directed to the patient.

A variety of pressure and flow transducers monitor internal gas flow, the output from the unit, and the gas return from the patient through the expiratory valve.

Controls and Alarms

A number of controls, monitors, and alarm settings are available on the Dräger E-4. Basically, the E-4 uses a single rotary knob, several hard touch pads on the side the computer screen, and the touch-sensitive soft knobs (cyber knobs) and soft pads (cyber pads) on the computer screen (Figure 12-25).

Peripheral Controls

Several controls used during normal operation of the ventilator are located on both sides of the screen. Those on the left side of the screen include the following: nebulizer, suction 100% O_2, inspiratory hold, print, and several blank keys for future upgrades. These controls are reviewed in the discussion of special functions later in this section.

On the immediate right side of the computer screen are touch pads that are used to select several operations. These pads include the following:

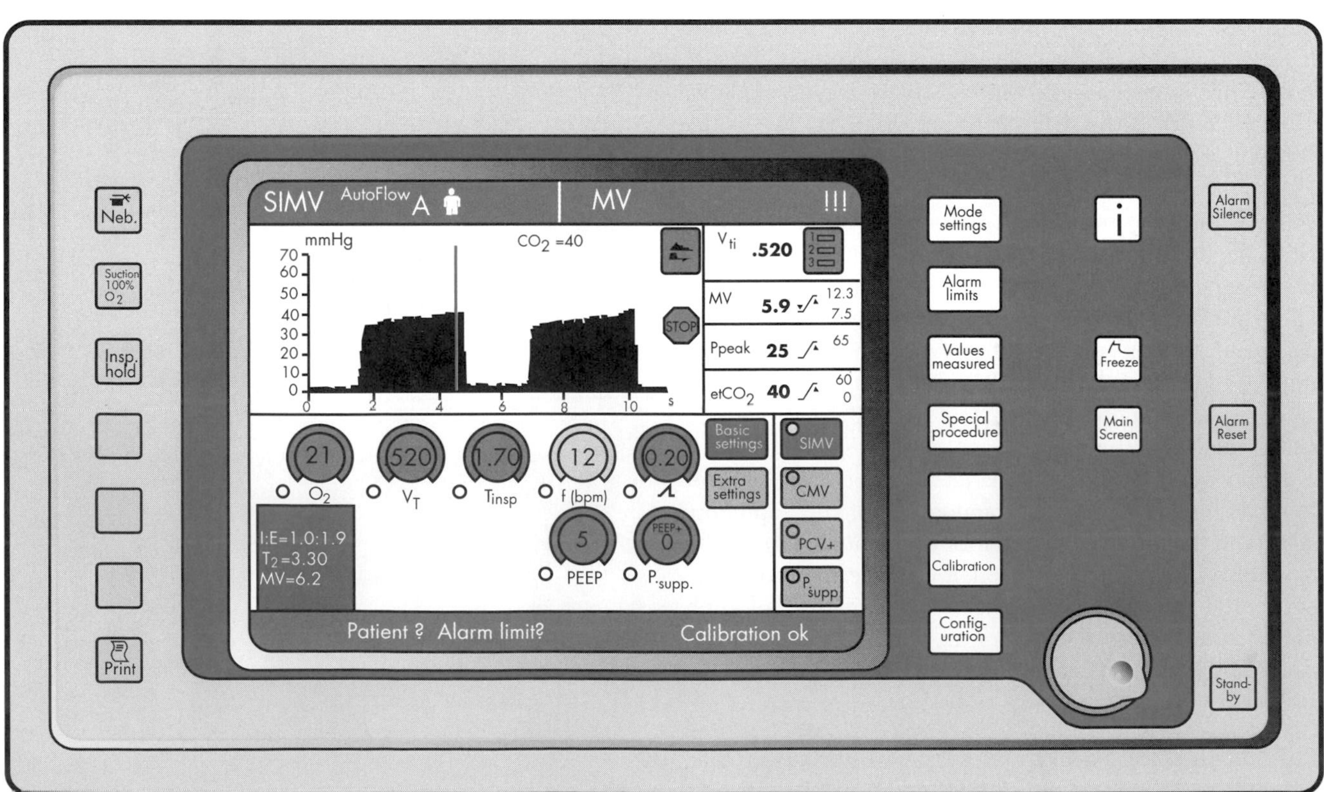

Figure 12-25 The front panel of the Dräger E-4 ventilator showing the touch pad controls, the rotary knob, and the screen in a standard ventilating mode.

1. MODE SETTINGS
2. ALARM LIMITS
3. VALUES MEASURED
4. SPECIAL PROCEDURE
5. A blank key (for future upgrades)
6. CALIBRATION
7. CONFIGURATION

The function of each will be covered as the various controls and alarms are described.

Three more touch pads and the rotary knob are to the right of these touch pads. These touch pads include an information key (i), a freeze control to freeze graphic waveforms, and a main screen pad for selecting standard menus to appear on the computer screen.

The knob can be rotated and pressed to select numerical values for parameters and activate the new parameters, respectively. It can also be used to move the cursor (vertical line) on the screen when it appears under certain functions.

On the far right side of the front panel are the following additional touch pads:

1. ALARM SILENCE (2 minutes)
2. ALARM RESET
3. STAND-BY (for switching between the stand-by and the operating modes)

Overview of Stand-by Controls

After the power switch is turned on, the unit runs a series of self-tests and a signal can be heard. After the tests are complete, the screen asks you to select adult, pediatric, or neonate (E-4 upgraded version 2.n software) by touching the desired soft pad (cyber pad) and entering the ideal body weight (IBW) of the patient (Figure 12-26). The available volumes and flows are different for each type of patient (Table 12-4). To set the IBW, touch the screen soft knob for IBW, which highlights the knob and changes its color to yellow. Rotate the dial knob to set the actual numerical value, which appears inside the screen soft knob. When the desired IBW appears, push the knob to set the selected value, which changes the soft knob from yellow to green to show that it has been set. These same actions (touching [soft knob or cyber pad], turning [rotary knob], and pushing [rotary knob]) are how most controls are set. The manufacturer refers to this sequence as "touch, adjust, confirm."

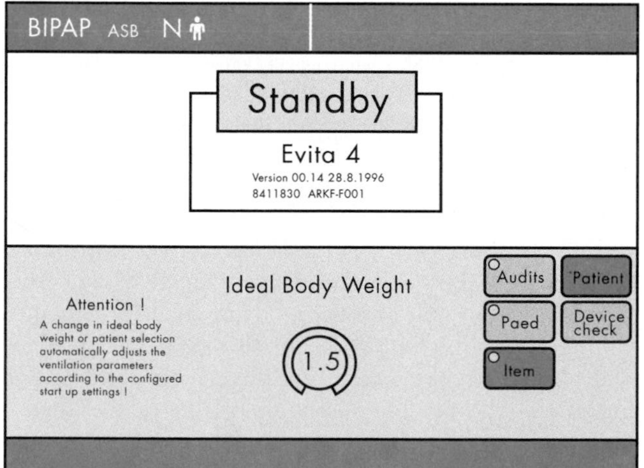

Figure 12-26 The screen during ventilator start-up on the Dräger E-4 version 2.n with Neoflow. (Redrawn from Dräger Corp, Telford, Penn.)

The unit requests the patient's IBW because the microprocessor is programmed at the factory to automatically begin ventilation using CMV with factory-set parameters. The factory default V_T is 7 mL/kg, based on the IBW of the patient. The respiratory rate is based on Radford's nomogram for the $\dot{V}_E$ of a person that size.[2] The mode and parameters may be reconfigured, but the operator can also do a standard ventilator set-up and select the mode and other appropriate parameters.

To have the unit automatically start ventilating a patient with programmed (configured) parameters, simply push the rotary knob. To set the unit up more specifically, touch the

Table 12-4 Ranges for parameters on the Dräger E-4

TIDAL VOLUME	
Adult	0.1 to 2 L
Pediatric	20 to 300 mL
Neonate	3 to 100 mL
FLOW	
Adult	6 to 120 L/min (to 180 L/min with Autoflow)
Pediatric	6 to 30 L/min (to 60 L/min with Autoflow)
Neonate	0.25 to 30 L/min
Neonate continuous flow	6 L/min
VARIABLE RANGES FOR ALL PATIENTS	
Respiratory rate	0 to 100 breaths/min 0 to 150 breaths/min with Neoflow
Inspiratory time	0.1 to 10 sec
Inspiratory pressure (set)	0 to 80 cm H_2O
Maximum pressure limit	0 to 100 cm H_2O
Percent oxygen	21% to 100%
PEEP	0 to 35 cm H_2O
Trigger sensitivity	1 to 15 L/min
Recommended	
Trigger sensitivity for neonates	0.3 to 5 L/min
Pressure support	0 to 80 cm H_2O
Rise time for PS	0 to 2 seconds

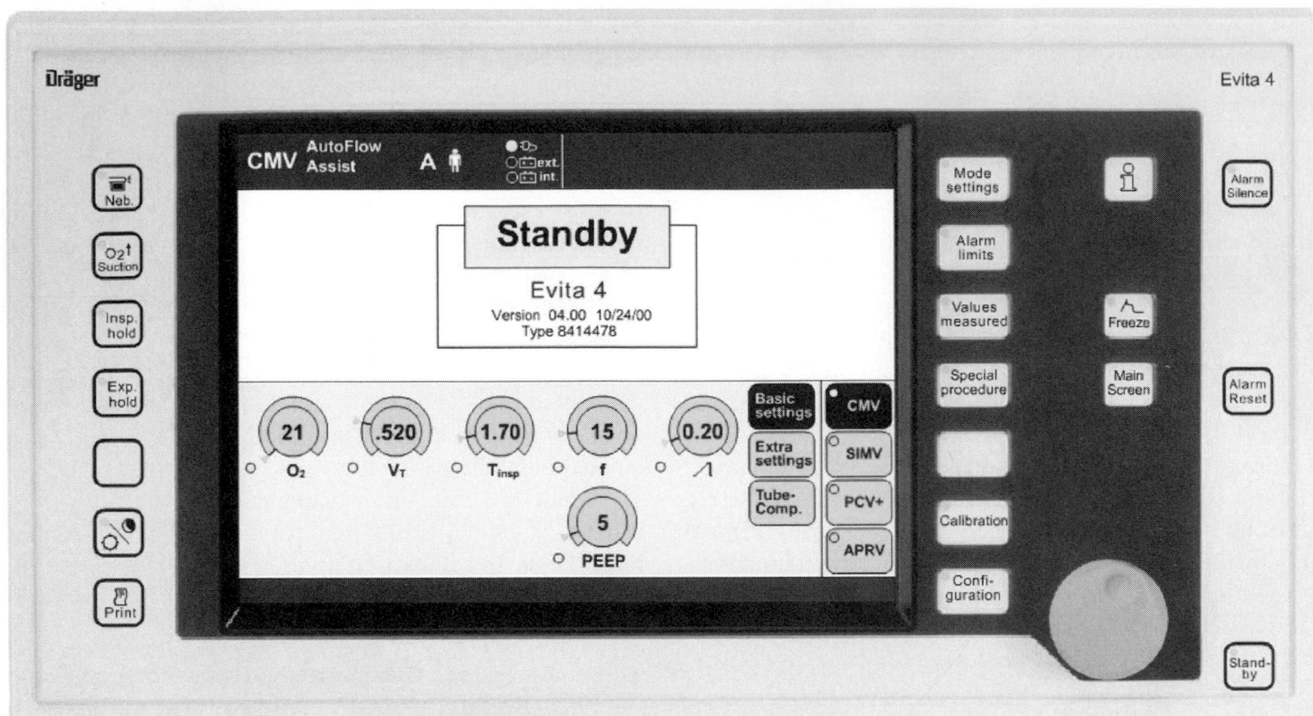

Figure 12-27 The Standby screen showing controls for setting up CMV ventilation. (Courtesy Dräger Corp, Telford, Penn.)

Box 12-28 Configuring the Ventilator, or Setting Parameters and Functions into Memory on the Evita-4

As with many computer programs, the Dräger E-4 microprocessor permits the operator to set a certain mode and its parameters. The operating manual provides a detailed description of each adjustment that can be made during configuration of the unit. A few examples are provided here.

To access the configuration function, press the configuration touch pad. The computer screen lists a menu of parameters or variables that you can select, including values, curves, trends, sound, screen, ventilation, and system defaults. To adjust any available screen, touch the desired soft pad. For example, if you wish to change the values measured screen, touch the values soft pad to bring up a menu of current available values (e.g., MV, Pplat, C, R, and f).

To replace one value with another, touch the appropriate soft pad to highlight the value to be deleted. A column of all the available measured and calculated variables appears to the left. Using the dial knob, select (highlight) the variable you want to be displayed. When it is highlighted, push the dial knob to replace the variable being deleted.

A similar procedure is available to change graphic waveforms, data trends, ventilation parameters, and system defaults. System defaults allow the unit to access specific external computer ports, such as the port that connects to a printer. System defaults also let you select computer variables, such as baud rate and parity check bits. System defaults provide a way to change the date, time, and language on the screen or the desired units of measurement (e.g., mbar [millibars] vs. cm H_2O).

If you want to change the ventilation mode and the parameters that automatically appear when the unit is turned on, you must enter an access code. This code is usually known by the individuals in the department who have the authority to change this set function (e.g., the clinical specialist or the department head).

Standby soft key and hold it down for about 3 seconds until the unit displays "Standby Activated." (Figure 12-27). The gas is shut off, but all adjustments can be made. Press the mode settings soft pad and make the desired settings. Touch the stand-by soft pad again, and the unit begins ventilation. *Note:* The programmed values can be changed by "configuring" the unit so that some other mode and parameters are available as soon as the unit is turned on (See the discussion of configuration in this section and Box 12-28.)

Because of the design of the E-4 unit, the control knobs that appear on the screen vary for each mode of ventilation selected. For example, if you wish to use the SIMV mode in volume ventilation, only the controls that are active in that mode appear on the screen. For this reason, it is easier to discuss the various controls as their uses or the specific modes are discussed. The available ranges for control variables are listed in Table 12-5. If you go beyond the range of normal ventilation for a parameter, the knob stops adjusting as you turn it. A message appears at the bottom of

Table 12-5 Commonly measured and displayed parameters on the Dräger E-4

Parameter	Definition	Range
Ppeak	Peak pressure	0 to 99 cm H_2O
Pplat	Plateau pressure	0 to 99 cm H_2O
Pmean	Mean pressure	0 to 99 cm H_2O
PEEP	Positive end expir. press	0 to 99 cm H_2O
Pmin	Minimum pressure	0 to 99 cm H_2O
MV	Minute ventilation	0 to 99 L/min
MVspn	Spontaneous MV	0 to 99 L/min
f	Total frequency	0 to 150 breaths/min
fspn	Spontaneous frequency	0 to 150 breaths/min
fmand	Mandatory frequency	0 to 150 breaths/min
VTE	Exhaled tidal volume	0 to 3999 ml
VTi	Inhaled tidal volume	0 to 3999 mL
F_IO_2	Fractional inspired O_2	15% to 100%
T	Temperature	18 to 51° C
R	Resistance	cm H_2O/L/sec
C	Compliance	mL/cm H_2O

the screen telling you what needs to be done to continue. For example, if you select a respiratory rate of 4 breaths/min in SIMV, and T_I (inspiratory time) is set at 1 second, the knob will freeze and the message at the bottom will read "I:E < 1:3 confirm," followed by an icon for the rotary knob. When you press the knob, the SIMV rate will go down to 4 breaths/min with a T_I of 1 second.

Monitors and Alarms

In every mode of ventilation, the E-4 provides monitored parameters at the top of the screen. There may be a graphic on the left side. On the top right are current values, such as O_2%, Ppeak, Pplat, and MV (minute ventilation). Although these are the variables most commonly selected, they can be changed by the institution according to the standards of the clinical site. Box 12-29 describes the selection of ventilator parameters for display.

Measured Values

The VALUES MEASURED touch pad brings up a screen that displays values being measured or calculated by the unit (see Table 12-5 and Figure 12-28), such as F_IO_2. The ventilator has a built-in oxygen analyzer and does an automatic oxygen calibration every 24 hours. The unit can optimally include a mainstream carbon dioxide analyzer that provides information on end-tidal carbon dioxide ($etCO_2$), CO_2/time, and single-breath CO_2 (CO_2/volume).

Box 12-29 Selecting Displayed Parameters

The E-4 allows graphed and digitally displayed information to be viewed. Available graphs include pressure, flow, volume, or end-tidal CO_2 graphed per unit of time. Any two graphs may be selected by touching the green soft (cyber) pad at the top right of the curve, and then touching the particular curve.

On the top right, digital measurements are displayed in three groups of four. Scroll through these measurements by touching the green soft pad at the top right of the measurements. O_2, V_T exhaled, MV, and f (frequency) are the most common. Pressures (Ppeak, Pplat, PEEP, and mean airway pressure) are the most common for Screen 2. End-tidal data are often placed on Screen 3.

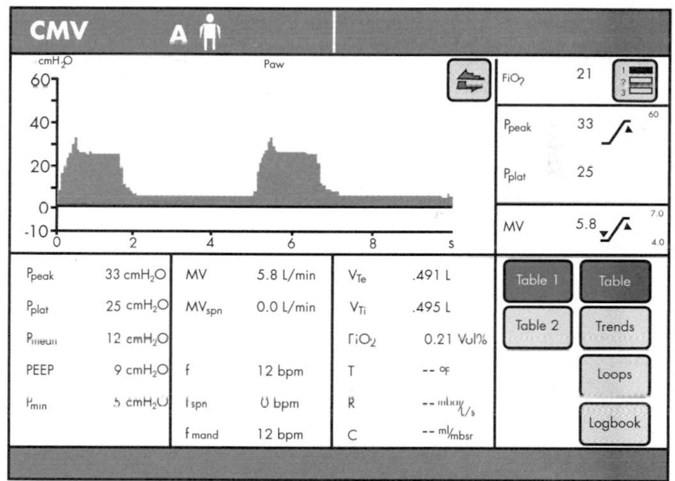

Figure 12-28 Example of a VALUES MEASURED screen on the Dräger E-4 ventilator. (Redrawn from Dräger Corp, Telford, Penn.)

Calculated values include carbon dioxide production ($\dot{V}CO_2$), deadspace (V_D), and V_D/V_T measurements. The analyzer is normally taken out of the circuit and calibrated before use. There is a special block built into the ventilator that allows zero and reference calibration of the carbon dioxide analyzer (see the operator's manual for instructions).[1]

Alarms

Alarms can be set by pressing the ALARM LIMITS soft pad, which provides a screen display allowing adjustment of the available alarm values (Figure 12-29). For example, to set the HIGH RATE alarm, touch the soft pad (cyber pad) adjacent to the respiratory rate (f_{spn}). The soft pad changes from green to yellow. Using the rotary knob, set the desired high rate; the number appears inside the soft pad. Press the dial knob to activate the new setting; the soft pad changes back to green. Table 12-6 lists the ranges for the adjustable alarms. The limits for O_2% are automatically set by the ventilator (see Table 12-6). The automatic alarm limit for low airway pressure is the set PEEP value plus 5 cm H_2O. For example, if PEEP is 5 cm H_2O, the low pressure limit is 10 cm H_2O and is not adjustable. When the upper Paw alarm limit is reached, an audio/visual alarm is activated and inspiratory flow delivery stops and the expiratory valve opens, dropping pressure to baseline. This alarm is functional in all modes of ventilation and is similar to the upper pressure limit on most ventilators. However, the Ppeak alarm is not to be confused with the Pmax pressure limit. The Pmax limit is not an alarm, but actually changes the way a breath is delivered during CMV, SIMV, and MMV ventilation. For this reason, Pmax is reviewed under the discussion of modes of ventilation.

There are basically three levels of alarm indicators on the E-4, as follows:

1. WARNING (top priority)
2. CAUTION (medium priority)
3. ADVISORY (low priority)

The function of each of these is listed in Table 12-7. After an alarm has been activated, the audible tone can be silenced with the ALARM SILENCE touch pad. The LED appears on the ALARM SILENCE pad when the audible alarms are inactive and is functional for 2 minutes. Once the problem is corrected, the alarm is reset by touching the ALARM SILENCE soft pad (LED off). Medium- and low-priority messages do not need to be acknowledged after the problem is solved, but high-priority messages must be acknowledged by the operator to verify that the problem has been resolved by pressing the ALARM RESET touch pad. The message leaves the screen and is stored in memory. (*Note*: Access to the LOGBOOK function is available on the ALARM LIMITS and the MEASURED VALUES screens to recall any stored, top-priority alarm messages.)

Examples of low-priority alarms include AIR SUPPLY LOW, FLOW MONITORING OFF, and INSPIRATORY HOLD INTERRUPTED. Examples of medium-priority alarms are AIR SUPPLY

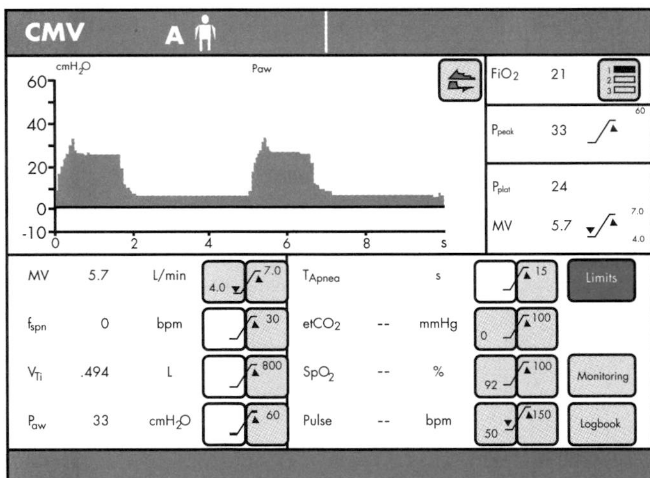

Figure 12-29 The ALARM PARAMETER screen on the Dräger E-4. (Redrawn from Dräger Corp, Telford, Penn.)

Table 12-6 Alarm ranges for the Dräger E-4

Parameter	Range
Minute ventilation	High MV 0.5-41 L/min
	Low MV 0-40 L/min
High fspn*	0 to 120 breaths/min
High VTi*	30 to 4000 mL
High Paw	10 to 100 cm H_2O
Apnea time	15 to 60 seconds
High end-tidal CO_2 ($etCO_2$)†	0 to 100 mm Hg
Low $etCO_2$†	0 to 99 mm Hg
NONADJUSTABLE O_2% ALARM	
O_2% <60%	Upper O_2% alarm is +4%
	Lower O_2% alarm is -4%
O_2% >60%	Upper O_2% alarm is +6%
	Lower O_2% alarm is -6%

*No lower alarm limit available.
†Only available when CO_2 analyzer (capnograph) is added.

Table 12-7 Displayed information with priority alarms on the Dräger E-4

Alarm light	Message* (on screen)	Message (background color)	Audio	Alarm level
Red flashing	Name of alarm followed by "!!!" (e.g., "APNEA!!!")	Red	Five tones; repeated twice every 15 seconds	Warning; top priority
Yellow flashing	Name of alarm followed by "!!" (e.g., "O_2 PRESSURE HIGH!!")	Yellow	Three tones; repeated every 30 seconds	Caution; medium priority
Yellow constant	Name of alarm followed by "!" (e.g., "FAN MALFUNCTION!")	Yellow	Two tones; occurs only once	Advisory; low priority

*Appears in the upper right corner of the screen.

Box 12-30 Modes of Ventilation on the E-4

CMV (continuous mandatory ventilation, an A/C mode)
SIMV (volume- or pressure-targeted)
SIMV+PSV
PCV+
PCV+PS
PSV
APRV
MMV
MMV/PSV
Apnea ventilation
Autoflow
PPS* (proportional pressure support)
Neoflow*

*Available on the upgraded version of the Dräger E-4.

PRESSURE TOO HIGH, CHECK SETTINGS, and PRESSURE LIMITED. Examples of top-priority alarms are numerous. A few examples are APNEA, DEVICE FAILURE, and LOW O_2 SUPPLY. The operator's manual provides a list of all alarms.[1] After any top-priority alarm, the operator must be absolutely certain that the patient is being ventilated. (*Note*: When a MIXER INOP. alarm occurs, the blender is defective and the manufacturer advises that the patient be manually ventilated and the unit removed from service until repaired by a service representative.)

Modes of Ventilation

Modes of operation available on the E-4 are listed in Box 12-30.

Standard Settings of Ventilator Modes

When the ventilator is first turned on, the standard mode that is programmed (configured) is CMV (i.e., an A/C mode using volume ventilation). The institution purchasing the unit can change this by reconfiguring the unit. To change the start-up mode, press CONFIGURE, then press the VENTILATION soft pad; enter the access code; touch MODES, select the desired start-up mode with the dial knob; and activate it by pressing the dial knob. The operator's manual provides a full description of configuring the start-up modes and alarm settings.

If the operator wants to change the mode of ventilation, pressing the VENTILATION soft pad provides a screen that lists the available modes. When the new mode soft pad is pressed, the parameters that can be set in that mode appear on the screen, and the MODE soft pad turns yellow. Parameters are set in a manner similar to the way in which

CLINICAL ROUNDS 12-8

You are setting up a patient on CMV with the Dräger E-4. The settings are as follows: V_T = 0.5 L (500 mL); f = 10 breaths/min; flow = 60 L/min; T_I = 2 sec; and the waveform is constant. Answer the following questions

1. What is the I:E ratio?
2. How long does it take the ventilator to deliver the volume?
3. If delivery time is shorter than the selected T_I, when does inspiration end?

See Appendix A for the answer.

alarm parameters are set. Touch the parameter soft knob that you want to change, for example V_T. The soft knob changes from green to yellow. Turn the rotary knob to obtain the desired numerical value, which appears in the center of the soft knob. Then press the rotary knob to activate this setting. The old mode continues to operate until the new setting has been selected. When it is selected, the new mode soft pad changes to black. Inactive modes appear green.

The Dräger E-4 provides flow-triggering in all modes of ventilation. The flow-trigger level is set by performing the following:

- Touching the EXTRA SETTINGS soft pad
- Touching the FLOW-TRIGGER soft pad
- Touching the FLOW soft knob
- Dialing in the desired flow-triggering value using the rotary knob
- Pressing the rotary knob activate the newly set flow trigger value

Trigger sensitivity can only be turned off in CMV. However, there are only rare situations in which sensitivity should be turned off. PEEP/CPAP and O_2% can be selected in any mode. (*Note*: If the power fails or STANDBY is selected, the settings that were in effect before the interruption are again in effect when the unit is reactivated.)

Continuous Mandatory Ventilation (CMV)

The CMV mode is an A/C volume ventilation mode. The operator sets V_T, flow, f, T_I, and desired alarm settings. Breaths are patient- or time-triggered, volume-targeted, and time-cycled. All breaths deliver the set V_T. Flow to the patient is restricted to the flow setting value. If the flow is high and the V_T is delivered before T_I is achieved, the inspiratory valve closes (the expiratory valve is already closed), and the breath is held. This can be identified by an inspiratory pause pressure in the pressure/time graph and flow returning to zero on the flow/time graph (See Clinical Rounds 12-8 and Figure 12-28). An inspiratory pause

Box 12-31 Pmax: Pressure-Limit Function

Pmax was the concept behind the first Evita ventilator. The manufacturer now believes that the Autoflow function is superior to Pmax and should be the option of choice for pressure reduction. In Pmax, the operator may manually adjust it to within 3 cm H_2O of the plateau. In Autoflow, the E-4 automatically brings Ppeak equal to or close to the Pplat, as timing allows. In Autoflow, the exhalation valve floats, but in Pmax it is closed. The manufacturer recommends that the Pmax be kept off in machine configuration.[3]

may also be identified by touching the I TIME or FLOW soft pad. When the pad is yellow, a blue **"smart window"** appears at the bottom left of the screen and displays the I:E ratio, T_E, and pause time. As the variable selected is changed, the new calculated values are displayed. For example, if the flow is decreased and T_I shortened, the pause time decreases.

The high peak pressures that occur with volume ventilation can be avoided by using the Pmax pressure limit function. When Pmax is used, the pressure and flow delivery characteristics of the unit change (see the following discussion and Figure 12-20 and Box 12-31).

Pmax Pressure Limit Function

Pmax operates in CMV, SIMV, and MMV modes. To configure Pmax, access CONFIGURE, then ventilation; enter the access code; touch MODES, and then PMAX. When Pmax is operational, the unit will guarantee the set V_T but limit the pressure delivered during the breath. The pressure in the circuit rapidly reaches the maximum pressure setting (PMAX), inspiration continues for the set inspiratory time (time-cycled), but the amount of pressure in the circuit does not go above this setting. Flow rises rapidly at the start of inspiration, and plateaus at the set value. It remains at the set value until the set Pmax is reached, at which point flow descends, maintaining the Pmax pressure throughout T_I (see Figure 12-20). The V_T will remain constant at the set value as long as flow drops to zero before the end of inspiration (i.e., a inspiratory hold). If flow does not drop to zero for the pressure being provided by the unit, the volume cannot be delivered and a VOLUME NOT CONSTANT alarm is activated.

It is recommended that the AutoFlow be used with this and any other volume mode so that patient flow is not restricted. When AutoFlow is used, it takes over the task of setting both INSP. FLOW and PMAX, and these screen soft knob controls are no longer displayed (See the discussion of AutoFlow later in this section).

SIMV and SIMV with Pressure Support Ventilation (SIMV + PSV)

As described in Chapter 11, SIMV provides a maximum number of mandatory breaths and allows the patient to breathe spontaneously between them. Spontaneous breaths can be provided using pressure support. Mandatory breaths can be patient- or time-triggered, volume-targeted, and time-cycled. Pressure-support breaths are described in the discussion on pressure support in this section. In the SIMV mode, either Pmax or AutoFlow can also be used. The flow-trigger ensures synchronous triggering of a mandatory breath with patient effort.

The function of SIMV on the E-4 is similar to its function on the Dräger Evita (see the discussion of the SIMV mode in the modes of ventilation section in the part of this chapter on the Evita). (*Note:* Software upgrades are now available that allow SIMV mandatory breaths to be pressure-targeted [PCV + SIMV].)

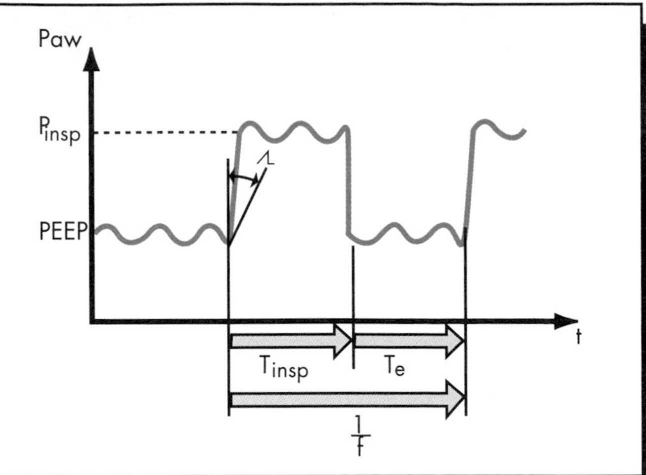

Figure 12-30 The pressure-time curve for a spontaneously breathing patient on PCV+. (Pinsp = inspiratory pressure setting; Tinsp = inspiratory time setting, and Te = expiratory time based on the total cycle time [TCT = 1 min/f, or 60 sec/f].) The angle drawn at the beginning of the first mandatory breath shows the potential for adjusting the slope using the RISE TIME control. See text for further explanation. (Redrawn from Dräger Corp, Telford, Penn.)

Pressure Control Ventilation Plus (PCV+)

In PCV+ the patient can breathe spontaneously between mandatory breaths, which means that the unit basically operates as SIMV. The patient can also breathe spontaneously during inspiratory flow delivery (Figure 12-30). Mandatory breaths are patient- or time-triggered, pressure-targeted, and time-cycled.

The operator sets a minimum respiratory rate and a flow-trigger. Time-triggering is determined by the set rate, and patient-triggering by the set flow-trigger. Pressure during a mandatory breath is equal to the PINSP pressure setting.

During PCV+ the unit functions as follows. When it is time for a mandatory breath and the patient makes an inspiratory effort, a mandatory breath is delivered. During this time, the set pressure is held relatively constant, but the patient can still breathe spontaneously by receiving flow on demand (see Figure 12-30). Spontaneous breaths that occur between mandatory breaths can be assisted with pressure support by setting the desired pressure-support level (PCV + PS). An elevated baseline (PEEP/CPAP) can also be set.

The RISE TIME control is used in this mode to slow flow and pressure delivery by using the soft knob with the symbol for an ascending ramp below it on the computer screen. Pressure rise is adjustable from 0 to 2 seconds and represents the amount of time it takes the ventilator to achieve the set pressure from the beginning of inspiration. A rapid rise is appropriate for a patient with a high peak inspiratory flow. A slow rise is more appropriate for a small pediatric patient with less of a high flow demand. In Figure 12-30, the arrow shown at the beginning of the first mandatory breath shows the potential changes in pressure delivery that can occur with a change in rise time. The rise can be rapid (arrow pointing to left line from baseline pressure) or slow (arrow pointing to right line from baseline pressure). In most clinical settings, the default rise time of 0.2 seconds is adequate; it is seldom necessary to go above 0.4 seconds. If rise time is being used, it will affect both mandatory and PS breath delivery.

Because V_T and $\dot{V}_E$ may vary in this mode, the operator needs to set $\dot{V}_E$ alarm limits carefully. As with SIMV volume ventilation, apnea ventilation can be activated during this mode as well, but Pmax and AutoFlow are not active during this mode because breath delivery is already pressure-targeted, and the ventilator controls these functions.

Pressure Support Ventilation (PSV)

The E-4 can provide PSV during SIMV, PCV, MMV, and spontaneous (CPAP) ventilation. The target pressure is set using the PSUPP. soft knob, which indicates the pressure above PEEP that will be delivered during a PS breath. PS breaths are patient-triggered, pressure-targeted, and flow-cycled (25% of peak for adults; 6% of peak for pediatric and neonatal settings). Patient-triggering can be based on the flow-trigger or the volume trigger when inspired volume exceeds 25 mL (12 mL in pediatric mode and 1 mL/32 msec for the neonatal setting)—whichever occurs first. Whenever PSV is active, the pressure rise time control is also functional.

If the patient actively exhales or fights the ventilator during the start of a PS breath, inspiratory flow ends. This is detected by the flow going to zero or less than zero. Inspiratory flow will also time-cycle at 4 seconds (1.5 for pediatric patients, but adjustable with the T_I control in neonatal patients). Prolonged T_I most commonly occurs if a leak is present. If the time-cycling criteria occur for three consecutive breaths, an alarm is activated to warn of a possible leak in the system.

Continuous Positive Airway Pressure (CPAP)

Spontaneously breathing patients often benefit from breathing at elevated baseline pressures (CPAP), which increases functional residual capacity. CPAP is available on the E-4 and can be provided with or without PSV. Simply turn the PSV level to 0 cm H_2O using its soft knob, and set the PEEP soft knob to the desired CPAP level (cm H_2O) if you wish to use CPAP alone.

Airway Pressure-Release Ventilation (APRV)

APRV is a mode of ventilation in which two levels of CPAP are set. It operates very much like PCV+, except that the "expiratory" interval is very brief in comparison (see Figure 12-23). After selecting the APRV soft pad, the upper pressure level is set using P_{high}, and the lower level is set using P_{low}. The unit also times the length of both pressure levels. T_{high} is the length of time that high pressure is provided, and T_{low} is the length of time that low pressure is provided. Both are intended for use with spontaneously breathing patients (see Chapter 11). The RISE TIME control can be used to taper the pressure change from P_{low} to P_{high}, but the length of rise time cannot be longer than the set T_{high} time. Apnea back-up ventilation is recommended when using this mode.

Mandatory Minute Volume Ventilation (MMV) and MMV with Pressure Support (MMV/PSV)

Mandatory minute volume ventilation (MMV) is set by selecting that soft pad and then setting the MMV you want the patient to accomplish using the V_T, flow, f, and T_I settings. A pressure support level should be set to ensure that the patient has adequate spontaneous tidal volumes. As described in Chapter 11, with MMV the patient can breathe spontaneously and contribute all of the $\dot{V}_E$ with only PSV or CPAP with no mandatory breaths; or the patient might contribute only a portion of the $\dot{V}_E$. The difference between the spontaneous and the set $\dot{V}_E$ is provided by mandatory breaths at the set volume. Pmax or AutoFlow can be used in MMV. (*Note*: It is important to set the high rate alarm to protect the patient from rapid shallow breathing that would result in an equivalent V_E, but would also increase work of breathing and provide an inadequate alveolar ventilation.)

Apnea Ventilation

Apnea ventilation supplies volume ventilation with a set respiratory rate and V_T in case the patient becomes apneic in any of the following modes: SIMV, PCV, CPAP, and APRV. If the patient stops breathing for the length of time set on the APNEA ALARM control, the alarm is activated and apnea ventilation begins. To set apnea ventilation, touch the EXTRA settings soft pad, then the APNEA VENT. soft pad, and then the ON soft pad. Set the desired volume and rate using the V_{TAPNEA} and F_{APNEA} soft knobs on the APNEA VENTILATION screen. When these parameters are set, press the dial knob for activation. The baseline pressure, O_2%, trigger sensitivity, and other alarm parameters remain as they are in the current mode.

AutoFlow

AutoFlow is a dual mode of ventilation similar to pressure regulated volume control and volume support in the Servo 300 ventilator. Use of AutoFlow provides pressure-targeted breaths with volume guarantee whenever volume ventilation (CMV, SIMV, MMV) is simultaneously selected (see Chapter 11). AutoFlow also alters the function of the inspiratory and expiratory valves, allowing patients to receive whatever inspiratory flow they demand—up to 180 L/min in any volume mode regardless of the volume settings. In addition, it makes the expiratory valve more interactive with the patient. For example, if the patient coughs or breathes during the set inspiratory time of a mandatory breath, the expiratory valve system allows the patient to inhale and exhale freely while maintaining the inspiratory pressure. There is very little build-up of resistance and pressure in the circuit when active patient breathing occurs. In AutoFlow, the circuit pressure rarely builds to the upper Paw alarm limit.

When AutoFlow is in use, the unit calculates the system compliance (C) and resistance (R) and establishes the minimum pressure needed to deliver the set volume.

To access AutoFlow, do the following:

- Select extra settings on the screen
- Touch the AutoFlow on soft pad
- Press the rotary knob to confirm that AutoFlow should be activated

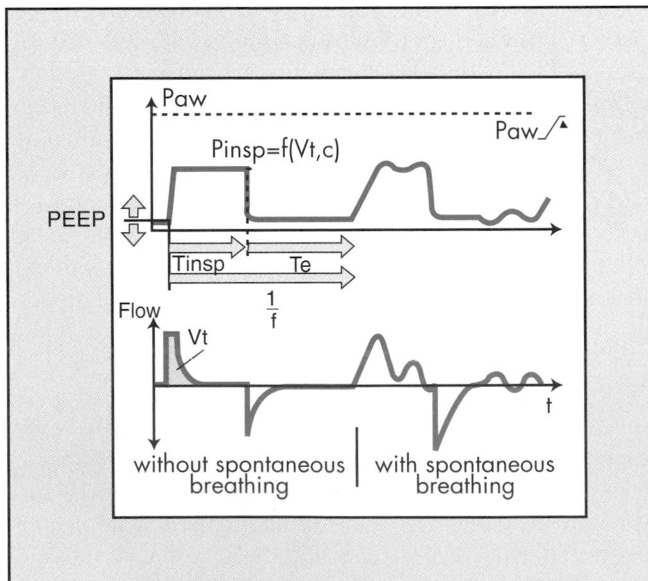

Figure 12-31 AutoFlow with a pressure-controlled, volume-guaranteed breath without spontaneous breathing (left). Flow drops to zero, and pressure delivery equilibrates with the pressure in the lungs. V_T has been delivered. During the second breath (right), the patient is spontaneously breathing during the plateau portion of the mandatory breath and afterward during the expiratory phase. (Redrawn from Dräger Corp, Telford, Penn.)

In AutoFlow the unit takes over the function of PMAX PRESSURE LIMIT and INSP. FLOW, and the soft knobs for those functions are deleted from the screen. When AutoFlow is started, the ventilator delivers a volume-targeted mandatory breath and measures the plateau pressure during that breath. The plateau pressure is used as the starting ventilating pressure for AutoFlow (Figure 12-31). The unit delivers plateau pressure, measures delivered volume, and calculates system C and R. If the delivered volume is lower than the set volume, it increases pressure delivery. If the delivered volume is too high compared to the set volume, it decreases pressure delivery. Pressure change between breaths is never greater than 3 cm H_2O. Volume delivery may also be higher than the set value if the patient is actively inspiring. If the operator wants to avoid exceeding a specific V_T, the V_{TI} UPPER LIMIT alarm can be used for this purpose. If the alarm is exceeded once, an advisory alert ("!") occurs and V_T delivery is limited. If the alarm is exceeded three times the following occurs:

1. A warning alarm is activated ("!!!," in red) with the message "exceeding Vti × 3."
2. V_T delivery is limited to the value of the V_{TI} UPPER LIMIT setting for all breaths.
3. The ventilator cycles into exhalation and drops airway pressure to the set baseline (set PEEP) if necessary for all breaths.

During spontaneous patient inspiratory efforts between mandatory breaths, the unit delivers whatever flow the patient demands. The patient can also breathe during the plateau phase of a mandatory breath (Figure 12-32). Inspiratory pressure is limited by the upper Paw limit setting minus 5 cm H_2O.

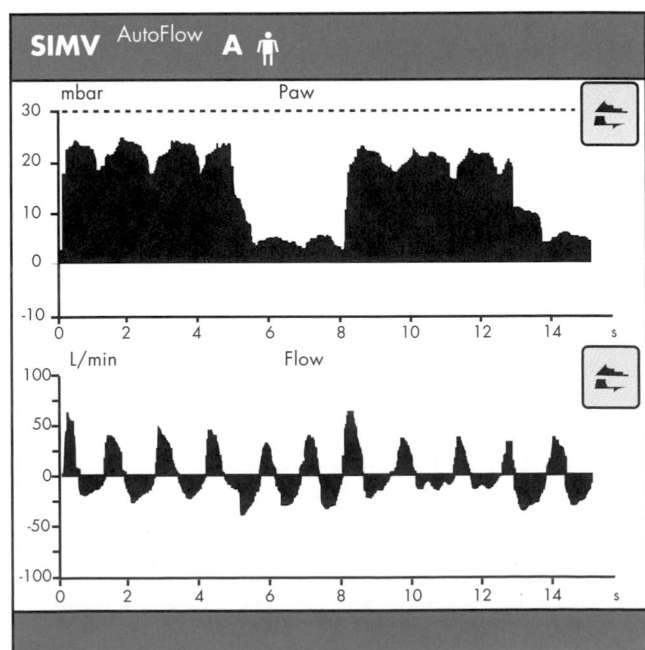

Figure 12-32 Volume-oriented SIMV with AutoFlow. Spontaneous breathing is possible in all phases. (Redrawn from Dräger Corp, Telford, Penn.)

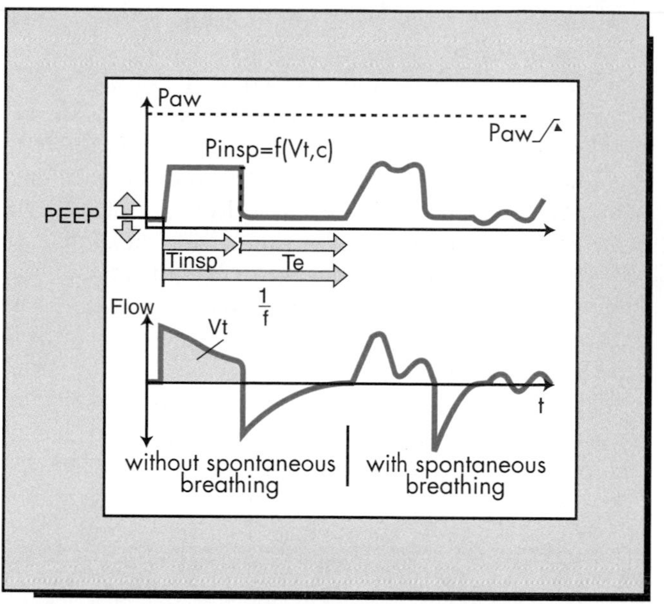

Figure 12-33 AutoFlow with a pressure-control breath in which flow does not drop to zero before inspiration ends. The set pressure does not equilibrate with the lungs. V_T delivery is lower because T_I was not long enough to deliver the pressure. Remember that this pressure is calculated to be what is required based on system C and R to deliver the set V_T. (Redrawn from Dräger Corp, Telford, Penn.)

When AutoFlow is used, there are several types of breath patterns that can occur, as follows:

1. If V_T is delivered and flow drops to zero before the unit time-cycles out of a mandatory inspiration, the ventilator ensures that the patient can breathe spontaneously during the remaining inspiratory time. During this time, however, the pressure being delivered by the unit is maintained.
2. If the patient breathes in and out during a mandatory breath, the plateau delivery stays constant and does not fluctuate significantly. Flow is provided as needed to meet patient demand. The expiratory valve opens during spontaneous exhalation to avoid pressure build-up and resistance to exhalation while still maintaining plateau pressure (Figure 12-33).
3. If inspiration ends before flow drops to zero, the volume will be delivered, but the pressure may be higher than the true plateau. The unit may have to step up pressure and flow to deliver V_T in a short T_I. The clinician may want to increase T_I to decrease pressure, but sometimes the pressure does not decrease (Clinical Rounds 12-9).[3]

It is strongly recommended that AutoFlow be activated whenever a spontaneously breathing patient is being ventilated—regardless of the volume mode chosen, CMV, SIMV, and MMV.

CLINICAL ROUNDS 12-9

A patient on AutoFlow has the following ventilator settings and monitored parameters: mode = SIMV; V_T (set) = 0.65 L (650 mL); f = 12 breaths/min; inspiratory pressure = 20 cm H_2O; T_I = 2 seconds; upper pressure limit = 30 cm H_2O.

The patient has done well on these settings for the past 4 hours. During the next hour, however, the respiratory therapist notices that inspiratory pause time (i.e., time when flow is zero) has become progressively shorter, and eventually there is no pause. Flow never goes to zero before the end of inspiration; inspiratory pressure is now 25 cm H_2O. What do you think the therapist should do in this situation?

See Appendix A for the answer.

Proportional Pressure Support (PPS)[4]

Proportional pressure support (PPS) is a proportional assist ventilation mode, described in Chapter 11, which is available on the upgrade of the Evita-4 ventilator (Software version 2.n). (*Note*: The company is currently awaiting Food and Drug Administration approval of PPS.) PPS provides a positive feedback system of respiration; that is, the more patients inspire, the more pressure they receive. The amount of pressure provided is based on the volume-assist and flow-assist set by the operator, which will be explained later in this section.

Key things to remember with PPS include the following:

1. There is no support if there is no inspiratory effort from the patient. Therefore the patient must have an adequate inspiratory effort and ventilatory drive.
2. It is important to set minimum $\dot{V}_E$ and apnea alarms, as well as apnea back-up ventilation in case the patient quits breathing. Upper Paw and upper V_T alarm limits are also set to protect against high pressures and volumes.
3. This is a positive-feedback system. The more actively patients inspire, the more assistance they receive from the unit, and vice-versa.
4. There must be no leaks in the system (cuff leaks, circuit connection leaks, or bronchopleural leaks).

When inspiration is strong during PPS, the unit supports the patient with a high pressure. With shallow, less forceful breaths, the unit provides a lower pressure. The amount of assistance provided during PPS is separated into the elastic (compliance) and the resistive components. Using VOL ASSIST, the operator decides how much work the unit will support for the elastic portion of the work of breathing. Using FLOW ASSIST, the operator determines how much work is provided by the unit to overcome resistive work.

To set PPS, the operator should perform the following procedure:

- Touch the PPS soft pad on the ventilator screen (standard screen for setting up ventilator modes)
- Touch the VOL ASSIST soft knob
- Set the desired value using the dial knob
- Press the dial knob for activation

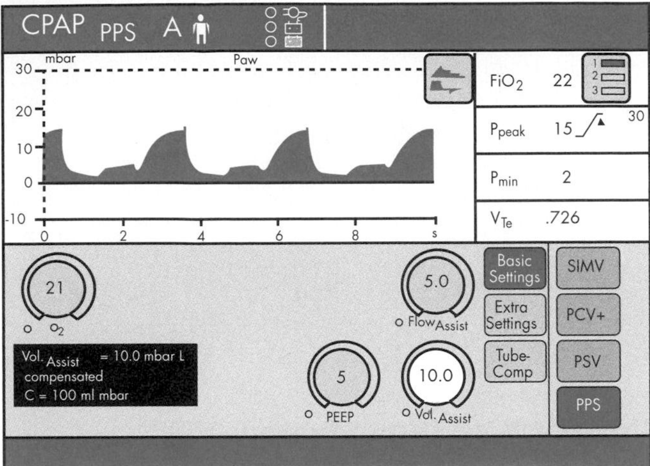

Figure 12-34 The screen during PPS on the Dräger Evita 4 (version 2.n). (Redrawn from Dräger Corp, Telford, Penn.)

- Touch the FLOW ASSIST soft knob and set the desired value using the dial knob (Figure 12-34)
- Press the dial knob for activation

The range of values for volume-assist and flow-assist are listed in Table 12-8. For example, if 10 cm H_2O/L is set, the unit compensates for the elastic work of breathing with a compliance of 100 mL/cm H_2O (Box 12-32). If 5 cm H_2O/L/sec is set for the flow assist, the unit will compensate for a resistance of 5 cm H_2O/L/sec (see Box 12-32). The ventilator calculates the amount of airway pressure it needs to provide for both the volume and flow assist portions of the breath.

PPS has the following limits: maximum Paw is equal to the upper Paw alarm limit minus 5 cm H_2O; maximum inspiratory V_T is equal to the upper alarm limit for V_{Ti};

Box 12-32 Calculating Compliance with PPS

The setting for volume assist is a pressure/volume measurement of elastance (cm H_2O/L). It is the inverse of compliance. In this example, if elastance = 10 cm H_2O/L; compliance = 1 L/10 cm H_2O, or 0.1 L/cm H_2O, or 100 mL/cm H_2O.

Flow assist is a measurement of resistance, where R = ΔP/flow. The setting for flow assist is cm H_2O/(L/sec).

Table 12-8 Proportional pressure support ranges of available settings on the E-4 with upgrade (version 2.n)

	Flow assist (cm H_2O/L/sec)	Increment (cm H_2O/L/sec)
Adult	0 to 30	0.5
(corresponds to a resistance compensation of 0 to 30 cm H_2O/L/sec)		
Pediatric	0 to 30	0.5
	30 to 100	5.0
(corresponds to a resistance compensation of 0 to 100 cm H_2O/L/sec)		
Neonatal	0 to 30	0.5
	30 to 300	5.0
(corresponds to a resistance compensation of 0 to 300 cm H_2O/L/sec)		
	Volume assist (cm H_2O/L)	**Increment (cm H_2O/L)**
Adult	0 to 24.9	0.1
	25 to 99.5	0.5
(corresponds to a compliance compensation of infinity to 10 mL/cm H_2O)		
Pediatric	0 to 99	1.0
	100 to 1000	10.0
(corresponds to a compliance compensation of infinity to 1 mL/cm H_2O)		
Neonatal	0 to 30	0.5
	30 to 300	5.0
(corresponds to a compliance compensation of infinity to 0.5 mL/cm H_2O)		

maximum T_I is limited to 4 seconds (1.5 seconds in pediatric patients; the neonatal setting is adjusted by the clinician with the T_I control [E-4 with Neoflow]). This is a new mode of ventilation in the United States, so its effectiveness will be evaluated as the results of its use in clinical studies are made available.

Neoflow[5,6]

Neoflow is an upgraded mode of ventilation that has been added to the Evita 4 ventilator, which allows it to be adapted for neonatal use (patient weight from 0.5 to 6 kg). Neoflow requires the installation of a flow sensor between the end of the endotracheal tube and the Y connector of the patient circuit. The other end is attached to the back of the ventilator unit. The flow sensor must be calibrated when first used and then at least once every 24 hours (see the operator's manual).

When the unit is turned on and the screen displays the STANDBY mode, the operator selects the NEO. soft pad for neonatal ventilation. In the neonatal mode, the unit can provide volume ventilation; AutoFlow; apnea back-up ventilation; pressure support with assisted spontaneous breathing (ASB); continuous base flow; and measurements of circuit leaks, airway pressure, and breath triggering (Table 12-9).

Flow Monitoring During Neonatal Ventilation

The addition of the flow sensor allows flow monitoring at the airway during neonatal ventilation. The unit is still functional if the sensor fails and cannot be replaced immediately. The flow sensor can be deactivated if a large leak is present. If flow monitoring is deactivated, however, neither volume ventilation nor patient-triggered breaths are possible. Minute ventilation cannot be monitored without the neonatal flow sensor.

Continuous Base Flow in Neonates

With the addition of Neoflow, the Evita 4 offers a continuous base flow of 6 L/min. Because the flow is continuous, the infant has the opportunity to obtain flow on demand. As soon as the patient begins inspiration, the unit delivers additional flow to maintain the baseline, thus keeping flow compatible with the patient's needs.

Table 12-9 Specifications for Neoflow on the Dräger E-4

Parameter	Range
Frequency	0 to 150 breaths/min
VT (inspiratory)	3 to 100 (max 2000) mL
Inspiratory pressure	0 to 80 cm H_2O
PEEP/CPAP	0 to 35 cm H_2O
PCV	0 to 80 cm H_2O
Trigger	0.3 to 15 L/min

Measurement of Leakage Flow in Neonatal Ventilation

The leakage flow that normally occurs around uncuffed endotracheal tubes in infants can be monitored with the flow sensor of the Evita 4 ventilator. The unit displays minute ventilation leakage (MVleak) on the front of the unit. MVleak represents the difference between inspiratory and expiratory flow averaged over time and displayed as a percentage of the delivered inspired minute volume. The unit assumes that any gas that does not flow back through the sensor from the patient must have escaped through a leak around the endotracheal tube and out through the patient's upper airway. The unit automatically corrects V_T (inspiratory and expiratory) and flow values based on its calculation of the leak.

Trigger Response in Neonates

The neonatal flow sensor detects the patient's inspiratory effort and is responsible for triggering any assisted breaths or patient-initiated gas flow from the unit. To avoid incorrect triggering due to leaks around the endotracheal tube, the E-4 takes into account the flow sensor signal (inspiratory flow) and the calculated leakage flow (MVleak). A trigger range of 0.3 to 3 L/min is recommended for neonatal ventilation.

AutoFlow in Neonates

AutoFlow as a volume entity with the Evita 4 is only available in neonates with the flow sensor. When the sensor is attached, AutoFlow is always active in CMV, SIMV, and MMV modes. Without the sensor, the ventilator will not volume ventilate, but will provide time-cycled, pressure-targeted ventilation and allow for spontaneous breathing throughout inspiration and expiration.

It is important to set the UPPER PAW ALARM limit so that if the patient's lung characteristics change or there is a sudden change in leakage, the patient will be protected from high pressures. When AutoFlow is initiated in neonates with the flow sensor attached, the unit provides two test breaths, first with a Paw of 5 cm H_2O and then with a Paw equal to 75% of that required to deliver the set volume. The third breath is at a pressure determined to be appropriate to achieve the set V_T.

Volume Ventilation in Neonates

Volume ventilation can be provided with CMV, SIMV, and MMV modes. When these are selected, AutoFlow is automatically active, allowing the patient to breathe spontaneously at any time.

Apnea Ventilation in Neonates

As in adult ventilation, the operator selects an apnea time. If this time is exceeded, an alarm is activated, and the ventilator switches to back-up ventilation. Unlike adult or pediatric back-up ventilation, apnea ventilation in the neonatal mode is pressure controlled ventilation. The operator selects apnea frequency (FAPNEA) and pressure above PEEP (PAPNEA). The I:E ratio is fixed at 1:2, and the F_IO_2 and PEEP levels remain the same.

The E-4 will also switch to back-up ventilation if a volume ventilation mode is in use and the flow monitor is either switched off or fails to monitor flow. In this situation, the pressure applied is the last mean pressure measured during a mandatory breath. T_I, f, O_2%, and PEEP remain the same.

Pressure Support (PS), or Assisted Spontaneous Breathing (ASB) in Neonates

Pressure support is also referred to as assisted spontaneous breathing (ASB) in some of the Dräger literature. As with adult and pediatric ventilation, PS is available with SIMV, MMV, and PCV modes, as well as for strictly spontaneous breathing. The pressure rise control is also operational. Maximum inspiratory time should also be set when using PS.

Special Functions

There are a variety of features on the Dräger E-4, some of which are similar to other ICU ventilators and others that are unique to this unit. These functions are reviewed here.

Sigh (Intermittent PEEP)

The E-4 provides sigh breaths in a format similar to the Evita and was described in that section. Sigh breaths are accomplished by increasing PEEP in the CMV mode. As with a sigh breath, the intended purpose of intermittent PEEP is to open up or keep areas of the lung likely to become atelectatic open. PEEP is increased to the set cm H_2O selected by the operator, which is added to the set PEEP for two breaths every 3 minutes (see Figure 12-18). Intermittent PEEP can be selected by touching the EXTRA SETTING soft pad on the screen and is set like other parameters. During the sigh interval, the VOLUME NOT CONSTANT alarm is deactivated. Because intermittent PEEP increases the baseline, it is advisable to appropriately set the Pmax pressure limit to avoid overdistention of the lungs during regular breath delivery (see Figure 12-18).

Intrinsic PEEP

An estimate of the amount of auto-PEEP as well as an estimate of the trapped volume in a patient can be determined by using the intrinsic PEEP (PEEPi) function. These measurements can only be performed as long as no active breathing by the patient occurs during the measurement.

To perform an auto-PEEP measurement, select the SPECIAL PROCEDURE touch pad. From the computer screen, touch the PEEPi soft pad. The maneuver is performed automatically, and the waveform display is frozen. On the screen, values for PEEP(set), PEEPi, and trapped volume (Vtrap) are shown. Using the dial knob and the screen cursor, the operator can select to view the auto-PEEP level at any time on the graph of pressure/time. The PEEPi values appear above the waveform.

Occlusion Pressure

Measurements of occlusion pressure (P0.1) are used to evaluate a patient's neuromuscular drive.[4] At the beginning of inspiration, the ventilator occludes the inspiratory and expiratory valves 0.1 second after the beginning of inspiratory flow. The pressure measured at that time is displayed. This procedure can be automatically performed by selecting the SPECIAL PROCEDURES touch pad, the P0.1 soft pad, and the START soft pad. The value for occlusion pressure is shown on the screen. The normal value is from about –3 to –4 cm H_2O. Values more negative than –6 cm H_2O may indicate impending exhaustion and respiratory muscle fatigue that may lead to respiratory failure, as in patients with chronic obstructive pulmonary disease. As with PEEPi, the waveform is frozen on the screen. Using the rotary knob and screen cursor the specific value for pressure from the pressure-time curve can be viewed at precise moments during the maneuver.

Special-Function Touch Pads

As mentioned previously, there is a set of touch pads to the left of the screen on the front panel of the E-4. Their function is explained here.

Neb Touch Pad

The nebulizer touch pad (NEB) switches on the nebulizer gas source and functions during adult ventilation only. Gas only flows through the nebulizer outlet during inspiration and automatically maintains the set $\dot{V}_E$ and approximates the set O_2%.

When the nebulizer is activated, the LED on the touch pad appears with a screen message: "Nebulizer on." The nebulizer continues to operate for 30 minutes or until the pad is touched again. After its use, a "flow calibration" message appears, showing that the nebulizer is off and the flow transducer is being automatically cleaned and recalibrated to preserve accuracy (Box 12-33).

Box 12-33 Clinical Note: Caution During Nebulization

1. Do not use a heat moisture exchanger (HME) during nebulization because it reduces medication delivery and may increase airway resistance by depositing medication on the HME.
2. Do not use filters on the nebulizer outlet because they may increase resistance and impair ventilation.

CLINICAL ROUNDS 12-10

Clinical note on suctioning:

1. If the patient is not disconnected after the suction 100% O_2 pad is pressed, the unit continues to ventilate the patient in the set mode but uses 100% O_2. After 3 minutes, the O_2 program is terminated and the alarms are reactivated.
2. To stop "suction 100% O_2", press the pad again. The LED will flash for 15 seconds and normal operation resumes. The oxygen enrichment cannot be restarted until the flashing stops.

Some institutions use closed-suction catheter systems and do not disconnect the patient prior to suctioning. Do you think that the clinician should still disconnect the patient to activate the oxygen enrichment function?

See Appendix A for the answer.

The expiratory flow sensor is a heated wire (see Chapter 8). To protect the sensor during the use of nebulized medications, a filter placed in-line before the sensor may be helpful.

Suction 100% O_2

The SUCTION 100% O_2 touch pad is used to provide100% O_2 for 3 minutes. When pressed, the LED on the pad is lit and the message "O_2 enrichment 180 s" appears at the bottom of the screen. The suction 100% O_2 control functions similarly to that on the Evita (See the discussion of this function in the section on the Evita). During the 3-minute suction interval, the low $\dot{V}_E$ alarm is turned off (Clinical Rounds 12-10). For 2 minutes thereafter, 100% O_2 is provided and the alarms are reactivated. (*Note:* If the patient is not disconnected after the 100% O_2 control is activated, the operator must touch the pad again to reactivate the alarm, or an undetected disconnect may occur.)

Inspir Hold

The INSPIR HOLD touch pad provides an inflation hold maneuver when pressed and held down for as long as the inspiratory pause is desired (maximum of 15 seconds). When activated, either the current inspiration is held, or a new mandatory breath is delivered and the inspiration is held. It functions in all modes except CPAP when pressure support is set at zero.

Print

The PRINT function allows the microprocessor to print if a compatible printer is attached.

Special Upgrades with Software Update 2.n

The Dräger E-4 has a software update version 2.n that includes the following few special features.

Compliance Compensation

The E-4 upgrade provides compensation for volume lost due to tubing compressibility. The unit adds the volume needed to compensate for the volume lost and subtracts this added volume from the measured expiratory volume to give a close measurement of the volume actually exhaled by the patient. The resistance and compliance of the patient circuit are determined when the patient circuit is changed (Standby mode) with the AIRTIGHT CHECK soft pad.

Support During Hose Change

When a patient circuit is changed, it is possible for the ventilator to check the hose for leaks by using the Standby mode (selecting the AIRTIGHT CHECK soft pad). In addition, the resistance and compliance of the circuit are also measured in order to provide compliance compensation for the volume lost due to tubing compliance (See the previous discussion of compliance compensation).

Automatic Tubing Compensation (ATC)

As a part of the breathing support package (software update version 2.n), an automatic tube compensation (ATC) feature has been added to the E-4 to compensate for the airway resistance associated with small artificial airways. ATC can be used with the PPS mode of ventilation, as well as with all other modes of ventilation. In CMV, SIMV, and MMV, tube compensation is active during expiration after a mandatory breath and during spontaneous breathing phases.

This ventilator function regulates airway pressure at the tracheal level (Box 12-34). When it is selected, the

Box 12-34 Calculation of the Tracheal Pressure on the Evita-4 Upgrade (version 2.n)

The Dräger E-4 (2.n software version) calculates and displays tracheal pressure based on a mathematical equation

$$P_{trachea} = Paw - K_{tube} \times Flow^2$$

where $P_{trachea}$ is the pressure in the trachea, *Paw* is the pressure at the Y connector of the patient circuit, K_{tube} is the tube coefficient (listed in the operating manual), and *Flow* is the patient flow (inspiratory flow is > 0, and expiratory flow is < 0). An example of a tube coefficient is 6.57 cm $H_2O/L^2/seconds^2$ for an endotracheal tube with an inner diameter (ID) of 8.0 mm.

For pressure support the equation is as follows:

$$\Delta Paw = Comp. \times K_{tube} \times Flow^2$$

where ΔPaw = pressure support at the tube, *Comp.* = degree of compensation (0% to 100%), K_{tube} = tube coefficient, and *Flow* is patient flow.

Box 12-35 Waveform Display on the Dräger E-4

1. Select the STANDARD PAGE computer screen by pressing the main screen touch pad. In the right field, four measured values are displayed. In the left field, two waveforms are displayed.
2. To select waveforms, touch the icon on the computer screen at the top right of the waveform area that looks like two tiny waveforms (Figure 12-25). Touch the screen key that indicates the waveform you desire.
3. To select loops, touch the VALUES MEASURED touch pad. The computer screen displays several selections on the lower right corner. Touch the loops soft pad on the screen. Two different loops appear on the lower left part of the screen. To change the loop parameters, touch the waveform icon between them.

ventilating pressure during all breaths compensates for the resistance associated with varying size endotracheal tubes. This compensation depends on the direction of air flow. The airway pressure is increased during inspiration and decreased during expiration. (*Note*: The expiratory portion can be switched off if the operator only wants to compensate for the inspiratory portion.) The pressure can be increased to a value equal to the upper Paw alarm limit minus 5 cm H_2O or reduced to a minimum of 0 cm H_2O.

To set the tube compensation function, the following should be performed:

1. During stand-by, select the TUBE COMP. soft pad.
2. Touch either the ET TUBE or the TRACH. TUBE soft pad, depending on the type of artificial airway in use.
3. Use the ID 0 soft knob to set the size of the tube's inner diameter (with the dial knob) and confirm it by pressing the dial knob.
4. Use the COMP. soft knob and the dial knob to set the percentage of compensation provided. For example, a reading of "70" inside the COMP. soft knob provides 70% compensation for the artificial airway.

Ventilator Graphic Waveforms

The graphics monitor with the E-4 is part of the main computer screen during standard operation. Additional waveforms can be viewed simultaneously, and different waveforms may be displayed during its normal function (see Box 12-29; Box 12-35). Timed graphics can be frozen by pressing the FREEZE touch pad on the right side of the unit's front panel. The operator can view a more specific measured numerical value for a given time on any graph by positioning the cursor on the computer screen and rotating the dial knob to the desired time on the curve. The value is shown on the screen above the waveform. The graph can be unfrozen by pressing freeze a second time.

The E-4 can also display trends of data. Select MEASURED VALUES and then TRENDS. In this setting, one can "zoom in" or "zoom out" to narrow or widen the time frame for the data trend by selecting those soft pads. Again, the operator can change the parameters being viewed or trended by touching the waveform icon. This function can also be analyzed by using the cursor with a link to the LOGBOOK.

Troubleshooting

The alarms and monitored information sections offer a great deal of assistance for solving the majority of problems that might occur with the E-4. In addition, the operator's manual contains a large troubleshooting section that alphabetically lists all the alarm messages, gives their priority level, provides common causes, and recommends remedies. Covering this extensive material is beyond the scope of this text. Users are advised to consult the operator's manual. For additional information about Dräger products check their website: http://www.draeger.com.

Dräger Evita 2 Dura

The Dräger Evita 2 Dura[1] is a modification of the Evita 2, a ventilator that was never marketed in the United States. The Evita 2 Dura is another in a series of three ventilators that includes the Evita and the E-4. All are manufactured by Drägerwerk (Lubeck, Germany) and represented in the United States by the Dräger Incorporated, Teleford, PA. There are a number of similarities between the units that will be mentioned as they are described.

The front panel of the Dura is divided into two main sections (Figure 12-35). The right side contains a majority of the ventilator settings touch pads and a primary control knob, which is called the dial knob. Settings are displayed in individual liquid crystal display (LCD) windows in this section. The left side contains a screen. The Evita 2 Dura uses either a high-contrast black and white or an optional color computer (LCD) screen. Although similar to the E-4, the Evita 2 Dura has a larger number of touch pads on the front panel. There are images or icons on the computer screen. All of the dials and knobs used to control the unit are discussed later in this section.

Below the front operating panel are the connections for the main inspiratory and expiratory lines, the expiratory valve, and the nipple connector for the nebulizer line (see Figure 12-35). The expiratory flow sensor is to the left of the

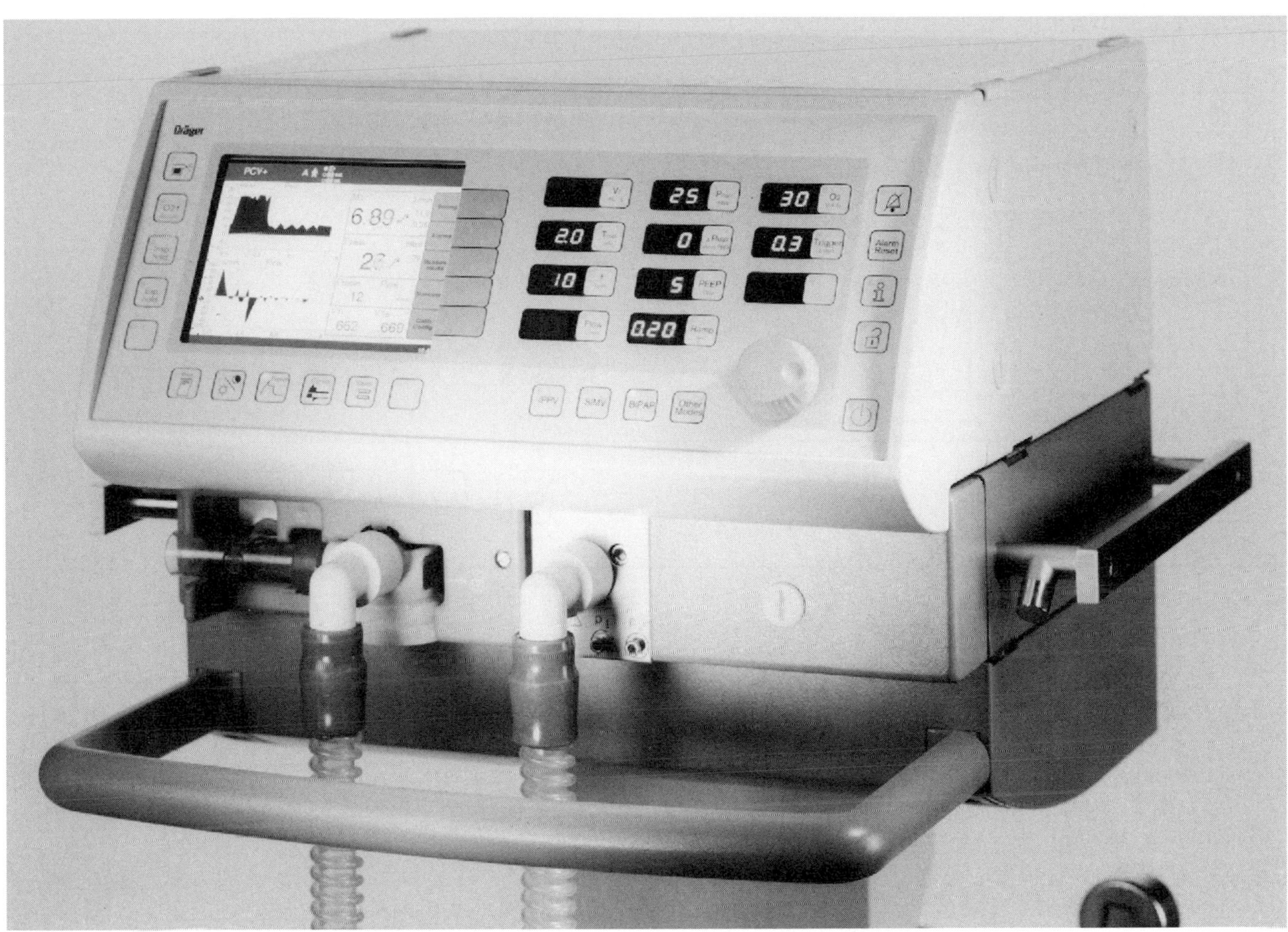

Figure 12-35 The Evita 2 Dura. (Redrawn from Dräger Corp, Telford, Penn.)

expiratory valve. On the far right side, below the unit's main control knob (dial knob), is a cover that protects the oxygen sensor and the ambient air filter.

Power Source

The Evita 2 Dura normally uses air and oxygen at high pressure (range 40 to 87 psig) as pneumatic power sources. A standard AC 120-volt outlet is used to power the microprocessor and electrical components. The unit can also operate with a single gas source, such as an air compressor; but this will alter the oxygen delivery capabilities. The on/off switch is on the back panel of the unit.

Internal Mechanism

The Evita 2 Dura has the same internal pneumatic components as the Evita 4 (see the discussion of internal mechanisms in the section on the E-4).

Controls and Alarms

The controls, monitors, and alarms are similar to those on the E-4. The Evita 2 Dura uses a single control knob or dial knob, several hard touch pads alongside the computer screen, and the touch-sensitive soft knobs and soft pads of the computer screen (see Figure 12-35).

Peripheral Controls

Several controls used during the normal operation of the ventilator are located around the screen (see Figure 12-35 and Figure 12-36). The controls to the left of the screen include the NEBULIZER, SUCTION 100% O_2 ENRICHMENT, and INSPIRATORY and EXPIRATORY HOLD. These are reviewed under the discussion of special functions in this section.

Below the computer screen are the following controls:

1. PRINTER to print material when the unit is attached to a compatible printer.

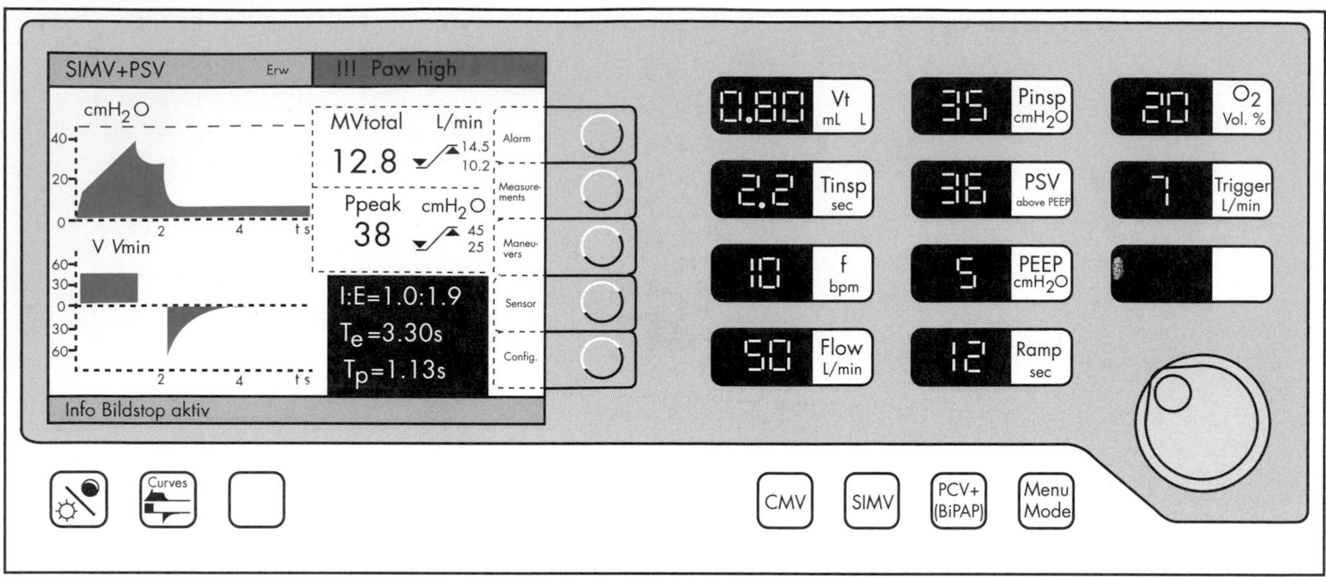

Figure 12-36 The front panel of the Dura, showing a typical monitoring screen and digital displays of the set parameters. (Redrawn from Dräger Corp, Telford, Penn.)

2. A touch pad with a symbol of a sun and new moon to set the screen backlighting bright or dark.
3. FREEZE SCREEN touch pad for freezing waveforms.
4. A "waves" key with symbols of waves on the touch pad to display a different pair of waveforms.
5. VALUES touch pad for displaying different combinations of measured values.
6. Blank touch pads for future use.

To the immediate right of the computer screen is a column of keys touching the side of the screen. When a menu screen appears, a column of items appears adjacent to these touch pads on the right of the screen. For example, Figure 12-37 shows the following list in the currently active screen: settings, alarms, measurements, maneuvers, and calibration configuration. The operator can touch MEASUREMENT, for example, and the unit will display a screen of all measured values in the current mode. Box 12-36 lists the specific functions for these touch pad controls.

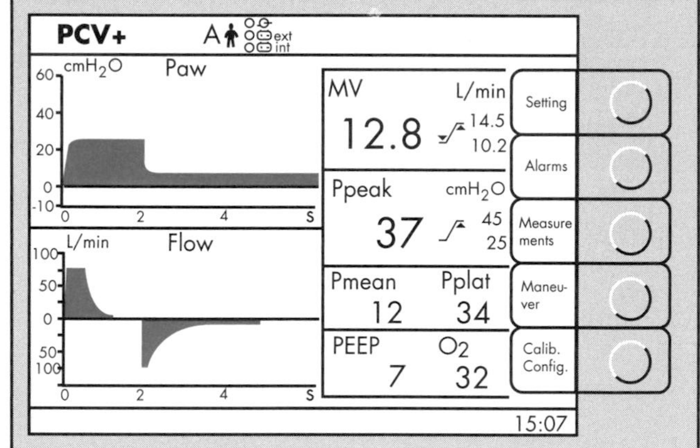

Figure 12-37 A close-up of the monitoring screen, showing the touch pads adjacent to the right side of the screen. (Redrawn from Dräger Corp, Telford, Penn.)

To the right of the screen and its adjacent keys are three columns of touch pads used to adjust several parameters (see Figure 12-36). These pads include the following:

1. Tidal volume (V_T; in milliliters or liters)
2. Inspiratory time (Tinsp; in seconds)
3. Respiratory rate (f; in breaths/minute)
4. Flow (in liters/minute)
5. Inspiratory pressure (Pinsp; in centimeters of water), for the pressure-control mode
6. Pressure support (Psupp above PEEP; in centimeters of water)
7. PEEP (in centimeters of water)
8. Pressure rise time (Ramp; ranges from 0.0 to 2.0 seconds), which adjusts the rate of rise in pressure at the beginning of a breath and is active for breaths during PCV and PS and when Autoflow is on
9. Oxygen percent (O_2%)
10. Trigger sensitivity (Trigger; in liters/minute)
11. Control or dial knob, which can be rotated and pressed to select numerical values for parameters and activate the new parameters, respectively

Immediately below this area are four more touch pads used to select ventilator mode screens (CMV, SIMV, and PCV+) and a touch pad for menu mode, which brings up a menu

Box 12-36 The Specifications for the Menu Keys at the Right Edge of the Evita 2 Dura Screen

ADDITIONAL SETTINGS is used for:

- Programming the other modes touch pad with one of the following available modes: CPAP/PSV, MMV, or other added options.
- Setting back-up ventilation parameters.
- Setting intermittent PEEP and the sigh control available during CMV ventilation.

ALARMS is used for:

- Displaying measured values with their alarm limits.
- Setting alarm limits.

MEASURED VALUES is used for displaying all measured values in the current mode. OPTIONS allows for the selection of lung mechanics maneuvers, loops, and any optional or additional controls added to the unit.

CALIBRATION/CONFIGURATION allows the following functions to be performed:

- Automatic calibration of O_2 or flow sensors.
- Turning monitor functions on/off.
- Setting audible alarm volume, screen contrast, date and time, language, measurement units, and configuring external interfaces under ventilator.
- Selecting two of the six available measured values for display.
- Selecting two sets of waveforms for display.
- Setting the default start-up ventilator parameters, alarm limits, and mode.

Box 12-37 Changing the Default (Programmed) Start-up Mode and Parameters

As with the E-4, the Evita 2 Dura can have the automatic start-up mode and its parameters and alarms changed. This is done by selecting CALIBRATION/CONFIGURATION, and proceeding through the selection of desired options, such as mode, V_T, and f. An access code must be entered to change these programmed default settings. Usually the clinical specialist or department head has the access code. (See the operator's manual for additional instructions.)[1]

screen. The ventilator modes are explained in the discussion of modes of ventilation later in this section.

To the far right of the front panel are five more touch pads. The first is an icon shaped like a bell with a cross line through it; this is the ALARM SILENCE touch pad (2-minute silence). The second is the ALARM RESET touch pad, which resets or acknowledges alarm messages. The third is the information key, "I." The fourth touch pad is a lock-shaped icon that can lock the controls to prevent inadvertent or unauthorized changing of ventilator settings. The fifth touch pad allows the unit to be placed in the STANDBY mode. To place the unit in STANDBY and stop ventilation, press and hold down the STANDBY touch pad for about 3 seconds, then press the ALARM RESET pad. To switch back to ventilation, press and release the STANDBY touch pad.

System Tests and Calibration

Before the unit is turned on and connected to a patient, a series of tests and calibrations is performed. First, the patient Y connector is connected to its "park" bracket on the right side of the ventilator. After the power switch is turned on, the unit runs a series of self-tests (for about 10 seconds). After the tests are completed, press and hold the STANDBY touch pad to switch the unit to standby. Silence any alarms with the ALARM RESET pad. After the unit is in standby, additional tests can be performed by pressing the MENU touch pad (on the right side of the screen) and following the instructions as they are provided by the screen display.[1]

If the CHECK CALIBRATION has been performed before the ventilator is brought to the ICU for use, then the Evita 2 Dura simply has to be turned on, and the self-tests run. After 30 seconds, the unit will automatically begin ventilation based on the programmed default parameters, alarms and mode. During these 30 seconds, however, the operator can select another mode and other parameters and activate these settings by pressing the dial knob (Box 12-37). Before it begins operation, the screen requires you to select adult or pediatric patient. Rotate the dial knob to choose the desired patient size, and press it to make a choice. The available volumes and flows are different for each type of patient. These values and other available parameter ranges are the same in the Dura as in the E-4 (see Table 12-4). To start ventilation with the default settings, press the dial knob again; ventilation begins immediately. The main screen is then displayed. Figure 12-37 shows an example of the computer screen during patient ventilation. The digital displays adjacent to the parameter touch pads display the selected setting. For example, next to the V_T touch pad the digital window will show the V_T setting (Figure 12-36).

Monitors and Alarms

The Evita 2 Dura normally provides two waveform selections on the left side of the monitor screen and the commonly viewed measured values such as airway pressure and minute ventilation on the right (see Figure 12-37). The values normally displayed can be changed by using the values touch pad below the screen. The waveform can be changed by using the waves touch pad. These two touch pads bring up additional sets of information that have been programmed into the unit. In addition, these selections can be changed using the configuration function so that any of the measured or calculated parameters and waveforms the operator chooses can be displayed.

Measured Values

To view MEASURED VALUES, touch the values measured touch pad to bring up a screen displaying a variety of values being measured or calculated by the unit, similar to those available with the E-4 (see Table 12-5 in the section on the Evita 4), including the MVleak measurement. With the measured values screen, a bar graph appears on the left that continually shows airway pressure.

Alarms

Alarms can be set by pressing the ALARM LIMITS touch pad on the right side of the screen, which provides a window allowing available alarm values to be adjusted (Figure 12-38). There is a diagonal line that is the symbol for alarm setting. The down arrow on this line indicates the lower alarm limit and the up arrow the upper alarm limit. For example, to set the HIGH RATE alarm, use the cursor and the dial knob to select "f_{spn} bpm" for spontaneous rate breaths/min alarm. Turn the dial knob to establish the desired high rate; the number appears next to the alarm symbol. Press the dial knob to activate the new setting. The adjustable alarms for $\dot{V}_E$, upper airway pressure, apnea time, high V_T, and high respiratory rate are the same as on the E-4 (see Table 12-6). The automatic alarm limit for low airway pressure is the set PEEP value plus 5 cm H_2O. For example, if PEEP = 5 cm H_2O, the low pressure limit is 10 cm H_2O and is not adjustable. See Clinical Rounds 12-11 for an example problem related to alarm settings.

As with the E-4, the Ppeak alarm is not to be confused with the Pmax pressure limit that is available on the Evita 2 Dura. The Pmax limit is not an alarm and is reviewed in the discussion of modes of ventilation later in this section.

The same three levels of alarm priority in the E-4 are used in the Evita 2 Dura. Table 12-7 lists and describes these alarms. After an alarm has occurred, it can be silenced with the ALARM SILENCE touch pad.

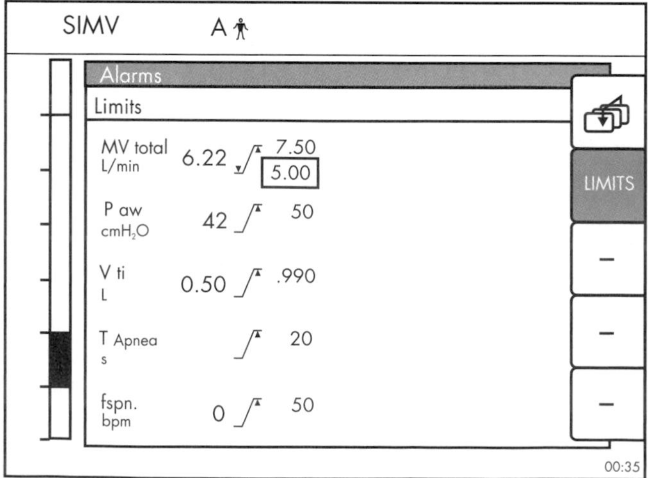

Figure 12-38 The alarm screen on the Evita 2 Dura. (Redrawn from Dräger Corp, Telford, Penn.)

When an alarm event occurs, exclamation points ("!," "!!," or "!!!") appear on the black and white monitor at the upper right corner of the unit. On a color monitor, a red or yellow light flashes, the color being determined by the alarm priority level. In addition, an alarm message is displayed at the upper right corner of the computer screen, providing information on the type of alarm limit that has been exceeded. If a low- or medium-priority alarm occurs and the problem is corrected, the alarm (lights, message, and sound) switches off. Warning messages ("!!!"), however, must be acknowledged by pressing the ALARM RESET touch pad. The sound is discontinued on a high-priority alarm, and the color returns to blue. The alarm wording is removed with the reset pad.

Modes of Ventilation

Modes of operation available on the Evita 2 Dura are listed in Box 12-38.

Standard Settings of Ventilator Modes

When the ventilator is first turned on, one of the following three types of patient ventilation will take place within 30 seconds:

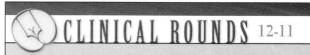

A respiratory therapist is trying to set the high respiratory rate alarm on the Dura. After using the cursor and the dial knob to select "fspn bpm," the desired value appears next to the alarm symbol on the screen. This, however, does not set the new alarm value. What is the problem?

See Appendix A for the answer.

Box 12-38 Modes of Ventilation on the Evita Dura

- **CMV:** Continuous mandatory ventilation
- **SIMV:** Synchronized intermittent mandatory ventilation (volume- or pressure-targeted)
- **MMV:** Mandatory minute volume ventilation
- **CPAP:** Continuous positive airway pressure
- **Psupp:** Pressure support
- **PCV+:** Pressure-control ventilation
- **APRV:** Airway pressure release ventilation
- Apnea ventilation
- Independent lung ventilation

1. If a system check has been performed, the default mode programmed into the unit becomes active.
2. If system checks have not been run since the unit was turned off, the ventilator automatically starts using the patient mode last used and the previously selected parameters. In this phase, the operator can change the ventilator settings to the default parameters by pressing the dial knob.
3. If the operator wants to change the mode of ventilation at the start time and does not want to use the default values, a new mode and appropriate parameters can be selected. After this is performed and the dial knob is pressed to confirm the new variables, the new mode is operational.

New parameters and modes can be selected when a ventilation mode is not currently active. A new parameter is adjusted by pressing the touch pad. For example, pressing the V_T pad allows selection of V_T. The LED on the V_T pad flashes, indicating that it can be changed. Turn the dial knob until the appropriate V_T value appears in the digital window next to the touch pad. After the desired value appears, press the dial knob to confirm selection of that value. If more than 30 seconds passes before the dial knob is pressed, the original value remains active. (*Note*: After the range limit of a parameter is reached, the indicated value does not change. A message appears at the bottom of the screen describing the problem and a possible solution.) To activate the mode keys, press and hold the key for about 3 seconds, or press the key once and then press the dial knob. The selected mode immediately becomes active.

If a mode besides the one set on the screen is desired, pressing the other modes key provides the option of selecting whatever has been programmed into the unit. To prevent unauthorized changes, press the LOCK touch pad. When its LED is lit, the parameter keys and ventilation mode keys are protected from being changed. To unlock, simply press the LED again.

Box 12-39 Autoflow and Pmax During CMV

Any problems related to flow restriction and high peak pressures, as well as most problems with pause time can be corrected using Autoflow. The understanding and use of Autoflow is paramount in the use of the Evita 2 Dura and the E-4.

Pmax is a system that originated with the first Evita and is not recommended in the Dura and E-4. Pmax pressure limit is also called pressure-limited ventilation (PLV) by the manufacturer.

The functions of Autoflow or Pmax with the E-2 Dura are the same as with the E-4 ventilator. For a description of AutoFlow and Pmax, see the appropriate discussions in the section on the Dräger E-4 ventilator.

Trigger Sensitivity

The Evita 2 Dura provides flow-triggering in all modes of ventilation. The flow-trigger level is set by performing the following:

- Touching the TRIGGER touch pad
- Turning to the desired flow-triggering value using the dial knob
- Pressing the dial knob to activate the newly set flow-trigger value

Trigger sensitivity can only be turned off in CMV, but probably should never be turned off. To deactivate flow-triggering, the value should be turned to <0.3, or >15 L/min; the display will show "—.")

PEEP/CPAP, and O_2% can be selected in any mode, but if the power fails or STANDBY is selected, the settings that were in effect before the interruption are in effect when the unit is turned on again.

Continuous Mandatory Ventilation (CMV)

The CMV mode is an A/C volume ventilation mode. The operator sets V_T, flow, f, T_I, and desired alarm settings. Breaths are patient- or time-triggered, volume-targeted, and time-cycled. All breaths deliver the set V_T. Flow to the patient is restricted to the flow setting value. If flow is high and V_T is delivered before T_I is achieved, the inspiratory valve closes (the expiratory valve is already closed) and a breath hold occurs. This can be identified by an inspiratory pause pressure in the pressure/time curve and by the flow returning to zero on the flow/time curve. This is similar to the function of the E-4 (see Figure 12-28). See Box 12-39 for a note on Autoflow and Pmax related to mode setting.

SIMV and SIMV with Pressure Support Ventilation (SIMV + PSV)

SIMV provides a maximum number of mandatory breaths and allows the patient to breathe spontaneously between the mandatory breaths (see Chapter 11). Spontaneous breaths can be provided using pressure support. Mandatory breaths can be patient- or time-triggered, volume-targeted, and time-cycled. Pressure-support breaths are patient-triggered, pressure-limited, and normally flow- cycled (see the later discussion of PS in this section). In the SIMV mode, Pmax or AutoFlow can also be used. Setting the respiratory rate (f) to zero turns the unit to spontaneous ventilation, and provides the selected CPAP. PCV-SIMV is now also available for the E-2 Dura and provides pressure-targeted mandatory breaths.

The flow-trigger ensures synchronous triggering of a mandatory breath with a patient effort. The function of SIMV is similar in the Dura, the Evita, and the E-4 (see the discussion of SIMV in the section on the Evita ventilator in this chapter).

Pressure-Control Ventilation Plus (PCV+)

Pressure control ventilation in the Dräger Evita 2 Dura is called "PCV+" "PCV+ with Psupp," and bilevel positive airway pressure by the manufacturer. The patient can breathe spontaneously at any time—even during the inspiratory inflation cycle. Due to the open expiratory valve system, the unit is similar in function to a high-flow CPAP device. Mandatory breaths are patient- or time-triggered, pressure-targeted, and time-cycled.

The operator sets a minimum respiratory rate, inspiratory pressure above PEEP (ΔP), and flow-trigger. The PCV+ mode in this ventilator is always a SIMV-based mode. That is, the patient can breathe spontaneously during the expiratory time. When f is 0, the patient is on CPAP, the spontaneous breathing mode. The PRESSURE RISE TIME control can be used in this mode to slow flow and pressure delivery at the beginning of a pressure breath. Pressure rise is normally set from 0.0 to 0.5 sec (range: 0.0 to 2.0 seconds) and represents the amount of time it takes the ventilator to achieve the set pressure from the beginning of inspiratory flow delivery.

Spontaneous breaths that occur between mandatory breaths can be assisted with pressure support by setting the desired pressure support level (PCV+ with Psupp). If pressure rise is being used, it will affect both mandatory and PS breath delivery. PEEP and F_IO_2 can be set when desired. The function of PCV+ of the Dura is identical to that mode on the E-4 (see Figure 12-30).

Because V_T and $\dot{V}_E$ may vary in this mode, the operator must carefully set $\dot{V}_E$ alarm limits. As with SIMV volume ventilation, apnea ventilation is available during this mode, as well, but activation of Pmax and Autoflow is not necessary during this mode because breath delivery is already pressure-targeted with the unit controlling these functions.

Pressure-Support Ventilation (PSV)

The E-2 Dura can provide PSV during SIMV, PCV+, and spontaneous (CPAP) ventilation. To set CPAP/PS on the Dura, the following steps are performed:

- Either go to a rate of 0 in SIMV or to the SETTINGS key pad
- Then go to the OTHER MODES key pad
- Select CPAP/PS as the other mode
- Activate it by either pressing the OTHER MODES key pad at the mode selections and holding it for 3 seconds or touching the OTHER MODES keypad and pressing the rotary dial for confirmation.

The target pressure is set by touching the PS key pad of the parameter selection keys. PS breaths are patient-triggered, pressure-targeted, and flow-cycled (25% of peak for adults, 6% of peak for pediatric patients). Patient-triggering is based on the flow-trigger. Whenever PSV is active, the pressure rise time control is also functional.

If the patient actively exhales or fights the ventilator during the start of a PS breath, inspiratory flow ends. This is detected by the flow going to zero or less than zero during the early portion of inspiration.

Inspiratory flow during PSV will also time-cycle at 4 seconds (1.5 seconds for pediatric setting). Prolonged T_I most frequently occurs if a leak is present. Apnea ventilation is available when PSV is selected.

Continuous Positive Airway Pressure (CPAP)

CPAP is available on the E-2 Dura by selecting SIMV, PCV+ or APRV modes and setting the respiratory rate to zero. It is set in the same manner as pressure support. Set the desired CPAP level (cm H_2O) if you wish to use CPAP alone. Set PS above PEEP if you want to assist spontaneous breaths with pressure support. Apnea ventilation is available when CPAP is selected.

Mandatory Minute Volume Ventilation (MMV) and MMV with Pressure Support (MMV/PSV)

As described in Chapter 11 and in the MMV section of the E-4, a patient can breathe spontaneously with MMV and contribute a portion of the overall $\dot{V}_E$. The difference between the spontaneous $\dot{V}_E$ and the set $\dot{V}_E$ is provided by mandatory breaths at the set volume. Autoflow or Pmax can be used in MMV ventilation.

MMV is made operational by pressing the SETTINGS key and then the OTHER MODES key. Highlight the MMV setting on the screen by rotating the dial knob, and then press the dial knob to activate the setting. To switch modes, press and hold the other modes control for 3 seconds. MMV then becomes the active mode. The operator selects V_T, flow (not necessary with Autoflow), f, T_I, trigger sensitivity, F_IO_2, and PEEP level. Pressure rise time can be used to taper pressure and flow delivery during PSV.

The frequency of a mandatory breath is determined by the level of spontaneous breathing. If the patient is providing sufficient spontaneous $\dot{V}_E$, no mandatory breaths occur. If spontaneous $\dot{V}_E$ falls below what the ventilator anticipates based on the set $\dot{V}_E$, however, mandatory breaths occur when the balance between set and spontaneous $\dot{V}_E$ becomes negative. The program for MMV ventilation is designed to allow for irregular patterns of spontaneous breathing with occasional short apnea intervals, and permits these irregularities without allowing too much time to pass with no breathe—either spontaneous or mandatory.

Apnea Ventilation

Apnea ventilation provides volume ventilation with a minimum respiratory rate in case the patient becomes apneic in any of the following modes: SIMV, PCV+, CPAP, and APRV (an upgrade feature). If the patient stops breathing for the length of time set on the apnea alarm control, the alarm is activated and apnea ventilation begins.

To set apnea ventilation, touch the SETTINGS touch pad, and then, using the dial knob, select the APNEA VENT. soft

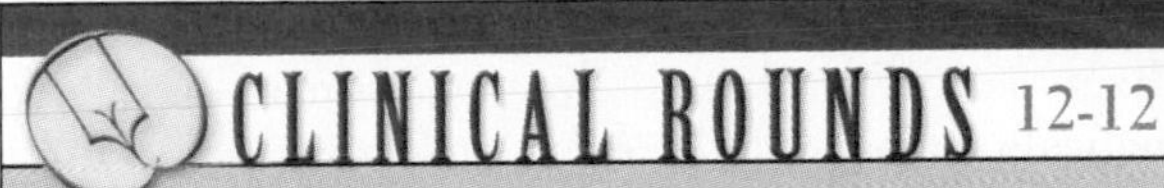

12-12

What is the primary difference between the APRV mode and the PCV+ mode on the Evita-2 Dura?

See Appendix A for the answer.

pad on the screen. Select and set the desired volume and rate using V_{TApnea} and f_{Apnea} on the screen using the dial knob. The baseline pressure, O_2%, trigger sensitivity, Autoflow, and other alarm parameters will remain as they are in the current mode if apneic ventilation becomes active.

If an apneic ventilation alarm occurs, apneic ventilation can be canceled by pressing the alarm reset touch pad. The unit continues to function in the original ventilation mode.

Airway Pressure-Release Ventilation (APRV)

APRV is a mode of ventilation that can be added to the Evita 2 Dura as an optional feature. It functions similar to the APRV mode in the Evita and the same as that in the E-4 (see the section on the E-4 and also Figure 12-23). (*Note*: APRV timing and pressure ranges have been expanded on the Dura and on the E-4 compared with those on the Evita ventilator.)

APRV is set in the following way:

1. Press the SETTINGS touch pad
2. Press the OTHER MODES touch pad
3. Select APRV on the screen by rotating the dial knob
4. Confirm by pressing the dial knob

The initials "APRV" appear in the upper right corner of the screen. The ventilator parameters are set in the same way, (i.e., by using the dial knob to adjust the number values and pressing it to confirm the new value).

An upper pressure level is set using P_{high} and a lower using P_{low}. The unit also times the length of both pressure levels. T_{high} is the length of time that high pressure is provided, and T_{low} is the length of time that low pressure is provided. Pressure rise can taper the slope from the low-pressure to the high-pressure level. The length of the pressure rise time, however, cannot be longer than the set T_{high} time. (Use of APRV is further explained in Chapter 11 and in other references[2] and it is not repeated here.) Clinical Rounds 12-12 presents a comparison of APRV and PCV+.

Apnea back-up ventilation is recommended when using this APRV. For Apnea ventilation, select SETTINGS, VENTILATION; then APNEA VENT. (dial knob); and choose the desired V_{TApnea} and f_{Apnea} with the dial knob.

Special Functions

The additional features on the Dräger E-2 Dura are similar to the same features on the E-4.

AutoFlow

AutoFlow is the same feature available with the E-4 ventilator that can be added to the Evita 2 Dura as a special feature with the ventilator plus upgrade and functions in the same manner. To select AutoFlow on the E-2 Dura, press the SETTINGS touch pad and then the Autoflow screen pad using the dial knob. When the mode is operating, a black dot appears in the upper left corner of the AutoFlow screen soft pad.

AutoFlow is available during CMV, SIMV, and MMV. It is strongly recommended that it be activated whenever a spontaneously breathing patient is being ventilated—regardless of the mode chosen. It allows for flow on demand and more rapid response of the inspiratory and expiratory valves. (*Note*: The function of AutoFlow in the Dura is identical with that in the E-4. For complete details of its operation, review the discussion of AutoFlow in the section on the E-4.)

Independent Lung Ventilation

As with the E-4, independent lung ventilation (ILV) can be programmed into the unit so that it can be coupled with another Dräger E-2 Dura or E-4. Used together, these ventilators can be employed for ILV in patients who are intubated with a double-lumen endotracheal tube. ILV synchronizes the function of the two units so that breath delivery to both lungs can occur simultaneously. ILV requires that the ventilators be connected by appropriate cables. ILV set-up is reviewed in the operator's manual and is not covered here.

Sigh (Intermittent PEEP)

As in the Evita and the E-4, the intermittent PEEP function on the E-2 Dura provides sigh breaths by increasing PEEP in the CMV mode (see Figure 12-18). Starting and setting intermittent PEEP increases end-expiratory pressure by the set value for intermittent PEEP for two consecutive mandatory breaths every 3 minutes.

Intermittent PEEP can be activated by touching the SETTINGS key and using the dial knob to select intermittent PEEP, as is done with other parameters. During the sigh interval, the VOLUME NOT CONSTANT alarm is inactivated. Because intermittent PEEP increases the baseline, it is advisable to set the upper pressure limit appropriately to avoid lung overdistention during regular breath delivery. Figure 12-18 shows the pressure-time graph of intermittent PEEP.

Intrinsic PEEP

An estimate of the amount of auto-PEEP present in a patient as well as an estimate of the trapped volume can be determined using the intrinsic PEEP (PEEPi) function. This is an added (optional) function. These measurements can only be performed when no patient activity occurs during the measurement.

To perform an auto-PEEP measurement, press the MANEUVER menu key, select PEEPi, and use the dial knob to select START soft pad on the screen. To start the measurement, press the dial knob. The maneuver is performed automatically, and the waveform display is frozen. Values for PEEP (set), PEEPi, and trapped volume (Vtrap), are shown on the screen. Using the dial knob and screen cursor, the auto-PEEP level at any time on the graph of pressure-time can be viewed. The PEEPi values appear above the waveform.

Occlusion Pressure

Measurement of occlusion pressure (P 0.1) is an added option to the Evita 2 Dura that functions the same way as in the E-4. This procedure can be automatically performed by selecting the MANEUVER menu touch pad, then the P 0.1 screen value (dial knob), and then the START screen soft pad using the dial knob. To start the measurement, press the dial knob. The maneuver is automatically performed, and the value for occlusion pressure is shown on the screen.

Carbon Dioxide Monitoring

Carbon dioxide monitoring (single-breath carbon dioxide analysis) can also be added to the Evita 2 Dura with the addition of the end-tidal carbon dioxide ($etCO_2$) option. As with the E-4, values for $etCO_2$, CO_2 production, and dead space can be analyzed, calibrated, and displayed. Dead space is measured as series dead space, a function of mechanical, not physiologic, dead space.

Special Function Touch Pads

As mentioned previously, there is a set of touch pads to the left of the screen on the front panel of the E-2 Dura. Their functions are explained here.

Nebulizer Touch Pad

The NEBULIZER control functions during any adult or pediatric ventilatory mode. Pressing the NEBULIZER touch pad turns the nebulizer gas source on, displays a nebulizer symbol and message on the screen, and lights the LED on the touch pad. Gas flows through the nebulizer outlet only during inspiration in the adult settings. In adult modes, it automatically maintains the set V_E and very closely approximates the set $O_2\%$ ($\pm 4\%$). During pediatric ventilation, nebulization is continuous and available during pressure-targeted modes of ventilation: PCV+, CPAP, PSV, PCV-SIMV, and APRV, as well as in all volume modes to which Autoflow is added.

The nebulizer continues to operate for 30 minutes or until the pad is touched again. After its use, a "flow calibration" message appears to indicate that the nebulizer is off and the flow transducer is being automatically cleaned and recalibrated to ensure accurate measurements.

O_2 Increase Suction

The 100% O_2 suction touch pad is used to provide 100% oxygen for 3 minutes in adults and uses the set $O_2\%$ plus 25% in pediatric ventilation. When pressed, the LED on the pad is lit and the message "O_2 enrichment 180 s" appears at the bottom of the screen. This function operates in the same manner on the Dura as it does on the Evita and the E-4 and is described in the section on the Evita ventilator.

Inspiratory Hold

The INSPIR HOLD touch pad provides an inflation hold maneuver when pressed. When held down, it provides an inflation hold for as long as the pause is desired, up to a maximum of 15 seconds. When activated, either the current inspiration is held, or a new mandatory breath is delivered and the inspiration held. It is functional in all modes except CPAP unless a pressure-support level above zero is set.

Expiratory Hold

An expiratory hold maneuver can be performed using the EXP. HOLD touch pad. This manually prolongs the expiratory phase for as long as it is pressed, up to 15 seconds. It can be used to estimate end-expiratory pressure during any mode of ventilation. (When the measurements screen is up, press the EXP. HOLD key and have the patient perform an MIP maneuver; the value is displayed as the minimum pressure value at the start of the next breath.)

Ventilator Graphic Waveforms

The graphics monitor on the Dräger E-2 Dura is part of the main computer screen during standard operation. Additional waveforms can be viewed simultaneously, and different waveforms can be displayed during normal function. Trends and loops can be added as options to the E-2 Dura package.

Troubleshooting

Press the "I" (information) touch pad to access on-screen help on operating the ventilator or troubleshooting. The alarms and monitored information sections provide a great deal of assistance for solving the majority of problems that might occur with the Dura. In addition, the operator's manual contains a troubleshooting section that alphabetically lists all the extensive alarm messages, tells their priority level, gives common causes, and recommends remedies. The user is referred to the manual for review of this information. Additionally, Dräger products information can be viewed check their website: www.draeger.com.

Hamilton AMADEUS^{FT}

The Hamilton AMADEUS^{FT} ventilator is an early generation ventilator produced by Hamilton Medical Incorporated. Because newer models, such as the VEOLAR^{FT} and the Galileo, are now available, the discussion on this model has been moved to the EVOLVE site for this text.

Hamilton VEOLAR^{FT}

Power Source

The Hamilton VEOLAR^{FT} is marketed by Hamilton Medical, Inc (Reno, Nev.) (Figure 12-39).[1-4] It requires a standard 115-volt AC electrical outlet and normally uses air and oxygen high-pressure gas sources for operation (ranging from 29 to 116 psig). It is a pneumatically powered, microprocessor-controlled ventilator used in the management of pediatric and adult patients.

Internal Mechanism

The basic internal mechanisms of the VEOLAR^{FT} are similar to the AMADEUS^{FT} (see figure of the internal circuit on the EVOLVE site: AMADEUS^{FT}).* Air and oxygen sources enter through high-pressure lines connected in the back of the unit and individually pass through separate filters and solenoids. Gas flow from these electronic solenoids is monitored and blended in an electronic mixer to match the desired F_IO_2. A differential pressure transducer monitors the flow generated while the gases leave this mixing area. Gases are delivered to an 8-L aluminum reservoir that is pressurized up to 350 cm H_2O. When the reservoir is filled to maximum pressure, the differential pressure transducer shuts down the flow of the blended gases. There is a pressure-relief valve on the reservoir set for 400 cm H_2O to avoid overpressurization. The advantage of the reservoir is that it permits the ventilator to provide high peak inspiratory flows to 180 L/min, thus doubling the rate of source gas mixing that occurs at levels up to 90 L/min.

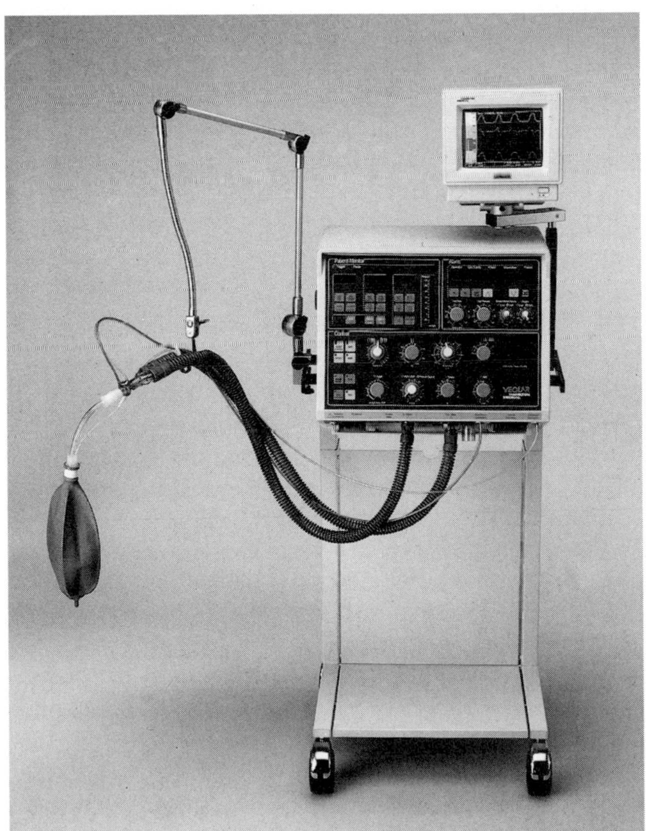

Figure 12-39 The Hamilton VEOLAR^{FT} (Courtesy Hamilton Medical, Inc, Reno, Nev.)

Gas passing from the reservoir is directed to the patient through a servo-controlled flow valve made up of an electromagnetically actuated plunger, a position sensor, and a differential pressure transducer (see Chapters 8 and 11). The motion of the flow valve is governed by the ventilator's electronic control processor, which takes information from the control panel about what it measures as flow demand and establishes how the gas will be delivered by the flow control valve. This ensures accurate volume and flow delivery to the patient.

After leaving the reservoir, the gas passes a pressure-release valve set at about 120 cm H_2O, and an antisuffocation valve, which opens if there is an emergency to allow the patient to breathe room air. There is also an oxygen-sensing fuel cell in this area through which the inspiratory flow of gas passes before entering the main inspiratory line of the patient circuit.

During exhalation, air leaves the patient and passes through the main expiratory line and finally through the expiratory valve. The expiratory valve contains a large silicon diaphragm with a big metal plate in the center to help stabilize the diaphragm. The movement of the expiratory valve is governed by an electromagnetic plunger. The plunger closes the valve during inspiration and controls the resistance through the valve on expiration to control the selected PEEP/CPAP levels.

**Many of the inner workings and features of the VEOLAR^{FT} are similar to those of the AMADEUS^{FT}. For a description of AMADEUS^{FT}, see the discussion on the EVOLVE site.*

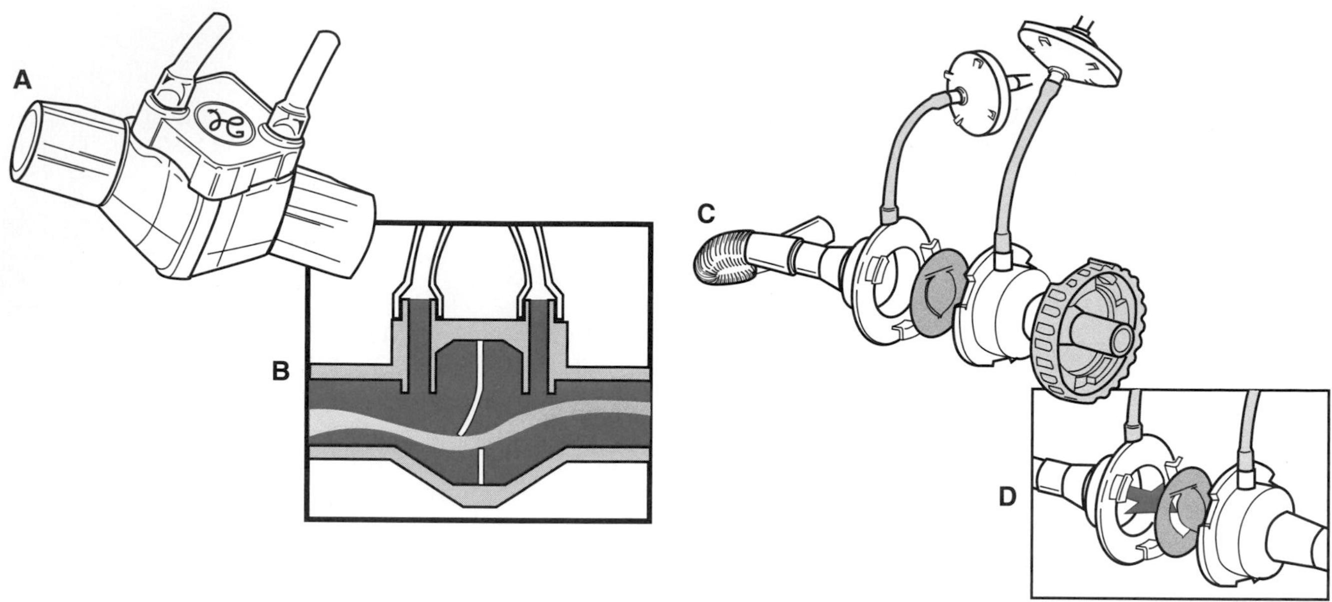

Figure 12-40 This series of drawings illustrates how a variable orifice pneumotachograph works. **A,** the variable orifice pneumotachograph used to measure flows and volumes at the patient Y connection on Hamilton ventilators; **B,** a cross-section through the pneumotachograph, or flow sensor; **C,** a line drawing of an early pneumotachograph used with the Hamilton VEOLAR^{FT}; **D,** a drawing that shows the displacement of the diaphragm during gas flow.

Proximal Pressure/Flow Monitoring Sensor

The VEOLAR^{FT} uses a flow sensor, which is a variable-orifice pneumotachograph. The flow sensor is placed at the patient's Y connector, to monitor flow, volume, and pressure (Figure 12-40). (See Chapter 8 for an explanation of the function of pneumotachographs.) This flow sensor, along with pressure transducers within the ventilator, gathers information for display in the monitoring section (See the following discussion of controls and alarms).

Controls and Alarms

The VEOLAR^{FT} ventilator's front panel is divided into three sections. The top two sections are for patient monitoring and alarms; the lower section contains the controls (Figure 12-41).

Control Panel

The control panel has two rows of control knobs and a set of eight touch pads (left side). The first row of knobs includes RESPIRATORY RATE (fSIMV and fCMV), V_T, and % cycle time (inspiration, pause, expiration, and flow pattern).

Two respiratory frequencies are controlled by the rate knob: CMV and SIMV frequency. The light-colored knob adjusts the rate in the CMV mode (from 5 to 120 breaths/min). This setting is also important because it determines the TCT for a mandatory breath. For example, if rate is 10 breaths/min, TCT is (60 sec)/(10 breaths/min), or 6 seconds. It is active in A/C, SIMV, PCV, sigh, and apnea back-up ventilation. The dark-colored knob sets the rate in SIMV (0.5 to 60 breaths/min). It is active in SIMV, PCV-SIMV, and apnea back-up. Suppose the following parameters are set:

- SIMV rate = 4 breaths/min
- CMV rate = 10 breaths/min (TCT = 6 seconds)

A mandatory breath occurs no more than every 15 seconds because the rate is set at 4 breaths/min. A complete mandatory breath time is 6 seconds; the patient has the remaining 9 seconds to breathe spontaneously.

The TIDAL VOLUME control can be adjusted from 20 to 2000 mL. The % CYCLE TIME knob is a dual knob similar to the RESPIRATORY RATE control that independently determines T_I, T_E, and pause time as percentages of TCT. (See Box 12-40 for an example and Clinical Rounds 12-13 and 12-14 for practice problems.) The last control in this row is the FLOW PATTERN control, which provides six different options (seven in older models) for inspiratory waveforms during volume ventilation (see Figure 12-41). Inspiratory flow patterns and peak flow are explained in Box 12-41.[1,2]

The second row of control knobs consists of the following: PRESSURE TRIGGER, PEEP/CPAP, and PINSP (SUPPORT), oxygen, and FLOW TRIGGER.

The PRESSURE TRIGGER control allows for pressure-triggered breaths (–1 to –10 cm H_2O, or off) when the FLOW TRIGGER control is off. When FLOW TRIGGER is on, an internal setting of –3 cm H_2O acts as a back-up to the flow trigger. The PRESSURE TRIGGER setting is the amount of pressure below baseline that must be generated by patient effort in order to trigger a breath.*

The pressure trigger is PEEP compensated.

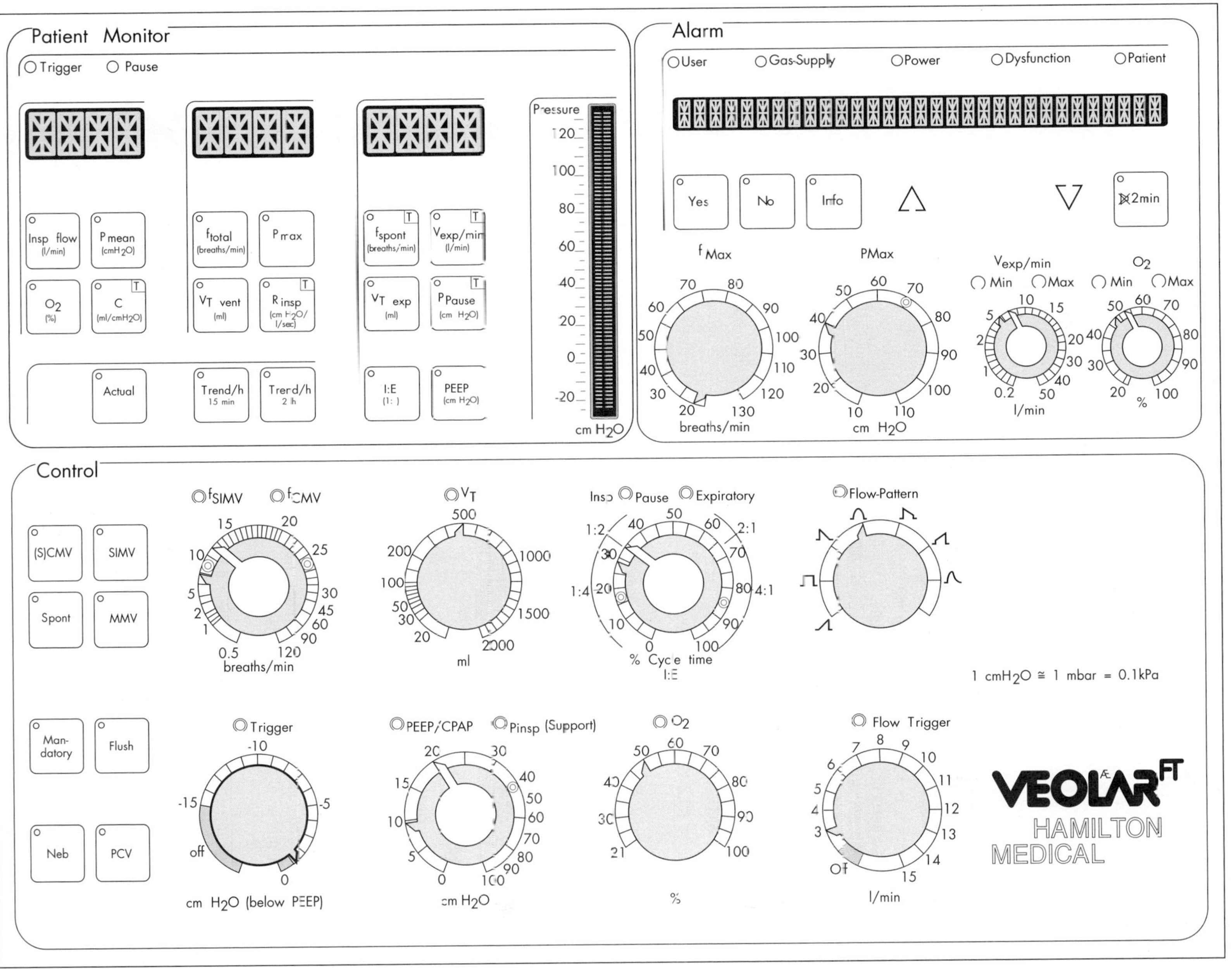

Figure 12-41 The operating panel of the Hamilton VEOLAR^{FT}. (Courtesy Yvon Dupuis.)

The PEEP/CPAP, PINSP (SUPPORT) control contains two control dials. The dark colored dial sets the PEEP/CPAP level (0 to 50 cm H_2O), and the light colored dial determines the inspiratory pressure for pressure-support breaths and is the difference between the set peak pressure (PIP) and PEEP. For example, if the dark colored pointer is at 10 cm H_2O, and the light-colored pointer is at 20 cm H_2O, then PEEP is 10 cm H_2O, pressure support is 10 cm H_2O, and PIP is 20 cm H_2O.

The oxygen control sets the desired oxygen percentage. The ventilator has a built-in oxygen analyzer that measures inspired oxygen levels and displays this value in the monitor section. The FLOW TRIGGER control sets the flow (in liters/minute) that the patient must draw from the expiratory base flow in order to flow-trigger a breath. The flow is measured by the flow sensor at the patient Y connector. The expiratory base flow in liters/minute is twice the FLOW TRIGGER setting. Base flow is only present at the end of expiration. Base flow is delayed at the beginning of exhalation to allow the patient to complete the expiratory phase without an increase in resistance.

A FLOW TRIGGER level of 5 to 6 L/min is recommended for most patients. Patients with minimal inspiratory effort may benefit by levels set at 3 to 4 L/min, which may also be more appropriate for pediatric patients. For patients with high inspiratory flow demands or with an air leak, a setting of 8 L/min or more may be more appropriate. Flow-triggering is available in all modes of ventilation. Even when flow-triggering is not selected, a base flow of 4 L/min is present during the end-expiratory phase to provide flow to patients as soon as they begin to make an inspiratory effort.

The left side of the control panel contains the touch pad controls. The first set of four are mode controls. The modes are reviewed in the discussion of modes of ventilation later in this section. The second set of touch pads contains the control for a fifth mode of ventilation, PCV. Also in this set of controls are touch pads for MANUAL, FLUSH, and NEBULIZER. The MANUAL touch pad delivers a manually triggered mandatory volume- or pressure-targeted breath based on the control panel settings. The FLUSH control allows for a rapid change in F_IO_2 by flushing the system with 60 L/min of fresh gas, based on the selected oxygen percentage setting.

Box 12-40 % Cycle Time Control

On the % CYCLE TIME, the dark-colored knob sets T_I for mandatory breaths. T_I is set as a percentage of TCT. For example, if TCT is 6 seconds (rate = 10 breaths/min) and %T_I is set at 20%, 20% of 6 seconds is 1.2 seconds (T_I).

The light-colored knob sets the point where inspiratory pause ends. For example, %T_I is 20%, and TCT is again 6 seconds. T_I is 1.2 seconds.

Pause (light-colored knob) is set at 30%. Pause time = 30% - 20% = 10% of TCT. Pause is 0.6 seconds.

Total T_I = T_I + pause = 1.2 seconds + 0.6 seconds = 1.8 seconds.

The resulting I:E ratio can be read on the outside scale of the % CYCLE TIME knob.

Box 12-41 Flow Patterns and Flow Rate of the VEOLAR[FT]

Flow Patterns of Waveforms

The six flow patterns include the following:

1. Constant (rectangular or square)—flow remains constant during inspiration.
2. Full descending ramp—flow begins at the highest value and decreases to zero when the V_T has been delivered.
3. Sine—flow begins and ends at zero; at mid-inspiration, flow is most rapid; at this point, one half of the V_T has been delivered.
4. 50% descending ramp—flow begins at a high value and falls linearly to 50% of the initial flow, at which point all the V_T has been delivered.
5. 50% ascending ramp—flow starts at a low value and increases to twice the initial flow, at which point all the V_T has been delivered.
6. Modified sine—similar to sine where flow begins slow, but here it accelerates more rapidly to a high value, at which time about $^1/_3$ of the V_T has been delivered; flow then descends to zero at end-inspiration.

The pure ascending ramp was omitted from the updated version because clinical research did not support its usefulness. (*Note*: If T_I is set at less than 0.5 seconds, the delivered flow waveform will always be constant, regardless of the flow waveform setting.)

Inspiratory Flow Rate

The patient monitor can display the peak flow measured by the servo-control valve. You can also calculate inspiratory flows from the set V_T, T_I, and flow pattern (flow = V_T/T_I).

For example, given the following settings:

- V_T = 1.0 L (1000 mL)
- Rate = 15 breaths/min (TCT = 60 seconds/15 = 4 seconds)
- %T_I = 25% seconds (T_I = %T_I × TCT = 0.25 × 4 seconds; T_I = 1 second)
- Waveform = constant

Flow = 1.0 L/1 second, or 60 L/60 seconds = 60 L/min.

Effect of Flow Pattern on Peak Flow

- For the full descending pattern, the peak flow is twice that of the constant flow.
- For the 50% descending or ascending flow patterns, peak flow will be 1.33 times that of the constant flow.
- For the sine wave, peak flow is 1.57 times that of the constant flow.

CLINICAL ROUNDS 12-13

The respiratory therapist sets the % cycle time control on the VEOLAR^FT as follows: T_I is 30% (tip of dark-colored control at 30%) and 45% (tip of light-colored control at 45%). What is the inspiratory pause time as a percentage of TCT? What percent of TCT is the T_E?

See Appendix A for the answer.

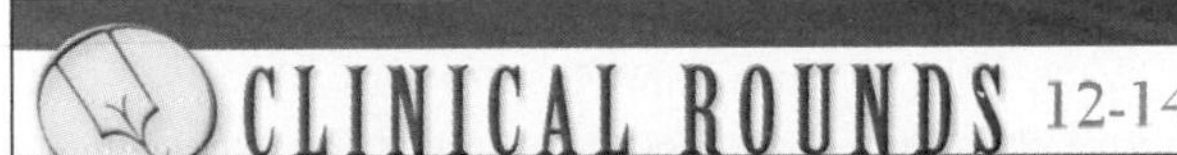

CLINICAL ROUNDS 12-14

A respiratory therapist is adjusting the controls for volume ventilation on an VEOLAR^FT. V_T is set at 0.7 L (700 mL), and rate at 10 breaths/min. The desired I:E ratio is 1:4. What setting should be selected on the % cycle time control?

See Appendix A for the answer.

The NEBULIZER control activates the nebulizer system. Blended gases at the set F_IO_2 are diverted from the internal pressurized reservoir to the nebulizer connector, which is a small nipple connector below the front panel near the other patient circuit connectors. It provides gas flow for 15 minutes, unless the NEB control is pressed again. The nebulizer gas flow slightly increases V_T delivery.

Monitor and Alarm Panel

The upper section of the operating panel contains monitored information and alarm controls (see Figure 12-41). The left side contains monitored information, and the right side contains alarm information and controls.

In the left section, directly under the words "Patient Monitor," are two lights. The TRIGGER light illuminates when the ventilator detects a patient's inspiratory effort, resulting in gas flow to the patient. The PAUSE light indicates that an inspiratory pause of at least 0.2 seconds is occurring.

The remainder of the patient display area contains three digital display windows and a vertical pressure bar graph. The operator can select the information seen in each display window. By pressing the appropriate touch pad below the window, the operator selects the variable to be displayed. When it is selected, the LED on the pad illuminates. For example, if the operator presses INSP. FLOW, the numerical value in the digital window will be the inspiratory peak flow in liters/minute.

The left window can display the following:

1. Peak inspiratory flow (INSP. FLOW, in liters/minute) for a mandatory or spontaneous breath
2. Mean airway pressure (PMEAN, in centimeters of water)
3. Oxygen percentage measured by the built-in oxygen analyzer (O_2 %)
4. Lung compliance (C, milliliters/centimeters of water)

A plateau pressure reading of at least 10% of the TCT is necessary to determine compliance (and also airway resistance). To obtain a plateau, simply separate the T_I% and T_E% dials on the % CYCLE TIME control.* The percent difference between the two is the % pause based on TCT. When the PAUSE LED flashes, this gives a plateau pressure measurement that the computer can use to calculate compliance and resistance. (Be sure to return the % CYCLE TIME dials to their original position.)

The central display window can provide information on the following:

1. Total respiratory rate (f_{TOTAL}, in breaths/minute)
2. Maximum pressure, or peak inspiratory pressure (PMAX, in centimeters of water)
3. Ventilator tidal volume (i.e., the volume that leaves the ventilator during a mandatory breath) (V_T VENT, in milliliters)
4. Airway resistance, calculated from the pressure change during inspiration and the average flow during inspiration (RINSP, in centimeters of water/liter/second)

A plateau pressure reading (minimum 10%) is also needed for the computer to calculate resistance.

The right window in the patient monitor area provides the following information:

1. Spontaneous respiratory rate (fSPONT, in breaths/min)
2. Expired minute volume measured at the patient's airway ($\dot{V}$EXP/min, in liters/minute)
3. Expired tidal volume measured at the patient's airway (V_T EXP, in milliliters)
4. Inspiratory pause pressure (PPAUSE, in centimeters of water)†
5. I:E ratio (Earlier versions of the VEOLAR^FT are labeled "I:E" and provide the I:E ratio reduced to a 1:__ value (i.e., if T_I = 2 seconds and T_E = 4 seconds, the I:E ratio is displayed as 1:2). Newer versions of the VEOLAR^FT are labeled INSP TIME, in seconds)
6. PEEP/CPAP display the baseline pressure (PEEP/CPAP, in centimeters of water).

There are three more touch pads beneath the first two patient monitor panels. When the pad is pressed, it displays the currently measured (actual) value of the parameter selected. When the TREND/H 15 min LED is pressed, the computer estimates a trend of what it expects to see over the

It is best to increase T_E% so that the peak flow does not change.

†Pause pressure can only be obtained with an inspiratory pause control during a mandatory breath in SIMV or CMV modes.

next 15 minutes based on the last hour of readings for fSPONT, $\dot{V}$EXP/min, C, and RINSP.

When TREND/H 2H is selected, the computer predicts a trend for the next two hours based on the last hour of calculations for the same parameters. Both touch pads automatically go back to current readings after 10 seconds.

The VEOLAR[FT] obtains monitoring information from the flow sensor at the patient's airway and from the internal pressure transducer. It uses the flow sensor at the patient's Y connector to determine expired volume and $\dot{V}_E$. Because of its location at the patient's airway, these volumes are the actual exhaled volumes and do not include volume compressed in the patient circuit. The value for expired $\dot{V}_E$ is based on the last eight breaths (updated breath by breath) and displayed in liters/minute. The volume that actually leaves the ventilator is monitored by the integral servo-control valve. These values can be monitored and displayed in the monitor panel.

The internal pressure transducer monitors peak, mean, and PEEP pressures, which can all be displayed on the monitor panel. Mean pressure is calculated based on the last eight breaths and is updated with every breath. The pressure manometer is a lighted, bar graph display vertically mounted in the central part of the upper panel. An optional pressure monitoring feature is also available and is described in the discussion of special features later in this section.

The alarm section contains adjustable control alarms, a row of control touch pads, a display window, and five LEDs (see Figure 12-41). The adjustable alarm specifications are listed in Table 12-10. The bottom row of control knobs includes HIGH RATE, HIGH PRESSURE, HIGH/LOW $\dot{V}_E$, and LOW/HIGH OXYGEN LIMITS. The $\dot{V}_E$ and oxygen knobs each contain two dials that allow high and low alarm limits ($\dot{V}_E$ and O_2%) to be set.

The row of touch pads provided include YES, NO, INFO, ALARM RECALL, up and down arrows, and a 2-MINUTE ALARM SILENCE. The YES and NO controls allow input to be given to the computer in response to messages in the message window. INFO, which is called ALARM RECALL on newer versions, can bring up information and alarm events during multiple alarm conditions. The up and down arrows can be used to give information to the computer during calibration, option set-up, and programming of modes (e.g., MMV and PCV). The ALARM SILENCE control quiets the audible alarms for 2 minutes when pressed; the LED on the pad illuminates. If pressed a second time, the alarms can reactivate. This control can also be used to prevent back-up ventilation from activating. For example, if the operator wants to disconnect the patient from the ventilator for some reason, this would normally cause several alarm conditions, as well as trigger apnea ventilation. By pressing the ALARM SILENCE button, apnea back-up ventilation is prevented for 2 minutes.

A display window is also located in the alarm section. A written message of an active alarm appears in this window. When more than one alarm is active, the operator can bring up alarms chronologically by pressing the INFO or the ALARM RECALL pad. When an important datum is available, such as "Flow Sensor Calibration Needed," this LED flashes. A continuously lit LED indicates that data or alarm information is available. Pressing the pad accesses the information that is displayed for 10 seconds. Information available besides alarm data include:

1. Patient circuit = pediatric
2. Flow sensor cal needed
3. Apnea back-up on
4. Apnea time = 40 seconds
5. No O_2 cell in use
6. Sigh on

The five diodes at the top of the alarm panel illuminate when one of these alarm parameters has been violated. These alarms include USER (OPERATOR), GAS SUPPLY, POWER, DYSFUNCTION (INOPERATIVE), and PATIENT. The USER or OPERATOR LED lights when the person operating the unit must take some action (e.g., reconnect the patient to the ventilator). An illuminated gas supply LED means that one or both of the high-pressure source gases has fallen to a pressure below 29 psig. The POWER LED lights up when electrical power has been lost. The DYSFUNCTION or INOPERATIVE LED means that an internal microprocessor error has occurred, and a technical fault number appears in the window. The PATIENT alarm is often caused by the patient (e.g., during a cough, which triggers a HIGH-PRESSURE alarm as well). When GAS SUPPLY, POWER, or DYSFUNCTIONAL (INOPERATIVE) alarms occur, the ALARM SILENCE button cannot silence the audible alarm, and the internal ambient valve opens to allow for spontaneous ventilation.

Table 12-10 Alarm specifications for the VEOLAR[FT]

Alarm	Range
High rate	20-130 breaths/min
High pressure	10-110 cm H_2O
Low expiratory $\dot{V}_E$	0.2-50 L/min
High expiratory $\dot{V}_E$	0.2-50 L/min
Low O_2 %	18%-103%
High O_2 %	18%-103%
Apnea	20 or 40 seconds
Fail to cycle	25 seconds
Disconnection	Two breaths (sensed by flow sensor)
V_T mismatch	Three breaths (flow sensor vs. setting error)
Flow out of range	Flow exceeds 180 L/min

Box 12-42 Nonadjustable Alarms on the VEOLAR^{FT}

- Loss of PEEP
- Apnea
- Failure to cycle
- Failure to set trigger
- Flow out of range
- Circuit disconnection from either the ventilator's or the patient's side of the flow sensor
- Mismatch of inspiratory or expiratory tidal volumes (flow sensor measurements vs. control setting of output)
- Flow sensor in wrong direction
- Low pressure for air or oxygen supplies or both
- Low internal reservoir pressure
- Inappropriate or absent power
- Various internal technical failure alarms

Nonadjustable alarms are also available and provide messages in the display window of the alarm panel. The nonadjustable alarms are listed in Box 12-42.

Modes of Ventilation

The VEOLAR^{FT} has the following modes available: A/C, SIMV, spontaneous (including pressure support), MMV, PCV, and SIMV/PCV. When a mode of ventilation is selected, the touch pad must be pressed for 2 seconds before a change occurs to prevent accidental mode changes. The LED on that touch pad then illuminates. Green LEDs adjacent to the knobs for specific controls (e.g., V_T) illuminate when the control is functional. For example, the LED for V_T illuminates when the A/C mode is selected, but not when PCV is selected.

Assist/Control (volume-targeted)

The A/C mode is a patient- or time-triggered, volume-targeted, time-cycled ventilatory mode. The controls for rate and V_T establish the minimum rate and set volume delivery. The % CYCLE control determines the I:E ratio and any pause setting desired. Trigger sensitivity is set to allow patient-triggering. (*Note*: A time period of 0.2 seconds must pass after expiratory flow begins before a patient can trigger another breath. This helps prevent breath stacking.) PEEP/CPAP (dark-colored control) can also be used to provide a positive-pressure baseline.

Synchronized Intermittent Mandatory Ventilation (SIMV) (volume-targeted)

The SIMV control provides volume-targeted SIMV ventilation. Breaths are patient- or time-triggered and time-cycled. A minimum number of volume-targeted mandatory breaths are set using the SIMV control. Spontaneous breaths occur from baseline pressure between the mandatory breaths. Spontaneous breaths can include pressure support. As with the A/C mode, there is a brief (0.2 second) period at the end of inspiration (beginning of expiratory flow) of a mandatory breath during which another mandatory breath cannot be triggered. It is important to set both the CMV rate, which establishes INSPIRATORY FLOW, RATE, and the SIMV RATE to determine minimum mandatory breath rate delivery (Box 12-43).

Box 12-43 Effects of CMV Rate and % Cycle Time in SIMV

While setting up SIMV ventilation, the initial CMV rate should be 15 breaths/min and the % T_I should be 33% to allow adequate flow for most patients. Setting CMV high increases the peak flow, but does not affect the maximum set SIMV rate. One should not set the CMV lower than 15 breaths/min in the SIMV mode unless very slow flows are desired, which is unlikely.

Spontaneous

In the spontaneous mode, the ventilator provides flow to the patient to maintain the baseline pressure and to continuously monitor the patient. The spontaneous mode also provides an apnea back-up ventilation mode. Spontaneous breaths can be assisted with pressure support. CPAP may also be added along with sigh breaths, if desired.

Pressure-Support Ventilation (PSV)

PSV is available for spontaneous breaths in spontaneous ventilation, PCV-SIMV, SIMV (volume targeted), and MMV. Breaths are always patient-triggered (pressure or flow). The mode is set by using the dual PEEP/CPAP and pressure-support [PINSP(SUPPORT)] control. The dark-colored dial sets the baseline pressure, and the light-colored dial sets the maximum inspiratory pressure above PEEP/CPAP. The amount of PS is the difference between the two settings.

During PSV, a rapid gas flow is directed into the patient circuit as soon as inspiration is detected. The ventilator reaches and sustains the target pressure until gas flow drops to 25% of the peak flow. The percentage at which flow cycling occurs can be changed. This option is set prior to ventilation (see Special Features/Dip Switch section, option 6). This option, which is also called the expiratory trigger sensitivity (ETS), determines when inspiration ends during pressure support or spontaneous breathing. This breath termination is based on end-inspiratory flow. For example, when ETS is "off," a spontaneous or PS breath flow cycles at 25% of measured peak inspiratory flow. When activated, the operator can select flow-cycling at one of the following settings: 12%, 18%, 31%, or 37% of peak inspiratory flow. Some clinicians favor lower cycling percentages for small pediatric patients. Patients with chronic obstructive pulmonary disease may benefit from higher percentage settings.

If a leak is present that prevents flow from dropping to the flow-cycling value, inspiratory flow will end after 3 seconds. If the patient circuit is disconnected, a LOW INTERNAL PRESSURE alarm may occur. This alarm occurs because the ventilator tries to increase the flow to maintain the set PS level. Because this cannot be done, the internal reservoir will lose pressure, and the alarm will sound.*

Minimum Minute Ventilation (MMV)

Minimum minute ventilation (MMV) is a patient-triggered, pressure-targeted, minute-volume–guaranteed mode of ventilation. As described in Chapter 11, this mode is a servo-controlled mode of ventilation used for weaning patients from ventilatory support. MMV is normally set at a value less than that provided during regular ventilation. When the patient's exhaled $\dot{V}_E$ drops below the set MMV level, the ventilator provides increased levels of pressure-support ventilation to spontaneous breaths until the exhaled $\dot{V}_E$ is maintained at the set MMV level.

To better understand how MMV operates on the VEOLAR^{FT}, the set up of this mode is reviewed. First, press the MMV touch pad. In the display window of the alarm panel, a flashing message appears: "X L/min." Use the up or down arrows in the alarm panel to set the desired MMV (in liters/minute), and press YES when you have the desired value. The unit then switches to MMV. It is also appropriate to set an inspiratory pressure level with the pressure support control that will achieve an acceptable V_T for the patient and reduce work of breathing.

As the patient initiates a pressure-supported breath, the ventilator monitors the patient's exhaled volumes, rate, and pressure-support level for eight breaths (updated breath by breath). If the predicted $\dot{V}_E$ is more than the level set on the MMV control, the ventilator does not interfere with the operation of the unit or the patient's breathing. If the predicted exhaled $\dot{V}_E$ based on these calculations falls below the set MMV, the ventilator begins to increase the PS level in increments of 1 cm H_2O. Any changes in pressure can be observed by watching the peak pressure display in the patient monitor section. As a result of pressure changes, each patient-initiated breath receives slightly more pressure, and thus more volume, until the minimum acceptable $\dot{V}_E$ and the MMV level are achieved. As the patient improves and the $\dot{V}_E$ becomes higher than the set MVV, the pressures decrease in increments of 1 cm H_2O.

There are safety limits of pressure within which the ventilator must operate during MMV. The pressure cannot go below the set pressure support level (plus PEEP). The absolute minimum is 5 cm H_2O of PEEP. It cannot go higher than the high-pressure setting, which should be set at 10 cm H_2O above the initial pressure-support value that provided an acceptable starting V_T.*

Another safety feature during MMV is the ventilator will not increase the PS level by more than 30 cm H_2O to a maximum of 50 cm H_2O (PS+PEEP). No mandatory breaths occur during MMV unless an apnea ventilation option is set and apnea is detected, at which time the apnea back-up ventilation mode initiates. Clinical Rounds 12-15 provides an example situation of the use of MMV on the Hamilton VEOLAR^{FT}.

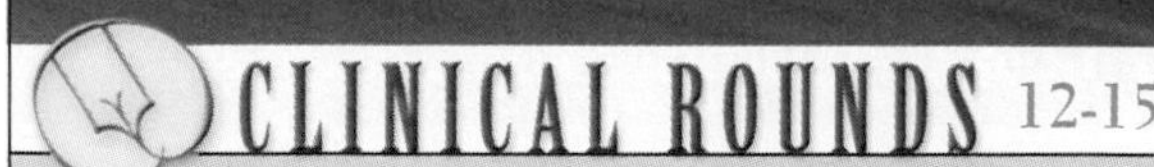

A respiratory therapist sets an MMV level of 6.0 L/min on a patient. Initial settings and monitored values are as follows:

- PS = 12 cm H_2O
- PEEP = 5 cm H_2O
- V_T exhaled = 0.6 L (600 mL)
- Respiratory rate (f) = 12 breaths/min
- $\dot{V}_E$ exhaled = 7.2 L
- Alveolar ventilation ($\dot{V}_A$ = 5.4 L/min

$[(V_T - V_D) \times f]$, where V_D = 150 mL

The patient develops a pleural effusion, exhaled V_T drops to 0.3 L, and respiratory rate increases to 18 breaths/min. Exhaled $\dot{V}_E$ drops to 5.4 L/min, and the patient's $\dot{V}_A$ has dropped to 2.7 L/min.

$(0.03 - 0.15) \times 18 = 2.7$

How will the ventilator respond to this situation? What is an important alarm to set when using MMV?

See Appendix A for the answer.

Pressure-Control Ventilation (PCV)

PCV is a patient- or time-triggered, pressure-targeted, time-cycled mode of ventilation. It is available for A/C (PCV-CMV) or SIMV (PCV-SIMV) breathing patterns. In PCV, setting T_I, pause time, and T_E is the same as in A/C.

To establish PCV on the VEOLAR^{FT}, select the PCV touch pad. When this is activated (LED lights), a message will appear in the display window of the alarm section: "PCV-CMV PCV-SIMV," one of which will be flashing. Use the YES and NO touch pads to select the desired option.

After this, the message display window provides a number (flashing) that is equal to the PEEP setting plus 20 cm H_2O. For example, if PEEP is 10 cm H_2O, the window will read 30 cm H_2O. Use the up or down arrows in the alarm section to increase or decrease the desired pressure value for PCV. For example, for PCV = 20 cm H_2O and PEEP = 5 cm H_2O,

*When you need to disconnect a patient on PSV, you should turn off PS first.

*Be sure to set a high rate alarm so that you will be alerted if the spontaneous rate becomes too high.

Box 12-44 Important Clinical Note about the PVC Mode

Because of variable tidal volumes during pressure ventilation, such as PCV and PSV, the clinician should set high and low $\dot{V}_E$ and high rate alarms carefully to provide an alert if the patient's lung condition changes.

The high-pressure alarm control should also be set 5 to 10 cm H_2O above the value in the windows. Just because the ventilator is in the PCV mode does not mean the pressure cannot be exceeded. If the patient coughs, for example, pressure increases. The high-pressure alarm control prevents circuit pressure from exceeding its set value (10 to 110 cm H_2O). If the set level is reached, inspiration ends. (*Note:* This control also adjusts a mechanical pressure release, which is automatically set 10 cm H_2O above the high-pressure alarm setting. If the pressure continues to rise for any reason [e.g., patient coughing], pressure is released through a separate outlet.)

scroll down to a value of 25 cm H_2O. Remember the value of the peak value setting includes PEEP and the PC pressure level. In this example, the target pressure in PCV is 20 cm H_2O plus 5 cm H_2O of PEEP, or 25 cm H_2O (Ppeak).

After the desired pressure is set, choose the YES touch pad to activate the PCV mode. The minimum PCV level is the baseline pressure (PEEP) plus 5 cm H_2O. To change the pressure, use the up or down arrows, and then push YES to activate. Pressing NO returns the key pad to the current setting so the operator can read the peak pressure above PEEP. Box 12-44 provides an important clinical note about this mode.

SIMV with Pressure-Control Ventilation

PCV-SIMV provides SIMV ventilation with pressure-targeted breaths. Settings are established in the same way as with PCV, except that PCV-SIMV is selected instead of PCV. Between mandatory breaths at the set pressure, the patient can breathe spontaneously from the set baseline pressure. Spontaneous breaths can also be pressure supported (PSV), in which case they are flow-cycled (see the discussion of pressure support earlier in this section). Pressure for PS breaths is set using the light-colored dial of the PEEP/CPAP-pressure-support control.

It is advisable to use graphic monitoring whenever possible. The VEOLAR^{FT} can connect to the Hamilton LEONARDO computer graphics package (Figure 12-42).

Special Features

A hinged panel or drawer just below the control panel on the right side of the ventilator contains several other controls (Figure 12-43).

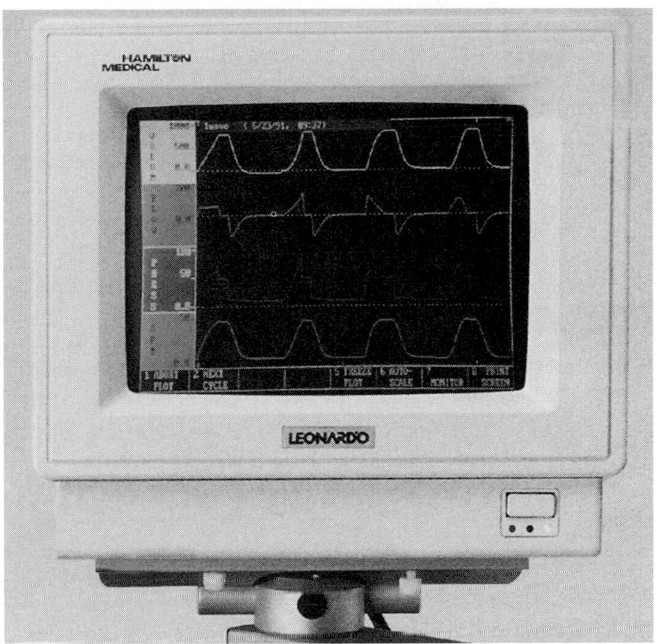

Figure 12-42 The Hamilton Leonardo Graphics Display Screen/Monitor. (Courtesy Hamilton Medical, Inc, Reno, Nev.)

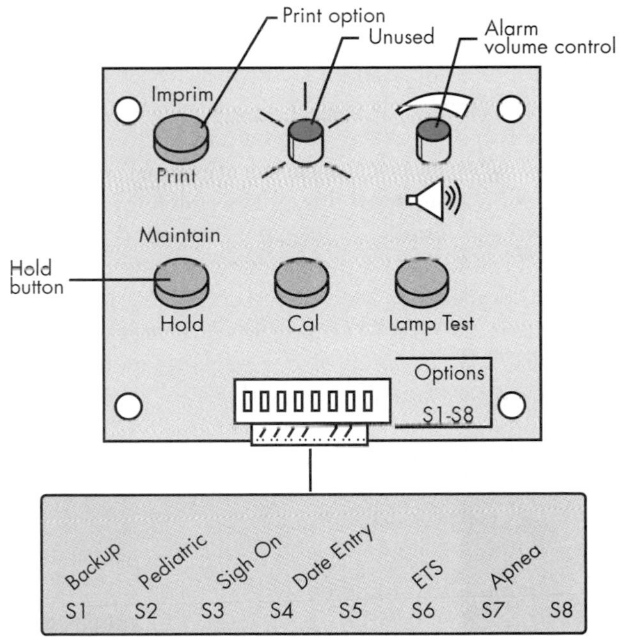

Figure 12-43 The additional controls under the front panel of the Hamilton VEOLAR^{FT}; see text for further explanation. (Courtesy Hamilton Medical, Inc, Reno, Nev.)

Additional Controls

The additional controls include an optional PRINT control; an unused control for future options; an ALARM VOLUME control; a CALIBRATION button, which initiates calibration (performed before patient use); a LAMP test, which illuminates the lamps on the control panel; and a HOLD control, which

Box 12-45 The Function of the Hold Control on the VEOLAR^{FT}

When HOLD is pressed during exhalation, it stops the delivery of the next breath (i.e., the valve closes when inspiratory flow is detected) and keeps the exhalation valve closed for measuring end-expiratory pressure or auto-PEEP.

To read this value, select the PEEP touch pad in the monitoring section. The HOLD button can also be used to estimate a patient's maximum inspiratory pressure (MIP). Again, press HOLD during expiration. When the expiratory valve closes (beginning of inspiratory flow), the PEEP display acts as a scrolling pressure manometer. The MIP is the most negative value seen.

Pressing HOLD during inspiration closes the expiratory valve at the end of inspiration and provides a reading of plateau pressure.

can measure a patient's plateau pressure, auto-PEEP, and spontaneous MIP (i.e., negative inspiratory force [NIF]) (Box 12-45).

DIP Switches

In addition to the controls described above, there are eight option or DIP switches that are used to access optional functions and must be set before the ventilator is turned on. The microprocessor identifies which switches are on and off when it boots up. It performs this search only once—during the first second after the ventilator is turned on.

The following are the options for the VEOLAR^{FT}:

1. Option 1 programs the unit to switch to apnea back-up ventilation if apnea is detected. Apnea is determined to be present if no flow is detected by the flow sensor for 20 or 40 seconds, or when the exhaled $\dot{V}_E$ is <1 L/min. When apnea is present, the VEOLAR^{FT} switches to a back-up mode, and an alarm is activated (Box 12-46).
2. Option 2 is the pediatric selection.
3. Option 3 is sigh.
4. Options 4, 5, and 8 are for service personnel and must be in the off position.
5. Option 6 is ETS (expiratory trigger sensitivity).
6. Option 7 is the apnea time control. To select 20 seconds, use the off position. The on position is for 40 seconds.

Optional Pressure Measurement

The VEOLAR^{FT} provides an optional monitoring port for measuring pressures in other locations, such as above the carina. The small connection for the optional pressure sensor, if installed, is installed below the front panel in the lower right corner where the tubing connections are located. This pressure port can only be used for monitoring and does not affect any functions. The operator can choose internal or optional pressure monitoring by using the installed option switch designed for that purpose.

Box 12-46 Back-up Ventilation on the VEOLAR^{FT}

The type of ventilation provided during apnea back-up ventilation depends on which mode was functioning when the condition occurred.

If the mode is set on spontaneous (with or without CPAP or PSV) or MMV ventilation, the ventilator switches to SIMV. If the mode is SIMV, then the ventilator switches to A/C. If the mode is PCV-SIMV, the ventilator switches to PCV (A/C form). The back-up V_T or pressure (PCV) is the set value. The back-up rate is either the fCMV rate or the fSIMV rate (rate control knobs).

CLINICAL ROUNDS 12-16

A respiratory therapist wants to add sigh breaths to the VEOLAR^{FT}, but repeated pressing of the sigh touch pad fails to set this control. What could be the problem?

See Appendix A for the answer.

In the off position, internal pressure is used for all functions. In the on position, the internal pressure sensor is used for control purposes, and the optional sensor is used for information presented in the patient monitor section. The microprocessor only looks at this switch when the unit is turned on, so it must be in the desired position beforehand. Using the sensor requires that a small-bore tube with filter be attached externally to the nipple adapter located below the front panel near the patient circuit connectors. The small-bore tube is then connected to the desired measurement port, for example, on a special endotracheal tube to measure pressures above the carina.

Troubleshooting

Occasionally the operator has problems starting normal ventilator operation after the power switch is turned on. This may be because of the position of the DIP or option switches, the function of which should be checked before the power switch is turned on (Clinical Rounds 12-16).

The VEOLAR^{FT} has two microprocessors that continually monitor each other's operation and the function of the unit. A behavioral error will give a technical error message to alert the operator that the ventilator must be changed and the problem diagnosed. The software contains a series of tests that can be accessed with the help of the service manual and can be used to troubleshoot virtually any problem that might occur.

The expiratory valve diaphragm is a silicon and metal disc that seals the system during normal operation. Sometimes a bent or malformed disc causes problems, which could include circuit leaks or difficulty maintaining PEEP/CPAP levels.

The miniature pneumotachograph or flow sensor is located so close to the patient that build-up of secretions or moisture in the connecting tubes or in the sensor itself occurs. A purge flow of 0.5 mL/min through the sensor lines helps to maintain the tubes patency. The VEOLAR[FT] also autocalibrates the sensor every 20 minutes while the unit is operating to avoid any problems.

Additional information can be found in the operator's manual and by checking the company's website: www.hamilton-medical.com.

Hamilton GALILEO[1]

The GALILEO is manufactured in Switzerland by Hamilton Medical and was first introduced in the United States in December 1998 (Figure 12-44). It is marketed by Hamilton Medical Inc., of Reno, Nev. The unit is currently intended for use with adults, pediatrics, and infants (weighing ≥ 3.0 kg). A recently released version of the GALILEO is referred to as the Galileo Gold. This version adds several new options that will be described later in this section.

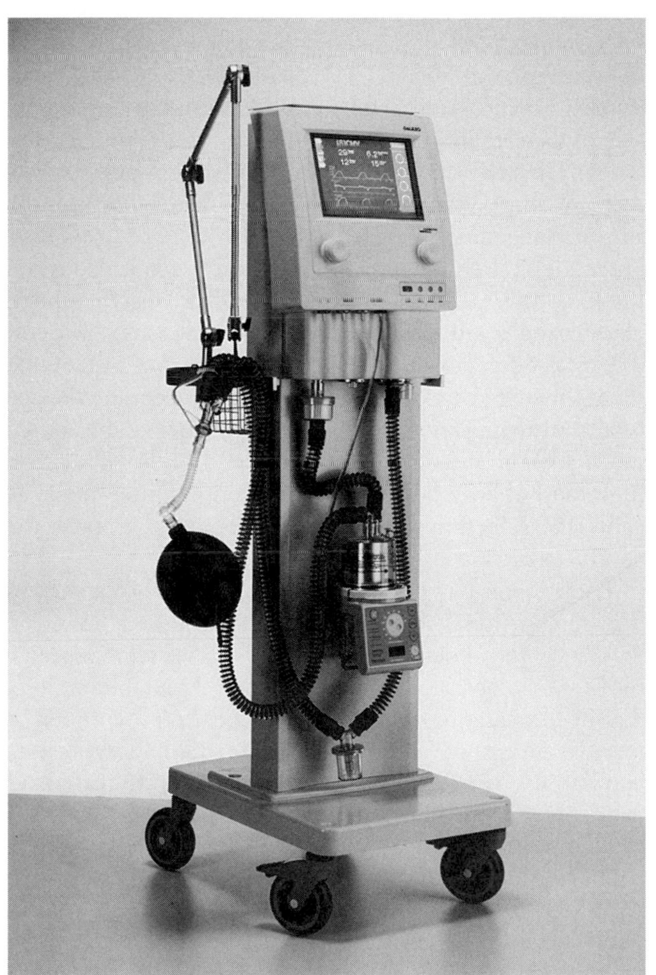

Figure 12-44 The Hamilton GALILEO. (Courtesy Hamilton Medical, Inc, Reno, Nev.)

Power Source

The GALILEO is a microprocessor-controlled unit that requires high-pressure gas and electricity for power. It normally operates from air and oxygen wall outlets (pressure range from 29 to 87 psig). An additional external compressor can be purchased as an option and can provide the required gas power source if no other sources are available. A 110-volt standard electrical outlet can provide the electrical power needed to operate the unit (range from 100 to 240 volt, alternating current). The main power on/off switch is on the back panel.

When the GALILEO is equipped with the new performance package, the ventilator contains an internal battery. If AC power fails, the ventilator automatically switches to internal battery power. This battery can provide about 1 hour of operating time when fully charged. Battery indicators provide information and the amount of charge remaining. A green indicator means the internal battery is full. A yellow indicator shows the battery is partially charged. A red indicator means the internal battery charge is low. An audible alarm will sound with a low battery charge. This alarm cannot be silenced. The ventilator needs to be connected to an AC power source. A battery test can be run to determine the charge level. This test should be performed before placing the patient on the ventilator.

The patient circuit has a proximal airway sensor that uses a variable-orifice differential pressure transducer to monitor and measure flow, volume, and pressure at the proximal airway (see Figures 12-40 and 12-45). The pressure transducer is a variable orifice pneumotachograph, the same type as that used in the VEOLAR[FT] (see also Chapter 8). The expiratory valve uses a variable-orifice expiratory threshold resistor that is also similar to those in the VEOLAR[FT]. The GALILEO has a built-in galvanic fuel cell for analyzing and monitoring delivered oxygen concentrations. Four small nipple connectors are close to the normal patient circuit main outlet and inlet (Figure 12-46). The two right adapters connect to the proximal airway pressure transducer. The next connector will power a small-volume nebulizer from a 15 psig independent compressor built into the ventilator. To determine if the GALILEO in use has the nebulizer, look at the setup screen. In the configure mode the nebulizer settings will be visible (different function screens will be reviewed later in this section).

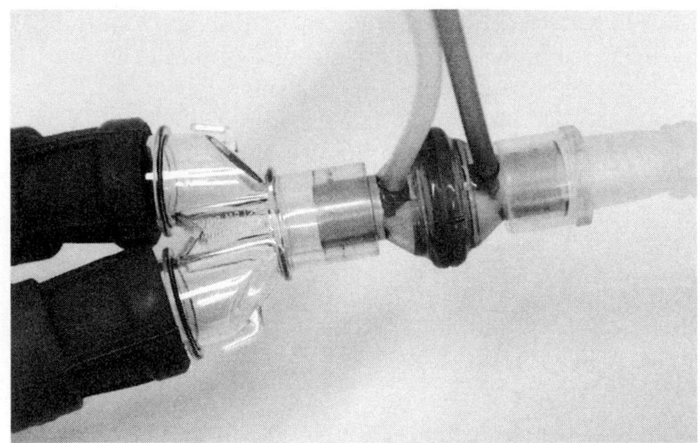

Figure 12-45 The flow sensor for the Hamilton GALILEO. (Courtesy Hamilton Medical, Inc, Reno, Nev.)

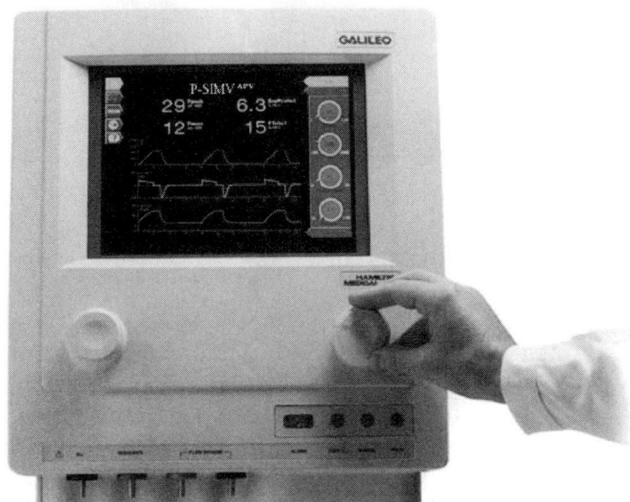

Figure 12-46 The front panel of the GALILEO. (Courtesy Hamilton Medical, Inc, Reno, Nev.)

When the nebulizer is available, it can provide 6 L/min of flow. (*Note*: The nebulizer should be placed in the inspiratory limb close to the Y connector. If it is placed between the flow sensor and the endotracheal tube, this will increase dead space ventilation.) Using the nebulizer results in a small increase in volume delivery, but does not affect F_IO_2.

The far left connector is for an auxiliary pressure line (Paux) that provides the option for adding an additional pressure monitor line for measurements such as carinal pressures or esophageal pressures. The auxiliary pressure line in the GALILEO is comparable to the optional (opt) pressure line in the VEOLAR^{FT}.

Internal Function

Two medical gas sources, air and oxygen, enter the internal circuit. Here their pressures are reduced. If one source becomes unavailable, the unit switches to the remaining gas source but remains operational. This affects F_IO_2 delivery, however. During normal operation, the gases are blended at the set F_IO_2 and stored under pressure in an internal reservoir tank that holds up to 8 liters under pressures of up to 350 cm H_2O. This pressurized gas allows for an uninterrupted flow, even at moments of high flow demand. After exiting the reservoir tank, gas is directed to an electromagnetic flow control valve. The flow control valve governs the pattern of gas delivery to the patient and is under the control of the microprocessor unit.

Modes and parameters selected by the operator are monitored, along with information received from the proximal airway monitor. This information governs the function of the flow control valve, the expiratory valve, and other internal operating mechanisms.

Controls and Alarms

The control panel for the GALILEO is a simple design. It uses two knobs for controlling the color-active matrix computer screen. The right knob is called the C (control) knob and the left is called the M (monitor) knob (see Figure 12-46). These knobs allow the operator to scan, select, and control all variables for operating and monitoring the ventilator.

Mode, control, and alarm are visible as a menu on the right side of the screen during normal operation (Figure 12-47). (*Note*: The active mode of ventilation appears at the top of the screen). As you scroll through the items listed on the screen using the C knob, each is highlighted in yellow. Once the desired option is highlighted, it is selected when the C knob is pushed. For example, if MODE is the option chosen and knob C is pushed, the unit opens a window displaying the ventilator mode screen listing all of the modes that are available (Figure 12-48). Select the desired mode by rotating knob C through this menu until the desired mode is highlighted. Push knob C to select the mode. You then must choose the CLOSE option on the same menu to verify the selection. This action automatically opens the controls window.

Each mode has its own CONTROL window (not shown) that contains only the parameters that can be adjusted in that mode. Initial default settings are displayed for the specific mode, so the operator can select and adjust all the variables that need changing. The controls appear on the screen as icons (drawings) of ventilator knobs. For example, in pressure ventilation using A/C, the operator has control over parameters such as $P_{CONTROL}$, RATE, PEEP, O_2%, and % I TIME. Just as with mode selection, scrolling through each parameter icon allows selection of the various functions.

When the desired knob icon is highlighted (yellow), select it by pushing control knob C. The icon then changes to activated (red). Once activated, change the numerical value of the parameter by rotating knob C either clockwise (to increase) or counterclockwise (to decrease). If, for example,

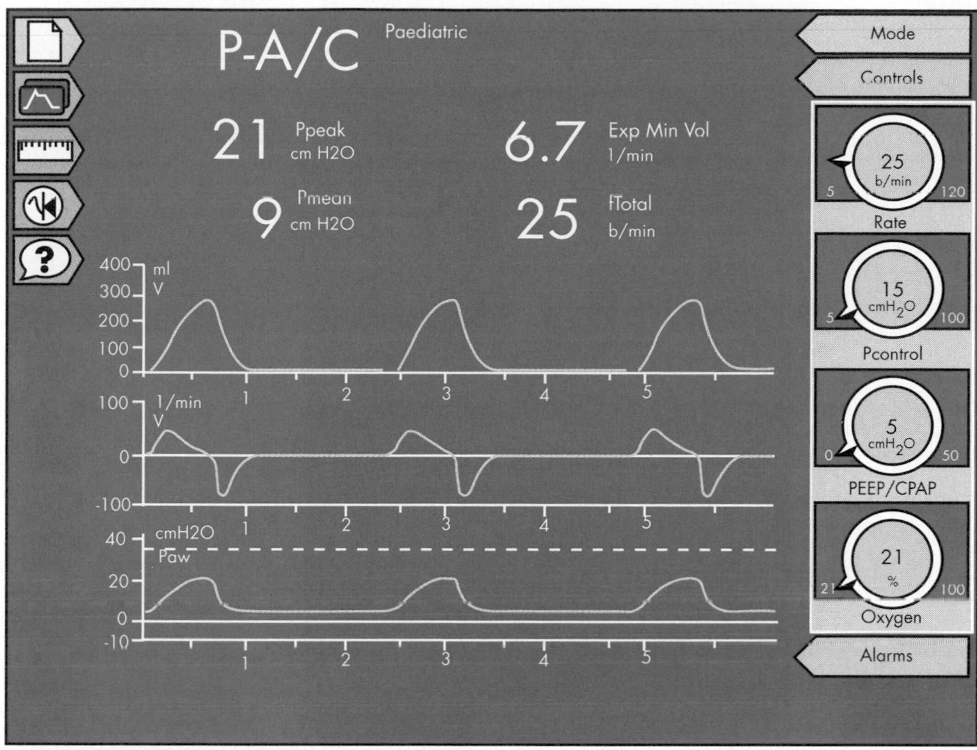

Figure 12-47 The normal operating window for P-A/C ventilation with the Hamilton GALILEO.

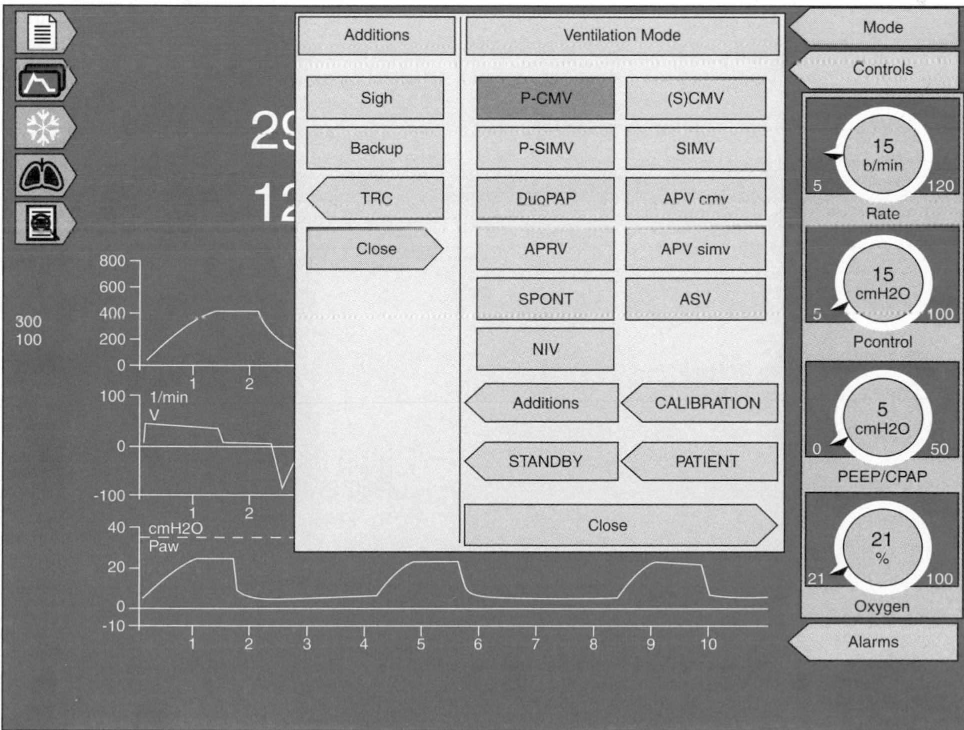

Figure 12-48 The Hamilton GALILEO Gold Version window showing the mode selections. The Gold version is a recent upgrade to the ventilator.

the pressure icon (knob) is highlighted, turning knob C can change its value from 5 cm H_2O to 100 cm H_2O. After the desired value is selected, it can be confirmed by pushing knob C. A selected control knob automatically deactivates after 60 seconds if the operator does nothing to change it (Box 12-47).

After the operator has adjusted all the control parameters, the CONFIRM icon must be selected to verify and activate the ventilator mode and parameters. The control window showing parameters for that mode disappears, and the new mode becomes active. (*Note*: The control window must be closed [CLOSE icon] before the new mode becomes active.)

Depending on the mode selected, from two to four parameter knob icons remain in a column on the right side of the normal operating screen. These icons display the parameters most often changed or manipulated in that mode of ventilation. For example, in the P-A/C (P-CMV) mode, respiratory rate, $P_{CONTROL}$, PEEP/CPAP, and O_2% appear (see Figure 12-47). This way the CONTROL window does not have to be reopened to make common changes. Box 12-48 summarizes the general rules for using knob C.

Box 12-47 Activating the New Mode

After any control menu has been chosen, the operator has a 60-second time limit. If knob C is not used and no selections are made within that time, the normal operating menu returns. In this way, the operator is not required to close a menu if no action is taken.

This rule also holds true for changing a parameter during ventilation. Suppose a respiratory therapist changed the set rate from 8 to 10 breaths/min. If she did not confirm the change, the change would not take place even though the numerical value on the rate icon went from an 8 to a 10. Without the change being activated, the ventilator screen returns to 8 breaths/min after 30 seconds, and the rate actually never changes.

Configuration of T_I, Peak Flow, or I:E

The GALILEO allows the user to program a basic function into the unit. This function relates to the cycling of a breath in volume ventilation modes. The operator can choose any of the following three options:

1. T_I
2. Peak flow
3. I:E ratio

Notice that each of these relates to the timing of breath delivery. For example, individuals who are used to ventilating patients with a set T_I would select the T_I option.

This programming option is only available during the start-up of the unit. The operator must press the M knob when the ON switch is turned on. The configuration screen appears and allows you to select one of the three options. After a choice is made and confirmed, the selected parameter

Box 12-48 General Rules for Using Control Knob C

Knob C is rotated to either highlight something on a menu or to change the numerical value of a parameter. It is pushed to select (activate) the highlighted option.

Operating controls that are yellow can be selected. Controls change from yellow to red when they are selected (by a push of Knob C) and are then active (i.e., the operator can change their numerical values). After the desired value appears on the screen near the active icon, pushing C again locks in that value.

The general rule is: rotate to locate, push to select, rotate to desired value, and push to confirm.

CLINICAL ROUNDS 12-17

Answer each of the following questions in relation to breath cycling.

1. The GALILEO is configured to keep T_I constant. The respiratory therapist is using volume-targeted A/C ventilation. The V_T is 0.5 L, rate is 10 breaths/min, and T_I is set at 25%. Calculate the T_I and the inspiratory flow (assume constant flow pattern).
2. Assume that the rate is increased to 12 breaths/min, but that V_T and T_I are the same as in the previous question. What is the new T_I and the new flow?
3. In this example, the GALILEO is configured to keep peak flow constant at the set peak flow during volume ventilation.
   - The respiratory therapist is using volume-targeted SIMV with a rate set at 15 breaths/min, and a V_T of 0.8 L. The peak flow is set at 60 L/min. What is the T_I?
   - The therapist switches the mode to P-SIMV. What is the new T_I?
4. The GALILEO is configured for I:E constant. The respiratory therapist is using PCV or P-A/C. I:E is 1:3, rate is 15 breaths/min, and $P_{CONTROL}$ is set at 15 cm H_2O.
   - What is the T_I?
   - What is the peak flow?
   - Imagine that an inspiratory pause of one-half second is added. Does the pause increase the T_I when the unit is configured for a constant I:E ratio? How would using a pause affect breath delivery in this case?

See Appendix A for the answer.

Box 12-49 Adjustable Control Variables for the Hamilton GALILEO

Rate Control

Sets the mandatory respiratory rate and determines the TCT for the mandatory breath.

Tidal Volume Control

Sets the desired volume delivery for a mandatory breath.

Pressure Control (Pcontrol)

Determines inspiratory pressure above baseline during inspiration for a mandatory pressure breath (e.g., pressure-targeted breaths in A/C and SIMV modes (range: minimum of PEEP + 5 cm H_2O, maximum of 100 cm H_2O).

Maximum Pressure Limitation

Sets the maximum pressure above baseline during adaptive support ventilation (ASV) and adaptive pressure ventilation (APV) modes.

Pressure Support (Psupport)

Establishes the pressure above baseline delivered during inspiration for PSV.

PEEP/CPAP Control

Adjusts the amount of positive baseline pressure that is applied to the patient's airway in all modes of ventilation.

Oxygen Control

Adjusts the percentage of inspired oxygen delivery.

I:E Control

Fixes the I:E ratio for mandatory breaths. This ratio is based on the relationship of the set rate, Ti/%Ti, and Pause/Tip, which establish the time cycling of a mandatory breath. Patient triggering can shorten T_E and modify the I:E ratio for that breath, but it does not change the set value (see Clinical Rounds 12-17).

Ti/%Ti Control

Determines the time allotted to deliver V_T. Ti/%Ti + inspiratory pause determines I:E ratio.

Inspiratory Pause (Pause/Tip) Control

Keeps the exhalation valve closed for the set time following V_T delivery.

Peak Flow Control

Sets peak flow delivery for volume-targeted breaths. Peak flow plus inspiratory pause determines the I:E ratio when the unit is configured for peak flow.

Flow Pattern (Flow-P) Control

Allows the selection of the desired inspiratory gas flow pattern during volume ventilation (four patterns available: constant, full ascending and descending ramps, 50% ascending and descending ramps, and sine).

Flow Trigger/Pressure Trigger/Trigger Off ($V'_{TR}/\Delta P_{TR}$/Trigger Off) Control

Allows the operator to adjust how sensitive the unit is to patient inspiratory effort. The measurement is performed at the proximal flow sensor (differential pressure transducer) located at the Y connector. An automatic leak compensation is linked with flow trigger. The flow trigger is linked to the expiratory base flow to initially satisfy flow demand by the patient.

Percentage Minute Ventilation (%MinVol) Control

Used to set the minimum $\dot{V}_E$ delivered by the ventilator. Total target $\dot{V}_E$ is calculated as 0.1 L/min/kg IBW for adults and 0.2 L/min/kg for infant/pediatric patients.

Ideal Body Weight (Body Wt) Control

Allows the operator to enter the patient's IBW in kilograms.

Target Volume (Vtarget) Control

Sets the desired (targeted) V_T delivered during a mandatory pressure-controlled breath in the APV addition.

Pressure Ramp (Pramp) Control

Determines the rise time of pressure delivery during pressure-targeted breaths (either pressure control or pressure support).

Expiratory Trigger Sensitivity (ETS) Control

Allows the operator to adjust the percentage of peak flow at which a pressure-support breath will flow-cycle (i.e., end inspiration). The range is 5% to 70% of measured peak inspiratory flow, in increments of 5%. For example, suppose peak flow during PSV is 100 L/min. If the operator sets ETS at 10%, inspiration will end when flow drops to 10 L/min.

becomes the control that appears on the normal operating screens.

For example, if T_I is selected, mandatory breaths are time-cycled regardless of the mode. If peak flow is selected, volume-targeted breaths in A/C and SIMV have their inspiratory flow determined by the peak flow setting, and in this case, T_I would be based on peak flow and tidal volume. (*Note*: If peak flow is chosen, T_I still operates in PCV [P-A/C] and SIMV pressure-targeted [P-SIMV] modes. Mandatory breaths in these modes remain time-cycled.) If I:E is selected, the I:E ratio remains constant in all volume modes, regardless of changes in flow or pause time (Clinical Rounds 12-17).

Adjustable Control Parameters

Knob C provides access to several adjustable control parameters for each mode of ventilation (Box 12-49).[1] After all the necessary control parameters have been selected and confirmed, the control parameter menu is closed and the normal operating screen reappears.

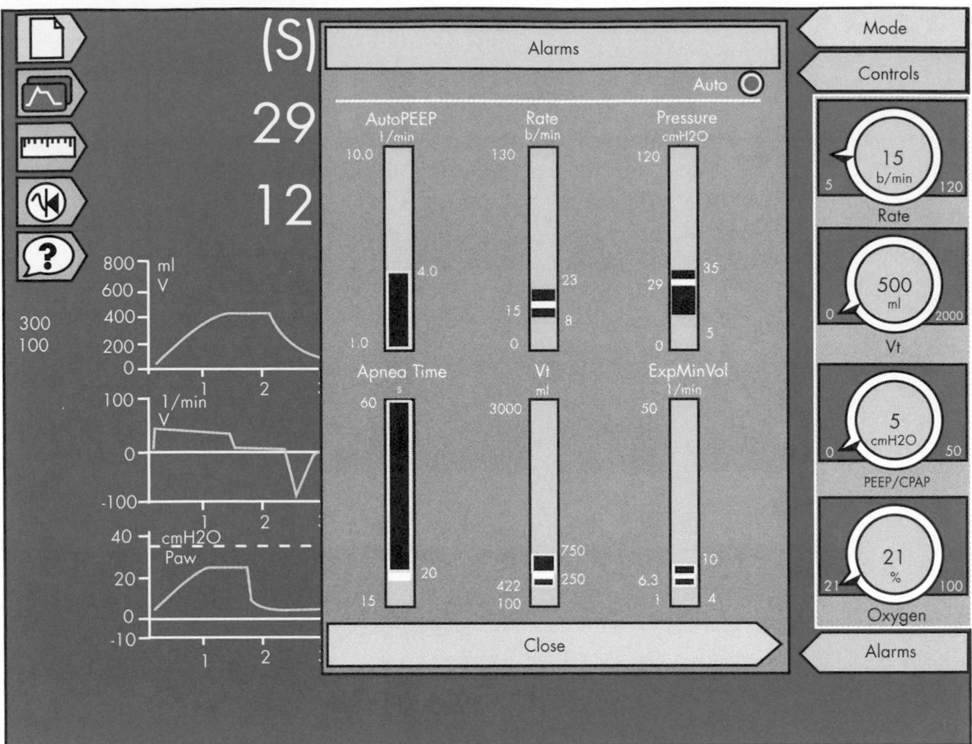

Figure 12-49 The alarm window on the Hamilton GALILEO. (See text for description.)

Alarms

When ALARMS is selected on the operating screen (controlled by C knob), the ALARM menu appears on the screen (Figure 12-49). Alarms can be automatically set by the ventilator. The operator simply selects and activates the term AUTO from the alarms menu. The computer is programmed to provide high and low alarm defaults for all available options in each mode.* The operator can choose to manually adjust high and low alarms to whatever value desired within the available range. The alarms appear on the menu as bar graphs. Selecting a particular alarm, such as low V_T, illuminates that bar graph (orange) to indicate it has been selected. Pushing knob C activates the selected alarm, changing it to red. After it is activated, turning knob C allows the alarm value to be adjusted to the desired numerical value. Pushing knob C when the desired number is present sets and verifies the alarm value.

For each alarm bar graph there is also a green horizontal line that appears on the graph (see Figure 12-49). This line (appears white in the figure) indicates the actual value measured for that parameter. Suppose that the HIGH-PRESSURE LIMIT alarm is selected, the green line shows the actual measured pressure value that is occurring for each breath. To the left of the green line, the numerical value for pressure also appears (green). This information is available whenever the alarm menu is active so that one can visually adjust the alarm range around the current value and also know the set value of each alarm parameter.

When an alarm occurs, an audible alarm sounds and the red indicator on the left side of the alarm silence key blinks. A message is displayed on the bottom of the screen (message bar), and the active alarm symbol is displayed. If more than one alarm limit was violated, the active alarm symbol will be visible on the screen. This indicates there are messages in the active alarm buffer. The operator can check what other alarms are active by selecting the alarm buffer. In earlier versions of the GALILEO the alarm buffer was an icon that looks like an "i" inside a folder. In the newer versions of GALILEO, the operator accesses the buffer by first closing any open window, selecting the active alarm symbol and pressing the M-knob.

The most recent alarm message will be at the top of the list. The alarm buffer will list up to six alarm conditions in order of occurrence and give the date and time of each alarm. The information about current alarms remains in the buffer as long as the condition that caused each alarm persists. If an alarm condition occurred and is corrected, it is stored into memory, and the GALILEO automatically resets the alarm. Information about active and reset alarms, along with other clinically significant events, is also stored in the event log.

Values for these are available from the manufacturer.

Table 12-11 Alarm specifications for GALILEO

Alarm System	Range
ADJUSTABLE ALARMS	
Low/high minute ventilation	0 to 50 L/min
Low/high pressure	0 to 110 cm H_2O
Low/high V_T	0 to 3000 mL
Low/high rate	0 to 130 breaths/min
Apnea time	15 to 60 seconds
Air trapping	1 to 10 L/min end expiratory flow
NONADJUSTABLE ALARMS	
High pressure during sigh	
Pressure not released	
Oxygen and air supply low	
Internal pressure low	
Check flow sensor tubing	
Disconnection on ventilator side	
Disconnection on patient side	
Oxygen concentration (high/low)	
No O_2 cell in use	
O_2 cell defective	
Turn the flow sensor (placed in the wrong direction)	
Oxygen supply, air supply (less that 28 psig)	
Loss of PEEP (3 cm H_2O below baseline for 10 seconds)	
Check settings (inappropriately set)	
Loss of power supply	
Ventilator inoperative	

Box 12-50 User Attention Messages

Flow sensor calibration needed
O_2 cell calibration needed
Check trigger
Check % MinVol/Pmax
Check rate
Check V_T
Check PEEP/Pcontrol
Check Psupport/Pcontrol
Check PEEP/Psupport
Check I:E
Check rate/T_I
Check V_T/T_I
Check T_I
Check %Ti
Check peak flow
Check Vtarget/Pmax
Check pause
Check flow pattern
Check Pramp
Check controls for sigh
Nebulizer inactive
Power alarm
If the message, "TECHNICAL FAULT" appears and is followed by a number, the ventilator is experiencing technical difficulties and needs to be replaced. The manufacturer's service engineer should be called and given the number of the technical fault.

Different priority alarms give different sounds, which helps the practitioner distinguish those requiring immediate attention from those that are less critical. Using the ventilator and listening to the various alarms helps the operator learn the different audible signals.

Adjustable and nonadjustable alarms are listed in Table 12-11. Box 12-50 lists user-attention messages for the GALILEO.

Upper Pressure Limit (Pmax)

Because of its importance in ventilator function, the high-pressure alarm and its setting are worth reviewing. It is common for respiratory therapists to set an upper pressure limit 10 to 15 cm H_2O above the peak ventilating pressure. This should be set for all modes—pressure- or volume-targeted. For example, in PCV the set pressure may be 40 cm H_2O, but what happens if the patient coughs? The pressure can rise above 40 cm H_2O (assuming that the high-pressure alarm is set above the PCV level). For safety purposes, always set the high-pressure limit about 10 to 15 cm H_2O above the ventilating pressures. When the high pressure limit is reached, inspiratory flow ends and the expiratory valve opens.

In the GALILEO, the high-pressure limit (Pmax) also serves another function when adaptive support ventilation (ASV) or adaptive pressure ventilation (APV) are selected. During the use of ASV or APV, the ventilator will not deliver pressures any higher than the upper pressure limit minus 10 cm H_2O (Pmax −10 cm H_2O). Pressures can become higher than Pmax −10 cm H_2O in the circuit if, for example, the patient coughs, but they can never go higher than the upper pressure limit setting (see the pressure bar graph in Figure 12-49 and "pressure" in Figure 12-50. Pmax is displayed with a color).

Monitoring

During normal operation, four parameters are always displayed on the screen: PEAK PRESSURE, MEAN AIRWAY PRESSURE, EXPIRED MINUTE VOLUME, and TOTAL RESPIRATORY

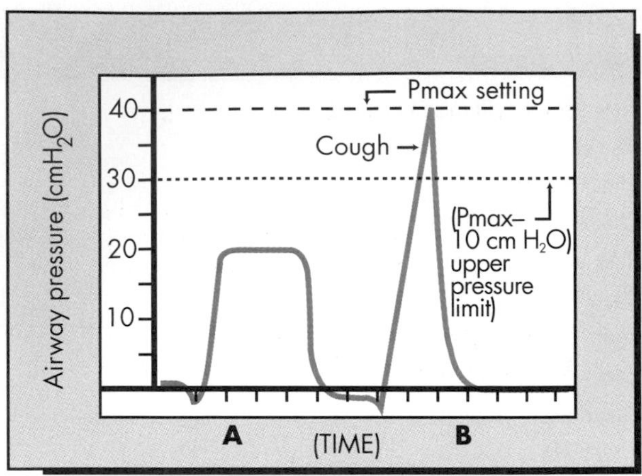

Figure 12-50 A pressure-time graph showing the Pmax pressure setting (dashed line), the upper pressure limit (Pmax minus 10 cm H_2O), a normal pressure breath **(A)** delivered during P-A/C + APV, and pressure during a cough **(B).**

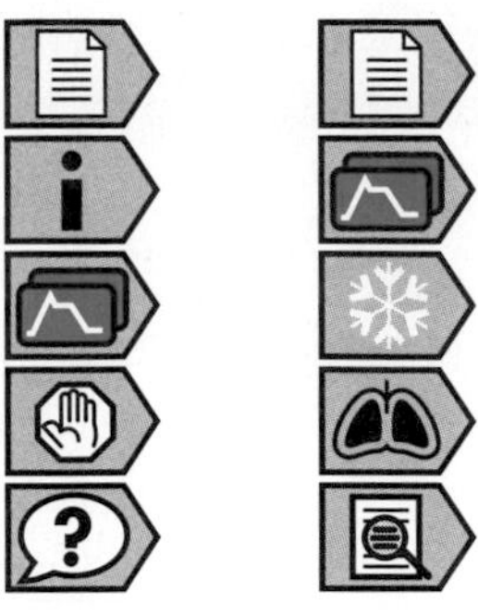

Figure 12-51 Monitor options on the Hamilton GALILEO and the GALILEO Gold version. **A,** original monitor options; **(B)** recently updated Gold version. (See text for description.)

RATE. In addition to these, several monitoring options appear on the upper left side of the screen (Figure 12-51) that are controlled by the M knob on the left side of the front panel (see Figure 12-46). The five main options appear as small icons in the monitoring menu. These options can be periodically changed by the manufacturer. The current available monitoring menu has the following: a sheet of paper, a waveform, a snow flake, a pair of lungs, and a paper with a magnifying glass over a sheet of paper.

When the sheet of paper icon is selected, its menu displays three icons: two sheets of paper, ASV, and a pressure icon (Paw/Paux). Selecting the sheets of paper provides information on the 26 parameters being measured and calculated including peak pressure, V_T, PEEP/CPAP level, $\dot{V}_E$, total respiratory rate, mean airway pressure, percentage of oxygen, static compliance, inspiratory airway resistance, pulmonary mechanics, pressure-time products, rapid shallow breathing index, I:E ratio, T_I, T_E, work of breathing (WOB), time constants, and so on. This screen lists the monitored parameters that are measured and calculated breath to breath but are not constantly displayed on the standard screen.

Paw and Paux are also available under this icon and provide monitored information on pressures measured from either the standard pressure measurements made with the flow sensor located at the Y connector (Paw) or the auxiliary pressure sensor connector. Recall that there is a small nipple connector (Paux) that allows a pressure monitor other than the one at the patient Y connector to be used. For example, the operator may want to monitor transpleural pressure using an esophageal balloon or carinal pressure using a special endotracheal tube or tube adapter. The user is advised to contact the manufacturer to find out the most appropriate auxiliary pressure monitoring equipment to use with the GALILEO.

The waveform icon in the monitoring menu pulls up a menu with four selections:

1. Real-time waveforms: pressure-, flow-, and volume-time scalars
2. Loops: pressure-volume, flow-volume, and flow-pressure. (*Note*: In the loops menu, you can also choose Paux or Paw vs. volume so that you can observe total pressures compared with volume and pressures in the airway or in the esophagus vs. volume.)
3. Trend curves
4. ASV target graphics screen: This screen provides information about adaptive support ventilation when the mode is operational. For example, in the ASV mode, the screen provides the target values for rate, V_T, $\dot{V}_E$, and inspiratory pressure above PEEP and displays actual measured V_T, rate, and $\dot{V}_E$. The target values can only be provided if the operator has selected ASV and completed the necessary set-up (see ASV in the discussion of modes of ventilation).

There is an icon for freeze frame (snowflake) that allows freezing of the current waveforms or trends and activates the cursor measurement.

The icon of the lungs has two items under its menu, a stop sign with a hand inside and a P/V (pressure/volume) curve icon. The stop sign allows selection of end-inspiratory and end-expiratory hold. Selecting the desired function results in the ventilator automatically performing the function. For example, in the inspiratory hold maneuver, it waits until the next inspiratory breath delivery to activate the hold. (*Note*: The ventilator will provide up to a 10-second hold [adults/pediatric patients] or 3 seconds for infants.) Selection of the P/V icon provides a pressure/volume curve maneuver (see Special Features section).

The magnifying glass icon opens the Event Log showing up to 1000 events, including alarms and setting changes. Earlier versions of the GALILEO monitoring menu had an "i" icon that was an information (help) menu.

Box 12-51 Parameters Monitored and Calculated in the GALILEO

PRESSURES*

Peak pressure (Ppeak), minimum pressure (Pminimum), plateau pressure (Pplateau), PEEP/CPAP pressure, and mean airway pressure (Pmean, calculated value).

FLOWS*

Inspiratory (Insp Flow) and expiratory (Exp Flow) flows.

VOLUMES*

Expiratory Tidal Volume (VTE)

Measured as exhaled air from the patient at the proximal airway pressure monitor.

Expired Minute Volume (ExpMinVol)

Measured at the airway; is the sum of eight consecutive measured breaths extrapolated to 1 full minute and updated after each breath.

Leakage Volume (VLeak)

This is the difference between inspired and expired V_T measured at the patient's airway.

BREATH-TO-BREATH MEASUREMENT

TIME

I:E ratio expressed as 1:X for normal I:E ratios and X:1 for inverse ratios, where X is the relative expiratory time for a measured breath and is updated with each breath. (Minimum is 1:9, and maximum is 4:1.)

fTotal† is the sum of spontaneous and mandatory breaths. fSpont† is the sum of only spontaneous breath frequency.

T_I is the actual inspiratory time (in seconds) for a mandatory breath, measured from the beginning of inspiration to the end of inspiratory pause. For a spontaneous breath, it is measured from the beginning of inspiration until the ETS (flow-cycling) criteria are met.

T_E is the actual expiratory time in seconds; it is the time between the beginning of exhalation and the start of inspiration.

Oxygen

Measured inspiratory oxygen concentration.

CALCULATED PARAMETERS (OTHER THAN MEAN AIRWAY PRESSURE)

Rinsp‡ (inspiratory airflow resistance) and Rexp‡ (expiratory airflow resistance) result from the patient's airway and the endotracheal tube and are measured in all modes and types of breaths.

Cstat (static lung-thorax compliance) is calculated using exhaled V_T (in liters) and measured pressures (in centimeters of water).‡

RCInsp (inspiratory time constant) and RCExp (expiratory time constant) are calculated from peak expiratory flow and volume.

WOBInsp (inspiratory work of breathing), auto-PEEP, P0.1 (occlusion pressure), PTP (inspiratory pressure-time product), and RSB (rapid shallow breathing index) are other calculated parameters.

*Breath-to-breath measurement.
†Measured for eight consecutive breaths and extrapolated to 1 minute. Updated after each breath.
‡Calculated using least squares fit.[2]

Real-Time Monitoring

The parameters measured by the proximal flow sensor and those calculated by the microprocessor are listed in Box 12-51.

Front Panel Touch Keys

At the lower right corner of the control panel are four touch controls (Figure12-46). The alarm touch pad (left) silences the audible portion of the alarm system for 2 minutes. It can be reactivated by touching it again. The highest priority alarms cannot be silenced with this control; that is, the audible alarm for the following cannot be silenced:

1. Loss of source gas pressure
2. Loss of electrical power
3. An internal technical error that can be life-threatening or cause catastrophic problems.
4. An apnea event (*Note*: Cannot be silenced until resolution of apnea.)

The next touch pad is the 100% O_2, which provides 100% oxygen for 5 minutes. This is useful in procedures such as oxygenation before suctioning. If pressed a second time, the set oxygen percent is quickly resumed.

The MANUAL touch pad delivers a manually-triggered mandatory (pressure or volume) breath. To avoid auto-PEEP after a manual mandatory breath, the unit waits until it recognizes a period of 0.2 seconds of no expiratory gas flow. In earlier versions of the GALILEO, the fourth touch pad was a print pad, which, when pressed, could print the current computer screen when the ventilator was connected to a compatible printer. In the latest version, the fourth key activates the nebulizer function described previously.

Modes of Ventilation

The modes of ventilation currently available for the GALILEO are listed in Box 12-52. A back-up rate is available whenever apnea is detected during any mode of ventilation with spontaneous breathing available. Whenever the mode screen is opened, in addition to a list of the modes, four items listed at the bottom of this menu can be used to open

Box 12-52 Modes of Ventilation

ADULT/PEDIATRIC
Assist/Control, A/C [(S)CMV]
P-A/C (P-CMV)
SIMV
P-SIMV
SPONT
APVcmv
APVsimv
ASV
DuoPAP
APRV
NIV (GALILEO Gold only)

INFANT
P-A/C (P-CMV)
P-SIMV
SPONT
APVcmv
APVsimv
ASV
DuoPAP
APRV

additional functions. They are as follows: ADDITIONS, CALIBRATION, STANDBY, and PATIENT. The ADDITIONS menu allows for the setting of SIGH breaths, BACK-UP VENTILATION and TUBING RESISTANCE COMPENSATION (TRC). These three will be reviewed later.

The STANDBY feature places the ventilator in a waiting mode that allows the operator to maintain current patient settings while the ventilator is not performing any ventilatory functions. The standby feature might be used if the patient is to be disconnected for any length of time.

The CALIBRATION function allows for calibration procedures which are performed before connecting the patient to the ventilator. Finally, the PATIENT selection menu allows for choosing between adult, pediatric and infant patient size.

Assist/Control (A/C)

This is a standard A/C volume-targeted mode that offers time- or patient-triggering (flow or pressure). The breath can be time- or volume-cycled. The term *volume-cycling* is used here to mean that inspiration ends when the measured flow and time are used to calculate that the set volume has been delivered (see Clinical Rounds 12-17). The parameters that can be adjusted in this mode are similar to other ventilators and include V_T, rate, peak flow, or $\%T_I$ or I:E, flow pattern, sensitivity (pressure- or flow-triggering), $O_2\%$, and PEEP/CPAP.

Box 12-53 Parameters That Can Be Adjusted by the Operator in SIMV (Volume or Pressure Ventilation)

Respiratory rate
V_T or Pressure (Pcontrol above PEEP)
PEEP/CPAP
$O_2\%$
I:E ratio or $\%T_I$ or peak flow in volume ventilation
Flow or pressure trigger ($V'_{TR}/\Delta P_{TR}$)
Pressure support (for spontaneous breaths)
Flow pattern and pause (in volume ventilation)
Pressure ramp (P_{ramp}; in pressure control and pressure support only)
Expiratory trigger sensitivity (ETS; in PSV only)
Target volume (in APV)

Synchronized Intermittent Mandatory Ventilation (SIMV)

As with most ventilators, the SIMV mode can be time- or patient-triggered and volume-targeted. Inspiration is time- or volume-cycled as in A/C. Breaths can be delivered with an elevated baseline (PEEP/CPAP). The patient can breathe spontaneously between mandatory breaths. PSV can be added to spontaneous breaths (see the discussion of the spontaneous mode). Box 12-53 lists parameters that can be selected on the CONTROL menu and adjusted by the operator in SIMV when this mode is activated.

In the GALILEO during SIMV, the mandatory breaths have a maximum TCT of 4 seconds, which is equal to a set rate of 15 breaths/min. If the rate is set higher, the TCT is shorter. For example at 20 breaths, the TCT is 3 seconds. If the rate is lower than 15 breaths/min, (e.g., 10 breaths/min [TCT = 6 seconds]), the TCT for a mandatory breath is still 4 seconds. A time of ≤ 4 seconds is used as a trigger window for the mandatory breath. If there is no triggering inside this 4-second window, a mandatory breath is delivered (time-triggered) at the end of the 4 seconds. If the ventilator is in a time-cycled mode, the T_I is also determined by the 4-second time frame. For example, in SIMV with a T_I set at 25%, T_I is 1 second. At a T_I of 50%, it will be 2 seconds. (*Note*: Expiratory time may vary. If a patient triggers a breath, this can shorten the T_E, the TCT is shortened as well.)

Spontaneous Mode (CPAP and PSV)

The spontaneous mode is used when the patient can breathe spontaneously but still requires some support or monitoring with alarms. The operator can adjust pressure support, CPAP, % O_2, triggering (flow- or pressure-), pressure ramp (PSV), and expiratory trigger sensitivity (ETS for PSV only). The ventilator provides flow to meet patient demand while maintaining the desired baseline pressure and pressure support.

In the GALILEO, PSV is set above the PEEP/CPAP level. For example, if the clinician sets 10 cm H_2O of pressure support and the patient is receiving 5 cm H_2O of CPAP, the pressure during inspiration will reach 15 cm H_2O (PS + CPAP). The ventilator provides 2 cm H_2O of pressure support within the system, even when PSV is set at zero. This is provided to reduce the work required by the patient to initiate flow from the demand system.

Another important feature of pressure-support ventilation that the GALILEO offers the user is the ability to adjust the flow percentage at which the unit cycles out of inspiration. This feature is called the expiratory trigger sensitivity (ETS). The GALILEO is preprogrammed to flow-cycle at 25% of peak for adults and 15% of peak for pediatric patients, but allows this value to be adjusted from 5% to 70% of peak flow.[1] For example, if the peak flow during a pressure-support breath is 100 L/min, and ETS is set at 30%, a PS breath will end inspiration when flow decreases to 30 L/min.

In case there is a leak in the system during PSV, a safety back-up is available. Inspiratory time cannot exceed 3 seconds. With the infant patient size, the maximum T_I is set by the operator. So that if there is a leak around the uncuffed endotracheal tube, there is not a problem with cycling. The GALILEO will also cycle out of a PS breath if the pressure reaches more than 2 cm H_2O above the set pressures.

Whenever pressure-targeted breaths are selected with either PSV or PCV, the GALILEO allows the operator to adjust the slope or rise of the pressure curve Pramp. The Pramp determines the amount of time it takes from the very beginning of inspiratory flow until the set pressure is reached. The pressure curve can be tapered so that pressure does not abruptly enter the upper airway. Pramp is available in PSV, PCV, PCV. APV, and ASV. (See Chapter 11 for more details about sloping or rise time.)

Pressure-Targeted Assist-Control Ventilation (P-A/C)

This mode, commonly called pressure controlled ventilation, is also referred to as pressure-targeted assist/control (P-A/C) in the GALILEO. In P-A/C, the ventilator is time- or patient-triggered (flow or pressure). The breath is pressure-targeted at the set pressure-control level and time-cycled out of inspiration. V_T varies with T_I, set pressure, patient effort, and changes in the patient's lung conditions. For this reason, it is especially important to set exhaled $\dot{V}_E$ alarm levels. As with PSV, the $P_{control}$ value is added to PEEP. For example, if $P_{control}$ is set at 15 cm H_2O, and PEEP is 10 cm H_2O, the maximum pressure generated by the ventilator during inspiration will be 25 cm H_2O. In this example, it is advisable to set the upper pressure limit (Pmax) between 30 and 35 cm H_2O to limit the amount of pressure that could build up in the circuit if the patient coughs or forcibly exhales. The amount of pressure control cannot be set lower than 5 cm H_2O above the baseline pressure (PEEP).

CLINICAL ROUNDS 12-18

A patient is being set up on P-A/C + APV on the GALILEO. The ventilator parameters are as follows: rate = 10 breaths/min, T_I = 1.5 seconds, PEEP = 5 cm H_2O, Pmax = 35 cm H_2O, F_IO_2 = 0.5, Vtarget = 0.6 L (600 mL).

A ventilating pressure of 25 cm H_2O is required to deliver the target volume for this patient. A few breaths after the mode is initiated, the respiratory therapist hears an audible alarm and sees a message indicating that ventilation is on "Pressure Limitation." What changes should the therapist make?

See Appendix A for the answer.

Pressure-Control Ventilation Plus Adaptive Pressure Ventilation (P-A/C + APV)

The operator can also select APV when using pressure control (P-A/C + APV). On the upper portion of the screen, "P-A/C^{APV}" is displayed. (*Note*: In newer versions of the GALILEO, this mode is called APV_{CMV} or pressure-controlled mandatory ventilation with adaptive pressure ventilation.)

With this selection the operator sets a target volume (VTarget) instead of a target pressure. This is a servo-control or closed-loop mode. Through the automatic control of inspiratory pressure and flow, the specified target volume is generated with the lowest pressure possible under the current lung conditions. The ventilator reaches and maintains pressure at the upper limit, and the breath time-cycles out of inspiration. If exhaled V_T is less than the set value (VTarget), pressure adjusts upward to deliver the desired volume. If V_T is more than VTarget, pressure is reduced.*

Maximum pressure is determined by the upper pressure alarm limit setting (Pmax). The upward adjustment in pressure that is performed by the ventilator to correct V_T cannot exceed Pmax –10 cm H_2O. (*Note*: The manufacturer currently recommends a high pressure alarm limit setting of at least 10 cm H_2O above the peak pressure.) The amount of pressure control cannot be set lower than 5 cm H_2O above the baseline pressure (PEEP). When the ventilator has to go beyond these pressure limitations to achieve VTarget, audible and visible alarms occur and a message appears at the bottom of the screen indicates that the ventilator has now reached "pressure limitations." The target volume may not be delivered with the current setting for Pmax. The clinician must then decide either to reduce the target V_T or increase Pmax, depending upon the patient's

**Pressure changes are made in increments of 1 to 2 cm H_2O.*

condition. (*Note*: P-A/C is similar to PRVC described in Chapter 11.) Clinical Rounds 12-18 provides a problem related to P-A/C + APV.

Pressure Control/SIMV (P-SIMV)

The GALILEO can provide SIMV using pressure-targeted mandatory breaths (P-SIMV). This mode is very similar to conventional SIMV. Mandatory breaths are patient- or time-triggered, pressure-targeted, and time-cycled. Tidal volumes vary depending on the set pressure, T_I, patient lung characteristics, and any patient effort that might be present. As with volume-targeted SIMV, a positive-pressure baseline (PEEP/CPAP) can be applied. Spontaneous breaths can be given aided with the use of pressure support.

Pressure Control/SIMV Plus Adaptive Pressure Ventilation (P-SIMV + APV)

P-SIMV can also be altered using the APV function. At the top of the screen "P-SIMV^{APV}" appears. (*Note*: Newer versions of the GALILEO also refer to this as APV_{SIMV}.) In P-SIMV + APV, mandatory breaths are still pressure breaths, but they become volume-targeted (set Vtarget). The ventilator adjusts pressure delivery during these mandatory breaths in order to achieve the volume target using the lowest possible inspiratory pressure. This is similar to P-A/C + APV. The primary difference is that a patient can breathe spontaneously between mandatory breaths at the set baseline and pressure-support level in P-SIMV + APV (see Box 12-53).

Adaptive Support Ventilation (ASV)

ASV is a servo-controlled (closed-loop) technique that functions using pressure-targeted breaths to assure a target minute ventilation while establishing protective lung strategies. The goal of ASV is to provide $\dot{V}_E$ and at the same time minimize the work of breathing, and avoid potentially detrimental patterns of breathing (rapid shallow breathing, excessive dead space ventilation, breath stacking and excessively large breaths[2]). (*Note*: At the time of this writing, ASV is not available in the United States.)

ASV adapts to the changing capabilities and lung conditions of the patient. The GALILEO automatically alters its performance to the patient's demands—from full support to spontaneous breathing. The more work the patient is able to perform, the less the ventilator provides. ASV can ventilate the patient from an acute stage to a weaning stage.

Normally, when respiratory therapists or physicians initially establish ventilation in a patient, they calculate initial settings of $\dot{V}_E$, rate, and V_T. These settings are calculated from equations that have been established through clinical research that use variables such as ideal body weight (IBW); patient height and sex; and any abnormal conditions that may be present.[3] For example, $\dot{V}_E$ may be based on body surface area calculated from patient weight and height and adjusted for abnormal body temperature.[3,4]

ASV also follows specific algorithms or formulas on which it determines optimum ventilation and the best way to deliver volume and rate. Some of these rules are *hard* and some are *soft*.[2] An example of a *hard* rule is the high pressure limit set by the operator. In ASV the ventilator will not exceed the high pressure limit, even if it is unable to achieve its set goals. *Soft* rules are based on clinician input and on the patient's respiratory mechanics. *Soft* rules usually have a range of variability and may change with time or with operator input. An example of a *soft* rule is establishing the low V_T limits that are equal to 4.4 mL/kg of IBW. The lower V_T limit assures that the minimum V_T will be at least twice normal dead space and is based on patient weight.[2]

ASV is such a new approach to ventilation that an explanation of its operation is divided into several different sections:

1. Ventilator programming to establish respiratory parameters in ASV
2. Setting up the ventilator for ASV
3. Initial test breaths
4. Variations in breath delivery

Ventilator Programming to Establish Respiratory Parameters in ASV

ASV is programmed to calculate an overall *minute ventilation* for the patient. It uses pressure-targeted breaths to accomplish delivery of the minute ventilation. Breaths are a combination of PC breaths (time-triggered and time-cycled breaths) and PSV breaths (any patient-triggered breaths are pressure-targeted and flow-cycled as with a PS breath). Both types of pressure-targeted breaths are also volume-guaranteed. The volume target is established by the ventilator, as is the respiratory rate and minute ventilation.

Some clinicians are concerned because the ventilator is performing many of the functions that are normally the clinician's purview. But the GALILEO uses well established equations and safe boundaries as guides for determining the minute ventilation, tidal volume and rate.[2-9] Each of the these parameters will be reviewed.

Minute Ventilation

The ventilator uses the following equations to calculate the minute ventilation:[4-9]

Equation 1

$$\text{IBW} > 15\text{ kg: } \dot{V}_E \text{ target} = 100 \times (\%\text{ MIN VOL}/100) \times \text{IBW(kg)}$$

Equation 2

$$\text{IBW} < 15\text{ kg: } \dot{V}_E \text{ target} = 200 \times (\%\text{ MIN VOL}/100) \times \text{IBW(kg)}$$

For example, an adult patient with an IBW of 70 kg set at 100% MIN VOL will have a target $\dot{V}_E$ of 7000 mL/min or 7.0 L/min. This $\dot{V}_E$ can be achieved using a number of

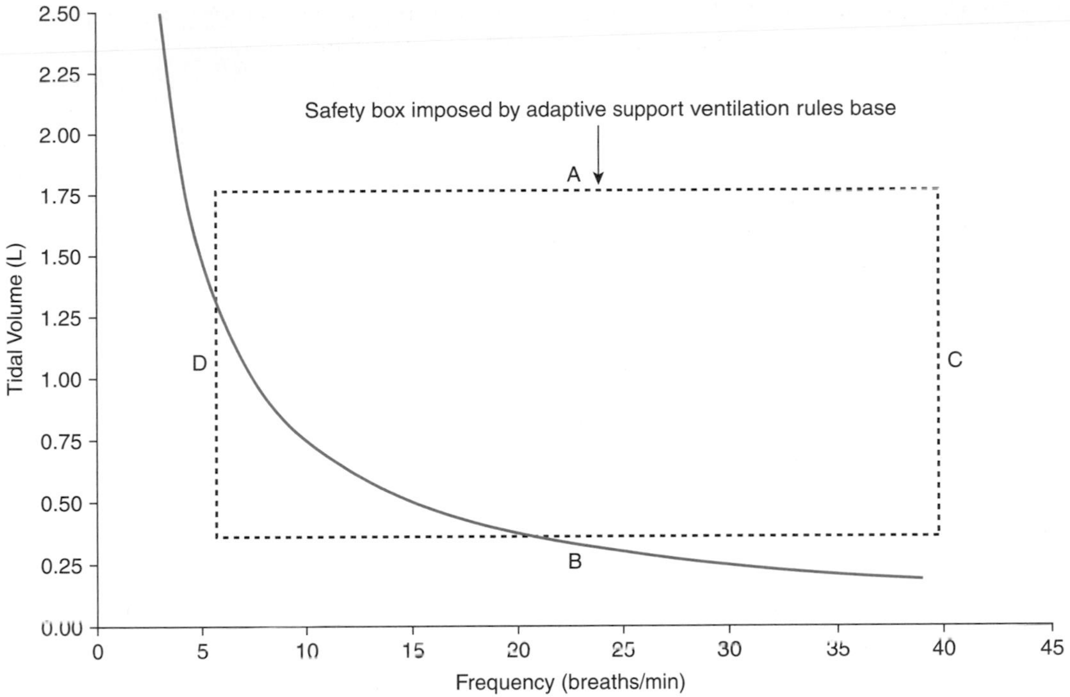

Figure 12-52 The dark line on the graph represents all the possible combinations of V_T and f that will result in a $\dot{V}_E$ of 7.0 L/min. The box *(dotted line)* within the graph represents the safest boundaries for protecting the lungs. The A boundary protects against high V_T and high pressures. The B boundary protects against hypoventilation. The C boundary helps to avoid hyperinflation or breath-stacking. The D boundary helps avoid apnea. (Redrawn from Branson et al, *Resp Care* 47:427, 2002.)

Box 12-54 Otis's Formula

Total respiratory frequency (f)

$$f = \frac{\sqrt{1 + 4\pi^2 RCe\left(\frac{\dot{V}_E - f \times V_D}{V_D}\right)} - 1}{2\pi^2 RCe}$$

Here *RCe* = expiratory time constant; $\dot{V}_E$ = minute ventilation; V_D = deadspace volume.

The GALILEO estimates dead space as 1 mL/pound IBW using Radford's nomogram.

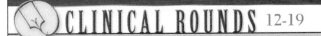

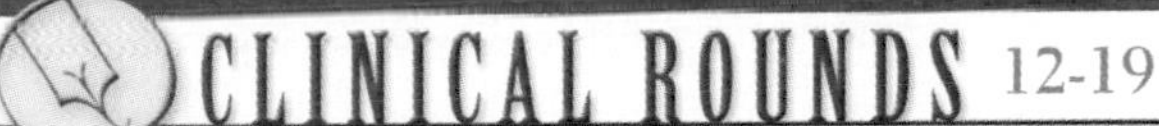

Problem 1:
An adult patient has an IBW of 60 kg. The operator sets $\dot{V}_E$ at 100%. What will be the $\dot{V}_E$ established by the ventilator for the patient?

Problem 2:
If an infant has an IBW of 5 kg, and the operator sets the $\dot{V}_E$ at 50%, what will be the $\dot{V}_E$ delivery for the infant by the ventilator?

See Appendix A for the answer.

combinations of V_T and f. However, not all combinations are safe for the patient. Figure 12-52 illustrates how the GALILEO places limits on the potential V_T and f combinations to make them safe for the patient. (*Note*: The operator always determines the absolute boundaries. For example, setting the high pressure alarm limit sets the boundary on high pressure.)

The $\dot{V}_E$ is divides into optimal targets for respiratory rate and V_T which is determined by using Otis's least work of breathing equation (Box 12-54).[5] The use of this equation and its operating premise makes the assumption that if the optimum breathing pattern results in the least work of breathing, it also results in the least amount of pressure during ventilation of a passive patient (Clinical Rounds 12-19).[2,5]

Tidal Volume

Establishing tidal volume limits is determined by both *hard* and *soft* rule boundaries.[2]

The *maximum* V_T can be established by using the *hard* boundary for low breath rate and the calculated $\dot{V}_E$. For example, a $\dot{V}_E$ of 7 L/min, with a minimum available rate of

Table 12-12 Safety limits in ASV

Parameter	Value
Minimum pressure	PEEP + 5 cm H_2O
Maximum pressure	PMax setting −10 cm H_2O
V_T minimum	4.4 mL/kg IBW (2 × V_D)
V_T maximum	22.0 mL/kg IBW (10 × V_D)
Minimum mandatory rate	5 breaths/min
Maximum mandatory rate	60 breaths/min
Minimum T_I	RCexp,* or 0.5 seconds
Maximum T_I	2 × RCexp, or 3 seconds
Minimum T_E	2 × RCexp
Maximum T_E	12 seconds

**RCexp*, Expiratory time constant.

5 breaths/min would establish *maximum* boundary for V_T at 1.4 L (1400 mL).

IBW is used to establish the *soft* boundaries for both high and low V_T.[2] High V_T is always less than 22 mL/kg. The lower V_T boundary assumes that V_T will be at least twice normal dead space, which is about 2.2 mL/kg. Thus the lower V_T limit is set at 4.4 mL/kg. For example in the 70 kg adult, a low V_T based on IBW would be 2.2 mL/kg × 70 kg = 308 mL.

High tidal volume would also be affected by the upper pressure alarm limit setting. If delivery of a high tidal volume violates this limit, the alarm would activate, ending inspiration and reducing V_T delivery.

Rate

The % Min Vol setting determines the *soft* rule for the maximum breath rate. Maximum breath rate is based on one of the following two equations:[2,7-8]

Equation 1

IBW >15 kg: Max f = 22 breaths/min × % Min Vol/100

Equation 2

IBW <15 kg: Max f = 45 breaths/min × % Min Vol/100

For example, the 70-kg patient described previously (target $\dot{V}_E$ = 7 L/min, 100% Min Vol setting) would have a *maximum* rate of 22 breaths/min.

A *hard* boundary for respiratory rate is set at 5 breaths/min for low rate and 60 breaths/min for maximum rate.[2] The low rate in turn affects the potential *maximum* V_T. For example, in a 70 kg patient, with % Min Vol set at 100%, maximum V_T would be the $\dot{V}_E$/5 bpm or 7.0 L/5 bpm = 1.4 L or 1400 mL $V_T$max.

Box 12-55 Static Compliance and Airway Resistance

The calculation of static compliance by the GALILEO does not require that the operator select an inspiratory pause (inflation hold) to get a static pressure reading. The static compliance is calculated mathematically using the least squares fit method. The unit performs 200 measurements/second of flow, pressure, and volume then does a linear regression calculation to estimate static compliance and airway resistance. The analysis of pressure, flow, and volume is based on a mechanical model of the respiratory system.[2]

As a safety feature to allow for sufficient time to exhale if respiratory rate is high, the ventilator measures the patient's expiratory time constant (RCexp) and makes sure that expiratory time is at least equal to 2 × RCexp.

Looking at Patient Lung Characteristics

In addition, the internal equations for $\dot{V}_E$, V_T and rate, ASV look at patient lung characteristics, which change with differences in pathology. For example, pulmonary edema results in reduced lung compliance. Low lung compliance is associated with a body's response of a higher rate and lower V_T. The ventilator makes an effort to reduce work of breathing by providing a rate and a V_T that reflects the patient's lung condition (lung compliance [C] and airway resistance [R]), but stays within its limitations (Table 12-12).

The ventilator is constantly analyzing T_I, T_E, total rate, inspired $\dot{V}_E$, expiratory time constant (RCexp), R, C, and ventilating pressures (Box 12-55).[9] It uses all this information, plus the input from the operator to establish an appropriate breathing pattern that at all times tries to reduce the work of breathing and to balance the patient's spontaneous and mandatory breaths.

Setting up the Ventilator for ASV

Before connecting the patient to the ventilator, as in all cases, the operator performs preoperational procedures and tests to assure optimum ventilator performance. The practitioner then provides some specific input information.

First, a high pressure alarm limit is set (ALARMS window). The manufacturer suggests a beginning high pressure limit of 45 cm H_2O. Maximum inspiratory pressure during ASV will always be 10 cm H_2O below the set high pressure alarm limit. At a set value of 45 cm H_2O, this would be a maximum of 35 cm H_2O.

Second, the operator enters the IBW of the patient (range 10 to 200 kg). IBW is used to determine the anatomic dead space of the patient at 2.2 mL/kg using Radford's nomogram.[4] Use of mechanical devices, like heat moisture exchangers (HME), will increase dead space and may also need to be considered when deciding on an IBW setting. As a rule of thumb, the operator should increase the body weight setting by 10% when using an HME.[2]

Third, the percent of minute ventilation (% MIN VOL) is set by the operator (range 10% to 350%). A safe starting point is 100%. If the patient is hyperthermic, the percentage may be increased by 5% per degree F (10% per degree C). In high altitude conditions, the % $\dot{V}_E$ may be increased by 5% per 500 meters above sea level.

Fourth, the operator can then select appropriate values for PEEP, trigger sensitivity, F_IO_2, Pramp and ETS, and confirm the initial settings. PEEP/CPAP and oxygen percentage aid in patient oxygenation. Trigger sensitivity adjusts the ease of breath triggering. Pressure ramp and ETS tailor PS breaths.

Initial Test Breaths

The GALILEO assesses the patient by providing three test breaths (pressure breaths), starting at a minimum pressure just above baseline and gradually increasing the pressure. (*Note*: During ASV pressure cannot go below PEEP/CPAP plus 5 cm H_2O or above the upper pressure limit alarm −10 cm H_2O.)

During the test breaths, the ventilator performs its measurements and calculations of V_T, f, C, R, and time constants. From these measurements, the ventilator can assess the elastic and resistive workload and establish the optimum breath pattern (i.e., the ventilatory pattern that represents the least work of breathing for the patient). Table 12-12 lists the safety limits autoprogrammed by the unit to avoid complications associated with mechanical ventilation, including auto-PEEP, lung tissue injury associated with excessive volume (volutrauma) and excessive pressure (barotrauma), apnea, and tachypnea.

After a stable breathing pattern is established, the operator needs to adjust alarm parameters appropriately.

Variation in Breath Delivery

The ventilator begins to deliver the optimum breathing pattern using pressure-targeted breaths.* It adjusts inspiratory pressure and mandatory rate to achieve a given minimal $\dot{V}_E$ based on Figure 12-53. In this graph the horizontal axis and vertical axis represent the measured respiratory rate and tidal volume, respectively. The bull's eye at the center is the optimum target for V_T and f. Each of the four quadrants represent the adjustments the GALILEO will make in inspiratory pressure (PI) and mandatory breath rate (fmand) to attain the optimum target.

- In the upper left quadrant, V_T is high and rate low. ASV will reduce P_I to reduce V_T and it will increase rate.
- In the lower left quadrant, V_T is low and rate is low. ASV will increase P_I and rate to correct the problem.

These breaths are like pressure-control breaths but are also volume-targeted to achieve the optimum calculated V_T.

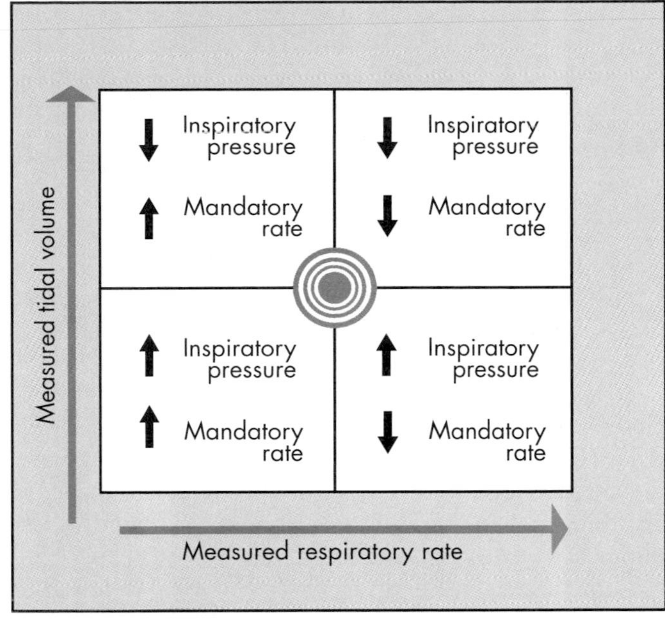

Figure 12-53 A graph representing the measured respiratory rate (x-axis), the measure VT (y-axis) and the target rate and volume (center bulls eye). Each quadrant shows how ASV will adjust ventilator parameters to bring the ventilator toward the target. (See text for explanation.)

- In the upper right quadrant, V_T is high and rate is high. ASV will reduce P_I and reduce rate.
- In the lower right quadrant, V_T is low and rate is high. ASV will increase PI and reduce rate.

If compliance, resistance, or spontaneous breathing efforts change, ASV measures these changes and readjusts the inspiratory support and rate to maintain protective lung strategies. It allows the patient to resume spontaneous breathing when able. Remember that although the mode provides a minimum selected $\dot{V}_E$, patients can achieve a higher $\dot{V}_E$ if they so choose.

Three common scenarios can occur that help to describe the function of ASV.

1. If the patient is not spontaneously breathing, P-SIMV breaths are delivered. The ventilator provides the % $\dot{V}_E$ set. Breaths are time-triggered and pressure-targeted to achieve the desired volume, as well as time-cycled. As lung conditions change, the pressure level is adjusted between minimum and maximum to deliver the calculated V_T with the least amount of pressure.

   If the patient assists a breath after having been apneic, the ventilator delivers a PS breath at the same pressure used for the pressure-controlled breath. This is logical because the ventilator has calculated this to be the pressure required to deliver the optimal V_T.
2. If the patient is providing some—but not all—of the work of breathing, patient-triggered breaths are

pressure-support breaths. Time-triggered breaths are pressure-control breaths. The ventilator calculates the difference between the spontaneous breathing rate and volume delivery, and the calculated rate (missing breaths) and volume delivery. The missing breaths are provided as added (time-triggered) pressure-controlled breaths designed to achieve the desired $\dot{V}_E$.

3. If the patient is spontaneously breathing and triggering all breaths, these will be pressure-support breaths with pressure adjusted to maintain optimum ventilation.

In spite of the advanced intelligence of the GALILEO's closed-loop ventilation with ASV, the clinician is still required to carefully monitor the patient. Such evaluate includes the review of arterial blood gas values, the patient's breathing pattern, and breath sounds, to name a few things.

Sometimes adjustments to the % MIN VOL will need to be made based the findings for arterial blood gases (ABGs). For example if ABGs are normal, % MIN VOL could remain the same, or weaning could be considered as long as the spontaneous breathing pattern was acceptable.

If pH is <7.30 and P_aCO_2 is high, the clinician might consider an increase in % MIN VOL while monitoring inspiratory pressure. If P_aCO_2 is low, the clinician might consider decreasing % MIN VOL as long as the spontaneous breathing pattern is acceptable.

With a low oxygen level (low PaO_2 and SpO_2), the clinician might considering an increase in PEEP/CPAP and F_IO_2. Many possibilities for abnormal ABGs and breathing patterns exist. The clinician needs to carefully evaluate the patient as well as ventilator parameters when making decisions about ventilator management.

To summarize ASV, it is a servo-controlled mode of ventilation that delivers pressure breaths targeted to achieve the desired, calculated volume. Time-triggered breaths are in PCV, and patient-triggered breaths are in PSV. The ventilator continually monitors patient lung characteristics and breathing patterns and calculates an optimum V_T with required pressure delivery and rate to optimize ventilation and minimize patient work of breathing. Patients may be completely controlled when first connected to the ventilator, but as they begin to recover and are able to spontaneously breathe, fewer mandatory breaths are required. Eventually patients breathe with only pressure-supported breaths. The ventilator continues to monitor all parameters and adjust its performance as needed.

Dual Positive Airway Pressure Mode (DuoPAP) and Airway Pressure Release Ventilation (APRV)

DuoPAP and APRV are similar forms of pressure ventilation designed to support spontaneous breathing on two levels of CPAP. These two modes were added to the Gold version of the GALILEO, which is a recent upgrade to the ventilator.

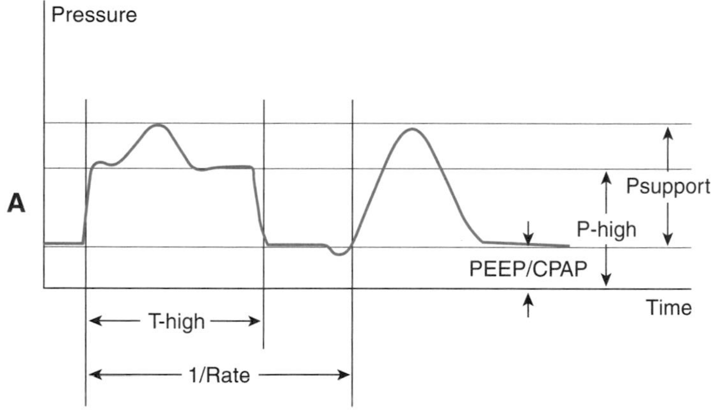

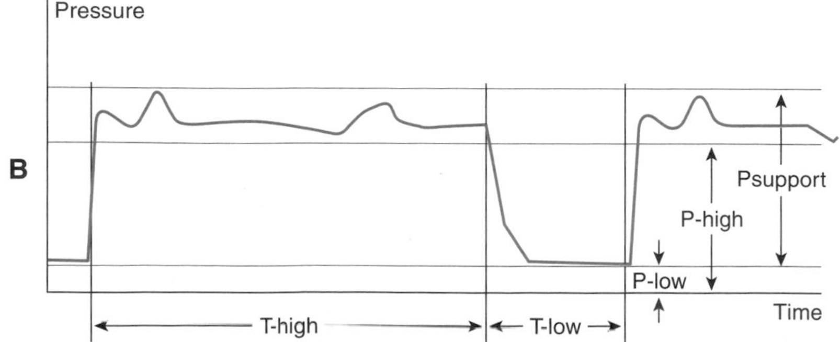

Figure 12-54 A pressure-time curves for DuoPAP, **A,** and APRV, **B.** See text for explanation. (Courtesy Hamilton Medical, Inc, Reno, Nev.)

DuoPAP

In DuoPAP the operator sets a P-high, the PEEP/CPAP (baseline pressure), T-high, and rate. P-high is the target pressure provided during the time frame set by T-high. The rate establishes the TCT. For example, suppose the following parameters are set: P-high = 20 cm H_2O, PEEP = 5 cm H_2O, T-high = 1 sec, and rate = 10 breaths/min. The TCT will be 60 sec/rate or 6 seconds. P-high of 20 cm H_2O will be applied to the airway for 1 second and PEEP of 5 cm H_2O for 5 seconds (TCT – T-high = remaining time). During either of these time intervals the patient can breathe spontaneously. Change from P-high to PEEP and PEEP to P-high can be either patient- or time-based.

With DuoPAP, pressure support can be added to the baseline (PEEP) setting. For example, if PS is set at 20 cm H_2O and PEEP is 5 cm H_2O, the peak pressure when the patient is breathing from baseline will be 20 + 5 or 25 cm H_2O (Figure 12-54).

Spontaneous breaths at the P-high level are only supported with PS when the PS setting is greater than P-high. In the previous example, with a P-high of 20 cm H_2O, if PS was at 20 cm H_2O, a spontaneous breath from the patient would result in pressure rising to 25 during peak spontaneous inspiration (5 cm H_2O above P-high; see Figure 12-54, *A*). Use of DuoPAP by clinicians will undoubtedly evolve as clinical research demonstrates its many potential uses.

APRV

APRV was described in Chapter 11. This mode, like DuoPAP, allows spontaneous ventilation at two levels of PEEP/CPAP. Using the GALILEO, the operator sets APRV by setting P-high and P-low with corresponding time intervals of T-high and T-low. As with DuoPAP, pressure support can be added and it follows the same pattern as described with DuoPAP above. That is, PS spontaneous breaths would only appear above the P-high plateau if PS + PEEP was > P-high.

In clinical use, APRV has most commonly been employed using long T-high times and short T-low times, establishing what is similar to an inverse I:E ratio. Spontaneous breathing is mostly done at the upper pressure level. There is usually a short T-low interval. As with DuoPAP, the change over from P-high to P-low to P-high can be based on either the set time or it can be synchronized with the patient's spontaneous breathing rate (Figure 12-54, *B*).

Noninvasive Ventilation (NIV)

NIV is available with the recently released GALILEO Gold version and was intended for use in the acute care environment, for adult and pediatric patients, but is not intended for home care use. NIV is designed for spontaneously breathing patients only using face masks or nasal masks as the interface with the patient. (*Note*: NIV should not be used for patients with irregular or absent breathing.)

The operator sets the spontaneous mode, baseline pressure (PEEP/CPAP), pressure support level, Timax, and ETS. Because leaks will be present, it is important to set breath cycling criteria and avoid long inspiratory times. It is probably more comfortable for the patient when the ventilator cycles based on the ETS setting (flow-cycle) rather than the Timax limit. A suggested starting point for ETS is 50%. ETS should probably not be set below 30%. However, because of leaks, the ventilator may never reach the flow-cycle criteria, even when ETS is set as carefully as possible. By setting a Timax, this function, available with the neonatal settings, forces the ventilator to cycle into exhalation even when a leak is present, thus avoiding a prolonged inspiratory phase. Timax should be sufficiently long (about 1.5 seconds) to give ETS the chance to cycle the ventilator.

The low V_T and EXPMINVOL alarms should be set low to avoid nuisance alarms. Because of leaks around the mask, the "Disconnection Pat.side" alarm, which is based on volume criteria, is disabled, as is the "Exhalation obstructed" alarm. The "Disconnection vent.side" alarm remains enabled.

Because NIV is a pressure-targeted mode, it is important to pay particular attention to the pressure alarms. The low pressure alarm should be set above PEEP/CPAP and within about 5 cm H_2O of the Psupport setting. If the PEEP and inspiratory pressures can be maintained, the ventilator is sufficiently compensating for leaks. It is recommended that the peak inspiratory pressure not exceed 28 cm H_2O because values higher may result in opening of the esophageal sphincter forcing gas into the stomach.[3]

Special Features

In the new Gold version of the GALILEO, there is an infant application for patients <10 Kg with the use of the new infant flow sensor. Another special feature that has been added to the GALILEO Gold package is the P/V tool, which is described below.

Three additional items available under the ADDITIONS menu are sigh, back up and TRC to the GALILEO Gold version. (*Note*: In the earlier version of the GALILEO the ADDITIONS menu listed sigh, standby, and nebulizer.)

Sigh

In all modes except ASV, a sigh breath can be applied every 100 breaths. In ASV it is applied every 50 breaths. In volume-targeted modes, the sigh function increases the V_T by 50% of the set value to a maximum of 2000 mL. In pressure-targeted modes, sigh increases inspiratory pressure by a pressure up to 10 cm H_2O as allowed by the maximum pressure setting (Pmax). In ASV, a sigh is delivered every 50 breaths at a pressure 10 cm H_2O higher than non-sigh breaths.

Back-Up Ventilation

Back-up ventilation also appears under the ADDITIONS menu and is recommended in all modes where spontaneous breathing is possible, but is actually not necessary in ASV. The operator has the opportunity to select the desired back-up ventilation (ADDITIONS menu) and apnea time (ALARMS window). If the set apnea time is exceeded, the APNEA BACK-UP VENTILATION (ABV) becomes active. A medium priority alarm sounds and the screen displays APNEA VENTILATION. Breath delivery in ABV is either volume- or pressure-targeted.

If ABV becomes active, the message CHECK BACK-UP CONTROLS is displayed. The operator can check the active settings for ABV by opening the CONTROLS window. Settings for ABV will be displayed for reviewing and confirming. To change a setting, the operator follows the procedure for making any parameter change described earlier in this section.

To prevent back-up ventilation from occurring when the patient is disconnected for suctioning or a similar procedure, the operator presses the ALARM SILENCE touch pad. This prevents ABV from becoming active for 2 minutes. In addition, whenever the ventilator mode is changed or ventilator calibration procedures are performed, back-up ventilation is automatically suppressed for 30 seconds.

Tube Resistance Compensation (TRC)

TRC is another feature listed in the ADDITIONS window. It is intended for use in spontaneously breathing patients. TRC can be set to reduce the patient's work of breathing associated with the flow resistance imposed by the endotracheal tube or tracheostomy tube. TRC is active during exhalation in volume modes and both inspiration and exhalation in other modes.

From the ADDITIONS window, the operator opens the TRC window. The selections for tube type include ET-tube (endotracheal tube) or Trache-Tube (tracheostomy tube) or Disable TRC. After a tube type is selected, the tube size can then be dialed in. A 100% compensation setting means the maximum practical compensation is provided. The percent compensated can be adjusted below this value. Pressing CONFIRM enables the TRC settings that were chosen. (*Note*: Setting TRC may result in auto-triggering of the ventilator requiring resetting of values or disabling of TRC.)

Pressure/Volume (P/V) Tool

The P/V tool is an automatic method for performing the super-syringe technique of evaluating pulmonary mechanics by using nearly static conditions (very low flow). The technique is used in spontaneously breathing patients who have such conditions as acute respiratory distress syndrome. It is contraindicated in patients with abnormalities such as open pneumothorax with chest tubes in place. When activated, the following occurs:[1]

1. The expiratory phase of the current mandatory breath is prolonged and pressure is reduced to zero to ensure complete lung emptying prior to P/V testing.
2. The breathing circuit is pressurized to a predefined peak pressure at the set ramp speed. Real-time pressure/volume values are plotted as the P/V technique is applied.
3. Pressure is released to baseline levels. The expiratory time is set to 3 × RCexp (value obtained from the previous breath).
4. Normal ventilation is resumed.

Review of the P/V curve allows the clinician to closely examine the patient's pulmonary mechanics.

Troubleshooting

The monitor, alarm, and message systems for the GALILEO provide important resources in solving common problems encountered during ventilation of a patient. The operator's manual also provides extensive and valuable information on troubleshooting common problems.

If a technical message appears, the operator should record the number indicated with the message and then contact Hamilton Medical technical support about the problem. Any ventilator with a technical error problem should immediately be removed from service and replaced by another unit.

Additional information can be found in the operator's manual and by checking the company's website: www.hamilton-medical.com.

Puritan Bennett 740

The Puritan Bennett 740 ventilator[1,2] is a relatively simple and inexpensive machine that is adaptable for pediatric and adult use in subacute and in acute care settings (Figure 12-55). Its lightweight, electrically powered design allows it to be used readily in patient transport within the hospital.

The update version, the 760, is identical in its platform. The internal mechanical systems, including the linear drive piston, are the same. The basic operating features are also the same. The main difference is the 760 has a slightly different operating panel (user interface). It also offers PCV as an optional mode. In addition, there are a few added features. These will be discussed separately in the section on the 760.

Readers who are familiar with the 7200 by Puritan Bennett will notice some similarities within this next generation of Puritan Bennett ventilators. What was the

"++" key on the 7200 has been replaced by a menu selection. The self-tests, POST, SST, and EST, are still available on the 740 and 760. In the 700 series ventilators, to activate new settings and modes the operator now presses "ACCEPT" rather than "ENTER" as in the 7200.

Power Source

The 740 is an electrically powered, microprocessor-controlled ventilator that does not require high-pressure gas to function. It normally uses a standard 120-volt AC outlet, but can also use the 2.5-hour internal battery or an optional 7-hour external battery. If an F_IO_2 above 0.21 is needed, the unit must be connected to a high-pressure oxygen source (40 to 90 psig). The power on/off switch is on the back panel of the machine, and the high pressure connector is on the right side.

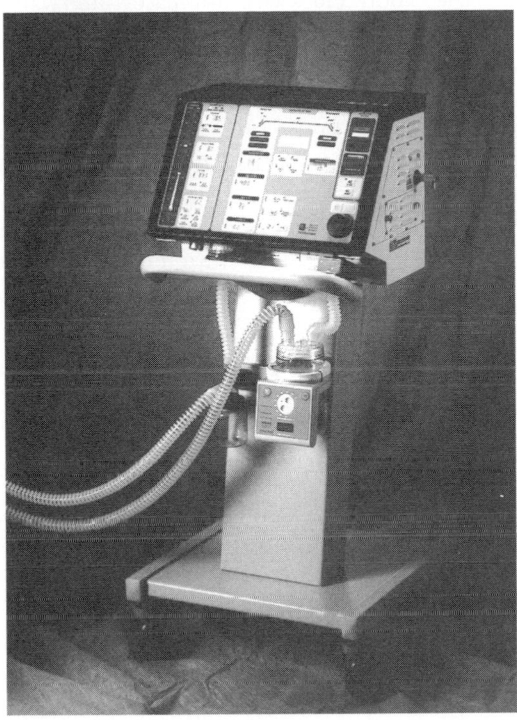

Figure 12-55 The Puritan Bennett 740 ventilator. (Courtesy Puritan Bennett, Inc, a division of Tyco Healthcare, Pleasanton, Calif.)

When the ventilator is first turned on, the message window shows "POST running ... ," and "PM Due:xxx." Post is the power-on self-test that checks the essential system functions and must be completed before the unit will operate. The "PM due" message indicates the number of hours until a routine maintenance check is due. After turning on the unit, the manufacturer recommends letting it warm up (run) for 10 minutes before connecting it to a patient so that the flow sensors respond with greater precision.

There is a more extensive test called the short self-test, or SST. SST should be run and alarms tested before using the unit on a patient (Box 12-56).

When the ventilator is not in use, it is appropriate to store the unit plugged into an AC electrical outlet in the *standby* mode. The standby mode is a waiting state during which the ventilator maintains its settings and the battery charges, thus assuring it will be charged for the next use. Box 12-57 provides instruction on entering the standby mode. Remember, *never* put the ventilator in the standby mode when a patient is connected. When the ventilator is in standby, the following indicators are illuminated: AC Battery Charging, Internal Battery Level, and Safety Valve Open.

Internal Mechanism

Information from the control panel is processed by a microprocessor and stored in the ventilator's memory. A second microprocessor responsible for breath delivery uses this information to control and monitor the pattern of gas flow to the patient.

The 740 uses a frictionless, linear drive piston that eliminates the need for a blender, compressor, or wall air

Box 12-56 Short Self-Test (SST) on the 740 Ventilator

1. Run the SST every 15 days, between patients, and when the patient circuit is changed.
2. Be sure a patient is not connected to the ventilator.
3. Turn the ventilator on. (If it's already on, turn it off and on again.)
4. Press menu and select SST.
5. Follow the instructions as they appear in the message window.
6. The ventilator runs the POST test.
7. Select the humidifier type: HME (heat moisture exchanger), dual heated wire (humidifier with heated wire on the expiratory limb or both inspiratory and expiratory limbs), and no heated wire (conventional humidifier without a heated wire circuit on the expiratory limb) when instructed.
8. Select the tubing type (adult or pediatric) when instructed.
9. Select the ET tube size. Enter the millimeter tube size when instructed. The pressure (flow) rise time is automatically adjusted based on the tube size.
10. When each test run during SST is displayed, press one of the following: ACCEPT, clear (to repeat), reset (to restart SST), and alarm silence (2 minutes) to stop the current test and skip to the end of SST.
11. When the last test is completed, the message "SST finished testing" is displayed along with the overall SST result.
12. Unblock the patient Y and press ACCEPT, and the ventilator reruns POST. After this, it is ready for ventilation.

Box 12-57 Entering the Standby Mode on the 740

1. Turn the ventilator on. If it is already on, turn it off and on again.
2. Press menu and use the control knob to select standby.
3. Press ACCEPT. The message window displays "Is pt disconnected? ACCEPT to proceed."
4. With the patient disconnected, press ACCEPT. The message window displays the confirmation message: "In standby mode. Clear to exit."
5. To exit, press CLEAR, and the POST will run.

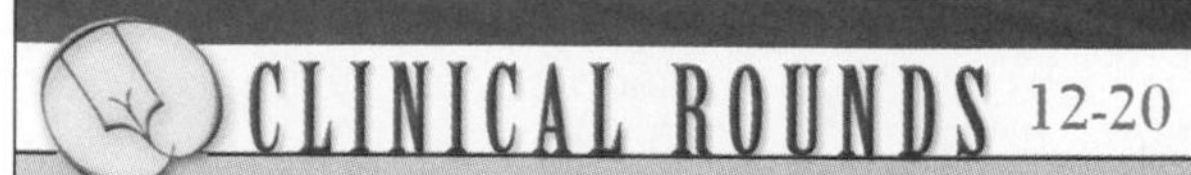

Because the 740 uses a linear drive piston, what waveform would you expect it to produce?

See Appendix A for the answer.

system (Figure 12-56). The piston/cylinder system is designed with a very thin gap (about as thick as a sheet of paper) between the piston and the cylinder wall to reduce friction between the piston and the wall and allow for a faster response than a sealed system. Understandably, a small amount of gas leaks through the gap between the piston and the cylinder. The software program compensates for this minimal leak, assuring accurate volume ventilation. During exhalation, the continuous forward motion of the piston is regulated and maintained to compensate for the leak and maintain set PEEP levels (Clinical Rounds 12-20).

When inspiration begins, the forward motion of the piston sends the gas past a galvanic oxygen sensor, a safety pressure-relief valve, a temperature thermistor, and finally into the patient circuit (see Figure 12-56). (*Note*: The percentage of measure oxygen is displayed in the message window. This $O_2\%$ can be turned on and off using the "oxygen sensor" subheading in the *menu* listing. More about the menu later.)

Controls and Alarms

The front panel of the 740 is grouped into the following three sections (Figure 12-57):

1. The ventilator settings section allows selection of the mode of ventilation, breath type, oxygen percentage, apnea parameters, and menu functions.
2. The patient data section displays monitored airway pressure information, breath timing, volumes, and current alarm settings.
3. The ventilator status section displays the current ventilator parameters and status including alarms, battery conditions, alarm silence, and alarm reset.

Clear, Accept, and Control Knobs

One of the most frequently used controls on the operating panel is the control knob. It is located at the lower right corner of the panel. Once a parameter is selected for change, it is the control knob that adjusts its value. This knob is also used when the menu key is selected to scroll through different items. When a setting value such as tidal volume flashes, this means the knob is linked to that setting. Turning the knob clockwise increases the value and counter-clockwise lowers the value (Box 12-58).

Just above the control knob are two buttons or keys: "CLEAR" and "ACCEPT." Pressing clear cancels recent setting changes and returns to the original settings or previously accepted settings. If it is pressed twice, the ventilator will return to its original operating state. Pressing "ACCEPT" activates new settings. If it is not pressed within 30 seconds of setting a new change, it will return the operating panel to its previous state.

Ventilator Settings

Within this section are controls for selecting the mode and basic parameters for ventilation.

Mode and Breath Selection Keys

On the 740 the touch keys for modes are located at the top center of the operating panel. The top left side of this section is labeled mandatory and the right, spontaneous. Available ventilator modes include A/C mode, SIMV, and spontaneous ventilation (SPONT), which can be supported with PSV. The area labeled VCV (volume-control ventilation) indicates that A/C and SIMV are volume-targeted mandatory breaths. Pressure control ventilation is available on the 760, but not the 740. The modes of ventilation and breath delivery are described later.

Support Pressure

On the right just below the Current/Proposed indicators is an active touch key for pressure support. The *Support Pressure* control sets pressure delivery for spontaneous breaths above the PEEP/CPAP baseline during spontaneous breathing. *Support pressure*, more commonly called pressure support (PS) can provide up to 70 cm H_2O of pressure. Inspiration ends in PS when the inspiratory flow delivery drops to 25% of the peak flow measured or 10 L/min, whichever is lower. For example, if the peak flow was 100 L/min, then 25 L/min would be the 25% point. Because 10 L/min is less than this, the flow stops at 10 L/min.

Although PS is normally flow-cycled out of inspiration, there are two safety back-up features to end the breath. If the pressure in the patient circuit exceeds the set PS by

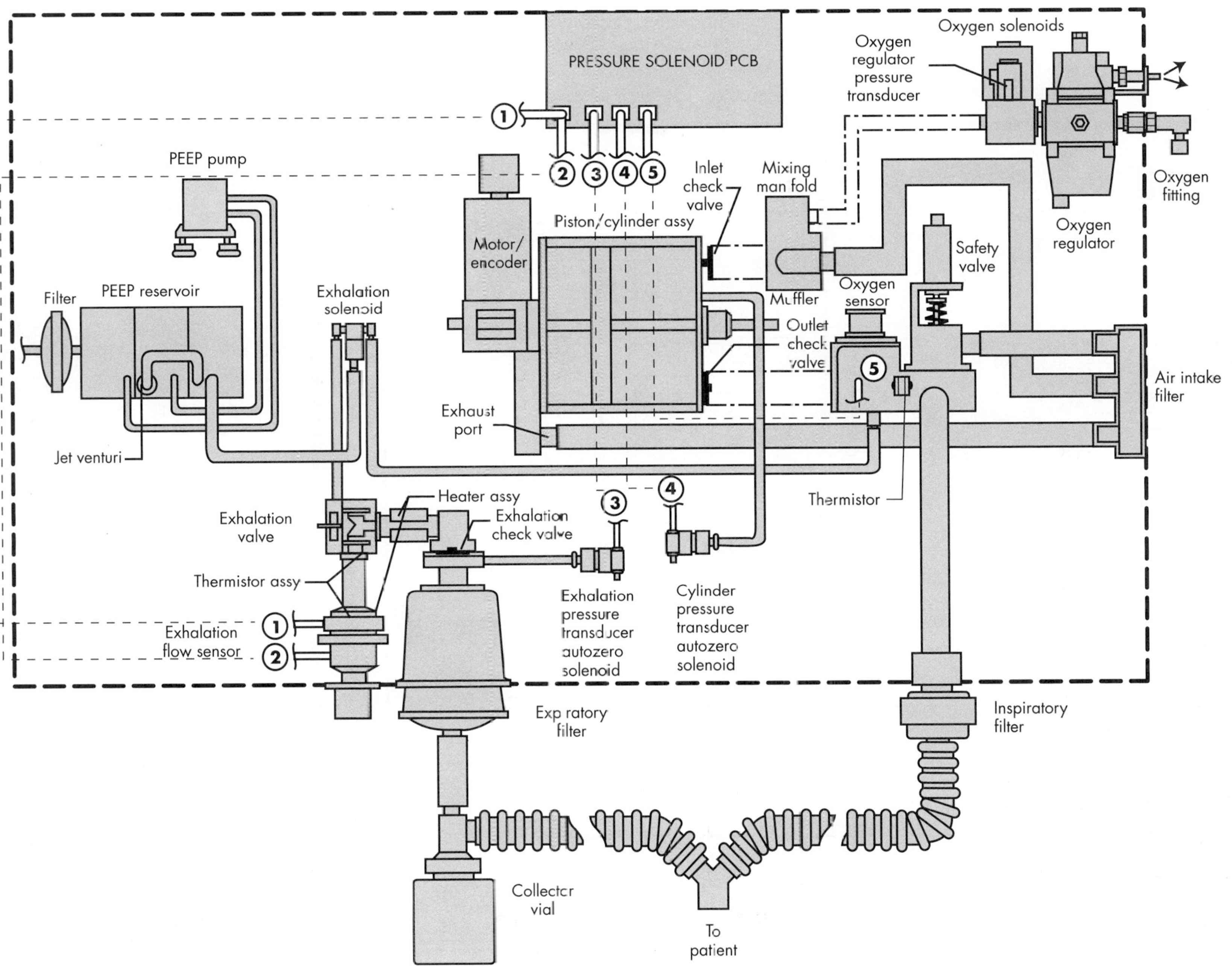

Figure 12-56 The internal pneumatic components of the Puritan Bennett 740. (Courtesy Puritan Bennett, Inc, a division of Tyco Healthcare, Pleasanton, Calif.)

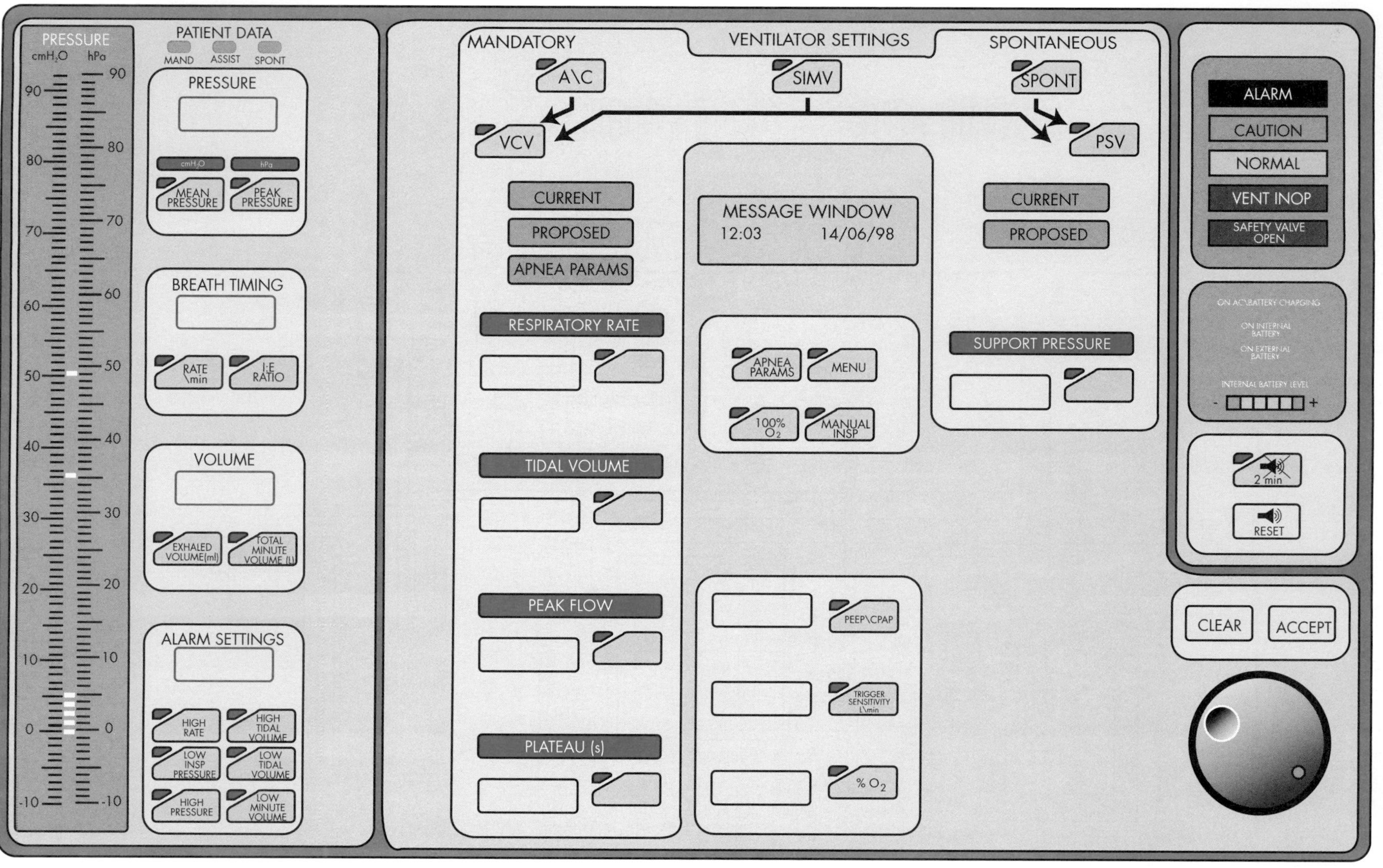

Figure 12-57 The front panel of the Puritan Bennett 740.

Box 12-58 Changing Ventilator and Alarm Settings on the 740[1]

1. Touch a setting key; the key lights, the selected setting flashes, and the message window shows the current setting.
2. Turn the knob to adjust the setting.
3. Repeat steps 1 and 2 for every setting you want to change. Press clear to cancel the most recent setting.
4. Press ACCEPT to apply the new setting. The key lights turn off, and the new settings are displayed. The message window reads: "Setting(s) accepted."

3 cm H_2O, inspiration ends. This could occur if a patient were trying to actively exhale. Inspiratory flow will also end if T_I becomes too long (T_I of 3.5 seconds for adults, 2.5 seconds in pediatric patients). This could happen if there were a significant leak in the circuit.

Indicators

Under the *mandatory* section are three indicator lights: current, proposed, and apnea parameters. *Current* illuminates when the ventilator is operating using the displayed settings. *Proposed* lights when the operator proposes a mode or breath type, but has not accepted it yet. *Apnea Params* lights when apnea ventilation is active. When this is illuminated, the "current" indicator will also light, showing the current, active apnea settings. When the operator is selecting new apnea ventilation settings, but has not accepted them yet, the *Apnea Param* and *Proposed* indicators light.

Under the "spontaneous" section of the Ventilator Setting panel on the right, there are two more indicators, *Current* and *Proposed*. These are active under spontaneous ventilation conditions or when spontaneous ventilation parameters are being set.

Parameter Settings

Several parameters keys are present in the ventilator setting section. The respiratory rate control (3 to 70 breaths/min) sets the guaranteed respiratory rate in A/C and SIMV. The tidal volume control (40 to 2000 mL) determines mandatory breath delivery in A/C and SIMV. Peak flow (range 3 to 150 L/min) delivers a peak flow of gas at the set rate during a mandatory breath. T_I is determined by V_T, flow, and rate. Plateau (0.0 to 2.0 seconds) provides an inspiratory pause at the end of a mandatory breath.

Message Window

At the top center of the operating panel is a window that displays information such as time and date or monitored oxygen percent. It can show up to four lines of information.

The first line is reserved for the highest priority alarm when one is present. On the 760, when no alarm is present, it displays the oxygen percent when the sensor is enabled. It can also provide information about the flow pattern during volume ventilation.

The second line provides information about menu functions or settings, the time remaining for an alarm silence, or current time and date. During normal ventilation it shows the flow in liters per minute (L/min).

The third and fourth lines are reserved for messages. For each breath the third line shows peak and end inspiratory flows. The fourth line shows end expiratory flow for PS breaths or PC breaths (760 only) to evaluate for air-trapping. A patient should have enough time for flow to return to zero before another breath begins. If he or she cannot, then air trapping is present.

Apnea Parameters, 100% O_2, Manual Inspiration and Menu Keys

Just below the message window are four more active keys. apnea parameters, 100% O_2, Manual inspiration, and Menu. The Apnea Params key allows the operator selects settings for apnea ventilation. Apnea ventilation is a back-up mode that becomes active when the set apnea time interval (Ta) has elapsed and the ventilator has not detected a patient inspiration. This feature is active in all modes of ventilation. On the 740 you set volume settings, such as tidal volume, rate and flow. In the 760 one can set either VCV or PCV parameters. For example, in PCV with the 760, the operator could select the inspiratory pressure, T_I or I:E fixed, and so on.

The apnea time internal is not set with the apnea key, but the menu key. Press the menu key and use the control knob to scroll to *User Settings*. Pressing "ACCEPT" once *User Settings* is highlighted accesses this submenu. Scroll to the Apnea Interval (Ta) and press "ACCEPT" to select this option. In the message window the ventilator displays this message: xx(10-60)s, Apnea Interval. Turn the control knob to select the length of the apnea interval from 10 to 60 seconds. For example if you select 30 seconds, the ventilator will wait 30 seconds to see a breath. If it does not see a breath, apnea ventilation begins. Just pressing "clear" eliminates the selection. To activate the new settings, the operator presses "ACCEPT."

To cancel apnea ventilation and return to normal ventilation, press the alarm reset pad located on the right side of the control panel in the ventilator status section. Apnea ventilation will also cancel if the ventilator detects the patient taking two spontaneous breaths.

The *100% O_2* key switches the delivered oxygen percent to 100% when pressed and gives 2 minutes at 100% O_2 then returns to the original setting. It takes a few breaths to get to the 100% delivery value. Please note that the 2-minute interval restarts every time the key is pressed. To stop this maneuver, wait the 2 minutes or press CLEAR.

The *Manual Insp* key delivers one mandatory breath to the patient based on the current settings when the A/C or SIMV modes are active. During spontaneous ventilation,

Table 12-13 Menu function summary

MENU Option	Function
More active alarms	Lists other active alarms in order of priority. (The highest priority active alarm is always displayed on the first line of the message window.) Turning the knob displays other active alarms. The ALARM RESET key clears (erases) this list. CLEAR returns to menu options.
Autoreset alarms	Lists alarms that have autoreset since ALARM RESET key was last pressed. Turning the knob lists other autoreset alarms. The ALARM RESET key clears (erases) this list. CLEAR returns to menu options.
Self-tests	Begins short self-test (SST) or extended self-test (EST).
User settings	(See text for description.)
Standby mode	Places the ventilator in a nonventilating waiting state.
Battery info	Displays the estimated operational time remaining on the internal and external batteries until they need recharging. (Available only when ventilator is operating on battery power.) CLEAR returns to menu options.
Software revision	Displays the version of software installed in the ventilator. CLEAR returns to menu options.
Oxygen sensor	Allows you to calibrate O_2 sensor, enable or disable O_2 sensor, and enable or disable O_2 display.
Service summary	Allows you to view estimates of oxygen sensor life remaining, internal battery operational time remaining, and the time until the next preventive maintenance is due.
Nebulizer	Allows you to start, stop, or view the current state of an EasyNeb™ nebulizer attached to the ventilator.

Courtesy Puritan Bennett, Inc, Pleasanton, Calif.

pressing the manual inspiration key delivers a mandatory breath based on the APNEA parameter settings.

The menu key can be used at any time to view other active alarms and autoreset alarms, to run the self tests, to access user settings, enter the standby mode, display battery information, check software version, control and calibrate the oxygen sensor, obtain a service summary, and use the nebulizer. Table 12-13 summarizes these menu functions. Menu information is displayed in the second line in the message window. (*Note*: The first item of information in the message window is always reserved for displaying any high-priority active or autoreset alarm.)

To access items in the menu, touch MENU, use the control knob to select the desired item, and press ACCEPT to ENTER that particular menu function. To exit the menu, press CLEAR, which also cancels the current function or display setting, or press any ventilator or alarm setting key. These actions cancel any change that was in progress but not completed.

User Settings

There are some special menu items that are unique and worth mentioning. These are under a subscreen that was added to the 740 (and 760) and is called "User Settings." To access this screen, touch the menu key and use the knob to scroll through the choices. When User Settings is highlighted, press the ACCEPT key. This submenu lists the following:

- Endotracheal tube
- Humidifier type
- Date and time set
- Apnea interval (Ta)
- VCV flow pattern
- Speaking valve setup
- Alarm volume

Two additional features are available on the 760, PCV timing setting and Volume LED bar, which will be described in the 760 section.

The *Endotracheal* (ET) tube selection, as other items in this submenu, is selected by using the control knob to scroll to and highlight this line, then pressing ACCEPT. When selected, an ET tube size is displayed in the message window. Use the knob to dial in the ET tube size used on the patient and press ACCEPT to activate this setting. This provides additional pressure and flow to the patient in PSV, and in PCV in the 760, to compensate the work imposed by the resistance of the ET tube.

The *humidifier* setting provides the opportunity to select the type of humidifier being used on the patient. Activating this option corrects calculations for spirometric values when the SST test is run. The operator can choose either heat moisture exchanger (HME), dual heated wire patient circuit, or no heated wire.

The date and time setting allows adjustment of the digital display for these values. Apnea interval (Ta) sets the length of time the ventilator will wait for a breath before beginning apnea ventilation.

VCV flow pattern allows the operator to select a square (constant) or a descending ramp for a flow pattern during volume ventilation. When selected the display screen reads:

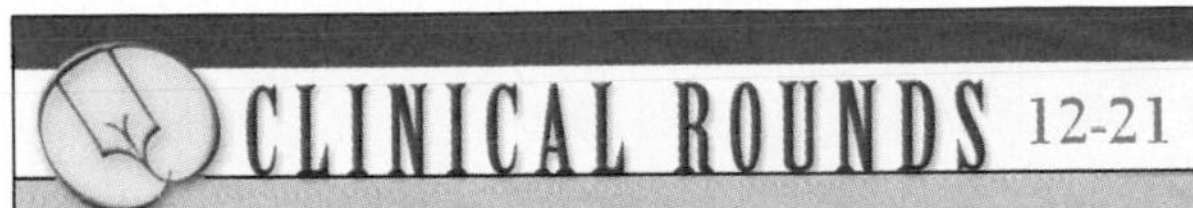

Changing Inspiratory Time in Volume Ventilation with Changing Flow Pattern

During volume ventilation, when changing from a square to a ramp flow pattern on the 740 or 760, you change the inspiratory time. Here's how that works. Suppose you select a square flow (constant flow) pattern to deliver a 500 mL tidal volume at a rate of 20 breaths per minute and your "peak flow" is set at 60 L/min. This flow, 60 L/min, is the same as 60L/60 sec or 1 L/sec = 1000 mL/sec.

Part I

First, what is the T_I, the T_E and the I:E ratio?

Part II

If the respiratory therapist switches the flow pattern from square to descending "ramp" but keeps all the other settings the same, will this affect inspiratory time?

See Appendix A for the answer.

"VCV Flow: square, Ti = 1.05 s. The *square* is the current flow pattern and the Ti is the current inspiratory time in seconds. Turn the knob to select "ramp" or "square." Using a descending ramp waveform can lengthen the inspiratory time. The "peak flow" is the setting on the control panel (Clinical Rounds 12-21). If the change in flow makes it impossible for the ventilator to deliver the volume in the time set, based on the rate, flow, and volume settings, an error message will appear: "Change not permitted." The flow will need to be adjusted.

Alarm volume allows for louder or softer audible alarms.

The Speaking valve setup is a unique feature for use when a special one-way valve that allows the patient to talk is added to the patient circuit. An example is the Passey Muir valve. Because the patient is exhaling into the room, volumes that normally pass through the exhalation volume measuring device do not do so. In this setting the ventilator actually uses the deliver volume to detect high and low V_T alarms. It turns off the low minute volume and disconnect alarms. Because the ventilator's ability to detect problems is reduced, the operator must be especially vigilant to the safety of the patient when a speaking valve is in use, paying particular attention to the instructions provided by the manufacturer of the valve. To select this feature from the User Settings menu, highlight it using the knob and press ACCEPT. The window will display "Speaking valve off" (assuming it is off). Turn the dial to select "Speaking valve on" and press ACCEPT. This function must be turned "off" after the valve is removed from the patient circuit to return the ventilator to normal operation. After the speak valve function is turned on, the screen will list a set of conditions that must be accepted:

- Volume alarms based on delivered volume
- Alarm DISABLED low minute volume
- Alarm DISABLED disconnect alarm

Accepting each of these statements tells the ventilator the operator is aware of the changes being made to the ventilator. It is suggested, while proceeding through the subsequent messages, that the PEEP be set at zero, a 10-second apnea interval be set and a low inspiratory pressure be set, which the ventilator can use to detect a disconnect. During normal operation with the speaking valve function on, the message window will read: "Disconnect disabled speaking valve on delivered volume ______ mL" (740 only). In the 760 using the speaking valve function disables the volume bar graph (more on this graph in the section on the 760). Be sure to return the ventilator to its normal operation when the speaking valve is no longer in use.

PEEP/CPAP, Trigger Sensitivity, and % O_2

At the very bottom center of the ventilator settings section of the control panel are three additional function keys: PEEP/CPAP, Trigger Sensitivity L/min, and % O_2. The PEEP/CPAP control sets the baseline between 0 and 35 cm H_2O and establishes the minimum pressure maintained during both inspiration and exhalation.

The 740 and 760 use flow-triggering to initiate all breaths. The TRIGGER SENSITIVITY control (1 to 20 L/min) establishes the trigger level. Unlike most ventilators, the 740 and 760 do not require a base flow to measure flow changes to provide flow-triggering. The microprocessor monitors flow coming from the piston. When the patient's inspiratory flow exceeds the set flow trigger level, inspiration begins.

The % O_2 key allows you to set the percent oxygen delivery to the patient to be set (21%-100%). After a new setting is selected, it may take several minutes for the O_2% to stabilize.

Patient Data Section

The patient data section of the keyboard allows the operator to view information on pressure, measured volume, rate, and alarm settings. To the far left, a pressure LED bar graph provides immediate readings of airway pressure. The highest sustained double bar of the pressure graph represents the high-pressure limit setting. The next double bar down is the current peak pressure, which is only displayed during exhalation. The last cluster of LEDs on this bar graph rise and fall synchronously with circuit pressure.

Also within the patient data section are monitoring indicators for regular ventilation parameters and common alarms. Table 12-14 lists patient data indicators or keys along with the function and range of each.

Patient Data Section Alarms

Within the patient data section are the common alarms for high rate, high and low pressure, low $\dot{V}_E$, and high and low

Table 12-14 The patient data section with indicators, functions, and ranges on the 740

Key/Indicator	Function	Range
PRESSURE		
MEAN PRESSURE	Shows the calculated value of ventilator breathing circuit pressure over an entire respiratory cycle. Updated at the beginning of each breath.	0 to 99 cm H_2O (0 to 9.9 kPa) Accuracy: ± (1 + 3% of reading) cm H_2O
PEAK PRESSURE	Shows the pressure measured at the end of inspiration (excluding plateau, if any). Updated at the beginning of each expiratory phase. (Default pressure display.)	0 to 140 cm H_2O (0 to 14 kPa) Accuracy: ± (1 + 3% of reading) cm H_2O
BREATH TIMING		
RATE/MIN	Shows the calculated value of the total respiratory rate, based on the previous 60 seconds or eight breaths (whichever interval is shorter). Updated at the beginning of each breath. (Default breath timing display.) The calculation is reset (and display is blank) when ventilation starts, when apnea ventilation starts or autoresets, and when you press the ALARM RESET key.	3 to 199 breaths/minute Accuracy: ± (0.1 + 1% of reading)/minute
I:E RATIO	Shows the ratio of measured inspiratory time to measured expiratory time. Updated at the beginning of each breath.	1:99 to 9.9:1 Accuracy: ± (0.1 + 2%)
VOLUME		
EXHALED VOLUME (mL)	Shows the patient's measured expiratory tidal volume for the just-completed breath. Corrected to BTPS and compliance-compensated. Updated at the beginning of each inspiration. (Default volume display.)	0 to 9 L Accuracy: ± (10 mL + 10% of reading)
TOTAL MINUTE VOLUME (L)	Shows the patient's measured expiratory minute volume, based on the previous 60 seconds or eight breaths (whichever interval is shorter). Updated at the beginning of each breath. The calculation is reset when ventilation starts, when apnea ventilation starts or autoresets, and when you press the ALARM RESET key.	0 to 99 L Accuracy: ± (10 mL + 10% of reading)
ALARM SETTINGS		
HIGH RATE	An active alarm indicates that measured respiratory rate is higher than the alarm setting.	3 to 100 breaths/minute Accuracy: ± (0.1 + 1% of setting)/minute
LOW INSP PRESSURE	An active alarm indicates that monitored circuit pressure is below the alarm setting at the end of inspiration. Inactive in spontaneous mode.	3 to 60 cm H_2O (0.3 to 6 kPa) Accuracy: ± (1 + 3% of setting)
HIGH PRESSURE	An active alarm indicates that two consecutive breaths were truncated because circuit pressure reached the alarm setting.	10 to 90 cm H_2O (10 to 90 kPa) Accuracy: ± (1 + 3% of setting)
LOW MINUTE VOLUME	An active alarm indicates that monitored minute volume is less than the alarm setting, based on an eight-breath running average.	0 to 50 L Accuracy: ± (10 mL + 10% of setting)
HIGH TIDAL VOLUME	An active alarm indicates that exhaled volume for three out of four consecutive breaths was above the alarm setting.	20 to 9000 mL Accuracy: ± (10 mL + 10% of setting)

Continued

Table 12-14 The patient data section with indicators, functions, and ranges on the 740—cont'd

Key/Indicator	Function	Range
LOW TIDAL VOLUME	An active alarm indicates that exhaled volume for three out of four consecutive breaths was below the alarm setting.	0 to 2000 mL Accuracy: ± (10 mL + 10% of setting)
OTHER INDICATORS		
Bar graph	Shows real-time pressures in centimeters of water (cm H_2O) or hectopascals (hPa). An LED shows the current high pressure alarm setting. During exhalation, LEDs show the peak pressure of the last breath.	-10 to 90 cm H_2O (-1 to 9.0 kPa) Resolution: 1 cm H_2O (1 kPa)
MAND	Lights at the start of each breath to indicate that a ventilator- or operator-initiated mandatory breath is being delivered.	Not applicable
ASSIST	Lights at the start of each breath to indicate that a patient-initiated mandatory breath is being delivered.	Not applicable
SPONT	Lights at the start of each breath to indicate that a patient-initiated spontaneous breath is being delivered.	Not applicable

Courtesy Puritan Bennett, a division of Tyco Healthcare, Pleasanton, Calif.

Table 12-15 Clinical alarm messages

Message	Meaning
APNEA	No patient effort detected for the set apnea interval
CONTINUOUS HI PRES	High pressure in circuit has not dropped below high pressure setting (SVO)
DISCONNECT	Exhaled $V_T \leq 15\%$ of set V_T for four breaths; resets if exhaled $V_T > 15\%$
HI EX TIDAL VOLUME	Exhaled $V_T > V_T$ set for 3 of 4 consecutive breaths
HI RESP RATE	Measured rate > high rate alarm set
HIGH PRESSURE	Circuit pressure > high pressure limit setting for two breaths; inspiration ends, and exhalation valve opens for each breath with excessive pressure
LOW EX TIDAL VOLUME	Measured $V_T <$ low V_T alarm set for three of four consecutive breaths
LOW EX MINUTE VOLUME	Measured $\dot{V}_E <$ set $\dot{V}_E$ alarm
LOW INSP PRESSURE	Circuit pressure < set low-pressure alarm during inspiration; active in A/C and SIMV modes only
O_2 % HIGH	Measured O_2 % > 10% of set O_2 % for ≥ 30 seconds
O_2 % LOW	Measured O_2 % < 10% of set O_2 % for ≥ 30 seconds
OCCLUSION	Patient circuit, inspiratory and/or expiratory filters occluded; ventilator detects abnormal differences in measured inspiratory and expiratory pressures; safety valve opens and ventilation is suspended
SETUP TIME ELAPSED	30 seconds or more have passed since you pressed a key or turned the control knob during power-on
PARTIAL OCCLUSION	Patient circuit, inspiratory and/or expiratory filters partially occluded. Ventilator detects abnormal differences in measured inspiratory and expiratory pressures. Ventilator continues normal ventilation.

V_T (see Table 12-14). The ventilator status section uses color indicators to specify the type of alarm occurring (i.e., high or medium priority). If the active alarm is an adjustable alarm, its key light also flashes and the message window is blank. (*Note*: An alarm setting can be changed even while the alarm is active.) The message window also shows additional alarm messages for both clinical and technical alarms. Table 12-15 lists the messages that appear for and the causes of common clinical alarms. Table 12-16 lists the technical alarm messages. When more than one alarm is or has been active, you can view these in the message window using the menu function.

Table 12-16 Technical alarm messages

Message	Meaning
AIR INTAKE ABSENT	Missing air intake filter
AIR INTAKE BLOCKED	High resistance on air intake filter
BAT NOT CHARGING	Battery voltage not increasing
CONTACT SERVICE	Ventilator service required
DELIV GAS HI TEMP	Room air temperature high
DELIV GAS LOW TEMP	Room air temperature low
EXH CCT HI TEMP	Differential pressure sensor temperature high
EXH CCT LO TEMP	Differential pressure sensor temperature low
FAN FAILED ALERT	Fan not operational or fan filter blocked
HI BBU TEMP ALERT	Internal power supply temperature high
HI SYS TEMP ALERT	Internal temperature of ventilator high
LOSS OF AC POWER	AC power disconnect
LOSS OF POWER	AC power lost and batteries are low
LOW EXT BATTERY	Low external and internal battery power
LOW INT BATTERY	Low internal battery power
LOW O_2 SUPPLY	O_2 line pressure low
REPLACE O_2 SENSOR	O_2 sensor missing or reading out of range*
SPEAKER FAILED	Main alarm speaker failed
SWITCH INT BATTERY	Power source has switched to internal battery

Courtesy Puritan Bennett, a division of Tyco Healthcare, Pleasanton, Calif.
*This message will not appear if O_2 alarm is disabled.

When the alarm condition corrects itself, the alarm will autoreset, and the alarm or caution indicators light steadily. The alarm condition that occurred is added to the autoreset alarm list.

Pressing ALARM SILENCE quiets the audible portion of the alarms for 2 minutes. If a new alarm condition occurs within the 2 minutes, the alarm sounds again. (*Note*: Pressing alarm silence during normal operation [no alarms] gives 2 minutes to perform bedside procedures without the audible alarm sounding. If an alarm occurs, the alarm or caution indicators flash, and the message window displays a message about the alarm.) Using the ALARM RESET key clears all alarm indicators and cancels the 2-minute alarm silence.

Ventilator Status Section

At the top right of the front panel, there is a section showing the current operating conditions of the ventilator, which are briefly described here.

Alarm

The alarm light flashes in red to indicate a high-priority alarm and gives an audible signal pattern of three beeps, then two beeps that repeat. The light is steadily lit when an alarm condition existed but has self-corrected (i.e., autoreset). The message window displays the alarm type that was present.

Caution

The flashing yellow caution light indicates a medium-priority alarm. It repeats a sequence of three beeps, and is lit steadily when the condition corrects itself (autoreset).

Normal

During normal operation, the normal light is constantly green.

Ventilator Inoperative

If a hardware failure or a critical software error occurs that could compromise safe ventilation of the patient, a ventilator inoperative condition occurs. The *Vent. Inop.* indicator light illuminates, a high-priority alarm sounds, and the safety valve opens (SVO), allowing the spontaneously breathing patient access to room air. The ventilator must be turned off and another means of patient ventilation established immediately. When the unit is turned on again, a trained individual must run an EST to establish the cause of the problem and correct it.

The ventilator remains in the SVO state until a POST verifies that the power levels to the ventilator are acceptable and that the microprocessors are functioning correctly. The ventilator settings must then be confirmed.

Safety Valve Open

A red indicator shows that the safety valve is open. This may indicate a ventilator inoperative condition or an obstructed patient circuit. If possible, the message window will display the cause and give the time that has elapsed since the last breath. If the condition is corrected and the *Vent. Inop.* indicator is off, press the alarm reset key to resume ventilation.

Internal/External Battery Indicators

In the battery charging section of the ventilator status panel, the indicator lights for the internal and external battery are located. These are explained earlier (see Table 12-14).

Alarm Silence and Reset

Below the battery indicators are the 2-minute alarm silence and alarm reset touch pads. The 2-minute silence quiets audible alarm sound for 2 minutes from the most recent time the key was pressed and it illuminates yellow when the silence is activated. The alarm reset does three things:

- Clears all alarm indicators.
- Cancels the alarm silence period.
- Resets the patient data displays.

The alarm will reactivate if the condition that caused the alarm is still present. This key will also cancel Apnea Ventilation if it is active. It also reestablishes previous settings and ventilation resumes. The only exception is a ventilator inoperative condition, which must be treated as a serious condition and the unit taken out of service.

Modes of Ventilation

There are three basic modes of ventilation in the 740 ventilator: A/C, SIMV, and spontaneous, each of which has a touch pad control on the front panel. In the A/C and SIMV modes, mandatory breaths are volume-targeted. When either A/C or SIMV is selected, the VCV pad LED lights, indicating that mandatory breaths are volume-targeted. Spontaneous breaths can be assisted with PS in the SIMV setting or the SPONT setting.

During ventilation, the active mode key is lit and settings are displayed. To change the mode, perform the same procedure as changing a setting. Select the mode by pressing the desired key. All of the available settings in that mode flash. For every flashing setting key, the operator must touch the key, and adjust the setting with the control knob before the new mode can be applied (Clinical Rounds 12-22). After all entries are completed, pressing "ACCEPT" activates the new mode.

Assist/Control

In A/C, the ventilator delivers volume-targeted breaths that are labeled as VCV breaths on the control panel. Breaths are patient- or time-triggered, volume-targeted, and volume-cycled. T_I can be extended by adding an inspiratory pause.

SIMV

In SIMV, mandatory breaths are patient- or time-triggered, volume-targeted, and volume-cycled. Spontaneous breaths are flow-triggered, pressure-targeted, and pressure-cycled unless PS is added.

Spontaneous

During spontaneous ventilation, the patient can breathe spontaneously from a zero baseline or from PEEP/CPAP. Breaths are flow-triggered, pressure-limited, and pressure-cycled. In addition, spontaneous breaths may be assisted using PS.

Pressure Support

With PS selected, patient-triggered spontaneous breaths in either the spontaneous or the SIMV mode receive the set pressure above PEEP/CPAP during inspiration. Breaths are patient-triggered, pressure-targeted, and flow-cycled. (See earlier discussion on support pressure.)

Apnea Ventilation

After all the parameters are set on a patient and the ventilator has started its normal operation, a message appears in the message window "Review Ta = 20 s" where Ta is the apnea interval and 20 is the current apnea interval in seconds. It is appropriate at this time to set the parameters for apnea ventilation.

Apnea back-up ventilation is an emergency mode of ventilation available in the spontaneous mode or with mandatory rates set at less than 6 breaths/min. It is triggered when the selected apnea interval time (Ta) elapses without a patient-detected breath. Box 12-59 outlines the procedure for setting apnea ventilation.

Troubleshooting

The message window and alarm package which are available with the 740 help to troubleshoot the majority of problems that may occur. The operator's manual provides more detail about the technical and clinical alarm conditions if special problems arise.

As with microprocessor-operated medical equipment, the Puritan Bennett 740 may be susceptible to certain transmitting devices such as cellular phones, walkie-talkies,

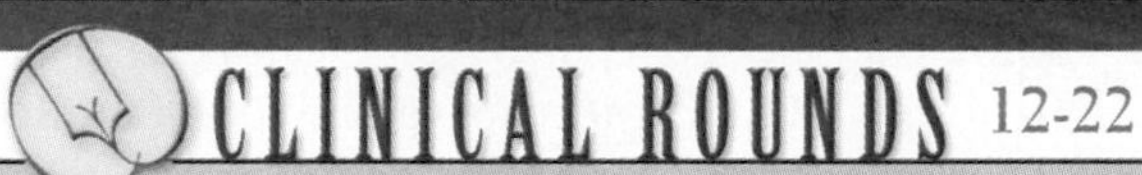

The respiratory therapist is setting up the A/C mode for a patient who will be ventilated with the 740. After selecting all of the settings he wants to change, he notices that the tidal volume key is flashing. What does this indicate, and what should he do?

See Appendix A for the answer.

Box 12-59 Setting Apnea Parameters on the 740

1. While the ventilator is in the spontaneous mode, or in A/C or SIMV with a rate less than 6 breaths/min, press *apnea params*. The apnea parameter key lights steadily.
2. The following key lights flash for apnea settings: respiratory rate, tidal volume, and peak flow. The message window displays "Apnea setup. Select a setting."
3. Each flashing light control must be touched. If necessary, adjust the setting as well. For example, touch the tidal volume key; it now lights steadily. Use the knob control to change the volume setting if desired and touch ACCEPT to have the new apnea V_T accepted.
4. Once all settings are set, press ACCEPT again to apply the new apnea settings. The message window will read "Setting(s) accepted."
5. If you press CLEAR before the settings have been accepted, the parameter is not updated. The apnea params key flashes. The message window shows: "All setup canceled. Update apnea."

cordless phones, and pagers. The radio frequency emissions from these devices are additive, so the ventilator must be located a sufficient distance from these to avoid interruption of its operation.

If an abnormal restart alarm occurs when the ventilator is turned on, the unit may be running on AC, but the battery is low.

There are some common errors respiratory therapists make when using the Puritan Bennett 740. These include the following:

- Failure to touch (address) each of the flashing settings buttons during startup and then connecting the patient and erroneously assuming the ventilator is operating appropriately.
- Not setting the low pressure alarm limit appropriate when using the "Speaking valve mode."
- Assuming that the battery will charge when the PB 740 is plugged in but turned off.

It is very important that therapists are familiar with all the aspects of safely operating the 740, as with any ventilator.

Puritan Bennett 760

As with the Puritan Bennett 740, the 760 ventilator is easy to operate, but still uses advanced technology (Figure 12-58). The 760 is nearly identical in its internal platform to the 740. For example, it also uses a linear drive piston and only requires an AC electrical power source to function. It is probably easiest to think of it as a 740 with additional options. The primary differences are the operating panel (user interface), the addition of the pressure control breath and a few additional features added to the menu.

It is assumed that the reader will have reviewed the function of the 740 before reading this section. The focus in this section will be the added options and the interface differences.

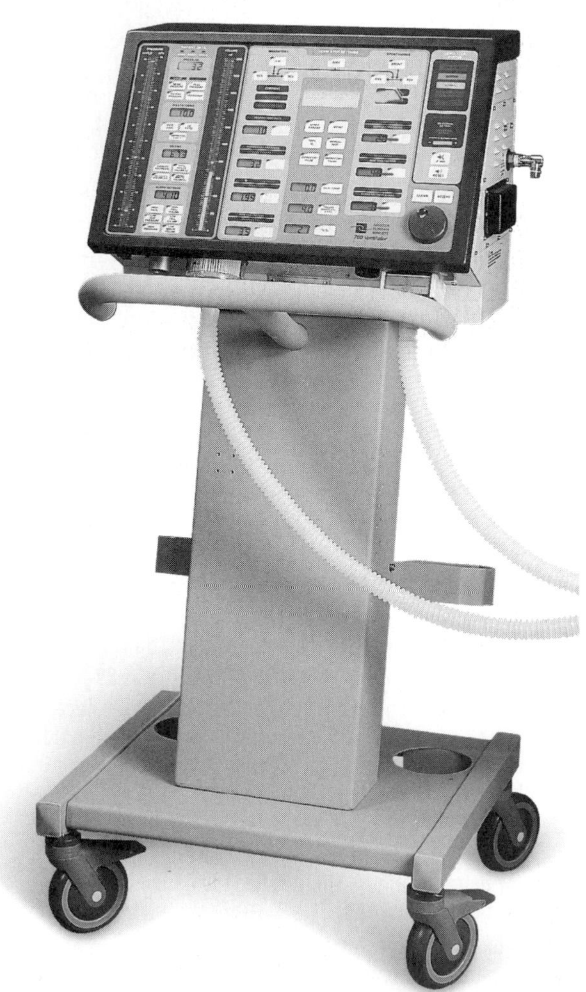

Figure 12-58 The Puritan Bennett 760 Ventilator. (Courtesy Puritan Bennett, Inc, a division of Tyco Healthcare, Pleasanton, Calif.)

Controls and Alarms

The 760 operating panel is also divided into three sections: the Ventilator Settings section, the Patient Data section, and the Ventilator status section (Figure 12-59).

Ventilator Settings Section

The 760 Ventilator Settings section contains the following added controls. In addition to A/C and SIMV volume ventilation, it also offers A/C and SIMV with pressure control ventilation (PCV) for the mandatory breaths. Settings and data display for PCV are added to the settings located in the left and right columns. These include inspiratory pressure, T_I or I:E ratio setting, rise time factor, inspiratory and expiratory pause, and exhalation sensitivity.

Inspiratory pressure sets the target pressure for PC breaths and is the pressure above PEEP delivered to the patient during inspiration (5 to 80 cm H_2O).

T_I/I:E Ratio displays the inspiratory time (T_I) and the I:E ratio and is located above the "peak flow" control. Which parameter is constant, T_I or I:E ratio, is determined by the setting the operator uses under the menu section called "user settings." (More information on this is provided in a later section.) The selected T_I or I:E ratio can be changed at any time during PC. After it is active, the selected value remains constant, even if the respiratory rate is changed. (Box 12-60 gives an example). To help set an appropriate inspiratory time during PCV, the message window displays peak inspiratory flow, end inspiratory flow and end exhalation flow in liters/minute. For example, if the operator wanted a slight pause at the end of inspiration (no flow period), T_I can be adjusted so that inspiratory flow ends at zero. To guard against auto-PEEP, be sure the flow at the end of exhalation is zero.

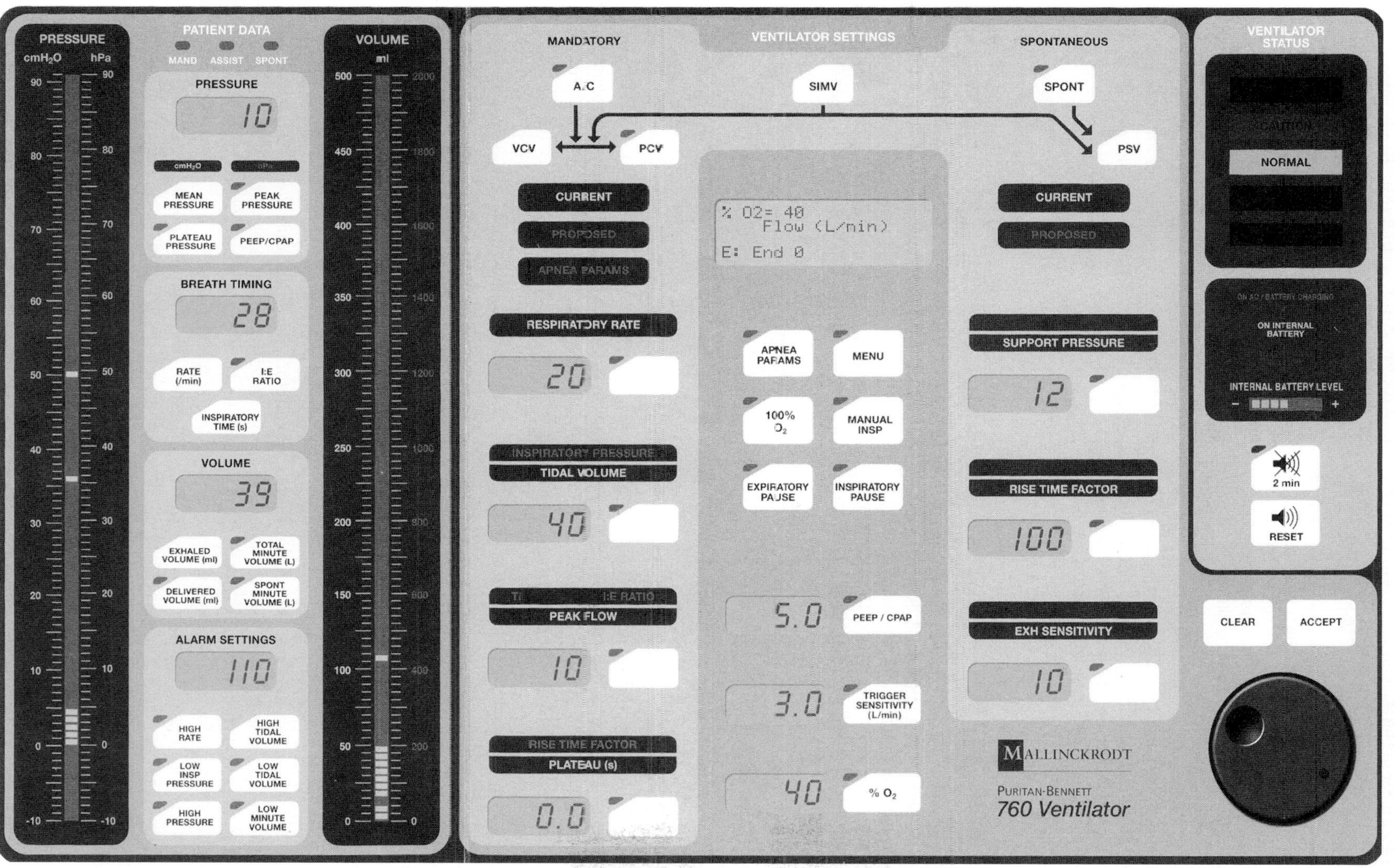

Figure 12-59 The Graphical User Interface (GUI) of the Puritan Bennett 760 Ventilator. (Courtesy Puritan Bennett, Inc, Pleasanton, Calif.)

Box 12-60 Using Constant T_I and Constant I:E Ratio on the 760

Suppose PCV is set with T_I constant and with a rate of 12 breaths/min. The total cycle time (TCT) will be 5 seconds. If T_I is set at 1 second, expiratory time (T_E) is 4 seconds (I:E = 1:4). T_E can vary and so can the I:E ratio when you change the rate. Suppose you increased the rate to 15 breaths/min. The TCT is now 4 seconds, T_I is still 1 second and T_E is now 3 seconds (I:E = 1:3).

You can change the selected T_I or I:E ratio, but the setting remains constant when you change the respiratory rate in PCV. Using our previous example, you can still increase the T_I when it is set as a constant. For instance, even with T_I set as the constant, you can increase T_I to 2 seconds at the set rate of 15 breaths/min. The new result will be a T_I of 2 sec, a T_E of 3 seconds and an I:E ratio of 2:3, or 1:1.5.

Suppose I:E is held constant at 1:4 with a rate of 12 breaths/min. T_I is 1 second and T_E is 4 seconds. If the rate is increased to 15 breaths/min with a constant I:E of 1:4, then T_I and T_E vary. T_I in this case is 0.8 seconds and T_E is 3.2 seconds (See Chapter 11 for equations). Again, you can change the I:E, even though it is constant. For example, if I:E is changed from 1:4 to 1:3 with a rate of 12 breaths/min, the T_I will be 1.25 seconds and the T_E 3.75 seconds.

There are two rise time factor controls on the 760 that allow rise time for PCV and PSV to be adjusted independently. *Rise Time Factor* for the PCV breaths is displayed above the PLATEAU control when PCV is the mandatory breath type. The control for setting Rise Time is located on the right side of the ventilator panel. Rise time is the amount of time it takes for inspiratory pressure to rise from 0% to 95% of the set pressure during PCV. It is adjustable from 5 to 100. A setting of 100 means it takes only 100 milliseconds (ms) to rise to the set pressure. This is a very rapid rise to the set pressure. The set pressure is delivered quickly so that the pressure is in the lungs for a larger part of the inspiratory time. When set at 5, it takes longer (2500 ms or 80% of T_I, whichever is less) to reach the set pressure. This is a very slow, tapered curve with the set pressure being in the lungs for a shorter period of time. Tapering the rate at which the pressure enters the lungs may be more comfortable for the patient (see Chapter 11, section on sloping or rise time for more information). When adjusting this setting, the actual time in seconds it takes to reach 95% of the target pressure appears in the message window.

The center section of the Ventilator Setting panel has the following items that are also present in the 740: apnea parameters, menu, 100% O_2, Manual inspiration, PEEP/CPAP, trigger sensitivity and %O_2. These were described with the 740. One additional feature with the apnea parameter settings on the 760 is the operator can select either PCV or VCV in the apnea ventilation (AV) settings. Using PCV in apnea ventilation allows rate, inspiratory pressure, and I:E Ratio or T_I to be set. Rise time factor is fixed at 50% in AV in the 760.

The three new items on the 760 control panel are the *Expiratory Pause* key, the *Inspiratory Pause* key, and the *Exhalation Sensitivity* key. These and the additional menu items will be reviewed.

Menu Items

In the 760 Menu under *User Setting* two features were added. The 760 User Setting menu includes a PCV timing variable and a volume LED bar enable/disable function. (*Note*: To enter the menu, press the "Menu" key and use the control knob to scroll to User Setting, then press "ACCEPT.")

PCV timing variable. When selecting *PCV Timing Setting*, the ventilator displays the currently selected item in the message window. It will display either "Timing variable = Ti" or "Timing variable = I:E." To change this variable, turn the control knob to highlight T_I or I:E. Press the "ACCEPT" key to activate the change. Pressing "CLEAR" allows the ventilator to remain with the current setting.

Volume LED. The *Volume LED bar* menu, also listed under user settings, provides two choices: Enable LED bar and Disable LED bar. The Volume LED bar itself is located in the patient data section of the operating panel and will be described later.

Expiratory Pause

Using Expiratory pause allows for measurement of auto-PEEP. The message window normally shows the end expiratory flow at the beginning of each breath. If expiratory flow is present when the ventilator delivers the next breath, auto-PEEP is present. At this point it would be appropriate to perform an expiratory pause.

It is assumed that the patient is not actively breathing when this measurement is done, because a stable reading cannot be made if the patient is trying to exhale or inhale during the maneuver. When Expiratory pause is activated, the exhalation valve closes at the end of the expiratory phase and the ventilator delays delivery of the next mandatory breath. The pause continues as long as the key is held down (maximum 20 seconds) and should last only until the expiratory pressure stabilizes. Five things can end the expiratory pause measurement: (1) releasing the key, (2) the patient initiates a breath, (3) an alarm occurs, (4) the pause lasts more than 20 seconds, or (5) the ventilator detects a leak.

After the maneuver, the auto-PEEP and total PEEP values are displayed in the message window for 30 seconds. The expiratory pause cannot be performed if the rate is set at less than 3 breaths/min.

Inspiratory Pause

The inspiratory pause key is used, as its name suggests, to pause at the end of inspiration. The data recorded are then used by the ventilator to calculate lung compliance and airway resistance. These values are displayed in the message window for 30 seconds after the test is performed. Again, as with end expiratory pause, the patient cannot be actively breathing if this test is to be successfully performed.

There are two ways to execute an inspiratory pause. First, the pause button is pressed once and the ventilator looks for a stable inspiratory plateau pressure reading. This method ends the pause when the plateau stabilizes or at the end of 2 seconds, whichever comes first. With the second method, after pressing the button the first time, the operator presses and holds the button after the pause has begun. The key must be held for at least 2 seconds. The pause can be lengthened for up to 10 seconds.

During this maneuver the ventilator closes the expiratory valve. When the button is activated the ventilator waits until the end of the inspiratory phase of the current breath. Or, it waits until next mandatory breath occurs. At the end of the inspiration, the pause is initiated. If the key is activated during spontaneous ventilation, the ventilator uses a mandatory breath based on the apnea ventilation settings for breath delivery before the pause.

You can press "clear" or release the INSP PAUSE key at any time to cancel the pause maneuver. An alarm occurring will also cancel the maneuver.

Exhalation Sensitivity

The final item on the Ventilator setting section included in the 760 is the *Exhalation Sensitivity* control. This adjusts the percent of the peak flow at which inspiratory flow ends during pressure support. Normally, a pressure support breath ends when the ventilator determines that the inspiratory flow to the patient has dropped to 25% of the measured peak flow or when the flow is 10 L/min, whichever is less (flow-cycled breath). On the 760, this percentage termination point is adjustable from 1% to 80% of peak flow. This applies to spontaneous as well as pressure supported breaths. Exhalation begins when the inspiratory flow is less than the set value. For example, if peak flow during inspiration is 100 L/min and exhalation sensitivity is set at 50%, exhalation will begin when the inspiratory flow drops to 50 L/min (50% of 100 L/min).

To help set the exhalation sensitivity appropriately it is important to watch the flow values displayed in the message window and to watch the patient. The patient should not be struggling to exhale; nor should their inspiratory times be too long. (*Note*: It is advisable to check that SST was recently run. This helps ensure the accuracy of these flows by ensuring that tubing compliance calculations are correct.)

Patient Data Section

As with the 740, the patient data section contains a pressure bar graph and digital windows that display pressure, breath timing, and volume monitored data. It also contains an alarm section that displays alarm settings. The 760 data section also contains a volume bar graph.

Plateau pressure and PEEP/CPAP touch pads have been added to the pressure section of the 760 so these values can also be displayed along with the mean and peak pressure. In the timing section, inspiratory time (seconds) has been added to the rate and I:E ratio displays of the 740. The operator can now obtain not only exhaled volume and total minute volume, but delivered volume and spontaneous minute volume as well. The delivered volume shows the measured inspiratory tidal volume for the last completed PCV or PSV breath.

The alarm section contains the same alarm parameters as the 740: high and low tidal volume, high rate, high and low inspiratory pressure, and low minute volume.

Volume Bar Graph

The volume bar graph (see Figure 12-59) shows real-time exhaled volumes in millimeters (mL). The scale is determined by the high tidal volume alarm setting. For example, for a high tidal volume alarm of less than 500 mL, the scale is 0 to 500 mL with 5 mL resolution. For high tidal volume alarms set higher than or equal to 500 mL, the scale is 0 to 2000 mL with 20 mL resolution.

The Volume Bar Graph can be enabled (turned on) or disabled (turned off) by using the User Setting menu accessible with the MENU key. LEDs indicate the current high and low tidal volume alarm settings. During exhalation, moving LEDs show the maximum exhaled volume for the last breath.

Ventilator Status Section

The Ventilator Status section on the right side of the operating panel are the same as those located on the 740, as are the control knob and the CLEAR and ACCEPT keys.

Modes of Ventilation

PC breath type is available on the 760. It can be selected as the mandatory breath in either A/C or SIMV. PC breaths in

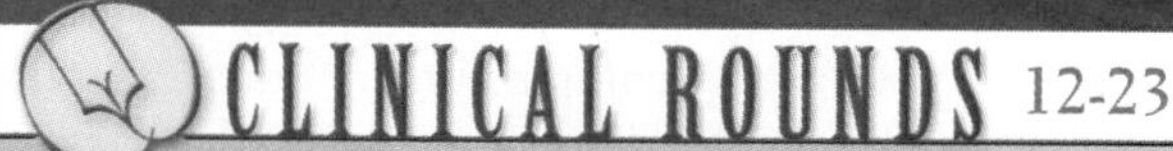

During A/C PCV ventilation using the 760, the respiratory therapist records the following data:

Inspiratory pressure = 18 cm H_2O, PEEP +5 cm H_2O, V_T exhaled = 350 mL (volume bar graph), rate = 16 breaths/min, T_I constant at 1.0 second, T_E = 2.75 seconds (I:E 1:2.75), end inspiratory flow = 5 L/min, end expiratory flow = 3 L/min.

Do you think the therapist should perform an inspiratory pause? An expiratory pause? What is your opinion of this information?

See Appendix A for the answer.

these two modes are patient- or time-triggered, pressure-targeted (inspiratory pressure setting), and time-cycled. After selecting either A/C or SIMV, the operator sets the variables that flash to select the parameters that must be set for the designated mode. Remember, as with the 740, all of the flashing controls must be set before pressing the "ACCEPT" key, which activates the mode. Along with rate, the operator can select T_I or I:E ratio as constants (PCV Timing Setting). These variables establish the inspiratory and expiratory time, and I:E ratio, which are displayed in the ventilator and data status sections of the operating panel. The operator must be sure to set the desired *PCV Timing Setting* from the User settings in the MENU. Rise time can be used to taper the beginning of the mandatory PC breath. See Clinical Rounds 12-23 for a problem related to PCV.

When SIMV is selected, the spontaneous breaths occur from the baseline pressure (PEEP/CPAP) and can also be supported with PS. The expiratory sensitivity can be set to adjust the termination point of inspiratory flow.

Puritan Bennett 840

The Puritan Bennett 840 (Figure 12-60) ventilator is owned and manufactured by Tyco HealthCare, a division of Tyco International.[1-3] It is designed to ventilate infant, pediatric and adult patients and is most commonly used in the acute care setting. The ventilator includes a Breath Delivery Unit (BDU) that controls ventilation and connects to the patient circuit. Above the BDU is a liquid crystal display (LCD) touch sensitive interface screen. The screen, called the Graphic User Interface (GUI) displays monitored patient data and ventilator settings and information.

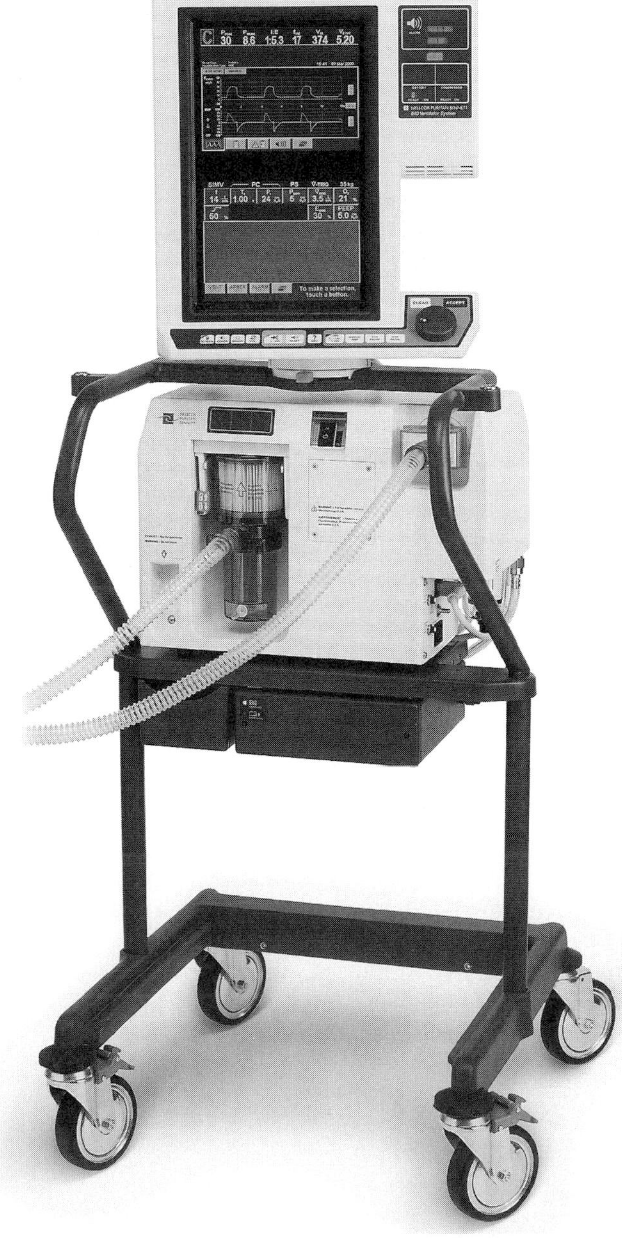

Figure 12-60 The Puritan Bennett 840 ventilator showing the graphic user interface, and the breath delivery unit. (See text for description.) (Courtesy Puritan Bennett, Inc, a division of Tyco Healthcare, Pleasanton, Calif.)

Power Source

The 840 ventilator is both electrically and pneumatically powered. It is electrically powered by a 120-volt AC. The on/off switch is located on the center front of the BDU. A green indicator lights adjacent to this when the unit is turned on. (*Note*: To turn the unit off, simply flip the switch off. No additional action is required.) There is a back-up battery power source as well. It is pneumatically powered by two gas sources, compressed air and oxygen (35 to 100 psig sources). The unit is intended for use with these two gases only.

Battery

The 840 has an internal back-up battery (802 Back-up Power Source) that provides power to the BDU and screen, but does not power the compressor (optional) or the humidifier. It is intended for emergency power if AC power is lost or falls below an acceptable minimum. Keeping the ventilator plugged in to an AC outlet between patient uses charges the back up battery (Box 12-61).

Patient Circuit

The patient circuit includes a main inspiratory line, patient connector and main expiratory line connected to an internally mounted exhalation valve. There are inspiratory and expiratory filters as well. The expiratory filter is heated and comes with a collector vial for liquid condensate from exhaled gas. The filter can be autoclaved for cleaning. The ventilator periodically checks the resistance through this filter during SST self-testing.

Box 12-61 Battery operation with the 840

The indicator for the battery or back up power source (BPS), is located in the upper right hand portion of the front panel in the status indicator section. A yellow light indicates the BPS is operating and the AC power is off or inadequate. A green light indicates the ventilator is operating and the BPS has at least two minutes charge available.

There are also battery charging indicators located on the BPS panel itself, below the breath delivery unit. When the ventilator is operating on main power, the top BPS charging indicator (green indicator next to gray battery icon) shows that the BPS is fully charged. When the bottom yellow indicator, next to gray battery icon, is illuminated, the BPS is still charging.

Compressor

A separate compressor can be purchased for the unit. It can provide up to 200 L/min flow and a minute ventilation of 50 L/min on room air. The compressor is attached to the ventilator by a high pressure air hose, data communication cable and electrical power cord. However, even if the compressor is attached, when the ventilator high pressure air connector is attached to wall or cylinder air, the ventilator switches to the wall air source. Indicators for the compressor are located in the Status Indicator Panel (SIP) on the upper right hand section of the GUI indicates compressor activity (Figure 12-61). There are two indicators for the compressor: "ready" and "on". When the green light is illuminated next to the "ready" indicator, the compressor is available. When the green light is on next to the "on", the compressor is supplying air to the ventilator.

Self Tests

Self tests on the 840 include the POST, EST and SST. For any self test, the ventilator MUST BE DISCONNECTED FROM THE PATIENT and the Y connector uncapped. Power on self test (POST) runs automatically to check the microprocessor when the ventilator is powered on. The extended self test (EST) is a more extensive test and is generally run by a qualified service technician.

The short self test (SST) takes 3 minutes and verifies proper ventilator operation, checks the patient circuit for leaks, measures circuit compliance and resistance, and checks the exhalation filter resistance. The SST should be run when a new circuit or humidifier is added, between patient uses and at least every 15 days during use. SST can only be run immediately after the ventilator is turned on. Box 12-62 provides further instructions. Following SST to begin normal ventilation the operator touches EXIT SST and then ACCEPT. The ventilator reruns POST and then displays the start up screen.

Box 12-62 Performing SST Testing with the Puritan Bennett 840

When the start up screen is displayed, the SST selection is pressed. (*Note*: The operator must be sure the patient connector is not capped or the ventilator will go into Safety Back-up Ventilation.) The operator must then press the TEST button on the side of the ventilator within 5 seconds. Waiting longer cancels SST.

When the Current SST Setup screen appears, the patient circuit is selected, such as adult or pediatric. Then the humidifier type is selected: HME (heat moisture exchanger), non-heated expiratory tube or heated expiratory tube. The operator sets the humidifier volume when applicable. Pressing "ACCEPT" begins SST and the screen provides instructions to the operator as it is being preformed. (*Note*: The operator must pay special attention to the messages in the lower right corner of the bottom screen. For example, part of the test requires connecting and disconnecting parts of the circuit and capping the patient Y connector.)

Following the test, the screen provides an alert about the ventilator's status. Should an error occur, a review of the operator's manual helps to determine what procedure needs to be followed. The operator's manual provides a table listing SST outcomes and how to proceed in each case.

Controls and Alarms

The controls and alarms are managed by the Graphic User Interface.

Graphic User Interface (GUI)

The Graphic User Interface has three basic sections: a touch sensitive screen, the status indicator section (upper right portion), and the control function keys and control knob along the bottom of the unit below the touch screen. Each of these will be reviewed.

DualView Screen

The "DualView" touch sensitive screen (see Figure 12-61) is visually divided into two sections. The upper screen displays patient data in both digital and waveform formats. The lower screen shows the actual settings, provides an information and instruction area and also has a "SandBox". The SandBox allows the therapist to select several changes at one time and view these before they are actually activated.

Upper Screen

The top screen holds patient information only and displays four areas: patient data, alarms and ventilator status, miscellaneous data and graphics (see Figure 12-61). No ventilator settings can be changed in this area.

The patient data at the very top of the GUI is provided in abbreviations. For example, $P_{I\ END}$ is the end inspiratory

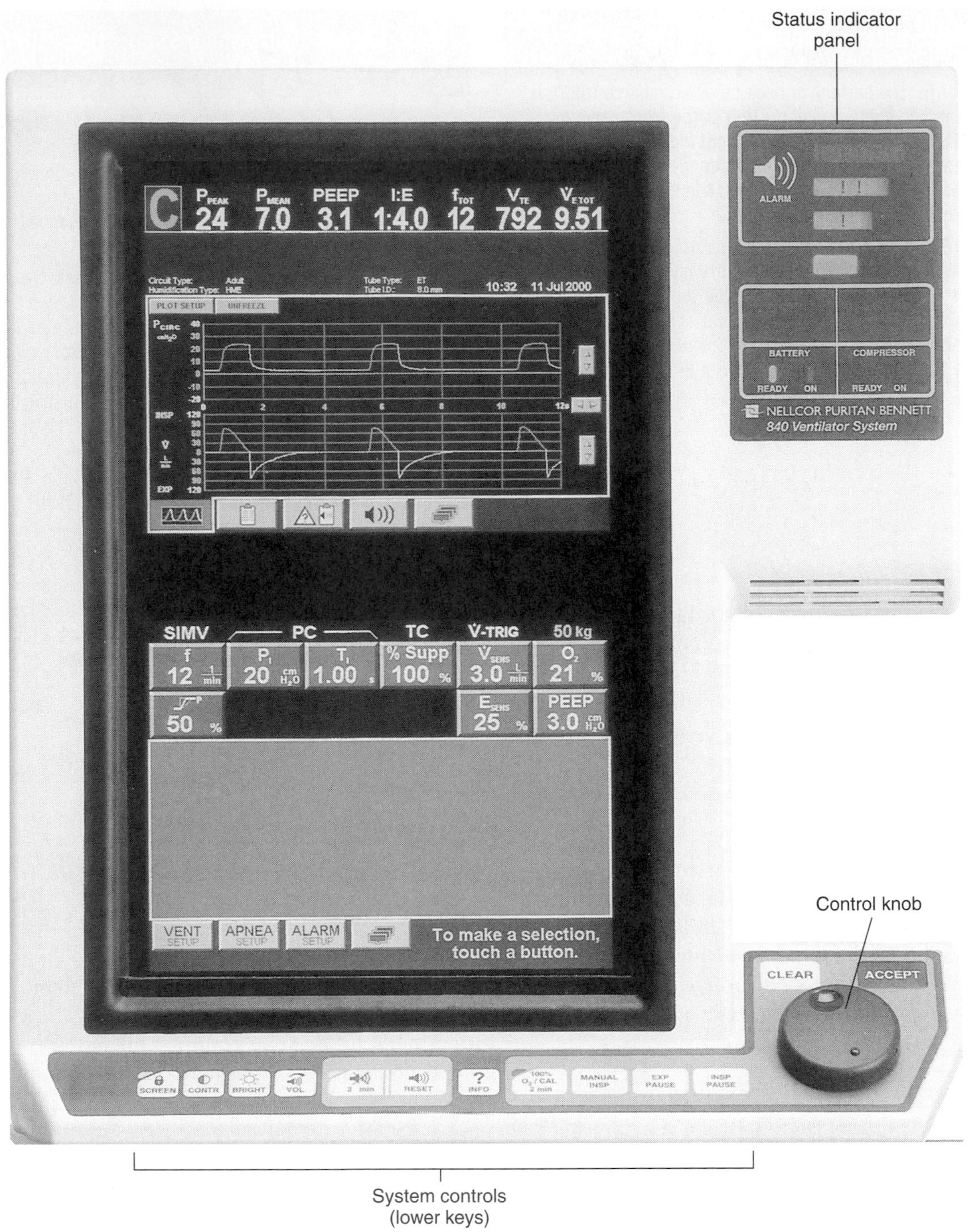

Figure 12-61 The Puritan Bennett 840 Graphic Interface Unit (GIU) with the DualView screens, the status indicator panel, the lower row of system control keys and the control knob. (Courtesy Puritan Bennett, Inc, Pleasanton, Calif.)

pressure. $\dot{V}_{ETOT}$ is total exhaled minute volume. (*Note*: $P_{E\ END}$ is displayed as PEEP on updated units.) The patient data area gives information about monitored parameters such as mandatory breath rate, I:E ratio, tidal volumes, PEEP, and peak flow. The manufacturer occasionally uses abbreviations that may be unfamiliar to the practitioner. Fortunately, these can be defined immediately by touching and holding the abbreviation for which information is needed. The full definition appears in a field at the bottom left corner of the lower screen. This disappears when the abbreviation is no longer being touched by the operator.

Below the monitored patient data on the top of the upper screen is a section that displays alarm messages when they occur. Alarms are grouped together by conditions that cause them and are accompanied by the help message with some suggestions to remedy the problem. For example, the "Circuit disconnect" alarm indicates there is "no ventilation," "check patient," and "reconnect circuit". These appear in

Box 12-63 A Spray of Particles

During a patient disconnect using earlier ventilators, like the 7200, the loss of pressure in the circuit, when PEEP was in use, resulted in the ventilator trying to compensate for the pressure drop. These ventilators would have a continuous surge of flow through the circuit to try to maintain pressure. The rapid flow would hit the water typically condensed in the circuit and create an aerosol that was then released into the patient's room. The risk was that everyone in the vicinity could inhale these potentially contaminated particles.

Table 12-17 Other Screens for Upper Data Window—Puritan Bennett 840

Diagnostic Code Log	Extensive History of Last 80 Alarms and the Results of the EST Test
Ventilator Configuration	Serial number and software version for the ventilator
Operational Time Log	Compressor time and total ventilator operation time
Test Summary	Displays last SST and EST
SST Results	Results of each test performed in SST

red and an audible high priority alarm simultaneously occurs. There is a digital timer that indicates the accumulated time of the non-ventilation period. During this alarm message, the gas flow in the circuit is reduced to 5 L/min. This is an "idle" mode. The reduction in flow helps prevent a spray of aerosolized particles from occurring (Box 12-63).

The alarm display section can list the two highest priority alarms at any time. Any others that might be present are displayed in another section called "more alarms" in the miscellaneous window (more on that later).

Below the alarms window is the graphics display area that typically monitors waveforms such as pressure-time and flow-time scalars. Additional graphs and loops are available below the display screen in a row of five icons (see Figure 12-61)

- Waveforms
- More information (a clipboard)
- Alarm log (a triangle and clipboard with picture of a speaker)
- More alarms (picture of a speaker)
- Other screens (picture of screens)

The *waveform* icon is the control that allows access to other scalars and loops. Under the more information *clipboard* one can see data not commonly displayed at the top of the screen such as spontaneous minute volume and measured oxygen percentage. The *alarm log* icon displays the last 80 alarm events. This section is deleted when a new patient is set up for ventilation. The *More alarms* icon displays active alarms not included in the upper alarm message section near the top of the screen that displays the top two alarms. Finally, the *other screens* contains items shown in Table 12-17.

Table 12-18 Four Function Keys on Lower Screen on the 840

Vent Setup	Used to activate the SandBox and make several changes at one time. Changes won't activate until the "ACCEPT" key is touched.
Apnea Setup	Allows changes to be made for the apnea ventilation mode. These include pressure or volume ventilation, tidal volume or set pressure, flow or inspiratory time (or I:E), flow waveform, oxygen percentage and apnea interval.
Alarm Setup	Shows actual values of a parameter and adjustable values on a bar graph scale. Alarms are automatically set up based on the patient's entered ideal body weight information, but can be adjusted.
Other Screens	Communication set-up for communicating with external devices. Time/Date changes, More settings: humidifier type, O_2 sensor enable/disable, and D_{sens} (disconnect sensitivity)

Lower Screen

The lower screen has five areas: the primary settings, the SandBox, the setup keys, the symbol definition area and the prompt area.

The primary settings appear at the top of this screen and are the current set parameters. They may include the trigger sensitivity, mode, mandatory rate, and volume, depending on the mode being used.

Below this is the subscreen area, which is accessed when the operator wants to change the mode or several settings all at one time. This is the SandBox which allows changes to be made without the changes becoming active until the ACCEPT key is pressed. The available ventilator modes for the 840 will be reviewed in a later section. (*Note*: Newer versions of 840 software allow batch changes to be made in the primary settings area as well.)

In the lower right hand corner is the Prompt screen. It is used to display information to guide use of the ventilator functions. In Figure 12-61 the prompt screen reads, "To make a selection touch a button" meaning a *screen button*. To the left of the prompt screen is a row of four screen buttons: Vent Setup, Apnea Setup, Alarm Setup and More Screens. Table 12-18 gives information about these four functions.

Status Indicator Panel

This separate panel, located to the right of the upper touch screen provides information about the status of the following: alarm indicators, ventilator inoperative condition, safety valve open, battery status and compressor status.

Alarm indicators show the level of alarm priority. High level alarms are indicated by the symbol "!!!" which is displayed in red, blinks rapidly and emits a tone during a high priority alarm situation. A medium alarm (yellow – "!!") beeps three times and blinks slowly if active. A low priority "!" alarm is a steady yellow light and the alert gives a two tone alert.

The "Vent Inop." Indicator means the unit cannot ventilate the patient and must be taken out of service. The safety valve open (SVO) means only a spontaneously breathing patient can breathe room air through this valve. During a "Vent Inop." condition, the operator must find an alternative method of ventilating the patient until the unit can be replaced.

System Controls Lower Keys

The touch keys across the bottom of the GUI, just below the lower touch screen, serve several important functions and are reviewed as they appear from left to right.

1. The Screen Lock Key appears yellow when the screen is in the locked position. When it is locked, touching the screen has no effect on the ventilator's function. This prevents accidental changes in settings and displays and allows for cleaning the screen. It can be unlocked by touching the control again. The screen automatically unlocks during alarm conditions.
2. The Display Contrast Key and the Display Brightness key alter contrast and brightness in the original black and white screen but have no function with the color GUI and are non-functional in newer versions of the GUI display.
3. The Alarm Volume Key can change alarm volume by holding down this key and turning the control knob.
4. The "2 min" Alarm Silence Key turns green and produces a two minute alarm silence period when it is touched. It will be reactivated in three conditions:
   - When the 2 minutes passes,
   - If the alarm reset key is pressed,
   - If a new high-urgency alarm condition occurs.
5. The "Reset" alarm key does four things. It clears active alarms, clears autoreset high-urgency alarms so they are no longer illuminated, cancels an active alarm silence and records any active alarms into memory. However, a "Device Alert" alarm cannot be reset, because of the danger to the patient. (More about these alerts later.)
6. The Question Mark (?) Key provides a display of basic operating information about the ventilator in the upper display window.
7. The "100% O_2/Cal 2 min" delivers 100% oxygen for 2 minutes when the ventilator is connected to an oxygen source. It lights up green during this period. Pressing it again restarts the 2-minute interval.
8. The Manual Inspiration Key delivers a manually-triggered breath based on the current mandatory settings. It can only be activated during the latter part of a mandatory exhalation to avoid breath stacking.
9. The Expiratory Pause Key is used to estimate end expiratory pressure and auto-PEEP (Box 12-64).
10. Inspiratory Pause Key is used to estimate the end inspiratory pressure. Pressing this key will pause inspiration for up to 8 seconds if held. This freezes the pressure-time waveform and shows the value for plateau pressure (P_{PL}), compliance (C) and resistance (R).
11. At the far right of the row of keys is the Control Knob. This is used to adjust the values for a setting, such as tidal volume. Once a parameter has been selected for change, touching the screen button for that item on the lower screen highlights the button. Once highlighted, turning the knob clockwise increases the value and counterclockwise decreases the value. Instructions appear in the lower right corner. Adjacent to the knob are two touch pads. The "clear" pad clears the change. The " ACCEPT" pad accepts the new setting and thereafter the ventilator operates using the new setting.

Breath Delivery Unit (BDU) Indicators

Besides the normal status indicator screen, there are also indicators on the front of the breath delivery unit (BDU) (see Figure 12-60). These illuminate red under serious conditions. The left indicator is a "ventilator inoperative" indicator. When active it cannot be reset. The ventilator must be taken out of service and another method of ventilating the patient provided. The middle alert is "safety valve open (SVO)," which indicates the patient is able to spontaneously breathe room air. This happens if the ventilator is inoperative, in which case the valve automatically opens. The right indicator alerts to a loss of the Graphic User Interface (GUI). When it illuminates red a malfunction is present in the GUI so that information displayed is unreliable. The ventilator must be taken out of service.

Alarms

The manufacturer refers to the alarm system as the SmartAlert system. The ventilator is equipped with the normal alarms such as high pressure, high and low tidal volume, high rate, prolonged inspiratory time, high and low oxygen percentage, apnea, power loss, and circuit disconnect. When these occur, a description of the alarm condition and possible remedies to the problem appear in the monitored data screen. The operator's manual provides a complete description of the available alarms.

An *apnea alarm* occurs when a patient's inspiratory efforts are not detected after a timed apnea period. The ventilator goes into Apnea Ventilation (AV) and the AV screen will be displayed. To resume normal ventilation, the reset button is pressed. Normal ventilation will also resume if the patient takes two spontaneous breaths.

Box 12-64 Expiratory Pause Key Function

The expiratory pause key is pressed to activate expiratory pause. Once the key is pressed, the ventilator waits until the end of the next mandatory inspiration and then closes the patient circuit. Closing the circuit involves closing the inspiratory and expiratory valves. An expiratory pause maneuver is begun.

For an automatic pause (key pressed and released), the ventilator performs the pause and waits until the pressure in the circuit stabilizes then takes a reading. The automatic pause lasts between 0.5 and 3 seconds.

For a manual pause (key pressed and held), the ventilator takes its measurement as soon as the pressure stabilizes or the pause ends. The pause cannot last longer than 20 seconds, at which time the patient circuit automatically opens. The manual pause is recommended for patients with suspected air-trapping or auto-PEEP.

On the screen, the graphics are displayed. This allows visualization of pressure stabilization. Of course, expiratory pause cannot be performed if the patient is making any ventilatory efforts or it will not be able to stabilize. At the end of the maneuver, the value for intrinsic or auto-PEEP ($PEEP_I$) and for total PEEP ($PEEP_{TOT}$ = set PEEP + [$PEEP_I$]) is displayed.

The *Device Alert* indicates that a background check detects a problem. This is a serious situation. The ventilator will only reset when an EST test is run and passed.

When a *procedure error* is detected, the ventilator begins "Safety Ventilation." For example, a procedure error is committed if a patient is attached to the ventilator before completing the setup, whereupon the procedure error alarm activates the Safety Ventilation function. A procedure error will also occur if power has been removed from the ventilator for 5 minutes or more.

Safety ventilation consists of pressure control mandatory breaths with a set pressure of 10 cm H_2O, a rate of 16 breaths/min, an inspiratory time of 1.0 seconds, an F_IO_2 of 1.0, and a PEEP of +3 cm H_2O.

To set the alarm limits, the alarm screen is selected (Alarm Setup button, lower screen). A window opens showing bar graphs, which indicate the current settings of the alarms and the measured value for the parameters (Figure 12-62). To change an alarm setting, the desired alarm screen icon is pressed. (*Note*: This icon is shaped like a box containing a speaker.) When the alarm is highlighted, the control knob is used to change the value. The "ACCEPT" button is pressed to activate the changes.

To view the alarm history, select the Alarm Log in the monitored patient data screen. To reset the alarms, touch the reset key at the bottom row of controls below viewing screen.

Basic Parameter Changes–Touch, Turn, and Accept

Making ventilator changes requires the therapist to view the lower screen and select a setting or mode. When the desired

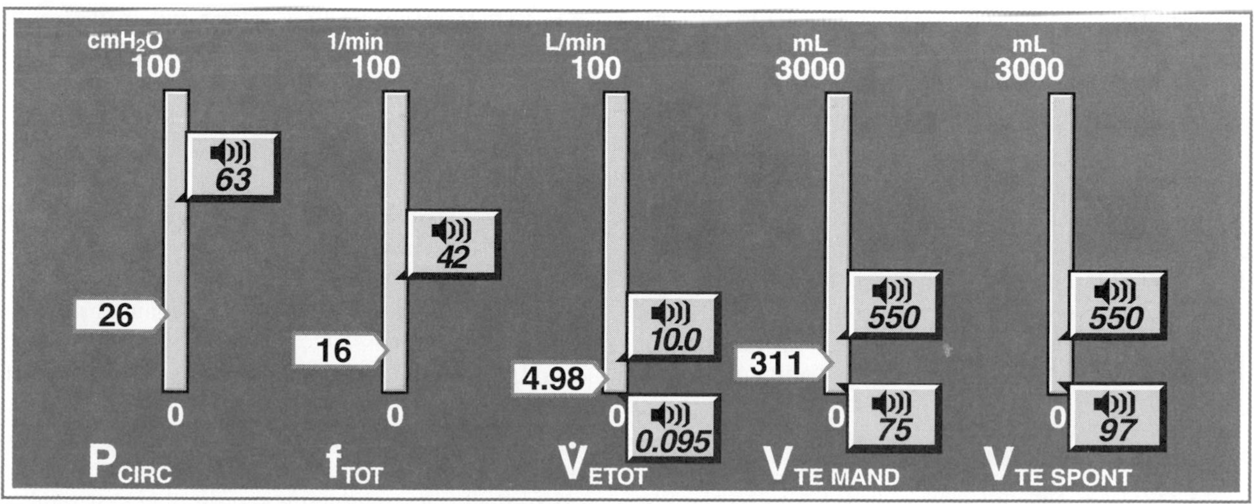

Figure 12-62 The Puritan Bennett 840 alarm setup screen which appears in the lower panel. Touching the alarm icon and turning the control knob adjusts the alarm level. The arrows to the left of the bars indicate the current value for that parameter. (See text for description.) (Courtesy Puritan Bennett, Inc, Pleasanton, Calif.)

Box 12-65 Calculating Ideal Body Weight (IBW)[5]

An estimate of IBW in pounds is as follows:

For males IBW = 106 + 6[Ht (inches) - 60] where *Ht* is the height

For example for a 5′ 8″ (68″) tall male: IBW = 106 + 6(68-60) = 106 + 6(8) = 154

To convert to kilograms, divide the weight in pounds 154 by 2.2, 154/2.2 = 70 Kg.

For females IBW = 105 + 5 [Ht (inches) - 60] where *Ht* is the height

For example for a 5′ 6″ (66″) tall female: IBW = 105 + 5(66-60) = 105 + 5(6) = 135.

To convert to kilograms, divide the weight in pounds 135 by 2.2, 135/2.2 = 61.5 Kg

parameter is on the lower screen, it is touched to highlight the item, the value is adjusted using the control knob and "ACCEPT" is pressed. The new setting becomes operational.

Starting a New Patient

After turning on the ventilator, a POST runs and the startup screen appears with the following items listed:

- Same patient (use previous settings)
- New patient
- SST

To begin a new patient, that selection is pressed. The practitioner is prompted to enter the patient's IBW. After this is entered, pressing the "continue" button on the screen brings up the next screen. Values for IBW are available in the operator's manual or can be calculated (Box 12-65).[5]

After IBW is entered by the operator, the mode is selected by touching the mode button and using the control knob to scroll through the options. The following modes are available: assist/control, SIMV, spontaneous, and BiLevel (optional). After mode selection, the operator choses mandatory breath type (VC, PC), or the spontaneous breath type (PS, none), where appropriate, and trigger sensitivity (pressure or flow). After the "continue" button is touched, the proposed settings then appear in the SandBox (lower screen). The SandBox allows access to the settings available for the mode and breath type selected. Values calculated by the computer based on the entered IBW appear. These values can be accepted or changed by touching the parameter and adjusting the value with the control knob. To begin ventilation once all the settings are selected, the operator presses the ACCEPT key. To cancel, the "RESTART" key is pressed.

Apnea Ventilation Screen Adjustment

After the ventilator is set up and the new patient is connected, it will begin ventilating using the assigned values. The next screen to appear is the Apnea Ventilation screen. The initial, IBW-based parameters are also automatically set in the AV mode. The therapist may wish to adjust the apnea time interval (T_A, range 10 to 60 seconds).

AV, a back-up mode, is activated when the apnea time interval has been exceeded without the ventilator delivering a breath. An AV display appears in the upper panel where the waveforms screen normally appears. The AV display is *not* an active touch screen. In addition to displaying AV parameters, this screen also displays two messages: one, how to adjust AV and two, how to deactivate the current apnea ventilation state. (*Note*: If the operator touches one of the icons, such as the graphics icon, the Apnea screen disappears.) To deactivate AV, press the alarm reset control. If the patient is still apneic, another alarm alert (!!) will occur. To quiet the alarm, the operator presses alarm silence.

Alarm Limits

The alarm limits to the patient are automatically adjusted based on the IBW. However, they should be checked to be sure they fit the desired values.

Making a Single Parameter Change

To quickly change a single parameter, the operator touches the screen button for the parameter in question. It will become highlighted and the "Breath Timing Bar" will appear on the screen (more information is provided in a later section). As the control knob is turned, the digitally displayed value of the setting changes. The numbers appear red to indicate that the value is different from what is currently active. After the value is set to the one desired, pressing the "ACCEPT" key activates the new value.

The Breath Timing Bar

The breath timing bar (Figure 12-63) shows the results of parameter setting changes on the I:E ratio. This allows a visual representation of the effect of the changes made. For example, if flow is increased, inspiratory time shortens for the same volume and rate, in volume ventilation (Figure 12-63, *A*). The green indicates T_I and the yellow indicates T_E. The actual value in seconds appears inside the bar for both T_I and T_E. Total cycle time is shown at the right end of the bar. The minute ventilation, based on set rate and tidal volume, appears above the bar (Clinical Rounds 12-24, Part I)

During pressure ventilation (Figure 12-63, *B*), three icons that look like locks appear above the breath timing bar. The left lock, if activated, makes T_I constant. (*Note*: Touching the lock activates it.) Any changes in rate may affect the I:E ratio and T_E, but T_I remains constant. If the second lock is activated, the I:E ratio becomes constant and T_I and T_E can change. The right lock, when activated, keeps T_E constant and T_I and I:E ratio vary. One possible reason for fixing T_E is if there is some concern that the patient might be air-trapping and the therapist wants to be sure T_E is long enough for complete exhalation. Clinical Rounds 12-24, Part II provides an exercise in pressure ventilation with T_I constant.

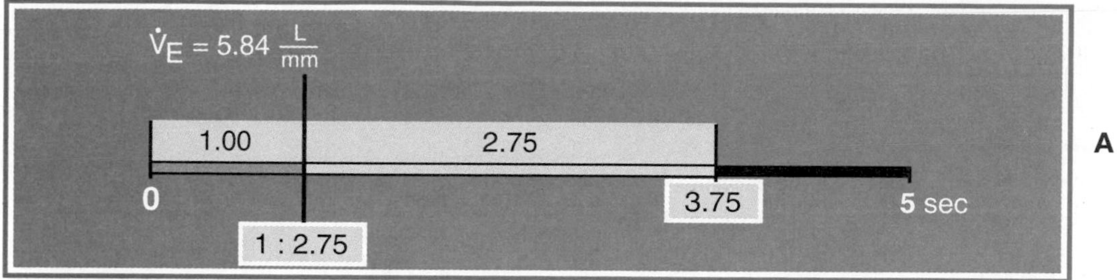

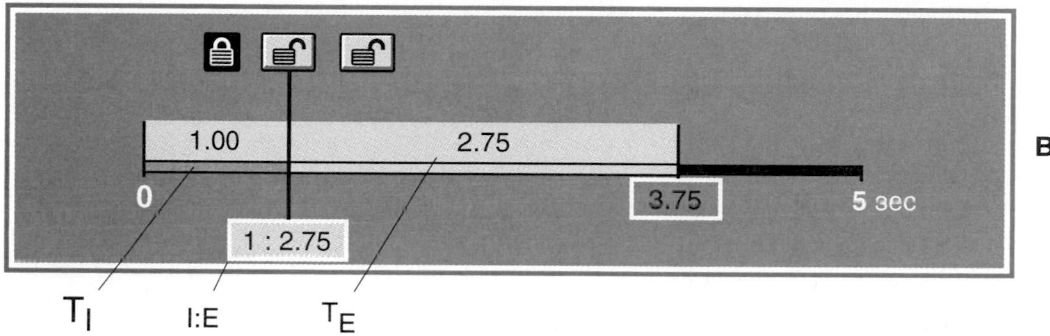

Figure 12-63 **A,** shows the breath timing bar for volume ventilation with a T_I of 1.0 seconds, a T_E of 2.75 seconds, and a TCT of 3.75 seconds on a time line of 5 seconds on a Puritan Bennett 840. The I:E ratio is 1:2.75 and the $\dot{V}_E$ is 5.84 L/min. **B,** shows the bar for pressure ventilation. In this picture, while values are the same as in **A,** the first lock above the bar is locked, so T_I is constant. (See text for description.) (Courtesy Puritan Bennett, Inc, Pleasanton, Calif.)

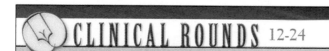

Breath Timing Bar

Part I

Assume that the current breath timing bar shows $T_I = 1.00$, $T_E = 2.75$, with a tidal volume (V_T) of 365 mL, a constant flow of 22 L/min, and a rate (f) of 16 breaths/min. Notice the total cycle time (TCT) is 3.75 seconds ($T_I + T_E = TCT$). What will the new values be for T_I and T_E if the flow is increased to 30 L/min?

Part II

During PC ventilation, the T_I is locked. T_I is 1.0 seconds long. The rate is 16 breaths/min with TCT = 3.75 second, T_E currently is 2.75 seconds. The respiratory rate is changed to 10 breaths/min. What will happen to T_I, T_E, and TCT? Then the T_I is changed to 2.0 seconds. Will this change occur with T_I locked?

See Appendix A for the answer.

Modes of Ventilation

The following section provides information about the modes available on the 840.

Assist/Control

Assist/Control ventilation is available as volume- or pressure-targeted. In this mode all breaths delivered have the preset volume (VC) or preset pressure (PC) delivered for every breath.

In volume A/C, abbreviated ASVC, breaths can be either time- or patient-triggered (pressure or flow), volume limited and volume-cycled (see Chapter 11). The following parameters can be set: V_T, mandatory rate, peak flow, flow waveform (square or descending ramp), trigger sensitivity (pressure or flow), PEEP, and F_IO_2. A plateau time (T_{PL}) for an inspiratory hold or pause may be selected, as can an upper pressure limit (Pcirc). The expiratory valve is closed during inspiration. This is different than the PC mode in which the expiratory valve floats. A cough results in a pressure rise in the circuit, which may go as high as the maximum pressure limit setting, at which point inspiratory flow ends.

In pressure A/C ventilation, abbreviated as PC, the breath is time- or patient-triggered (pressure or flow), pressure-limited and time-cycled. The following parameters are set: inspiratory pressure (P_I), mandatory rate, inspiratory time (T_I), F_IO_2, trigger sensitivity (pressure or flow), PEEP, rise time % (sloping), upper pressure limit, and one of the following can be set as a constant: T_I, T_E, or I:E ratio. (See discussion on breath timing bar earlier.)

Synchronized Intermittent Mandatory Ventilation (SIMV)

SIMV can have mandatory breaths that are either volume- or pressure-targeted. These breaths have the same parameters set as in assist/control. For the spontaneous breaths, the patient can breath at a zero baseline, or with PEEP/CPAP added. Spontaneous breaths can also be aided with pressure support (PS) ventilation. For PS the following additional parameters are set: support pressure (P_{SUPP}), rise time percent (RT%), and expiratory sensitivity (E_{SENS}). The last two are described in the section on special features.

Spontaneous Modes

Selecting a spontaneous mode setting allows the operator to provide the desired F_IO_2, sensitivity, baseline pressure (PEEP/CPAP), rise time %, expiratory sensitivity, and high pressure limit. Spontaneous breaths, as in SIMV, can be aided with pressure support. When PS is not applied, each spontaneous breath receives pressure support of 1.5 cm H_2O above PEEP to reduce work of breathing. For apnea ventilation, VC or PC with associated parameters must be chosen.

BiLevel Ventilation

BiLevel ventilation is a form of augmented pressure ventilation similar to APRV, which was described in Chapter 11. The pressure scalar for BiLevel resembles SIMV-PC. BiLevel can also be used for noninvasive ventilation with a mask interface.

BiLevel allows for unrestricted spontaneous ventilation and synchronization of breathing with the patient's inspiratory and expiratory pattern. The operator selects BiLevel as the mode of ventilation using the control knob. As with APRV, it provides two levels of PEEP or CPAP, designated $PEEP_H$ for the high level of PEEP with a range of 5 to 90 cm H_2O, and $PEEP_L$ for the lower level with a range of 0 to 45 cm H_2O. $PEEP_L$ must be set at least 5 cm H_2O lower than $PEEP_H$. These two pressures are independent. For example, if $PEEP_L$ is 5 and $PEEP_H$ is 10, the highest pressure reached is 10 cm H_2O.

The operator also sets the breath rate and the amount of time that $PEEP_H$ and $PEEP_L$ are applied, using the

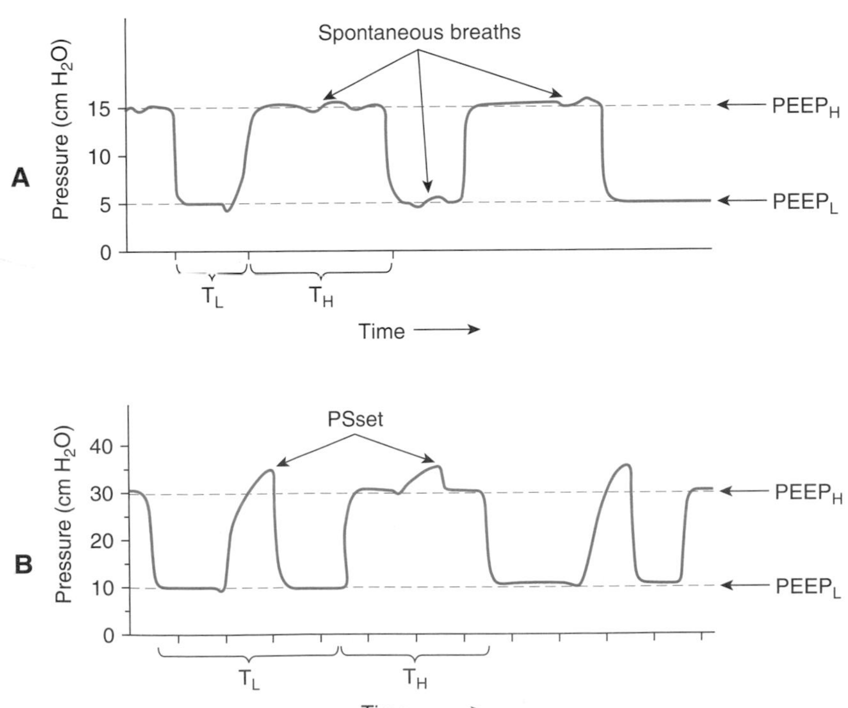

Figure 12-64 A, A Puritan Bennett 840 pressure/time curve during BiLevel ventilation showing spontaneous breaths superimposed over $PEEP_H$ and $PEEP_L$ levels. **B,** Pressure support set (PSset) at 35 cm H_2O with $PEEP_H$ of 30 cm H_2O and $PEEP_L$ of 10 cm H_2O. Notice how PSset is clearly visible in T_L time-frames, but is superimposed on the $PEEP_H$ during T_H time-frames.

Box 12-66 Potential Advantages of BiLevel Ventilation[1]

Increased patient comfort
Reduced requirements for sedation
Improved monitoring of all volumes, spontaneous and mandatory
Prevent alveolar collapse and over distention

CLINICAL ROUNDS 12-25

The following waveform appears on the upper screen. What change to the graph would you make?

See Appendix A for the answer.

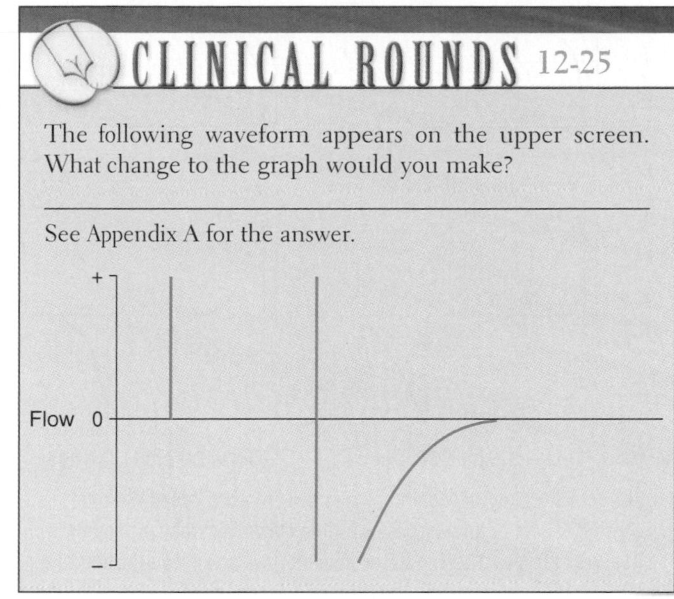

abbreviations T_H and T_L, respectively. For example, when setting up BiLevel to function as APRV, T_H might be set at 2 seconds and T_L at 1.0 second.[5,6] PEEP levels would be targeted to keep alveoli open using $PEEP_L$, but at the same time $PEEP_H$ would be set to avoid overinflation. Figure 12-64, *A*, shows how spontaneous breathing can occur at both levels of PEEP. When no pressure support is set, a spontaneous effort receives 1.5 cm H_2O of pressure to reduce the work of breathing.

In addition, spontaneous breaths can also be augmented with pressure support. If the pressure support level is set higher than $PEEP_H$, the upper portion of the pressure support breath will actually appear above the $PEEP_H$ level (Figure 12-64, *B*). During $PEEP_L$, the PS breath can be seen as it most commonly appears. Box 12-66 lists some of the potential benefits of BiLevel ventilation.

Special Features

There are several features available with the Puritan Bennett 840 that will be reviewed here. They include graphics, respiratory mechanics, rise time percent, an active exhalation valve, and expiratory sensitivity

Graphics

In the upper screen, there is a section that displays scalars and loops. This area can display one or two scalars, or one loop. In this same screen at the top left corner is a "plot set up" screen button that allows the operator to change the current graphics (see Figure 12-61, top screen). To the right of this screen button is a "freeze" button that freezes the current screen.

Touching the "plot set-up" screen button allows the operator to change the graphic display. The subscreen allows selection of Plot 1, the top graph, and Plot 2, the bottom graph. Selecting only one graph using Plot 1 results in an enlarged graph that fills the screen. The control knob is used to change the graph. "Continue" on the graphics screen is then selected to activate the new waveform. There is no need to press "ACCEPT" because ventilator settings are not being changed.

The operator can change the vertical (size) and horizontal (time) scales by using the arrows to the right of the waveforms. The "freeze" function actually captures 48 seconds of data. By changing the time line (horizontal scale) one can visualize the entire 48 seconds. In this same freeze frame, the graphs can be changed. For example, changing a pressure-time to a flow-time scalar, results in the flow-time scalar to appear in the window. This flow-time scalar will represent the same time period as the previous pressure time scalar. Touching "unfreeze" unlocks the waveforms (Clinical Rounds 12-25).

The baseline position of a pressure-volume loop is automatically set at the current PEEP setting. If the PEEP setting is changed, the baseline for the loop resets to the new PEEP level.

The baseline can also be manually moved to another position. To move the base line, the operator touches the baseline pressure button and uses the control knob to position the baseline where desired.

Respiratory Mechanics

The 840 can perform measurements of static compliance, resistance, plateau pressure, total PEEP ($PEEP_{TOT}$), and auto-PEEP or intrinsic PEEP ($PEEP_I$). Static compliance (C) is measured when an inspiratory pause maneuver is performed. Airway resistance (R) can also be calculated during an inspiratory pause when the constant flow waveform is selected during volume-controlled ventilation. $PEEP_{TOT}$ and $PEEP_I$ are measured when the expiratory pause is activated. Some conditions can interfere with accurate expiratory pressure readings and will result in error messages. These conditions include such things as leaks in the circuit, active patient breathing efforts, and unstable plateau pressure readings. For example, if a patient is actively breathing during an expiratory pause maneuver,

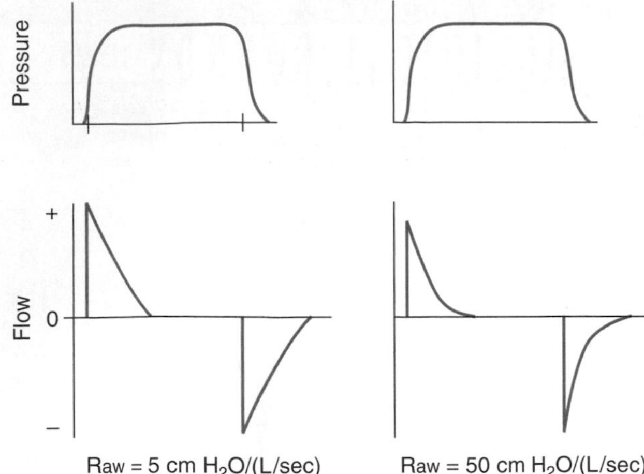

Figure 12-65 Using the sloping or rise time feature called rise time percent (RT%), an optimum pressure-time curve is established on the Puritan Bennett 840. The ventilator adjusts flow to achieve the pressure-time curve even when airway resistance (Raw) changes. Compare the right to the left curve. Notice how flow delivery is lower in the right-hand curve. This may affect volume delivery. Monitor V_T. (See text for further explanation.)

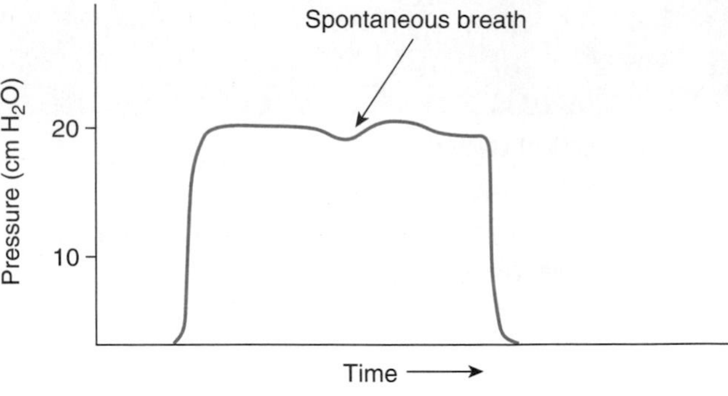

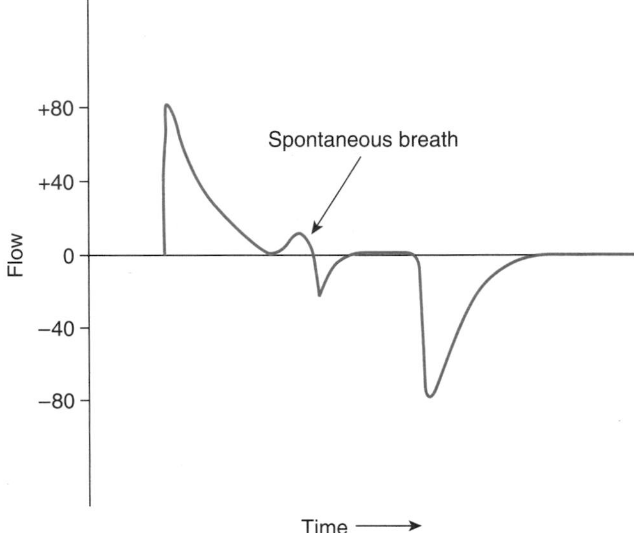

Figure 12-66 The active exhalation valve of the Puritan Bennett 840 can accommodate pressure changes in the patient circuit during pressure-targeted breaths. (See text for description.)

the algorithm will wait up to 2 minutes for the patient's respiratory rate to decrease so the ventilator can perform the expiratory phase maneuver.

Rise Time Percent

Another feature of the 840 is rise time percent (RT%) this is the same as sloping or rise time described in Chapter 11. RT% is available for PC and PS breaths.

RT% works as follows. The available range of settings is 1% to 100%. If the operator sets the percentage at 50%, the ventilator takes the first 50% of the breath to reach the set pressure for the pressure-targeted breath (PC or PS). The set pressure is then maintained the last 50% of T_I. If the percentage is set at 1%, the operator wants the ventilator to be at the set pressure only 1% of the time; which means it takes the other 99% of T_I to reach the set pressure. This is a very short time. Too slow of a delivery of pressure may actually reduce tidal volume delivery and should be avoided. If the percentage is set at 100%, the ventilator will rise quickly to the set pressure so that the total inspiratory time is spent at the desired pressure.

Slowing the rate at which the pressure enters the airways and lungs may be more comfortable for the patient. On the other hand, a quicker rise to the set pressure may give areas of the lungs that have different compliance values (time constants) a better opportunity to inflate more evenly.

If the rise is too fast, an overshoot of the pressure curve may appear. This is called chatter, ringing, or oscillation (see Figure 11-86 in Chapter 11). An appropriately adjusted RT% may reduce work of breathing and reduce asynchrony of ventilation. These adjustments should be monitored carefully.

The RT% screen button only appears when a pressure-targeted mode (PC, PS, or spontaneous) is selected. The programming of the 840 includes Smart Pressure rise algorithms. Based on evaluation of resistance, compliance, and the pressure curve, the ventilator can automatically adjust to achieve an algorithm-driven pressure-time curve (Figure 12-65), or the operator can adjust the RT% rate he or she wishes.

Active Exhalation Valve

The exhalation valve on the 840 is designed so that the set pressure, for example in pressure ventilation, is not only being delivered through the inspiratory line to the patient, but is also powering the exhalation valve. If the pressure in the patient circuit exceeds the set pressure during inspiration, as when a spontaneous breath or cough occurs, the exhalation valve allows either increased flow to the patient for the spontaneous breath or venting of the excess pressure during a cough (Figure 12-66). This helps provide better breath synchrony and prevents high pressures from being generated and potentially harming the patient. This feature is active in pressure breaths (PC and PS), but is currently not available in volume-controlled breaths.

Expiratory Sensitivity

As mentioned in Chapter 11, pressure support ventilation is normally flow-cycled and some ventilators offer adjustable flow cycling percentages. On the 840, this feature is called expiratory sensitivity (E_{SENS}). E_{SENS} represents the percent of peak inspiratory flow at which the ventilator cycles in spontaneous breaths, such as PSV and is adjustable from 1 to 45%. The higher the E_{SENS}, the shorter the T_I. It should be adjusted to match the patient's spontaneous inspiratory phase. If the breath ends too soon, V_T delivery is compromised. If T_I is too long, the patient may actively exhale, increase expiratory work resulting in patient/ventilator dyssynchrony. T_I in PSV may also be too long if there is a leak in the system (Figure 12-67).

NeoMode Option

The 840 Ventilator NeoMode option can provide ventilation with tidal volumes from 5 to 315 mL, which allows ventilation in the IBW range of 0.5 to 7.0 kg (1.1 to 7.7 lb). It provides a flow sensitivity of 0.1 to 10 L/min even in the presence of leaks. Inspiratory times of 0.2 to 8.0 seconds are available in PC and flows of 1.0 to 30 L/min in VC with a square or descending ramp pattern. Mandatory rates can be selected from 1 to 150 breaths/min. The NeoMode accommodates high rates, leaks, and small endotracheal tubes. No proximal airway sensor is required for this special option designed specifically for the newborn infant.

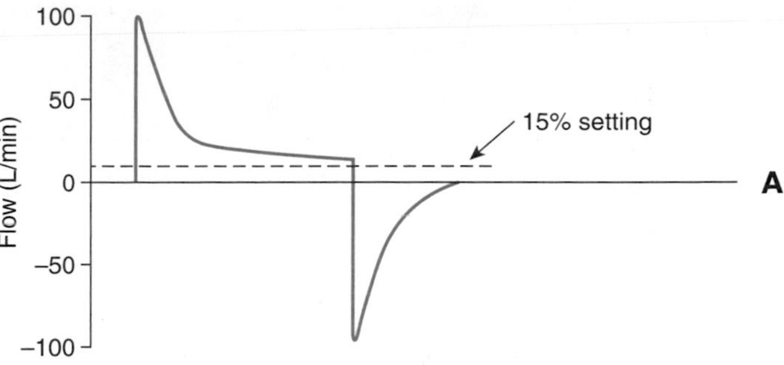

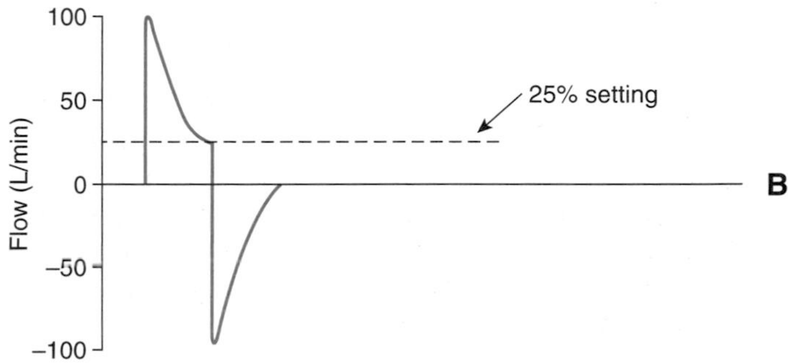

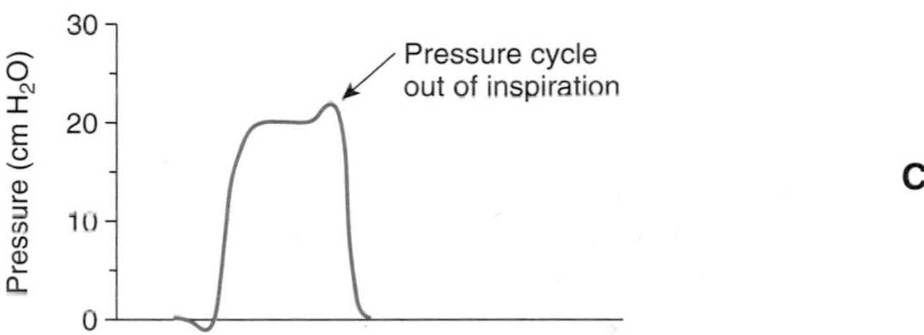

Figure 12-67 These Puritan Bennett 840 scalars represent PS ventilation. **A** shows a flow-time scalar with a prolonged T_I due to a leak in the circuit and a low expiratory sensitivity setting of 15%. **B** demonstrates how increasing the percent setting to 25% has shortened T_I to a more reasonable value. **C** shows a P/T curve in which pressure rises slightly during PS due to the active exhalation of the patient. This causes a pressure-cycling out of inspiration.

Troubleshooting

Common alarm errors are easily solved by reading the alarm messages that provide suggestions about the alarm situation. This provides a rapid method of troubleshooting.

A common problem for individuals who are just beginning to use the 840 is remembering to press the "ACCEPT" key. If a parameter has not changed after adjusting the value, the most likely cause is forgetting to press "ACCEPT."

The operator's manual provides an extensive alarm and troubleshooting section to assist the user in solving problems related to operation of the Puritan Bennett 840.

Puritan Bennett 7200

The Puritan Bennett 7200[1,2] was one of the first ventilators to provide microprocessor control of its electrical functions (Figure 12-68). It was originally released in 1983 and has since gone through a series of upgrades, which included two different front control panel changes to improve ease of use. The third and current front panel version is the one described throughout this section. The 7200 is intended for pediatric and adult patient use in the acute care setting.

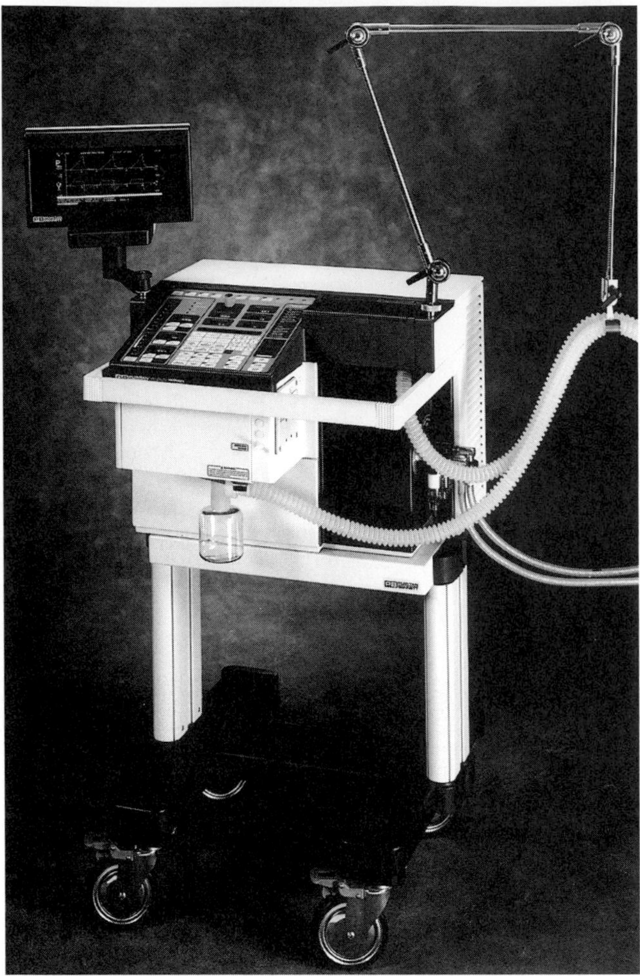

Figure 12-68 The Puritan Bennett 7200 and graphics monitor. (Courtesy Puritan Bennett, Inc, a division of Tyco Healthcare, Pleasanton, Calif.)

Power Source

The unit requires both pneumatic and electrical power sources to operate. It normally uses air and oxygen high-pressure sources (35 to 100 psig) for pneumatic functions, but it can also operate from a single gas source or a high-pressure compressor. The latter two options will, of course, alter oxygen delivery. A standard 115-volt AC 60 Hz outlet provides the electrical power source. (*Note*: If the ventilator is disconnected from the power source, it will stop operating. It does not have an internal battery source to power the ventilator.)

Internal Mechanism

The internal mechanism is shown in Figure 12-69. The air and oxygen sources flow through inlet filters to regulators (*A* and *B*), which reduce and balance pressure to 10 psig (about 700 cm H_2O). The gases are then conducted through flow transducers (*D* and *E*) to the electrically operated, microprocessor-controlled proportional solenoid (metering) valves (*F1* and *F2*). These valves regulate the amount and pattern of gas flow to the patient based on settings and microprocessor control. The crossover solenoid (C) powers the PEEP control using air or oxygen, depending on which is available.

As gas passes from the solenoid valves, it flows through the following:

1. A pressure transducer (G), which acts as an internal barometer
2. A safety/check valve that serves two functions:
   - As an overpressure-relief valve (H) that opens at 140 cm H_2O.
   - As an antisuffocation (safety) valve (*I*) that opens during the start up self-test and if pneumatic or electric power is lost.

Gas flow to the expiration valve is controlled by a solenoid (*J*). During a mandatory breath, this solenoid opens, allowing gas to be directed through the expiratory line and closing the expiratory valve (*K*). During expiration, the expiratory solenoid (*J*) closes and gas flows from the PEEP regulator (*L*) and the PEEP Venturi (*M*) to the back of the expiratory valve. This produces the set level of PEEP/CPAP during expiration.

There are two differential pressures transducers: one measures PEEP (*N*), and one measures airway pressure (*O*). Exhaled patient air passes through the expiratory flow transducer (*P*), which provides information for measuring and calculating V_T and $\dot{V}_E$, as well as monitors and provides some alarm functions.

Controls and Alarms

The three front panels designed for the 7200, beginning with its original design in the 1980s and progressing to the most recent version in 1994 (Figure 12-70), are divided into three basic sections, as follows:

1. ventilator settings (controls)
2. patient data (monitoring information)
3. ventilator status (alarm information)

Box 12-67 describes the function of each section. Although the positioning of these controls has changed somewhat, the overall design stayed consistent. Table 12-19 lists the specifications for the updated (Enhanced) version of the 7200.

Self-Test

When the ventilator is first turned on (power switch on the left side), the microprocessor starts the POST. The POST usually lasts about 5 seconds, depending on the version used. Like most microprocessor-controlled ventilators, the 7200 must complete these essential tests before it becomes functional. POST actually runs in the following situations:

1. When the ventilator is turned on
2. When EST is run
3. When power is interrupted
4. When ongoing checks detect a system error

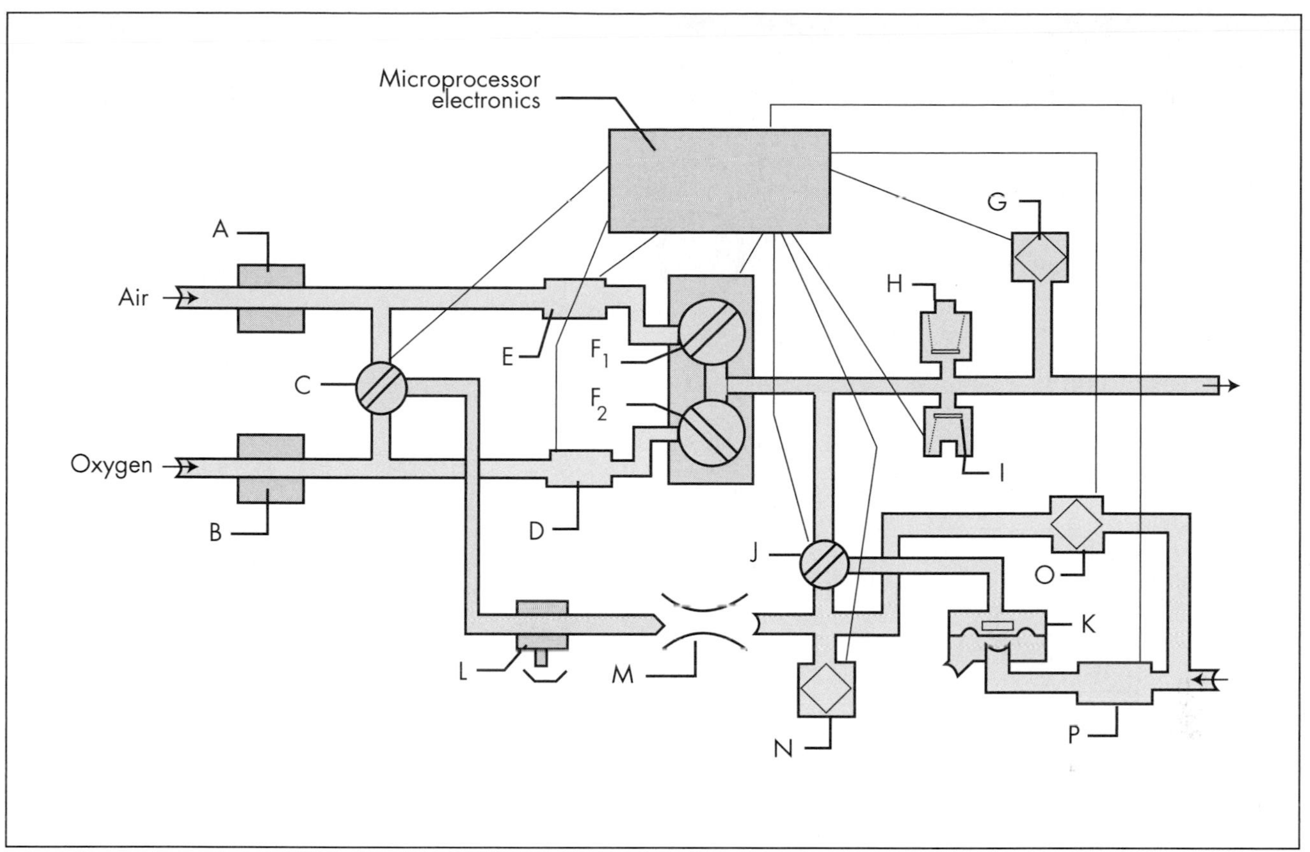

Figure 12-69 The Puritan Bennett 7200 interval schematic. (From Pilbeam SP: Mechanical ventilation. In Burton GG, Hodgkin JE, Ward JJ, editors: *Respiratory care: a guide to clinical practice*, ed 4, Philadelphia, 1997, JB Lippincott.)

After POST, all previous ventilator settings are recalled from memory and activated (Box 12-68). If POST fails, the back-up ventilation mode becomes operational. (The discussion of special functions later in this section provides an explanation of back-up ventilation.) In addition, the message window gives all error codes that need to be recorded for the service representative. A replacement ventilator should be provided immediately.

Two additional ESTs, called QUEST and TEST, can also be selected. (*Note*: No EST or POST should be run while the ventilator is connected to a patient.) The quick extended self-test (QUEST) executes 26 tests and takes about 2 minutes. To run QUEST, the operator presses the EST button on the side panel and ENTER on the front panel, then ENTER again when the window reads "PAT TUBING OFF- ENTER." (*Note*: This instruction is to ensure that the patient is not being ventilated while the test is being run.) The instructions provided in the display window should be followed as they appear. QUEST should be run whenever the patient circuit is changed.

The total extended self-test (TEST) executes 60 tests and takes about 3 to 5 minutes. It is part of the normal maintenance procedure and is routinely performed by biomedical personnel. As with QUEST, it is accessed by pressing the EST and ENTER buttons After the "PAT TUBING OFF-ENTER" instruction, ENTER is pressed, and in response to "QUICK EST," the key labeled "↓ ↓" is pressed. Finally, ENTER is pressed again. As with QUEST, the operator then simply follows the instructions sequentially displayed in the window. (*Note*: The explanation for canceling EST and responding to error messages is beyond the scope of this text and is really intended for ventilator maintenance. The reader is referred to the operator's manual if these procedures are required.)

Initial Start-Up

After the machine is turned on and the POST is completed, the message "Review Apnea Params" appears in the window as a reminder to ensure that the apnea parameters are appropriate for the patient and, then, the mode selected (see the discussion of special functions later in this section). Automatic sigh parameters also need to be checked to be sure they are set as desired for the new patient; otherwise, old values stored in memory will become operational. The operation of sigh is described in the discussion of additional control parameters in this section. In addition, it is important to look at the PEEP control because it may have been set on the last patient and not returned to the zero position after use.

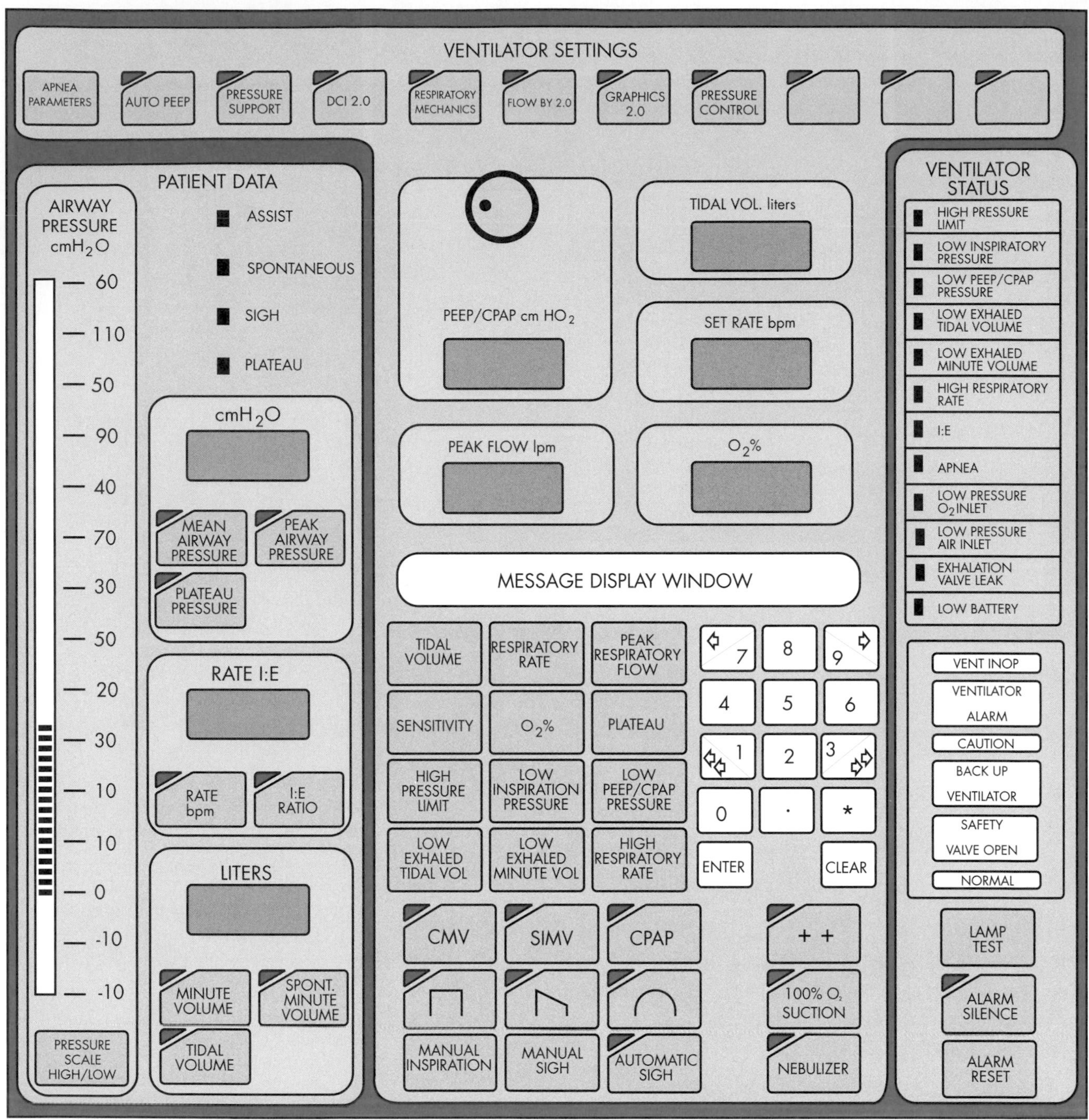

Figure 12-70 Third-generation control panel for the Enhanced Plus 7200 ventilator. (Redrawn from Puritan Bennett, Inc, a division of Tyco Healthcare, Pleasanton, Calif.)

General Setting of Parameters

The ventilator is operated using the touch pads on the front panel. With the exception of the PEEP/CPAP control knob, all parameters are set using these function keys.

To view the set value for any parameter, the appropriately named function key is pressed. There are some function keys that display the parameter value at all times, including the following:

- Tidal volume
- Respiratory rate
- Peak inspiratory flow
- Sensitivity
- O_2%

There are also function keys for alarm variables. These are reviewed in the discussion of monitors and alarms.

When the operator presses a key pad, the current set value for that variable appears in the message display window

Box 12-67 Description of Keyboard Sections

Patient Data Section

Displays monitored patient information, such as pressure, volume, rate, I:E ratio, and breath type.

Ventilator Settings Section

Contains the keys that allow one to set values for specific parameters and alarms. It contains a message window that displays values for set parameters and allows selection of special functions, such as manual inspiration, manual sigh, and 100% O_2 suction. Use of the key in this section, along with the numeric key pads, provides access to supplemental functions, such as pressure control and flow-by. (*Note*: Some of these functions are also available by pressing the labeled keys at the top of the front panel [see Figure 12-70].)

Ventilator Status Sections

Contains 12 alarm indicators and six status display indicators that notify the operator if there is an alarm condition. Three key pads additionally allow for testing of the front panel lights, such as alarm silencing, alarm reset, and lamp test.

on the central portion of the panel. Changing the value requires several steps, which are outlined in Box 12-69 and can be followed using the algorithm in Figure 12-71.

Ventilator Settings

Establishing appropriate settings includes setting breath parameters and additional control parameters.

Breath Parameter Keys

The V_T control is functional in volume-targeted modes (CMV and SIMV) and provides a range of 0.10 to 2.5 L. The range for respiratory rate is adjustable from 0.5 to 9.9 breaths/min in increments of 0.1 breaths/min and from 10 to 70 breaths/min in increments of 1.0 breaths/min. The rate control functions in CMV, SIMV, and PCV. The peak inspiratory flow (10 to 120 L/min) only operates during volume ventilation.

Breaths are volume-cycled during volume ventilation; that is, a breath ends when the ventilator determines that the flow provided over a specific time has delivered a specific volume (V_T = flow × inspiratory time).* If a flow is selected that cannot deliver the set volume within a time that provides an acceptable I:E ratio, a message reads "DECR RESP RATE FIRST." The ventilator microprocessor knows that reducing the rate allows a longer T_I. Of course, increasing the flow also solves the problem and will not change $\dot{V}_E$. Box 12-70 provides examples of situations in which this message occurs, and Clinical Rounds 12-26 gives an exercise for calculating the volume, rate, and flow that would result in an error message.

This can also be called flow cycling; see Chapter 11.

Table 12-19 Specifications for the Puritan Bennett 7200 microprocessor ventilator

Modes	
A/C (CMV) (volume control)	
A/C (CMV) (pressure control)	
SIMV (volume control)	
SIMV (pressure control)	
SIMV (volume control) + PSV	
SIMV (pressure control) + PSV	
CPAP (with PSV)	
CPAP (without PSV)	
Breath type	Range
Breath type—mandatory	
Volume control	
Volume (mL)	100-2500
Rate (breaths/min)	
A/C (CMV)	0.5-70
SIMV	0.5-70
Peak inspiratory flow (L/sec)	10-120
Flow waveform	Square, descending ramp, sine
Plateau (sec)	0-2.0
Inspiratory hold (sec)	0.0-2.0
Pressure control	
Inspiratory pressure (above PEEP) (cm H_2O)	5-100
Inspiratory time (sec)	0.2-5
Rate (breaths/min)	
A/C (CMV)	0.5-70
SIMV	0.5-70
I:E ratio	1:9.0-4:1
Breath type—spontaneous	
Pressure support (cm H_2O)	10-70
PEEP/CPAP (cm H_2O)	0-45
Common Parameters	
Oxygen percentage	**21-100**
Inspiratory trigger	
Pressure (below PEEP, cm H_2O)	0.5-20
Flow (L/min)	1-15
Other Featured Parameters/Functions	
Manual inspiration	
Manual sigh	
Automatic sigh	

Continued

Table 12-19 Specifications for the Puritan Bennett 7200 microprocessor ventilator—cont'd

100% oxygen suction (2 min)
Nebulizer
Apnea interval and ventilation
Flow-by (flow-triggering)
Clock/calendar set
Auto-PEEP
Digital communications interface
Respiratory mechanics
Graphics
Trending
Pulse oximeter
Display screen
Metabolics (integrated)
Alarm indicators
High and low pressure
Apnea
I:E ratio
Power loss
Exhalation valve leak
Low volume
Low exhaled minute volume
Ventilator inoperative
Low pressure oxygen/air inlet
High rate
Low CPAP/PEEP
Low battery

From Pilbeam SP: Mechanical ventilation. In Burton GG, Hodgkin JE, Ward JJ: *Respiratory care: a guide to clinical practice*, ed 4, Philadelphia, 1997, JB Lippincott.

Pressure sensitivity (0.5 to 20.0 cm H_2O) is adjusted with the key pad and numerical controls. However, flow-triggering is also available when the flow-by function is selected. Flow-by and flow-triggering in the 7200 are described in the discussion of special functions in this section. The available % O_2 ranges from 21% to 100%. There is no built-in oxygen analyzer to test the F_IO_2 delivery.

Use of the plateau control closes the inspiratory and expiratory valves at the end of inspiration for the amount of time selected (from 0.0 to 2.0 seconds). An inspiratory plateau is only functional during a volume breath. The inspiratory phase is increased by the amount set.

Box 12-68 Back-up Memory Battery

The memory that contains previous set parameter values is powered by batteries. This helps prevent loss of information if electrical power is interrupted (e.g., the machine is accidentally unplugged while in use). If the battery fails, the message "1401 ERR" indicates that the 7200 is using the default parameters that are programmed into the read-only memory (ROM) of the microprocessor. The operator should review all settings immediately, per the following list of default parameters:

- Mode CMV
- Constant flow waveform
- V_T of 0.5 L
- Rate of 12 breaths/min
- Flow of 45 L/min
- Sensitivity of −3 cm H_2O below baseline
- 100% O_2
- High-pressure limit of 20 cm H_2O
- Low-pressure limit of 3 cm H_2O
- Apnea interval of 20 seconds

The following functions are off or disabled: 100% O_2 suction, sigh, nebulizer, low PEEP/CPAP alarm, low V_T alarm, low $\dot{V}_E$ alarm, and low rate alarm.

Box 12-69 Changing the Value of a Parameter

To change the value of any variable (e.g., tidal volume), the operator must do the following:

1. Press the key pad with the variable on it.
2. Press the desired numerical value using the number keys located below the message window.
3. Press the ENTER key to place the new value in memory.

An acceptable setting is confirmed by two beeps. If the entry is outside the range of the parameter, four beeps will sound and the display screen displays an error message: "INVALID ENTRY." For example, a tidal volume of 3.0 L is outside the range of the unit (see Table 12-19) and therefore invalid. The operator must press CLEAR and try again.

If it takes more than about 20 to 30 seconds for the change to occur, the unit reverts back to the previous setting. (*Note*: The new setting is never activated until the ENTER key is pressed.)

Additional Control Parameters

In addition to the variables and settings already described, there are three more areas of the front panel (see Figure 12-70) where functions can be set and settings monitored:

1. The lower central portion of the front panel, below the alarm function keys and the numerical pad
2. A row of controls across the top of the panel
3. A set of display screens that show current settings

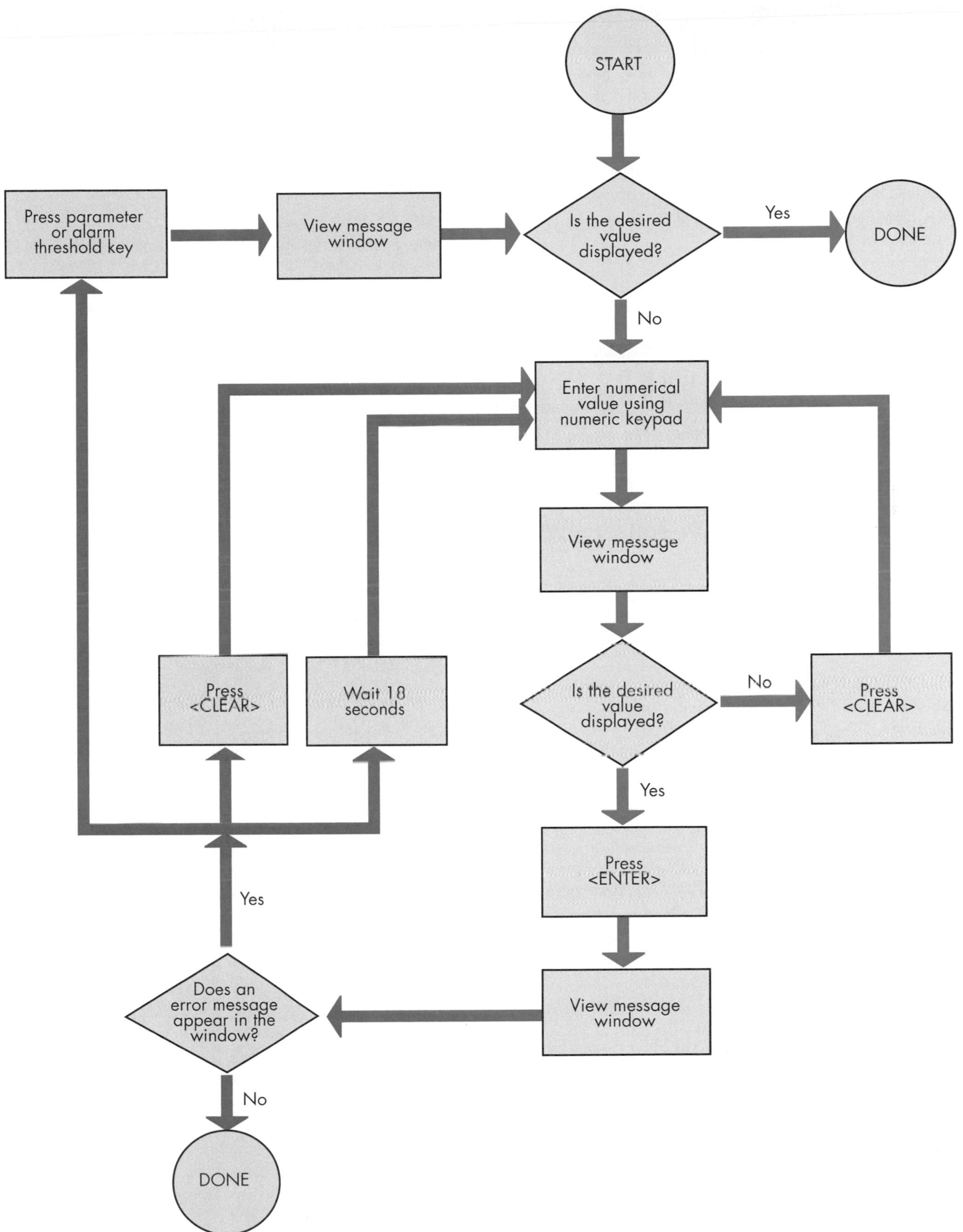

Figure 12-71 An algorithm for viewing and changing Puritan Bennett 7200 ventilator parameter values. (Redrawn from Puritan Bennett, Inc, a division of Tyco Healthcare, Pleasanton, Calif.)

Box 12-70 Message: "DECR RESP RATE FIRST"

This message appears when a new value for V_T, peak inspiratory flow, or plateau or flow waveform is selected that results in lengthening the T_I to ≥75% of TCT based on the rate setting. Therefore the ventilator gives preference to T_I to lengthen TCT, so it is suggested that the rate be reduced. Of course, one could also increase inspiratory flow, alter the plateau time, or change the waveform pattern.

(*Note*: During PCV, T_I can be ≥80% of TCT to allow for inverse ratios up to 4:1 in this mode.)

CLINICAL ROUNDS 12-26

A respiratory therapist selects the following settings on the 7200 ventilator during a laboratory test with the machine: V_T = 1.0 L (1000 mL), rate = 20 breaths/min, flow = 30 L/min, and flow waveform = constant. Will the "DECR RESP RATE FIRST" message appear with these settings?

See Appendix A for the answer.

The controls directly below the alarm function keys are discussed first. The first three functional keys are used for selecting CMV, SIMV, and CPAP. Pressing the desired key pad and then pressing ENTER to activate a new mode (see the discussion of modes of ventilation in this section).

Next are the three function keys that determine the flow waveform in volume-targeted breaths. The available waveforms are constant (rectangular), descending ramp, and sine wave. The amount of flow delivered during each type of waveform is determined by the peak flow setting. For example, with a constant (rectangular) waveform selected, the flow is constant at the value set on the peak flow control. For a descending ramp, the starting flow is the peak flow setting, and the ending flow is 5 L/min. For a sine curve, the flow begins and ends at 5 L/min, and the flow rises to the peak flow setting at the middle of inspiration.

Because breaths are volume-cycled in the 7200, changing the peak flow and/or the waveform also changes the I:E ratio. To keep the I:E ratio the same when changing a waveform from constant to descending, the peak flow is doubled. When changing from constant to sine, the peak flow setting must be increased to 1.5 times the current setting.

The next function pads are manual inspiration, manual sigh, and automatic sigh. Selecting manual inspiration delivers a breath based on the selected parameters. Manual sigh delivers a sigh breath based on the settings selected for automatic sigh. Pressing the automatic sigh function key allows the operator to select sigh parameters. The display window requests entry of sigh parameters, which are described in Box 12-71.

Box 12-71 Sigh Parameters

After pressing the automatic sigh key, follow the instructions in the message window.

Sigh TV (tidal volume)—0.1 to 2.5 L

Sigh HIPL (high-pressure limit)—10 to 120 cm H_2O

Sigh Events—1 to 15 (corresponds to a sigh every 4 to 60 minutes)

Multiple Sighs—1 to 3 sighs per event.

After all new entries are complete, press ENTER when the window message is "UPDATE PARAMS-ENTER." This updates the sigh parameters. Finally, press ENTER when the window reads "AUTO SIGH ON-ENTER" to complete the entries and turn on the automatic sigh function.

To clear the sigh function, press the automatic sigh function key. When "AUTO SIGH OFF-ENTER" appears in the window, pressing the ENTER key turns off the sigh function.

Below the numeric key pads are three more function keys, as follows:

1. + +
2. 100% O_2 suction
3. nebulizer

The + + key allows the operator to select certain functions and options and operates like a computer menu. When it is pressed, the number of the last function selected appears in the window (Table 12-20). To scroll to the desired option, press the + + key to go forward, or the * key to go backward. Another way to access a specific function is to press the numbers representing the desired option and then ENTER. After an option or function is selected, the directions in the message window are followed. For example, apnea parameters are Option 1. The message "1 APNEA PARAMETERS" appears. Pressing ENTER when that message appears results in the message, "APNEA INT XX SEC." The operator uses the number keys to set the desired apnea time interval and again presses ENTER. The operator follows the directions in the next window that appears. This continues until all the necessary parameters have been selected and "UPDATE PARAMS-ENTER" is displayed. Pressing ENTER updates all the selected apnea parameters and activates them.

Selecting the 100% O_2 suction key causes the ventilator to deliver 100% O_2 for 2 minutes. The message window flashes to indicate that delivered oxygen is different than the set value (as long as the set O_2 is <100%). Choosing this option does not deactivate alarms, so if the patient is disconnected for suctioning, alarms will occur (e.g., low pressure alarm).

Table 12-20 List of + + key options and functions for the Puritan Bennett 7200

Number	Function or Option
Function 1	Apnea ventilation*
Function 2	Clock-calendar reset
Function 3	Patient data
Function 4	Auto-PEEP
Option 10	Pressure support
Option 20	Digital communications interface (DCI)
Option 30/40	Respiratory mechanics*
Option 50	Flow-by (flow trigger)*
Option 60	Graphics
Option 80	Pressure-control ventilation
Option 90	Pulse oximetry

Courtesy Puritan Bennett, Inc, a division of Tyco Healthcare, Pleasanton, Calif.

*Covered in the discussion of special functions in this section.

Box 12-72 Conditions When Nebulizer Function is Suspended

1. Excessive nebulizer flow—checked every eight breaths; "NEB DISCONNECT" is in the display window; excessive flow can be caused by leaks or disconnects in the nebulizer tubing.
2. During apnea and disconnect ventilation.
3. When the Respiratory Mechanics/Monitoring option is selected.
4. If low oxygen or air inlet pressure alarms occur.
5. If the operator selects any combination of peak flow and O_2% that yields less than 10 L/min through the solenoid supplying the nebulizer circuit, the microprocessor senses the low flow and deactivates the solenoid supplying the nebulizer. The light on the nebulizer key remains lit.

(*Note*: If Flow-by is on, it is turned off when the nebulizer is activated. Be sure to turn Flow-by back on when nebulization is complete.)

The nebulization key allows a gas flow at the set O_2% to exit the nebulizer connector for 30 minutes after it is activated. It automatically turns off the flow-by function and only works during inspiratory flow when the flow is greater than 10 L/min (mandatory or spontaneous breaths). Box 12-72 lists conditions when the nebulizer function is suspended. If the nebulizer function is suspended, the nebulizer key's light goes off, and the key does not work. However, the 30-minute clock continues to run. When the condition has been corrected, nebulizer flow resumes.*

The top row of controls in the ventilator setting section was added to the most recent version of the 7200 (Enhanced key board) and allows direct access to many of the functions and options listed under the + + key. By pressing one of these keys, the display window immediately accesses that function. The operator simply follows the directions for setting up or operating the selected option, in the same way as accessing the function through the + + key. (*Note*: Some of the key selections allow access to more than one function, such as the respiratory mechanics option.) The controls in this row include the following:

1. Apnea parameters
2. Auto-PEEP
3. Pressure support
4. DCI 2.0
5. Respiratory mechanics
6. Flow-by 2.0
7. Graphics 2.0
8. Pressure control

Items 1, 5, and 6 are covered in the discussion of special functions later in this section. Items 3 and 8 are included in the discussion of modes of ventilation, and 7 is reviewed in the discussion of ventilator graphic waveforms. Of the remaining keys, two blank touch keys for future upgrades appear on the right, and the two remaining keys, auto-PEEP and DCI 2.0, provide additional special functions.

The auto-PEEP key is Function 4 and is now a standard feature on every Enhanced 7200 ventilator (7200ae, 7200spe, and 7200e). It is used to estimate end-expiratory pressures. The unit measures total PEEP at end-exhalation and estimates auto-PEEP by subtracting the set (extrinsic) PEEP from the total PEEP.

The DCI (digital communications interface) function provides data reports that include data logs, chart summary reports, ventilator status reports, and host reports.

Finally, the top central portion of the ventilator setting section has digital display screens for showing the values of the current settings of the following parameters:

1. PEEP/CPAP (in cm H_2O)
2. Tidal volume (in liters)
3. Set rate (in breaths/minute)
4. Peak flow (in liters/minute)
5. O_2%

Monitors and Alarms

The Puritan Bennett 7200 has two main sections for providing information about monitored values and alarm displays. The monitored values are provided in the patient data section of the front panel, and the alarm display is in the ventilator status section. Alarms are set using the control

**If flow-by was used before giving a nebulizer treatment, the operator must be sure to turn it back on.*

Box 12-73 Pressure Monitoring on the 7200 Ventilator

1. Mean airway pressure—airway pressure averaged over all measurements made during an entire breath (I + E) for mandatory or spontaneous breaths; updated and displayed at the end of each subsequent breath cycle; negative values reported as zero.
2. Peak airway pressure—measures peak airway pressure at the end of inspiration for a mandatory breath.
3. Plateau pressure—measures plateau pressure. The ventilator reads the average of the last four pressure sample measurements made during a plateau and displays this average at the end of a plateau; otherwise, display window is blank.
4. PEEP/CPAP—displayed continuously on the right of the patient data panel on the enhanced key board; based on the amount of pressure applied to the ventilatory side of the exhalation valve multiplied by the area ratio. (*Note*: The area ratio is computed every time a self-test is run. The value, however, changes little.)

Box 12-74 I:E Ratio

The set value for I:E may not equal the actual value if the set value is based on a volume-targeted breath using volume flow and rate or on a pressure-targeted breath using T_I and rate. For example, during SIMV or CMV, the I:E ratio may vary even though the ventilator settings do not change if the patient triggers a breath during the T_E.

pads for the alarms in the lower portion of the ventilator setting section just below the key pads that control breath delivery. The patient data section is reviewed first, then setting of alarms is discussed, and then monitoring of alarm information in the ventilator status section is presented.

Monitors: Patient Data Section

The patient data section of the front panel includes monitoring displays for the following:

1. Breath type
2. Pressures
3. Rates
4. I:E ratio
5. Volumes

Each of these sections provides calculated or measured patient information that is digitally displayed. All of these displays are blank during a POST. Measured data is obtained from sensors for flow, pressure, and temperature (both inspiratory and expiratory). The microprocessor uses the measurements to calculate and display the information.

Breath Type

Small LEDs at the top right of the patient data section light up depending on the type of breath delivery. There is an LED for a patient assist when the patient triggers a mandatory breath, an LED for a spontaneous breath, one for a sigh breath, and one to indicate that a plateau maneuver is being performed. If a mandatory breath is time-triggered, no light illuminates.

Pressures

On the left side of the section is a dual-scale, pressure-reading bar graph that displays airway pressure in centimeters of water. The other available selections require pressing the desired variable from the three available and then its value is displays in the pressure window. The three available pressures are shown in Box 12-73, along with the measurement for PEEP/CPAP.

Respiratory Rates and I:E Ratio

The operator can select either the measured respiratory rate or the I:E ratio to be displayed. Respiratory rates (in breaths/minute) are digitally displayed in the assigned window. Rates are read as the average rate of breathing calculated for a patient's 10 previous breaths (spontaneous or mandatory). The I:E ratio is only for mandatory breaths and is the actual measured value displayed as "1:X.X." For example, an I:E of 1:4 is a normal value, and a reading of "1:0.5" represents an inverse ratio of 2:1. The X.X term is calculated by dividing the time for exhalation by the time for inhalation (X.X = T_E/T_I). (*Note*: T_E is calculated by subtracting T_I from the TCT, where TCT is the TCT measured from beginning of inspiration to the end of exhalation. The end of exhalation is not simply the end of expiratory flow [which may have occurred before this], but is also considered the beginning of the next breath.) During CPAP, the I:E ratio displayed is the one retained from the last mandatory breath delivered (Box 12-74).

Volumes

The digital display in the volume window provides readouts of measured values in liters for V_T, $\dot{V}_E$, and spontaneous $\dot{V}_E$. The operator simply selects which value to be displayed. These values are corrected to BTPS (body temperature, ambient pressure, saturated) as well as for tubing compliance. (*Note*: This discussion is exclusive to the Enhanced [newest] keyboard and does not apply to the basic keyboard. On the basic keyboard, the exhaled volume is displayed on an analog meter, but this reading is not corrected for BTPS or tubing compliance. As a result, the analog volume reading and the digital volume reading [corrected for both] differ on the basic keyboard.)

Spontaneous V_T is displayed on a breath-by-breath basis. The mandatory breath V_T displayed is usually an average of eight breaths. If a breath is 50 mL different than the average volume for the eight mandatory breaths, the digital display only shows that breath—not the average.

Box 12-75 Compensation for Compressible Volume

During an extended self-test (EST), the 7200 determines the compliance of the patient circuit. Whenever a mandatory volume-targeted breath is delivered, the machine measures PIP and increases or decreases the delivered volume of the next breath to ensure that the set V_T is the volume that reaches the patient's lungs. This is accomplished by holding the T_I constant, when it is based on V_T and flow settings, but slightly increasing flow delivery to increase the volume delivered.

Each exhaled volume is corrected as well. The microprocessor simply subtracts the volume added during inspiration from that measured during exhalation at the expiratory valve. Thus the exhaled volume reading is also corrected so that it shows the amount that is theoretically delivered to the patient's lungs. This amount is theoretical because any leaks in the system affect delivered volumes. Clinical Rounds 12-27 provides a sample problem.

CLINICAL ROUNDS 12-27

A patient is being ventilated with the 7200 with a set V_T of 0.6 L (600 mL), a constant (square) flow pattern, and a flow of 60 L/min. The tubing compliance (C_T) was calculated during the last EST as 2 mL/cm H_2O, and the PIP for the last breath was 30 cm H_2O. What will be the amount of volume added to the delivered breath? What will be the exhaled V_T reading, assuming that there are no leaks?

See Appendix A for the answer.

Both mandatory and spontaneous $\dot{V}_E$ are based on an eight-breath projected running average or a 1-minute sample, whichever occurs first.[1] The mandatory and spontaneous $\dot{V}_E$ are calculated separately at the end of each complete breath, and are also displayed at the end of a breath.*

Correction for Compressible Volume

The 7200 compensates for volume that is compressed in the patient circuit so that the amount of air reaching the patient's lungs is very close to the value for V_T delivery set by the operator (Box 12-75 and Clinical Rounds 12-27).

Setting of Alarms

Setting the alarm limits is done similarly to setting the ventilation parameters (see Box 12-69 and Figure 12-71).

*When spontaneous $\dot{V}_E$ is used, the type of breath is displayed on the large graphics window.

Table 12-21 Permissible ranges for alarm thresholds

Alarm	Range
High-pressure limit	10 to 120 cm H_2O
Low inspiratory pressure	3 to 99 cm H_2O
Low PEEP/CPAP pressure	0 to 45 cm H_2O
Low exhaled V_T	0.00 to 2.50 L
Low exhaled $\dot{V}_E$	0.00 to 60.0 L/min
High respiratory rate	0 to 70 breaths/min

Courtesy Puritan Bennett, Inc, a division of Tyco Healthcare, Pleasanton, Calif.

Box 12-76 Low Battery and I:E Ratio Alarms

When either a low battery or an I:E event condition occurs, the ventilator lights up the corresponding alarm indicator but does not light up the alarm display or provide an audible alarm. Each alarm resets to a normal display when corrected.

Table 12-21 provides a list of the key pad alarms and ranges. (*Note*: The low inspiratory pressure alarm parameter only applies to mandatory breaths.)

When alarm limits are violated, the following three events generally occur:

1. An audible alarm is activated.
2. A visual indicator and the ventilator alarm display in the ventilator status section flash.
3. A message appears in the message window to describe the alarm condition. If the alarm condition is corrected by the next breath, the audible alarm is silenced; but, the caution light is continuously lit, and the appropriate LED indicator changes from flashing to continuous. These are turned off by touching the ALARM RESET key pad. The advantage is if the operator is away from the ventilator when an alarm condition occurs, the data from the event is kept for later reference. Box 12-76 gives two exceptions to this general condition, and Clinical Rounds 12-28 provides a troubleshooting exercise.

Events that reduce supply gas make the ventilator inoperative or severely compromise its ability to function. For example, if both gas supplies are lost, an audible alarm sounds, SVO illuminates, and the valve opens. In addition, both the low air and low O_2 LEDs flash. The opening of the safety valves provides a route from which a spontaneously breathing patient can receive room air.

If the microprocessor systems find a major fault that prevents safe ventilator operation, the following two red alarm indicators flash:

1. Ventilator Inoperative
2. Safety Valve Open

If the gas system is still working but the electronics are not, the red BUV (back-up ventilator) indicator flashes, and an audible alarm sounds. This provides back-up ventilation as is presented in the discussion of special functions in this section. The section on special functions also describes the indicators for the various alarm conditions.

CLINICAL ROUNDS 12-28

A patient is being ventilated with the 7200 ventilator using volume ventilation. The mode is switched from CMV to SIMV. The mandatory V_T is 0.7 L (700 mL), and the rate is set at 5 breaths/min. The spontaneous rate is 10 breaths/min, and spontaneous V_T is 0.4 L (400 mL). The low V_T alarm keeps activating even though it is set at 0.6 L (600 mL) and there are no leaks in the circuit. What is the problem?

See Appendix A for the answer.

Ventilator Status

The ventilator status display has three basic sections: the top provides an LED display of any current or recent alarms (Table 12-22); the second section contains the ventilator status display (Table 12-23); and the bottom section has three touch pads (LAMP TEST, ALARM SILENCE, and ALARM RESET). Pressing LAMP TEST and ENTER initiates a test that checks lamps, displays, and meters that are located on the front panel, as well as the audible alarm and the remote alarm if installed. In addition, it cancels the alarm silence function. The ALARM SILENCE key quiets audible alarms for 2 minutes to allow for undisturbed bedside procedures. It also cancels displays of self-test error messages. The ALARM RESET clears all alarm indicators, initiates a battery test, and also, as with the LAMP TEST, cancels ALARM SILENCE.

Modes of Ventilation

The 7200 offers three primary modes of ventilation: CMV, SIMV, and CPAP (spontaneous), as well as two optional modes: PCV and PSV. The touch keys for CMV, SIMV, and CPAP are on the lower central portion of the front panel. CMV and SIMV are commonly selected to provide volume ventilation, but if PCV is in use, these key pads also establish breath triggering and pattern for pressure ventilation. That is, PCV can be as A/C (CMV) or PCV in the SIMV mode.

Table 12-22 Types of alarms and events that may occur with the 7200

Type of Alarm	Triggering Event
High pressure limit*	Measured peak airway pressure $>$ set limit; ends inspiration and opens exhalation valve
Low inspiratory pressure	Airway pressure $<$ set minimum for one mandatory breath cycle
Low PEEP/CPAP pressure	Airway pressure is $\leq$ the set minimum for $>$ 1 sec, or 5 L/min of gas flow is delivered during a spontaneous breath
Low exhaled V_T	In CMV, value for mandatory breaths (4-breath running average) $<$ set; in SIMV and CPAP, value for spontaneous breaths (4-breath running average) $<$ set
Low exhaled minute volume	Sum of minute volume for mandatory and spontaneous breaths $<$ set minimum (based on 8-breath projected running total, or on a 1-minute sample, whichever comes first)
High respiratory rate	Breath rate $>$ set maximum (for 10-breath running average)
I:E	Length of mandatory inspiration including plateau time $>$ 50% of length of total breath cycle
Apnea	No exhalation detected during set apnea time
Low-pressure O_2 inlet*	Pressure at O_2 inlet $\leq$35 psig, O_2 % set $>$22%
Low-pressure air inlet*	Pressure at air inlet $\leq$35 psig when connected to wall outlet or $<$7.5 psig when connected to compressor
Exhalation valve leak	Volume of gas measured by exhalation valve sensor during inspiration is $<$10% of the delivered V_T or 50 mL, whichever is greater
Low battery	Internal battery power is not adequate to provide 1 hour of audible alarm and battery back-up memory

Courtesy Puritan Bennett, Inc, a division of Tyco Healthcare, Pleasanton, Calif.

*Minute ventilation and oxygenation may be seriously affected if one of these alarm conditions persists.

Table 12-23 Function of the alarm summary display

Display	Function
Ventilator inoperative	Red display. When lit, the microprocessor has determined that the ventilator is not functional due to a system fault. Coincides with illumination of safety valve open display. Back-up ventilation is not provided.
Ventilator alarm	Red display. Signals that an alarm has been triggered and has not autoreset. Usually, one or more of 12 indicators flashes to identify it.
Caution	Yellow display. Signals that an alarm was activated and automatically reset. Steady illumination of one or more of the 12 indicators identifies the alarm that was active.
Back up ventilator	Red display. Lights when the back-up ventilator (BUV) emergency mode is active. When the ventilator is in BUV, factory-preset breath parameters are used.
Safety valve open	Red display. When lit, the patient circuit is opened to room air and the patient breathes unassisted by the ventilator. The ventilator enters this mode when all connected gas supplies are lost, POST is running, a system fault is detected, or AC power is lost. Safety valve open is employed temporarily during POST and is canceled after POST is completed successfully.
Normal	Green (or blue) display. When lit, the ventilator is operating within acceptable ranges and no alarm conditions exist. If an alarm is reset with the alarm reset key, this display lights instead of the caution display.

Courtesy Puritan Bennett, Inc, a division of Tyco Healthcare, Pleasanton, Calif.

Continuous Mandatory Ventilation (CMV)

CMV is an A/C mode of ventilation in which breaths are patient- or time-triggered, volume-targeted (PCV not set), and volume-cycled. Press the CMV pad once, then select the desired V_T, flow, respiratory rate, flow waveform pattern, trigger sensitivity, and alarm thresholds. Pressing the CMV pad a second time activates the new mode.

Synchronized Intermittent Mandatory Ventilation (SIMV)

In SIMV, mandatory breaths can be patient- or time-triggered and are volume-targeted (PCV not set) and volume-cycled, as in CMV. Spontaneous breaths are patient-triggered (pressure or flow). With the added option of PSV, spontaneous breaths can be assisted with the selected pressure level. Box 12-77 and Figure 12-72 describe the synchronization of mandatory breaths with spontaneous breaths. Clinical Rounds 12-29 provides an exercise in problem solving related to the SIMV mode.

Spontaneous/Continuous Positive Airway Pressure (CPAP)

The CPAP mode is a purely spontaneous mode. All breaths are patient-triggered and can be at a zero baseline or at a positive baseline (CPAP). They can also have PSV added.

Box 12-77 Synchronization of SIMV and Spontaneous Breaths on the 7200 Ventilator

Whether a patient-triggered breath is mandatory or spontaneous is determined by when the patient effort occurs in the SIMV cycle. The SIMV cycle is composed of two phases, as follows:

1. Patient-initiated mandatory phase (PIM phase)
2. Spontaneous phase

In the PIM phase, patient-triggering results in a mandatory breath. After breath delivery, the PIM phase ends and the spontaneous phase begins. In this phase, patient-triggering results in a spontaneous breath. At the end of the spontaneous phase, the SIMV cycle ends and the next one begins with a new PIM phase. For example, with a rate of 10 breaths/min, the SIMV cycle is 6 seconds long. A PIM breath could occur at anytime during the 6 seconds. Once the patient triggers the breath and the mandatory breath is delivered, the remainder of the time can be spent in spontaneous ventilation.

If no PIM breath is triggered, the spontaneous phase never begins and PIM continues through the next SIMV cycle. At the start of the next SIMV cycle (12 seconds later in this example), the ventilator time-triggers a mandatory breath (see Figure 12-72). If no patient effort is detected, mandatory breaths follow the beginning of each subsequent SIMV interval.

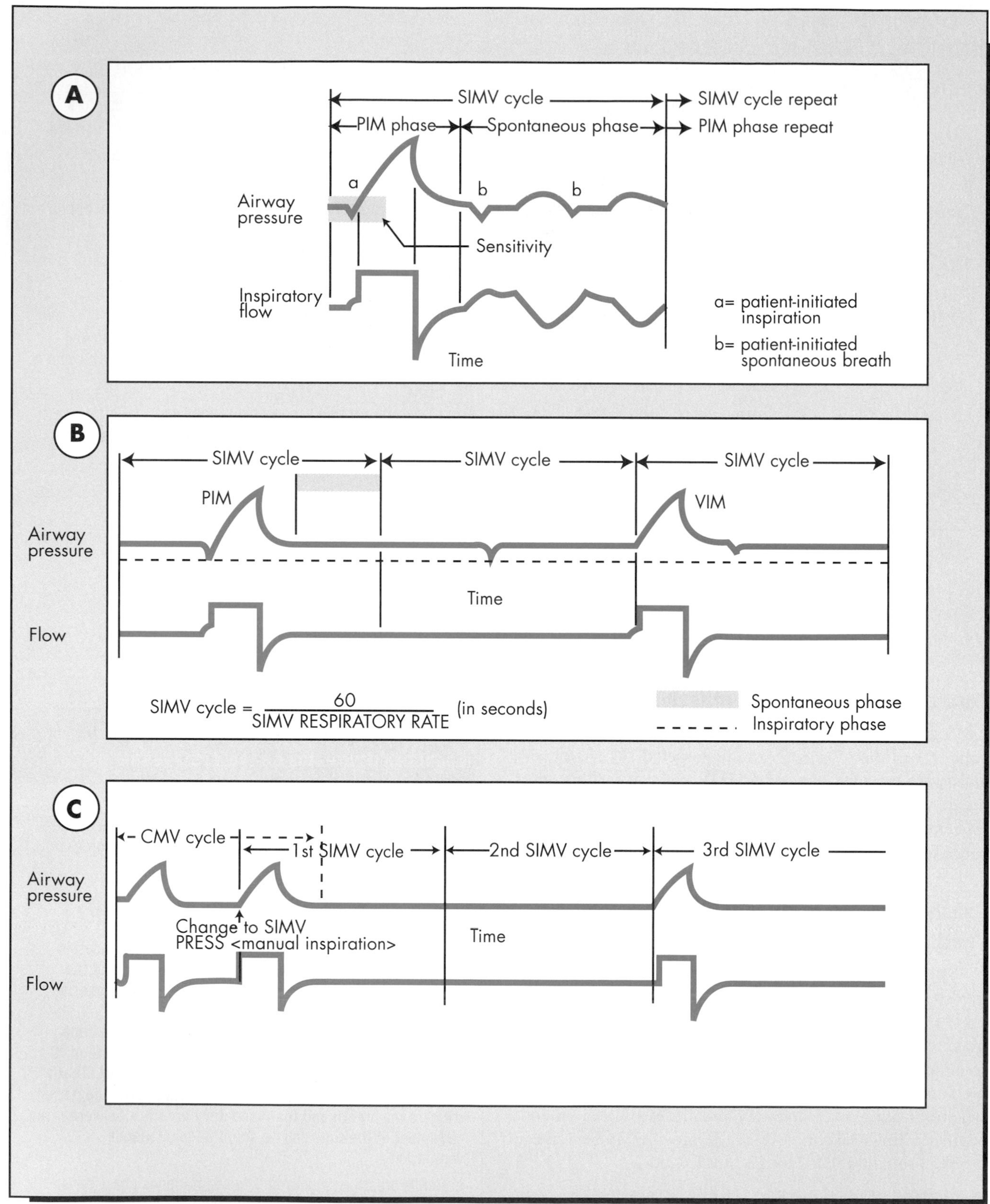

Figure 12-72 Breath patterns during SIMV on the Puritan Bennett 7200. **A,** an adequate inspiratory effort that triggers a mandatory breath and is followed by a spontaneous phase. **B,** no adequate inspiratory effort is sensed; two SIMV cycles pass, and a time-triggered mandatory volume-targeted breath (VIM) occurs. **C,** the switch from CMV to SIMV; the ventilator automatically begins timing the first SIMV cycle (any time remaining from the CMV cycle is ignored). (Redrawn from Puritan Bennett, Inc, a division of Tyco Healthcare, Pleasanton, Calif.)

Pressure Control Ventilation (PCV)

PCV is an added option (80) that can be accessed using either of the following two ways:

1. By pressing the PCV pad at the top of the front panel
2. By activating Option 80 under the key (Box 12-78).

PCV provides pressure-targeted mandatory breaths in the CMV and SIMV modes. Table 12-24 lists the range of variables available in PCV. This option allows selection of either T_I or the I:E ratio as a constant based on respiratory rate (Option 82). Because selecting these can be confusing the first time they are used, a detailed explanation is given in Table 12-25. Usually when an inverse ratio is desired, a constant I:E is set. With normal I:E ratios, it may be more appropriate to set T_I constant. When changing the respiratory rate, a message appears as a reminder of which parameter (I:E or T_I) is currently constant. Clinical Rounds 12-30 gives an example of initiating PCV and selecting T_I or I:E as constant.

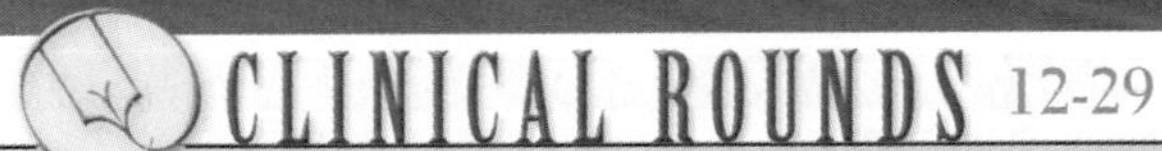

A patient on SIMV has been successfully ventilated for 24 hours at a rate of 2 breaths/min with the 7200 ventilator. Suddenly, the patient becomes apneic. How long could the patient remain unventilated?

See Appendix A for the answer.

Unlike other modes of ventilation, during PCV or PCV apnea ventilation, the message window provides a continuous sequence of messages to advise that PCV—not volume-targeted ventilation—is in use. The messages are preceded by an asterisk and, in general, list the following:

1. Mode
2. Pressure
3. T_I
4. I:E ratio

The 7200 even provides for pressure-targeted mandatory breaths in apnea ventilation when PCV is the operating mode (see apnea ventilation in the discussion of special functions in this section). Option 81 is the apnea ventilation option for PCV and has parameter ranges similar to those for normal PCV. An apnea interval of 10 to 60 seconds is available, although setting an interval >20 seconds is unusual.

Error messages that can occur in PCV, their causes, and possible solutions are listed in Table 12-26. It is very important to set the upper pressure limit in PCV. Although the selected inspiratory pressure is the maximum that can be provided by the ventilator, if the patient coughs, circuit pressure can rise above this value. Just as in volume ventilation, if airway pressure is greater than or equal to the upper pressure limit, inspiration ends.

The plateau function is not operational during PCV. An inspiratory pause can be obtained by increasing T_I (see Chapter 11). Sighs are also not operational during PCV.

Pressure Support Ventilation (PSV)

PSV (Option 10) provides pressure-targeted, spontaneous breaths in the SIMV and CPAP modes. PS breaths are

Box 12-78 Initiating Pressure-Control Ventilation

1. Press the pressure control key (at the top of the front panel) or the + + key, and then press 80 and ENTER.
2. "80 PCV" appears in message window; press ENTER.
3. "INSP PRESS YYY CMH$_2$O" appears; enter the desired pressure value for mandatory breaths and press ENTER.
4. "<I>E X.XX/XXX" appears. <I> indicates that the inspiratory component may be changed if desired. Select the desired value and press ENTER. The message "<I>/E Y.YY/XXX" appears, indicating Y.YY as the new inspiratory component.
5. Press ENTER and "I/<E> Y.YY/XXX" appears. XXX is the expiratory component. If the inspiratory component is anything but 1, <E> must be 1. If you try to enter something other than 1, T_I is automatically changed to 1. (*Note*: The numerical values entered for I and E components cannot be less than 1.0. For example, rather than 1:0.25, 4:1 is entered; you cannot type in 0.25.
6. The I:E ratio displayed in the message window appears as "X.XX/1.00 (IRV)" or "1:X.XX" for normal I:E ratios. The Patient Data display for I:E, however, is calculated using monitored data and is always displayed as "1/XX" for normal ratios and IRVs.
7. <E> must be ≤ 9. If <E> is >9, the message "E >9 SET INSP TIME" appears to indicate you have set E >9.
8. Key in the desired expiratory component and press ENTER. The message becomes "I/<E> Y.YY/YYY," where Y.YY/YYY represents the new I:E ratio. Press ENTER. "INSP TIME X.XX" is the T_I (in seconds) based on the requested I:E ratio and the set rate.
9. Values that result in an I:E ratio >4:1 cause the message window to read "DECR RESP RATE FIRST" or "CHANGE RR-I/E-IT."
10. Press ENTER. The message "NEW I/E = Z.ZZ/ZZZ" appears if you changed the I:E ratio, with Z.ZZ/ZZZ being the new ratio based on T_I and rate.
11. Press ENTER. "UPDATE PARAMS-ENTER" asks you to press ENTER again if you want to use the new settings. Press CLEAR to cancel.
12. Press ENTER. "REVIEW FUNCTION 81" appears to prompt you to update the PCV apnea parameters under function 81.

patient-triggered, pressure-targeted (1 to 70 cm H_2O in newer version; 1 to 30 cm H_2O in earlier version), and flow-cycled ($\leq$ 5 L/min). As a safety back-up feature, PSV also cycles out of inspiration when airway pressure is 1.5 cm H_2O above PSV + PEEP, or if T_I is $\geq$ 5 seconds.

The pressure setting in PSV is added to the CPAP level. For example, if CPAP is 5 cm H_2O and PSV is 10 cm H_2O, PIP is 15 cm H_2O. PSV is set by selecting the PRESSURE SUPPORT key pad at the top of the front panel or by selecting Option 10 using the + + key and following the instructions in the message window to select desired settings. (*Note*: PSV cannot be used when older versions of Flow-by (Option 50) are activated, but it is functional with Flow-by version 2.0.)

Special Functions

There are a wide variety of options and functions available for the 7200, several of which have already been discussed. A few more important features, including the following, are presented here:

1. Three emergency modes of ventilation: apnea ventilation, back-up ventilation, and disconnect ventilation
2. Respiratory mechanics and Flow-by

Whenever certain alarm conditions occur or the ventilator detects certain faults or system errors, the ventilator automatically starts one of the three emergency ventilation modes. When apnea or disconnect ventilation occur, the ventilator uses the operator-selected parameters set for apnea ventilation.

Because the PEEP/CPAP control is not part of the electronics, it is active at its current setting during any emergency mode of ventilation. The displays may not be functioning properly in an emergency situation. Therefore, the operator should not change the PEEP setting when an emergency mode is active.

Table 12-24 Range of parameters for PCV

Pressure Control Ventilation Parameter	Range	Increment
Inspiratory pressure	5.0 to 100 cm H_2O	1 cm H_2O
I:E Ratio	($4\geq I\geq 1$, $9\geq E\geq 1$) (one component must be 1)	0.1 for each component
Respiratory rate	0.5 to 9.9 bpm	0.1 bpm
	10 to 70 bpm	1 bpm
Inspiratory time	0.20 to 5.00 sec	0.02 sec
O_2	21% to 100%	1%

Courtesy Puritan Bennett, Inc, a division of Tyco Healthcare, Pleasanton, Calif.

CLINICAL ROUNDS 12-30

Here are two example problems about changing the rate in PCV:

Problem 1—In PCV on the 7200, the rate is set at 10 breaths/min and the I:E ratio is 1:1. What is T_I? Assuming T_I is constant, and the rate is changed to 15 breaths/min, what will the new I:E be?

Problem 2—If the ratio rather than T_I is constant (1:1), and the rate is increased from 10 to 15 breaths/min, what will be the new T_I?

See Appendix A for the answer.

Table 12-25 Choosing the constant parameter of TI or I:E in PCV

Operator Action	Message Window Response	Comments
Select Option 82	82 PCV I/E CONSTANT	The I:E ratio is being held constant.
Press ENTER	CONSTANT IT-PUSH CLR	Press clear to hold T_I constant, or press ENTER to keep I:E ratio constant.
Press CLEAR	82 PCV I-T CONSTANT	The T_I is now held constant when set respiratory rate is changed.
		-or-
Select Option 82	82 PCV I-T CONSTANT	T_I is being held constant.
Press ENTER	CONSTANT IE-PUSH CLR	Press clear to hold the I:E ratio constant, or press ENTER to keep T_I constant.
Press CLEAR	82 PCV I/E CONSTANT	The I:E ratio is now held constant when set respiratory rate is changed.

Courtesy Puritan Bennett, Inc, a division of Tyco Healthcare, Pleasanton, Calif.

NOTE: Messages may differ slightly on the 7202 display. Press * at any point in the sequence to review the previous parameter or message. Press the + + key at any point in the parameter set-up to exit the function.

Table 12-26 Error messages provided in PCV on the 7200

Error Message	Explanation	Operator Action
CHANGE I/E/FIRST	This message appears when a change in set respiratory rate would cause a T_I of less than 0.2 second or more than 5 seconds (and Function 82 is holding I:E ratio constant).	Change the I:E ratio through function 80, change the respiratory rate, or change parameter control through Function 82.
CHANGE PF/TV/RR	This message appears when changing from PCV to volume ventilation and the current settings fail the I:E ratio check.	Check for the appropriate peak flow, V_T, or respiratory rate before changing to volume ventilation. Check also waveform and plateau settings.
DECR INSP TIME FIRST	This message appears when a change in set respiratory rate would cause the I:E ratio to exceed 4:1 (and Function 82 is holding T_I constant).	Decrease T_I, change the respiratory rate, or change parameter control through Function 82.
CHANGE RR/I/E-IT	This message appears when a change in the set I:E ratio causes the ventilator to calculate an invalid T_I.	Change the I:E ratio, T_I, or respiratory rate.
DECR RESP RATE FIRST	This message appears when a change in T_I would result in the I:E ratio exceeding 4:1.	Decrease the set respiratory rate or change T_I.
E>9 SET INSP TIME	This message appears when the requested expiratory component is greater than 9 for the set I:E ratio. To achieve a larger expiratory component, set the T_I.	Enter an expiratory component less than 9. Or, change the T_I to achieve an expiratory component greater than 9.

Courtesy Puritan Bennett Inc, a division of Tyco Healthcare, Pleasanton, Calif.

Apnea Ventilation

Whenever an apneic period exceeds the set apnea time, the ventilator initiates apnea ventilation using the apnea parameters set by the operator (Table 12-27). These can be set for either volume- or pressure-targeted ventilation. When the unit is in CMV or SIMV, apnea ventilation has no low inspiratory pressure alarm. "Alarm" illuminates in the alarm summary display, and the message "Apnea Ventilation" appears. Only the ALARM SILENCE and ALARM RESET keys are operational. The machine will reestablish ventilation if the patient triggers two consecutive breaths. After ventilation is restored, pressing the RESET key clears alarm indicators.

Back-Up Ventilation

Back-up ventilation (BUV) occurs whenever POST fails, the ongoing checks detect three system errors within 24 hours, or the AC voltage is <90% of the rated value. Audible and visible alarms occur. Under these circumstances, the pneumatic system of the ventilator is controlled by an analog circuit that is separate from the microprocessor systems. BUV uses the following factory-preset parameters to ventilate the patient:

1. Rate = 12 breaths/min
2. V_T = 0.5 L (whether volume or pressure ventilation was previously set)
3. Constant flow delivery at 45 L/min
4. Current PEEP setting
5. 100% O_2 (if available)
6. High-pressure limit about 30 cm H_2O above PEEP

Table 12-27 Parameter ranges for volume- and pressure-targeted apnea ventilation

Range of Selection	Default Value
FOR BOTH	
Apnea interval: 10 to 60 seconds	20 seconds
Breath rate: 0.5 to 70 breaths/mi	12 breaths/min
Oxygen percentage: 21% to 100%	100%
FOR VOLUME VENTILATION	
Tidal volume: 0.1 to 2.5 L	0.5 L
Peak flow: 10 to 120 L/min	45 L/min
FOR PRESSURE VENTILATION	
Default to volume settings	
Inspiratory pressure: 5 to 100 cm H_2O	
Inspiratory time: 0.5 to 50 seconds	
I:E ratio: 1:9 to 3:1 (4:1 in PCV)	

Courtesy Puritan Bennett, Inc, a division of Tyco Healthcare, Pleasanton, Calif.

The BUV indicator lights in the alarm summary section. All other displays are blank, and all functions except the PEEP/CPAP are nonfunctional. If BUV occurs, provide another means of ventilating the patient as soon as possible and have the ventilator serviced.

In pediatric patients, the patient is protected from excessive volume or pressure provided by BUV by two factors. First, small endotracheal tubes increase resistance to inspiratory flow. Second, the pressure limit of about 30 cm H_2O prevents pressures from getting too high.

Disconnect Ventilation

Whenever the microprocessor detects inconsistencies in airway pressures, PEEP, and gas delivery pressure in the pneumatic system, the disconnect emergency mode activates.[1] Tubing disconnects or plugged tubing can cause these conditions. The machine uses the apnea ventilation setting, but the sensitivity setting is not recognized. When disconnect ventilation activates, the following alarm indicators are turned on:

1. Alarm (in alarm summary display)
2. High peak pressure
3. "Airway press disconn." (in message window)

Only the ALARM RESET and ALARM SILENCE keys are operational. Disconnect ventilation does not automatically reset itself. After the problem that caused the alarm is corrected, pressing RESET restores the ventilator to its previous state.

If something prevents the 7200 from initiating an emergency ventilation mode, the safety valve opens to allow a spontaneously breathing patient access to room air.

Respiratory Mechanics

The Puritan Bennett 7200 can measure, calculate, and display the following respiratory mechanics when Options 30 and 40 have been added:

1. Maximum inspiratory pressure (negative inspiratory force)
2. Vital capacity
3. Airway resistance (static and dynamic)
4. Compliance (static and dynamic)
5. Peak flow (spontaneous)

MIP, which is called negative inspiratory pressure (NIP) on the 7200, measures the maximum negative pressure generated by the patient against an occluded airway during a 3-second interval. The maneuver ends when the patient begins to exhale and MIP (NIP) is displayed.

The vital capacity function does not measure forced vital capacity, but slow vital capacity. Before the patient begins a maximal inhalation, the message window must read "VC MNVR ACTIVE." The maneuver is successful and vital capacity is displayed when the patient begins a breath after the vital capacity-maneuvered breath.

Activation of a static mechanics maneuver causes the ventilator to deliver a volume-targeted breath with a constant flow, followed by a plateau measurement. Calculated values for Raw and C_S are displayed in the message window at the beginning of the next breath (Box 12-79). The dynamic mechanics for C and Raw measured during active flow delivery are determined by sampling the instantaneous values for pressure, volume, and flow at numerous intervals during inspiration for a mandatory breath. Using the equation of motion discussed in Chapter 11, the microprocessor determines and calculates the various values.

Peak spontaneous flow (Option 41) is measured, calculated, and displayed (in liters/minute) for spontaneous breaths. The operator can select either an eight-breath average or have the most recent breath displayed.

Box 12-79 Static Mechanics Measurements

If a message followed by an asterisk appears in the display window after a static mechanics measurement (e.g., "SM CMP 40* RES 23*"), then a stable plateau was not obtained during the maneuver. Accuracy of these values depends on whether airway pressure stabilizes during inflation hold and the exhaled values fall to zero (baseline) at the end of the breath cycle.

Blank displays mean that the calculation was out of acceptable range (CMP [compliance], 0 to 500 mL/cm H_2O; RES [resistance], 0 to 100 cm H_2O).

Flow and Flow-By Triggering

Flow-by (version 1.0) was first introduced as a method to provide a continuous flow of air past the upper airway, similar to a continuous-flow IMV circuit (see Chapter 11). To accomplish mandatory breath triggering with the flow-by feature, the manufacturer had to make the unit flow- rather than pressure-triggered. In addition, the original version of flow-by (version 1.0) was only active in CPAP and SIMV and only when pressure support was *not* selected.

It is now known that flow-by actually reduces the work of breathing associated with breath triggering.[2] With continuous flow in the patient circuit, fresh gas is available to patients as soon as they begin to inspire. This reduces the delay between the patient's demand for flow and the beginning of flow from the internal flow valve.

The introduction of flow-by version 2.0 made flow-triggering available in all modes of ventilation, including PSV.

To operate flow-triggering when flow-by is selected, the operator first selects flow-by using the + + key and selecting Option 50 or by pressing the flow-by function key on the top row of controls on the front panel. The message window prompts the operator to set the base flow and the flow-trigger level.

The base flow is the continuous gas flow present in the patient circuit during the expiratory phase. During mandatory inspiration and during inspiration in PSV, the base flow is suspended. At the beginning of exhalation, the base flow is

Table 12-28 Recommended base flow and flow sensitivity settings for the 7200

Base Flow Setting	Range of Allowed Flow Sensitivity
5 L/min	1 to 3 L/min
6 to 9 L/min	1 L/min to 1/2 of base flow set
20 L/min	1 to 15 L/min

Courtesy Puritan Bennett, Inc, a division of Tyco Healthcare, Pleasanton, Calif.

always 5 L/min—regardless of the base flow set. This eliminates resistance to exhalation when it begins. The manufacturer has programmed the 7200 to require base flow to be about twice the flow-trigger or flow sensitivity setting (Table 12-28). For example, if a flow-trigger of 4 L/min is selected, a base flow of 8 L/min would be appropriate.

Base flow is monitored by the expiratory flow transducer. When the base flow drops by the trigger flow amount, inspiration begins (Box 12-80). The lower settings for flow sensitivity require less work for the patient to trigger a breath. For example, triggering is easier with a trigger of 1 L/min than it is at a trigger of 3 L/min. During flow-triggering, the manufacturer recommends the following settings:

1. 1 L/min for small patients (<25 kg)
2. 2 L/min for patients between 25 and 50 kg
3. 3 L/min for large patients (>50 kg)

Because flow-triggering is so sensitive, the operator needs to watch for auto-triggering.

Flow-by is not available during nebulization. The older version of flow-by must be turned off during nebulization and then reactivated after the treatment. With the newer versions (2.0), the unit automatically switches to pressure-triggering when nebulization is activated, but the operator has to restart flow-by when nebulization is complete.

Ventilator Graphic Waveforms

The graphics 2.0 option allows the operator to select several waveforms to be viewed during ventilation and provides the following monitoring capabilities:

1. Waveforms (Function 60), including scalars and loops
2. Trending waveforms (Function 61)
3. A curser for trending curves
4. Freeze/print (Function 62) to freeze a waveform on the screen or print it with an attached compatible printer
5. Changing of patient number and room (Function 3)
6. "Plethysmogram" is another available waveform but requires Option 90: pulse oximetry

Box 12-80 Range of Flow-Trigger Variables

In flow-by version 1.0, the flow sensitivity or trigger range is 1 to 10 L/min. In flow-by version 2.0, the range is 1 to 15 L/min. The minimum base flow for both is 5 L/min, and the maximum is 20 L/min. If the base is set too high, it can cause inadvertent PEEP and increase airway pressures.

Box 12-81 Systems Evaluated to Verify Proper Function of the 7200 Ventilator

1. Microprocessor and associated electronics during POST program
2. Pressure and flow transducers
3. Expiratory valve
4. Patient circuit
5. PEEP regulator
6. BUV
7. Safety valve with associated over pressure

The waveforms menu allows two waveforms or loops to be displayed at one time (e.g., the scalars pressure, flow, and volume per unit time, and the loops pressure-volume and flow-volume). Selecting the + + key and Option 60 accesses the graphics package. Pressing the graphics 2.0 key at the top of the front panel also accesses graphics. The bottom of the graphics screen allows viewing of graph selections and the directions for selecting those choices.

Option 61 brings up the trending menu on the graphics screen with appropriate directions for setting up trending plots. Currently, there are 39 parameters available for trending, including regularly measured values such as V_T and rate, and added options including the pulse oximeter and the metabolic monitor.

Troubleshooting

The alarms and monitors on the 7200 provide a wide variety of methods to solve and detect problems. In addition, the extensive series of self tests and the continuous automatic testing verify the functional readiness of every subsystem of the ventilator, including those items listed in Box 12-81.

One problem occasionally encountered by clinicians operating the 7200 is auto-triggering. The operator has to carefully balance trigger sensitivity with patient effort. On one hand, one does not want the patient making excessive effort to trigger the unit. On the other hand, auto-triggering resulting from leaky circuits or slight dips in pressure when PEEP is set at moderately high levels is also undesirable.

Another note of caution is indicated when slow SIMV rates are set. First, when switching from CMV to SIMV, the operator should give a manually-triggered breath. This prevents any delay that might occur with mandatory breath delivery. It is important to ensure that apnea time and low V_T alarm limits are set appropriately (see the discussion on SIMV earlier in this section).[1]

As with most medical equipment that is microprocessor controlled, the use of walkie-talkies, portable cellular phones, and other transmitting devices may interfere with their operation. Manufacturers are aware of this problem and have begun devising methods to protect against it. However, unless one is sure about the equipment, the use of such transmitting devices should be avoided.

Puritan Bennett Adult Star

The Adult Star ventilator has two models, the 1500 and the 2000. These units are designed for pediatric and adult use primarily in the acute care settings. Puritan Bennett (a division of Tyco Healthcare) is no longer making this ventilator. However, because some units are still in use, the operation of the Adult Star has been placed on the EVOLVE site for this text.

Newport Breeze E150

The Newport Breeze E150 is a general purpose ventilator that can be used for neonatal, pediatric, or adult patients (Figure 12-73).[1] The Duoflow system permits mandatory and spontaneous inspiratory gas flows to be controlled separately.

Power Source

This microprocessor-controlled ventilator is both pneumatically and electrically powered. It requires high-pressure air/oxygen gas sources (35 to 90 psig, optimum of

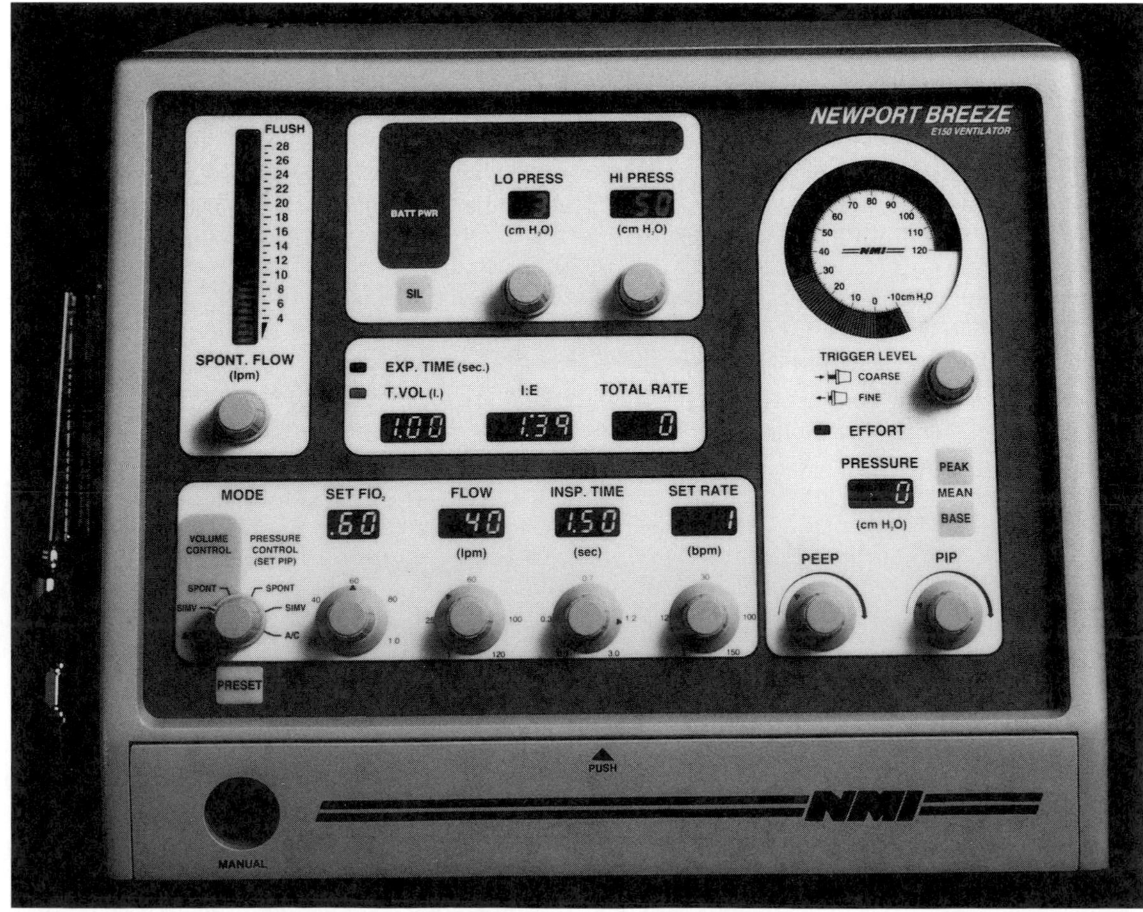

Figure 12-73 The Newport Breeze E150 ventilator. (Courtesy Newport Medical Instruments, Inc, Newport Beach, Calif.)

50 psig) and a standard AC electrical outlet (110 or 240 volts). The ON/OFF power switch is behind a drop-down door on the lower section of the front control panel. When the power switch is turned on, a temporary alarm sounds. This is followed by a brief self-test.

There is an internal battery that normally charges when the unit is plugged into an AC power source, usually a standard wall outlet. The internal battery acts as a back-up source of electrical power during power outages or if the AC power cord is disconnected. When fully charged, the battery lasts up to 1 hour.

The air and oxygen high-pressure hoses are connected to the back of the unit. The Breeze E150 operates from a single gas source if one becomes disabled, but this may affect the percentage of oxygen delivered. (*Note:* If both gas sources fail, the spontaneously breathing patient can obtain room air through the internal emergency intake valve, which requires an inspiratory effort of about –2 cm H_2O.)

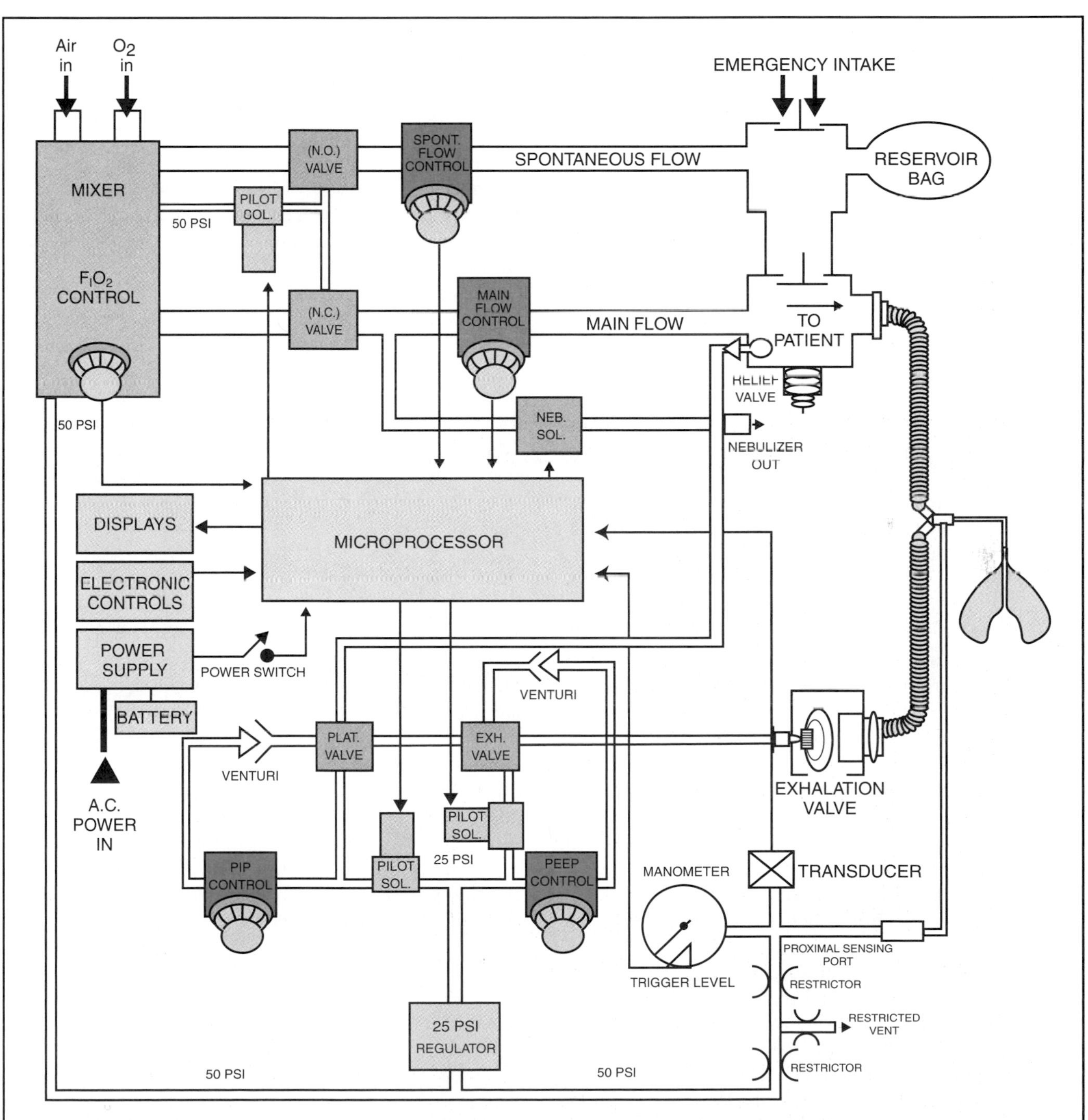

Figure 12-74 A pneumatic diagram of the Newport Breeze E150 internal circuit (see text for explanation). (Courtesy Newport Medical Instruments, Inc, Newport Beach, Calif.)

Box 12-82 Control Valves that Govern Gas Flow in the Breeze E150

1. A spontaneous to mandatory flow-switching pilot solenoid valve
2. Spontaneous and mandatory inspiratory control pneumatic interface valves
3. Spontaneous and mandatory flow-regulating needle valves
4. Mandatory breath inspiratory and expiratory pressure-switching valves
5. Inspiratory (pressure control only) and expiratory pressure-regulating needle valves
6. A mushroom balloon type of exhalation valve

There is no built-in internal oxygen analyzer, but an optional one is available. F_IO_2 should be checked regularly by the operator.

An optional flowmeter that can be attached to the side of the unit can be used to supply mixed gas for either a resuscitation bag or an external small-volume nebulizer.

Internal Mechanisms

The internal mechanisms are shown in Figure 12-74. High-pressure air and oxygen enter the ventilator through a mixer (blender) inside the back of the unit. The mixer regulates inlet gas pressures, then blends the gases to the set O_2%. Blended gas then flows to two separate internal pathways: the main flow circuit and the spontaneous flow circuit. A series of control valves (Box 12-82) governs the gas output from these circuits.

When a mandatory breath is triggered, this activates the pilot solenoid valve, which generates a pneumatic signal that opens the normally closed (n.c.), mandatory (main) inspiratory control pneumatic interface valve. Gas is then directed from the blender through the mandatory flow-regulating needle valve into the patient circuit. If volume-targeted A/C, A/C plus sigh, or SIMV modes are selected, the mandatory breath trigger also causes an electronic signal, resulting in complete closure of the mushroom/balloon-style exhalation valve during inspiration. If pressure-targeted, A/C, or SIMV is selected, the mandatory breath trigger causes an electronic signal that allows the set PIP control to determine the maximum pressure in the patient circuit by establishing the pressure in the exhalation valve.

During mandatory breath exhalation, the spontaneous inspiration pneumatic interface valve is turned on and the main flow off. The PEEP solenoid valve causes the set PEEP level to be established at the patient circuit exhalation manifold. In the Breeze E150, as in the Wave E200 (without compass monitor), there is an externally mounted expiratory valve that must be connected to the exhalation valve small nipple-connector outlet to function.

Controls and Alarms

The front panel of the Newport Breeze E150 is visually divided into five distinctive sections: a flowmeter, an alarm and indicator panel, a digital display panel, a breath control panel, and a pressure control panel (Figure 12-75). The controls that govern breath delivery will be reviewed first, and then the monitor and alarm sections are discussed.

Spontaneous Flow (Digital Flowmeter Panel)

The digital flowmeter to the left of the panel displays and controls the flow during spontaneous breaths for the SIMV and spontaneous modes (1 to 28 L/min calibrated, 58 L/min at flush setting). This flow is used also to stabilize baseline pressure between mandatory breaths in A/C.

In A/C, the operator sets spontaneous flow at 4 L/min and adjusts it as necessary to maintain the baseline pressure level (PEEP/CPAP). The spontaneous flow is only operational between mandatory breaths in the A/C and SIMV modes.

Spontaneous flow should be set to meet patient demand. A reservoir bag is available and should be added to the circuit if a patient's inspiratory efforts result in significant pressure deflections on the pressure gauge. The bag serves as a reservoir for mixed gas that a patient can access if the peak inspiratory flow exceeds the spontaneous flow setting. Clinical Rounds 12-31 provides an exercise in adjusting flow settings. The spontaneous flowmeter also provides gas flow to the patient, if an electronic ventilator malfunction is detected.

Breath Control Panel

The breath control panel contains the adjustments for mode, F_IO_2, flow, T_I, and rate. The mode control allows selection of either volume-targeted (volume control) or pressure-targeted (pressure control) ventilation. (Modes of ventilation are reviewed later in this section.) F_IO_2 is adjustable from 0.21 to 1.0. The FLOW CONTROL knob sets the constant gas flow for mandatory breaths (3 to 120 L/min). T_I varies from 0.1 to 3.0 seconds. The mandatory rate setting can be adjusted from 1 to 150 breaths/min.

Pressing the PRESET touch pad (membrane switch) below the mode control causes the digital displays to illuminate, showing set parameters. This is useful in switching from a spontaneous to a mandatory ventilator mode.

Pressure Display Panel

The pressure display relies on pressure sensing through a proximal airway pressure line connecting the outlet on the lower right side of the ventilator to an adapter at the Y connector in the patient circuit. This line is purged with gas flow to reduce the risk of line obstruction from water or contaminants. Use of a bacterial filter in this line is also advised. Pressures are measured internally through an integral pressure transducer.

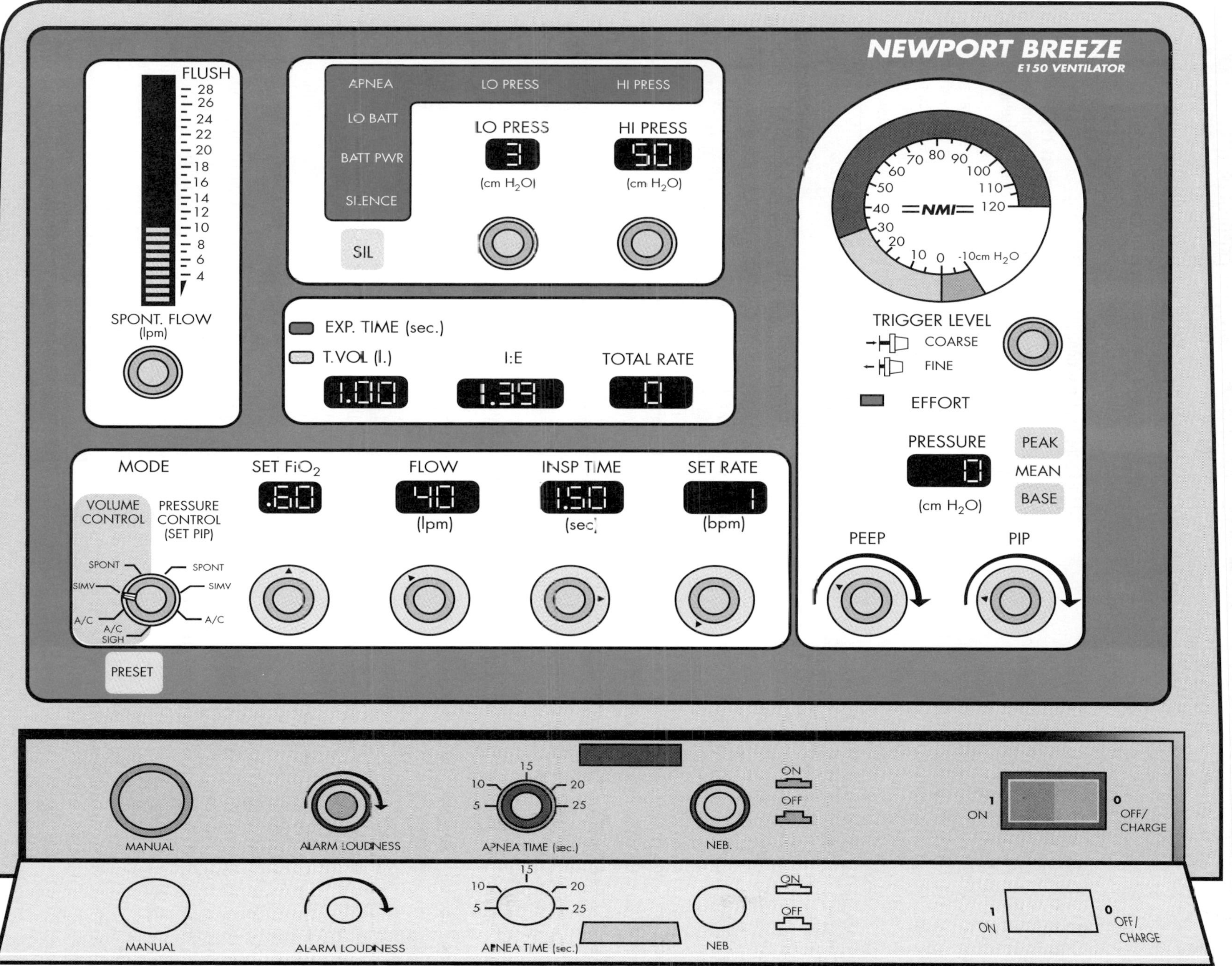

Figure 12-75 The front panel of the Newport Breeze E150.

CLINICAL ROUNDS 12-31

Problem 1

During SIMV ventilation of a patient on the Breeze E150, the respiratory therapist notes that the pressure gauge dips to –8 cm H_2O during the inspiratory phase of spontaneous breaths. What should the therapist do to correct this problem?

Problem 2

A patient is on 10 cm H_2O of CPAP on the Breeze E150 ventilator. The respiratory therapist notices that the airway pressure is 10 cm H_2O during inspiration but rises to 15 cm H_2O during expiration. What should the therapist do to correct this problem?

See Appendix A for the answer.

Box 12-83 Trigger Sensitivity on the E150

If the knob is in the coarse position when the ventilator is turned on, the trigger level will be from –10 to +60 cm H_2O. Its precise value depends on the position of the knob.

If the trigger knob is pushed in for the fine-tuning position, the trigger level will be from –5 to –10 cm H_2O, depending on the knob position.

If the effort light will not illuminate, check to be sure the trigger has been adjusted to reflect the baseline pressure setting. If the trigger level is set very close to baseline pressure, but the patient effort does not cause the light to illuminate, it may be necessary to reduce the spontaneous flow setting. With too much flow in the circuit, the ventilator may not sense the patient effort. Also check for circuit leaks. With too little flow, the patient may generate significant negative pressures in order to breathe spontaneously.

Pressure Gauge

An electronic pressure gauge at the top of this panel displays measured airway pressures (–10 to 120 cm H_2O). It is a backlit LCD that lights up in green to indicate the current pressure changes at the airway, peak pressure for the breath, baseline pressures, and trigger sensitivity setting.

Trigger Level and Effort Indicator

A small visual indicator, EFFORT, illuminates when a patient effort is detected. This is based on the trigger setting. There is a knob that allows adjustment of trigger sensitivity (about –10 to 60 cm H_2O). Coarse adjustment brings the trigger level within 5 cm H_2O of the desired setting. Fine adjustment allows the operator to set the trigger to respond to minimal patient effort without resulting in auto-triggering. Box 12-83 explains some additional information on setting trigger sensitivity.

Digital Pressure Indicator

The digital pressure window displays peak, mean, or baseline airway pressure. Peak or baseline pressure readings can be displayed for 30 seconds by pressing either the PEAK or the BASE touch pads. After 30 seconds, the display automatically returns to mean pressure. (*Note:* Pressing the PRESET touch pad, will return the display to mean pressure at any time.)

PEEP and PIP Controls

The PEEP control adjusts baseline pressure from 0 to 60 cm H_2O. PIP adjusts pressure delivery during pressure-targeted mandatory breaths (0 to 60 cm H_2O). It is *not* additive to the baseline or PEEP setting.

Data Display Panel

The data display panel shows the calculated V_T (liters) when the Breeze E150 is set to deliver volume-targeted breaths and displays T_E when set to deliver pressure-targeted breaths. The I:E ratio is the calculated value based on the settings for mandatory breaths. If the I:E ratio becomes inverse, the colon in the ratio flashes. When the maximum I:E ratio is exceeded (maximum is 4:1), the entire T_I display flashes.

Alarm and Indicator Panel

The alarm and indicator section at the top of the front panel allows the setting of both a HIGH-PRESSURE (10 to 120 cm H_2O) and a LOW-PRESSURE (3 to 99 cm H_2O) alarm. If the HIGH-PRESSURE alarm setting is exceeded, the ventilator goes into the expiratory phase. The LOW-PRESSURE alarm activates if the proximal airway pressure fails to exceed the LOW-PRESSURE alarm setting during a mandatory breath. The LOW-PRESSURE alarm also serves as a low CPAP alarm in the spontaneous mode (see the discussion of the apnea alarm later in this section). Indicators within this same panel illuminate for APNEA, LOW and HIGH PRESSURE, LOW BATTERY, BATTERY POWER, and ALARM SILENCE (60 seconds).

The apnea alarm receives its information from the PATIENT TRIGGER EFFORT setting in all modes. The APNEA TIME INTERVAL control (5, 10, 15, 30, or 60 seconds) is behind a drop-down door in the lower section of the front control panel. If this control is set at 5 seconds during spontaneous ventilation, the trigger level indicator no longer monitors spontaneous breaths. Instead, the LOW-PRESSURE alarm acts as a low CPAP alarm, suggesting the presence of a disconnection or leaks (Box 12-84).

Power Source Failure Alarms

The two audible alarms for power source on the E150 are the GAS SUPPLY SOURCE FAILURE and the POWER FAILURE alarms. If one gas supply is lost or the inlet gas pressure drops too low, a pneumatic crossover valve opens to allow the ventilator to continue operating. A reed alarm on the

Box 12-84 Setting a Low CPAP Alarm

In the spontaneous mode, only a low CPAP alarm is available in place of the apnea alarm. To set the CPAP alarm, place the apnea alarm delay in the first position (5-second). This inactivates the apnea alarm and activates the low CPAP alarm. Then set the low-pressure alarm just below the CPAP level (about 2 cm H_2O below). If the pressure in the patient circuit drops below the low CPAP alarm level for 4 seconds, the low press alarm is activated.

rear of the air/oxygen mixer activates to alert the operator of the condition. $O_2\%$ delivery to the patient may vary in this situation. If both pressurized gas sources fail, the ventilator gives a continuous audible alarm and the safety valve opens allowing the spontaneously breathing patient access to room air.

When the internal battery goes into operation, the battery power indicator illuminates. When only about 15 minutes of battery power remain, a quick pulse alarm activates, and the low battery indicator lights up. If an electrical or mechanical failure is detected, a continuous alarm sounds. The operator should be sure the patient has ventilatory support.

Modes of Ventilation

Using the mode selector knob, the operator can choose either volume or pressure-targeted ventilation. With either of these, A/C, SIMV, or spontaneous modes can be used. One can also choose volume-targeted A/C with sigh. In the spontaneous mode, the existing settings can be checked by pressing the PRESET touch pad (below the mode control switch).

Volume-Targeted Breaths

Volume-targeted mandatory breaths are available in A/C, A/C plus sigh, and SIMV.

Assist/Control

In the A/C volume-targeted mode, breaths are time- or patient (pressure)-triggered, volume-targeted, and time-cycled. Mandatory flow delivery is constant at the set value. V_T delivery is determined by the flow and T_I settings. For example, if the flow is set at 60 L/min, and T_I is 1.0 seconds, the V_T is 1.0 L (1000 mL). The I:E ratio is based on respiratory rate and T_I. Continuing with this example, if the rate is 10 breaths/min, TCT is 6 seconds (60 sec/[10 breaths/min]). T_I is 1 second, T_E is 5 seconds, and the I:E ratio is 1:5.

Assist/Control with Sigh

This mode functions like regular volume-targeted A/C, except that a sigh breath equal to 1.5 times the V_T is delivered every 100 breaths. During a sigh breath, T_I is extended to 1.5 times the set T_I.

CLINICAL ROUNDS 12-32

A respiratory therapist is setting A/C, pressure-targeted breaths for a patient being ventilated by the E150. Settings are as follows: rate = 12 breaths/min, T_I = set at 0.5 seconds, flow = 30 L/min, PIP = 30 cm H_2O. During inspiration, the therapist notices that the pressure rises slowly during inspiration and peaks at 27 cm H_2O. What is causing the problem of achieving the target pressure delivery?

See Appendix A for the answer.

Synchronized Intermittent Mandatory Ventilation (SIMV)

During volume ventilation in the SIMV mode, mandatory breaths are the same as described previously. Spontaneous breaths are from the spontaneous flow source, which is described later in this section.

Pressure-Targeted Breaths

Pressure-targeted mandatory breaths are available in A/C and SIMV modes.

Assist/Control–Pressure-Targeted

Mandatory breaths are patient (pressure)- or time-triggered, pressure-targeted, and time-cycled. Pressure during inspiration is based on the PIP setting. The PIP control determines the pressure in the exhalation valve, which in turn determines the maximum pressure in the patient circuit. Flow output from the ventilator is provided at the mandatory flow setting in the form of a square wave, but flow entering the airway tends to be more of an exponential descending waveform. The length of inspiration is based on the T_I setting. As expected, volume and flow delivery to the patient vary with changes in compliance and resistance.

Maximum available flow for most adult ventilators is based on the flow setting. In the E150 flow is slightly different. If the operator sets a low flow value, it takes longer for the ventilator to achieve the set PIP. On the other hand, a high-flow setting achieves the set PIP more quickly, functioning similarly to the slope or rise control on other ventilators. A steeper slope (faster rise) results from a higher flow setting. A slower slope (slower rise) results from a lower flow. Ideally, the flow should be set to achieve the fastest pressure rise possible to attain the greatest volume delivery during the early part of inspiration. Clinical Rounds 12-32 provides a problem along these lines.

SIMV–Pressure-Targeted

SIMV–pressure-targeted mandatory breaths are delivered as described previously. The mandatory breath rate is set by

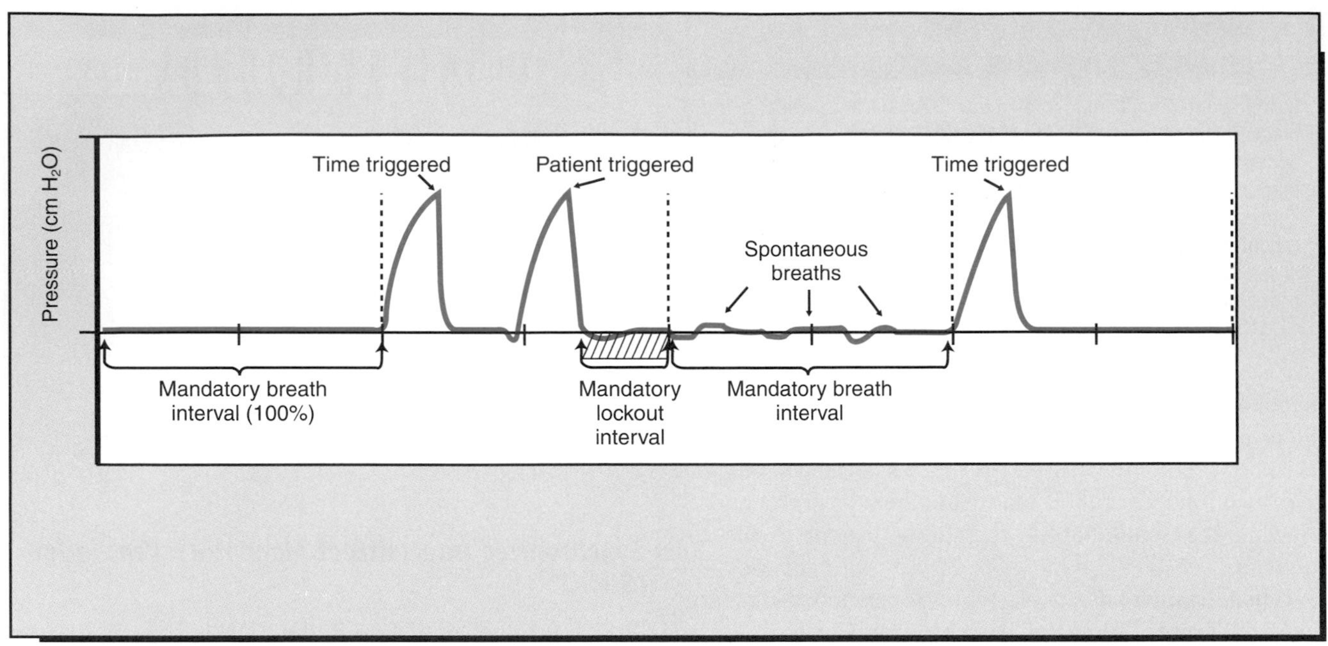

Figure 12-76 The timing of mandatory and spontaneous breaths in SIMV with the Breeze E150. The dotted vertical lines indicate mandatory breath intervals (see text for explanation).

the rate control and the length of inspiration is based on T_I. Spontaneous breaths receive flow from the spontaneous flowmeter. The reservoir bag acts as a mixed gas reservoir accessible to the patient. (*Note:* The flowmeter must be turned on with SIMV and spontaneous modes to provide gas flow to the patient during spontaneous breathing efforts.)

Both breath types are synchronized with a patient's spontaneous efforts based on the sensitivity setting. Figure 12-76 shows how mandatory breaths are timed.

The mandatory breath interval (MBI) is 60 seconds/set rate. For example, if the rate is 20 breaths/min, the MBI is 3 seconds. No patient effort was detected in the first MBI in Figure 12-76 shown as a dotted line. Therefore, at the beginning of the next MBI, a time-triggered mandatory breath is delivered. During the next MBI after the time-triggered breath, a patient triggers a mandatory breath. The patient can breathe spontaneously during the remaining time of the MBI. In the third MBI, a mandatory breath is not delivered because the patient received one in the second MBI, and the patient is now spontaneously breathing In the fourth MBI, a time-triggered breath is delivered because a complete MBI has just preceded it with no patient-triggered mandatory breath (Box 12-85).

Spontaneous

In the spontaneous mode, the patient receives air exclusively through the spontaneous flowmeter and reservoir bag. The operator can select the spontaneous setting under either the volume or pressure controls. The only difference will be in how a manual breath is delivered (see Special Features section).

Box 12-85 A Mandatory Breath Lockout Interval in SIMV with the Breeze E150 Ventilator

Whenever a mandatory breath is patient-triggered during SIMV, a mandatory breath lockout interval is activated. This limits the mandatory breath rate to the set rate. Note the second mandatory breath interval (MBI) in Figure 12-76 *(second dotted line)*. The lockout interval starts at the end of inspiration of a patient-triggered mandatory breath. A time-triggered breath is not delivered at the beginning of the third MBI because a patient-triggered breath occurred in the preceding interval. The patient can breathe spontaneously during the lockout interval.

Graphic Display Screens

Newport originally offered the Navigator Graphics Monitor as an option for viewing and printing graphic data. A description of this monitor is included in the section on the Newport Wave. This unit is no longer for sale. Newport Medical Instruments now offers the Beacon GM350 Monitor internationally, however, it is not available in the United States at this time.

Special Features

A few special features are available with the E150. Controls for these features are located behind a drop-down door in the lower section of the front control panel. In addition to these, the function of the pressure relief valve will also be reviewed.

Lower Control Panel

The MANUAL control on the left allows manual triggering of a positive-pressure inflation in any mode. When it is pressed, gas is delivered based on the breath type (pressure or volume control) and the current settings. F_IO_2 remains the same.

In all modes, on the volume side of the mode control switch, a manual breath is delivered at the mandatory flow setting until one of the following occurs:

1. The button is no longer pressed.
2. The high-pressure alarm is violated (cycles into exhalation).
3. The maximum time limit (2 seconds) elapses.

In all modes, on the pressure control side of the mode switch, a manual breath delivers a pressure-targeted inflation using the set mandatory flow and PIP settings. Inspiration ends based on the three criteria just listed.

As many as 150 manual inflations, per minute, can be delivered. (*Note:* If the pressure-relief valve setting is reached before the HIGH-PRESSURE alarm limit during a manual inflation, the pressure will plateau but inspiration will not end until one of the three criteria is met.)

The ALARM LOUDNESS control adjusts the sound level of audible alarms.

The nebulizer control (NEB) provides gas flow through the nebulizer outlet with the set F_IO_2. Flow through the nebulizer outlet delivers approximately 6 L/min in addition to the flow provided during regular ventilation. This volume is added to the digital volume display so the volume displayed is accurate. With a T_I <0.4 seconds, it may be advantageous to use an external flowmeter to power the nebulizer because there is not enough time for nebulization through the machine outlet itself.

The APNEA TIME control has settings for 5, 10, 15, 30, and 60 second intervals and is active in all modes. When the specified apnea interval elapses without a time- or patient-trigger breath being detected, an alarm is activated.

Pressure-Relief Valve

On the back panel of the E150 is a pressure relief valve that limits pressure delivery through the patient circuit during any mode, but does not end inspiration. It is adjustable from 0 to 120 cm H_2O. During normal operation, it is set at a value above the high-pressure alarm setting as a safety pop-off device.

To set the pop-off pressure prior to patient use, the operator turns the high-pressure alarm limit to 120 cm H_2O and caps the patient Y connector. The mode selector is then set to volume-controlled, A/C and the MANUAL control is pressed. The pressure gauge is observed and the pressure-relief valve rotated until the pressure plateaus at the desired relief pressure.

(*Note:* Recently a software package has become available that is a teaching aid for the Newport Breeze E150. The software provides a visual screen showing the ventilator's controls along with a description of their function. This program uses mouse interaction to control the ventilator screen knobs, thus demonstrating how using one control affects another. Users of this software can also simulate attaching the patient circuit. The manufacturer currently has this software available online [www.newportnmi.com] or will be able to provide E150 users with CD versions.)[4,5]

Troubleshooting

When patients are unable to take in a deep breath, they may be unable to receive adequate flow from the reservoir system. For patients who cannot generate an inspiratory pressure of at least −1 cm H_2O, it is probably better to cap the position where the reservoir bag normally attaches using the reservoir bag cap. If the patient is able to take in a deep breath and the reservoir bag has been replaced with a cap, the patient will be able to open the emergency intake valve. The patient can then draw in room air when their spontaneous inspiratory flows exceed the set spontaneous flow. This is a situation in which the operator must carefully monitor the patient to determine which action is appropriate: using the cap or using the reservoir bag.

The operator's manual contains an extensive table of common problems and their causes and solutions. Users are advised to follow that guide during use of the ventilator. Table 12-29 lists a few of the problems presented in the manual.

Because this unit is microprocessor-controlled, operators need to be cautious with radio frequency emitting devices, such as cellular phones, pagers, and walkie-talkies. These types of devices should not be used in the vicinity of the ventilator.

Table 12-29 Additional examples for troubleshooting on the Newport E150 Breeze

Problem	Possible Cause(s)
Inaccurate F_IO_2 delivery	Faulty analyzer, problems with mixer
Reservoir bag deflates during a spontaneous inspiration	Spontaneous flow too low, leak in circuit or bag
Ventilator stops cycling	Blown fuse, electrical malfunction, gas source failure
Airway pressure dips below selected PEEP/CPAP pressure first, before stabilization	Faulty exhalation valve or diaphragm, or spontaneous flow does not meet patient's demand
Pressure builds too slowly during manual inflation	Flow setting too low, or leak in circuit

Courtesy Newport Medical Instruments, Inc.

Newport Wave E200

The Newport Wave E200[1-4] is a general-purpose ventilator designed for use in neonatal, pediatric, and adult patients (Figure 12-77). An additional accessory, the Compass Expiratory Monitor, can be added to enhance ventilator capabilities. The Navigator Graphics Monitor was available on earlier models. Air compressors are also available to power this unit.

Power Source

The E200 Wave is a microprocessor-controlled, pneumatically, and electrically powered ventilator. It requires high-pressure air and oxygen gas sources (35 to 90 psig, optimum of 50 psig) and a standard AC electrical outlet (110 or 240 volts).

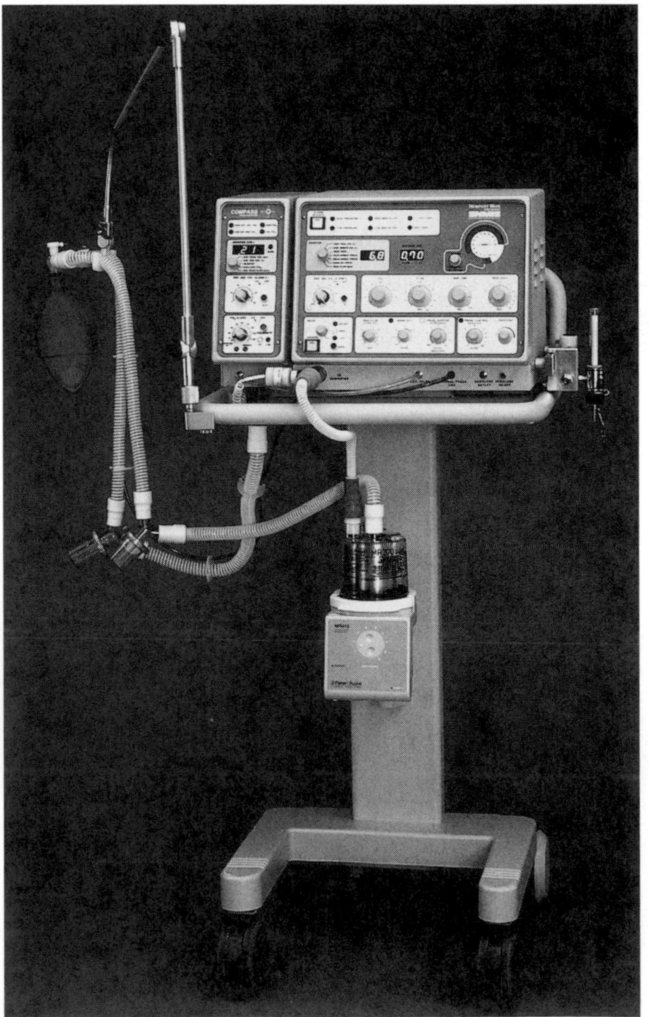

Figure 12-77 The Newport Wave E200 ventilator. (Courtesy Newport Medical Instruments, Inc, Newport Beach, Calif.)

The air and oxygen high-pressure hoses are connected to the back of the unit. The E200 operates from a single gas source if one becomes disabled, but this may affect oxygen delivery. (*Note:* If both gas sources fail, the spontaneously breathing patient can obtain room air through the internal emergency intake valve. This requires an inspiratory effort of about –2 cm H_2O. In such a situation the patient should be immediately ventilated by another method.)

The electrical ON/OFF power switch is on the back panel of the machine. When the power switch is turned on, a temporary audible alarm sounds. This is followed by a brief self-test.*

Internal Mechanisms

Internal mechanisms are shown in Figure 12-78. Source gases (air and oxygen) enter the internally mounted gas mixer. Blended gas leaving the mixer (28 psig) enters an accumulator tank and is pressurized to 2 atmospheres. The accumulator helps provide a high gas flow to meet the patient's peak inspiratory flow needs during spontaneous breathing—with or without pressure support. From the accumulator tank, flow is directed to the high-speed servo-control valve, which is also called a metering valve. This valve is an electromagnetic poppet valve (see Chapter 11). Its function is controlled by a microprocessor, which establishes the pattern of flow to the patient based on ventilator settings on the control panel. From the servo-control valve, gas is directed through a flow sensor, which is a differential pressure transducer, and then to the patient.

If the optional Compass monitor is not in use, the expiratory valve is mounted externally and is connected to the main unit's exhalation valve connector by a small-bore tube. The exhalation valve is a balloon diaphragm. The internal pressure on the balloon is determined by gas from the main flow manifold or by the flow from the PEEP control valve. Pressure within the exhalation valve is monitored by an electronic pressure transducer.

Controls and Alarms

The front panel is divided into several sections (Figure 12-79). The top portion contains monitors, alarm indicators, and the high- and low-pressure alarm settings. The central portion houses the controls for ventilator settings and the $\dot{V}_E$ alarm control. The bottom section includes the connectors to the patient circuit and the nebulizer control button. Adjacent to many of the controls are LEDs that light up to alert that the control is activated.

**When the operator turns the ventilator off, the alarm silence button needs to be pushed to silence the alarm that results.*

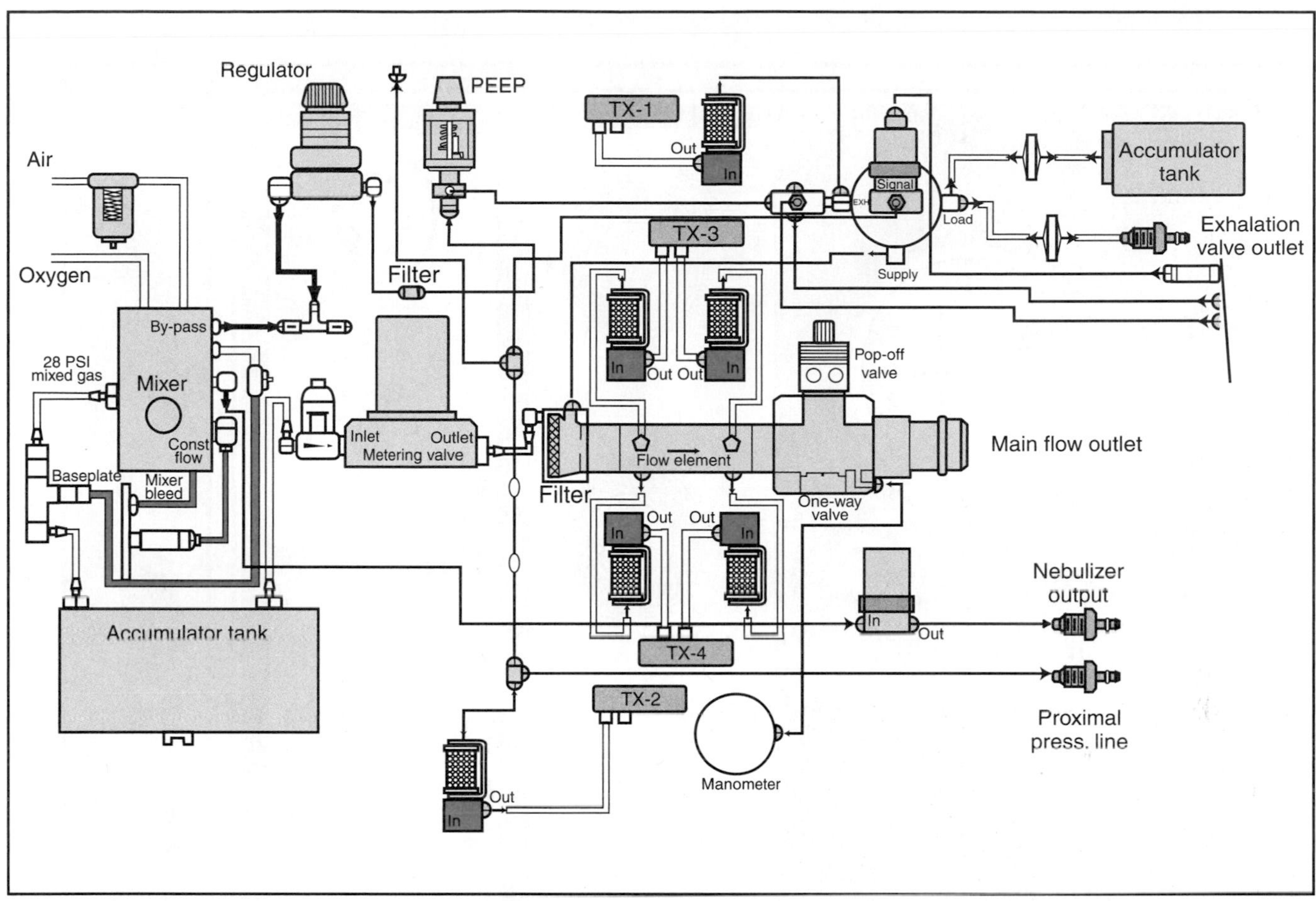

Figure 12-78 The internal circuit of the Newport Wave E200 (see text for explanation). (Courtesy Newport Medical Instruments, Inc, Newport Beach, Calif.)

Ventilator Settings Section

Mode

At the left of the bottom row is the control for selecting a ventilator mode (spontaneous, SIMV, A/C, and A/C + sigh).

There is a manual breath button in this section as well. Pressing the manual button delivers gas flow at the set flow value for as long as the button is pressed (maximum 3.8 seconds). Pressure is limited to the pressure-relief valve setting, or, if pressure control is engaged, the set pressure target—whichever is lower. If the inflation causes the airway pressure to reach the upper pressure limit alarm setting, the unit cycles into exhalation.

Bias Flow

BIAS FLOW (expiratory) provides flow in the circuit during the expiratory phase (0 to 30 L/min). Bias flow washes out any exhaled carbon dioxide, making fresh gas immediately available when the patient inhales. In addition, it reduces the ventilator's response time for pressure-triggering a breath.

Immediately after delivery of a breath (either mandatory or spontaneous), there is a brief period of no bias flow. The absence of bias flow at this time allows the patient to exhale without added resistance. When pressure in the circuit is within 2 cm H_2O of baseline, the bias flow resumes at the flow rate set. (*Note:* Any time airway pressure is elevated more than 2 cm H_2O above baseline, there is no bias flow.)

A recommended starting level for bias flow on adult patients is 2 to 5 L/min. The adult range is marked in green. For neonatal and pediatric patients, the starting level is about 2 to 3 L/min. In general, it is recommended that the least amount of bias flow possible be used. If it is set too high, it is more difficult for a patient effort to be detected by the trigger sensor.

Sensitivity

The sensitivity setting adjusts the airway pressure change required for a patient to trigger a mandatory or spontaneous breath (−5 to 0 cm H_2O). The sensitivity setting is also used to detect all breaths for monitoring. The total rate count is displayed in the monitor section. (*Note:* If a patient effort is not detected by the trigger sensitivity, it will not be counted in the monitored total rate, and the inspiratory V_T and the $\dot{V}_E$ will not be measured and displayed. If the Compass

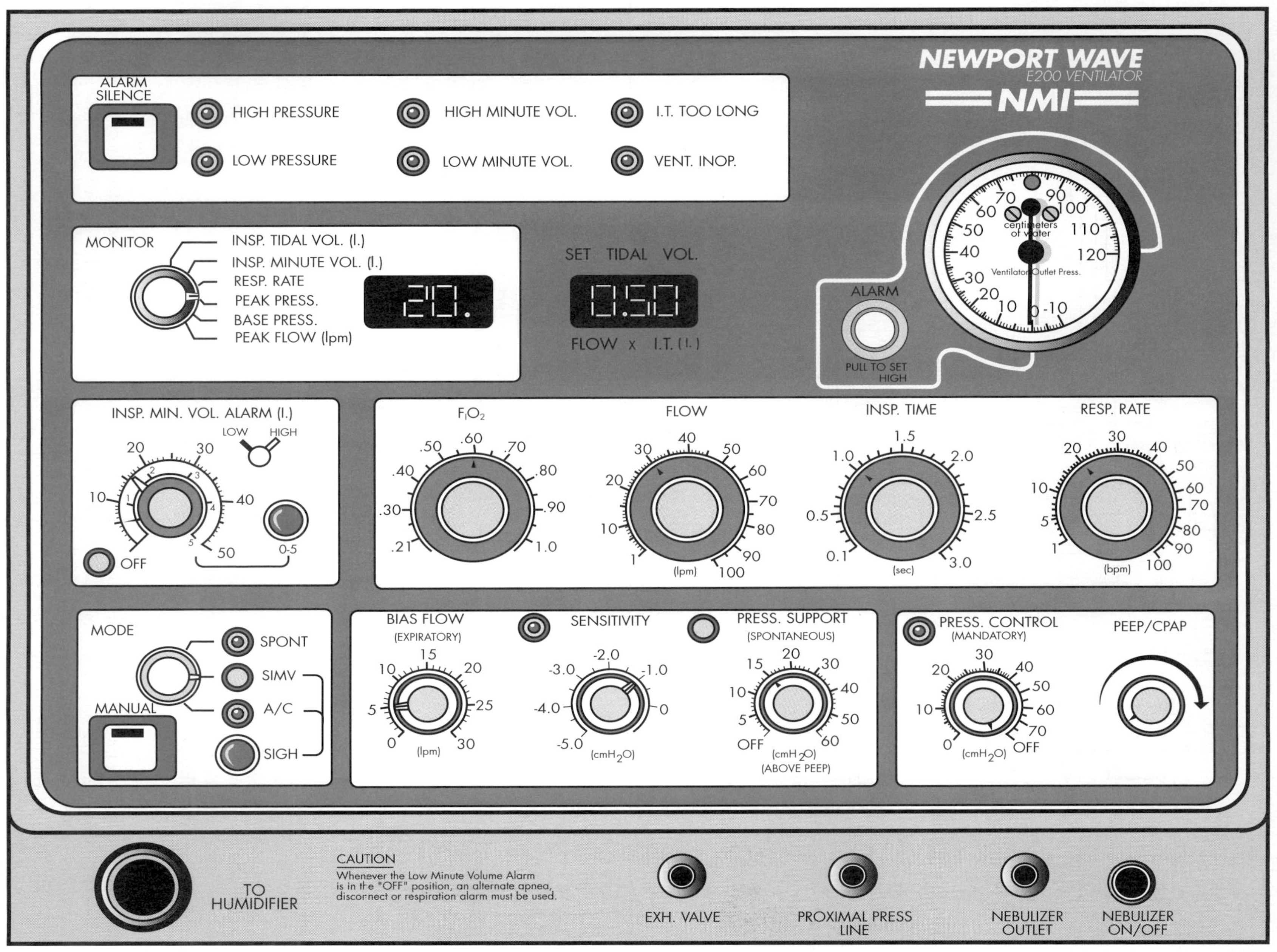

Figure 12-79 The front control panel of the Newport Wave E200 (see text for description).

monitor is in use and the expiratory V_T and the $\dot{V}_E$ are not measured and displayed, the bias flow is set too high or the sensitivity trigger setting is set too low.)

Sometimes patients have leaks around the endotracheal tube, such as occurs with uncuffed infant tubes. In this situation it is recommended that the bias flow be increased to help compensate for the leak and stabilize the baseline pressure. First, however, the integrity of the patient circuit should be confirmed by performing a leak check. Sometimes, even when the patient circuit is not leaking, but a small airway leak is present, the ventilator appears to auto-trigger, and the baseline pressure may be unstable. In this situation, set the trigger sensitivity to –0.5 cm H_2O and increase the bias flow in 1 L/min increments until the auto-trigger condition ceases. A severe leak may require that the ventilator be made less sensitive to auto-triggering by reducing the trigger sensitivity to a more negative value.

Box 12-86 The Inspiratory Minute Volume Alarm–Wave E200

This alarm is based on the rate of volume delivered from the ventilator, not including bias flow. When the bias flow is on, the LOW MIN. VOL alarm may sound if the patient's efforts do not cause the Wave to trigger because it will not measure any volume. For the alarm to work effectively, bias flow should be set as low as possible or at about 2 to 3 L/min.

For example, suppose the bias flow is set at 15 L/min, and the patient is in the spontaneous mode with a CPAP level of 10 cm H_2O. With so much flow passing, if the patient's efforts do not cause enough of a pressure drop to meet the trigger sensitivity setting, the ventilator will not "see" the patient's V_T and, therefore the low $\dot{V}_E$ may be violated.

Pressure Support (Spontaneous)

Use of the PRESS. SUPPORT (spontaneous) setting provides PSV for spontaneous breaths in the spontaneous and SIMV modes. Pressure support in the Wave E200 offers automatic inspiratory slope control, as well as a self-adjusting, variable breath termination (cycling-off criteria). The pressure range settings for PSV can be up to 60 cm H_2O, or off. This pressure setting is additive to the baseline or PEEP/CPAP level (see the discussion of modes in this section).

Pressure Control (Mandatory)

The PRESS. CONTROL (PC) knob adjusts the pressure provided during inspiration for pressure-targeted mandatory breaths (ranges 0 to 75 cm H_2O, or off). When activated, all mandatory breaths in A/C and SIMV are pressure-targeted. If the FLOW is set to the maximum level during PC, the unit automatically manages the inspiratory slope of all mandatory breaths (see the discussion of modes in this section).

PEEP/CPAP

The baseline pressure is adjusted using the PEEP/CPAP control. Because it is not numbered, the operator must watch the pressure displayed in the monitor window to view the selected baseline level. Baseline pressure ranges from 0 to 45 cm H_2O.

Inspired Minute Volume Alarm

The INSP.MIN.VOL.ALARM control is the first one on the left in the next row of the ventilator setting section. It is used to adjust for both high and low $\dot{V}_E$ alarms (in liters/minute). This knob is a dual control with the higher (white) portion setting the high $\dot{V}_E$ and the lower (black) portion setting the low $\dot{V}_E$ alarm. The minute volume alarm has two possible ranges. With the 0-5 button unlit (i.e., not pressed) the range is from 0 to 50 L/min. When the 0-5 button has been pushed and is green, the range is from 0 to 5 L/min. See Box 12-86 for further explanation of this alarm. Expiratory $\dot{V}_E$ alarms are located on the Compass monitor.

The high $\dot{V}_E$ alarm can detect a leak or a disconnection in the patient circuit if the baseline pressure is set to a positive value. When proximal pressure drops due to a leak or disconnection and the drop in pressure repeatedly activates the trigger, the measured inspiratory $\dot{V}_E$ may increase in comparison with the patient's actual $\dot{V}_E$.

The low $\dot{V}_E$ alarm can be used to detect apnea when the spontaneous ventilation mode is in use or obstructions occur in the airway during pressure-targeted ventilation.

F_IO_2

Oxygen delivery can be adjusted from 0.21 to 1.0. The delivered oxygen concentration should be checked using an oxygen analyzer. There is one included in the optional Compass monitor.

Flow

The flow (1 to 100 L/min) provides a constant gas flow at the set value during volume ventilation and sets the maximum flow available during pressure-targeted mandatory breaths. It is recommended that the flow be set to the maximum (100 L/min) during pressure-targeted ventilation so that the Wave's microprocessor can automatically adjust the inspiratory rise (slope) during mandatory breath delivery.

Inspiratory Time

Mandatory breaths, either pressure- or volume-targeted, are time-cycled. The T_I setting ranges from 0.1 to 3.0 seconds.

Respiratory Rate

This control sets the rate for mandatory breath delivery in either A/C or SIMV modes. Rate ranges from 1 to 100 breaths/min.

Alarms and Monitors

In addition to the $\dot{V}_E$ alarm already reviewed, the top panel has a high- and low-pressure alarm control located adjacent

CLINICAL ROUNDS 12-33

The following are the pressures and pressure alarms set on the Wave for a patient receiving volume ventilation:

- Peak pressure = 30 cm H_2O
- PEEP = 10 cm H_2O
- High-pressure alarm = 40 cm H_2O
- Low-pressure alarm = 25 cm H_2O
- Trigger sensitivity = –0.5 cm H_2O (below baseline)

The low-pressure alarm activates. You note the pressure gauge reads 7 cm H_2O during exhalation, and peak pressure is now 28 cm H_2O. The sensitivity trigger light flickers on, even though the patient does not appear to be inhaling. What do you think is causing the pressure drop? Why has the low-pressure alarm activated?

See Appendix A for the answer.

to the pressure gauge (–10 to 120 cm H_2O). The high- and low-pressure alarm settings are indicated by lit green segments on the pressure gauge. (*Note:* The low-pressure alarm segment turns dark when its set value is exceeded by the current airway pressure level.) Rotating the knob to its normal position sets the low- and high-pressure alarms in tandem. To set only the high alarm, pull the knob out before rotating it. If the pressure does not exceed the low pressure setting during a mandatory inspiration, an audio-visual alarm occurs. The low-pressure alarm is also violated if the airway pressure drops below the sensitivity pressure setting for 3 seconds in any mode or for half of T_E for two consecutive breaths in the SIMV mode, whichever is shorter. Clinical Rounds 12-33 presents a problem about this situation.

The pressure displayed on the pressure gauge must reach the HIGH PRESSURE alarm setting for the HIGH PRESSURE alarm to occur.* When patient circuit pressure reaches the set value, the ventilator cycles into exhalation. For the HIGH PRESSURE alarm, the pressure is measured near the main flow outlet port just inside the ventilator. If a HIGH PRESSURE alarm event occurs and the patient circuit pressure does not drop to at least 5 cm H_2O above baseline, no more mandatory breaths are delivered. An additional safety feature is the pressure-relief valve, which is reviewed in the discussion of special features later in this section.

At the top left corner of the front panel is a section containing an ALARM SILENCE button (60 seconds) and six LED indicators. Conditions resulting in illumination of these indicators are listed in Table 12-30.

Figure 12-79 shows a rotating knob with a list of measured and calculated parameters as well as a digital display window in the upper portion of the front panel. Box 12-87 lists each parameter.

There is a window in the central portion of the E200 that displays the set V_T during volume-targeted breaths. This is based on flow and T_I settings and is not a measured value. The measured inspiratory V_T is displayed in the monitor window and the measured expiratory V_T is displayed in the monitor window of the optional Compass monitor.

There are some built-in automatic high-pressure alarms as well.

Table 12-30 Alarm indicators on the E200 Wave

Alarm	Triggering condition
High pressure	Airway pressure exceeds set high-pressure alarm setting
Low pressure	Airway pressure does not achieve low-pressure alarm setting during a mandatory breath
High $\dot{V}_E$	Measured inhaled $\dot{V}_E$ exceeds set high $\dot{V}_E$ alarm
Low $\dot{V}_E$	Measured inhaled $\dot{V}_E$ is lower than low $\dot{V}_E$ alarm
T_I too long	T_I has exceeded setting based on I:E ratio limit setting of switch on back panel (manufacturer uses "IT" to abbreviate inspiratory time)
Vent. Inop.	Microprocessor has detected a malfunction. The ventilator goes into exhalation. (Sometimes turning the unit off and then back on allows it to reset. If it does not, find another machine to ventilate the patient and call a service representative.)

Courtesy Newport Medical Instruments, Inc.

Box 12-87 Monitored Parameters

Measured Values

Inspired tidal volume (0 to 9.99 L)

Inspired minute volume (0 to 99.9 L/min)

Respiratory rate (0 to 999 breaths/min)

Peak airway pressure (0 to 120 cm H_2O)

Base pressure (0 to 120 cm H_2O; measured at the exhalation valve)

Peak inspiratory flow (0 to 999 L/min; spontaneous and mandatory)

Calculated Value

Mean airway pressure (0 to 120 cm H_2O)

Circuit Connections and Nebulizer Control

Just below the main front panel are the connections for ventilator output to the humidifier, the exhalation valve line connector, the proximal airway pressure monitoring line (receives purged gas to reduce obstruction), and the nebulizer line connector. Each connection is color-coded and sized differently to avoid accidental interconnection of lines. The NEBULIZER ON/OFF control is on the far right side.

Turning on the nebulizer control results in about 6 L/min (15 psig) of gas coming from the nebulizer outlet during each mandatory volume-targeted inspiration. The nebulizer does not function with PSV, PCV, or spontaneous breaths.

While the nebulizer is on, the flow from the ventilator is reduced by the amount delivered through the nebulizer line. This is to keep actual V_T and $\dot{V}_E$ delivery constant. The operator must remember to turn off this control when the treatment is finished.

Back Panel Controls

Back panel controls are described in Box 12-88. Two additional, nonadjustable alarms are the mixer alarm, which sounds continuously if the air or oxygen inlet gas pressure drops below 31 psig, and the power supply alarm. If the AC power is lost or disconnected, this alarm is continuous for 5 minutes. A continuous alarm sounds that may be silenced with the ALARM SILENCE button if the ventilator is turned off.

Modes of Ventilation

Modes of ventilation available on the E200 include A/C (either volume- or pressure-targeted), SIMV (either volume- or pressure-targeted), and spontaneous (including PSV).

Volume-Targeted Ventilation

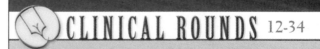

During volume ventilation the V_T is determined by the set flow and T_I. For example, if the flow is set at 80 L/min (1.33 L/sec) and the T_I is 0.5 seconds, V_T is 0.667 L (667 mL). The V_T value appears in the set tidal volume display. The I:E ratio is based on respiratory rate and T_I. For example, if the rate is 20 breaths/min, TCT is 3 seconds (60 sec/[20 breaths/min]). If T_I is 0.5 sec, T_E is 2 sec, and the I:E ratio is 1:4. Clinical Rounds 12-34 gives an example of a problem related to V_T adjustment on the Wave.

Pressure-Targeted Ventilation

If the PRESS. CONTROL knob is not turned off, mandatory breath delivery is pressure-targeted. The set tidal volume digital display will read "—." As one would expect, flow is delivered in a descending, exponential manner as pressure at the airway increases toward the set value. Volume delivery varies with changes in patient lung compliance and airway resistance. Real-time V_T and $\dot{V}_E$ should be monitored.

If there is a slight leak in the circuit during pressure ventilation, the leak supplement function activates. With this function, the ventilator increases flow to maintain the set pressure. The operator should be sure to carefully monitor and assess the patient, as well as ventilator parameters to ensure that volume and pressure delivery are adequate during PCV.

The maximum available flow during PCV is based on the flow setting. If a low flow value is set, it takes longer for the ventilator to achieve the set PIP. A high flow setting achieves the set PIP more quickly. As mentioned, for best results the highest flow value is set. This allows the microprocessor to see the automatic slope control to adjust the rise time or slope.

If the flow is set manually, it must be set high enough to achieve the set pressure before the end of inspiration. In addition, as T_I is increased, the amount of time that the pressure plateaus during inspiration increases (see Chapter 11). This will increase mean airway pressure.

High-Pressure Alarm in Pressure Ventilation

When pressure is set on the PRESS. CONTROL dial, an automatic high-pressure alarm limit is set at 10 cm H_2O

Box 12-88 Back Panel Controls

Inspiratory Pause Control

Can be set at 0% (off), 10%, 20%, and 30% of T_I.

(*Note:* During a pause, T_I for the Wave is constant at the value set on the front panel. Therefore using inspiratory pause does not increase T_I, but encroaches on the time during which inspiratory flow occurs. As a result, flow actually increases over the set value, and peak pressures may increase.)

I:E Ratio Switch

Allows I:E ratios of up to 3:1 or limits I:E ratios to 1:1 before alarming.

Audible Alarm Volume Control

The respiratory therapist is attending a patient being ventilated by the Wave E200. Current settings are as follows: mode = A/C, flow = 60 L/min, T_I = 0.75 sec, pressure control = off, rate = 10 breaths/min, F_IO_2 = 0.5, bias flow = 4 L/min, and PEEP = 5 cm H_2O. Current blood gases are: pH = 7.38, $PaCO_2$ = 44 mm Hg, and PaO_2 = 56 mm Hg.

The physician wants to improve oxygenation and asks the therapist to increase T_I to increase mean airway pressure. How would the therapist respond to this request?

See Appendix A for the answer.

above that value and terminates inspiration when exceeded. If pressure fails to fall to ≤5 cm H_2O below baseline during exhalation, no additional mandatory breaths are delivered. (*Note:* In PCV, an obstruction of the endotracheal tube cannot be detected by the high-pressure alarm system during inspiration. An obstructed tube does not require much flow to achieve the pressure, so there would not be a high-pressure alarm. An obstructed tube is detected as a drop in the minute ventilation and activates the LOW MINUTE VOL. alarm. However, a HIGH PRESSURE alarm is activated if the patient tries to actively exhale during inspiration with PCV.)

Low-Pressure Alarm in Pressure Ventilation

During pressure-targeted ventilation (PRESS. CONTROL set), an automatic LOW PRESSURE alarm is set at half of the set pressure value. If the airway pressure does not exceed this value during inspiration, the alarm activates. The LOW PRESSURE alarm also activates if the airway pressure falls and remains below the trigger sensitivity pressure setting for 3 seconds in any mode or half of the expiratory time for two consecutive breaths in the SIMV mode—whichever is shorter. This usually indicates a leak in the circuit.

Assist/Control

In A/C, breaths are patient- or time-triggered, volume- or pressure-targeted, and time-cycled. All breaths are mandatory.

Synchronized Intermittent Mandatory Ventilation[3]

In SIMV, mandatory breaths are patient- or time-triggered, volume- or pressure-targeted, and time-cycled. Spontaneous breaths are patient-triggered, pressure-limited, and pressure-cycled. PSV can be added to spontaneous breaths.

In SIMV, mandatory breaths are synchronized with a patient's spontaneous efforts based on the sensitivity setting. Figure 12-76 shows how mandatory breaths are timed. The MBI equals 60 seconds/(set breaths/min). For example if the rate is 20/min, the MBI is 3 seconds. In the first MBI in Figure 12-76 (dotted line), no patient effort is detected; therefore, at the beginning of the next MBI, a time-triggered mandatory breath is delivered. During the next MBI after the time-triggered breath, the patient triggers a mandatory breath. The patient can breathe spontaneously throughout the remaining time of the MBI. In the third MBI, a mandatory breath is not delivered because the patient received one in the second MBI. In the fourth MBI, a time-triggered breath is delivered because a complete MBI has just preceded it with no patient-triggered mandatory breath (see Box 12-85).

Spontaneous

In the spontaneous ventilation mode, bias flow, F_IO_2, PEEP/CPAP, pressure support, and sensitivity are set. The patient breathes gas provided by either the bias flow control or demand flow. The patient can also obtain gas at the set pressure when PSV is active. No mandatory breaths are delivered. If the patient's effort causes airway pressure to decrease by the amount set on the sensitivity control, the ventilator provides additional flow or pressure support. Once the breath is detected, the internal servo-control flow valve delivers whatever flow the patient demands or whatever flow is needed for pressure support, up to 160 L/min. For this reason, it is important to set the sensitivity appropriately so the patient's work of breathing is not increased (Box 12-89). Spontaneous breaths that are detected are counted and displayed by the rate monitor.

Box 12-89 Setting Bias Flow and Sensitivity in the Spontaneous Mode

It is very important to carefully adjust both bias flow and sensitivity in the spontaneous mode. The patient's inspiratory effort must exceed the sum of the pressure produced by the bias flow and the pressure required to trigger the sensitivity, or the internal flow valve will not open.

If a high bias flow is set, this may provide a substantial part of the patient's flow requirements. In this case, the pressure at the airway opening may not decrease. The potential problem is that the patient's efforts may not meet the trigger sensitivity setting, and the internal flow control valve will not open. No pressure support would be available. If this is a problem, the bias flow should be set lower.

In the spontaneous mode, only the HIGH PRESSURE alarm can be activated. When CPAP is applied, the LOW PRESSURE alarm is automatically set based on the reading from the proximal pressure line. If the patient circuit pressure falls below the trigger sensitivity level for 3 seconds or longer, the low-pressure alarm sounds.

Pressure Support

The PRESS. SUPPORT control adjusts the PSV level for spontaneous breaths in the spontaneous and SIMV modes. The LED lights up when this mode is active. In either volume- or pressure-targeted SIMV mode, PSV is available between mandatory breaths.

PS breaths are patient-(pressure) triggered, pressure-targeted, and flow-cycled. The flow that ends inspiration in PSV is calculated by the microprocessor. This calculation is based on a formula using target pressure, maximum flow delivered, and time. The longer any PS breath lasts, the higher the percentage of peak flow required to end (cycle) the breath. Inspiratory flow during PSV also ends if one of the following conditions occurs:

1. V_T reaches 4.0 L
2. PIP is 2 cm H_2O > PSV pressure setting
3. T_I is longer than 3 seconds

Sigh

The Wave E200 can provide sigh breaths in either volume- or pressure-targeted ventilation. The sigh function is selected by pressing the small green SIGH button next to the mode selector (active, lit; inactive, unlit). A sigh breath is given every 100 breaths when it is selected. For volume-targeted ventilation, the V_T delivered during a sigh breath is 1.5 times the set V_T. For pressure-targeted ventilation, the set peak pressure is achieved, just as with a normal breath. For either volume- or pressure-targeted ventilation, T_I during a sigh breath is 1.5 times the set T_I. The HIGH PRESSURE alarm limit does not change for the sigh breath. The operator may want to take this into account when setting this alarm and the sigh function.

Graphic Display Screens

The Navigator Graphics Monitor can no longer be purchased as a separate unit but was previously available with the Wave E200 or the Breeze E150 ventilators. Some ventilators still have the Navigator Monitor so it will be described here.

In addition to providing real time scalars of volume, flow, and pressure over time and loops for flow-volume and pressure-volume, the monitor can also automatically perform measurements of compliance and resistance. It also monitors respiratory rate, inspiratory and expiratory $\dot{V}_E$, inspiratory and expiratory V_T, peak inspiratory and expiratory flows, inspiratory and expiratory times, leak percent, and dynamic compliance and resistance. Alarm functions are also available for respiratory rate, $\dot{V}_E$, PIP, and apnea.

Box 12-90 Procedure for Suctioning with the E200

1. Press and hold the ALARM SILENCE key for 3 seconds; beep will sound.
2. During the next 10 seconds, the alarm silence light is on, and the ventilator continues to function normally as it waits for a circuit pressure change.
3. When airway pressure drops below the trigger sensitivity pressure during exhalation or when a low-pressure alarm condition occurs during a mandatory breath, the E200 switches into the suction stand-by mode.
4. In this mode, the following occur:
   - The LOW-PRESSURE alarm indicator flashes.
   - The alarm silence lamp remains lit for 60 seconds, after which the audible alarm sounds.
   - Bias flow is delivered through the circuit. When the high-range minute volume alarm is set, flow is 20 L/min. When the low-range minute volume alarm is set, flow is 10 L/min.
   - Pressure-targeted breaths (PC and PS) are disabled.
5. Reconnecting the patient and eliminating major leaks from the circuit cancels the suction standby mode and returns the ventilator to normal operation.

(*Note:* If suction standby is enabled by pushing the ALARM SILENCE button for 3 seconds, but the circuit is not disconnected, nothing happens. After 10 seconds, the alarm silence is canceled.)

Special Features

A few special features are available with the Newport Wave E200 ventilator and are reviewed here.

Suctioning a Patient

The E200 has a special feature that allows the ventilator to be placed into temporary standby for suctioning the patient. Box 12-90 lists the steps involved in this procedure.

Pressure-Relief Valve

On the side panel of the E200 is a pressure-relief valve that limits pressure delivery through the patient circuit during any mode, but does not end inspiration. This safety pop-off is adjustable from 0 to 120 cm H_2O. Turning the knob clockwise increases the pressure limit; turning it counter clockwise lowers it.

During normal operation the operator should set the pop-off pressure about 10 cm H_2O above the high-pressure alarm setting. This control must be set before patient use. To do this, the following procedure is performed:

1. The PRESS. CONTROL knob is set to the "off" position.
2. Flow is set to a normal level for the patient.
3. The high-pressure limit is set at 120 cm H_2O.
4. The patient Y connector is occluded.
5. The manual button is pressed and the operator observes the pressure gauge.
6. The pressure-relief valve is rotated until the pressure plateaus at the desired value.
7. Ventilator controls are returned to the proper settings.

Remote Alarm Silence

The E200 has a REMOTE ALARM SILENCE control, which is a long cable that connects to the back panel. The button on the end of the cable can be used to silence alarms for 60 seconds. This is helpful when suctioning the patient from the side of the bed opposite the ventilator.

Newport Compass Ventilator Monitor

A separate monitor unit, called the Compass, can be attached to the Wave E200 to monitor expired gases. The unit can be mounted directly onto the left side of the ventilator. The analyzer for F_IO_2 can be hooked directly into the patient circuit or into the optional flush valve that mounts on the other side of the Wave E200. The Compass contains a heated, filtered exhalation system with its own exhalation valve. When it is in use, there is no need for the externally mounted valve. Instead, the expiratory valve line on the Wave is attached to a small connector near the bottom of the Compass. The exhalation system provides alarms for high- and low-expired $\dot{V}_E$, high and low F_IO_2, and monitors expired V_T, $\dot{V}_E$, I:E ratio, F_IO_2 (analyzed), and expired peak flow.

Troubleshooting

In addition to the alarms, monitors, and indicators available, the operating manual contains additional tips on troubleshooting. There is also a laminated card containing this information that can be hung on the side of the ventilator. The Wave E200 performs self-zeroing on all sensors and transducers at timed intervals and whenever it is turned on, although it still may be possible for a component to require calibration. Malfunctions of electrical components or transducers can occur when such devices are out of calibration or failing. Keeping a regular maintenance schedule is essential to avoiding such problems. The user should refer to the service manual in such circumstances or contact a service representative.

Because the Wave is microprocessor-controlled, avoid the use of radio frequency-emitting devices, such as cellular phones, pagers, and walkie-talkies, in the vicinity of the ventilator.

Pulmonetic Systems LTV 1000 Ventilator[1-4*]

The LTV 1000 Ventilator is an electrically powered unit that uses an internal rotary compressor to generate gas flow to the patient (Figure 12-80). The lap top ventilator (LTV) currently comes in four models, the LTV 1000, 950, 900, and 800. The 1000 has a built in oxygen blender and can provide PCV. The 950 does not have a built in blender but does provide PCV. The 900 has flow-triggering, volume ventilation, and pressure support, but neither the blender nor PCV. The 800 is strictly a pressure-trigger, volume-controlled ventilator. In general, the 800, 900, and 950 are used in home care and skilled nursing facilities, whereas the 1000 can be used in a variety of settings, including the intensive care unit. This discussion will be restricted to the LTV 1000. The 800, 900, and 950 models will be mentioned when appropriate.

On the left side of the unit are the connecting ports for the ventilator (Figure 12-81). These include a power cord connector (1), a *patient assist* call cable or a remote alarm port (2), a communications port (3), and an oxygen hose connector (4). On the same side are two vents. The ventilator uses room air and oxygen to provide gas flow to the patient. The room air enters the ventilator through a large opening covered by a filter (5). This opening must not be blocked or flow to the patient will be restricted. The second smaller opening allows air to be drawn in to cool the internal components of the unit (6). It also must be kept unblocked.

The oxygen connecting port can be attached to either a high-pressure or a low-pressure oxygen source. An example of a high-pressure source is wall oxygen (40 to 70 psig). For low-pressure oxygen sources, such as an oxygen concentrator, a female DISS oxygen adapter is available that allows connection to regular oxygen tubing. Other low pressure O_2 sources might include an O_2 flowmeter attached to a wall outlet or an O_2 cylinder with a regulator and flowmeter attached. (*Note:* the internal oxygen blender is only available on the LTV 1000.) Oxygen enters the ventilator and blends with room air in the mixing chamber, which is called an Accumulator/Silencer. This chamber both blends the gas and acts as an acoustic silencer to reduce compressor noise.

Power Source

The LTV series ventilators are designed to run on AC or DC (12 volt) power. Although the unit normally uses an AC power cord adapter, more recently released LTV models have a 6-inch pigtail adapter (see Figure 12-81). When connected to an AC power outlet, the internal battery is continuously charged.

For DC power, the LTV can use either its own internal battery or one of two available external DC batteries. The internal battery can last about 60 minutes when fully charged (Box 12-91). The fully charged large external battery can provide up to 8 hours of power, the smaller battery about 3 to 4 hours. It takes up to 8 hours to recharge the large external battery when it is completely depleted. (*Note:* An optional auto lighter adapter is also available for using the LTV ventilator while in a car.)

Patient Circuit

On the right side of the ventilator are the connections for the patient circuit and a small opening for the alarm sound (Figure 12-82, #1). This alarm opening should not be covered or the alarm volume will be reduced. There is a 22 mm connector for the main inspiratory flow line (Figure 12-82, #2), and a small connector for the exhalation valve line (#3) that powers the external exhalation valve.

There are also two flow transducer connectors located on the right side (Figure 12-82, #4). Two small-gauge gas lines are attached to these connectors and to the two connectors located on the patient Y adapter. The transducer located by the patient Y connector is used for flow, volume, and pressure monitoring. A pulse of gas is sent through these lines with each breath during the first minute of ventilation and then once a minute thereafter. This helps keep the lines clear.

In addition to closing the patient circuit during inspiration, the exhalation valve of the LTV also controls the PEEP levels. This is done by pushing the PEEP valve lock with one hand and rotating the valve with the other to increase and decrease PEEP levels (Figure 12-83, *detail* A).

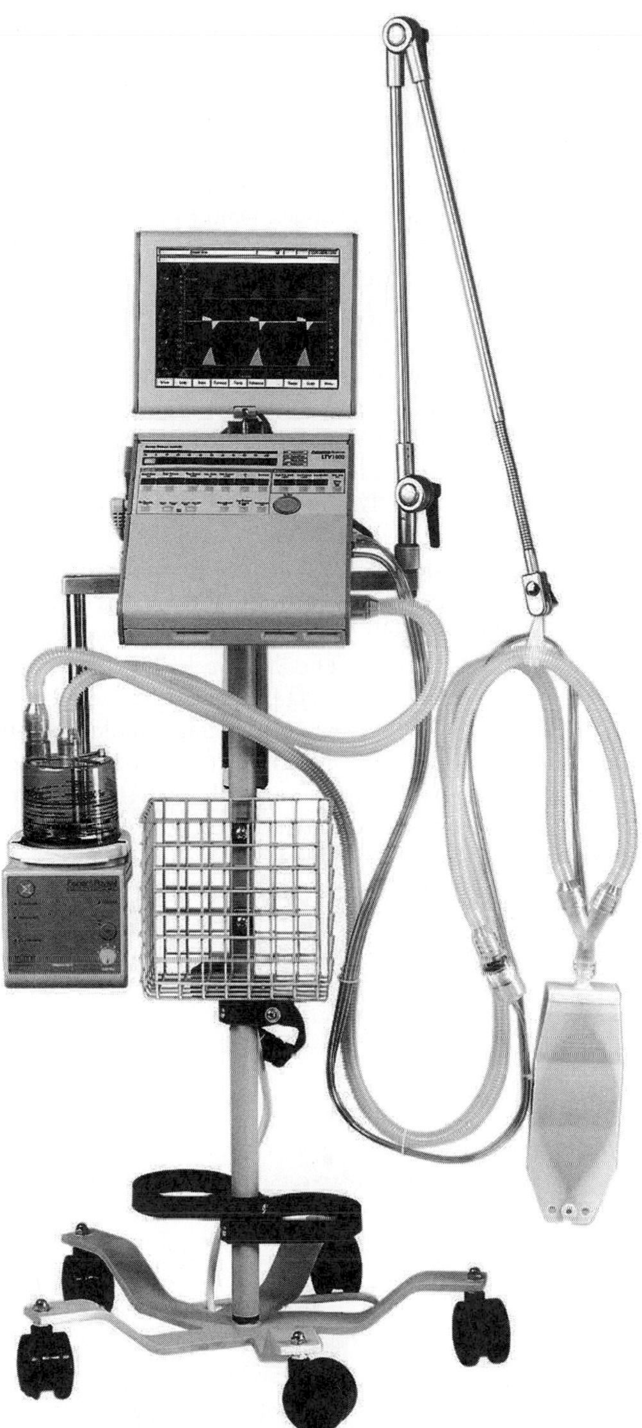

Figure 12-80 The LTV 1000 ventilator with patient circuit, humidifier and monitoring screen. (Courtesy Pulmonetic Systems, Colton, Calif.)

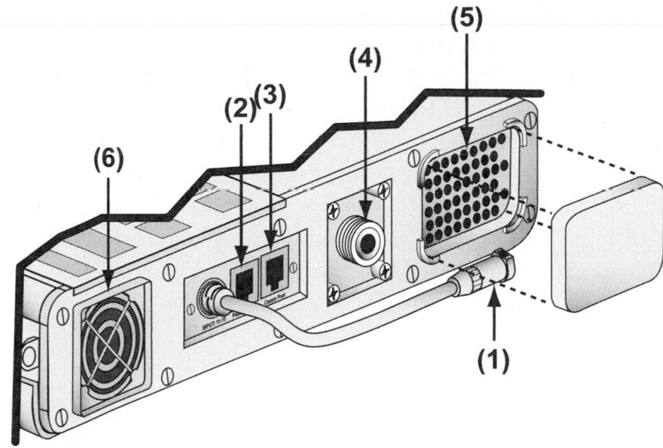

Figure 12-81 The left side of the LTV ventilator panel showing the following: *(1)* power connecting port, *(2)* remote alarm port, *(3)* communication port, *(4)* O_2 hose connector, *(5)* vent and filter for gas intake to compressor, and *(6)* vent and filter for gas going to fan to cool components (see text for more detail). (Courtesy Pulmonetic Systems, Colton, Calif.)

Box 12-91 Internal Battery–AC Power not Connected

When the internal battery is operational, the battery level indicator illuminates. The color code provides information about available charge time remaining.

LED Color	Internal Battery Level	Approximate Battery Time*
Green	Acceptable	60 minutes
Yellow	Low	30 minutes
Red	Critically low	7 minutes

*Approximate value.
Available time depends on currently active ventilator settings. To conserve power, the other screen displays go blank. Only the pressure manometer remains illuminated.

Controls and Alarms

The commonly used controls are located on the front panel of the LTV. As with many of the newer ventilators that use built-in microprocessors, some controls are menu driven and are not located on the panel itself but are pulled up on the display window when needed.

Before using the ventilator on a patient, a number of checks are used to test the system's functions. This procedure is described in the troubleshooting section at the end of this section.

Front Panel Controls

The front panel (Figure 12-84) contains controls, alarm, and monitoring displays. The controls are divided into two rows. The bottom row contains main function buttons or touch pads, and the upper row contains parameter setting buttons.

Above the row of parameter controls is a display window, which has two main functions. It displays current ventilator data and provides access to additional control functions. To the right of the controls, alarm setting keys are located. Just below the alarm keys is a SET VALUE knob.

The ON/STANDBY button turns the ventilator on and illuminates the LED above it (Box 12-92). The ventilator automatically begins to ventilate the patient using the last settings. To place the ventilator into STANDBY, the operator presses and holds the button for 3 seconds. As long as the unit is plugged into an AC outlet and placed in STANDBY, the internal battery will be charged.

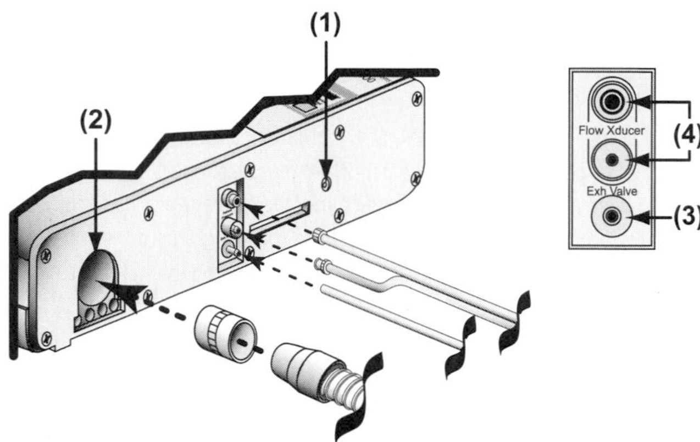

Figure 12-82 The right side of the LTV ventilator panel showing the following: *(1)* alarm sound port, *(2)* main outlet port to patient circuit, *(3)* exhalation valve line connection, and *(4)* connections for transducer lines (see text for more detail). (Courtesy Pulmonetic Systems, Colton, Calif.)

The SELECT (volume/pressure) button allows the operator to choose either volume- or pressure-targeted breaths. Pressing the button toggles between the two choices. The currently active breath type is continuously illuminated. Pressing the button causes the new selection to flash. A change in breath type is confirmed by pressing the button again. If the button is not pressed to confirm, the ventilator simply remains in the current breath type. (*Note:* The LTV 800 and 900 models have only volume-targeted mandatory breaths.)

Between the breath-type button and the mode button is an indicator labeled NPPV for noninvasive positive pressure ventilation. This illuminates when the NPPV mode has been selected from the EXTENDED FEATURES Menu. A noninvasive interface, such as a mask, can be used to connect a patient to the LTV ventilator during any mode of ventilation. However, when NPPV is enabled, some of the alarms are deactivated. (See Modes of Ventilation.)

The mode control SELECT provides the options of assist/control or SIMV/CPAP. To select a mode, the operator presses the SELECT button. The flashing LED is the mode that will become active if the SELECT key is pressed again.

The INSP/EXP HOLD (inspiratory/expiratory hold) button allows the operator to perform either of these two functions. The operator presses the button and reads the display window (monitoring screen), which will show one of the following: INSP HOLD, EXP HOLD. Pressing the INSP/EXP HOLD button scrolls through the choices on the screen.

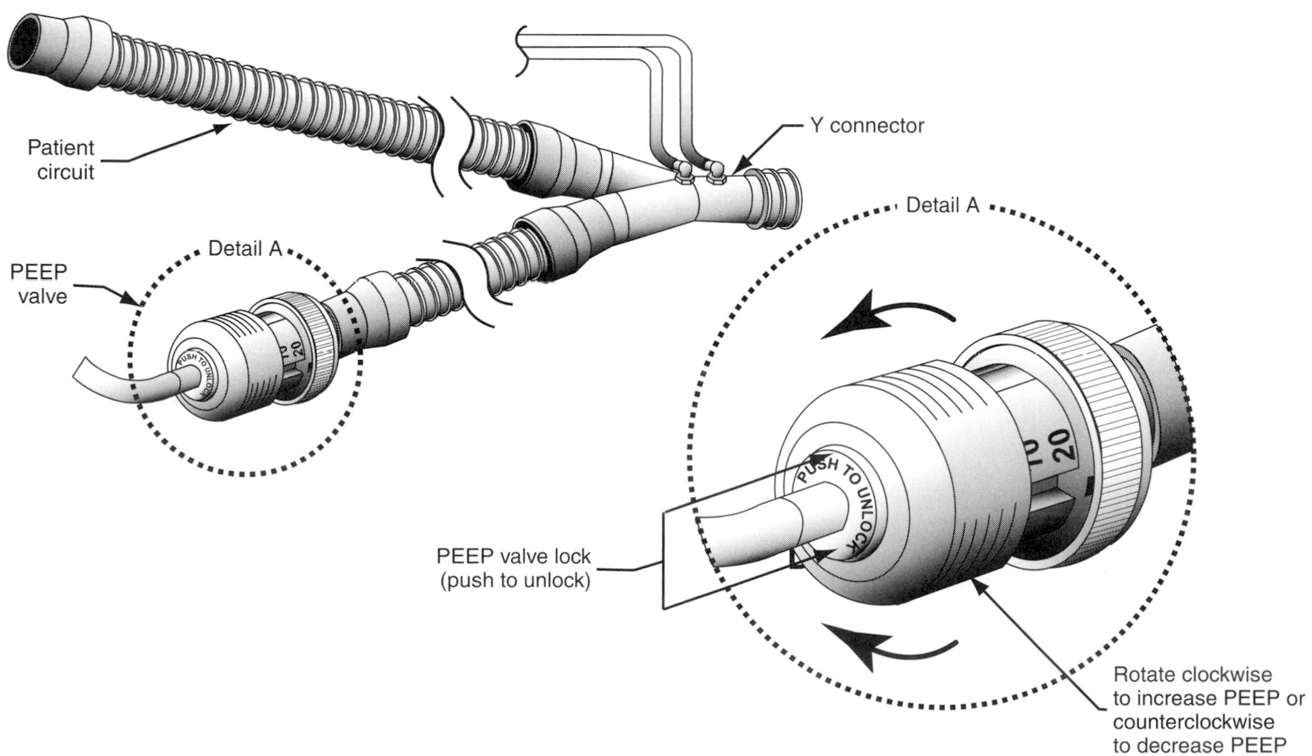

Figure 12-83 Patient circuit for the LTV ventilator with enlarged detail (*A*) showing exhalation valve with PEEP mechanism. (Courtesy Pulmonetic Systems, Colton, Calif.)

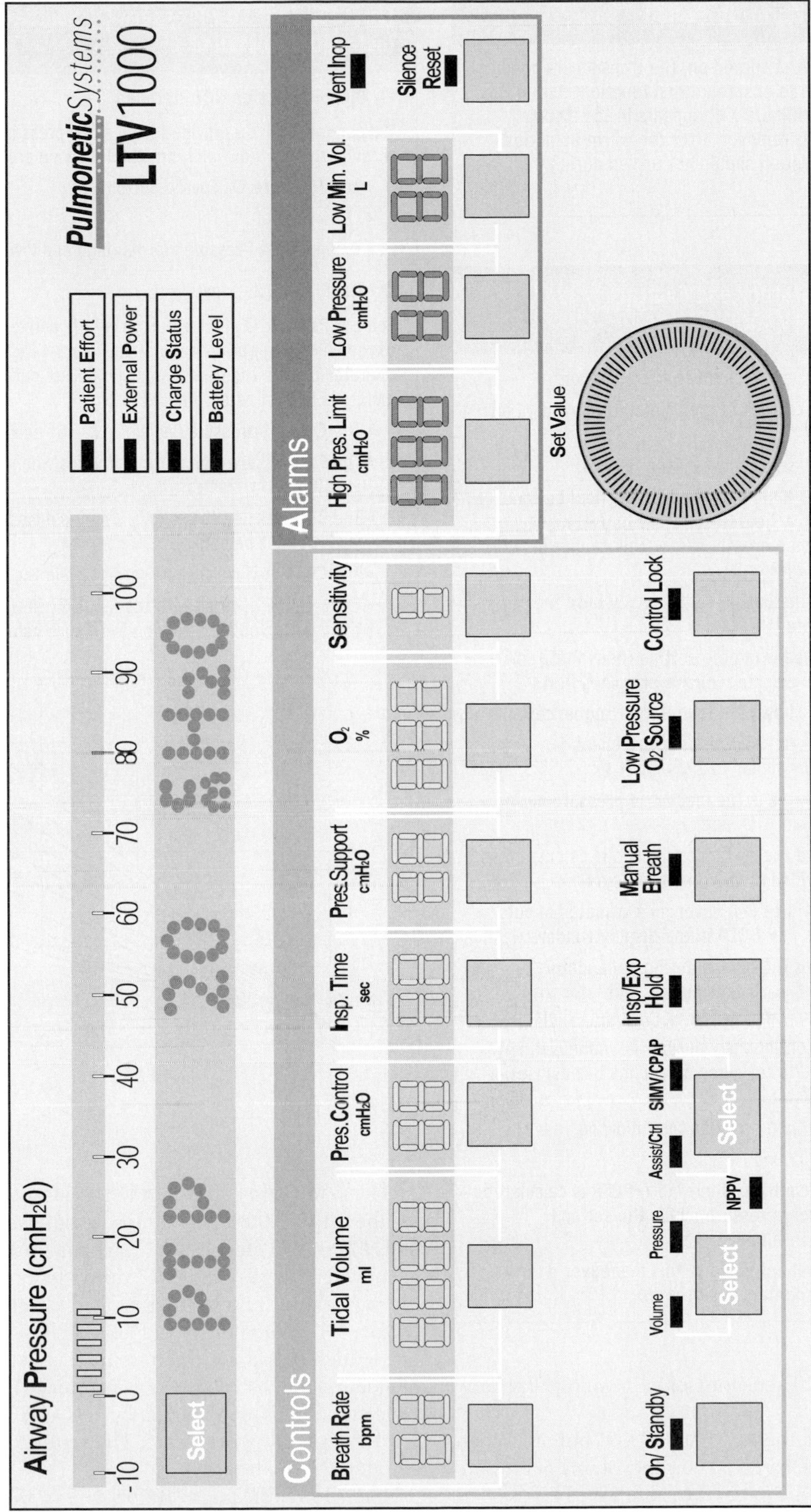

Figure 12-84 The front panel with controls, displays, alarms and indicators for the LTV 1000 (see text for detail). (Courtesy Pulmonetic Systems, Colton, Calif.)

Box 12-92 The Warm-Up Period

When the ventilator is first turned on, the transducers need 60 seconds to warm-up to ensure normal function. During this period the message "WARMUP XX" appears in the display window. This message is removed after the warm-up period. The leak test and calibration should not be run during this period.

Box 12-93 Inspiratory and Expiratory Hold Procedures in the LTV 1000

To complete an INFLATION HOLD maneuver, the operator:

1. Scrolls through the choices in the display window until insp hold appears.
2. The LED above the INSP/EXP HOLD button flashes.
3. The operator pushes and holds the INSP/EXP HOLD button to perform an inspiratory hold (inspiratory pause) maneuver during the next volume breath. (*Note:* This cannot be done during pressure ventilation.)
4. The operator holds the button continuously until the maneuver is completed.
5. The button is released when the setting reads **P Plat** or when 6 seconds has elapses, whichever comes first.
6. The display window shows the following in sequence:
    - **Δ Pres** xx, where xx is the pressure change or plateau pressure minus PEEP in cm H_2O,
    - **P Plat** xx where xx is the measured pressure during the plateau in cm H_2O, and
    - **C Static,** where the static compliance is calculated as set volume divided by Δ Pres, in mL/cm H_2O.

To perform an EXPIRATORY HOLD maneuver for estimates of auto-PEEP, the operator sets EXP HOLD in the display window.

1. The operator presses the button during a mandatory volume or pressure breath causing the ventilator to perform an expiratory hold at the end of that exhalation.
2. The button is held continuously during the maneuver, until the display reads **P Plat** or when 6 seconds has elapses, whichever comes first.
3. The display window then provides the following values:
    - **P Exp** in cm H_2O and
    - **Auto-PEEP** in cm H_2O, where Auto-PEEP is calculated as end expiratory pressure minus the set and monitored PEEP value.

(*Note:* The ventilator will not perform this maneuver during a pressure support or a spontaneous breath.)

Box 12-93 describes the procedure for performing inspiratory and expiratory hold.

The next control is the MANUAL BREATH button. When pressed a manual breath based on current volume or pressure settings is delivered to the patient. In addition, a bolus of air purges the flow sensor line.

Box 12-94 Low Pressure O_2 Source–Not Installed or Installed

O_2 Blending Option NOT installed

Oxygen may still be provided from a low pressure O_2 source through the low flow inlet, but the following are inactive:

- Low Pressure O_2 Source button
- O_2% control
- Oxygen Inlet Pressure alarms (high and low)

O_2 Blending Option Installed

The LOW PRESSURE O_2 SOURCE button is only active when the oxygen blending option is installed. To activate this option, the operator pushes the LOW PRESSURE O_2 SOURCE button until it is on and its LED illuminated. While it is on:

- The O_2 inlet pressure low alarm is NOT active
- The O_2 pressure high alarm activates when the O_2 source is >10 psig
- The %O_2 display shows only dimmed dash lines and the %O_2 cannot be set.
- The O_2 inlet flow must be set to obtain the desired O_2%
- O_2% delivery varies with the input O_2 flow (L/min) and the minute volume based on the figure below.

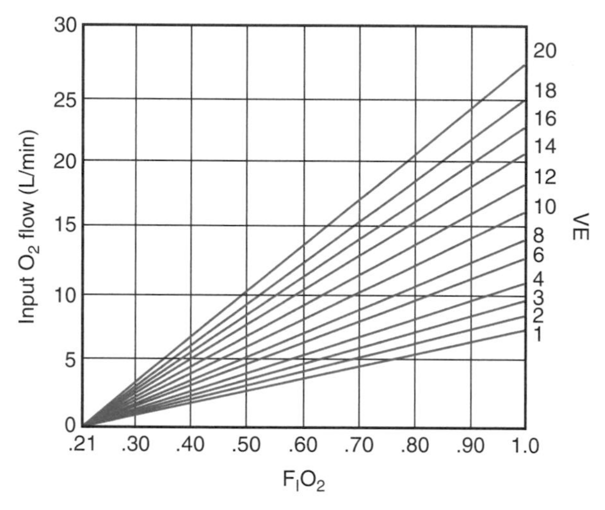

The LOW PRESSURE O_2 SOURCE is a feature only available for the LTV 1000. (This button is not available with the 800, 900, or 950 models.) Certain changes in alarm features occur when oxygen is supplied from a low pressure/low flow O_2 source and the LOW PRESSURE O_2 feature is activated (Box 12-94). When the LOW PRESSURE/O_2 SOURCE is NOT on, a high-pressure oxygen source is expected and gas blending is done within the ventilator. The delivered O_2 concentration is determined by the O_2% setting on the ventilator's front panel. (*Note:* The ventilator does not have a built-in O_2 analyzer.)

The CONTROL LOCK button allows the screen to be locked so that the settings cannot be accidentally changed.

Pushing once turns the lock on. The LED above the control lock illuminates (panel locked). If the operator tries to change a setting when the panel is locked, the display window reads LOCKED and the LED flashes. Pressing the CONTROL LOCK button again unlocks the screen.

The *hard* method of locking should be used when children or others may have access to the ventilator such as in the patient's home. The operator selects CTRL UNLOCK from the Extended Features menu (reviewed later in this section). If *hard* lock has been selected in this menu, the operator must press the CONTROL LOCK button for 3 seconds to unlock the control panel.

The upper row of controls contains the parameter settings such as rate and tidal volume. The procedure for changing the variables in this row, and in the alarms, is basically the same. The parameter button is touched to make a change. This action brightly illuminates the set value for the parameter and dulls the displays for all other parameters. The SET VALUE knob is rotated until the value desired appears in the display above the parameter button. The change is immediately active, if the SET VALUE knob is pressed again or after 5 seconds.

The number in the window above each parameter represents the value set for that parameter. Numbers appear bright when the parameter is active in the current mode and breath type. They appear dim when they are not. A parameter's digital display will also brighten if it is selected for changing. All others then dim. Three parameters—sensitivity, pressure support, and respiratory rate—can be turned off. The respective display for any of those three parameters will be blank ("- -") when it is turned off.

When the LTV is being powered by the internal battery, after 60 seconds all the digital displays turn off, if no button has been pushed or control changed. The displays can be re-illuminated by pushing any button or turning the SET VALUE knob. Flashing displays will also occur (Box 12-95).

Box 12-95 Conditions When Displays Will Flash

1. When the limit has been reached for a value as the operator is adjusting that value, the display will flash. For example, when setting tidal volume, if the V_T is set too high for the available peak flow based on the set T_I, the V_T display will flash.
2. A flashing display results when alarm conditions are occurring or an alarm has just occurred.
3. If a control display flashes, a special condition has occurred. For example, pressure support (PS) breaths are normally flow-cycled. If a time-cycled PS breath occurs, the pressure support indicator will flash.
4. The message "Locked" will flash in the display window if someone has tried to change the controls when the panel is locked. It will flash for 3 seconds.

The BREATH RATE control sets the minimum mandatory breath rate (breaths/min). It can be turned off ("- -"). The rate range is 1 to 80 breaths/min. The TIDAL VOLUME button controls volume delivery during volume-targeted ventilation (Range 50 to 2000 mL). INSPIRATORY TIME (T_I) sets the length of inspiration for volume- and pressure-targeted breaths (range 0.3 to 9.9 sec). Inspiration cannot be shorter than 300 milliseconds. When V_T or T_I is being adjusted, the calculated flow ($\dot{V}$calc) is shown in the display window. The peak flow is based on the setting of T_I and V_T (Box 12-96).

PCV is a feature available in the LTV 1000 and 950 models. The PRESS. CONTROL button establishes the inspiratory pressure for pressure-targeted breaths. The operator pushes the PRESS. CONTROL button and uses the SET VALUE knob to change to the desired inspiratory pressure (range 1 to 99 cm H_2O). This pressure is *not* added to the baseline PEEP. PEEP/CPAP is set mechanically using the expiratory/PEEP valve.

PRESS. SUPPORT establishes the target pressure above *zero* baseline for pressure-supported spontaneous breaths [Range: off ("- -"), or 1 to 60 cm H_2O.) PS is available for spontaneous breaths with SIMV in either pressure- or volume-targeted ventilation and for CPAP breaths (see Modes of Ventilation.)

The O_2 % button establishes the percent O_2 delivery when it is on and a high pressure oxygen source is available. (*Note:* The LOW PRESSURE O_2 button must be in the off position.)

The SENSITIVITY button is used to set the flow-trigger sensitivity level for assisted or spontaneous breaths. The range is off ("- -") and 1 to 9 L/min. The most sensitive setting is 1 L/min. The base flow is preset at 10 L/min and requires no setting by the operator. When a trigger is detected, the Patient Effort LED illuminates.

There are only a few clinical circumstances where turning off the sensitivity might be appropriate. One example might be in a patient has a large air leak through a bronchopleural fistula (BPF). For example, if the leak resulting from the BPF is more than 15 L/min, even with the sensitivity at 9 L/min (least sensitivity) and leak compensation available (newer models compensate a 6 L/min leak), air may still leak from the system. Large air leaks can prolong inspiration

Box 12-96 Flow Pattern and Peak Flow in the LTV

The flow pattern is automatically set as a descending ramp for all volume-targeted breaths. The peak flow at the beginning of inspiration is calculated by the ventilator such that the tidal volume can be delivered during the set T_I and inspiration ends when flow drops to 50% of the peak or 10 L/min, whichever is highest. The range of available flow is 10 to 100 L/min for a mandatory breath.

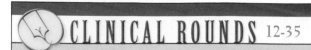

Problem 1

During A/C volume-targeted ventilation with a set rate of 8 breaths/min, the operator notices that the actual rate is 8 breaths/min, but the airway pressure bar graph shows frequent dips in pressure between –5 and –10 cm H_2O. The Patient Effort indicator is not illuminated. The patient shows significant use of the sternocleidomastoid muscle and supraclavicular retractions. What should the respiratory therapist do?

Problem 2

The RT XDCR DATA menu shows a LEAK measurement of 1.32 L/min. What would an appropriate sensitivity setting be in this patient?

See Appendix A for the answer.

Box 12-97 Low Pressure Alarm Settings: All Breaths versus Mandatory Breaths

Assume the ventilator is set with the inspiratory pressure at 25 cm H_2O in SIMV pressure-targeted ventilation with a pressure support of 15 cm H_2O.

If ALL breaths are monitored for low pressure, the operator would set the low pressure alarm to a value lower than the PS level. In this case it might be about 10 cm H_2O. If the circuit pressure does not rise to 10 cm H_2O for any breath, the alarm will sound.

If only mandatory breaths were monitored, the operator might set the low pressure alarm at about 20 cm H_2O. The alarm would only occur if a mandatory breath's pressure dropped below 20 cm H_2O. The alarm would not be active for spontaneous breaths.

and also result in accidental early triggering of a breath during exhalation (auto-triggering). The leak is falsely seen as a patient effort. In this case it may be appropriate to set a mandatory breath rate and turn the sensitivity off.

In addition to flow-triggering, there is a back-up pressure sensing trigger that will pressure-trigger a breath in the following circumstances:

- When sensitivity is set between 1 and 9 L/min,
- The ventilator is in exhalation,
- A minimum expiratory time has elapsed (300 milliseconds), and
- The airway pressure drops below –3 cm H_2O.

The *leak compensation* feature in newer models is constantly measuring for leaks and adjusting the baseline of the ventilator in order to compensate for leaks (up to 6 L/min). For example, if the operator sets the sensitivity to 2 L, the ventilator would normally trigger a breath when a 2 L change in baseline (bias flow) was detected during expiration. Suppose a 4 L/min leak exists with a 2 L/min sensitivity setting. The ventilator identifies the 4 L/min leak and adjusts the baseline flow so that the required patient effort is still only 2 L/min to trigger a breath and auto-triggering is avoided.

In earlier models of the LTV, which do not have leak compensation, the sensitivity is usually set higher than the leak measurement. The operator can check the current leak measurement by going into the RT XDCR DATA menu and selecting the LEAK measurement displayed. For example, if the LEAK is measured at 2.38 L/min, an appropriate sensitivity setting would be 3 L/min. The difference would represent the trigger (3 – 2.38 = 0.62). An effort of 0.62 L/min would have to be inhaled by the patient from the bias flow to trigger the next breath (Clinical Rounds 12-35).

Alarms

The alarm controls and settings are to the right of the parameter controls. The first alarm is the HIGH PRESS. LIMIT (cm H_2O). This control establishes the maximum pressure allowed in the patient circuit. If the set value is reached, an audible alarm sounds, the display window reads "HIGH PRES," inspiration ends, and the exhalation valve opens. If a high-pressure condition continues for more than 3 seconds, the internal turbine stops rotating and circuit pressure empties to the atmosphere. The audible alarm automatically stops when the pressure drops to the high-pressure limit minus 5 cm H_2O, or drops to a circuit pressure of 25 cm H_2O, whichever is less. To set the HIGH PRESS. LIMIT, the button is pressed and the SET VALUE knob rotated to the desired value (range 5 to 100 cm H_2O).

To set the LOW PRESSURE alarm value (cm H_2O), the operator pushes the LOW PRESSURE button, and rotates the SET VALUE knob. The actual value appears in the display window. The knob is rotated until the desired value is seen (range 1 to 60 cm H_2O). The LOW PRESSURE alarm has two possible functions. The LTV can apply the low pressure alarm to all breaths, both spontaneous and mandatory (ALL BREATHS selection) or to mandatory breaths only (VC/PC ONLY selection). The mandatory breaths can be pressure- or volume-targeted.

The operator accesses the extended menu functions (discussed later in this section) to set the low pressure alarm for either all breaths or for mandatory breaths only (Box 12-97). When the LPPS (low peak pressure *spontaneous*) alarm is turned off, the message "LPPS OFF" appears in the display window. Spontaneous breaths have no low pressure alarm. This is an informational message only. (*Note:* The operator can remove the LPPS Off message from the screen by activating the scroll feature of the display window [Box 12-98].)

Box 12-98 The Scroll Feature

Double clicking (pressing twice) on the SELECT button adjacent to the display window results in a scrolling of ventilator parameters in the window. For example, peak airway pressure, PEEP, respiratory rate, and other ventilator parameters appear consecutively in the window. Each parameter remains in the window with the current measured value for 2 seconds and then the next parameter appears.

When scrolling is active, the "LPPS off" message appears for 2 seconds as well, notifying the operator that LPPS (low peak pressure spontaneous) is off.

If the operator wants to stop the scrolling to freeze a particular parameter in the window, he or she would press the SELECT button once when the desired parameter is in the window. This allows continuous monitoring of a specific parameter such as respiratory rate. To reactivate scrolling, simply press the SELECT button twice.

When scrolling is active and the low minute volume alarm is off, the "LMV Alarm off" message appears in the message window in the sequence of ventilator parameters.

The LOW MIN. VOL. alarm sets the minimum expected exhaled $\dot{V}_E$ [Range: Off ("- -") or 0.1 L to 99 L]. If $\dot{V}_E$ drops below the set value, an audible alarm sounds and the message "LOW MIN VOL" appears in the message window. If the low $\dot{V}_E$ alarm is turned to the off ("- -") position, a message will appear saying LMV-off alarm off in the display window after 60 seconds. It is an informational message only. The operator can resume scrolling of parameters by pressing the SELECT button twice (see Box 12-98). (*Note:* The LMV alarm is not active in NPPV.)

The message LMV LPPS OFF appears in the window, if both the low $\dot{V}_E$ and low peak pressure for spontaneous breath alarms are off (Clinical Rounds 12-36). The message appears in the window following the disabling of the alarm(s) as a safety feature and at all times, unless scrolling is active. If scrolling is active, the message becomes one of the scrolled parameters.

The VENT INOP indicator just right of the alarm controls is illuminated only when the ventilator is in the inoperative state. This occurs under the following conditions:

1. The ventilator has been put into Standby (ON/STANDBY button held 3 seconds)
2. The power sources, either internal or external, are insufficient to operate the ventilator,
3. The ventilator has been turned off,
4. A condition exists which renders the ventilator unable to provide patient ventilation and is unsafe.

When an ventilator inoperative alarm occurs, the inspiratory flow stops, the exhalation valve opens allowing the patient to breath spontaneously from room air, the oxygen blender solenoids close, the INOP LED is RED and an audible alarm sounds continuously. Another mode of ventilating must be provided for the patient immediately.

CLINICAL ROUNDS 12-36

A Respiratory Therapist turns the LTV 1000 on to begin ventilating a new patient. The patient is to receive CPAP at 10 cm H_2O and 90% O_2. The therapist notices a message in the display window: "LMV LPPS OFF." What does the message mean and what should the therapist do?

See Appendix A for the answer.

The SILENCE/RESET button is used to silence an alarm for 60 seconds. This button can also be used to start a 60 second alarm silence period, for example, before disconnecting the patient for some procedure or when the ventilator is placed in STANDBY. After an alarm condition has been resolved, this button can also be used to clear the visual alarm displays. The SILENCE/RESET button also silences the VENT INOP audible alarm, but the VENT INOP LED will remain lit for at least 5 minutes.

In addition to the alarms described, additional alarms conditions may occur and present an alarm message in the display window. These alarms and a description of their condition are presented in Table 12-31.

The SET VALUE Knob

This knob allows adjustment of the numerical values of the ventilator parameters and alarms and it scrolls through menu items that appear in the display window.

Airway Pressure Bar Graph and Display Window

At the very top of the operating panel is the AIRWAY PRESSURE display. This horizontal bar graph displays the pressure in the patient circuit (Range: minus (−) 10 to (+) 108 cm H_2O).

The display window displays monitored data, alarm messages and the Extended Features Menu. During normal operation, the monitored data are presented sequentially. Table 12-32 shows the sequence of monitored data and how the values are calculated. Each item is displayed for 3 seconds.

The SELECT Button–Display Screen

The SELECT button to the left of the display screen has several functions. It is used to stop the normal scrolling of monitored ventilator parameters. Pushing the button once while the normal data scan is active halts the screen with the current parameter data showing. Each time the button is pushed after that, the next data item in the list is displayed. Scanning can be resumed by pressing the button twice within 0.3 seconds.

The Extended Features menu is selected by pushing the SELECT button for 3 seconds. The first menu item is displayed in the window (see Extended Features section).

Table 12-31 Additional Alarms on the LTV Ventilator Series*

Message	Description
BAT EMPTY	Occurs when operating on internal battery power and the charge level falls below empty threshold. The message cannot be cleared.
BAT LOW	When operating on internal battery power and the charge level falls below the low threshold, this alarm occurs.
DEFAULT	"Default" message flashes in display window. During POST, if the ventilator detects an invalid stored setting, the DEFAULTS alarm occurs and the affected settings are set to the present default values. (See operator's manual for more detail on default settings.)
DISC/SENSE	"Disc/Sense" message flashes in the display window. The breath is terminated. This occurs when the ventilator detects a sense line that is pinched or blocked or disconnected.
HIGH O_2 PRES	"High O_2 Pres" message is flashed in the display window. The O_2% control display is flashed. Occurs when inlet pressure is >75 psig (assumes Low Pressure O_2 source is off). Not available in NPPV modes.
HW FAULT	"HW Fault" flashes in display window. This occurs when the ventilator detects a hardware problem such as the cooling fan is not operating. (See operator's manual for a list of hardware problems.)
LOW O_2 PRES	"Low O_2 Pres" flashes in the display window. This occurs when the oxygen inlet pressure is less than 35 psig (assumes Low Pressure O_2 source is off). Not available in NPPV modes.
NO CAL DATA	"No Cal Data" flashes in the display window. Ventilator continues to operate. The following values are displayed as NO CAL: Vte, PIP, MAP, PEEP, and VE. This occurs when the ventilator detects invalid or missing calibration records on power up. Default calibration values are used. Push "Silence/Reset" twice. This clears the alarm and allows continued ventilator operation. However, the NO CAL message remains. Take the unit out of service and perform calibration procedures. (See operator's manual for more details on procedures.)
POWER LOST	"Power Lost" message flashes in display window. The external power and the charge status LEDs are off. The Battery Level LED is lit showing battery charge level. Ventilator begins operating from the internal battery. After 60 seconds, the displays are turned off to conserve battery power.
POWER LOW	"Power Low" message flashes in display window. External power LED displays yellow. This occurs when the ventilator is operating on external power and the voltage drops to the low level.
RESET	"Reset" message flashes in the display window. This occurs when the ventilator detects a condition that makes safe ventilator operation uncertain. It reinitializes itself to allow POST to be performed. If the POST does not detect any further problem, the ventilator resumes operation and a "RESET" message is posted. If the POST detects a problem that is considered unsafe, a ventilator "INOP" message and alarm occurs. In this case, remove the ventilator from service. An error code is written to the Event Trace indicating the type of problem detected. Check the Event Trace for information (see operator's manual for error codes).
XDCR FAULT	"XDCR Fault" appears in the display window. This occurs when a transducer autozero test fails. The autozero for the transducer is scheduled at periodic intervals during ventilator operation. If an autozero test fails, it will automatically run again on the next breath. The alarm/message remains active until a valid autozero is performed. If the problem persists, remove the unit from use and contact a service technician.

*All these alarm conditions have an audible alarm and message. The audible alarm can be silence by pressing the "Silence/Reset" button either once or twice. Problems that involve patient safety can be temporarily silenced, but the alarm message stays in the window. The problem must be corrected and the alarm reset.

Front Panel Indicators

To the right of the pressure manometer are four indicators. The PATIENT EFFORT indicator illuminates when the ventilator detects a patient's inspiratory effort based on the sensitivity setting. The EXTERNAL POWER illuminates when the unit is operating from an external power source. This can be an AC power source or an external battery. The adjacent LED is green when power is adequate and yellow when external power is low. Table 12-33 and Box 12-91 provide information on the battery charging status and related indicator color.

Extended Features

Table 12-34 illustrates the options available under the Extended Features Menus. Box 12-99 describes how to navigate the Extended Features menu. Besides the alarms available on the operating panel, the Extended Features

Table 12-32 Monitored Data

Parameter	Description
PIP	Peak inspiratory pressure (cm H_2O). Greatest pressure measured during inspiration and the first 300 msec of exhalation.
MAP	Mean airway pressure (cm H_2O). Calculation of mean airway pressure for the last 60 seconds, displayed in 10 second intervals.
PEEP	Positive end-expiratory pressure (cm H_2O). The measured pressure at the end of exhalation.
f	Total respiratory rate per minute based on the last 8 breaths. Updated every 20 seconds. Includes all breath types.
Vte	Measured exhaled tidal volume. Measured and displayed at the end of each exhalation.
VE	Minute volume monitor displays the exhaled tidal volume for the last 60 seconds as calculated from the last 8 breaths. Recalculated and displayed every 20 seconds or the completion of every exhalation, whichever occurs first.
I:E	Displays the calculated ratio inspiration to expiration with the smaller of the two reduced to a value of 1. Displays regular and inverse ratios.
$\dot{V}$calc	The calculated peak flow, which occurs at the beginning of the breath for a volume-targeted breath (not included with pressure ventilation). The calculation is based on set V_T, T_I and a predetermined minimum flow at the end of inspiration. Flow normally drops in a descending ramp fashion to 50% of the calculated peak or 10 L/min, whichever is greater.

Table 12-33 Battery Charge Status and LED Color Indicators (Charge Status LED)

LED Color	Charge Status
Flashing yellow	The ventilator is performing precharge qualification testing of the internal battery before beginning the charging procedure. Occurs when the external power is first applied to the unit. Takes from a few seconds to an hour on a very depleted battery.
Green	Internal battery fully charged.
Yellow	Internal battery is being charged but has not reached a full charge level.
Red	The internal battery cannot be charged. The ventilator has detected a charge fault or internal battery fault. Remove from service and contact a certified service technician.

menu accesses additional alarm controls. These are described in Table 12-34 along with the controls and options available in the ventilator operations section of the Extended Features Menu.

Several other functions are available through this menu. Users are advised to follow the ventilator maintenance procedures outlined in the operator's manual provided by the manufacturer for viewing the following: transducer Autozero, real-time transducer data, event trace, and ventilator maintenance.

Breath Types and Modes of Ventilation

As with other ventilators, the LTV ventilator series distinguishes breath-type and mode. For example, breaths can be volume or pressure targeted. Each of these breath types is available in the assist/control mode or SIMV mode.

Breath Types

As described in Chapter 11, the terms trigger, limit, and cycle are used to describe breaths. The trigger variable begins inspiration. The limit describes what variable controls delivery of inspiration and the maximum value for that variable, either pressure or volume in this case. The variable that ends inspiration is called the cycle variable.

There are four breath-types in the LTV ventilator: volume control, pressure control, pressure support, and spontaneous. To select volume or pressure breaths, the operator toggles the SELECT – VOLUME (or) PRESSURE button to establish breath type (bottom row of controls).

Volume controlled breaths are either patient- (flow or pressure), time-, or manually triggered. The limiting value

Table 12-34 Extended Features Menu Items—Alarm and Ventilator Operations

Message	Description
ALARM OPERATIONS	
ALARM VOL	Sets the loudness of the alarm volume
APNEA INT	Sets the apnea interval in seconds—the maximum time allowed between the beginning of one breath and the beginning of the next (range 10-60 sec)
HP DELAY	High-pressure delay selects for either immediate or delayed audible notification of a high-pressure alarm. NO DELAY or DELAY 1 BRTH or DELAY 2 BRTH
LPP ALARM	The low peak pressure alarm in this menu is used to select the type of breaths to which the LPP alarm applies. When ALL BREATHS is selected, the low peak pressure alarm setting applies to all mandatory (pressure or volume) and spontaneous breaths. When VC/PC ONLY is applied, only mandatory breaths (pressure or volume) have the low peak pressure alarm active. Spontaneous breaths would have no LPP alarm in this setting. (*Note:* the actual pressure value for the low peak pressure alarm in cm H_2O is set with the low-pressure alarm on the operating panel.)
EXIT	Press the select button while EXIT is displayed to return to the top of the Alarm op menu.
VENTILATOR OPERATIONS	
RISE TIME	As with the ramping or sloping feature on other ventilators, this Variable Rise Time option adjusts the rate of pressure and flow delivery at the beginning of a pressure-targeted breath (Pressure Control, Pressure Support). Range is 1 through 9, with 1 being the fastest rate of rise.
FLOW TERM	Flow termination is the percent flow of the measured peak inspiratory flow at which the ventilator will cycle a pressure support breath. Range is 10% to 40%, with 25% being the default flow-cycling percentage. When PC FLOW TERM is enabled, this flow-cycling function also applies to pressure control breaths (PC breaths are then flow- or time-cycled).
TIME TERM	The variable time termination feature selects the maximum time for cycling the inspiratory phase of pressure support breaths (0.3 to 3.0 seconds). PS breaths are time-cycled if the set time termination is reached before the flow-cycling termination point has been reached. Thus, PS breaths can be flow- or time-cycled.
PC FLOW TERM	Enabling this feature allows PC breaths to be flow-cycled, if the flow termination point set under (FLOW TERM) occurs before the set T_I elapses.
LEAK COMP	This feature tracks the baseline flow. In the presence of a stable leak and when no auto-cycling is present, the system adjusts to maintain set sensitivity even when a small leak is present. The maximum leak value that can be compensated is 6 L/min.
NPPV MODE	This selection enables or disables the non-invasive positive pressure mode setting.
CTRL UNLOCK	Use the Control Unlock option to select the *Easy* or *Hard* unlocking option. When *Hard* is selected, unlocking requires the operator to push and hold the LOCK button for 3 seconds. Normal *Easy* lock just requires pushing the button once.
LANGUAGE	Selects the language for use in the display window. Includes: English, Dansk, Deutsch, Espanol, Francais, Italiano, Portugues, and Svenska.
VERxxxxxxxx	Displays the software version installed in the ventilator.
USAGE xxxxx	Displays the number of hours of use of the ventilator.
COM SETTING	This option allows modification of the communication setting. Options: data, monitor, printer, and modem.
SET DATE	View or set the current date with this option.
SET TIME	Sets the time.
DATE FORMAT	Formats the date.
PIP LED	Use this option to turn the PIP LED on or off. When enabled, the airway pressure display LED representing PIP of the previous breath remains lit during exhalation.
LTVxxxxxxxx	Model number of the LTV ventilator
Vhomexxx	Allows viewing of the LTV flow valve's home position. This is set during manufacturing or when the flow valve is displaced.
EXIT	Push the SELECT button when EXIT is displayed to return to the top of the VENT OP menu.

Box 12-99 Navigating the Extended Features Menu

- To access this menu, push and hold the SELECT button for 3 seconds. Be sure the screen is unlocked.
- To view the next item on the menu, turn the SET VALUE knob clockwise. Turning it counterclockwise allows viewing of the previous item.
- To enter a menu item or select a setting, push the SELECT button.
- To exit the menu, turn the SET VALUE knob until EXIT appears in the window, then push SELECT.
- To toggle an option on or off, push the SELECT button.

is the set tidal volume. Flow is delivered in a descending ramp waveform. The cycling method is time (T_I). The operator can also set breath rate, $O_2\%$, and sensitivity.

Pressure controlled breaths are also patient-, time-, or manually triggered. (*Note*: the LTV 900 and 800 do not have pressure control.) The target inspiratory pressure is set with the PRESS. CONTROL button (cm H_2O). The target pressure is the maximum pressure delivered by the ventilator during inspiration and is NOT additive to PEEP. PEEP is set by the mechanical PEEP valve located on the expiratory valve. For example if the pressure control is set to 25 cm H_2O and the PEEP is at 5 cm H_2O, the normal pressure reached during inspiration will be 25 cm H_2O. Baseline pressure will be 5 cm H_2O. The usual cycle mechanism for a pressure control breath is time. Breath rate, T_I, $O_2\%$, and sensitivity are also set.

If desired, the operator can select flow-cycling for PC breaths rather than time-cycling by activating the flow termination percent feature using the Extended Features menu. Flow-cycling percent can be adjusted from 10% to 40% of peak flow. The default setting is 25%. For example, if the peak flow during inspiration is 50 L/min and the flow-cycling setting is 25%, inspiratory flow ends when the flow drops to 12.5 L/min (25% of 50 L/min). A pressure controlled breath will time-cycle unless the flow termination setting occurs before the set inspiratory time elapses. If a long T_I is set, such as 1.5 seconds, it is more likely that the flow will drop to the set flow termination point before 1.5 seconds has elapsed.

A Rise Time profile can also be set with pressure control to taper pressure and flow delivery at the beginning of inspiration. This is also selected using the Extended Features menu. The default setting for Rise Time is Profile 4. (*Note*: The fastest rise time setting is #1 and the slowest is #9.)

Pressure support breaths are patient-triggered, pressure-limited and flow-cycled. As with pressure control breaths, pressure support assumes a zero baseline, so the set value is not added to the PEEP pressure as in most other ventilators. Flow-cycling can be adjusted using the flow termination

CLINICAL ROUNDS 12-37

During PSV with an SIMV rate of 6 breaths/min, the peak flow measured by the ventilator is 25 L/min. The flow-termination is set at 10%. At what flow will inspiratory flow end?

See Appendix A for the answer.

CLINICAL ROUNDS 12-38

A physician wants his patient weaned from mandatory breaths and orders a pressure support of 12 cm H_2O plus a PEEP of 3 cm H_2O for a total inspiratory pressure of 15 cm H_2O. How would the therapist adjust these values on the LTV?

See Appendix A for the answer.

feature described above. A default of 3 L/min is preset so that inspiratory flow cannot drop lower than 3 L/min (see Clinical Rounds 12-37).

Pressure support breaths are time-cycled if T_I exceeds the Time Termination Limit (range 0.3–3 sec), which is set through the Extended Features menu. PS breaths will also time-cycle if T_I exceeds the length of two breath periods. The PRESS. SUPPORT display will flash briefly when a breath is time cycled. As with pressure control, the Rise Time profile may be selected from the Extended Features menu for PSV.

Spontaneous breaths are designed to meet patient demand and maintain the circuit pressure at the measured PEEP value from the previous breath. The breath is cycled when the flow drops below 10% of the maximum flow measured during inspiration or 2 L/min, whichever occurs first. Spontaneous breaths will also time-cycle if the breath time exceeds 2 breath periods.

Modes of Ventilation

The LTV series ventilator provides the following modes of ventilation: control, assist/control, SIMV, CPAP, apnea backup ventilation, and noninvasive positive pressure ventilation (NPPV).

Control and Assist/Control are available when the "Assist/Ctrl" LED is illuminated near the mode SELECT button. Control is considered active, by the manufacturer, when the sensitivity is set to off ("–"). However, there is seldom a good reason to make a ventilator insensitive to the patient (see previous discussion on sensitivity setting).

Assist/control is considered active when a value greater than zero sensitivity is set. The breath type is established by the breath-type SELECT button (volume- or pressure-targeted). The rate is set by the BREATH RATE control. In Assist/Control the set rate can be the minimum rate setting. The patient can trigger additional mandatory breaths.

The SIMV mode is active when the "SIMV/CPAP" LED is illuminated near the mode SELECT button. The BREATH RATE (1 to 80 breaths/min) establishes the minimum mandatory breath rate. Patients can spontaneously breathe between mandatory breaths. Spontaneous breaths can be from the set baseline pressure (zero or PEEP) and can also be supported with pressure support.

CPAP is considered the active mode if the "SIMV/CPAP" LED is illuminated and the BREATH RATE is off ("—"). In CPAP, spontaneous breaths can be from the baseline pressure and can also be given pressure support (see Clinical Rounds 12-38).

Apnea backup ventilation is available should the patient become apneic. The apnea interval is set using the Extended Features menu. The ventilator begins apnea backup ventilation in the assist/control mode based on the current settings. The active controls are displayed at full intensity and others are dimmed. If the set breath rate is ≥12 breaths/min, the apnea breath rate is the set breath rate. If the set breath rate is <12 breaths/min, and the breath rate is not limited by other control settings, the apnea breath rate is 12 breaths/min. If the set breath rate is limited to <12 breaths/min, because of tidal volume, flow and T_I settings, the apnea breath rate is the highest allowed rate. Normal ventilation resumes when two consecutive patient-triggered breaths occur or when the operator resets the apnea alarm using the SILENCE/RESET control.

Box 12-100 Alarms Available During NPPV*

High pressure	Internal battery low
Apnea alarm and Apnea backup ventilation	Internal battery empty
Sense line disconnected	Vent Inop
External power low	Defaults

*All other alarms are disabled. The displays for low minute volume and low peak pressure are set to dimmed dashes showing they are not active.

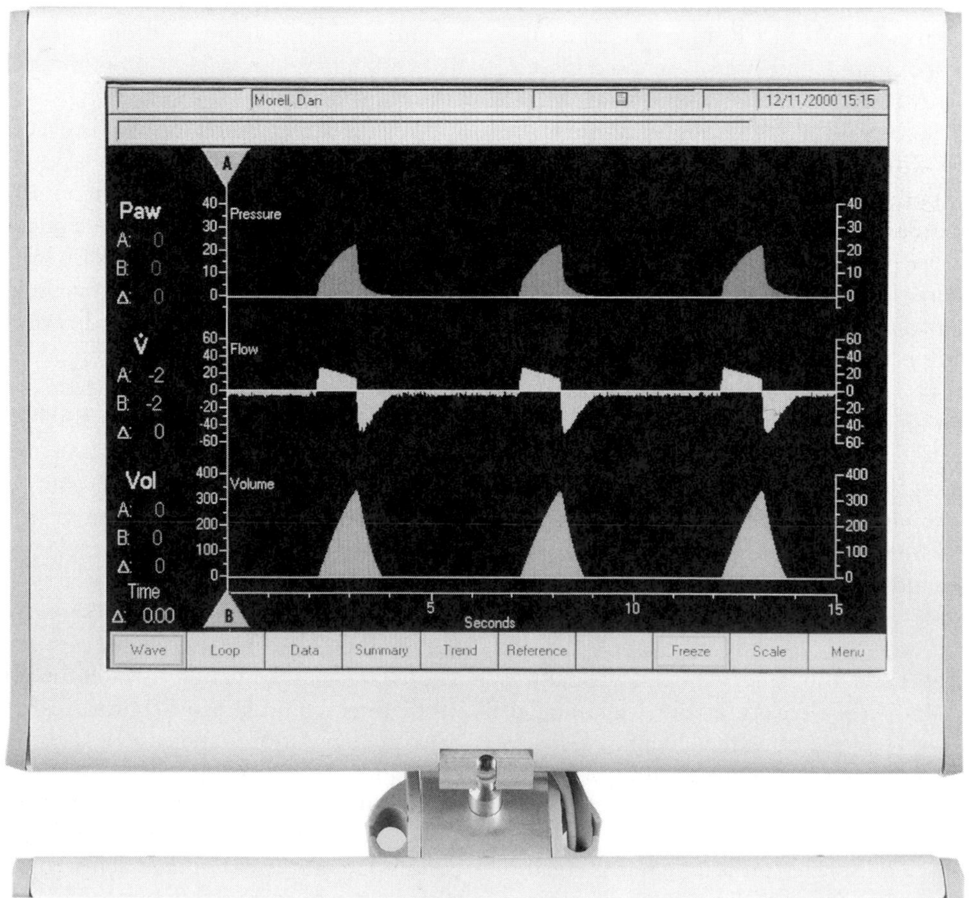

Figure 12-85 The monitor screen of the LTV ventilator series showing the scalars for pressure, flow, and volume. (Courtesy Pulmonetic Systems, Colton, Calif.)

Box 12-101 Ventilator Checkout Tests

To perform the ventilator checkout tests, the following steps are performed.

1. The ventilator is turned on, and is placed in standby by pushing and holding the ON/STANDBY button for 3 seconds.
2. Next, the operator pushes and holds the SELECT button and simultaneously pushes the ON/STANDBY button once.
3. The operator continues to hold the SELECT key until the Power On Self Tests (POST) is completed.
4. The words *Vent Check* appear in the monitor window.
5. The ventilator check goes through the following sequence of items: alarm, display, control, leak, and exit. (*Note:* When this menu is entered, the words REMOVE PTNT [remove patient] appear next in the display window as a reminder to disconnect the patient from the unit. To clear this alarm and verify to the microprocessor that the patient has been removed, the SILENCE/RESET button is pressed.)
6. The first test, *alarm*, is then displayed in the window. Pressing the SELECT button runs this test and should result in the audible alarm sounding. To end the alarm test, simply press SELECT again.
7. Each subsequent test is run in a similar fashion. The next menu item will appear, in this case *Display*. The operator presses SELECT to run this test and verify that all displays are working. All panel LEDs will illuminate.
8. Pressing SELECT following this test brings the next test, *Control*, into the window. The control test verifies that the ventilator buttons and the SET VALUE knob are working.
9. To run the control test, the operator pushes SELECT while *Control* is displayed in the window. The window then reads *Select*.
10. To test each control, push the desired button. For example, push the BREATH RATE button and *Breath Rate* appears in the window.
11. This sequence is followed until all buttons have been tested.
12. The SET VALUE knob is tested by turning it clockwise and counterclockwise. The direction of rotation is displayed in the window. Pressing SELECT button exits the test.
13. The final ventilator check item is the LEAK test. It is used to test the patient circuit for leaks. The patient Y connector is blocked. The Leak test is accessed by pressing the SELECT key when "LEAK" is displayed in the window, pushing the SELECT button again and the leak test is performed. (*Note:* The ventilator will not run the leak test until it has been on [running] for 60 seconds. This is the required warm-up period for the transducers before leak testing.)
14. At the end of the test, the display window shows either "leak passed" or "leak failed" and gives the amount of the leak in L/min. The leak test will fail if the leak is greater than 1 L/min.

NPPV is provided as a secondary mode that may be selected in addition to the primary ventilation mode. NPPV is selected using the Extended Features menu and specific alarms are available (Box 12-100). When activated, ventilation is delivered according to the selected mode and breath type that are currently active. The NPPV LED is lit when it is on. The number of alarms in NPPV is limited when it is active.

Special Features

One of the optional features of the LTV series is a monitor screen that provides several display windows including scalars, loops, and data. Figure 12-85 shows the waveform screen with scalars for pressure-time, flow-time, and volume-time displayed. The screen can be frozen to view an event, or scaled to size the waveforms. Another screen provides pressure-volume and flow-volume loops.

The data screen displays information normally scrolled in the display window of the operating panel. The data include PIP, PEEP, Vte, MAP (mean airway pressure), f, $\dot{V}_E$, I:E, $\dot{V}$calc, and peak flow. The right side of the data screen lists information on current parameter and alarm settings and also settings of the items available in the Special Features Menu such as flow termination and rise time. The obvious advantage of having a monitoring screen is the easy and immediate access to information, including trends.

Troubleshooting

To avoid difficulties in ventilator operation, it is appropriate to run the ventilator checkout tests prior to using the LTV on a new patient and or following a circuit change. Before running the checkout tests, the patient circuit and all related components are attached. The patient is disconnected from the unit during testing. Box 12-101 describes the ventilator checkout test procedure.

General Troubleshooting

The exhalation valve is cleaned during regular maintenance. This valve is delicate and needs to be handled carefully. If apparent leak problems occur and the circuit does not pass the leak test, the operator should be sure the exhalation valve diaphragm is correctly seated.

The operator's manual contains a section on troubleshooting that is symptom based. For example, suppose a control does not operate. The manual explains that the control may not be active in the current mode or breath-type. Or, the controls could be locked. Or, perhaps the control has not been "selected" by pushing the associated button. The user is advised to review the suggestions listed in the troubleshooting section of the operator's manual for more detail.

Esprit Ventilator (Respironics)[1]

The Esprit is a microprocessor-controlled ventilator intended for use with adult or pediatric patients (minimum V_T 50 mL) in acute or subacute facilities (Figure 12-86). It can be used for either noninvasive or invasive ventilation.

Power Source

The Esprit is electrically powered and selects its power source based on the following priority: AC power, external battery (if present), optional back-up battery. If the unit is disconnected from AC power, the battery indicator illuminates yellow.

Before turning on the unit, the operator must be sure the main circuit breaker is in the "on" position. (*Note:* When the ventilator is not in use, the manufacturer recommends that the ventilator remain plugged into AC power and the main circuit breaker be "on." This helps to maintain the expected life of the lead acid back-up battery.)

To provide variable oxygen concentrations, the Esprit requires connection to a high pressure oxygen source (40-90 psig).

Internal Mechanism

The internal pneumatic system is based on a three-stage blower capable of providing pressure and gas flow to the patient (100 cm H_2O pressure, 3 to 140 L/min, max. 200 L/min, respectively). The blower eliminates the need for using an air compressor or high pressure air source. When the unit is operating and is disconnected from an AC power (battery indicator yellow), the blower will continue to operator from the battery, allowing the unit to be used in transport. A fully charged backup battery will power the Esprit for about 30 minutes, depending on the ventilator settings. (*Note:* A change in blower sound occurs, which results from the change in RPM [revolutions per minute] of the blower [>60 cm H_2O Hi Press or <60 cm H_2O Hi Press].)

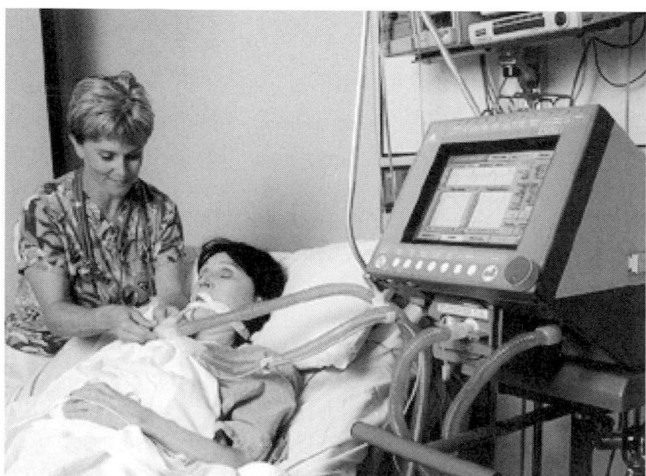

Figure 12-86 The Esprit ventilator with patient circuit. (Courtesy Respironics Inc, Murrysville, Pa.)

Controls and Alarms

All the major operational controls for the Esprit are located in the front panel, which is divided into a top section and a smaller bottom section (Figure 12-87). The top section contains all the indicators, the touch sensitive display screen and the controls. The lower section contains the connections for the patient circuit, the heated expiratory valve filter, and the on/off switch.

Front Panel Indicators

Across the top of the ventilator just above the screen are the indicators for the operational status and alarm conditions of the Esprit (see Figure 12-87). These LED indicators begin on the left with the NORMAL indicator, which illuminates when the ventilator has been turned on and no active or auto-reset alarms are present. The ALARM HIGH indicator, next in line, flashes red during a high-priority alarm. The ALARM MED/LOW indicator flashes yellow to indicate a medium alarm and continuously when a low-priority alarm exists, respectively. These two alarm indicators will show a continuous yellow light if an alarm condition had occurred, but was corrected (auto-reset).

When the ventilator inoperative (VENT INOP) indicator is illuminated, the Esprit has established that a hardware malfunction has been detected and the unit is not capable of supporting ventilation. It should be removed immediately from use and another method provided to ventilate the patient.

The SAFETY VALVE open (SVO) alert is illuminated whenever any of the following conditions exist:

- An occlusion in the circuit is detected
- Oxygen and air sources are no longer operable
- A hardware malfunction is detected and the ventilator inoperative state (VENT INOP) is activated.

In SVO, the safety valve opens, the exhalation valve remains open and the air and oxygen valves close. A high-priority alarm occurs, the SAFETY VALVE indicator lights and the normal indicator is turned off. The ventilator does not provide support to the patient, so another immediate method to ventilate the patient should be provided.

The alarm silence icon is yellow when the audible alarm has been disabled. It stays illuminated for 2 minutes when the ALARM SILENCE button (bottom row) is pressed. If a new alarm condition occurs while it is active, the visual alarm function will be activated. Pressing the ALARM RESET button in the bottom row of controls clears the alarm silence and audible alarms can again be heard.

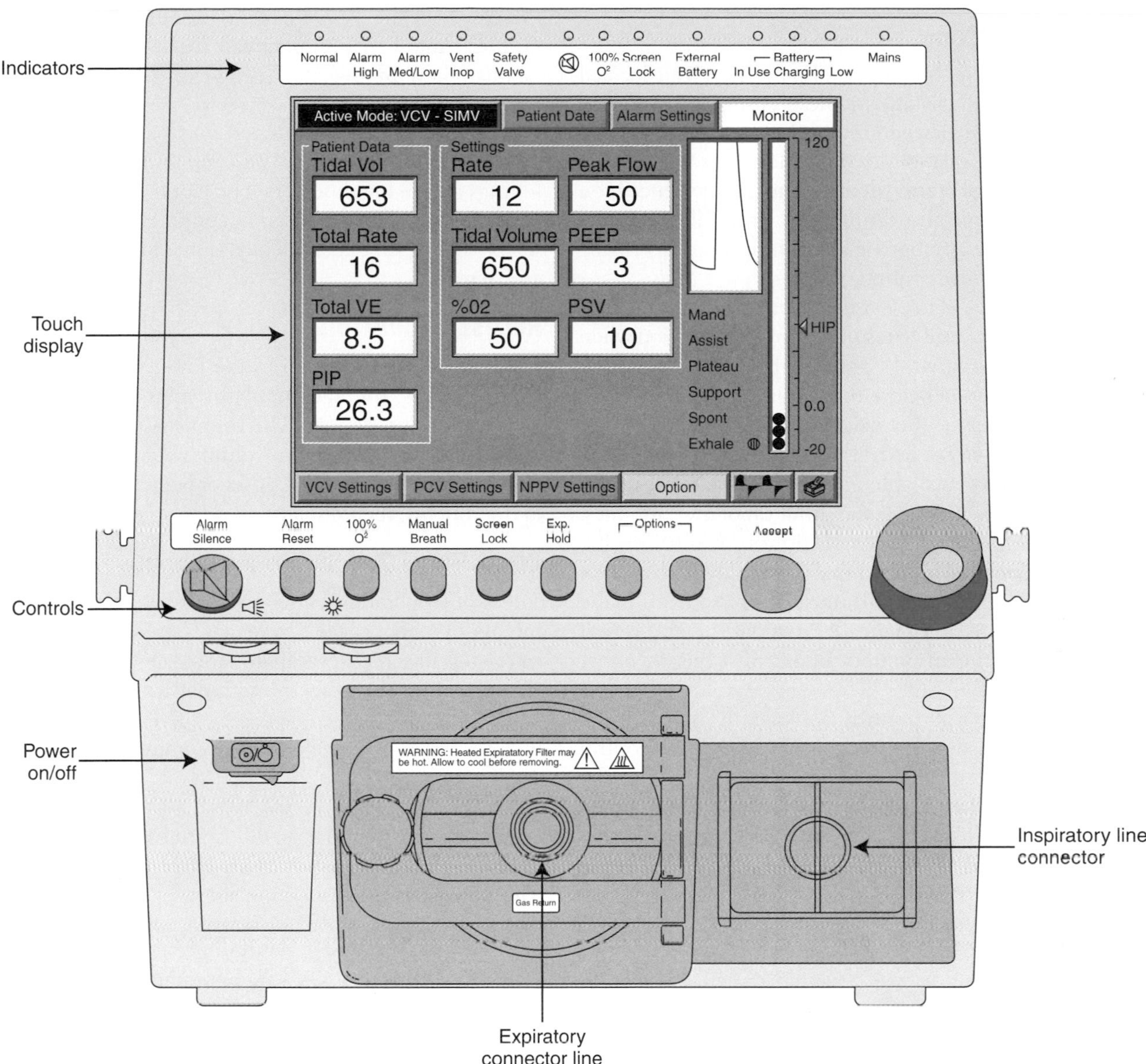

Figure 12-87 A diagram of the front panel of the Esprit ventilator showing: *(1)* indicators, *(2)* touch display with monitoring screen, *(3)* controls, *(4)* power on/off switch, *(5)* connector line for exhalation line-to-heated exhalation filter, and *(6)* inspiratory line connector.

The 100% O_2 indicator is only active when the control button on the front panel labeled 100% O_2 has been pressed and 100% O_2 is being delivered to the patient. The indicator remains illuminated for the two minutes of oxygen delivery. The 100% O_2 indicator is not related to the percent oxygen delivery. In other words, if the operator sets the inspired %O_2 setting to 100%, the 100% O_2 indicator does not light. It lights only when the 100% O_2 front panel key has been pressed.

The SCREEN LOCK indicator lights green when active. A screen lock prevents inadvertent changes to the keys on the touch sensitive screen.

The EXTERNAL BATTERY indicator has been reserved for future release in the Esprit and is not currently an available option for use.

BATTERY has three indicator positions. BATTERY IN USE lights yellow to show the ventilator is running from the back-up battery. BATTERY CHARGING lights yellow when the back-up battery is charging. Charging can take up to 10 hours. The indicator will turn off when the battery is fully charged. BATTERY LOW flashes red when about 5 minutes or less of power remains in the back-up battery. The operator should immediately connect the ventilator to an AC power source.

The MAINS indicator illuminates green when the ventilator is connected to an AC power source and the main circuit breaker is on.

Front Panel Buttons

The front panel control buttons (see Figure 12-87) are located just below the screen. Many of these controls correspond with the indicators reviewed previously.

Pressing the ALARM SILENCE button on the far left provides 2 minutes of alarm silence. The alarm silence icon at the top of the unit also illuminates. If an alarm occurs during this time, the appropriate alarm indicator will visually appear, but the silence continues.

ALARM RESET is used to clear the visual indicators for auto reset alarms. It is also used to resume normal ventilation when apnea back-up ventilation is present. Pressing this button also ends alarm silence before the 2 minutes is completed.

100% O_2 increases the oxygen percent to 100% for 2 minutes. After it is pressed, it cannot be canceled. If an oxygen source is not available and this button is pressed, a low O_2 alarm will be active for the duration of the 2 minutes.

Pressing the MANUAL BREATH button results in the delivery of an operator-initiated mandatory breath based on the current ventilator settings. It must be pressed during the expiratory phase of a breath. A manual breath is not permitted during the inspiratory phase of a breath, either mandatory or spontaneous.

The SCREEN LOCK control locks and unlocks the graphics or touch screen. Using the screen lock control helps to prevent accidental or inadvertent changes in the screen function. When the screen is locked, all on screen keys are disabled and the screen lock indicator in the top row illuminates. Only the following controls remain active when the screen lock is on:

- Manual breath
- 100% O_2
- Exp. Hold
- Alarm reset
- Alarm silence

The expiratory hold (EXP HOLD) button is used to estimate end expiratory pressure for the determination of auto-PEEP. It is only active at the end of a mandatory breath and is not available in NPPV or during emergency ventilation modes. When pressed, an exhalation hold function begins following exhalation for the currently active breath, and the "expiratory hold maneuver" subscreen appears on the regular screen (Figure 12-88). The air, O_2, and exhalation valves are closed. No gas flow goes into or out of the patient circuit to allow for equilibration of the pressure in the circuit and the patient's lungs.

The subscreen graphic allows viewing of the pressure-time curve and digitally displays the pressures. After a stable reading is achieved, the unit can calculate and display end-exhalation pressure, exhalation pause pressure, and auto-PEEP. If the button is held continuously and exhalation exceeds 5 seconds, the ventilator automatically ends exhalation and begins a new inspiratory period.

Auto-PEEP is calculated using the following equation: (Auto-PEEP = Exhalation Pause Pressure – End Exhalation Pressure). If the Auto-PEEP is calculated as a negative number Auto-PEEP display will read "–." There is also a "status: abort by operator" message if the software is not installed.

The OPTIONS buttons are reserved for future use. Finally, the ACCEPT button allows the operator to activate selected settings on the touch screen. The Control Knob to the right of the ACCEPT button is used in conjunction with the touch screen to enter operator-selected values for ventilator settings and alarms.

Recessed Controls

Just below the front panel in the lower left corner are two control knobs, the audible alarm volume (icon), and the display brightness (icon). The volume control can lower the audible sound of the alarm volume, but cannot turn it off. The brightness control increases or decreases the brightness of the touch screen display.

Front Panel Touch Screen Display

The front operating panel (graphic user interface) is an infrared touch sensitive screen. There are two different categories of screens: ventilator and diagnostic. The former appears when the machine is functioning as a ventilator. The diagnostic screen appears when the Esprit is not functioning as a ventilator and is running self-tests.

Diagnostic Mode

Similar to other ventilators, the Esprit has several diagnostic functions including a power on self-test (POST) that runs when the unit is turned on, a short self-test (SST), and an extended self-test (EST). Diagnostics are available to perform the following:

- Run tests that can only be run when a patient is not attached

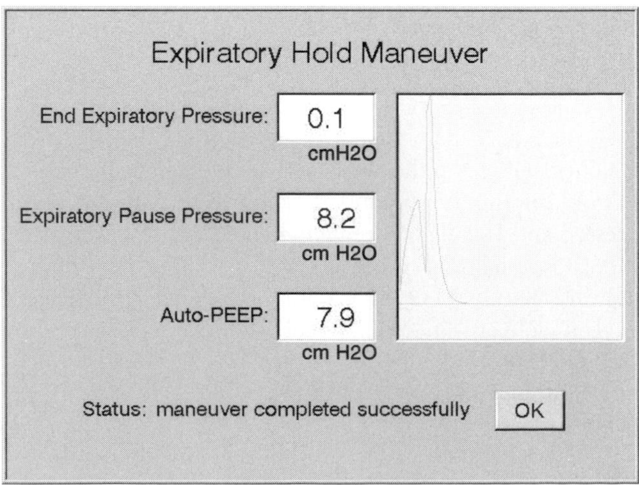

Figure 12-88 Expiratory hold maneuver window (see text for description). (Courtesy Respironics Inc, Murrysville, Pa.)

- Determine the circuit compliance (enabled or disabled)
- Set altitude, time, date
- Perform more detailed service and maintenance functions

Calibrate the inline oxygen sensor during EST

(*Note:* During the preoperational procedure, if time is found to be incorrect more than once, the internal battery may need to be replaced.)

Short Self Test (SST)

The SST is usually run between patients, and when the circuit is changed. SST verifies the patient circuit is free of major leaks. If major leaks are present in the patient circuit the ventilator will not run. The integrity of the system requires a tight circuit during SST and EST or these tests will fail. Performance of the SST also measures the leak rate and the circuit compliance. It tests critical hardware components including the safety valve, flow sensors and the auto-zero solenoids. If SST passes, the ventilator and attached components are ready for patient use. A ventilator that has failed SST should not be used without verifying the operational safety of the unit by other methods. (*Note:* The SST will provide a text prompt to remind the clinician to be sure the patient is not connected during SST because the high pressures generated to the patient circuit can injure a patient.) The SST is run using the diagnostics screen (Box 12-102).

Extended Self Test (EST)

EST is a more comprehensive system test normally run only by qualified personnel, such as a field service technician, trained in its use. EST verifies the overall functional integrity of the ventilator by testing all the critical hardware subsystems and components. It is run as part of the regular maintenance of the machine to verify performance, particularly if performance of a unit is in question.

As with the SST, the patient should never be connected when the test is run. As with SST, EST is also accessed through the diagnostics screen. If a ventilator fails to pass the EST, the ventilator should not be used with a patient.

The User Configuration Screen and Tubing Compliance

Also available on the diagnostics screen is the user configuration screen. This screen allows the operator to set the date and time, the altitude at which the ventilator is operating and to enable or disable the tubing compliance compensation feature. "USER CONFIG." is pressed to access the user configuration screen. In this screen, there is a soft pad labeled COMPLIANCE. Circuit compliance is enabled when the COMPLIANCE soft pad has a white background. When active the exhaled volumes reported by the Esprit are compensated for tubing compliance. Compensation is based on the circuit compliance calculated during the last SST. (*Note:* After completing SST or EST or user configuration screen, the ventilator must be turned off to get back to a set-up screen.)

Front Panel Touch Screen Display

In the touch screen (see Figure 12-87), menu items appear across the top and bottom of the screen. The center portion of the screen contains the data relevant to the breath type and mode that has been selected (Box 12-103). The menus also include patient data, alarm settings, and monitor. Touching one of these labels brings up a new screen.

The elements that are common to all ventilator screens (nondiagnostic) include a top bar, a bottom bar, and a manometer. The top bar lists: the currently active mode and breath type, PATIENT DATA, ALARM SETTINGS, and MONITOR. The bottom bar lists the following:

- VCV SETTINGS—displays VCV settings screen that allows the operator to view and change settings for volume-targeted breath delivery.
- PCV SETTINGS—displays and allows changes in settings for pressure-targeted breath delivery.

Box 12-102 Running the SST Test

The operator should:

1. Be sure the patient is disconnect and the ventilator is off.
2. Press and hold down the ALARM RESET and 100%O_2 buttons for 5 seconds while turning on the ventilator.
3. The diagnostic screen appears and a message in the center reads:
   "WARNING: Entering Diagnostics Mode. Verify that the patient is disconnected prior to proceeding. -OK."
4. Press "OK."
5. Press the SST key at the top, left corner of the screen, then press "Start" to begin the test.
6. Prompts will appear instructing the operator to unplug and plug the patient Y following the prompts.
7. When the test is completed, the calculated patient circuit compliance will appear on the screen.

Box 12-103 Breath Type and Ventilator Mode

In the Esprit ventilator, the manufacturer distinguishes between breath type and mode in the following manner. VCV (volume control ventilation), PCV (pressure control ventilation), and NPPV (noninvasive positive pressure ventilation) are designated as breath types.

VCV and PCV are available in the following mode settings: assist/control (A/C), synchronized intermittent mandatory ventilation (SIMV), and continuous positive airway pressure (CPAP).

NPPV is available in two modes: spontaneous (Spont), and spontaneous/timed (Spont/T).

- NPPV SETTINGS—displays the NPPV settings and allows changes for noninvasive ventilation (Spont and Spont/T).
- OPTION—this touch pad is for future use.
- Graphics (icon)—displays the waveforms and loops screen if this option has been installed in the unit. (*Note:* The graphics are available if the waveform picture appears black against a gray background. The graphics are not available if this key is gray-on-gray.)

When VCV-SIMV is the active mode, ACTIVE MODE: VCV-SIMV (top, left, Figure 12-87) will be highlighted, indicating it is the currently active mode. Also visible are the current settings for that mode, and centrally located patient data.

The pressure manometer is located on the right side of the screen. The abbreviation HIP, which appears along side the pressure manometer, marks the high pressure alarm setting. When this value is reached, the inspiratory phase ends. The operator can touch the HIP soft pad and the HIGH PRESSURE subscreen appears. This screen is used to change the high-pressure setting. The alarm screen can also be used to set the high-pressure limit. When the high pressure is set at >60 cm H_2O, the blower motor RPM increases to provide the necessary pressure increase. Table 12-35 describes the various symbols used within the bar graph of the manometer to indicate the breath type currently present.

Setting Screens

In general, the process by which a patient is set up includes selecting the breath type, modes, presetting the parameters, alarms, and activating the changes. During ventilator normal operation, all parameter, mode, and alarm limit settings are selected using the same three-step procedure. First, the parameter is selected by touching the appropriate screen pad. Next a screen insert appears on the operating screen (Figure 12-89). The current set value appears in the digital window. For example, in Figure 12-89, the value for peak flow is 30 liters per minute (LPM). Up and down arrows on the adjacent bar to the right of the value allow the operator to increase or decrease the value. This can also be done with the control knob. A bar graph on the extreme right shows the setting range and current setting. In this case, "3 to 140 LPM" of peak flow is available and 30 is the current setting. Pressing the ACCEPT pad in the screen insert or pressing the ACCEPT button on the front panel activates the change. Pressing CANCEL returns the ventilator to the previous setting.

The soft pads in the main screen have an active and an inactive state. Active settings have a gray background with black letters. Inactive settings have a gray background with gray letters and are not being used by the ventilator to control ventilation or as an alarm limit. Box 12-104 gives an example of an exception.

Selecting Settings For a New Patient

The breath type, either VCV, PCP, or NPPV, is selected and the screen for the selection appears. Specific parameters, such as peak flow in VCV, are then set by touching the parameter soft pad. The subscreen for that parameter allows adjustment to the desired setting (see Figure 12-89).

Table 12-35 Breath Indicator

Breath	Symbol	Description
Mand	●	Operator or ventilator triggered mandatory breath.
Assist	◡	Patient triggered mandatory breath.
Plateau	◉	Inspiratory hold, can be set at the end of the inspiratory phase of a VCV breath type.
Support	◓	Patient triggered spontaneous breath with PSV > 0, or IPAP > EPAP.
Spont	○	Patient triggered spontaneous breath, PSV = 0, or IPAP = EPAP.
Exhale	⏀	Indicates exhalation phase of any breath.

(Courtesy Respironics, Inc, Carlsbad, Calif.)

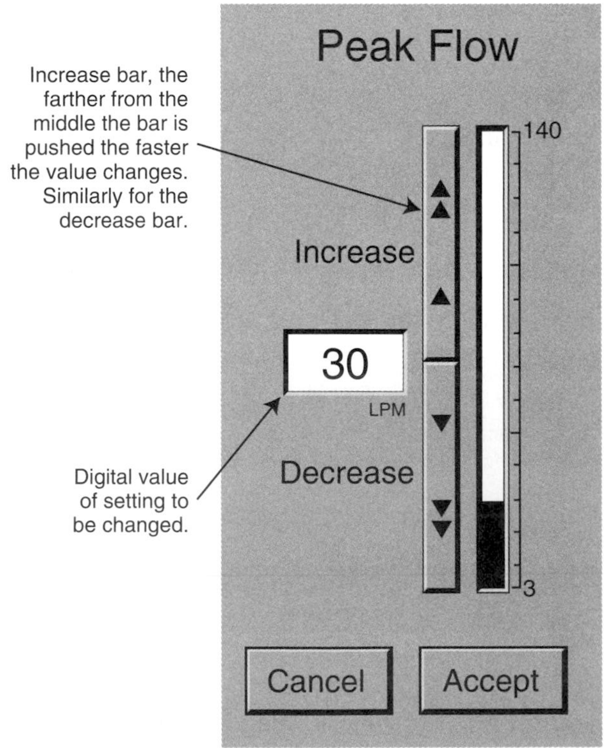

Figure 12-89 The subscreen window for setting peak flow when that parameter has been selected (see text for description). (Courtesy Respironics Inc, Murrysville, Pa.)

Some subscreens display not only the selected parameter, but also the calculated data based on the setting. For example, during VCV, the rate subscreen displays the calculated minute volume that results from the set rate and volume. In PCV when rate is displayed, the calculated value for the I:E ratio is also displayed.

Box 12-104 Active Keys Even When They Are Not

Some setting keys will appear active even though they are not being used in the current **active mode.** This is because the setting of these keys is used in Apnea Ventilation or when the manual inspiration key is pressed. For example, if CPAP is selected as the active mode, tidal volume (VCV) or inspiratory pressure (PCV) are not active. However, the operator needs to include one or the other, depending on the mode, in case the patient becomes apneic and apnea ventilation begins. One should choose a value appropriate for the patient being ventilated for any active key that appears on the screen.

When a new breath type is selected, the mode available for that breath type can also be selected (see Box 12-103). Figure 12-90, A, shows the ventilator currently active in VCV-A/C. The VCV SETTING pad on the bottom menu has been pressed. Some of the parameters are gray lettering on a gray background (PSV, E-trigger, Rise Time) indicating they are not currently active. However, the operator can use the grayed keys to change the settings as needed for going into PCV, for example. Table 12-36 lists the patient data parameters available and their definition.

Pressing the ACTIVATE key at the top right corner of the screen brings up a prompt that asks "Change to ________ control ventilation?" Pressing "OK" in response to this prompt activates the new breath type and all the new settings. Figure 12-90, *B*, shows an example of the prompt window when PCV has been selected as the new mode.

Pressing "Review Alarms" in the prompt window brings up the subscreen for adjusting the alarms for the new mode (see Alarm section). If "cancel" is pressed, nothing changes and the screen returns to the active mode screen.

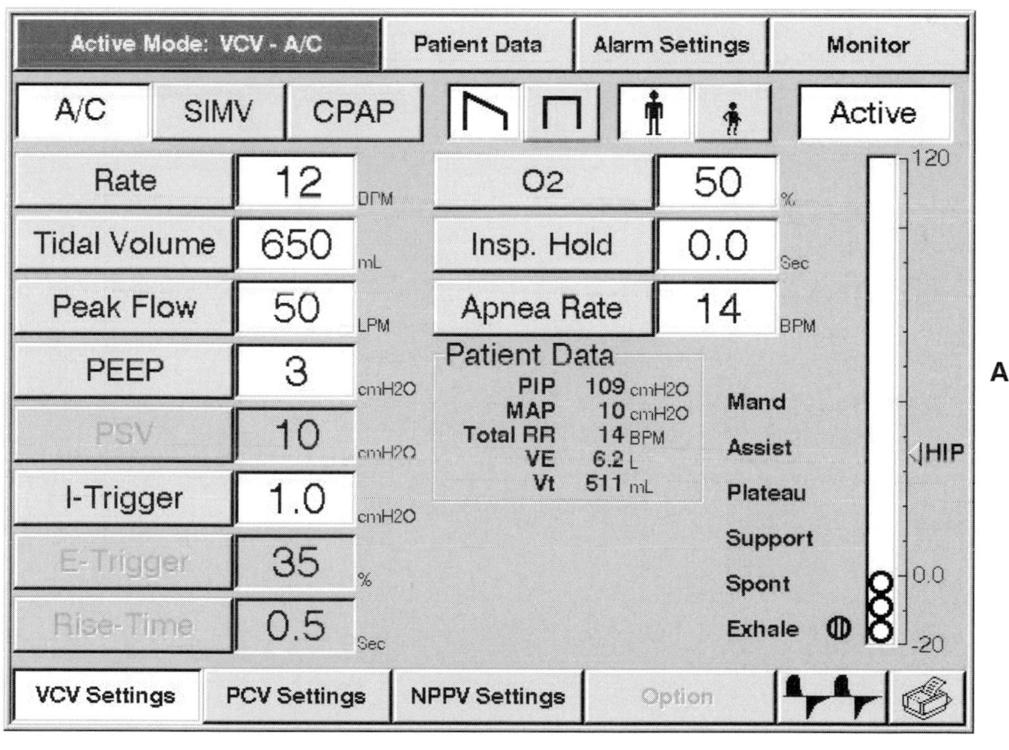

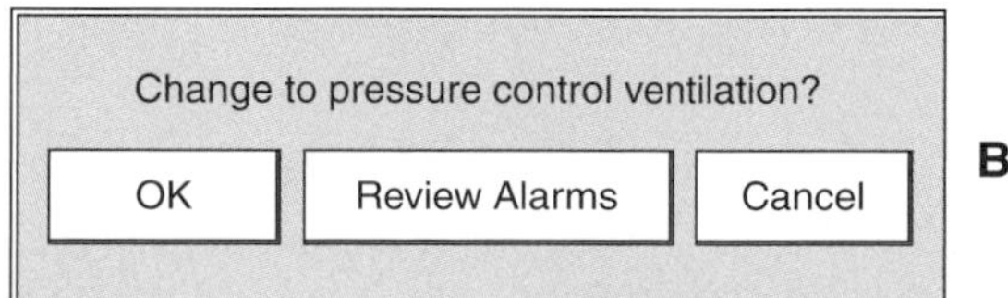

Figure 12-90 **A,** The VCV setting screen during the active mode VCV-A/C. **B,** Example of a prompt window when "Activate PCV" has been pressed in the setting screen and settings have been selected (see text for explanation). (Courtesy Respironics Inc, Murrysville, Pa.)

Table 12-36 Patient Data Parameters and Definitions

Parameter	Description	Range
PIP	Peak inspiratory pressure (maximum pressure during inspiration)	-20.0 to 130 cm H_2O
MAP	Mean airway pressure (average airway pressure during the total breath cycle)	-20.0 to 130 cm H_2O
Pe End	Pressure at end-expiration (pressure measured at end expiration)	-20.0 to 99.9 cm H_2O
Pi End	Pressure at end inspiration (pressure measure at end inspiration or at the end of an inspiratory hold)	-20.0 to 130 cm H_2O
Tidal Vol	Exhaled tidal volume (compliance compensated if enabled)	0 to 999 mL
Spont VE	Spontaneous minute volume	0 to 99.9 L/min
Total VE	Exhaled minute volume	0 to 99.9 L/min
%O_2	Delivered O_2 (1 second average of O_2 readings if O_2 sensor is installed)	0.0 to 110%
Spont Rate	Spontaneous respiratory rate	0 to 150 breaths/min
Rate	Total respiratory rate	0 to 150 breaths/min
F/Vt	Rapid shallow breathing index (ratio of respiratory rate to exhaled tidal volume for spontaneous breaths)	0 to 500 breaths/min/L
I:E Ratio	Ratio of inspiratory time to expiratory time	9.9:1 to 1:99

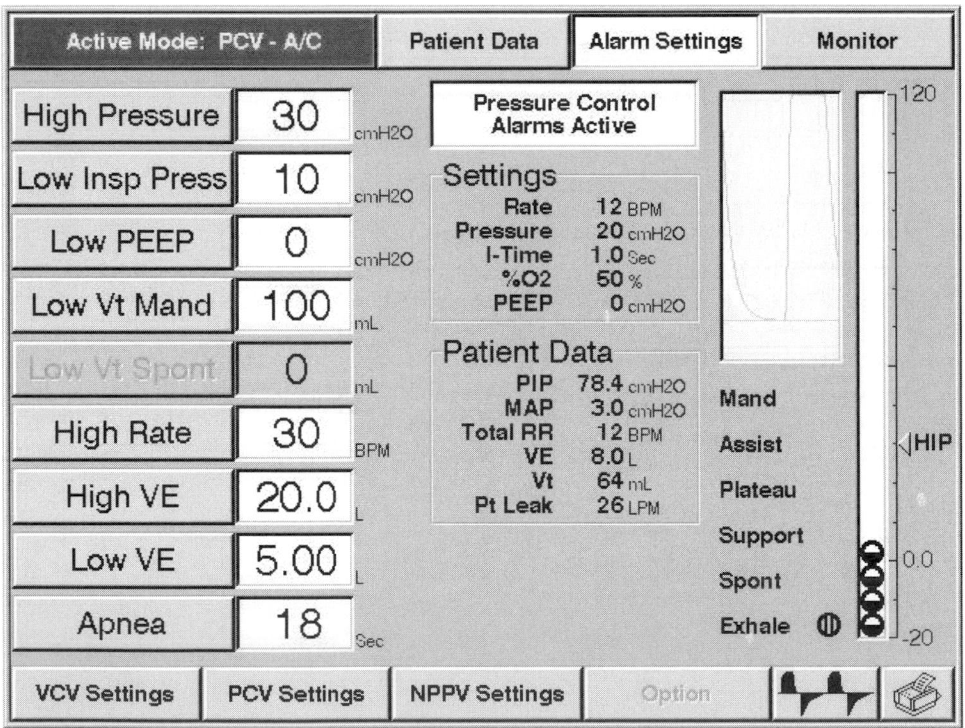

Figure 12-91 The alarm setting screen displaying the various alarms available for setting. The active mode is PCV-A/C and the screen is for setting PCV alarms (see text for explanation). (Courtesy Respironics Inc, Murrysville, Pa.)

Patient Data Section

Touching PATIENT DATA accesses the screen that lists all the current monitored ventilator parameters (see Table 12-36). The format for this screen is the same in VCV, PCV, and NPPV breath types.

Monitor Screen

The monitor screen (see Figure 12-86) is the default screen and automatically displays if the screen has not been touched in 15 minutes. Pressing the MONITOR touch pad also brings it into view. This screen varies depending on the breath type being delivered.

Alarms Settings

After set-up of breath type and mode, it is appropriate to adjust the alarm settings. Pressing the "Alarm Settings" touch pad displays the available alarm settings (Figure 12-91). This screen can also be accessed during the process of changing the mode.

To adjust the alarm, the operator touches the pad for that alarm. For example, during VCV when the operator touches LOW V_T MAND., the subscreen for that alarm appears. As with setting a parameter, the arrow keys or control knob can be used to increase or decrease the displayed value. Press "ACCEPT" to activate the new alarm setting.

The high-pressure alarm subscreen can be activated either by this method or by touching the HIP key adjacent to the pressure manometer in PCV or VCV settings. In NPPV the high-pressure limit is automatically set at 10 cm H_2O above the IPAP setting.

Active Alarm Conditions

In most cases alarms have a visual indicator, an audible sequence of tones, and a screen alert window with a message. Alarms have three priority levels. High-urgency alarms illuminate a red indicator and emit a sequence of 5 tones. These types of alarms require immediate attention. Medium-urgency alarms give a yellow flashing indicator with a sequence of three tones. These alarms require a prompt response. Low-urgency alarms give a continuous yellow indicator with no audible tone.

The audible alarm for a medium or high level alarm will stop when the alarm condition that caused them has ended (auto-reset). A window in the lower center screen labeled "Alerts" lists the current alarms in bold print and auto-reset alarms in normal print. The operator must reset the alarms to clear the visual indicators. The ALARM RESET button clears the visual indicators for currently active or auto-reset alarms. If the condition occurs again, the visual indicator turns on again. Pressing ALARM SILENCE gives a two-minute silence.

Only a few alarms cannot be silenced. They are so urgent that they require immediate resolution of the problem to avoid endangering the patient. They include the following:

- Gas supplies lost—SVO
- Low back-up battery
- Backup battery on (not currently available)

Some alarms cannot be manually reset. The operator must be sure the problem has been resolved rather than trying to reset the alarms. These alarms include the following:

- Occlusion—SVO
- Low O_2 (*Note:* The alarm range is ± 6% of the set value. Although the actual percent change within the delivered gas is almost immediate, it takes time for the software to reset the measured value. As a result a low or high %O_2 alarm occurs after about 30 seconds when the set O_2% is changed.)
- High O_2
- Low O_2 supply

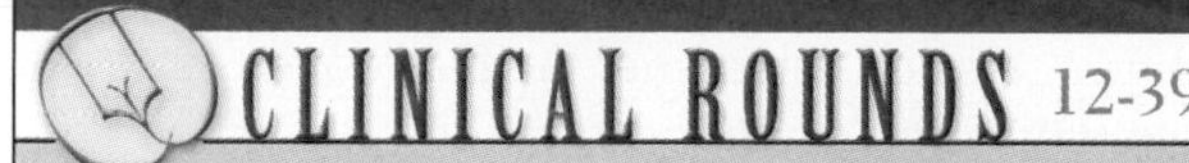

An adult patient is being ventilated with VCV-SIMV at a rate of 4 breaths/min and PSV is set at 10 cm H_2O. An "I-Time Too Long" alarm occurs. What condition could have caused the alarm to occur?

See Appendix A for the answer.

The Esprit has the same traditional alarms that are present in all ventilators including high and low inspiratory pressure, low PEEP, high rate, high and low minute volume, low V_T (spontaneous, mandatory), apnea, high and low O_2, low O_2 supply, gas supplies lost (safety valve open), low back-up battery, and battery back-up on. Unusual alarms include low EPAP for NPPV mode, I-Time too long, and Occlusion (SVO).

Low EPAP in the NPPV modes indicates that pressure has dropped below the low alarm level during exhalation. There may be a leak in the circuit or patient interface (mask). I-Time that is too long is a medium-priority alarm to indicate that a spontaneous pressure supported breath has exceeded the maximum time allowed. For adults the maximum time is 3.5 seconds (averaged over three breaths); for pediatric patients, it is 2.5 seconds (also averaged). Prolonged T_I might occur when a leak is present during PSV (see Clinical Rounds 12-39).

If the patient circuit becomes crimped or blocked, or the expiratory filter occluded, inspiration will end and the unit goes into exhalation. This results in an Occlusion-SVO (safety valve open) alarm. The air and oxygen valves close and the exhalation and safety valves open. A spontaneously breathing patient can obtain room air through the open valves. The ventilator resumes normal operation when it is determined that the obstruction has been cleared. The operator may need to clear the patient circuit and check the expiratory filter and humidification devices to be sure they are not obstructed or causing too much expiratory flow resistance.

Modes of Ventilation

The modes provided by the Esprit for VCV and PCV, include A/C, SIMV, and CPAP. These are intended for the intubated patient. NPPV is available for patients who have interfaces such as a nasal mask, a full face mask, nasal pillows, or a mouthpiece with a lip seal. NPPV can be spontaneous (Spont) or provide a back-up breath rate (spontaneous/timed settings). In addition, there is a back-up mode called Apnea Ventilation.

Before selecting the mode of ventilation, it is appropriate to select the patient size: Adult or pediatric keys. (Figure 12-90, A, top right screen). Selecting one or the other adapts the ventilator's breath delivery algorithms to suit the patient type for compliance and resistance. The patient type selected determines the flow output at various rise time settings for pressure-targeted breaths (PCV, PSV, and IPAP). In addition, the "I-Time too long" alarms for spontaneous pressure supported breaths are set (3.5 seconds for adults and 2.5 seconds for children; averaged over three breaths).

Mode Selection

After selecting breath type, the available modes for that breath type appear in the top left portion of the screen. To select a mode, the operator must be sure to touch MONITOR or the ACTIVE MODE. If VCV or PCV breath types are active, A/C, SIMV, or CPAP can be selected. If NPPV is active, the operator selects SPONT or SPONT/T. The ventilator asks for mode confirmation by bringing up a screen message. For example, it might say "Change mode to SIMV? Yes – No."

A/C and SIMV–Volume Control Ventilation (VCV)

If VCV is selected for either A/C or SIMV modes, the mandatory breaths are either time- or patient-triggered (pressure or flow), flow-limited and time-cycled. (*Note:* This can also be considered volume-cycled. That is, flow is delivered over a specific time based on the rate.) In A/C, all breaths are mandatory. In SIMV, the minimum mandatory rate is set and the patient is able to breathe spontaneously between mandatory breaths from the baseline pressure (PEEP/CPAP).

In A/C or SIMV for the mandatory breath, the operator can select rate, tidal volume, peak flow, PEEP, PSV, I-trigger (sensitivity), expiratory trigger, rise time, O_2, inspiratory hold, apnea rate, and either constant (square) or descending (decelerating) ramp for the flow waveform. The selected waveform is highlighted in the VCV screen. Pushing the desired waveform pad activates that flow pattern. (*Note:* The waveform pattern cannot be set in PCV or NPPV modes.) Also available are the % oxygen, inspiratory hold and apnea rate.

Machine sensitivity to a patient's inspiratory effort is adjusted using the I-TRIGGER control. Touching the I-TRIGGER pad in VCV, PCV or NPPV SETTINGS window brings up the inspiratory trigger subscreen. The operator can select either pressure- or flow-triggering for PCV and VCV. NPPV is always flow-triggered. The trigger works by measuring the drop in either pressure or flow (whichever is active) in the patient circuit. Inspiration begins when the trigger level is detected. A suggested initial setting for pressure is 1-3 cm H_2O. (*Note:* The operator should monitor for auto-cycling, particularly if PEEP is increased.) For flow-trigger, a flow of 1-2 L/min is recommended. The bias flow is automatically set by the ventilator to 3 L/min above the threshold trigger setting. For example, for a trigger of 1 L/min, the bias flow is 4 L/min.

For support of spontaneous breaths in SIMV, PSV can be added. Pressure supported breaths are patient-triggered, pressure-limited and flow-cycled. The flow-cycling is adjustable from 10% to 45% of the peak flow measured during inspiration. The parameter labeled E-TRIGGER (expiratory trigger) is the control that adjusted the flow cycling percentage. For example, if E-trigger is set at 45%, the pressure support breath ends when the inspiratory flow drops to 45% of the measured peak flow. This setting will result in a shorter inspiration than will a setting of 10% (see Chapter 11).

A/C and SIMV–Pressure Control Ventilation (PCV)

When PCV is selected, either A/C or SIMV is available. The mandatory breaths are time- or patient-triggered (pressure or flow), pressure-limited and time-cycled. The following are set: rate, pressure, inspiratory time (I-time), PEEP, PSV, inspiratory trigger, expiratory trigger, rise time, oxygen percent, and apnea rate (Box 12-105). As with VCV, in A/C all breaths are mandatory and in this case are pressure-limited. In SIMV, mandatory breaths are pressure-limited and the patient can breathe spontaneously between these breaths from the established baseline (PEEP/CPAP) and with PS added, if desired.

CPAP Mode

CPAP can be activated during VCV or PCV breath type. The selection of CPAP assumes a mandatory breath rate of zero breaths/min. However, one should still set a rate in case apnea occurs for establishing the rate during apnea ventilation. The baseline can be adjusted above zero to 35 cm H_2O. All patient-triggered breaths are spontaneous and can be supported with pressure support. Triggering is based on the I-trigger setting with either pressure or flow selected.

NPPV

In NPPV the operator sets parameters for spontaneous ventilation mode or spontaneous/timed ventilation mode. In *spontaneous ventilation* mode (Spont), inspiratory positive airway pressure (IPAP), and expiratory positive airway pressure (EPAP) are set. IPAP must be greater than or equal to EPAP. All breaths are patient-triggered using

Box 12-105 Rise Time Percent

Whenever a breath is pressure-targeted the rise time percent can be set. This parameter is active in PCV, PSV, and NPPV. It allows sloping or tapering of the curve during the beginning of inspiration. Rather than rising to the set pressure as rapidly as possible, the ventilator slows delivery of the pressure. It is adjustable from 0.1 to 0.9 second. The shorter the time, the more rapidly the pressure rises to its set value. (See Chapter 11 under "Initial operator selection of parameters" for more information on sloping.)

flow-triggering (I-Trigger). Rise time percent can be used to taper the beginning of the breath. Exhalation (EPAP) begins when the inspiratory flow drops to a percentage of peak flow measured during inspiration. The percentage is determined by the *E-Trigger* setting.

In spontaneous/time ventilation (Spont/T), the patient can breathe spontaneously or receive time-triggered breaths from the ventilator, with a set inspiratory time and rate. This minimum rate setting guarantees that the patient will receive at least the set number of breaths per minute. In earlier versions of the Esprit, these breaths are synchronized with the patient's inspiratory effort (flow-triggered). If no patient effort is detected, time-triggering occurs based on the set rate. Again, the high inspiratory pressure (HIP) limit is automatically adjusted by 10 cm H_2O above the current IPAP setting in NPPV.

In Rev. 4.0 of the Esprit, some alternations have been made to the Spont/T mode.[2] The Spont/T mode no longer delivers patient-triggered mandatory breaths. In Rev. 4.0 the patient either breathes spontaneously or receives ventilator time-triggered breaths. Spontaneous patient-triggered breaths receive the set IPAP level and T_I based on the E-trigger setting. An intra-breath period timer is active and resets with every patient-triggered breath. If the patient does not trigger a spontaneous breath within the time limit, the ventilator begins delivering time-triggered breaths at the set inspiratory time, rate and IPAP level.

Apnea Ventilation (AV)

As with most ventilators, the operator can set an apnea time interval (10 to 60 seconds). This setting is available on the alarm setting screen. If the ventilator fails to detect a patient breathing effort within this time frame, an alarm occurs and apnea ventilation begins. "Apnea" will appear in the Alerts window. The Esprit will deliver breaths using the A/C mode with either PCV or VCV, depending on which is set. The machine defaults to the settings for VCV or PCV. For example, in VCV, it bases apnea ventilation breath delivery on the set V_T, flow, PEEP, $O_2\%$, and so on. The breath rate is established by the operator set apnea rate, which is set in the breath setting screen. There is an exception to this. The set apnea rate cannot be set lower in AV than the rate selected for the normal ventilating mode. If attempts are made to set it lower, a window appears stating, "Apnea Rate must be greater than or equal to set rate." The ventilator will automatically change the rate to equal the set rate (Clinical Rounds 12-40).

When AV occurs in NPPV, the ventilator delivers only mandatory breaths at the set apnea rate or in response to patient effort. The AV settings in NPPV include rate, IPAP, EPAP, I-time, rise time, I-trigger, E-trigger, $O_2\%$, and Apnea rate.

To return to normal ventilation, the operator presses the ALARM RESET button below the screen. Normal ventilation will also resume if the ventilator detects two consecutive inspiratory efforts from the patient.

> **CLINICAL ROUNDS 12-40**
>
> An adult patient receiving VCV-SIMV ventilation has a set rate of 8 breaths/min. The apnea ventilation rate is set at 4 breaths/min. If the ventilator goes into apnea ventilation, what will the actual mandatory breath rate be?
>
> See Appendix A for the answer.

Special Features

There are currently two options available for the Esprit, the oxygen sensor and the graphics software package.

An optional oxygen sensor may be installed to allow monitoring of inspired oxygen concentrations. O_2 sensor calibration is performed during EST. Sensors should be calibrated and replaced as needed based on the manufacturer's specifications. To prevent contamination of the O_2 sensor, it is placed between the ventilator gas output port and the inspiratory bacterial filter before being connected to the main inspiratory line of the patient circuit.

An optional graphics package is also available. This software adds a graphics screen that displays flow-time, pressure-time, and volume-time scalars. In addition flow-volume and pressure-volume loops are displayed. The graphics screen allows the operator to rescale the graphic, freeze a graphic display, and save and overlay an image. The latter feature can be used for pre- and post-bronchodilator comparison. The freeze function provides additional scrolling and identification of all parameter displayed values for both waveforms and loops.

Troubleshooting

The alarms previously described help to point out problems during ventilation. In addition, there are also messages that appear on the screen when the operator tries to set up parameters that are outside the available limits of ventilation. For example, in A/C volume ventilation, the I:E ratio is limited to a maximum of 3:1. If a peak flow, tidal volume, inspiratory hold, waveform, or apnea rate setting results in an I:E ratio of greater than 3:1, a message appears that reads "I:E Ratio must be less than 3:1. Check V_T, Peak Flow, Insp. Hold, (or apnea rate)." Also in A/C, the inspiratory time cannot exceed 9 seconds or a similar message appears.

In PCV, the I:E ratio cannot exceed 4:1. A message similar to the one mentioned previously will occur if the settings result in an inverse I:E ratio that is >4:1. The operator should check the inspiratory time, apnea rate, or rise time to be sure they are set appropriately. In NPPV, the I:E ratio is also limited to 4:1 or less. In NPPV the operator would adjust apnea rate, I-Time rate or breath rate to correct an I:E ratio problem.

A common error that operators make when they first begin to use the ventilator is in setting the flow sensitivity. If a flow of 2 L/min is set, the ventilator will trigger inspiratory flow when the flow through the circuit at end exhalation drops by 2 L/min (see Chapter 11, flow-triggering). The bias flow is automatically set by the ventilator 3 L/min higher than the trigger flow. For example, with a 2 L/min setting, the bias flow will be 5 L/min. If the patient is struggling to trigger the ventilator, the operator should check the appropriateness of the I-trigger setting.

Another item that is easy to forget is to press the "Activate ..." when the breath-type is changed.

The Esprit is not designed for operation near magnetic resonance imaging equipment and should be kept away from such equipment.

Siemens Servo 900C

The Servo 900C ventilator[1-4] was released in the United States in 1981 and was designed for use in infant, pediatric, or adult ventilation (Figure 12-92). It consists of a pneumatic section that sits over the electronic control section containing the operating controls and control panel and regulates gas flow to the patient.

Power Source

The Servo 900C requires a gas source and a standard electrical outlet for operation. It is pneumatically powered and electronically controlled, but does not use a microprocessor. It can be operated using either a high-pressure or a low-pressure gas source because both types of gas inlets are provided.

Internal Mechanism

The internal mechanism is shown in Figure 12-93. Compressed gases are blended to the desired F_IO_2 and enter the ventilator through either the high-pressure or low-pressure inlet one-way valve, although both can be used simultaneously. The high-pressure unit is usually powered by a blender that connects to high-pressure air and oxygen. The low-pressure port can be used to operate the ventilator without a high-pressure gas source. It is also used to administer anesthetic gases. From the inlet port, gas passes through an oxygen analyzer (O_2 cell), a bacterial filter, and into a plastic, spring-loaded bellows (see Figure 12-93).

The spring-loaded bellows provides the working pressure and is capable of delivering pressures up to 120 cm H_2O

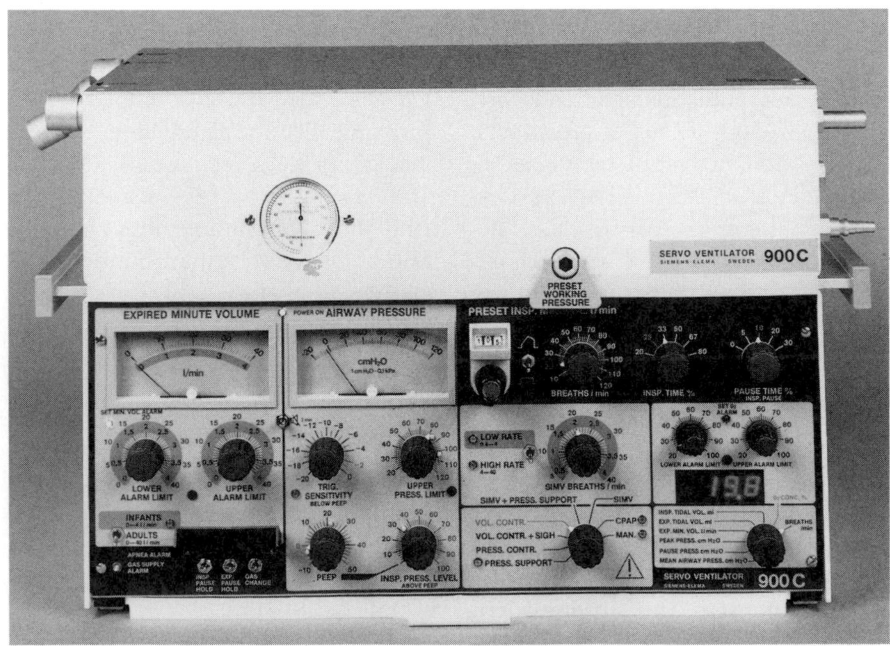

Figure 12-92 The Siemens-Elema Servo 900C. (Courtesy Siemens Medical Systems, Inc, Danvers, Mass.)

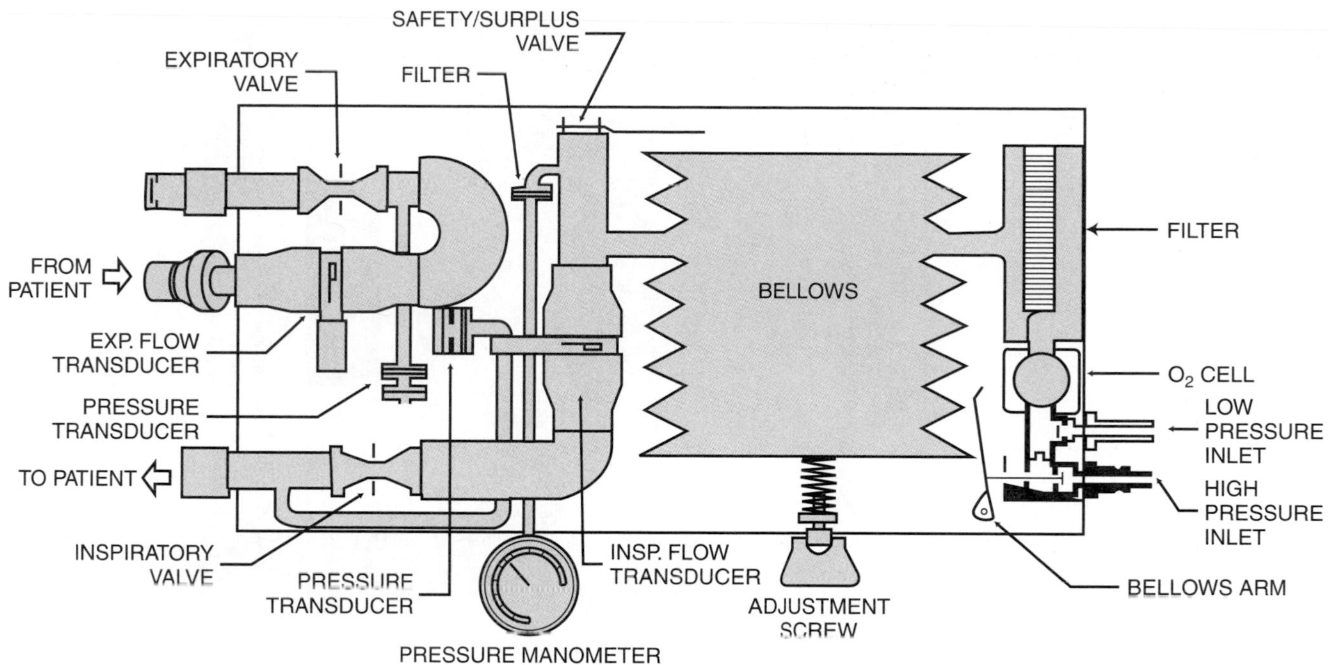

Figure 12-93 A view from above the pneumatic unit of the Servo 900C (see text for explanation). (Courtesy Siemens Medical Systems, Inc, Danvers, Mass.)

into the patient circuit (Box 12-106). Tension on the spring is adjusted by using a control adjustment marked preset working pressure, as shown in Figure 12-94. Spring tension determines the operating pressure within the bellows. During inspiration, gas from the bellows is directed into the patient circuit by way of an inspiratory servo valve that is composed of an inspiratory flow transducer and a scissor-like valve controlled by a stepper motor (see Figure 11-17). Gas passes through the flow transducer, where it is measured, and flows into the main inspiratory line of the patient circuit. At the same time, the expiratory servo valve is closed. The expiratory valve movement is controlled by an electromagnetic solenoid (pull-magnet). During exhalation, the expiratory valve opens and the patient exhales freely through the main expiratory line.

Controls and Alarms

The front control panel for the Servo 900C is divided into an upper and lower portion (see Figure 12-94). The front adjustment screw on the pneumatic section is used to control the working pressure, which is set above the peak pressure required to ventilate the patient. On the face of the pneumatic unit is a manometer that provides a reading of the working pressure inside the bellows. The lower portion (control interface) contains the remaining primary operating controls, alarms, monitors, and the mode setting control.

The left section of the control panel contains the HIGH- and LOW-$\dot{V}_E$ alarms, the EXPIRED $\dot{V}_E$ monitor, and several other alarms and indicators. At the lower left corner of the $\dot{V}_E$ monitor is a light that is illuminated when the limits for the $\dot{V}_E$ alarm have not been set. At the upper right of the $\dot{V}_E$ monitor there is a light indicator that is activated when the electric power is connected and is deactivated when power is disconnected (Box 12-107). The ALARM SILENCE button is located at the lower right corner of the $\dot{V}_E$ monitor. A switch at the lower left corner of the left panel governs the range of the $\dot{V}_E$ monitor settings. The adult settings for this switch range from 0 to 40 L/min; the infant settings range from 0 to 4 L/min (Clinical Rounds 12-41).

Three other alarm indicators are in this panel section: EXPIRED $\dot{V}_E$, APNEA, and GAS SUPPLY. The EXPIRED $\dot{V}_E$ alarm lights and sounds when the set alarm limits are exceeded (Table 12-37). The APNEA alarm gives an audio/visual signal if the time between two breaths (spontaneous or mandatory) is more than 15 seconds. The GAS SUPPLY alarm indicates an inadequate source gas pressure to maintain ventilation.

In the lower left section of the control panel, under a small panel cover are three special function buttons: INSPIRATORY PAUSE HOLD, EXPIRATORY PAUSE HOLD, and GAS CHANGE. When the INSPIRATORY PAUSE HOLD button is depressed, both inspiratory and expiratory valves close at the end of the inspiration, but before exhalation begins, and remain closed until the button is released. The unit automatically delays the next mandatory breath, which provides a manually controlled inspiratory hold or pause maneuver for estimating plateau pressure. Depressing the EXPIRATORY PAUSE HOLD button closes both inspiratory and expiratory valves at the end of exhalation for a prolonged expiratory pause and allows measurement of end-expiratory

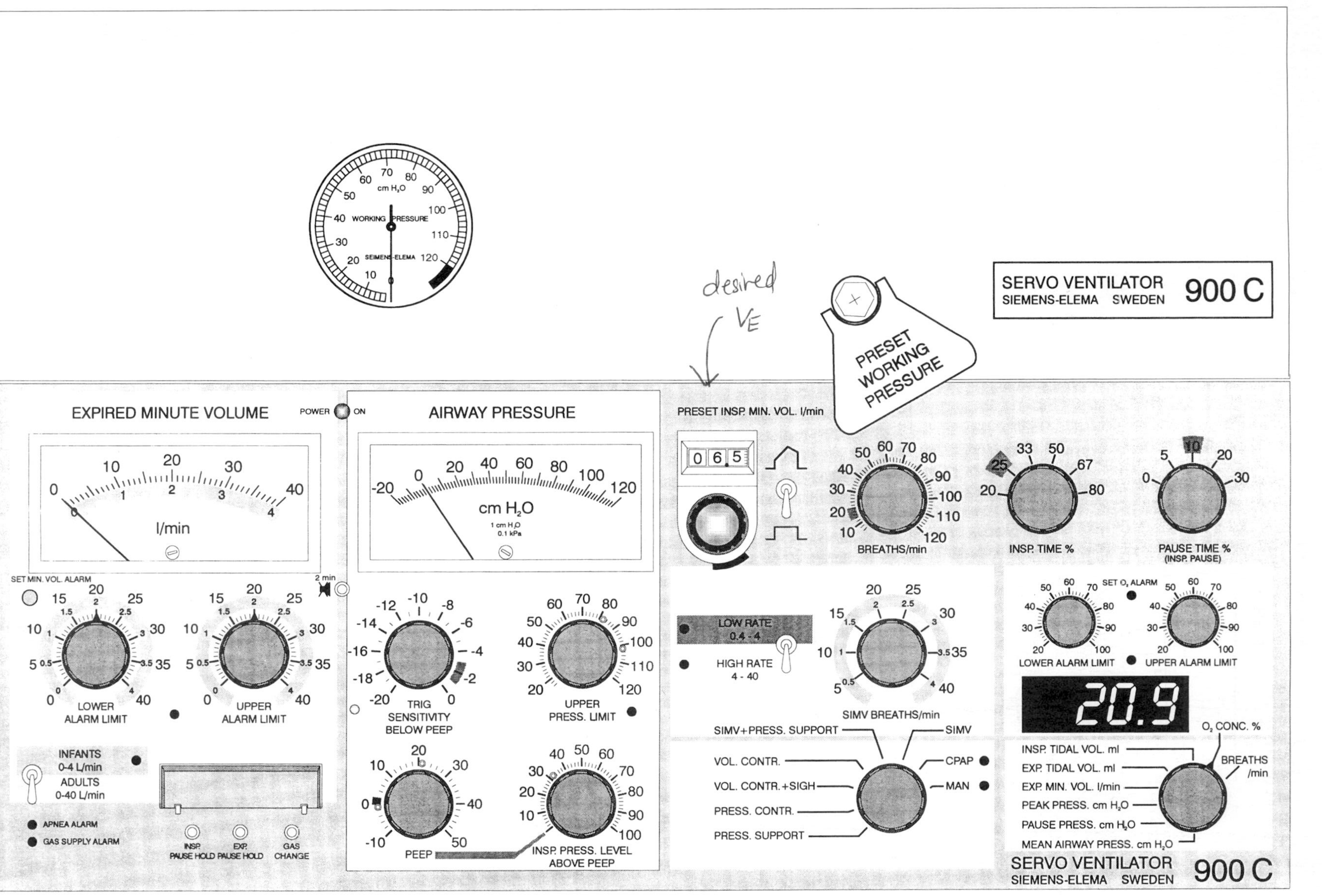

Figure 12-94 The control panel of the Servo 900C (see text for explanation). (Courtesy Yvon Dupuis.)

Box 12-106 Important Clinical Note

The bellows of the Servo 900C must have a pressurized gas source to fill and compress the spring, or the ventilator cannot operate (see Chapter 11, Figure 11-13).

Box 12-107 Important Clinical Note

The green power on light goes out if the ventilator is turned off (on/off switch on back of ventilator) or if the electrical power is disconnected. An audible alarm occurs, as well. To stop the sound, the alarm silence button must be pushed and held down for several seconds. If nothing is done, the sound will eventually stop on its own (in 5 to 10 minutes).

pressures (auto-PEEP). Pressing the GAS CHANGE button opens both valves and allows the bellows to empty its volume through the patient circuit. Gas continues to flow from the gas inlet through the bellows and the circuit as long as the button is depressed (Clinical Rounds 12-42). This allows for a rapid change of the O_2%. For example, the operator could use this control to flush the circuit with the desired O_2% before connecting the patient to the ventilator. In this way, the O_2% in the circuit is at the desired value as soon as the patient is attached.

The airway pressure panel contains the pressure manometer for monitoring inspiratory gas pressure. Below this manometer are four knob controls. The top left control is TRIG. SENSITIVITY BELOW PEEP, which establishes how much effort the patient must make to pressure-trigger inspiration. The UPPER PRESS. LIMIT is the next control. It sets the maximum pressure that can occur during inspiration. If this value is reached, inspiration ends (pressure-cycling). The next control is the PEEP control, which establishes the positive pressure baseline. The control marked INSP. PRESS. LEVEL ABOVE PEEP establishes the ventilating pressure for pressure-targeted ventilation in PCV and PSV. This control is only functional when either of those modes is selected (i.e., pressure control, pressure support, and SIMV + pressure support).

The right side of the operating panel has a row of controls across the top used for establishing volume delivery and respiratory rate. The first control is the PRESET INSPIR. MIN. VOL. L/(0.5 to 40 L/min). The front dial of this control is used to select the desired $\dot{V}_E$. Next to this is a STET switch to select either a constant flow pattern or what the manufacturer calls an accelerating inspiratory flow pattern. The flow patterns are only available during volume ventilation. To the right of the flow switch is the rate control knob (BREATHS/MIN). The setting on this control and the $\dot{V}_E$ setting determine the V_T ($V_T = \dot{V}_E$/rate). The INSP. TIME %

CLINICAL ROUNDS 12-41

An audible alarm sounds during initiation of ventilation for an adult patient with the 900C. The clinician notices a visual alarm between the $\dot{V}_E$ setting controls; however, the rate and volume of ventilation seem appropriate for the patient (6 L/min), and the patient is being ventilated. Examination of the patient reveals that breath sounds are present with good chest wall excursion. What could be the problem?

See Appendix A for the answer.

Table 12-37 Alarm Limits for the Minute Ventilation Alarm on the Servo 900C

	Adult	Infant
Upper alarm limit	3 to 43 L/min	0 to 4.3 L/min
Lower alarm limit	0 to 37 L/min	0 to 3.7 L/min

Courtesy Siemens Medical Systems, Inc.

CLINICAL ROUNDS 12-42

A patient will require hyperoxygenation prior to suctioning of the airway. What is a simple method for providing 100% oxygen to the patient through the ventilator?

See Appendix A for the answer.

(20% to 80%) and the PAUSE TIME % (0% to 30%, or inspiratory pause) controls determine the length of inspiration. The sum of these two settings represents T_I. T_I cannot exceed 80% of the TCT when TCT is based on the breaths/minute setting (Box 12-108).

The $\dot{V}_E$ control and T_I % can be used to calculate inspiratory gas flow when the constant flow waveform is selected. Multiplying the $\dot{V}_E$ by (100%/T_I%) equals the gas flow. Look at the following example:

$\dot{V}_E$ is 10 L/min

T_I % is 20%

10L/min × (100%/20%) = 10 L/min × 5 = 50 L/min

Box 12-108 Inspiratory Time and Total Cycle Time on the Servo 900C

T_I, T_E, and I:E are determined by the settings of the BREATHS/MIN, INSP.TIME %, and PAUSE TIME % controls.

Example

Suppose that the BREATHS/MIN control is set at 10, INSP. TIME % is 33%, and PAUSE TIME % is 0%.

$$TCT = 60 \text{ seconds/rate}$$

$$TCT = 60 \div 10 \text{ breaths/min, or 6 seconds}$$

$$T_I = TCT \times (\text{insp. time \%* + pause time \%*})$$

$$T_I = 6 \text{ seconds} \times 0.33^* = 2 \text{ seconds}$$

$$T_E = TCT - T_I = 6 \text{ seconds} - 2 \text{ seconds} = 4 \text{ seconds}$$

$$I{:}E = 1{:}(T_E/T_I) = 1{:}(4/2) = 1{:}2$$

Example

Suppose that BREATHS/MIN is set at 15, INSP. TIME % is 20%, and PAUSE TIME % is 10%.

$$TCT = 60 \text{ seconds/rate}$$

$$TCT = 60 \div 15 \text{ breaths/min, or 4 seconds}$$

$$T_I = TCT \times (\text{insp. time \%* + pause time \%*})$$

$$T_I = 4 \text{ seconds} \times 0.30 = 1.2 \text{ seconds}$$

$$T_E = TCT - T_I = 4 \text{ seconds} - 1.2 \text{ seconds} = 2.8 \text{ seconds}$$

$$I{:}E = 1{:}(T_E/T_I) = 1{:}(2.8/1.2) = 1{:}2.33$$

Example

Suppose the BREATHS/MIN is set at 12, the INSP. TIME % is 67%, and the PAUSE TIME % is 20%.

$$TCT = T_I + T_E, \text{ or 60 seconds/rate}$$

$$TCT = 60 \div 12 \text{ breaths/min, or 5 seconds}$$

$$T_I = TCT \times (\text{insp. time \%* + pause time \%*})$$

$$T_I = 5 \text{ seconds} \times 0.87^* = 4.35 \text{ seconds}$$

$$T_E = TCT - T_I = 5 \text{ seconds} - 4.35 \text{ seconds} = 0.65 \text{ seconds}$$

$$I{:}E = 1{:}(T_E/T_I) = 1{:}(0.65/4.35) = 1{:}0.15 \text{ or } 6.7{:}1$$

In this example, how would the ventilator respond? What is wrong with this situation?

See Appendix A for the answer.

*Changed from a percentage to a fraction.

Box 12-109 Adjusting Flow by Using the SIMV Rate

A patient is being ventilated in the volume-control mode with the 900C. The rate is set at 12 breaths/min, $\dot{V}_E$ is set at 6 L/min, T_I% is 20%, and pause % is 0%. The flow waveform is set on constant (rectangular). What is the V_T? What is the estimated inspiratory flow?

$$V_T = (6 \text{ L/min}) / (12 \text{ breaths/min}) = 0.5 \text{ L}$$

$$6 \text{ L/min} \times (100\%/20\%) = 6 \text{ L/min} \times 5 = 30 \text{ L/min}$$

The patient has a high inspiratory flow demand, and the respiratory therapist must increase flow to the patient. T_I% is already at its shortest rate. How could this be done without changing $\dot{V}_E$?

The therapist could change to SIMV at the same rate (12 breaths/min). Then he or she could increase the breaths/min rate and the $\dot{V}_E$ settings to higher values that would still give a 0.5 L (500 mL) V_T. For example, 24 breaths/min at a $\dot{V}_E$ of 12 L/min provides a V_T of 500 mL (or 48 breaths/min at $\dot{V}_E$ of 24 L/min provides a V_T of 500 mL).

For these two examples, calculate the new flow:

Example 1: 12 L/min × (100%/20%) = 60 L/min

Example 2: 24 L/min × (100%/20%) = 120 L/min

Will these changes alter the rate or the $\dot{V}_E$? No. The rate is now established by the SIMV rate control, which is at the original rate of 12/min. V_T is still 500 mL. The parameters that have changed are the T_I, which changed the flow, and the mode, which is now SIMV. The guaranteed $\dot{V}_E$ is still the same.

(*Note:* It could be argued that changing to SIMV may not be appropriate. A patient with a high inspiratory demand may also need a higher $\dot{V}_E$. The problem with switching to SIMV is that not every patient effort will be fully supported with a mandatory breath as with A/C.)

What will happen if the T_I% is increased to 50%? Will the flow increase or decrease for the same $\dot{V}_E$? See the following equation:

$$10 \text{ L/min} \times (100\%/50\%) = 10 \times 2 = 20 \text{ L/min}$$

If T_I% is longer with the same $\dot{V}_E$, flow will be slower. Box 12-109 shows how using SIMV rate control can help the clinician increase flow without changing V_T or $\dot{V}_E$.

Below the $\dot{V}_E$ and rate settings is another set of controls. The first two controls are for setting the respiratory rate during SIMV ventilation. On the right is the SIMV BREATHS/MIN knob, which is exclusively for controlling the respiratory rate in the SIMV mode. On the left is a toggle switch for selecting the range in which the SIMV BREATHS/MIN knob operates. In the up (LOW RATE) position, the rate ranges from 0.4 to 4 breaths/min. When it is down

(HIGH RATE position), the rate range is active, providing from 4 to 40 breaths/min. These two controls are active whenever an SIMV mode is selected (SIMV and SIMV + pressure support). In SIMV, the SIMV BREATHS/MIN control establishes the mandatory breath rate and must be set lower than the BREATHS/MIN control. If it is set higher, the ventilator defaults to the BREATHS/MIN control for rate and overrides the SIMV BREATHS/MIN setting. For example, if BREATHS/MIN is set at 10, and SIMV BREATHS/MIN is set at 12, the ventilator will deliver 10 breaths/min.

The knob for ventilator modes on the lower panel of this section determines which mode is active. The eight available positions on this knob are included in the following discussion of modes of ventilation.

Finally, the far right section of the operating panel contains the knobs for setting the oxygen alarm (SET O_2 ALARM, LOWER ALARM LIMIT, UPPER ALARM LIMIT), and a digital window displaying various measured and calculated parameters. These parameters can be displayed by rotating the knob just below the digital window, which allows the practitioner to view the following:

- MEAN AIRWAY PRESS. (cm H_2O)
- PAUSE PRESS. (cm H_2O)
- PEAK PRESS. (cm H_2O)
- EXP. MIN. VOL. (L/min)
- EXP. TIDAL VOL. (mL)
- INSP. TIDAL VOL. (mL)
- O_2 CONC %
- BREATHS/MINUTE

Modes of Ventilation

The Siemens Servo 900C can provide eight different modes of ventilation through its mode selection switch (see Figure 12-94).

Volume-Control

A/C volume ventilation is available under the control marked VOL. CONTR. The inspiratory $\dot{V}_E$ is set as desired and the BREATHS/MIN control is set to the desired rate to establish the desired V_T. For example, if the $\dot{V}_E$ is set to 5 L/min and the rate to 12 breaths/min, the V_T will be 600 mL (V_T = [5 L/min]/[12 breaths/min]).

The following additional parameters may also be set in A/C:

- Inspiratory time percentage
- Trigger sensitivity
- PEEP
- F_IO_2
- Inspiratory pause

Breaths are patient- (pressure-) or time-triggered, volume-targeted, and time-cycled. For the rate just presented, set the insp. time % at 33% and the flow waveform on constant. The TCT will be 5 seconds (60 seconds/12 breaths/min), and the T_I will be 33% of 5 seconds, or 1.65 seconds.

Volume Control + Sigh

Volume control plus sigh provides patient- or time-triggered, volume-targeted, time-cycled ventilation with a sigh breath every 100 breaths. The T_I and V_T are doubled for a sigh breath. When the mode switch is moved to this setting, the sigh breath occurs on the second breath, giving the clinician an opportunity to evaluate peak pressure for a sigh breath.

Pressure Control

PCV provides patient- or time-triggered, pressure-targeted, time-cycled breaths. The inspiratory pressure setting determines the pressure level above PEEP (baseline). Both working pressure and the upper pressure limit need to be set appropriately, as with any mode of ventilation. A breath will pressure-cycle if the upper pressure limit is reached. This helps to avoid dangerously high pressures.

Pressure Support

PSV is patient- (pressure-) triggered, pressure-targeted, and flow-cycled. As with pressure control, the target pressure is set using the inspiratory pressure control (above PEEP). The main difference between PCV and PSV is when the flow decreases to about 25% of the peak flow measured during inspiration, PSV is flow-cycled out of inspiration. As a safety feature, inspiratory flow also ends if the airway pressure rises 3 cm H_2O above the set pressure or if T_I exceeds 80% of the TCT based on the set rate on the BREATHS/MIN control (Clinical Rounds 12-43).

Synchronized Intermittent Mandatory Ventilation

SIMV on the Servo 900C is similar to that on other ventilators. The rate is determined by the SIMV BREATHS/MIN control knob, which is set lower than the BREATHS/MIN knob. The BREATHS/MIN knob determines the time of a

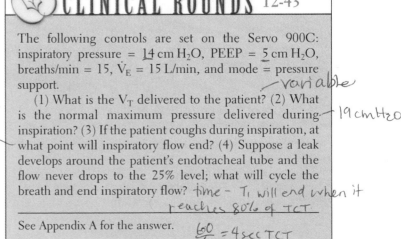

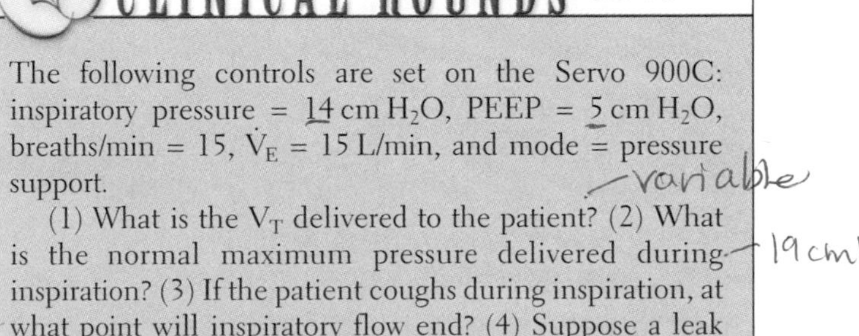
CLINICAL ROUNDS 12-43

The following controls are set on the Servo 900C: inspiratory pressure = 14 cm H_2O, PEEP = 5 cm H_2O, breaths/min = 15, $\dot{V}_E$ = 15 L/min, and mode = pressure support.

(1) What is the V_T delivered to the patient? (2) What is the normal maximum pressure delivered during inspiration? (3) If the patient coughs during inspiration, at what point will inspiratory flow end? (4) Suppose a leak develops around the patient's endotracheal tube and the flow never drops to the 25% level; what will cycle the breath and end inspiratory flow?

See Appendix A for the answer.

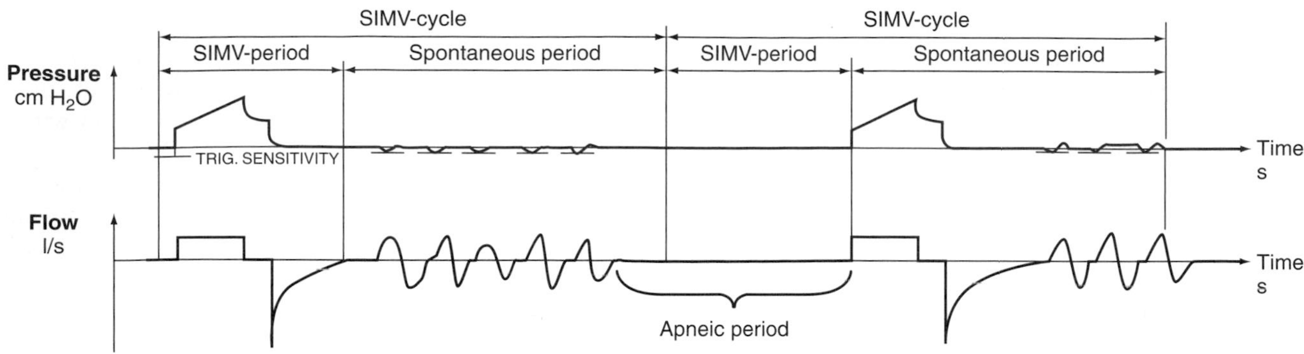

Figure 12-95 The SIMV cycle (see text for explanation). (Courtesy Siemens Medical Systems, Inc, Danvers, Mass.)

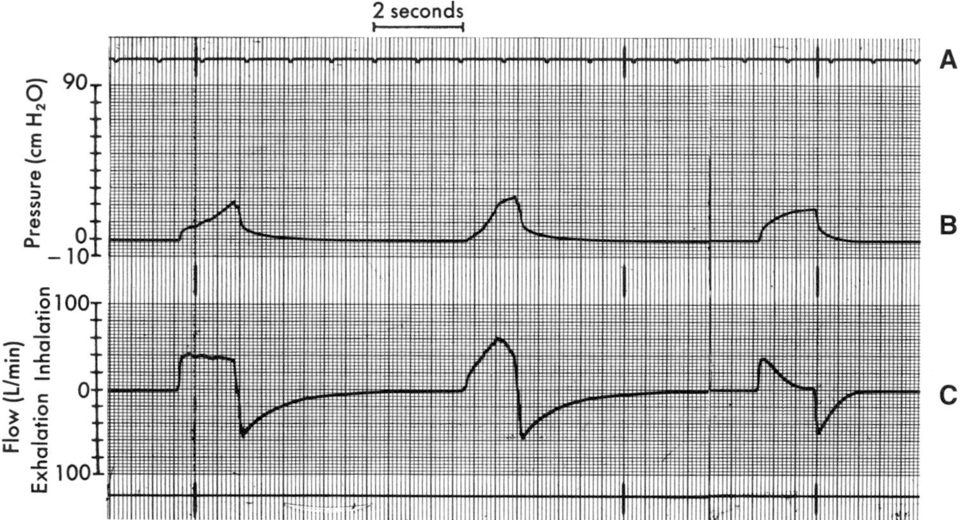

Figure 12-96 Flow and pressure patterns for the Servo 900B. Lung analog is set for 50 mL/cm H_2O compliance and 5 cm H_2O/L/sec resistance. **A,** the flow waveform is constant (rectangular). **B,** The flow waveform is a sine-wavelike pattern. **C,** Working pressure is reduced to 20 cm H_2O, and the lung analog is set for 10 mL/cm H_2O compliance and 5 cm H_2O/L/sec resistance. Note the descending shape of the flow curve with increased load and reduced working pressure. (Courtesy Siemens Medical Systems, Inc, Danvers, Mass.)

mandatory breath delivery. V_T is still determined by the set $\dot{V}_E$ and the BREATHS/MIN rate setting. This mode is divided into different time frames (Figure 12-95), as follows:

1. An SIMV-cycle, which is the period of time between mandatory breaths (SIMV-cycle = 60/SIMV-rate setting)
2. An SIMV-period, which is the time allotted for each mandatory breath (SIMV-period = 60/BREATHS/MIN knob setting)
3. A spontaneous breathing period, which equals the SIMV-cycle minus the SIMV-period

For example, with the BREATHS/MIN knob set at 15 breaths/min and the SIMV rate is set at 6 breaths/min, the following are true:

- SIMV-cycle = 60/6 = 10 seconds
- SIMV-period = 60/15 = 4 seconds
- Spontaneous breathing period = 10 seconds − 4 seconds = 6 seconds

Figure 12-95 helps show the spacing of breaths in SIMV. When the patient triggers a breath, the ventilator delivers a volume-targeted, time-cycled breath. The patient can then breathe spontaneously at the baseline pressure. The SIMV-cycle is timed from the beginning of the mandatory breath. When this time has elapsed, the ventilator waits for a patient effort during the SIMV period that follows. An effort sufficient to trigger a breath during this period will deliver the set volume. If the patient fails to take a breath during this period, the ventilator will time-trigger a mandatory breath.

SIMV + Pressure Support

SIMV + pressure support is the same as SIMV described above except that spontaneous breaths are pressure-supported at the level indicated on the INSP. PRESS. ABOVE PEEP control.

Continuous Positive Airway Pressure (CPAP)

CPAP is a purely spontaneous mode that provides the option of a positive-pressure baseline (0 to 50 cm H_2O).

Manual

The manual mode is generally restricted to use in the operating room in conjunction with an anesthesia bag and a manual ventilation valve (accessory equipment). The manual ventilation valve is attached to the ventilator's outflow port and is connected to the inspiratory line of the patient circuit, similar to an anesthesia system. When circuit pressure rises above 4 cm H_2O during manual inflation, the expiratory valve closes and gas goes to the patient. When pressure drops below 4 cm H_2O during expiration, the expiration valve opens. When circuit pressure is less than 2 cm H_2O, demand flow fills the bag. The amount of flow into the bag is determined by the preset $\dot{V}_E$. The apnea alarm does not work in this mode. A patient can breathe spontaneously from the circuit as long as the inspiratory effort is great enough to open the valve (–2 cm H_2O).

Troubleshooting

The flow pattern on the 900C can only be maintained when adequate working pressure is set. Driving force can be reduced so that the peak pressure generated during a mechanical breath is nearly equal to the working pressure inside the bellows. Flow will then decrease or taper during inspiration, and V_T will be variable (Figure 12-96).

Use caution when reducing the breaths/min rate. As the rate drops, the V_T increases. For example, if the $\dot{V}_E$ is 5 L/min and the rate is 10 breaths/min, V_T is 0.5 L. Decreasing the rate to 6 breaths/min raises the V_T to 0.83 L. For this reason, it is usually advisable to reduce volume before rate when making a $\dot{V}_E$ change.

There is a troubleshooting section in the operating manual to help identify common problems.

Siemens Servo 300

The Servo 300 Ventilator[1-3] is manufactured by the Siemens-Elema AB Medical Systems Corporation (Solna, Sweden) primarily for use in the intensive care unit for neonatal, pediatric, or adult patients. It consists of two sections connected by a 2.9-meter cable. One section is the control or operating panel. The other is the patient unit, which connects directly to the patient circuit. The patient circuit consists of a main inspiratory and a main expiratory line.

The control panel contains the electronic circuits that control ventilator function (Figure 12-97). It also contains the touch pads and dials with which the operator selects specific patient settings. The control panel provides illuminated information about selected parameters (green digital display) and measured parameters (red digital display). The patient unit controls the flow of gas to the patient. Flow and pressure are continually measured within the patient unit and compared with the control panel settings and adjusted as needed. Practitioners often purchase the graphics monitor and an end-tidal carbon dioxide module as important additional items for monitoring patients.

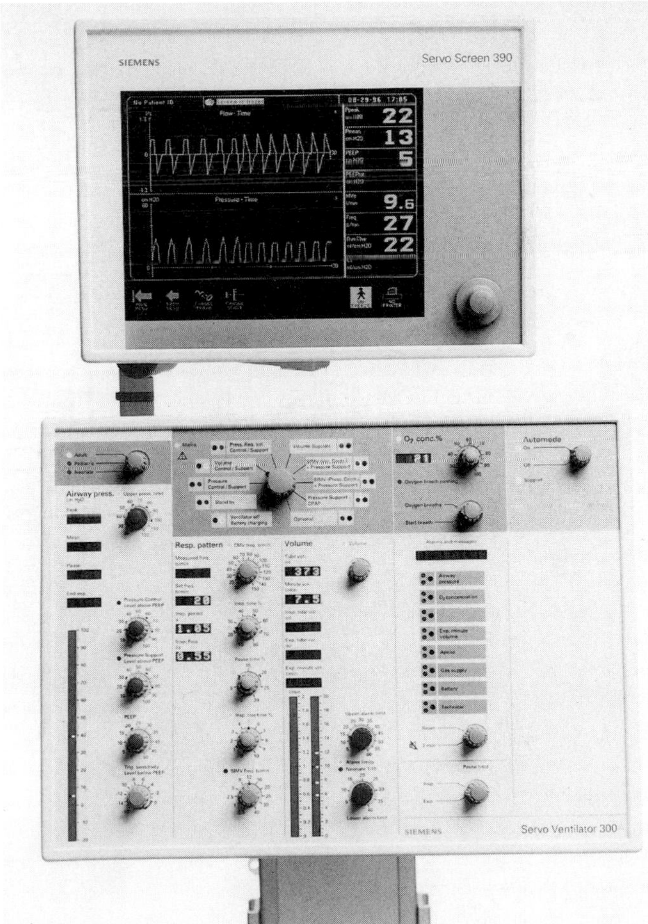

Figure 12-97 The Servo 300A with the graphics monitor on top. (Courtesy Siemens-Elema AB, Solna, Sweden.)

Power Source

A standard 110- or 120-volt electrical outlet provides power to the display unit and the microprocessor-control unit. Two 50-psig (range from 29 to 94 psig) gas sources for air and oxygen are also normally used to power the Servo 300 and to provide the flow to the patient (single-circuit ventilator). (*Note:* The unit can function with a single high-pressure gas source, but O_2% delivery may be altered.) This ventilator also contains two internal 12-volt batteries that provide back-up electrical power. The discussion of alarm features in this section reviews ventilator operation when either the electrical power or the gas supply fails.

The ON power switch is on the front panel at the top center of the ventilator control panel and is the same control that allows the operator to switch modes of ventilation (see Figure 12-97). Switching to any of the ventilator modes activates the ventilator. Switching it from any mode back to the VENTILATOR OFF BATTERY CHARGING setting turns the ventilator off, but also activates an audible alert. In older models, the FAB (failure alarm box) alarm control was on the top, left side of the ventilator and was pressed to

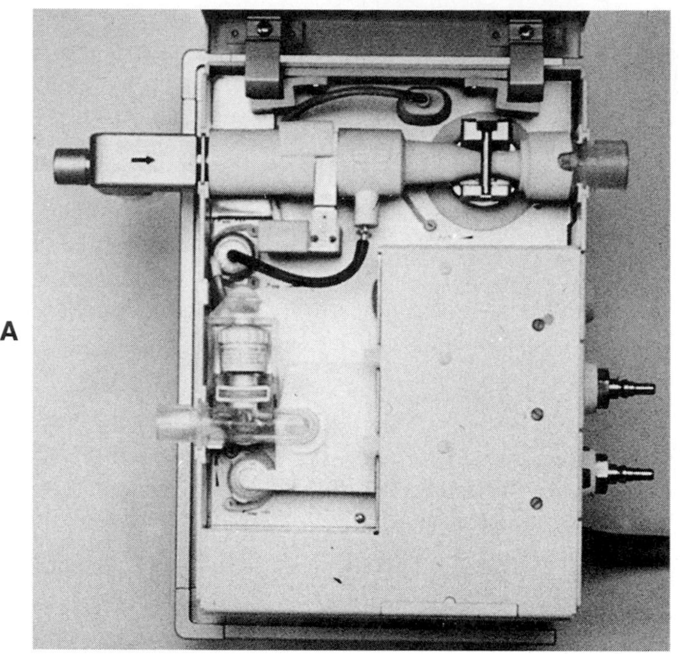

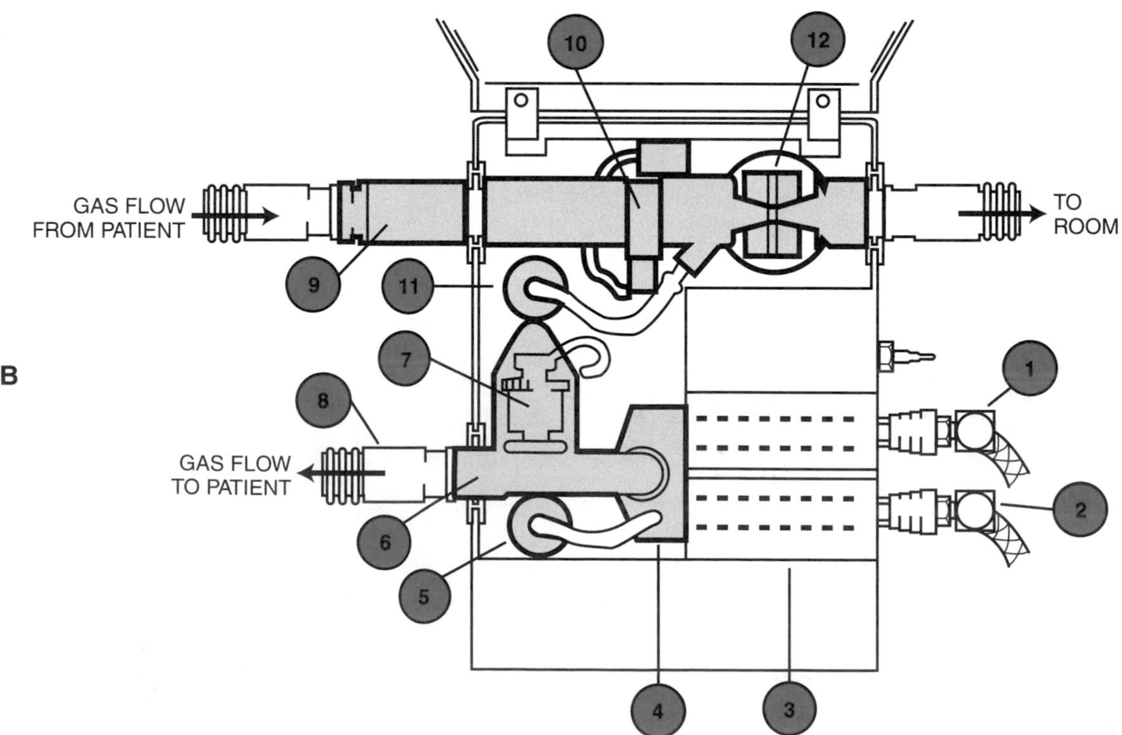

Figure 12-98 Internal components of the Siemens Servo 300. **A,** Photograph of the internal components. **B,** Diagram of the internal components (see text for explanation). (**A,** Courtesy Siemens-Elema AB, Solna, Sweden.)

deactivate. In newer models, the FAB alarm is internal and does not require deactivation.

Internal Mechanism

The flow delivery of gas to the patient is controlled by a high-performance, rapid-response (4 to 6 milliseconds) solenoid valve. Figure 12-98 shows the internal components of the Servo 300. The air and oxygen sources enter through separate gas inlets (1 and 2). They pass through bacterial filters and enter the gas modules where pressures are monitored (3). The two gas sources leave their respective modules and enter a mixing chamber, and pressure is again measured (4). Knowing the pressures within the modules and mixing chamber, the flow solenoid can determine the operation of the pin or needle valve that controls gas flow into the unit. The exiting gas is again measured for pressure (5) as it enters the inspiratory line (6). The inspiratory line houses a pressure release or a safety valve (120 cm H_2O maximum), the housing for the oxygen analyzer (7), and the main outlet for gas going from the ventilator to the patient (8).

The patient's expired gas passes into the ventilator through the connector for the main expiratory line (9), where expiratory gas flow (10) and pressure (11) are measured. (*Note:* Patient circuit pressures are monitored by both the inspiratory [5] and the expiratory [11] pressure transducers. Transducers also monitor flow for flow-triggering.)

Gas then passes through the expiratory valve (12), which helps control the phasing (inspiration/expiration) of a breath and the level of PEEP present in the expiratory line. The expiratory valve, also called a gate valve, contains a soft, compressible tube that passes between two rollers. These rollers float and come together to adjust resistance to expiration when PEEP is employed and also open and close to allow phasing of a breath. The gas then passes out of the ventilator through the expiratory one-way valve.

Controls and Alarms

The control panel contains nine sections (Figure 12-99), which include the following: 1) PATIENT RANGE SELECTION; 2) AIRWAY PRESSURES; 3) MODE SELECTION; 4) RESPIRATORY PATTERN; 5) VOLUMES; 6) OXYGEN CONCENTRATION; 7) ALARMS, MESSAGES, and ALARM SILENCE/RESET; 8) PAUSE HOLD; and 9) AUTOMODE.

Patient Range Selection

The patient range selection knob at the upper left corner lets the operator pick the appropriate setting based on patient size: ADULT, PEDIATRIC, or NEONATE. This selection affects several ventilator parameters (Table 12-38).

Airway Pressures

The left panel contains four pressure controls, one control for trigger sensitivity, four digital monitors of airway pressure, and a bar graph display of monitored pressure. The four pressure controls are as follows:

1. UPPER PRESS. LIMIT (16 to 120 cm H_2O)
2. PRESSURE-CONTROL LEVEL ABOVE PEEP (0 to 100 cm H_2O)
3. PRESSURE-SUPPORT LEVEL ABOVE PEEP (0 to 100 cm H_2O)
4. PEEP (0 to 50 cm H_2O)

The UPPER PRESSURE LIMIT is for patient safety and limits the maximum airway pressure in all modes of ventilation. If the UPPER PRESSURE LIMIT is reached during breath delivery, inspiration ends and an audible alarm activates. The pressure control knob is active in two modes of ventilation: Pressure control and SIMV (PRESS.CONTR.) + pressure support. The pressure support knob is active in three modes: pressure support, SIMV (VOL.CONTR.) + pressure support, and SIMV (PRESS.CONTR.) + pressure support. These are discussed in the following section on mode selection. PEEP sets pressure during exhalation in any mode currently available.

The TRIG. SENSITIVITY LEVEL BELOW PEEP is the knob that determines the patient effort required to trigger a breath and is active in all modes. It provides flow- or pressure-triggering. Pressure-triggering is set by turning the knob counterclockwise to the indicated pressures (0 to –17 cm H_2O). This reduces the sensitivity, making triggering more difficult. The flow-triggering setting is indicated by the green and red (most sensitive) markings on the dial. With flow-triggering selected, a low flow of gas passes through the patient circuit only during the expiratory phase and is monitored by both the inspiratory and expiratory flow transducers. Flow-triggering of a breath occurs when the expiratory flow transducer measures a drop in flow (see Chapter 11, flow-triggering). The set bias flow in the Servo 300 is based on the size of patient selected (adult, pediatric, or neonatal; see Table 12-38). For example, when adult is selected on the patient selection switch, 2 L/min flows through the circuit during exhalation. The flow-trigger range for an adult is 0.7 to 2 L/min, depending on where the operator sets the triggering sensitivity dial. The closer the dial is set to the red area, the less the amount of flow that must be removed and the more sensitive the triggering.

The airway pressure monitors provide illuminated red digital readouts of measured values for peak, pause, and end-expiratory pressures and a calculated value for mean pressure. PIP is the highest pressure reached during inspiration, as measured by the inspiratory pressure transducer. It is displayed on the pressure bar graph, which is described later in this section. The upper pressure limit uses this value for its operation, but the digital display value of PIP is the pressure measured by the expiratory pressure transducer.

Mean pressure is a calculated value based on the pressure measured during each complete breath cycle (inspiration plus expiration).

Pause pressure displays the pressure measured by the expiratory pressure transducer when a pause time is selected

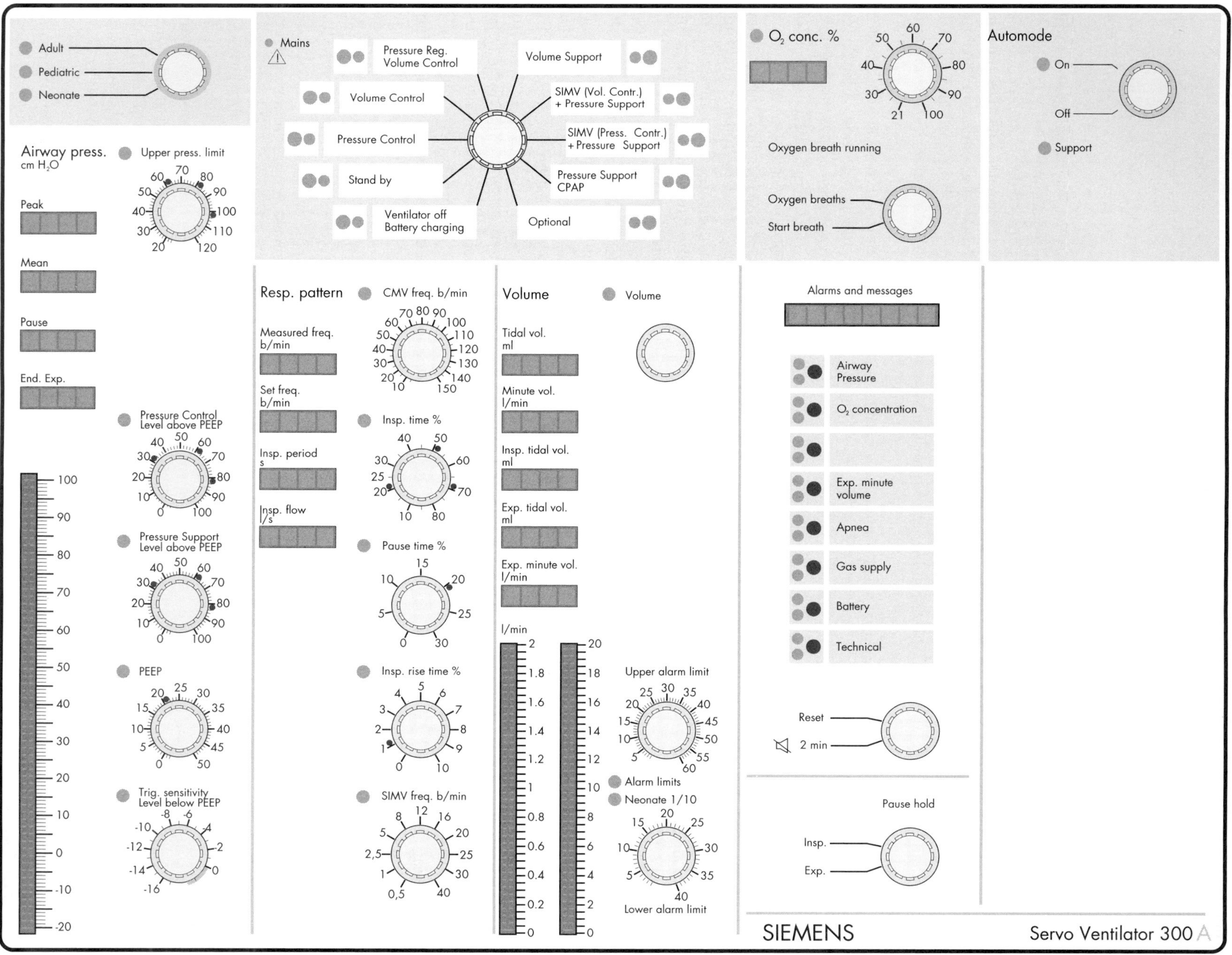

Figure 12-99 The front control panel of the Siemens Servo 300A (see text for explanation). (Courtesy Yvon Dupuis.)

Table 12-38 Parameters and Functions Affected by Patient Range Selections

CONTINUOUS FLOW THROUGH THE CIRCUIT DURING EXHALATION	
Adult setting	2 L/min
Pediatric setting	1 L/min
Neonatal setting	0.5 L/min
MAXIMUM INSPIRATORY PEAK FLOW	
Adult setting	200 L/min
Pediatric setting	33 L/min
Neonatal setting	13 L/min
MAXIMUM MEASURED TIDAL VOLUME	
Adult setting	3999 mL (range 0 to 4000 mL)
Pediatric setting	399 mL (range 0 to 400 mL)
Neonatal setting	39 mL (range 0 to 40 mL)
APNEA ALARM TIME	
Adult setting	20 seconds
Pediatric setting	15 seconds
Neonatal setting	10 seconds
FLOW TRIGGER RANGE	
Adult setting	0.7 to 2.0 L/min
Pediatric setting	0.3 to 1.0 L/min
Neonatal setting	0.17 to 0.5 L/min
UPPER ALARM LIMIT–MINUTE VENTILATION	
Adult setting	0 to 60 L/min
Pediatric setting	0 to 60 L/min
Neonatal setting	0 to 6 L/min
LOWER ALARM LIMIT–MINUTE VENTILATION	
Adult setting	0.3 to 40 L/min
Pediatric setting	0.3 to 40 L/min
Neonatal setting	0.06 to 4 L/min

Courtesy Siemens Medical, Inc.

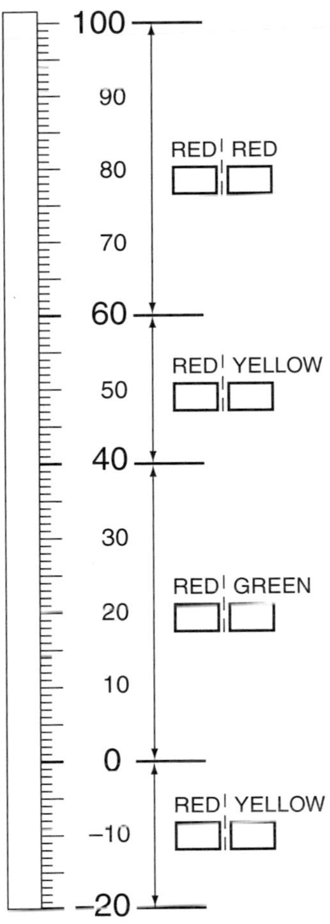

Figure 12-100 An airway pressure bar graph for the Servo 300 ventilator. This is an enlargement of the lower left hand section of the main panel (see text for explanation). (Courtesy Siemens-Elema AB, Solna, Sweden.)

on the PAUSE TIME % control or when the manual inspiratory pause (INSP.) is held during inspiration long enough for a pause to occur. It can be activated whenever a mandatory volume or pressure breath occurs in SIMV or A/C modes. The end-expiratory pressure display shows the pressure at the end of each breath and is also measured by the expiratory pressure transducer. When an expiratory pause is manually activated, both the inspiratory and expiratory valves close and this window display shows the value for total PEEP ($PEEP_I + PEEP_E$) as measured by the ventilator.

The airway pressure bar graph has flashing diodes of various colors, which monitor several pressure values. The diodes on the left side are red. The diodes on the right have different colors, depending on the pressure level. The right diodes are yellow for values less than 0 cm H_2O, green for values from 0 to 40 cm H_2O, yellow for values from 40 to 60 cm H_2O, and red for values from 60 to 100 cm H_2O. The upper pressure limit is indicated by four diodes (two on the left, two on the right) that flash when the pressure limit is reached or when it is set above 100 cm H_2O. The lower diodes on the bar graph indicate the pressure settings.

The actual airway pressure is shown by two side-by-side flashing diodes. The left one shows pressure measured by the inspiratory transducer and the right one shows that measured by the expiratory pressure transducer. Because they are measured at different places, the operator will see separations occurring between the two when they reflect pressure variations such as the rebound of pressure within the patient circuit or resistance to expiratory flow in the circuit. The value for the peak pressure digital display corresponds to the right illuminated diode (Figure 12-100). The pressure-control, pressure-support, and PEEP settings are shown by two diodes. If pressure support is set higher than pressure control, the diodes indicating both controls start flashing. PEEP is the lowest set of diodes because PC and PS are additive to the set PEEP value.

A patient-triggered breath is indicated on the bar graph by two red and yellow flashing diodes that appear on the bottom right.

Mode Selection

At the top center of the control panel is a rotating knob with nine different positions (see Figure 12-99). These include VENTILATOR OFF BATTERY CHARGING, STAND BY, PRESSURE CONTROL, VOLUME CONTROL, PRESSURE REG VOLUME CONTROL, VOLUME SUPPORT, SIMV (VOL.CONTR.) + PRESSURE SUPPORT, SIMV (PRESS.CONTR.) + PRESSURE SUPPORT, PRESSURE SUPPORT—CPAP, and OPTIONAL.

VENTILATOR OFF BATTERY CHARGING is the off position for the ventilator. Keeping the ventilator plugged into an electrical outlet with the knob in this position recharges the internal battery. The manufacturer recommends this as the best option for the ventilator when it is not in use. When the ventilator is in the STANDBY position, the electrical circuits are supplied with power and the expiratory flow transducer can warm up to its operating temperature (104° F, 40° C). Patient settings can be selected for use while the ventilator is in STANDBY. The seven ventilator modes are described in the discussion of modes of ventilation later in this section.

The OPTIONAL position of the mode knob has no function, but can be used to add future upgrades.

Respiratory Pattern Settings

Below the panel that contains the modes selection control is a panel that governs the respiratory pattern and digitally displays the selected and measured values. There are a total of five control knobs: CMV FREQ. B/MIN, INSP.TIME%, PAUSE TIME %, INSP.RISE TIME%, and SIMV FREQ.B/MIN. There are also four digital display panels: MEASURED FREQ. B/MIN, SET FREQ.B/MIN, INSP. PERIOD S, and INSP. FLOW L/S.

The control marked CMV FREQ. B/MIN sets the number of mandatory breaths per minute when volume control, pressure control, or pressure-regulated volume control are set on the mode selection knob (5 to 150 breaths/min). These modes are described as control modes by the manufacturer in relation to the new feature Automode (see modes of ventilation). It is recommended that the CMV FREQ. B/MIN knob always be set appropriately for the patient being ventilated because it determines the TCT (breath cycle time) for all modes. The ventilator does not permit T_I to exceed 80% of this TCT. In addition, CMV FREQ.B/MIN is the back-up rate for volume support, if the patient becomes apneic.

INSP. TIME % determines the percentage of time spent providing inspiratory gas flow (10% to 80%) based on the TCT. All mandatory breaths in either volume- or pressure-control ventilation are time-cycled in either A/C or SIMV modes.

> **CLINICAL ROUNDS 12-44**
>
> The respiratory therapist decides to use IRV on a patient who is difficult to oxygenate with the Servo 300 in volume control. The INSP. TIME % control is turned to 80%, and the PAUSE TIME % to 10%. The yellow light next to the PAUSE TIME % control begins to flash. What does this indicate?
>
> See Appendix A for the answer.

PAUSE TIME % (0 to 30% of TCT) provides an inspiratory pause (no inspiratory gas flow) and increases the length of inspiration for a volume-controlled breath. The sum of inspiratory time and pause time can never exceed 80% of the total cycle time, as determined by the rate set on the CMV FREQ. B/MIN knob—regardless of the ventilator mode (Clinical Rounds 12-44). If the sum of these two settings exceeds 80%, the adjacent yellow indicator light flashes.

INSP. RISE TIME % determines the time (% of TCT) in which the flow or pressure will gradually rise to the set value in any mode of ventilation. INSP. RISE TIME % is considered a patient comfort feature in adults and a lung protective strategy in newborns because it prevents pressure overshoots. As long as the value is set above zero (range 0% to 10% of TCT), the delivery of pressure and flow is tapered and does not instantly increase to the set value at the beginning of inspiration. Figure 12-101 shows how sloping affects pressure and flow delivery. At the zero setting there is no sloping, and pressure and flow rise rapidly. This can be uncomfortable for a patient and can cause oscillations or ringing in the patient circuit (see Figure 11-86). The maximum rise time setting of 10% gives the maximum time for tapering flow and pressure delivery as well as a more gradual rise to the set parameters.

SIMV FREQ. B/MIN determines the minimum number of breaths per minute when either SIMV mode is selected (range 0.5 to 40 breaths/min). It must be set at a value lower than the CMV FREQ. B/MIN control, or the ventilator will default to the frequency set on the CMV FREQ. B/MIN and the yellow light adjacent to the SIMV FREQ. B/MIN control will flash.

The display panels in this section provide information about the respiratory pattern. MEASURED FREQ. B/MIN indicates in red the total of all breaths (spontaneous and mandatory) measured by the ventilator. SET FREQ. B/MIN shows the set rate in green for A/C and SIMV modes. INSP. PERIOD S. provides the calculated T_I (in seconds) for mandatory breaths. INSP. FLOW L/S shows the calculated flow (in liters per second) based on the TCT, set volume, and T_I for mandatory volume breaths.

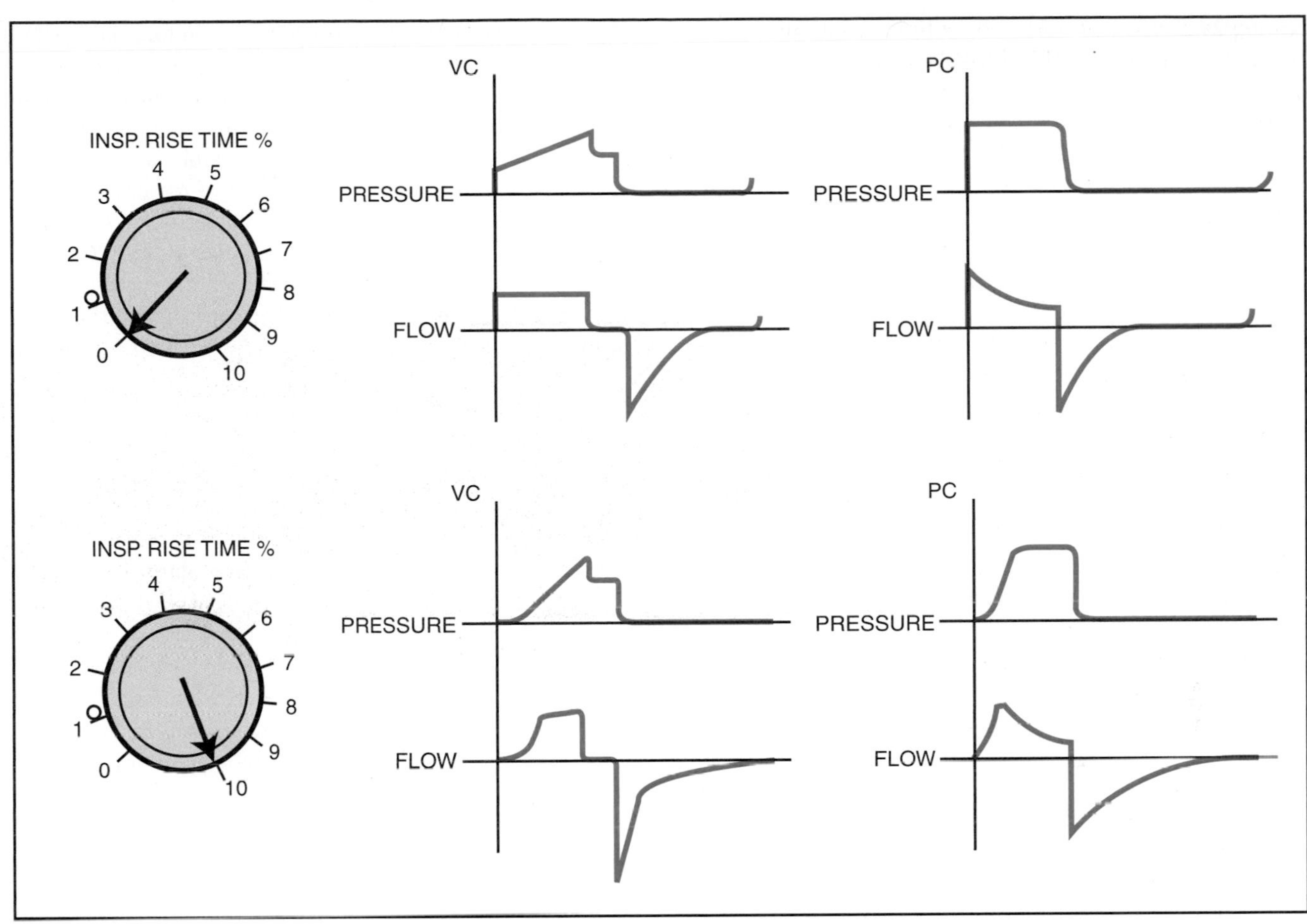

Figure 12-101 Inspiratory rise time percentage. During volume-control ventilation *(left curves)*, flow is normally constant when the inspiratory rise time percentage is set at zero *(top left)*. The use of inspiratory rise time tapers the beginning of the flow curve *(bottom left)*. During pressure ventilation *(right curves)*, flow is normally a descending ramp *(top right)*. Use of an inspiratory rise time percentage above zero tapers the beginning of the flow curve *(bottom right)*.

The TCT, flow (in liters/min), and the set I:E ratio can be obtained from the ventilator without manual calculations. Simply touch the pad next to the STANDBY setting, and immediately touch the pad next to the mode setting selected for the patient. (*Note:* You don't have to press hard on these touch pads because they are light-sensitive, not touch- or pressure-sensitive.) This causes the digital display windows in this panel to read as follows:

1. SET FREQ. B/MIN will show "(t)s" alternating with a numerical display of the calculated TCT (in seconds).
2. INSP. PERIOD S will show "I:E" alternating with a numerical display of the set I:E ratio.*
3. INSP. FLOW L/S will show "/min" alternating with a numerical display of the calculated flow (in liters/minute). (This is only shown when volume ventilation modes are in use.)

In addition to these readings, the yellow light indicators adjacent to functional controls in the selected mode will flash. To return to the normal display function, touch the STANDBY touch pad again. The normal display will also resume if a minute passes without any operator intervention.

**This is the set ratio and not a measurement of the I:E ratio. If the patient triggers a breath, this can shorten T_E and alter the set I:E ratio.*

Volume Settings and Displays

The V_T and $\dot{V}_E$ are set using the volume control, which is active during the following modes: volume control, pressure regulated volume control, volume support, and SIMV (VOL.CONTR.) + pressure support. The available V_T range can vary depending on the size of the patient selected (see Table 12-38). All measured flows and set and indicated volumes are referenced to standard conditions (1013 mbar, 760 mm Hg). To obtain a reading of ambient conditions, the operating manual provides the required conversion calculations and necessary tables. This provision might be significant at high-altitude environments (e.g., 5,000 to 10,000 ft), and the reader is referred to the operator's manual.

There are two volume reading displays for the set values. TIDAL VOL. ML shows the set V_T (mL) as a green digital number. MINUTE VOL. L/MIN shows the set $\dot{V}_E$ (in liters/

minute; as a green number) for volume ventilation in A/C ("volume control") or SIMV ("SIMV [Vol.Contr.] + pressure support"). Also provided are values for $\dot{V}_E$ (green) in pressure-regulated volume control (PRVC) and volume support modes of ventilation.

Measured volumes are provided by the following three windows that give digital values illuminated in red:

1. INSP. TIDAL VOL. ML provides the volume of each breath as measured by the inspiratory flow transducer during delivery from the ventilator outflow port. Monitored range is 50 to 3999 mL for adult settings, 10 to 399 mL for pediatric settings, and 2.0 to 39 mL for neonatal settings. If the measured value exceeds the range for the patient size selected (see Table 12-38), the number flashes and an over-range alarm occurs (see the discussion of alarms later in this section).
2. EXP. TIDAL VOL. ML displays the volume measured by the expiratory flow transducer for each breath coming back through the ventilator's expiratory port connection. Monitored ranges are the same as those for inspired V_T. As with inspired volumes, if the value exceeds the set range, the number flashes. When no leaks are present, inspiratory and expiratory values are approximately equal.
3. EXP. MINUTE VOL. L/MIN indicates the measured exhaled $\dot{V}_E$ in red numbers. The display range is from 4.0 to 60 L/min for adults, 1.0 to 5.0 L/min for pediatric patients, and 0.20 to 1.50 L/min for neonatal patients (Box 12-110). (Expired $\dot{V}_E$ is calculated by using a digital low-pass filter of the expiratory flow with time constants: 10.5 seconds in adults, 4.9 seconds in pediatric patients, and 3.4 seconds in neonates.)

In this same section of the control panel are indicators and controls for the minute ventilation alarms. There are upper and lower minute volume alarm controls, the scale of which varies depending on the patient range (according to size) selected (see Table 12-38). There is also a volume bar graph that provides indicators for various minute ventilation parameters. Colored diodes are red on the left side of the bar and green on the right. The set upper alarm limit is indicated by two red and two green diodes and is read at the lower two diodes. When the upper minute ventilation limit is set above 20 L/min, the lower two diodes start flashing. When the upper $\dot{V}_E$ alarm is exceeded, all four diodes flash. The monitored (measured) $\dot{V}_E$ is shown by one red and one green flashing diode. The set $\dot{V}_E$ is shown by one red and one green nonflashing diode. The measured $\dot{V}_E$ is superimposed on the set $\dot{V}_E$ when these values are equal. The lower $\dot{V}_E$ alarm limit is indicated by two red and two green diodes at the bottom of the volume bar graph. When the set lower alarm limit is violated, the diodes flash. (*Note:* The lower $\dot{V}_E$ alarm functions as the disconnect alarm. If the measured $\dot{V}_E$ falls below the lower alarm limit, the diodes flash.)

Oxygen Concentration

In the upper right section of the control panel is a control knob for adjusting the F_IO_2 delivery (0.21 to 1.0). Upper and lower F_IO_2 alarms are automatically set internally by the microprocessor at 0.06 (6%) above and below the selected F_IO_2. The absolute minimum alarm limit is 0.18 (18%). There is a digital display of the set oxygen concentration. An internal oxygen analyzer continuously monitors oxygen delivery.

Near the oxygen control is a knob marked OXYGEN BREATHS/START breath. When the switch is turned to OXYGEN BREATHS, the ventilator provides 100% oxygen for 20 breaths or for 1 minute—whichever comes first, and switches back to the present oxygen delivery setting. A yellow indicator light labeled "OXYGEN BREATH RUNNING" lights up when this control has been activated, and the display window reads "O_2 CONC. %." This 100% oxygen delivery can be canceled by turning the switch to OXYGEN BREATHS again before 20 breaths or 1 minute has passed (Box 12-111).

The other side of this knob is the START BREATH control, which is similar in some ways to the manual breath control on other ventilators. When activated, a breath based on the set control values is delivered. In the SIMV mode, this activates a mandatory breath. It is important to allow the patient time to exhale before activating this breath delivery.

Alarms, Messages, and Alarm Silence/Reset

The ALARM section is on the right side of the patient control panel. Small lights in this section are yellow or red. A steady yellow light indicates two possible conditions: either a high-

Box 12-110 Important Clinical Note

The Servo is primarily a $\dot{V}_E$-based ventilator. This affects V_T delivery when the rate ("CMV FREQ.B/MIN") is adjusted. For example, suppose $\dot{V}_E$ = 5 L/min (V_T = 0.5 L and f = 10 breaths/min). If you decrease f to 5 breaths/min, V_T will increase to 1.0 L to maintain $\dot{V}_E$. When you need to reduce the mandatory rate, it is recommended that you reduce the V_T (by 1/2 to 1/3) first.

Box 12-111 Important Clinical Note

When "Oxygen Breaths" is activated, the following alarms are silenced for a maximum of 55 seconds:

- Oxygen alarm
- Expired $\dot{V}_E$ alarm
- Apnea alarm
- Technical alarm for overrange

Table 12-39 All High-Alarm Functions in the Servo 300 (in Order of Priority)

Technical errors—try restarting unit	
Power failure test	
Internal RAM (random access memory) test	
Internal ROM (read-only memory) test	
Internal CPU (central processing unit) test	
Ref and timing micro module (MM) error	
Mixer MM error	
Panel MM error	
Range switch error	
Mode switch error	
Operating error	**Check function**
Airway pressure	Airway pressure too high
Apnea	Apnea alarm
Expired $\dot{V}_E$	$\dot{V}_E$ too low/high
O_2 concentration	O_2 concentration too low/high
O_2 cell disconnect	O_2 sensor
No battery capacity left	No battery capacity
Limited battery capacity left	Limited battery capacity
High battery voltage	Internal battery voltage too high
Mains failure	Battery
Pressure transducer error	Check tubing
Power failure	Technical error (see operating manual)
O_2 potentiometer error	Technical error (see operating manual)
Out of gas	Check pneumatic power source
Gas supply air	Check pneumatic power source
Gas supply O_2	Check pneumatic power source
High continuous pressure	High continuous pressure
CMV potentiometer error	Technical error (see operating manual)
Servo Control Module (SCM)	Technical error (see operating manual)
Microprocessor error	
Overrange	Overrange: select pediatric/adult
Barometer error	Technical error (see operating manual)
Regulation pressure limited	Limited pressure

priority alarm condition has been corrected, and the alarm condition has been stored in memory; or certain alarm limits have been overridden, and the alarm has been turned off manually. Another indicator is an audible caution (ticking) sound that occurs under a few special conditions and acts as a reminder to the user. For example, ticking occurs under the following conditions:

- The oxygen cell is disconnected.
- An error is detected in either a flow or a pressure transducer.
- The ventilator is placed in the stand-by mode.
- The ventilator is operating on battery power.
- Only one high-pressure gas source is being used.

A red flashing light and a sound signal a high-priority alarm condition requiring immediate attention. Table 12-39 lists the high-priority alarms in order of importance.

There are seven alarm indicators—eight in some versions (CO_2 concentration)—in this section of the control panel: AIRWAY PRESSURE, OXYGEN CONCENTRATION, EXPIRATORY MINUTE VOLUME, APNEA ALARM, GAS SUPPLY, BATTERY, and TECHNICAL. The message display window at the top of this panel provides information about a current or recent alarm. This window normally displays the measured oxygen concentration.

If more than one alarm is active at a time, the highest priority alarm is displayed. The operator can display the alarm text for any of the seven alarm indicators by touching the light diode to the left of the desired alarm indicator. For example, if a yellow light next to an alarm indicator is constantly lit, a recent alarm condition for this parameter may have occurred. A message will appear in the display window showing the reason for the caution, but will alternate with the oxygen concentration reading.

If more than one yellow light is present, the operator can sequentially select each illuminated light and check the alarm memory for that parameter. The lights can be turned off by using the RESET control or changing to another ventilatory mode.

Alarm conditions for the other seven parameters are listed in Table 12-40, which describes the more common causes for such conditions. Historical Note 12-1 provides a description of one of the original alarms. Box 12-112 provides information about the safety switches on some of the control knobs.

Besides resetting visual alarms, the RESET/2 MIN control can be used to silence some high-priority alarms by turning it to the 2 MIN position for more than 2 seconds, thus providing 2 minutes of silence. If the knob is turned to RESET before the end of 2 minutes, the alarm sounds again. For example, before disconnecting a patient for suctioning or a similar procedure, turn the RESET/2 MIN control to 2 MIN. A short beep and the message "Alarms muted" indicate that the alarms are silenced. The audible alarms for MINUTE VENTILATION, OVERRANGE, and APNEA can be silenced for 2 minutes in this manner. (The UPPER PRESS. LIMIT alarm cannot be silenced with the 2 MIN. knob.)

Pause Hold

At the lower portion of the right section is a manual control used to provide an inspiratory or an expiratory pause. When

Table 12-40 Servo 300 alarm parameters, messages, and causes

Alarm	Cause
AIRWAY PRESSURE	
Upper Press. Limit	Set upper pressure limit has been reached and inspiration ends.
Airway Pressure Too High	Airway pressure exceeds the upper pressure limit.
Limited Pressure	Inadequate pressure to deliver volume support or pressure-regulated volume control breaths.
High Continuous Pressure	Continuous pressure $>$15 cm H_2O plus PEEP level; continuous for more than 15 seconds.
OXYGEN CONCENTRATION	
O_2 CONC TOO LOW/HIGH	FiO_2 measured at above or below 0.6 of set F_IO_2, or $F_IO_2 < 0.18$; alarm inactive during and for 1 minute after oxygen breaths are activated.
O_2 SENSOR	Oxygen cell is not connected.
EXPIRED $\dot{V}_E$	
(Must be set correctly for each patient size: adult, pediatric, neonatal.)	
EXP MINUTE VOLUME TOO HIGH	Expired $\dot{V}_E$ exceeds alarm setting.
EXP MINUTE VOLUME TOO LOW	Expired $\dot{V}_E$ is below alarm setting.
APNEA ALARM	
APNEA ALARM	No breaths (spontaneous or mandatory) detected; Adult = 20 seconds, pediatric = 15 seconds, neonatal = 10 seconds.
GAS SUPPLY ALARM	
AIR SUPPLY PRESSURE TOO LOW/HIGH AIR:X.X BAR O_2 X.X BAR	Air supply is out of range ($<$29 to $>$100 psig). Ventilator defaults to use available gas source.
O_2 SUPPLY PRESSURE TOO LOW/HIGH AIR:X.X BAR O_2 X.X BAR	Oxygen supply is out of range. Ventilator defaults to use available gas source.
AIR SUPPLY PRESSURE TOO LOW O_2 SUPPLY PRESSURE TOO LOW HIGH AIR:X.X BAR O_2 X.X BAR	Both gas sources have failed. Internal safety valve and expiratory valve open so patient can breathe room air if able.
BATTERY	
If the main power source fails, the ventilator switches to battery power and this alarm activates (yellow light). The graphic screen turns off.	
LIMITED BATTERY CAPACITY LEFT INTERNAL: XX V	High-priority alarm if voltage remaining $\leq$23 volts.
NO BATTERY CAPACITY LEFT	Voltage $\leq$ 21 volts; cannot be silenced.
SEE OPERATING MANUAL	At 18 volts, safety valve opens.
TECHNICAL ALARMS	
These are generally corrected by the technical staff. The alarm listed here can be corrected by the clinician.	
CHECK TUBINGS	Inspiratory/expiratory pressure difference $\geq$25%, or at least 5 cm H_2O for 20 seconds. Causes: disconnected pressure transducer tubings, transducer error, clogged bacterial filter, or any blockage in breathing system

an INSP. PAUSE HOLD is activated, the inspiratory and expiratory valves close at the end of inspiration, preventing expiratory gas flow. The valves remain closed until the control is released or held for a maximum of 5 seconds. Using this control gives an opportunity to check plateau pressure during this pause time. When EXP. PAUSE HOLD is activated, the inspiratory and expiratory valves close at the end of exhalation, just when another mandatory breath would have occurred. The valves remain closed as long as the control is held or up to a maximum of 30 seconds. This extended expiratory time allows expiratory pressure to be measured, which may facilitate estimation of the auto-PEEP level.

When a Servo 300 includes the available graphic monitor screen (see Figure 12-97), the inspiratory and expiratory pause controls can be used to have the microprocessor

HISTORICAL NOTE 12-1

In the original version of the Servo 300, a separate back-up alarm was available that mounted on the left side of the ventilator and was called the failure alarm box (FAB).

If there was a 24-volt power failure, or if the ventilator mode control was turned to the ventilator off position, this audible and visible (red) alarm was activated and could not be silenced until the button on the FAB was pressed. This alarm also became activated briefly as a self-test when the ventilator was first turned on, and after a few seconds, became silence on its own.

This failure alarm prevented the electrical power from being disconnected or the ventilator from being turned off—either accidentally or deliberately—unless done by someone who was familiar with the FAB alarm who knew how to silence it.

In newer versions of the Servo 300, the FAB alarm is incorporated internally and is self-tested when the unit is turned on. When the ventilator is turned off, this alert "chirps," and then is silenced automatically.

Box 12-112 Descriptions of the Safety Features on the Servo 300

Measured values are shown as red digital displays. Set values are shown as green digital displays.

Yellow lights that are constantly illuminated indicate active controls that must be set by the operator in the selected mode. A flashing yellow light indicates that a control has been set incorrectly.

Safety catches are indicated by small black markings that appear on the number scale of certain control knobs or dials (e.g., UPPER PRESS. LIMIT, PRESSURE CONTROL LEVEL ABOVE PEEP, PRESSURE SUPPORT LEVEL ABOVE PEEP, PEEP, INSP. TIME %, and O_2 CONC.). To turn a dial past a safety catch, the operator must push in the top of the knob while rotating it past the safety catch.

calculate a patient's static compliance (Cs). To perform this procedure, the operator turns the inspiratory pause control until the graphic screen displays the message "Measuring Static Compliance" at the top center. Immediately the inspiratory pause is switched to the expiratory pause position for a few seconds and then it is released. After a few seconds the calculated Cs value appears on the graphic screen. This calculation takes into account the PEEP level, but not the tubing compliance factor.

Modes of Ventilation

The mode of ventilation is set with the mode selection switch. There are two ways in which appropriate settings for

Box 12-113 Steps of Using the Set Parameter Guide (SPG)

1. Before connecting the patient to the ventilator, use the mode selection switch to set the standby mode.
2. Touch the light diode next to the desired mode (e.g., next to the volume control). It will illuminate the controls or parameters to set for that mode.
3. Touch the light diode a second time; the first control parameter that needs to be set will flash, and the others will be off. For example, the light next to the patient range selection switch will flash, telling you to set that control.
4. Touch the light diode next to the mode (e.g., volume control) again, and the next control that needs to be set (e.g., upper pressure limit) will flash.
5. Continue setting controls when they flash and touching the light next to the desired mode until you have set all appropriate parameters.
6. Upon completion of the SPG, the ventilator will beep three times to indicate that you have completed the process. The mode is now ready to be operational or active.

(*Note:* If the patient is already connected to the ventilator and the clinician decides to use the SPG feature, any control that is active in the current mode of ventilation will be immediately changed. For example, a patient is in volume control mode with a rate of 12 breaths/min. The clinician uses SPG to switch the patient to SIMV at a rate of 12 breaths/min. If the CMV frequency knob is turned to 30 breaths/min so that it is higher than the SIMV frequency, the rate immediately goes to 30 breaths/min.)

a mode can be achieved. First, if the patient is not yet connected to the ventilator, the patient settings can be selected (using the Set Parameter Guide [SPG]) while the mode selection switch is in the standby position (Box 12-113). The second method of mode selection is commonly used when the patient is already being ventilated and the operator wants to switch the mode. The operator touches the light diode to the left of the desired ventilator mode. The light next to the desired mode flashes, the parameters that are set for the desired mode illuminate, and those for the current active mode are turned off. When the pad next to the desired mode is touched a second time, the same sequence as the SPG cab be followed, which essentially walks one through each control that needs to be set in the desired mode. To actively change to the desired mode, the operator turns the mode control switch to the new mode.

A word of caution needs to be added because changing any parameter or control that is active in current mode takes effect immediately. To distinguish between the active and inactive controls, those that are currently active flash rapidly, and those that will be active in the new mode flash at a normal speed. For example, the INSP. TIME % control adjusts T_I in both volume and pressure control mode. In either of these two modes, if the inspiratory time is

Box 12-114 A Note of Caution

It is strongly recommended that whenever a patient is connected to a Servo 300 for the first time, all appropriate parameters should be selected from the start-up. For example, even if volume ventilation is going to be used, the appropriate inspiratory pressure for pressure control and pressure support settings must still be set. This way, even if the mode switch is accidentally changed, the parameters appropriate for the patient will already be within a reasonable setting range and will pose no danger to the patient.

increased while following the SPG, the T_I increases as soon as it is adjusted (i.e., changes do not wait for the new mode to be activated). Box 12-114 provides a word of caution.

The mode selection switch has a left half and a right half. Modes on the left (PCV, VCV, and PRVC) are A/C modes and provide a clinician-selected volume or pressure for every patient breath. Modes on the right (VS, SIMV(VC) + PSV, SIMV(PV) + PSV, and PSV/CPAP) allow for spontaneous breaths. Not all patient-triggered breaths are mandatory.

Remember that regardless of the mode selected, there are certain things that are always true. Pressure cannot exceed the UPPER PRESS. LIMIT setting. If the limit is reached, volume delivery is reduced. T_I cannot exceed 80% of TCT (based on the CMV frequency setting). Flow and volume delivery can vary if a patient's active inspiration drops pressure below the baseline. For example, during pressure ventilation, such as during pressure control, the flow pattern is commonly a descending flow curve, and flow and volume delivery can vary. During volume ventilation, flow is usually constant, and there is no control knob with which to select a particular inspiratory flow curve (e.g., constant flow or a descending flow waveform) during volume ventilation. The only control the operator has over the flow waveform is the sloping or tapering feature provided by the INSPIR. RISE TIME % control. The patient, however, can obtain as much flow as desired (up to 180 L/min) during any mode of ventilation when airway pressure drops below the baseline (PEEP setting). This results in a flow-time curve that varies depending on patient demand. Because a patient can obtain increased flow, volume can vary—even during volume ventilation. For example, using the volume control mode, the selected volume is normally delivered, and this represents a minimum volume. If the patient so desires, additional volume can be obtained with an active inspiration.

Each of the modes is reviewed, with particular emphasis on some of the newer ventilatory methods available with the Servo 300.

Pressure Control

Pressure control allows patient- or time-triggering and provides pressure ventilation that is time-cycled based on the T_I %. Inspiratory pause cannot be used in this mode. Flow delivery usually follows a descending curve, and minimum respiratory rate is set with the CMV frequency control.

Volume Control

Volume control is patient- or time-triggered and provides volume-targeted ventilation with time-cycling. Flow delivery is normally constant. V_T is calculated based on CMV frequency and $\dot{V}_E$ settings, as follows:

$$V_T = \dot{V}_E/f.$$

Minimum respiratory rate is set with the CMV frequency control. T_I is determined by the inspiratory time % and the pause time % controls.

Pressure-Regulated Volume Control

Pressure-regulated volume control (PRVC) is a servo-control (closed-loop) mode of ventilation that is very similar to the pressure-control mode. Breaths are patient- or time-triggered, pressure-targeted, and time-cycled. The main difference is that the ventilator can guarantee volume delivery while still using pressure ventilation. It does this by constantly calculating system and patient compliance, volume delivery, and the pressure limits within which it has to operate. The following will explain how the Servo 300 performs its function in PRVC.

When PRVC is activated, the ventilator begins by giving a breath with an inspiratory pressure of 10 cm H_2O (5 cm H_2O on older models). It then measures the volume delivered and calculates system compliance. The next three breaths are delivered to provide a pressure that will deliver approximately 75% of the set V_T.* For each subsequent breath, the ventilator calculates compliance of the previous breath and adjusts the inspiratory pressure level to achieve the set V_T on the next breath (Figure 12-102).

For example, suppose the set volume is 500 mL and the measured volume is 525 mL at a pressure of 23 cm H_2O (C = 22.8 mL/cm H_2O). In this case, the pressure might drop to 22 cm H_2O to deliver the 500 mL. The pressure is reduced until the set and the monitored volumes are the same. On the other hand, if the measured volume is too low, the pressure level is increased. The ventilator will not change the pressure more than 3 cm H_2O from one breath to the next. This protects the patient from large changes in pressure. The maximum pressure that can be delivered is equal to the upper pressure limit setting minus 5 cm H_2O. The minimum pressure limit is the baseline setting. If the pressure reaches the UPPER PRESS. LIMIT − 5 cm H_2O, the message window will read "LIMITED PRESSURE," and an alarm sounds. The operator must then decide whether to increase the UPPER PRESS. LIMIT and thus allow the ventilator to increase pressure to achieve the set V_T, or to

**The V_T is determined by the minute ventilation and rate settings, and is displayed in the V_T window.*

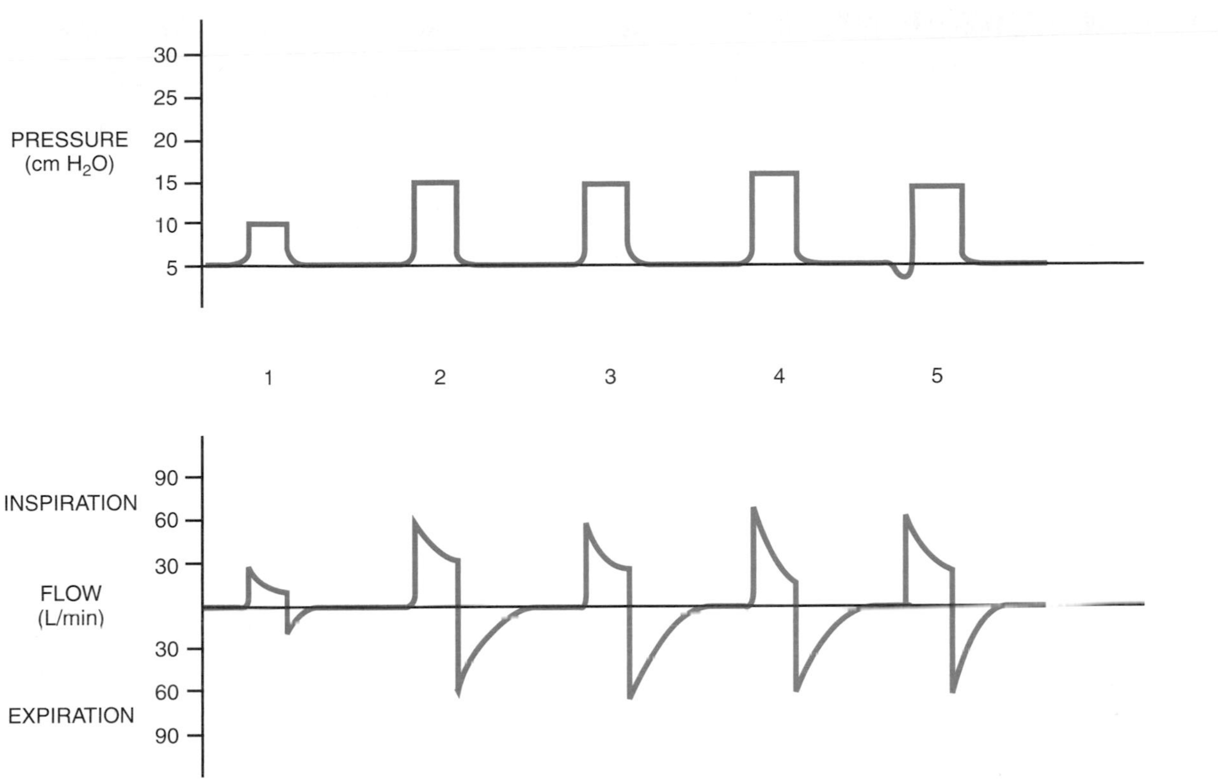

Figure 12-102 Test breaths in PRVC (see text for explanation).

accept a lower V_T setting to prevent pressure from going too high.

One reason PRVC was designed was to provide the advantages of PCV, such as a descending flow ramp waveform to help improve gas distribution, an inspiratory flow rate that can vary with patient demand, and a limited pressure to prevent excessive pressures in the lungs. More important, however, PRVC provides another valuable feature: it guarantees a volume delivery.

Suppose a patient is being ventilated with volume control and the operator wants to switch to PRVC. The following should be performed:

- Ensure the UPPER PRESS. LIMIT is set appropriately. A starting value about 5 to 10 cm H_2O above the patient's current plateau pressure might be appropriate. This is a safe range and could be readjusted if necessary once PRVC is activated.
- As long as no changes to other parameters are indicated, (e.g., T_I, V_T, f, baseline pressure, or F_IO_2), they can remain the same.
- The mode control switch is rotated to PRVC to activate the mode, and the ventilator self-regulates within the parameters set.

As long as safe limits for pressure and other parameters have been set, the patient will be safe. Some respiratory therapists and physicians are hesitant to use PRVC in part because of the uniqueness of the concept and their reluctance to try something different. Undoubtedly, as clinical trials of this mode are evaluated, its use will reflect its success in managing ventilated patients.

Volume Support

Volume support (VS) is also a servo-control mode that might be considered the weaning counterpart to PRVC and volume control. It is a mode of ventilation that provides breaths that can best be compared with pressure-support breaths. That is, they are normally patient-triggered, pressure-targeted, and flow-cycled (5% of measured peak flow). The flow waveform is normally a descending-ramplike curve. The primary difference is that like PRVC, a minimum V_T can be guaranteed. Also, as in PRVC, the ventilator runs a series of test breaths beginning with one breath at 10 cm H_2O (5 cm H_2O in older models). It then gives three breaths at approximately 75% of the pressure calculated to deliver the V_T. Finally, the pressure is provided to give the appropriate volume.

As with PRVC, breaths are constantly monitored, and pressure increases when the volume reading is low or decreases if the volume reading is high in increments of no more than 3 cm H_2O. Also as in PRVC, pressure can rise as high as the upper pressure limit setting minus 5 cm H_2O to deliver the set minimum volume. If the pressure reaches this limit, the message: "LIMITED PRESSURE" appears in the message window, and there is an audible alarm. Baseline pressure represents the minimum pressure level.

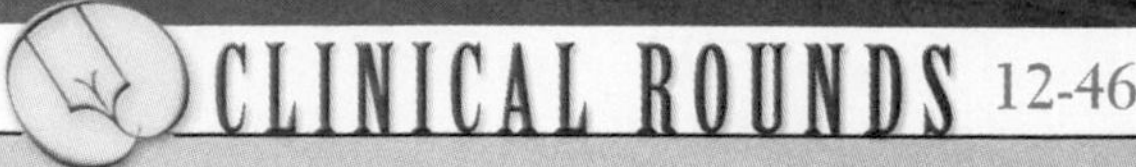
↑ press ∴ ↑ V_E
V_E can be higher then set value → not lower

CLINICAL ROUNDS 12-45

A patient is on volume support; the rate is set at 12 breaths/min, and the minute ventilation is at 6 L/min. V_T is targeted at 500 mL. The ventilator is able to maintain this volume within the pressure limitations, but the patient's spontaneous rate drops. How will the ventilator respond to the drop in the patient's respiratory rate (to 8 breaths/min)?

See Appendix A for the answer.

CLINICAL ROUNDS 12-46

A patient on SIMV (VOL. CONTR.) + pressure support has a set CMV frequency of 15 breaths/min and an SIMV frequency control setting of 3 breaths/min. What are the SIMV cycle time, the SIMV period, and the spontaneous period for these settings?

See Appendix A for the answer.

There are a few important differences between volume support and PRVC. First, there is no back-up rate in VS. If the patient becomes apneic, the ventilator automatically switches to PRVC, and the light diode next to that mode flashes. An alarm sounds, and the message window indicates that apnea has been detected. For this reason only spontaneously breathing patients who have intact respiratory centers should be placed on this mode. Another important difference has to do with the minute ventilation setting. The Servo 300 tries to maintain the minute ventilation that the operator has set on the ventilator. Clinical Rounds 12-45 provides an exercise with an example of how the ventilator responds in volume support.

Because volume-support breaths are really pressure support breaths, one might wonder why volume support is used. The reason, of course, is that the ventilator can guarantee a minimum volume delivery. If a patient is ready for pressure support, volume support is also appropriate. An advantage of VS is the operator does not have to constantly adjust pressure levels, as sometimes occurs with PSV. The ventilator adjusts the pressure as the patient's condition changes. In addition, if the patient becomes apneic, the ventilator switches to a mode that provides continuous ventilation (e.g., PRVC).

Synchronized Intermittent Mandatory Ventilation (SIMV Vol. Contr.) + Pressure Support

The SIMV (vol. control) + pressure support (SIMV VOL. CONTR. + PSV) mode provides mandatory breaths similar to those in volume control. During SIMV, the mandatory rate and SIMV cycle time are determined in the following way. The SIMV frequency control must be set lower than the CMV frequency to correctly establish the desired SIMV mandatory breath rate. If it is not, the ventilator defaults to the CMV FREQ. B/MIN setting, and the yellow indicator next to the CMV frequency control flashes. Cycling times are determined as follows: the SIMV cycle time is calculated by dividing the SIMV frequency into 60 seconds. For example, with the SIMV FREQ. B/MIN set at 4 breaths/min, the SIMV cycle time is 15 seconds. The SIMV cycle time has two phases. The first phase is the SIMV period, and the second is the spontaneous period. The SIMV period equals the CMV FREQ. B/MIN setting divided into 60. For example if the CMV frequency is set at 10 breaths/min, the SIMV period is 6 seconds. The spontaneous period is equal to the SIMV cycle time minus the SIMV period (e.g., 15 seconds – 6 seconds = 9 seconds).

When a mandatory breath is triggered, the SIMV cycle begins. After delivery of the mandatory breath, the patient has 9 seconds to breathe spontaneously without receiving a mandatory breath (spontaneous period). At the end of 9 seconds, the 6-second SIMV period begins. The patient has 6 seconds in which to make an inspiratory effort and get a mandatory breath. If the patient fails to take a breath, then a time-triggered breath occurs at the end of the 6 seconds. This is very much like SIMV in the Servo 900C (see Figure 12-95). Clinical Rounds 12-46 provides a problem related to SIMV.

SIMV (Press. Contr.) + Pressure Support

SIMV (PRESS. CONTR.) + pressure support is SIMV in which mandatory breaths are pressure-control breaths. Pressure support can be added for spontaneous breaths. The only difference between SIMV (VOL. CONTR.) and SIMV (PRESS. CONTR.) is that mandatory breaths are volume-controlled in the former and pressure-controlled in the latter. The operator sets the pressure control level above PEEP.

Pressure Support-CPAP

The pressure support-CPAP setting is intended for spontaneously breathing patients. Breaths are patient-triggered when spontaneous breaths can be detected at a set baseline pressure (0 to 50 cm H_2O). Pressure support can also be set for all spontaneous breaths. The pressure is added to the baseline pressure (pressure support level above PEEP). At PS greater than zero, inspiration is pressure-limited and flow-cycled at 5% of the measured peak flow. No minimum guaranteed rate or volume is provided in this mode.

Automode[2]

In late 1997 a new feature was introduced in the United States called Automode. The ON/OFF control for this mode

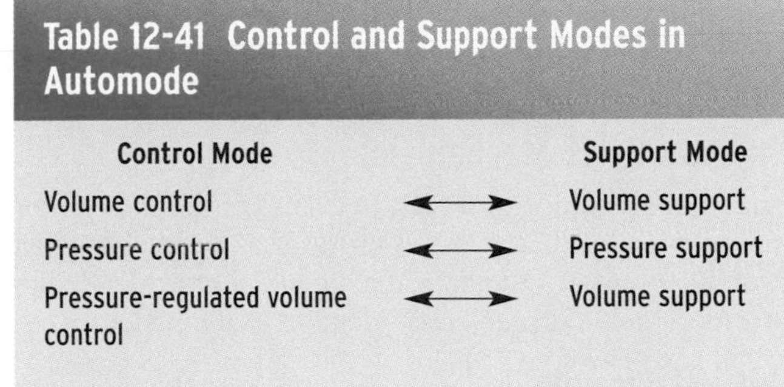

Table 12-41 Control and Support Modes in Automode

Control Mode		Support Mode
Volume control	⟷	Volume support
Pressure control	⟷	Pressure support
Pressure-regulated volume control	⟷	Volume support

is at the upper right corner of the updated operating panel (see Figures 12-97 and 12-99). This mode is designed to switch from a control mode to a support mode of ventilation if the patient triggers two consecutive breaths. The ventilator remains in the support mode as long as the patient keeps triggering breaths. Table 12-41 shows the control and support modes that are operational in Automode.

Automode works as follows. Suppose the patient is in the PRVC mode, and Automode is on. When the ventilator detects two consecutive patient efforts, it delivers one more PRVC breath on the second breath, and the next (third) breath is in volume support.

If the patient is in volume control and the same conditions occur, the ventilator switches to volume support in a similar fashion. The first volume-support breath in this situation (volume control to volume support) is delivered at a pressure level equal to pause pressure. If no pause time is set, the ventilator uses the following formula to determine the inspiratory pressure for volume support:

$$\text{set P} = [(\text{PIP} - \text{PEEP}) \times 0.5 + \text{PEEP}].$$

The ventilator does not run through the series of test breaths it normally performs when the mode switch is turned to volume support.

If the patient is in pressure control with Automode and two patient efforts are detected, the switch to pressure support occurs on the third breath. The operator must have previously selected a pressure-support level above PEEP because that is the pressure that will be delivered by the ventilator when it switches to pressure support.

The purpose of Automode is to adapt ventilator status to a patient's spontaneous inspiratory efforts. The benefit of Automode obviously lies in its ability to monitor patient breathing effort. For this reason, it is essential that triggering sensitivity is set appropriately, and that auto-triggering is not occurring. Auto-triggering would be detected as a patient-initiated breath and might cause the ventilator to cycle into a support mode. There is a back-up safety feature if this occurs. If the ventilator does not detect a patient effort within a fixed time period while Automode is on, it switches from the support mode back to the control mode. In the adult setting, this period is 12 seconds; in the pediatric setting, it is 8 seconds; and in the neonatal setting, it is 5 seconds.

At this time, Automode is a new feature of the Servo 300A. Additional clinical experience will help provide more information about its benefits and uses.

Graphics Display Screens

The graphics display screen provides the standard graphs for flow-time, volume-time, and pressure-time, in addition to several loops, including flow-volume and volume-pressure. From one to four different graphs can be viewed at any time. The right side of the graphic display has spaces for digital display of parameters, including peak pressure, mean pressure, dynamic compliance, and static compliance. Static compliance can be measured by using the PAUSE HOLD control, described in the earlier discussion about ventilator controls. Data screens on which the operator can custom design the monitored parameters to be displayed are also available. An example of an available option is the I:E ratio, which is the actual value on this screen as measured by the ventilator.

A carbon dioxide analyzer module can be attached to the Servo 390 graphics screen to display capnographic waveforms and calculations, including end-tidal carbon dioxide, carbon dioxide production, and dead space.

Troubleshooting

As noted previously, whenever the mandatory breath rate is reduced in a volume-controlled mode, the V_T delivery is increased because the ventilator is designed to deliver a specific $\dot{V}_E$. It is recommended that the volume be reduced by about one-half before any large decrease in rate is performed.

Because many of the safety features base their function on clinician-selected settings, it is advisable to set all available parameters and alarms before instituting ventilation on a patient. For example, the ventilator will never allow the T_I to exceed 80% of the TCT. This is the TCT based on the CMV frequency. The ventilator has many safety features to limit this type of error that were reviewed in the discussion of controls and alarms in this section.

The operating manual contains a section that reviews common alarms and associated problems. Radio frequency interference (RFI) and electromagnetic frequency interference (EMI) can affect the function of medical devices using microprocessors. The Servo 300 is specially shielded to ensure protection against RFI and EMI interference. This shielding meets current safety standards.

Special Features

The manufacturer has a module for the delivery and measurement of nitric oxide that is currently in use in Europe and may soon be available in the United States. Because of the ability to add to the microprocessor unit, adding new modes of ventilation as they are developed is always within the scope of future planning.

Newly Released Ventilators

Four recently released ventilators have been added to this chapter. They include the Dräger Savina, the Siemens Servo^{i}, the Viasys Avea, and the Newport e500. It is difficult to determine how abundant and successful these ventilators will be until sufficient time has passed to determine the merits of each in the clinical setting. The basic operation of each ventilator will be reviewed.

The reader should keep in mind that newer ventilators are computer operated. Software for these ventilators is frequently upgraded, and these upgrades may include changes in some functions and addition of optional software functions. The operator should check the ventilator in use and determine what software version is operational and what options have been included.

The Dräger Savina[1-2]

The Dräger Savina (Figure 12-103), introduced in the United States in 2001, is an intensive care ventilator for use in adult and pediatric patients where available tidal volumes start at 50 mL (range 50 to 2000 mL). The ventilator can be used in recovery rooms, intensive care units, subacute care facilities, and transport in and outside the hospital.

Power Source

The Savina is pneumatically and electrically powered. The ventilator normally operates from an AC power source that provides power to an internal turbine and electronic components. The ventilator also connects to a high-pressure oxygen supply that allows for variable oxygen concentrations. An internal battery (DC power supply) is used for back-up power in the event of an AC power disconnect. There is also a DC adapter on the back panel for connection to an external battery.

Indicators on the lower right corner of the front panel provide information about the current power source (Figure 12-104). Normally the LED for AC power is illuminated (green) to indicate connection to an AC power source. The EXT. LED illuminates when the ventilator is operating from an external DC battery. This power source might be used during air or ground transportation. The INT. LED illuminates when the internal battery is the power source. The internal and external battery LEDs are yellow when charging and green when fully charged. Using two fully charged external batteries can power the Savina for up to 7 hours.

When the ventilator switches from AC to DC source, a message on the front panel information window reads "!! Int. battery activated." The internal battery can provide about 1 hour of operating power to the ventilator, when fully charged. An "!!! Int. batt. almost discharged" message warns that an alternative source of power must be supplied to avoid interruption of ventilation.

Internal Drive Mechanism

An internal turbine provides the air pressure source for normal breath delivery. When the Savina is also connected to a high pressure O_2 source, air and oxygen are blended to provide variable oxygen concentrations to the patient.

Patient Circuit

Connections for the patient circuit are located just below the front panel (see Figure 12-104). The inspiratory line, located on the right, should be installed with an inline bacterial filter in place. Either a heated humidifier or an HME can be used with the Savina. (*Note*: The operator should never use the two together.) The expiratory line connection is below the front panel on the left. During normal maintenance, the expiratory valve assembly is removed for cleaning, but should not be disassembled beyond removing the expiratory diaphragm.

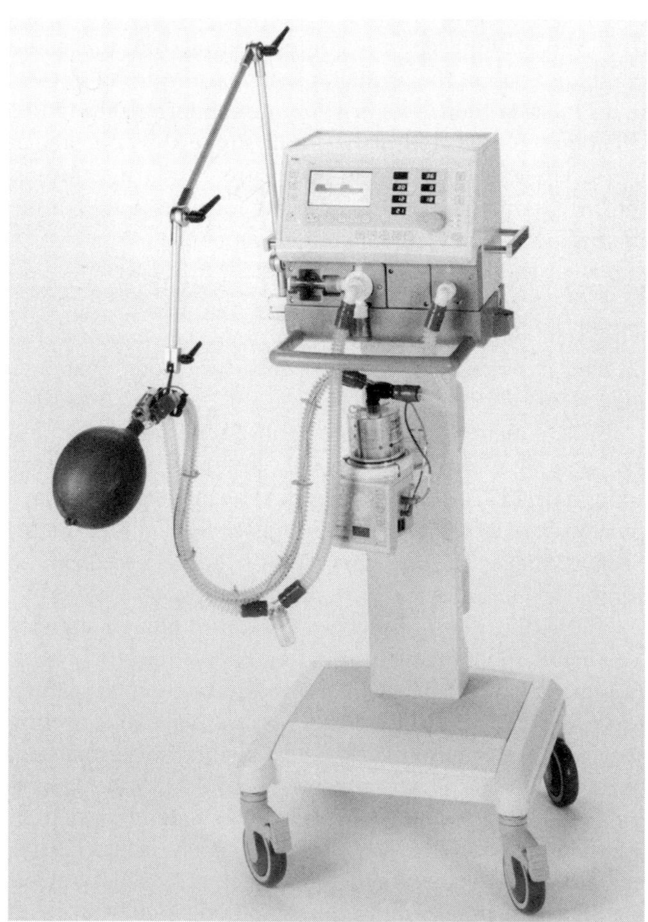

Figure 12-103 The Savina from Dräger Medical showing the support arm with the patient circuit and a heated humidifier attached. (Courtesy Dräger Medical, Telford, Penn.)

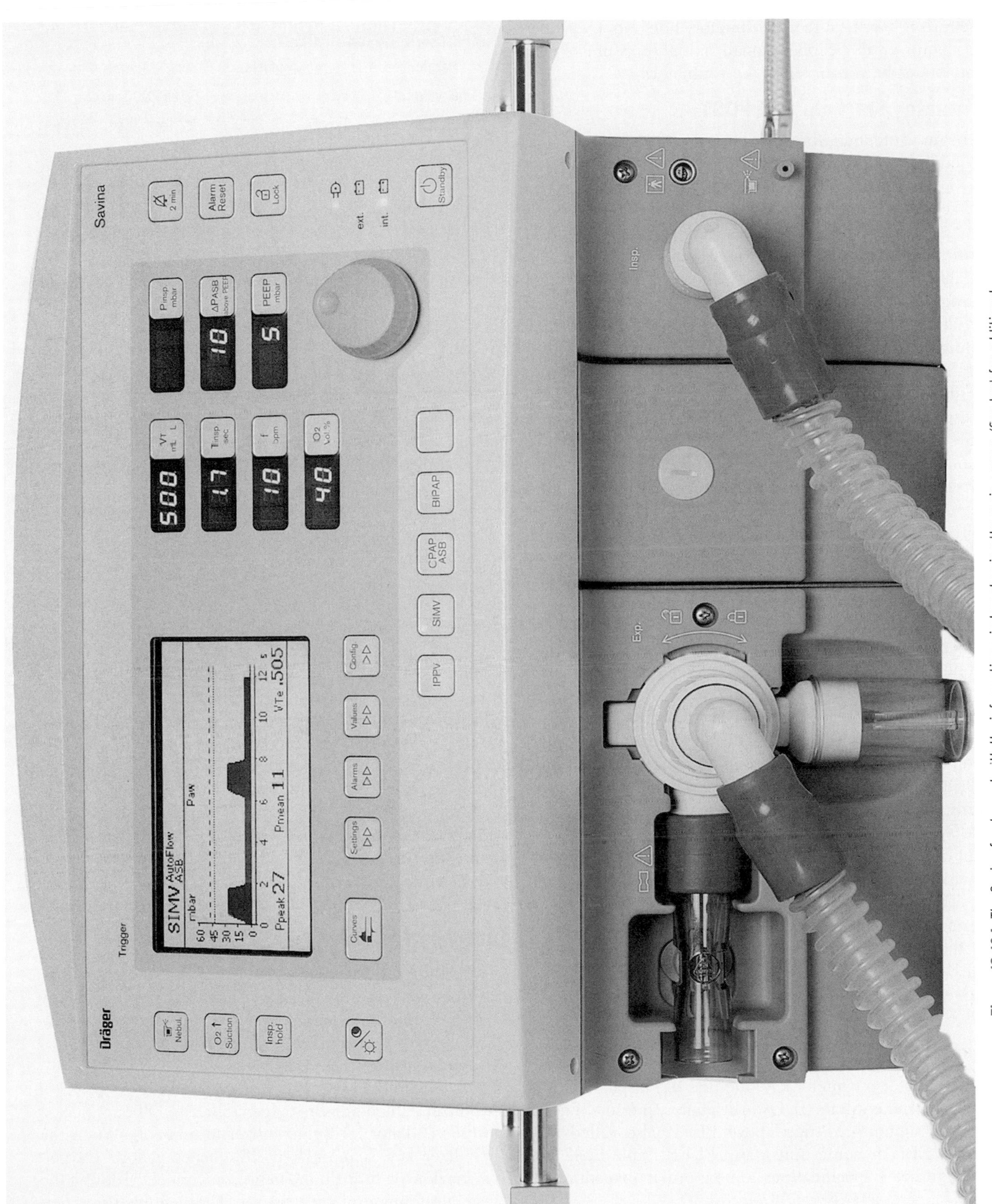

Figure 12-104 The Savina frcnt panel with the information window showing the main screen. (See text for additional information.) (Courtesy Dräger Medical, Telfcrd, Penn.)

An expiratory flow sensor is located to the left of the expiration line connection. There is a connector for attaching a nebulizer hose next to the inspiratory line port. (*Note*: For the nebulizer to be operational, a high-pressure oxygen source must be connected to the ventilator.)

Ventilator Start Up and POST

To begin ventilation, the power switch on the back panel is turned on and the Savina performs a power-on self test (POST). After the POST, the LEDs illuminate along with the keys and status lights and the audible alarm sounds briefly. The operator can use these alarms and indicators to confirm LED and audible functions. After POST, the ventilator automatically starts ventilation using the last settings.

Before using the ventilator on a new patient, some additional tests should be run. For the testing procedure, a test lung is connected at the patient Y-connector. The ventilator is turned on, POST is run, and the operator then sets specific parameters and performs a series of checks to verify ventilator function. (*Note:* This information can be found in the operator's manual.[1]) After the test procedures are completed, the ventilator is ready for use on a new patient.

To suspend ventilation until new settings have been selected, the operator presses the STANDBY key after power on. Then the "Alarm Reset" key is pressed to confirm that the ventilator is not connected to a patient. Ventilation parameters can be changed during standby. After parameters are set, pressing the STANDBY key again starts ventilation at the new settings.

Controls and Alarms—Front Panel Controls

The front panel of the Savina is divided into several sections (see Figure 12-104). The information window is toward the left side of the front panel. The window provides data, waveforms, and instructions depending on the screen selected. The ventilator parameter control keys are located to the right of the window. To the left of the information window are auxiliary function keys. Below the window are touch keys for selecting a display screen to appear in the information window. Along the bottom of the front panel are the mode selection keys and, to the right, the control dial. On the far right side of the front panel are four frequently used keys: ALARM SILENCE, ALARM RESET, LOCK, and STANDBY.

Ventilator Parameter Control Keys

The ventilator parameter keys include V_T, inspiratory time (Tinsp), respiratory rate (f), O_2%, inspiratory pressure (Pinsp), pressure support (ΔPsupp above PEEP, also called P_{ASB} above PEEP on some units), and PEEP. Table 12-42 lists the parameter specifications. The normal procedure for setting a parameter is as follows:

- Touch the desired parameter key. The yellow LED for that parameter illuminates.

Table 12-42 Ventilator Parameter Specifications—Savina

Parameter	Abbreviation	Range
Tidal volume	V_T	50 to 2000 mL
Inspiratory time	Tinsp	0.2 to 10.0 sec
Respiratory rate	Rate	2 to 80 breaths/min
Oxygen concentration	O_2	21% to 100%
Inspiratory pressure	Pinsp	0 to 100 cm H_2O
Pressure support	ΔPsupp. above PEEP	0 to 35 cm H_2O above PEEP
Positive end-expiratory	PEEP	0 to 35 cm H_2O

- Rotate the control dial until the value displayed in the window adjacent to the key is the desired parameter value.
- Press the control dial to confirm the new value. The yellow LED in the key will no longer be illuminated.

The new setting immediately becomes effective.

Certain ventilator settings are limited during the initial setting. For example, PEEP is limited to a threshold value of 20 cm H_2O, although PEEP up to 35 cm H_2O is available. When the PEEP pressure is adjusted up to 20 cm H_2O a message appears at the lower right portion of the screen "PEEP >20 cm H_2O—Confirm." To go beyond the threshold value, in this case 20 cm H_2O, the operator must press the control dial, turn the control dial to the new value, and press the dial again to confirm the new setting.

One of the ventilator controls that does not have an immediate value change is the oxygen concentration. It takes approximately 3 minutes for the oxygen percent to reach the newly set value after the value has been changed. This might cause the "High O_2" or "Low O_2" alarm to activate.

Auxiliary Function Keys

The control keys to the left of the window include a nebulizer key (optional feature), an oxygen increase and suction key (labeled "100% O_2" for Europe, and "O_2 ↑suction" for the United States), a manual inspiration key (Insp Hold), and a key for adjusting screen brightness.

The nebulizer key activates a gas source to power a nebulizer. A high-pressure oxygen source must be connected to the ventilator for the nebulizer to function. When the nebulizer key is pressed, it illuminates yellow. Oxygen begins flowing through the nebulizer connector during the inspiratory phase of each breath. The nebulizer function lasts for a period of 30 minutes. During this time a message is present on the information window, "! Nebulizer On."

Box 12-115 Suctioning and Increased Oxygen Function

After depressing the "O_2 ↑Suction" (100% O_2) key for about 3 seconds the display will read "O_2 enrichment" and will start counting down from 180 seconds. The remaining time is continuously displayed in the information window along with the message "O_2 enrichment 100% 180 s."

At any time during those 180 seconds, should the operator disconnect the patient to suction, a new message "Execute suction and reconnect" will appear and a new time countdown starting at 120 seconds will appear. The flow through the patient circuit will diminish to prevent excess water spray.

All alarms will be suppressed for this time. During the 120 seconds when the patient is reconnected, the Savina will sense the reconnect and resume ventilation with the message "Final O_2 enrichment 100%" and count down from 120 seconds. In this final stage the audible alarms for low MV and high Paw will be suppressed.

Use of the nebulizer affects the F_IO_2 during the treatment, but delivered minute ventilation remains constant. An inspiratory flow of 18 L/min is needed to trigger the nebulizer gas supply. For this reason, use of the nebulizer is recommended for adults and larger children, but *not* for infants or small children. The ventilator's flow sensor is automatically heat-cleaned after the 30-minute treatment. (*Note*: The nebulizer function is designed for nebulizers requiring flows of 6 L/min. Use of other types nebulizers may result in discrepancies in minute ventilation readings.)

The key labeled "O_2 ↑suction" or "100% O_2" provides 180 seconds of 100% O_2 when pressed. This function automatically increases baseline pressure to 4 cm H_2O of PEEP if the baseline is <4 cm H_2O. The PEEP allows the Savina to detect a disconnection for suctioning. The suctioning procedure may actually last for up to 7 minutes (Box 12-115; see the section on suctioning described with the Evita earlier in this chapter for more details.)

The "Insp.Hold" key is used to deliver a breath or provide an inspiratory hold (increased T_I) to the patient. It can be activated either during a ventilator breath, prolonging the breath by increasing T_I or between mandatory ventilator breaths to give extra breaths based on current settings. The operator can press the "Insp.Hold" key during a breath to provide inflation hold for up to 15 seconds. Inspiratory hold is available in all modes except CPAP without pressure support. (*Note*: In the CPAP [spontaneous breathing] mode, if PS is more than zero, inspiratory hold delivers the set PS level.)

Screen Pages

The five control keys below the information window are used to select the screen page to display in the window. The screen pages (see Figure 12-104) are all formatted in a similar fashion. At the top left area the ventilation mode appears. At the top right is an alarm message field that displays information during an alarm event (not pictured). The large center area of the screen displays waveforms and measured values. The two bottom rows of the screen display measured values and an information bar.

The first key on the left under the screen is called "Waveforms" and changes the screen display to the main screen page. The waveforms screen also allows switching between the waveforms displayed (flow-time or pressure-time). The next key, "Settings," displays ventilator parameters and allows for setting ventilation parameters (Box 12-116). The "Alarms" key displays the current alarm limits and allows for setting new values. Setting alarm limits is done in the same way as setting ventilator parameters (see Box 12-116). The "Values" key displays the page of measured values (Table 12-43). Finally, the configuration key on the right allows access to system settings such as the language used on the screen, the volume of the alarms, and the measured parameters displayed in the measured values field (Box 12-117).

Box 12-116 "Settings" Screen

The Settings screen displays the following:

- An analog bar of airway pressure (Paw)
- A menu for setting the supplementary ventilation parameters "Trigger," "FlowAcc," and "AutoFlow"
- A setting menu for apnea ventilation with parameters for "V_{TApnea}" and "f_{Apnea}"
- A setting menu for sigh

The operator uses the control dial to scroll through the selections on the screen. When the desired setting is highlighted (bold frame), the control dial is pressed to activate that parameter for setting. To set the parameter, the operator uses the control dial to change the value or the setting (on/off) and presses the dial to confirm the value or setting selected.

Box 12-117 Configuration Screen

The Configuration screen has a total of four pages. The screen allows the adjustment of the following parameters:

- Screen contrast
- Alarm volume
- Measured values displayed
- Manual calibration for O_2 sensor
- F_IO_2 and flow monitor (on/off)
- Pmax (on/off)
- Plateau (on/off)
- Language, date, and time
- MEDIBUS protocol

Table 12-43 Measured Values Displayed

Value	Abbreviation
Peak pressure	Ppeak
Plateau pressure	Pplat
Mean airway pressure	Pmean
PEEP	PEEP
Exhaled tidal volume	VTe
Minute volume	MV
Spontaneous minute volume	MVspn
Inspiratory hold time interval	Tplat
Total respiratory rate	ftot
Spontaneous respiratory rate	fspn
I:E ratio	I:E
Fractional inspired oxygen	F_IO_2
Temperature	Temp (Celsius)
Peak flow	$Flow_{peak}$

Settings Screen

The parameters that can be selected for setting are listed in Box 12-116. Several of these warrant further discussion, including trigger, flow acceleration, AutoFlow, and sigh.

The trigger variable adjusts for patient-triggering of breaths using flow-triggering. In the "Settings" screen, the operator selects "trigger" and uses the control dial to adjust the trigger sensitivity. The least sensitive is the "off" position. A low value represents a high sensitivity, with a range of 1 to 15 L/min. For example, a value of 2 L/min would represent a sensitive setting requiring little patient effort to trigger a breath. (See Chapter 11 for additional information on flow-triggering.)

The flow acceleration feature is similar to the sloping or rise time feature used in other ventilators (see Chapter 11). Flow acceleration influences the rate of pressure and flow delivery at the beginning of inspiration. A greater value results in a steeper (faster) increase in pressure and flow. The available range is 5 to 200 cm H_2O/sec. A setting of 100 cm H_2O/second represents a reasonable starting point. Flow acceleration must be adjusted to suit an individual patient's needs. Flow acceleration is used in both pressure- and volume-targeted breaths. During volume ventilation, the faster the flow, the quicker the delivery of V_T. The resulting value for peak flow may be observed by bringing up page two of the "Measured Values" screen.

AutoFlow is a unique mode adaptation that can provide pressure-targeted ventilation for any of the volume modes available on the Savina. AutoFlow was described extensively in the section on the Dräger E-4 ventilator in this chapter. Box 12-118 provides a brief explanation of its function. When AutoFlow is enabled, the high airway pressure and high tidal volume limit must be set appropriately in the event that these two variables increase due to a change in patient compliance.

Box 12-118 AutoFlow

AutoFlow provides pressure-targeted breaths with volume guaranteed and can be activated in any volume-targeted modes (CMV, SIMV, MMV) (see Chapter 11 discussion of PRVC).

AutoFlow is enabled in the "Settings" screen. When AutoFlow is activated, the first breath the ventilator delivers is a volume-targeted breath. The ventilator then measures the plateau pressure during that breath. The ventilator calculates the system compliance (C) and resistance (R) and establishes the minimum pressure needed to deliver the set volume. If the V_T is lower than the set V_T, the Savina increases pressure delivery. If the delivered volume is too high compared to the set volume, it decreases pressure delivery. Pressure adjustment between breaths is never greater than 3 cm H_2O.

Volume delivery may also be higher than the set value if the patient is actively inspiring. The operator can avoid exceeding a specific V_T by using the V_{Ti} upper limit alarm for this purpose.

AutoFlow allows patients to receive whatever inspiratory flow they demand—up to 180 L/min in any volume mode regardless of the volume settings (Figure 12-31). In addition, AutoFlow makes the expiratory valve more interactive with the patient. For example, if the patient coughs or breathes during the set T_I of a mandatory breath, the expiratory valve system allows the patient to inhale and exhale freely while maintaining the inspiratory pressure. In AutoFlow, the maximum available pressure is the set high pressure limit minus 5 cm H_2O.

If the set V_T is reached (flow = zero) before T_I has elapsed, a plateau pressure phase is maintain without additional volume or flow delivery. The patient can breathe spontaneously during the plateau phase (Figure 12-31). (See Dräger Evita 4 in this chapter for additional information on using AutoFlow.)

A sigh breath is only available in the CMV A/C modes. The sigh is operated as it is in the Dräger E-4. When activated, the end-expiratory pressure increases by a value equal to the set PEEP plus the intermittent (sigh) PEEP, which is set by the operator. This value can be up to a total of 35 cm H_2O for two mandatory breaths every three minutes, thus providing sigh breaths (increased FRC). For example, with a PEEP of 5 cm H_2O and a sigh pressure of 15 cm H_2O, the pressure during a sigh breath will be 20 cm H_2O.

Alarm Silence, Alarm Reset, Lock, and Standby

The alarm silence key provides 2 minutes of audible alarm silence when pressed. The alarm silence key LED illuminates during this period. Box 12-119 describes the alarm priority system of the Savina. After an alarm condition has been corrected, the audible alarms are automatically switched off as is the illuminated LED in the upper right corner of the front panel. Pressing the "alarm reset" key removes any messages from the window.

To protect current settings from changes, the operator presses the LOCK key. The yellow LED illuminates. This prevents changes in parameter keys, mode keys, and screen settings. To unlock, press the LOCK key again.

Setting Alarm Limits

Table 12-44 lists the alarms that can be set along with their available ranges. The "Alarms" screen page allows alarm limits to be set. As with other screens, the operator uses the control dial to highlight the desired alarm (outlined in bold). Pressing the control dial selects the alarm. Using the control dial again allows the operator to set the desired value. Pressing the control dial then activates the newly set alarm limit.

Three commonly used alarms are not adjustable: LOW AIRWAY PRESSURE and the HIGH and LOW O_2 ALARMS. The low airway pressure alarm limit is automatically adjusted based on the PEEP setting. A lower airway pressure alarm will occur when an airway pressure equal to the set PEEP + 5 cm H_2O is not exceeded for at least 0.1 seconds for two consecutive mandatory breaths.

The high and low oxygen concentration alarms are also automatically set. For set F_IO_2 values less than 0.6, the upper and lower O_2 alarm limits are 4% above and below the set O_2%. For set F_IO_2 values greater than 0.6, the upper and lower O_2 alarm limits are 6% above and below the set O_2%. Several other nonadjustable alarms are also listed in Table 12-45. Most alarm conditions provide explanatory messages in the information window to assist the operator in determining the cause of the alarm.

Box 12-119 Alarm Categories

Three alarm priorities are provided: top priority, medium priority, and low priority.

- Top priority alarms result in a top priority message in the information window with a warning describing the alarm that was activated, followed by three exclamation points (!!!). A red LED flashes in the upper right corner of the front panel and a five-tone audible sequence occurs twice and is repeated every 7.5 seconds.
- Medium priority alarms provide a message stating the alarm condition. This is followed by two exclamation points (!!). A yellow LED flashes in the upper right corner of the front panel. A three-tone audible alarm activates every 20 seconds.
- Low priority alarms provide a message in the window stating the cause of the alarm. This message is following by one exclamation point (!). A yellow LED illuminates in the upper right corner of the front panel and does not flash. A two-tone audible alarm sounds only once.

Table 12-44 Alarms and Alarm Ranges for the Dräger Savina

Alarm	Setting Range
Upper Pressure Limit (Paw)	10 to 100 cm H_2O
High Minute Ventilation (MV↑)	2.0 to 41.0 L/min
Low Minute Ventilation (MV↓)	0.5 to 40.0 L/min
Apnea Time (T_{Apnea})	15 to 60 seconds
High Respiratory Rate (ftot)	10 to 120 breaths/min
High Inspiratory Tidal Volume (V_{Ti})	0.06 to 4.0 L

Table 12-45 Nonadjustable Alarms

Alarm	Condition
High Ambient Temperature	Ambient temperature >30° C.
Gas Supply Failure	Loss of high-pressure oxygen source.
Ambient Pressure High	The measured atmospheric pressure exceeds the acceptable range for the ventilator or a pressure sensor is faulty.
Ambient Pressure Low	The measured atmospheric pressure is less than the acceptable range for the ventilator or a pressure sensor is faulty.
Breathing Gas Temperature High	Breathing gas temperature >40° C.
Check Settings	Result of an internal data loss. The Savina continues operating using factory default settings until the ventilator is checked and adjusted.
Device Failure XX.YYYY	Ventilator fault. If Alarm reset does not remedy, remove ventilator from service and provide ventilation to the patient.
Exp. Valve Failure	Expiratory valve faulty or not properly installed.
	Possible faulty flow sensor.
Fan Failure	Cooling fan has failed. Remove ventilator from service and provide ventilation to the patient.

Modes of Ventilation

Along the bottom of the front panel are the keys used for selecting the ventilation mode. These include CMV A/C (IPPV internationally), SIMV, PCV+ (BiPAP internationally), and CPAP/PS (CPAP/ASB internationally).

Setting Ventilator Parameters in Advance When Changing Modes

Before changing a mode, it is appropriate to set all the desired variables for that mode before switching to the new mode. To perform this procedure, the operator presses the desired mode key (yellow LED flashes). In the area of the front panel containing the ventilator parameters, the LEDs for any additional parameters required for the new mode will start flashing. Each of the flashing parameter keys is set by pressing the key, using the control dial to select the desired value and pressing the control dial to confirm the selection. After all the parameters are set, the operator presses the control dial to activate the new ventilation mode. (*Note*: Two other methods can be used to activate a new mode. Pressing the mode key for 3 seconds will activate the new mode. Or, pressing the mode key briefly and then pressing the control dial will activate the mode.)

The Savina can also be used for NPPV by using an appropriate patient interface, such as a mask. During NPPV, the Savina provides leak compensation. The operator may want to turn off or readjust the following alarms during NPPV: high V_T, low MV, low airway pressure (delay), and apnea alarm.

CMV A/C

CMV and CMV Assist/Control in the Savina are represented as two modes: CMV or controlled ventilation and CMV A/C or assist/control ventilation. As described in Chapter 11, controlled implies no patient-triggering. Assist/control allows patient-triggering to occur if the patient has some spontaneous effort. This discussion will focus on CMV A/C because deliberately turning off a ventilator's sensitivity (trigger) to a patient's effort is generally ill-advised.

CMV A/C is a volume-targeted mode of ventilation in which all breaths are delivered at the set V_T. Inspiration is time- or patient-triggered (flow-triggering), volume-targeted, and volume- or time-cycled. For CMV A/C the operator sets V_T, rate, inspiratory time, and PEEP. Trigger and FlowAcc can also be enabled using the "Settings" Screen. (*Note*: When trigger is enabled, the mode at the top left of the window will read "CMV assist" ["IPPV assist" internationally].) In CMV A/C a minimum breath rate is set, but the patient may trigger additional breaths at the set volume. The set V_T is delivered for each breath.

Two types of *inspiratory cycling* can be programmed to end inspiration. The plateau feature "on" and the plateau feature "off." When the plateau feature is enabled, inspiration is time-cycled and consists of two parts. First, the inspiratory flow, adjusted with flow acceleration, delivers the set tidal volume. Second, when inspiratory flow stops after delivery of V_T, the exhalation valve remains closed until the set T_I has elapsed. This results in an inspiratory pause during which the airway pressure drops to a plateau representing lung distending pressure (Figure 12-105, *breath 1*). When plateau is enabled, the set T_I is an adjustable parameter.

When the plateau feature is disabled, inspiratory time cannot be set. Inspiratory time depends on the set V_T and the flow acceleration setting. The Savina switches to exhalation after the set tidal volume has been delivered (volume-cycling) (Figure 12-105, *breath 2*).

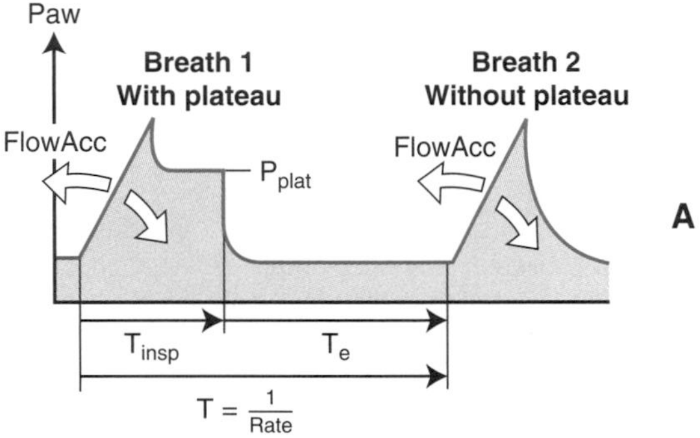

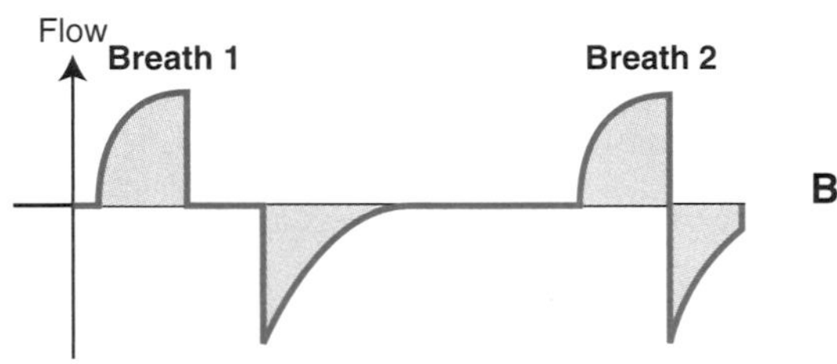

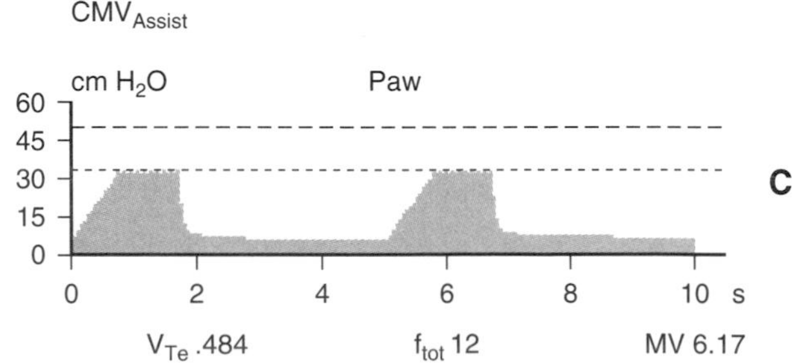

Figure 12-105 In breath **1** (parts A and B), the plateau feature is "on." CMV ventilation with flow acceleration (FlowAcc) adjusted for a ramp in pressure at the beginning of inspiration. After V_T delivery, flow ends, the expiratory valve closes and a plateau pressure results. In breath **2** (parts A and B), the plateau feature is "off" during CMV ventilation. FlowAcc is enabled. Volume-cycled breaths occur. Notice T_I is shorter than in breath **1.** In **C,** CMV A/C (assist) with Pmax is illustrated. The pressure limit set at 30 cm H_2O. The dashed horizontal line at approximately 50 cm H_2O represents the upper pressure limit at which an alarm will activate and inspiration will end. (Courtesy Dräger Medical, Telford, Penn.)

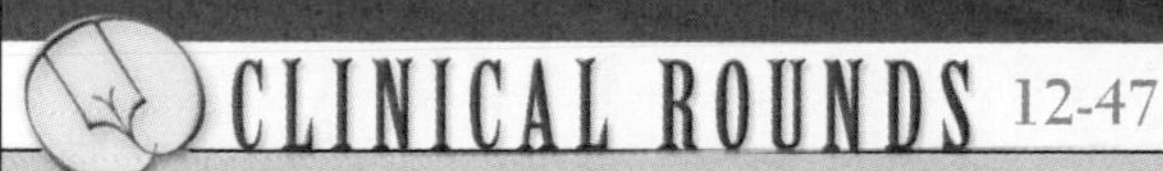

A respiratory therapist observes the flow-time waveform during CMV A/C ventilation and notes that the inspiratory flow drops to zero before the patient begins exhalation. What information does this provide to the therapist about the cycling of the breath and about the patient's lung compliance?

See Appendix A for the answer.

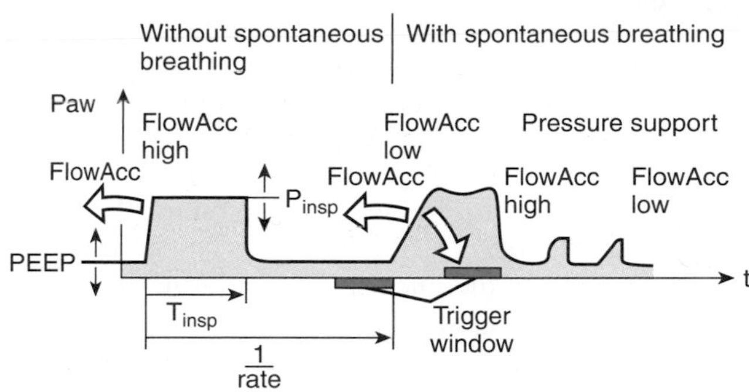

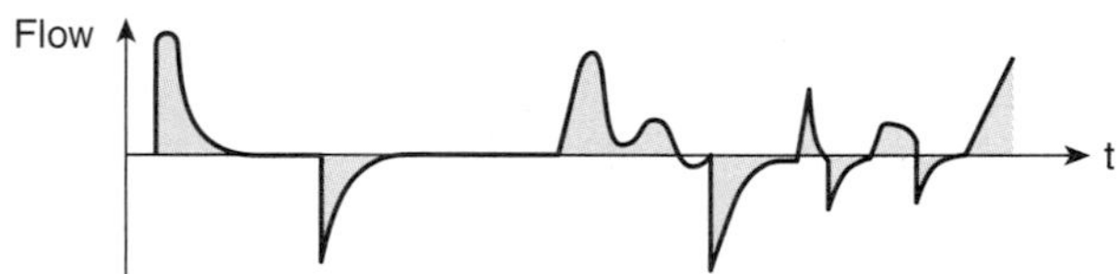

Figure 12-106 This figure shows PCV+ ventilation. The breath on the left is a pressure-targeted breath without spontaneous breathing. The Pinsp key sets the pressure for the mandatory PCV+ stroke. Spontaneous breaths occur at the baseline pressure (PEEP set). Flow acceleration (FlowAcc) is set for a rapid flow delivery. Inspiratory pressure (Pinsp) is delivered during the set inspiratory time (Tinsp). The next breath (right) occurs with spontaneous breathing. The trigger window illustrates the time during which the ventilator will wait for a patient's inspiratory effort. Flow acceleration is set lower for the mandatory breath compared to the previous breath. The patient can breathe spontaneously during a mandatory breath or between mandatory breaths. Pressure support is also set. One spontaneous breath shows a high FlowAcc delivery and the next a low FlowAcc delivery. The flow curve shows the variation in flow delivery to accommodate patient demand. (See text for further description.) (Courtesy Dräger Medical, Telford, Penn.)

CMV A/C can also be pressure-limited by enabling the maximum pressure limit feature (Pmax). The intended use of Pmax is to avoid high pressures during volume ventilation. Pmax is enabled using the configuration screen. The desired pressure limit is set with the Pinsp parameter key on the front panel.

When Pmax is operational, the ventilator targets the set V_T but limits the pressure delivered during the breath. When the pressure in the circuit reaches the pressure setting (Pinsp), inspiration continues for the set inspiratory time (time-cycled), but the amount of pressure in the circuit does not go above Pinsp (Figure 12-105, C). The V_T delivery remains constant at the set V_T as long as flow drops to zero before the end of inspiration; in other words, an inspiratory hold occurs. If flow does not drop to zero by the end of the set T_I, the volume cannot be delivered and a volume a "V_T low" message appears (Clinical Rounds 12-47). The volume can be increased either by increasing Pinsp, T_I, FlowAcc, or some combination of the three.

SIMV, SIMV/PS

Synchronized intermittent mandatory ventilation, as described in Chapter 11, provides a maximum number of mandatory breaths at set intervals based on the set rate. Mandatory breaths can be time- or patient-triggered and are volume-targeted and volume- or time-cycled (see CMV A/C, plateau feature enabled). Between mandatory breaths the patient can breathe spontaneously from the baseline pressure. Spontaneous breaths can be assisted with pressure support. As with CMV, volume breaths can be pressure-limited using the Pmax feature. FlowAcc is also available for both mandatory breaths and spontaneous breaths supported with PSV.

PCV+ (BiPAP International Version)

"Pressure control ventilation plus" (PCV+) is an optional ventilation mode similar to PC-SIMV plus PEEP. PCV+ is intended for use in spontaneously breathing patients. This mode provides two levels of pressure, with each pressure level (high and low) being delivered for a set time frame. The patient can breathe spontaneously at either pressure level (Figure 12-106).

The lower level pressure is set with the PEEP control key, whereas the upper pressure level is set with the Pinsp control key. The steepness of the increase from PEEP to Pinsp can be adjusted using the "FlowAcc" function. The time pattern is set using the rate and inspiratory time controls. During the lower pressure phase, spontaneous breaths can also be supported with PS (ΔPsupp above PEEP control key). (*Note*: The operator must set an appropriate trigger, so that the patient's efforts are detected by the ventilator.)

Tidal volume delivery varies depending on patient effort, patient lung characteristics, and the pressure difference between the two CPAP levels (PEEP and Pinsp). Tidal volume will also be affected by PS setting.

A patient can be weaned with PCV+ by gradually reducing Pinsp or the rate as the patient is able to maintain a greater amount of the work of breathing. Because V_T and $\dot{V}_E$ are not set in PCV+, the operator must exercise caution in setting alarm limits for tidal volume and minute ventilation.

CPAP/PS

Continuous positive airway pressure and the pressure support modes are intended for use with spontaneous breathing patients only. CPAP elevates the baseline pressure. PS provides a patient-triggered, pressure-targeted, flow-cycled breath. The trigger setting determines the patient effort required to trigger inspiratory flow. The "Psupp.above PEEP" control sets the target pressure during inspiration. "FlowAcc" can be used to adjust the rate of inspiratory pressure and flow delivery at the beginning of the breath.

Inspiration normally ends when the ventilator detects a drop to 25% of measured peak flow. Inspiratory flow will also end if the patient actively exhales resulting in airway pressure higher than the set value, or if inspiration exceeds 4 seconds.

Apnea Ventilation

In the event of a spontaneously breathing patient becoming apneic during SIMV, CPAP/PS, or PCV+ ventilation, apnea ventilation (AV) provides safety back-up volume ventilation with a minimum breath rate. For example, if no patient effort is detected, the Savina activates an alarm after the set apnea time (T_{Apnea}) has elapsed. The f_{Apnea} and V_{TApnea} set in the "Settings" screen become the active rate and tidal volume settings. The I:E ratio is set at 1:2.

To set AV, the operator selects the "Settings" screen and enables AV by turning the control dial so that "Apn.-Vent.Off." is highlighted, then presses the control dial. This enables the AV feature (apnea ventilation on) and allows setting f_{Apnea} rate (must be set > 2 breaths/min) and V_{TApnea}. The apnea time delay (T_{Apnea}) is set in the "Alarms" screen page.

A patient can breathe spontaneously between mandatory breaths during AV. To end AV when it has become active, press the "Alarm Reset" key. The Savina returns to the original set mode of ventilation.

Troubleshooting

The alarm messages that appear in the information window provide direction regarding the possible cause of an alarm condition. The majority of problems are easily solved. In situations in which an immediate solution is not available, the operator should find another means to ventilate the patient until the problem can be remedied. Clinical Rounds 12-48 provides an example of a problem situation.

Servo^{i} Ventilator System[1-2]

The Servo^{i} Ventilator system (v.1.1, Siemens Medical Systems, Inc.) consists of two main parts, a patient unit where gases are mixed and delivered to the patient and a user interface (front panel) where the ventilator settings are selected and information monitored (Figure 12-107). The ventilator can be used in acute care facilities and for in-hospital transport and is intended for patients ranging in size from newborns (0.5 to 30 kg) to adults (10-250 kg).

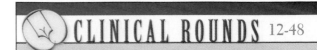

Problem 1

The message "!!! Int. batt. Almost discharged" appears in the window at the same time that a 5 tone alarm sounds and an LED in the top right corner of the front panel illuminates red. What should the respiratory therapist do to solve this problem?

Problem 2

The message "!!! Device Failure XX.YYY" appears in the window at the same time that a 5 tone alarm sounds and an LED in the top right corner of the front panel illuminates red. What should the respiratory therapist do to solve this problem?

See Appendix A for the answer.

Three different configurations can be purchased which differ primarily by the modes included. The Servo^{i} Infant includes SIMV(pc) + PS, PS/CPAP, and PC (modes will be reviewed later). The Servo^{i} Adult has SIMV(VC) + PS, PS/CPAP, and VC. The Servo^{i} Universal includes all modes as well as PRVC. VS-Automode and the nebulizer feature are optional on all platforms. A software package is available for a lung recruitment strategy that can be used for tracking compliance, peak pressures, and other parameter changes during lung recruitment.

Power Source

The Servo^{i} is electrically and pneumatically powered. The electrical power sources for the Servo^{i} ventilator include AC power and 12-volt DC internal batteries (optional). The status indicator for the power source is a STATUS pad located at the upper right corner of the touch screen. Besides indicating the current power source, this STATUS pad also serves additional functions (Box 12-120).

If the main power fails, the ventilator automatically switches to battery operation. The battery capacity is displayed on the battery module and is also displayed under the STATUS MENU touch pad. If no battery module has been inserted or connected, a high-priority alarm occurs and the inspiratory and expiratory valves open to allow for spontaneous breathing from room air. Box 12-121 describes the battery module.

The Servo^{i} has two gas modules, one for a high-pressure air source and one for high-pressure oxygen. (*Note*: During operation if the air and O_2 pressure is too low, the safety valve and the expiratory valve open and an alarm occurs.)

All ventilator settings are made using the front panel, also called the User Interface. The ventilator can be operated using the touch screen and the main rotary dial or the direct access knobs when applicable.

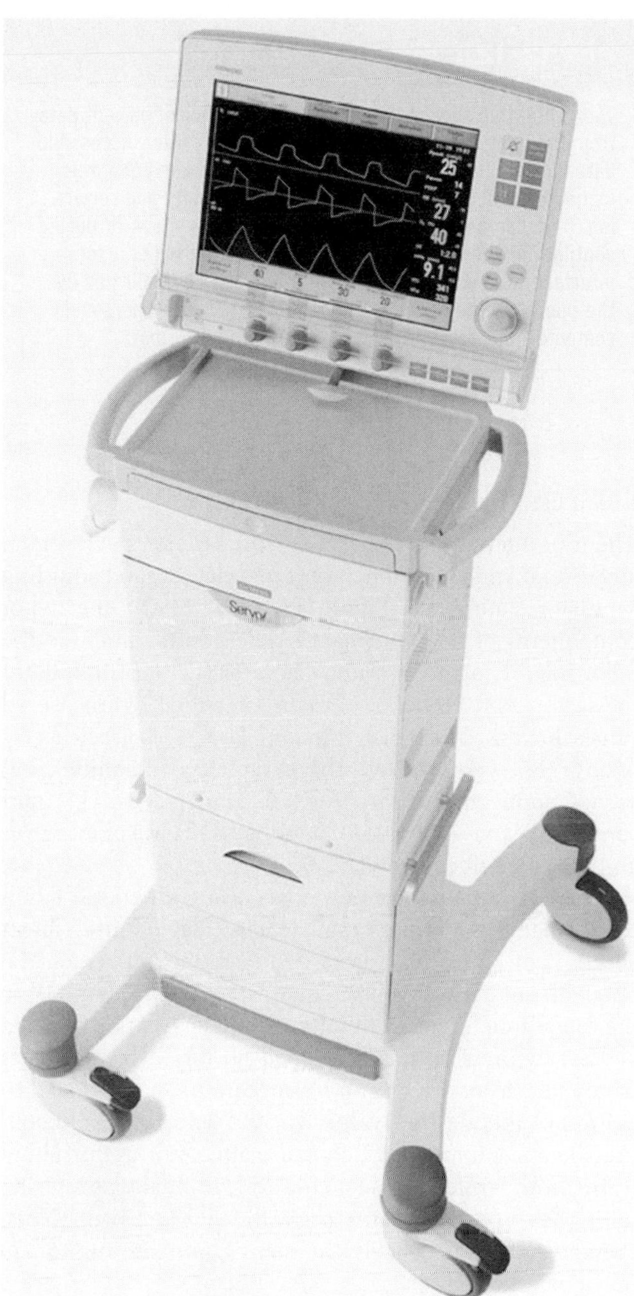

Figure 12-107 The patient unit and user interface *(top)* of the Servo^i. (Courtesy Siemens Medical Solutions, Inc., Danvers, Mass.)

Internal Drive Mechanism

The internal drive mechanism of the Servo^i is the same as the Servo 300 described previously in this chapter. The modules for air and O_2 regulate the gas flow into the ventilator. The gas flow is then directed into the inspiratory mixing section. The O_2 concentration and the gas pressures are measured. The gas mixture is then directed through the main inspiratory channel to the inspiratory limb of the patient circuit.

Box 12-120 Status Window

When the STATUS pad in the upper right corner of the touch screen is pressed, a list appears showing:

- General system information
- Status of O_2 cell
- Status of expiratory cassette
- Status of modules
- Installed options
- Status of pre-use check

Box 12-121 Battery Module

The Servo^i has an external battery module capable of holding six 12 volt rechargeable and interchangeable batteries. These batteries are automatically charged when the ventilator is connected to an AC power supply.

The battery module is used as a back-up power source should AC power fail, and can also be used during transport. Each battery provides approximately 30 minutes of power. When fully discharged each battery requires 3 hours to fully recharge. The batteries are charged in consecutive order one at a time.

An indicator on the battery module shows the amount of charge remaining. The operator presses the button adjacent to the battery power indicator to illuminate the scale (25%, 50%, 75%, or 100%). The touch screen of the front panel of the Servo^i also displays the number of minutes remaining battery back-up time.

Exhaled gases from the patient pass into what the manufacturer refers to as an expiratory cassette. As exhaled gas enters the cassette, a moisture trap collects condensate from the exhaled air. Within the expiratory cassette, expiratory flow is measure by ultrasonic transducers and expiratory pressure by pressure transducers. (*Note*: The expiratory cassette can be exchanged between Servo^i ventilators. However, a pre-use check should be performed after exchanging the cassette.) Inspiratory and expiratory flow and pressure are continuously measured with transducers and controlled by the feedback system within the patient unit. Information is compared to front panel settings. Differences between set and measured values result in adjustment of gas delivery based on the set target variable (flow, volume, pressure)

Setting up a New Patient

Whenever the Servo^i is going to be used on a new patient, pre-use checks, described in the Operator's manual and shown on the User Interface during the operation, are performed. When the pre-use check window appears on the screen, it provides a "yes" or "no" option. Running the checks feature evaluates internal technical functions such as pressure

Box 12-122 Compensate for Circuit Compliance "Yes" or "No?"

Some circumstances require that the compensation for circuit compliance feature be turned off.

First, the feature is not needed in pressure-targeted breaths because volume is variable anyway and must be monitored. These include pressure control, pressure support and SIMV (PC).

Second, in instances where infants with uncuffed endotracheal tubes are being ventilated with small volumes, the low expired minute ventilation alarm may activate, even when set at its lowest value. This is because in the presence of system leaks, low volumes, and tubing compensation active, the flow through the expiratory channel is very low and may be detected as a low $\dot{V}_E$ situation. The manufacturer suggests turning the circuit compliance compensation feature off.

Box 12-123 Ventilation Record Card

The ventilation record card allows the transfer of patient data from the ventilator system to a personal computer. Accessible data include: patient name, patient identification code, the logged events, trends, technical log, test results and service log. Data can be copied to the card in standby mode or during ventilation. The card is inserted into the front panel (user interface). Copying of the information must be confirmed by the operator. The card can then be inserted into a personal computer and accessed using Windows Excel format.

and flow transducers, O_2 cells, the safety valve, internal battery, internal leaks, and the patient circuit for leaks and for circuit compliance. The screen lists the 11 tests performed and advises the operator what needs to be performed. For example, for part of the test the operator is instructed to occlude the patient Y-connector. As each consecutive test is passed, the screen indicates the "passed" status.

It is during the precheck test that the operator can elect to activate the tubing compliance function. This function, when enabled, adjusts delivered V_T in volume modes for loss of volume associated with the compressibility of the patient circuit (Box 12-122). See Chapter 11 for an explanation of tubing compressibility.

After testing is completed, new patient data can be entered. Touching the PATIENT DATA or ADMIT PATIENT pad in the top bar of the screen allows the operator to enter patient information. These include: patient name, identification number, date of birth, date of admission, body height, and body weight. (*Note*: The operator must be sure to save the previous patient's data to a Ventilator Record Card [a computer memory disc] to avoid erasing data [Box 12-123].) As a privacy issue, the operator needs to be aware that if a patient's name is entered, that name will appear at the top of the operating screen. It may be more appropriate to use an identifying number.

After entry of patient data, a window appears that allows the operator to select a patient category: "Infant" or "Adult." Selecting the appropriate patient size affects parameter ranges and default categories based on patient size. For example, the default mandatory breath rate in SIMV for infants is 20 breaths/min and 5 breaths/min for adults. As another example, the inspiratory rise time default setting is 0.05 seconds for both infants and adults. The range is 0 to 0.2 seconds for infants and 0 to 0.4 seconds for adults.

A quick method for admitting and entering patient data is to use the pad located in the top row of the touch panel controls (Figure 12-108).

Controls

The user interface or front panel consists of a touch screen and several knobs and touch keys for selecting and adjusting ventilator parameters. Figure 12-108 illustrates the major components of the front panel. The controls include the following: (1) a menu touch pad area, (2) text and alarm messages, (3) fixed keys, (4) main rotary dial, (5) measured values boxes, (6) special function keys, (7) direct access knobs, (8) on/off switch (back panel of machine), (9) service connector, (10) mains indicator (green), (11) start ventilation/stop ventilation (standby), (12) waveform area, and (13) patient category.

The Servo[i] uses four ways of accessing functions: touch screen panel functions, main rotary dial control, direct access knobs, and fixed keys. Using the touch screen the operator can activate a particular menu by simply pressing the menu touch pad. Ventilator parameters can be selected and set by pressing the touch pad on the screen (enables parameter; turns white), and using the main rotary dial to "turn to" the desired value for the selected parameter. Pressing the parameter touch pad again confirms the setting (turns from white to blue). However, to finally accept the setting, the operator must press the ACCEPT pad. (*Note*: Pressing CANCEL cancels the setting and returns to the previous value.)

The items located on the touch screen can also be set by using the main rotary dial. Turning the dial causes the items on the screen to be sequentially highlighted, like scrolling through a computer menu. After the desired parameter is highlighted, pressing the dial confirms the selection. Turning the dial again changes the parameter value. To enter the selected value the operator presses the main rotary dial. To activate the new setting, the dial is turned to highlight ACCEPT on the screen and again press the dial.

Just below the screen is a bottom row of controls beginning with the START VENTILATION/STOP VENTILATION (STANDBY) key (left side), four direct access knobs located directly underneath the touch screen, and four special function keys on the right.

The START VENTILATION/STOP VENTILATION key can be used to place the ventilator in a standby condition for allowing

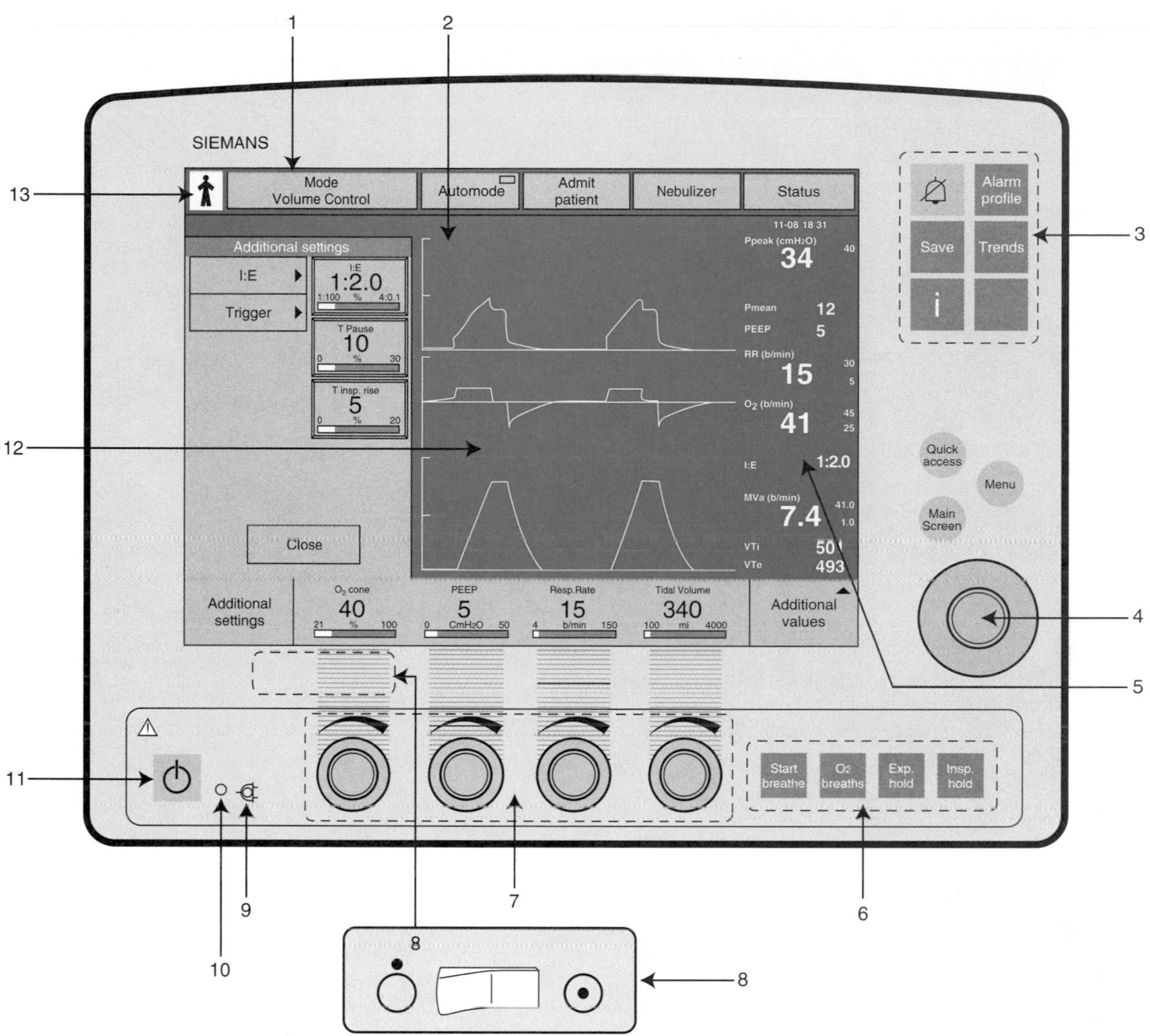

Figure 12-108 The Control panel/User Interface of the Servo[i] ventilator. (See text for further description.)

warm-up of the ventilator electronics or after a pre-use check has been completed. Pressing START VENTILATION/STOP VENTILATION and then the "yes" pad stops ventilation. Pushing the key again begins ventilation.

The direct access knobs are for immediate adjustment of ventilator parameters. When a specific mode of ventilation is in use, four parameter boxes related to that mode appear in a row at the bottom of the screen just above the direct access knobs. They include O_2 concentration, PEEP, rate, and volume or pressure. The knob just below each parameter allows the operator to change the setting. Color-coding of the set value provides information about the parameter limits. White is considered a safe setting range. Yellow is an advisory to indicate that the setting is too low or too high for what is considered safe limits. Red indicates a setting outside of safe limits and the patient's response should be monitored closely. The color indicator for each setting is to advise the user that he or she is setting a level that should be monitored closely because it could lead to lung damage or inappropriate ventilation.

The special function keys to the right of the direct access knobs include START BREATH, O_2 BREATHS, EXPIRATORY HOLD, and INSPIRATORY HOLD. Pressing the START BREATH key results in a manually activated breath using the set parameters. The O_2 BREATHS key provides 100% O_2 for 1 minute or until the key is pressed again. When EXPIRATORY HOLD key is pressed, an expiratory hold results at the end of expiration for as long as the key is pressed up to 30 seconds. Pressing the INSPIRATORY HOLD key provides an inflation hold that begins at the end of inspiration and lasts as long as the key is pressed (maximum 30 sec.).

Fixed keys are located in the upper right corner of the front panel. There are two kinds of fixed keys: those used for short-cuts to a function or screen and those that start special

Table 12-46 Items Contained in the Menu Screen

List of Contents That Appears on Screen	Details
Alarm	Alarm profile, alarm history, and alarm mute
Review	Accesses trends and recorded waveforms
Options	Lists installed optional features
Compliance circuit compensation	Indicates compensation for circuit compliance when performed during pre-use check
Copy data	Copies data to ventilation record card
Biomed	Provides access to display of default configurations
Panel lock	Locks panel settings, for example during transport; can be unlocked using MAIN SCREEN control
X	Changes patient category

An *arrow* next to a screen item indicates that submenus are present and will open when the screen item is touched.
A *sheet icon* next to an item on the list indicates that there is no submenu for that item.

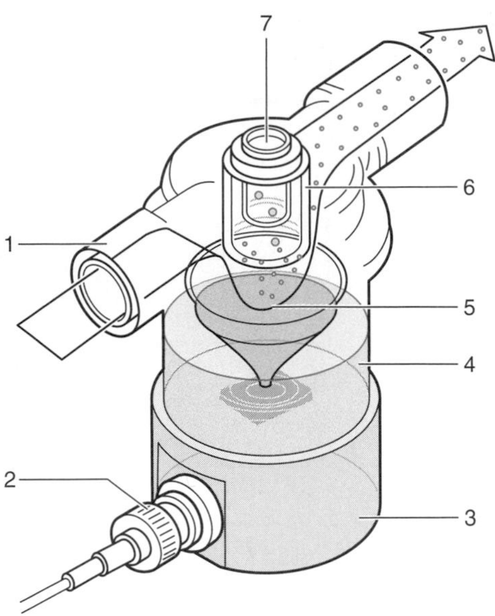

Figure 12-109 The Servo Ultra Nebulizer assembly of the Servo[i] showing *(1)* main gas flow connector (from the ventilator to the patient), *(2)* the power cable from the ventilator, *(3)* the ultrasonic generator, *(4)* the water chamber (couplant cup), *(5)* the medication cup, *(6)* a T-piece adapter containing baffles, and *(7)* the injection membrane. (See text for further description.) (Courtesy Siemens Medical Solutions, Inc, Danvers, Mass.)

ventilator functions. The latter require continuous direction by the operator when used.

Fixed Keys

The fixed keys include an ALARM SILENCE KEY, ALARM PROFILE, SAVE, TRENDS, INFORMATION (I), and a blank key. Pressing ALARM SILENCE provides 2 minutes of silence to all alarms except high-priority alarms for Paw high, and No battery capacity. Pressing ALARM PROFILE results in the alarm screen appearing. This screen displays the upper and lower alarm limits settings for all applicable alarms. The alarm screen can also be used to change alarm settings. Additional information about alarms is provided later.

The TRENDS key when pressed displays a screen showing trended values. Trends can be recorded for up to 24 hours with values being saved every 60 seconds. All saved events and system changes, such as running pre-use ventilator checks, are shown as event "stamps" on the screen. The TRENDS screen provides controls for locating the time and type of an event, scrolling up and down the screen between event graphs, finding a explanation of an event, changing the resolution of the time axis, and closing the window.

Three round keys are located just below the square fixed keys. The three include a MAIN SCREEN key, a MENU key and a QUICK ACCESS key. Pressing the MAIN SCREEN key is a shortcut to return to the main view screen. The MENU key brings up a list of items when pressed (Table 12-46). Pressing the QUICK ACCESS key brings up a menu for loops, and scales.

Touch Screen Controls

The touch screen area contains several areas for controlling functions and viewing information. Across the top is a row containing the following from left to right (Figure 12-108):

- Patient category—displays current selection (infant or adult).
- Current mode of ventilation.
- X Automode [on/off] (an option)—Pad that turns Automode on and off.
- Admit patient/enter patient data—A quick access to the patient data field.
- X Nebulizer [on/off] (an option)—Pad that turns the nebulizer function on and off (see the following section).
- System status—indicates the current source of power.

Automode and the nebulizer are optional features.

Nebulizer

The Servo[i] ventilator comes equipped with an optional ultrasonic nebulizer for the delivery of medications. For the nebulizer to function the ventilator must be operating from an AC power source. Pressing the nebulizer pad brings up a TIME pad on the touch screen. The operator sets the time for the treatment by using the main rotary dial. Pressing the

ACCEPT pad begins nebulization. After it is enabled, the nebulizer operates continuously regardless of the mode of ventilation or settings. No extra gas volume is added to the tidal volume, so F_IO_2 and minute ventilation remain unchanged.

The nebulizer assembly is fitted into the patient circuit with a T-piece (Figure 12-109). Medications are placed in a medication cup through an injectable cap. The medication cups are designed so that the airflow in the inspiratory limb of the patient circuit passes through the area where medications are being nebulized. The bottom of the medication cup sits within another chamber that contains sterile water. The water is in direct contact with the ultrasonic generating crystal and the bottom of the medication cup. (*Note*: The nebulizer cannot be used without sterile water in contact with the ultrasonic generator crystal or the crystal may break.) Chapter 4 includes an explanation of ultrasonic nebulizer technology.

Just below the top row of functions is a second row containing two fields. On the left is a box that provides text messages. When a purple symbol (a "I" in a circle) appears near the area of this box, the most recent breath was patient-triggered. The field on the right is the area for displaying alarm messages.

Below the two top rows is a large area of touch screen. The left is for displaying the real-time waveforms, and the right shows measured values and set alarm limits.

Waveforms

Three scalars are show simultaneously within the operating screen: pressure-time (yellow), flow-time (green) and volume-time (light blue). The sweep and vertical axes can be individually or automatically adjusted. (*Note*: To bring up loops, the operator presses the QUICK ACCESS pad and then the LOOPS pad.) When the ventilator is equipped with the optional CO_2 monitor module, a fourth scalar can also show the CO_2 measured as a graphic.

Measured Value Boxes

Measured values boxes are normally displayed numerically on the right side in the touch screen. The values that appear can be customized by the operator (Table 12-47). They can be either a measured or a calculated value such as V_T, Paw, PIP, and so on. Also located in this area are the lower and upper alarm limits. If a value in the box is outside the acceptable range three asterisks appear in the box.

In the lower right-hand corner of the touch screen is an ADDITIONAL (MEASURED) VALUES control that can be used by the operator to selected preferred values for display.

On the lower left corner of the touch screen is a box for ADDITIONAL SETTINGS. This control provides a shortcut for adjusting parameter values. When the ADDITIONAL SETTINGS pad is pressed, the touch screen brings up a window showing all available settings for the current mode. As with other parameters, colors indicate a suggested level of safety of the parameter setting (white, yellow, and red).

Parameter Controls

When a mode is selected, a touch screen window appears showing only the parameters available in that mode. Available parameters include rate, tidal volume, pressure control above PEEP (PC above PEEP), pressure support above PEEP (PS above PEEP), inspiratory rise time, I:E ratio, pause time, trigger sensitivity, PEEP, inspiratory cycle-off, breath cycle time, SIMV rate, trigger timeout, and O_2 concentration.

A few of the more unique parameters will be described.

Inspiratory rise time

This control adjusts the rate of rise to full inspiratory flow or pressure at the beginning of a breath. This function is similar to sloping or ramping in other ventilators (see Chapter 11).

Table 12-47 Shown Measured Values

DEFAULT VALUES	
P_{peak}	Maximum inspiratory pressure
P_{mean}	Mean airway pressure
PEEP	Total positive end expiratory pressure
RR	Respiratory rate
$\dot{V}ee$	End expiratory flow
I:E	Inspiratory-to-expiratory ratio (only during controlled ventilation)
Ti/T_{tot}	Duty cycle or ratio of inspiration time to total breathing cycle time (only during spontaneous breathing)
O_2	Oxygen concentration in percentage
MV_e	Expiratory minute volume
VT_i	Inspiratory tidal volume
VT_e	Expiratory tidal volume
ADDITIONAL MEASURED VALUES	
P_{plat}	Pressure during end-inspiratory pause
$PEEP_{tot}$	Intrinsic positive end expiratory pressure
MV_i	Inspiratory minute volume
C*static*	Static compliance, respiratory system
E	Elastance
C *dyn*	Dynamic characteristics
R_i	Inspiratory resistance
R_e	Expiratory resistance
WOB*p*	Work of breathing, patient
WOB*v*	Work of breathing, ventilator
Tc	Time constant
SBI	Shallow breathing index

Courtesy Siemens Medical.

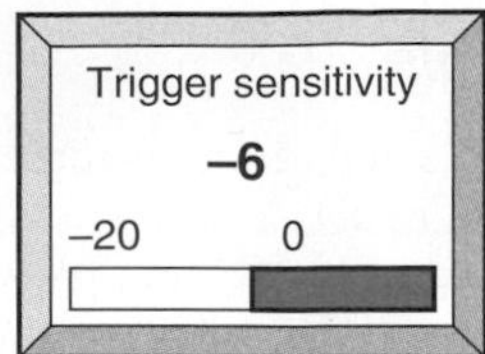

Figure 12-110 The trigger sensitivity box on the Servo[i]. (See text for additional information.) (Courtesy Siemens Medical Solutions, Inc, Danvers, Mass.)

Box 12-124 Trigger Sensitivity Bar

When the trigger sensitivity bar (Figure 12-110) is displayed colors are also displayed but are different from those of ventilator parameters. If the trigger sensitivity bar is green, this indicates a normal setting for flow-triggering. If the bar is red, the risk of self-triggering is present (overly sensitive). If the bar is yellow, pressure-triggering is being used.

Inspiratory rise time can be adjusted either as a percentage of the total cycle time or in seconds.

Trigger Sensitivity

The Servo[i] uses flow- and pressure-triggering to respond to patient's inspiratory efforts. The trigger sensitivity box that appears on the touch screen displays a horizontal bar graph (Figure 12-110, Box 12-124). This bar graph provides a visual indicator of the required patient effort.

When sensitivity is set above zero, breaths are flow-triggered. The more the bar appears to the right side, the more sensitive the flow-trigger function. The sensitivity bar is green for normal settings and red for settings that are very sensitive (auto-triggering possible.)

When sensitivity is set below zero (to the left side of the bar), the ventilator becomes pressure-triggered rather than flow-triggered. A yellow bar indicates pressure triggering is set. The negative pressure required to begin inspiration appears as a digital value in the trigger sensitivity box.

Inspiratory Cycle-Off Function

In supported modes of ventilation, such as pressure support, inspiration is flow-cycled. The flow-cycling variable is adjustable from 1% to 40% of the peak flow measured.

Breath Cycle Time

Breath cycle time is the total cycle time in a mandatory breath in SIMV (inspiratory time plus pause time plus expiratory time). It is set in seconds.

Trigger Timeout

Trigger timeout is the maximum allowed apnea time in Automode. After this time period has elapsed, the ventilator switches back to a control ventilation mode. Trigger timeout is not a constant amount of time, but varies depending upon how much spontaneous breathing the patient is doing. The more consecutive spontaneously triggered breaths that occur, the longer the timeout becomes. This means that for the spontaneously triggering patient, the timeout increases successively during the first ten breaths. (See Automode later in this section.)

Alarms

All alarms on the Servo[i] are audible and visual. The three alarm categories are high priority, medium priority, and low priority. High-priority alarms result in a red background. The background turns yellow after the alarm condition ceases but the alarm message remains on the screen until manually reset. Medium-priority alarms are indicated with a yellow background, as are low-priority alarms. The latter can be cleared from the screen even if the alarm condition remains.

Alarm limits are set by first pressing the ALARM PROFILE key, which brings up control pads on the touch screen for adjustable alarm limits. The operator presses the alarm limit desired, turns the main rotary dial to select the new value, and confirms the setting by pressing the parameter touch pad or by pressing the main rotary dial. Table 12-48 lists the available alarms and their defined values. The operator can use a recommended set of alarm limits in VC, PC, and PRVC modes by pressing Autoset. Pressing the ACCEPT key activates the new alarm limits. (*Note*: Autoset cannot be used during standby. The function needs to obtain patient values in order to propose values from calculated patient data.)

Pressing the DISPLAY CURRENT ALARMS key (bell icon) results in the appearance of a screen list of current alarm conditions in order of priority.

Modes of Ventilation

The modes of ventilation available on the Servo[i] are the same as those available on the Servo 300 with the addition of SIMV PRVC + PS. Only changes made to the Servo[i] regarding the modes will be included in this section.

The Servo[i] modes include four basic mode categories: controlled ventilation, supported ventilation, spontaneous ventilation, and combined ventilation. A special feature called Automode is also available and is the same feature as Automode available with the Servo 300e. The apnea criteria can be set and the Automode feature is activated after one breath, rather than two breaths with the Servo 300A. Trigger timeout also adds an additional safety to be sure the patient is ready for Automode. The timeout setting represents the maximum apnea time permitted during Automode. The control and assist/control (A/C) modes are volume control (VC), pressure control (PC), and PRVC. The support modes are VS and pressure support (PS). The SPONTANEOUS BREATHING/CPAP represents the spontaneous mode. The combined modes are SIMV modes that incorporate mandatory breaths based on VC, PC, and PRVC.

Table 12-48 Alarms and Alarm Ranges

Alarms	Range
AIRWAY PRESSURE (UPPER)	
Adult	16 to 120 cm H_2O
Infant	16 to 90 cm H_2O
High continuous pressure	Set PEEP + 15 cm H_2O exceeded for >15 sec.
O_2 concentration	Set value ± 6% or ≤18%
EXPIRED MINUTE VOLUME (UPPER ALARM LIMIT)	
Adult	0.5 to 60 L/min
Infant	0.1 to 30 L/min
EXPIRED MINUTE VOLUME (LOWER ALARM LIMIT)	
Adult	0.5 to 40 L/min
Infant	0.1 to 20 L/min
APNEA	
Adult	15 to 45 sec
Infant	5 to 15 sec
Gas supply	Below 2.0 kPa × 100 and over 6.5 kPa × 100
Respiratory rate	1 to 160 breaths/min
Battery	Limited battery capacity: 10 minutes
	No battery capacity: less than 3 minutes
Low end-expiratory pressure	0 to 47 cm H_2O. Setting alarm to zero is alarm off position
Technical	See Operator's Manual chapter on Patient Safety
AUTOSET (ALARM LIMITS) SPECIFICATIONS	
High airway pressure	Mean peak pressure plus 10 cm H_2O or at least 35 cm H_2O
Upper minute volume	Expiratory minute volume plus 50%
Lower minute volume	Expiratory minute volume minus 50%
Upper respiratory rate	Breathing frequency plus 40%
Lower respiratory rate	Breathing frequency minus 40%
Low end exp. press.	Mean end expiratory pressure minus 3 cm H_2O

Activating a Mode

To select a mode of ventilation, the operator touches the mode pad twice (the pad that shows the current mode setting). A menu of available modes appears on the touch screen. Pressing the touch pad for the desired mode results in all the related parameters for that mode appearing on the screen. Parameter variables can then be selected and adjusted. (*Note*: the direct access knobs at the bottom of the screen are inhibited when the parameter window is open from the mode menu.)

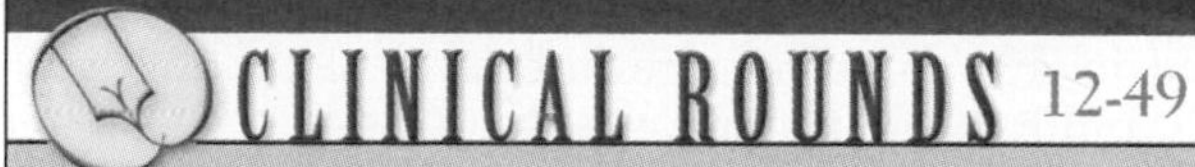

A patient on volume control ventilation using the Servo^{i} is actively inspiring during mandatory breath delivery. The set V_T is 600 mL, the rate is 10 breaths/min and the I:E to 1:2. The flow curve rises sharply after the flow-triggering of the breath, then flow plateaus. After the plateau the flow rises and falls like a sine wave and plateaus again. Inspiratory flow then ends.

Question 1: Why is the flow not constant during breath delivery?

Question 2: What will cycle the breath out of inspiration in this situation?

Question 3: Will the set V_T be delivered?

See Appendix A for the answer.

Volume Control

Volume control is similar to assist/control with a volume target. During volume ventilation on the Servo^{i} the flow is normally constant based on V_T, rate, and inspiratory time (based on I:E ratio). If no patient effort occurs during inspiration, flow remains constant. However, if a patient effort is detected during inspiration, the ventilator switches to pressure support to satisfy the patient's flow demand. Thus the patient can actually receive a volume higher than the set value and additional flow.

Clinical Rounds 12-49 provides an example of the application of volume control.

Pressure Control

Pressure control is similar to pressure control on the Servo 300. All breaths are delivered at a set pressure and can be time- or patient-triggered and time-cycled. The rate of inspiratory flow and pressure delivery can be adjusted using inspiratory rise time. PEEP can be used to elevate the baseline pressure

Pressure Regulated Volume Control

PRVC is available on the Servo^{i} and functions in the same manner as it does on the Servo 300. (See Chapter 11 and the Servo 300 earlier in this chapter for a review of PRVC.) The difference is in the Servo^{i} the first breath of a start sequence is a volume breath, using the set V_T, with a 10%

pause time. The plateau pressure measured during the pause is used to determine the pressure level of the following breath. In PRVC each inspiration is delivered at a constant pressure (pressure-targeted). However, the pressure can change from one breath to the next because the Servo^i endeavors to achieve the set tidal volume as its target. Changes occur in 3 cm H_2O increments up to a maximum pressure equal to the upper pressure limit minus 5 cm H_2O. Breaths can be patient- or time-triggered. Inspiratory flow and pressure delivery can be adjusted using the inspiratory rise time feature. Inspiration is time-cycled based on the set inspiratory time.

Volume Support

Volume support (VS) is a patient initiated breathing mode. Volume support on the Servo^i is based on V_T. The operator does not set minute volume when setting up the mode, so VS is not the same as on the Servo 300. The inspiratory pressure level is constant during a single breath. The pressure changes from one breath to the next to achieve the set V_T (increments of 3 cm H_2O). All breaths are patient-triggered. The rate of inspiratory flow and pressure delivery can be adjusted using inspiratory rise time. Inspiration is flow-cycled based on the set percent of peak inspiratory flow. An alarm occurs if the pressure level required to achieve the set V_T reaches the upper pressure limit minus 5 cm H_2O.

In VS (and in PS) it is advisable to set an appropriate apnea time and to set the low and high rate and expired minute volume alarms for the patient in the event that spontaneous breathing changes significantly.

Pressure Support

PS is similar to PS on the Servo 300 except that the flow-cycling variable can be adjusted using the inspiratory cycle off control ("Inspir cycle off"). Breaths are patient-triggered, pressure-targeted, and flow-cycled. Inspiratory pressure and flow delivery can be adjusted with the inspiratory rise time function.

Spontaneous Breathing/CPAP

Spontaneous breathing will occur under three conditions:

1. In VS when the target volume is maintained without requiring an added pressure from the ventilator. In other words, the patient's inspiratory effort triggers the ventilator to deliver flow to meet his or her demand. This flow requirement may result in a V_T delivery greater than the set value at a pressure near baseline.
2. In PS when the inspiratory pressure is set at zero.
3. When "X" is the function in Automode when either of the above conditions is met.

A spontaneous breath ends when flow decreases to the set percent of peak flow or if the upper pressure limit is exceeded (Clinical Rounds 12-50). The Servo^i also offers a low PEEP alarm.

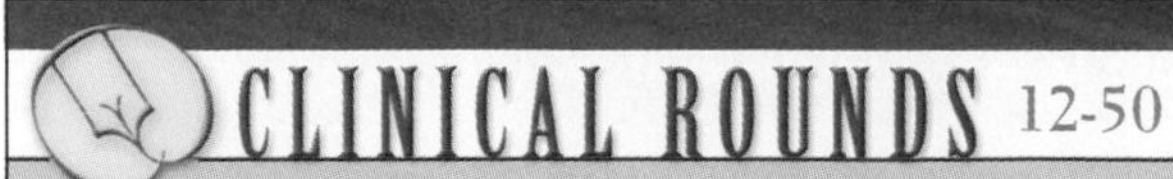

CLINICAL ROUNDS 12-50

A patient is switched from pressure support to volume support using the Servo^i ventilator. Settings are: V_T = 450 mL, upper pressure limit = 40 cm H_2O, PEEP = 3 cm H_2O, sensitivity to flow-trigger, F_IO_2 = 0.3. After the first few minutes, the respiratory therapist notices the pressure being maintained at 3 cm H_2O with no significant rise in pressure during inspiration. Spontaneous respiratory rate is 12 to 14 breaths/minute. What does the therapist know about the patient's spontaneous tidal volume based on this information? ______

See Appendix A for the answer.

SIMV

As with other ventilators, SIMV on the Servo^i provides mandatory breaths at a set rate and the patient can breath spontaneously between mandatory breaths. Mandatory breaths can be synchronized with the patient's spontaneous effort. In the Servo^i during SIMV, the mandatory breaths can be of three different types: PRVC, VC, or PC. Each of these breath types function was described earlier. Spontaneous breaths are from the baseline pressure (PEEP/CPAP) and can be supported with PS.

Automode

The Automode feature is similar to the Servo 300 Automode. The ventilator adapts to the patient's breathing pattern. Initially the ventilator starts in a control mode (VC, PC, and PRVC). If the patient triggers a breath, the ventilator reacts by delivering a support mode. In VC, the ventilator switches to VS, in PRVC it switches to VS and in PC it switches to PS. In the Servo^i, Automode is activated when the patient triggers one breath, whereas with the Servo 300 the ventilator waits to see two consecutive breaths before switching to the support mode.

If the patient is adequately maintaining ventilation, the support mode continues. However, if the patient fails to make an inspiratory effort, the ventilator switches back to the control mode.

When a spontaneously breathing patient regularly initiates breaths, the ventilator allows more time to elapse before it will deliver a mandatory breath if no patient effort is detected. This is called the "trigger time out" described earlier. The operator can set a maximum "trigger time out." (*Note*: If the patient meets a 10-cycle criteria and is still spontaneously breathing, the ventilator then uses an apnea time set by the operator to determine switching back to a control mode if the patient becomes apneic.)

Back-up Ventilation

In case the set apnea time is exceeded (adult, 15 to 45 sec; infant, 5 to 15 sec) in volume or pressure support modes, a safety back-up mode is enabled. Back-up ventilation uses default settings. In VS the ventilator switches to VC. In PS/CPAP the ventilator switches to PC. Default settings used are an I:E ratio 1:2, a rate of 15 breaths/min in adults and 30 breaths/min in infants, and an inspiratory rise time of 0.05 sec. For pressure support switching to pressure control, the back-up pressure level is either the set PS above PEEP or 20 cm H_2O, whichever is higher.

Special Features

The user interface of the Servo^i is significantly different from the Servo 300. The graphic display module has been incorporated directly into the front panel. The user interface can be attached directly to a patient's bed, as can the patient unit giving the Servo^i portability characteristics.

Along with the usual printed material available to purchasers of the ventilator, the Servo^i also has submitted a computer CD to the Food and Drug Administration (FDA). The CD is intended to provide interactive features, video clips and menu items that give additional instructive information. This CD is pending FDA approval.

Troubleshooting

The majority of alarm events that occur are easily solved using the displayed messages that provide a description of the problem involved. For example, the "Respiratory Rate: Low" message suggests the patient's respiratory rate has fallen below the alarm limit. The operator's manual contains a complete description of each alarm message, possible causes, and remedies, which is beyond the scope of this text. The reader is referred to that manual for additional information.

VIASYS AVEA Ventilator[1-3]

The AVEA ventilator was developed by VIASYS Healthcare, Critical Care Division, Palm Springs, Calif (Figure 12-111). The critical care division includes Bird, Bear, and Sensormedics products, previously part of the Thermo Respiratory Group. The AVEA is a servo-controlled, software-driven ventilator designed for neonatal to adult size patients. The user interface is a full color, active matrix LCD touch screen. Membrane buttons surrounding the touch screen give access to various screens and enable special functions. AVEA can be used for conventional invasive or noninvasive positive pressure ventilation.

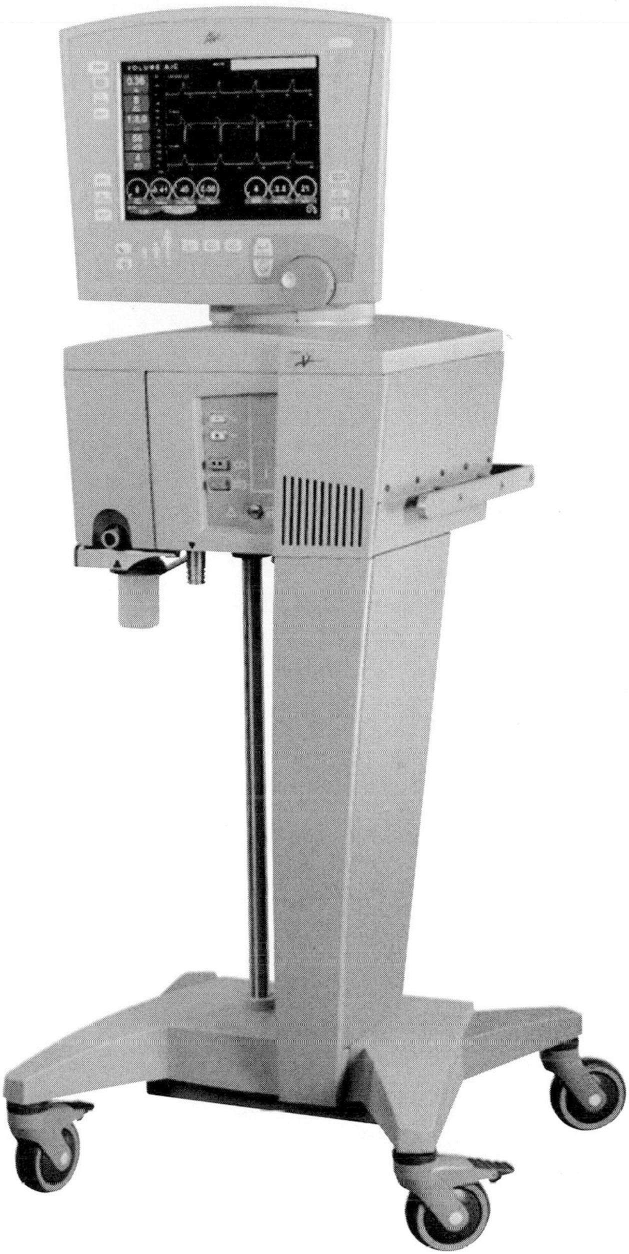

Figure 12-111 The AVEA ventilator. (Courtesy VIASYS Healthcare, Critical Care Division, Palm Springs, Calif.)

Power Source

AVEA is electrically and pneumatically powered. Gas power can be provided by external high-pressure wall gas or by an internal compressor. Electric power is provided by a standard 110 volt AC power source. Emergency back-up power is also available from an internal battery or from an optional external battery source. Box 12-125 and Figure 12-112 describe and illustrate the indicators used to provide information about the main power and battery charge status.

Internal Drive Mechanism

High-pressure gas input to the ventilator is by way of two gas sources: air and oxygen. A rigid accumulator serves as an internal reservoir to supply flow on demand to the patient.

When no high-pressure air source is available, the internal compressor operates to supply air flow. The internal scroll pump compressor was designed using technology similar to

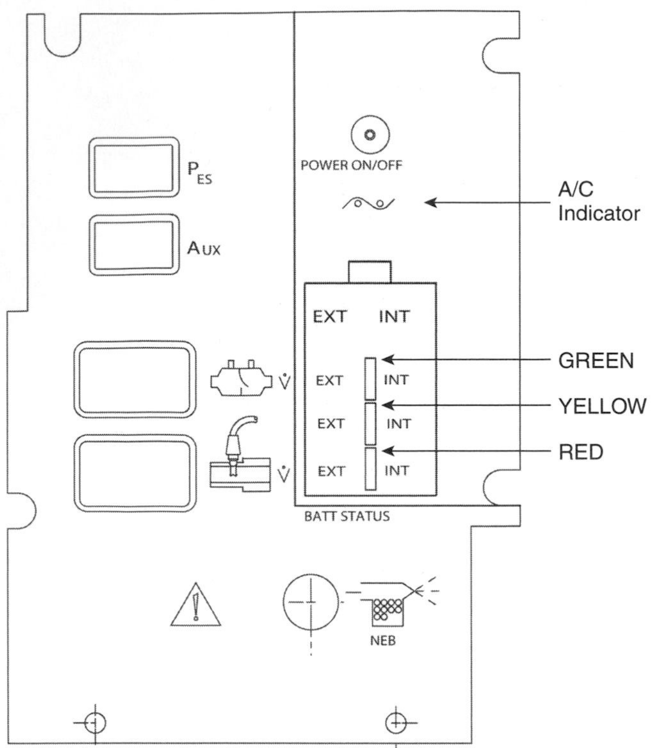

Figure 12-112 Front Panel Display area located in the unit below the display screen, containing connectors for pressure and flow/volume monitoring as well as battery indicators. (See text for further description.) (Courtesy VIASYS Healthcare, Critical Care Division, Palm Springs, Calif.)

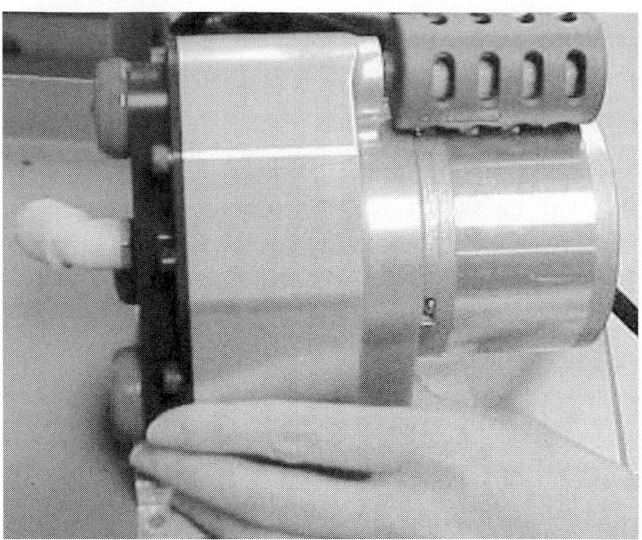

Figure 12-113 The compressor of the AVEA containing the scroll pump. (Courtesy VIASYS Healthcare, Critical Care Division, Palm Springs, Calif.)

Box 12-125 Main Power and Battery Status Indicators

Visual indicators are located on the front panel provide information about the electrical power source (Figure 12-112):

- **Power On—green indicates power on and a power source is available. (*Note*: The on/off switch itself is located on the back panel.)**
- **AC Power Indicator—The green AC indicator is on whenever the ventilator is connected to AC power. It displays whether the power switch is on (I) or off (0).**
- **External Battery Indicator—Illuminates whenever the external battery is the primary power source.**
- **Internal Battery Indicator—Illuminates when the internal battery is the primary power source.**
- **Battery Status Indicator—Illuminates incrementally depending on the available charge remaining in the battery source (internal or external). Green is >80% charge remaining, yellow is 40 to 80% charge remaining and red is <40% of charge remaining.**
- **Order of Power Consumption—The order of power consumption for all available power sources is AC power, External Battery Power, and Internal Battery Power.**

refrigerator compressors (Figure 12-113). In a cross-sectional view the scroll pump looks like a nautilus shell on the inside. The scroll pump can be described as an orbital compressor in which one half is stationary and the other half moves in a circular fashion. When operating, the gas is drawn into the compressor and, as it rotates, the gas is moved farther into the scrolls within until it reaches the center, where it exits the compressor to power the ventilator. When the internal compressor is active, the symbol of the nautilus shell, located on the front panel below the user interface module, will illuminate.

Controls

The User Interface Module (UIM) contains all software and electronic control mechanisms for the ventilator and communicates with the gas delivery engine via cable connection on the rear panel. Other connections on the rear panel of AVEA include two DISS gas inlet fittings—one for air and one for oxygen—analog input/output for synchronized independent lung ventilation (Figure 12-114) and input of up to two external signals to be displayed on the main screen of the user interface. A remote nurse call connection, the O_2 sensor cell and external battery connection are also found on the rear panel. The DISS connectors can be changed to adapt for helium-oxygen delivery. When the helium connector is added, the ventilator software adapts for the change in density and viscosity of the lighter gas so that parameter displays such as flow and volume are corrected.

Patient monitoring from AVEA includes esophageal, tracheal, and proximal airway pressure monitoring. Proximal airway flow sensing, with either variable orifice or hot wire flow sensing technology is available for measuring

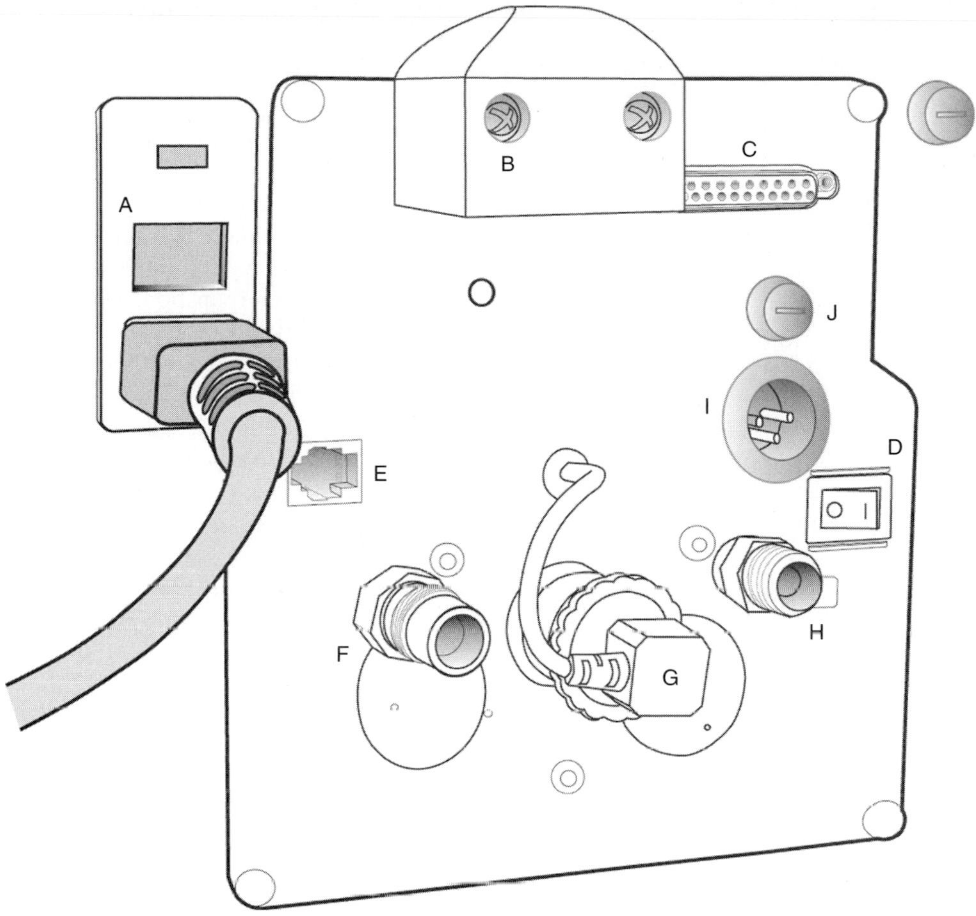

Figure 12-114 The rear panel of the ventilator showing the following: *A*, AC power connector; *B*, UIM connector; *C*, analog input/output/ILV port; *D*, the Power on/off switch; *E*, a nurse call system connector; *F*, air DISS fitting; *G*, oxygen sensor; *H*, oxygen DISS fitting; *I*, external battery connector; and *J*, external battery fuse. (See text for further explanation.) (Courtesy VIASYS Healthcare, Critical Care Division, Palm Springs, Calif.)

tidal volume delivery at the patient Y-connector (see Figure 12-112). Connections for each of these devices are color-coded, labeled, and keyed to avoid incorrect attachments.

Located in this same section of the ventilator cabinet are indicators for AC and DC power supply and the nipple connection for the internal nebulizer. Underneath the touch screen are connections for an external printer, a separate external display device (SVGA connector), an MIB port (medical information buss), and two RS-232 interface connections for data input and output.

Except for the on/off power switch located on the rear panel of the unit, all operator controls are located on the front panel of the user interface. Before using the ventilator on a new patient or when the patient circuit is changed, a number of checks need to be performed to ensure the proper function of the ventilator. Two different test series are run. The first verifies general operations and the second verifies alarm function.

Ventilator Set Up

After start-up testing, the clinician can choose to either "Resume Current" and continue ventilation at current control settings, or select "New Patient," which clears previous data (trends and saved loops). Ventilation begins at default values for the currently selected patient size (neonatal, pediatric, or adult) when "New Patient" selection is accepted. The operator selects the appropriate patient size and, once accepted, the ventilator SET UP screen appears (Figure 12-115).

The SET UP Screen allows the clinician to enable certain features that include automatic tube compensation (ATC), leak compensation, and circuit compliance compensation (see Chapter 11 for an explanation of tubing compliance and its calculation), BTPS (body temperature pressure saturated) correction for active (heated humidifier) or passive (heat moisture exchanger) humidification systems, and an EST (electronic self-test). Patient weight and a 24-character patient ID can also be entered. (*Note*: The patient weight

A

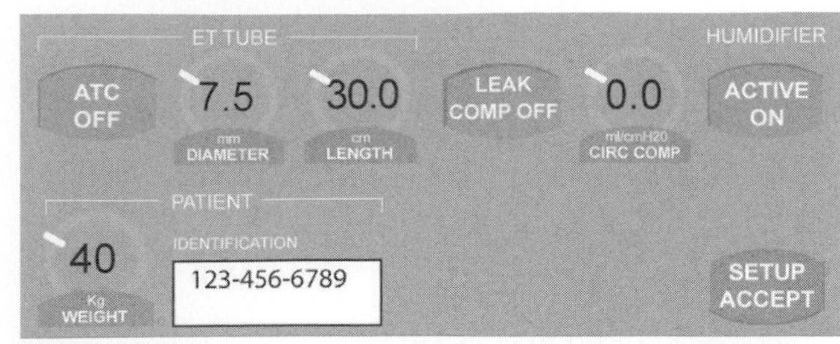

B

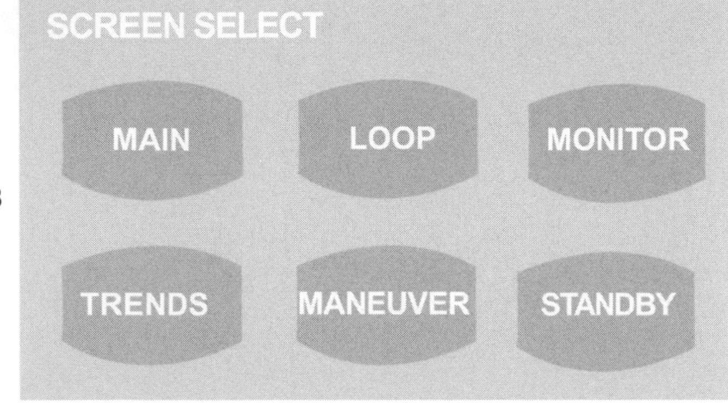

Figure 12-115 **A,** The Ventilation Setup window of the AVEA Ventilator which allows selection of automatic tube compensation (ATC), leak compensation, circuit compliance, humidifier type, and patient weight and identification number. **B,** the Screens Selection window which allows displaying of the following screens: main, loop, monitor, trends, maneuver, and standby. (See text for explanation.) (Courtesy VIASYS Health Care, Critical Care Division, Palm Springs, Calif.)

information is used to correct displayed monitored values for patient weight.) After all selections have been made, the operator presses SET UP and "ACCEPT," and ventilation begins.

Membrane Buttons and LEDs

Figure 12-116 shows the membrane buttons and LEDs labeled 1 through 23 moving counterclockwise around the screen.

1. This LED flashes in the presence of high- and medium-priority alarms.
2. The Alarm Silence button provides a 2-minute audible alarm silence.
3. The Alarm Reset button cancels visual indicators of resolved alarms.
4. The Alarm Limits button opens and closes the Alarm Limits window where operator adjustable alarm settings are located.
5. The Manual Breath button delivers a single mandatory breath using current settings when pressed during the exhalation phase of a breath.
6. The Suction button with LED Indicator initiates a "Disconnect for Suction" maneuver (Box 12-126).
7. The Increase O_2 button increases O_2% for 2 minutes: (increase to 100% in adult and pediatric patients; and increase to 20% above the set $O_{2\%}$ or 100%, whichever is less for neonates). If pressed again during the 2-minute interval, the maneuver is cancelled and the ventilator resumes its prior O_2% settings.
8. A Data Dial is used to change a highlighted field or control on the touch screen.
9. The "ACCEPT" button activates proposed changes to highlighted field or controls.
10. The "CANCEL" button causes the ventilator to disregard proposed changes and revert to the previous settings, still in effect.
11. The Expiratory Hold (EXP HOLD) button allows measurement of end expiratory pressure for auto-PEEP determination. The hold is up to 20 seconds in adult/pediatric patients and 3 seconds in neonates. (See Chapter 11 for an explanation of auto-PEEP.)
12. The Inspiratory Hold (INSP HOLD) button can be used to determine plateau pressure (maximum 3 seconds).
13. The Nebulizer button provides nebulization for 30 minutes synchronized with the inspiratory phase. Powering the nebulizer requires attachment of a high-pressure air source and a total flow to the internal nebulizer of >15 L/min. (See Box 12-127 for further information.)
14. Patient Size LED indicators show the currently selected patient size. There is no associated membrane button.
15. The Panel Lock button (LOCK) disables all front panel controls except manual breath, increase % O_2, alarm reset, alarm silence, and the panel lock button.
16. Pressing the PRINT button prints current screen displays to an external printer.
17. The SET-UP key opens and closes the Ventilator Set-up screen.
18. The ADV SETTINGS button opens and closes an advanced settings window for feature activation or parameter adjustment.
19. The MODE button opens and closes the Mode menu. The Mode Indicator can also be used to access the Mode menu.
20. The EVENT button opens and closes a menu of event markers such as "arterial blood gas" that can be placed on the trend display.
21. The FREEZE button suspends real-time update of data on the current graphics screen display until it is pressed again. With the screen frozen, the data dial can be used to scroll a cursor through waveform or loop graphics for examination of specific data points.
22. The SCREEN button opens and closes the Screen menu. The Screen Indicator can also be used to access this menu.
23. The MAIN button returns to the main screen display from any screen.

Primary Breath Controls

Primary breath controls are rate, tidal volume, inspiratory pressure, peak flow, inspiratory pause, PEEP, pressure support,

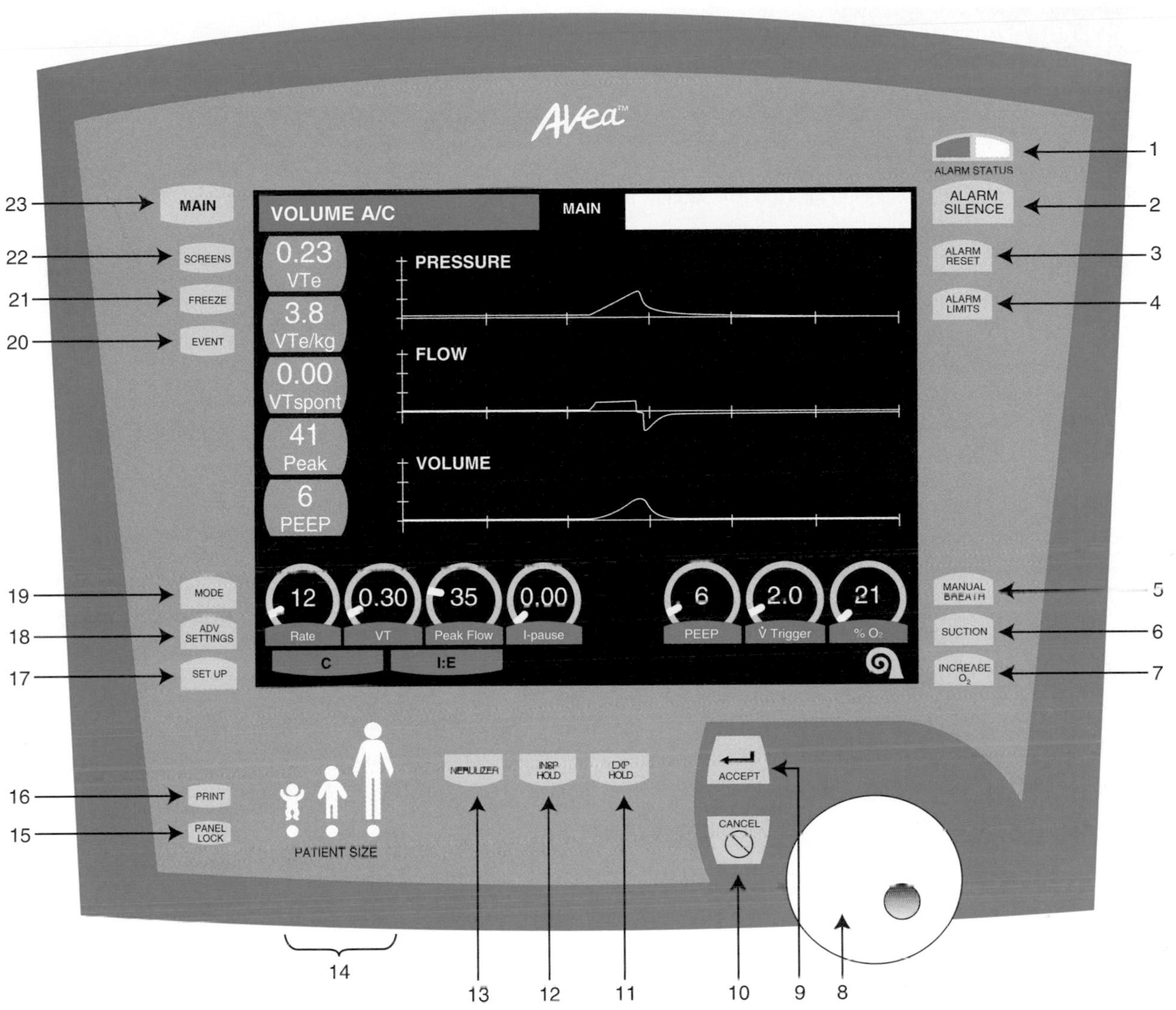

Figure 12-116 The front panel (User Interface Module) of the AVEA Ventilator showing the membrane buttons, the LEDs and indicators, the DATA DIAL and the touch screen displaying the normal operating screen. (See text for explanation.) (Courtesy VIASYS Healthcare, Critical Care Division, Palm Springs, Calif.)

Box 12-126 Disconnect for Suctioning Maneuver

When the Suction button is pressed the ventilator will:

1. Enable "Increase % O_2" maneuver for 2 minutes (See Increase O_2 button)
2. Disable the demand system on loss of PEEP
3. Silence all alarms for 2 minutes

If the Suction button is pressed again during the 2 minutes, the maneuver is cancelled.

Box 12-127 Nebulizer Function

When the internal nebulizer is used, the ventilator decreases the flow to the patient by 6 L/min to compensate for the nebulizer output. However, because the internal nebulizer flow can be as high as 8 L/min, use of the nebulizer may still impact the tidal volume delivery. This needs to be monitored closely, particularly in neonatal patients.

Use of an external flow meter to power the nebulizer is not recommended since it would have no compensation for volume, is constant during both inspiration and exhalation and could affect percent oxygen delivery.

flow trigger, and F_IO_2. These controls are displayed along the bottom of the touch screen (see Figure 12-116). Only controls active for the current mode of ventilation are visible. For example, if Volume Assist Control is selected, tidal volume is available as a primary control but not inspiratory pressure. Table 12-49 lists all the primary breath controls and their description.

To change a primary breath control, the operator touches the screen directly over the control. The control highlights

Table 12-49 Primary Breath Controls AVEA Ventilator

Display control (units)	Description
Rate (bpm)	Breath rate shown in breaths/min. 1 to 150 bpm (neo/ped), 1 to 120 bpm (adult)
V_T (mL)	Tidal volume in mL (100 to 2500 mL, adult; 25 to 500 mL, peds; 2 to 300 mL, neonate)
	When operating only on the internal compressor, the maximum available V_T is 2000 mL
Insp Press (cm H_2O)	Inspiratory pressure, 0 to 100 cm H_2O (adult/pediatric), 0 to 80 cm H_2O (neonate). Used during pressure ventilation as the target pressure
Peak Flow (L/min)	Sets the peak inspiratory flow during volume ventilation. 3 to 150 L/min (adult), 1 to 75 L/min (peds), 0.4 to 30 L/min (neonate)
Insp Time (sec)	Inspiratory time, 0.2 to 5.0 sec (adult/pediatric), 0.15 to 3.0 sec (neonate). Sets the maximum inspiratory time for all mandatory breaths and ends inspiration if the normal cycling criteria have not been met and when the time limit is reached
Insp Pause (sec)	Sets inspiratory pause after volume delivery 0.0 to 3.0 sec. Adds to the set inspiratory time
PSV (cm H_2O)	Pressure support ventilation, 0 to 100 cm H_2O (adults/peds), 0 to 80 cm H_20 (neonate)
PEEP (cm H_2O)	Positive end-expiratory pressure, 0 to 50 cm H_2O
Flow Trig (L/min)	Flow trigger sensitivity. Sets the inspiratory flow trigger in L/min, 0.1 to 20 L/min. When enabled, sets a bias flow through the patient circuit during part of the expiratory phase
% O_2 (%)	Controls the percentage of oxygen delivery—21% to 100%
Pres High (cm H_2O)	In APRV sets the maximum pressure target, 0 to 100 cm H_2O
Time High (sec)	In APRV sets the time during which maximum pressure is maintained, 0.2 to 30 sec
Time Low (sec)	In APRV sets the time during which minimum pressure is maintained—0.2 to 30 sec
Pres Low (cm H_2O)	In APRV sets the minimum pressure target, 0 to 45 cm H_2O

(changes color) showing that it can now be changed. To change the setting, the operator turns the DATA DIAL clockwise or counterclockwise to increase or decrease the value. After the desired setting appears, touching the control again or pressing the "ACCEPT" button accepts the change. The control will return to its normal color and ventilation continues with the new setting in effect. If the operator presses the CANCEL button, rather than the ACCEPT, or if he or she does not accept the change within 15 seconds, the control returns to its normal color and ventilation continues at previous settings. The technique of using touch, turn, and accept applies to almost all user interactions with the touch screen display.

Modes of Ventilation

As with many currently available ventilators, AVEA offers a selection of modes and breath-types. At the time of this writing, AVEA offers volume and pressure A/C, volume and pressure SIMV, PRVC in A/C and SIMV modes, airway pressure release ventilation (APRV), and time-cycled pressure-limited (TCPL) in A/C and SIMV ventilation. CPAP and pressure support ventilation (PSV) are also available. (*Note*: See Chapter 11 for a description of the basic function of each of these modes.)

Selections are made from the Mode menu, which is accessed by pressing the Mode button or the Mode Indicator. The menu will display only the modes and breath-types available for the currently selected patient size. Figure 12-117 shows the adult/pediatric mode menu *(A)* and the infant mode menu *(B)*.

Assist/Control Ventilation

During A/C ventilation, the set breath rate establishes the minimum breath rate. The patient can receive additional breaths above this set amount, but all breaths are mandatory (i.e., at the set pressure or volume). Breaths may be time- or patient-triggered. Flow-triggering is the usual patient-trigger. A/C breaths are pressure- or volume-targeted. When pressure-targeted A/C is selected, the breath is commonly time-cycled based on the set inspiratory time (T_I). When volume-targeted A/C is selected, the common cycling mechanism is volume.

During a mandatory breath (pressure- or volume-targeted), the demand system is active and can provide additional flow or volume if demanded by the patient. Volume A/C is also the default mode for adult/pediatric patients. It is automatically set when a new patient is selected if no other mode is activated.

A

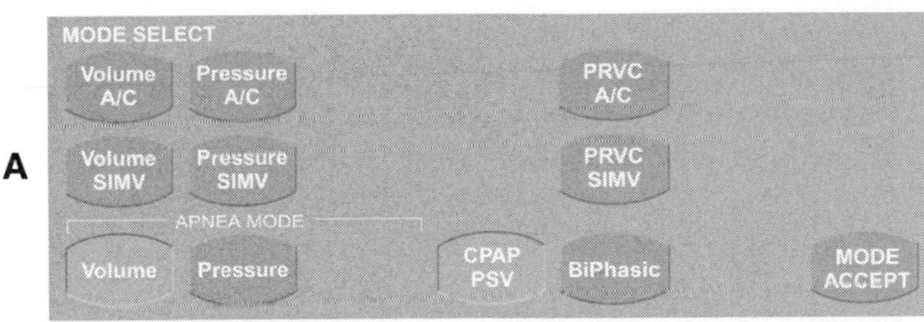

B

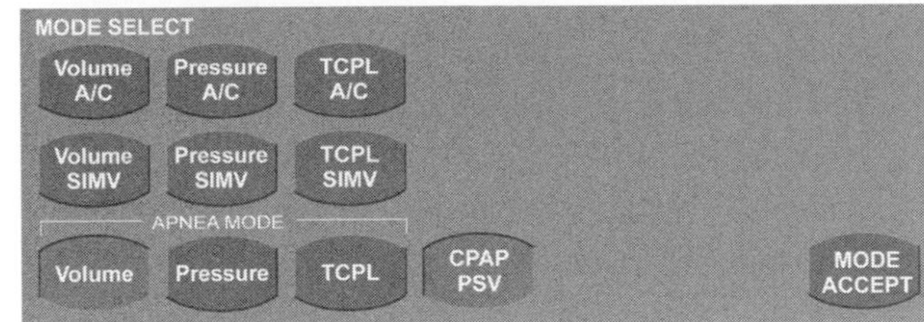

Figure 12-117 The Mode Select Screens for adult/pediatric patients (**A**) and for neonatal patients (**B**). In the Adult/Pediatric screen the term BiPhasic has been recently replaced with APRV. (See text for more detail.) (Courtesy VIASYS Healthcare, Critical Care Division, Palm Springs, Calif.)

SIMV

The SIMV mode provides mandatory breath deliver at the set breath rate and allows for spontaneous breathing from the baseline pressure between mandatory breaths. Mandatory breaths can be time- or patient-triggered, as with A/C ventilation. Mandatory breaths can be either pressure- or volume-targeted. Pressure-targeted mandatory breaths are usually time-cycled and volume-targeted mandatory breaths are usually volume-cycled. Spontaneous breaths in SIMV can be from a zero baseline or from a baseline with PEEP/CPAP added. Spontaneous breaths are also supported with PSV.

Pressure Regulated Volume Control (PRVC)

PRVC is a pressure-targeted A/C form of ventilation that adjusts pressure delivery to guarantee a set tidal volume. Mandatory breaths are time- or patient-triggered, pressure-targeted and time-cycled. The volume setting is done through the Special Features screen. The first breath is volume-targeted. This breath is evaluated by the ventilator to measure system compliance and resistance and provide a pressure target for the next breath. From that point on, breaths are pressure-targeted. Adjustments are made in the pressure if the ventilator is not achieving the set volume. Pressure changes are made up or down in steps of 3 cm H_2O. (See Chapter 11 for a further description of PRVC.)

Airway Pressure Release Ventilation (APRV)

APRV allows the patient to spontaneously breathe at two preset pressure levels. These two levels are set using PRES HIGH and PRES LOW settings. The values for these are selected based on the patient's optimum PEEP/CPAP value to prevent both lung injury (PRES HIGH) and avoid alveolar collapse (PRES LOW). The duration of the high pressure is established by the TIME HIGH setting. The duration of the low pressure is based on the set TIME LOW value. Thus breaths are both time-triggered and time-cycled.

This mode has very specific clinical uses and patients must be monitored carefully when it is used. APRV is not available in the neonatal patient size setting. Apnea Back-up Ventilation is also not available during APRV ventilation.

Time-Cycled Pressure Limited (TCPL)

TCPL ventilation is only used for neonatal patients. TCPL ventilation can be used in A/C or SIMV modes. With TCPL-A/C, mandatory breaths are time- or patient-triggered, pressure or volume-targeted, and time-cycled. With TCPL-SIMV, mandatory breaths are time- or patient-triggered, pressure- or volume-targeted, and time-cycled. Spontaneous breaths are similar to those with standard SIMV, patient-triggered, pressure-targeted, and flow-cycled.

The CPAP/PSV mode is used for patients who are spontaneously breathing. CPAP breaths are patient-triggered, pressure-limited, and flow-cycled, as are PS breaths. If CPAP or PSV pressures are set at zero, 3 cm H_2O of PS is given during spontaneous breathing. This helps reduce work of breathing by the patient through the system.

The default flow-cycle settings called "PSV cycle" are 25% (adult/ped) and 10% (neo). The PSV flow-cycle can be adjusted from 5% to 45% using the Advanced Settings menu. As a safety back-up, PS breaths will time-cycle out of inspiration if the T_I becomes too long. Time-cycling is based on the PSV Tmax setting. The default values for PSV Tmax are 0.5 seconds (adult/ped) and 0.35 seconds (neo). Adjustments to PSV Tmax are also made in the Advanced Settings window described below.

Noninvasive Positive Pressure Ventilation (NPPV)

NPPV can be performed using any mode and with the dual limb patient circuit (adult, pediatric and neonatal sizes). Leak compensation must be turned on using the ventilator set-up screen when non-invasive is selected. A nasal mask or face mask is connected to the patient as the non-invasive interface.

Apnea Back-up Ventilation (ABV)

ABV is active in all SIMV and CPAP/PSV modes. When CPAP/PSV is selected, the operator must select the breath type and mode for ABV and set the primary controls. If the set apnea time elapses before a breath is detected, apnea ventilation is initiated. After ABV begins, the ventilator delivers a mandatory breath. If no spontaneous effort is detected, the ventilator continues to delivery breaths. The audible alarm can be temporarily silence, but not reset until apnea ventilation ceases. Resuming ventilation requires that two consecutive patient-triggered breaths be detected by the ventilator. If apnea continues, the operator would need to change the rate or the mode of ventilation to keep the patient appropriately ventilated. (*Note*: The operator should also check the apnea time to be sure it is set correctly.)

Advanced Settings

Advanced settings are controls that allow the clinician to refine breath delivery beyond the scope of the primary breath controls. The ADV SETTINGS membrane button opens and closes the Advanced Settings window. (*Note*: Advanced settings are associated with specific primary controls. However, not all primary controls will have an associated advanced setting.)

1. Volume limit (Vol Limit) is a feature active in pressure-targeted modes of ventilation including A/C Press, SIMV Press, TCPL, and PSV breaths. In neonatal ventilation this requires the use of a proximal flow sensor that connects at the patient Y-connector. When volume limit is activated, pressure-targeted breaths also become volume-limited. That is, if the set volume limit (a *maximum* volume) is reached before the normal time-cycle or flow-cycle criteria for a breath, the breath is terminated (volume-cycled.) If the set V_T is not delivered before the normal cycling mechanism (T_I set in A/C and SIMV Press vent, or the flow-cycle limit in PSV), ventilation continues at the set pressure and ends inspiration using the normal cycling criteria. The potential advantage of this feature is protection of the lungs from excessive volume delivery in the face of changing lung characteristics during pressure ventilation.
2. Machine volume (Mach Vol) is another volume criterion that establishes a *minimum* volume delivery. It is active in pressure-targeted A/C and SIMV, TCPL, and PS breath. When the "Mach Vol" feature is set, the machine delivers the set pressure and monitors volume delivery through the internal flow sensor. If the set "Mach Vol" is achieved during inspiration, the ventilator mode cycles via its normal cycling mechanism. If Mach Vol is NOT achieved before the set cycling criteria, the ventilator delivers the minimum tidal volume by transitioning to a continuous inspiratory flow to achieve the set volume within the set T_I. As a result of the increased flow requirements, airway pressure increases as well. The ventilator adjusts flow and thus, pressure, to achieve the Mach Vol (minimum volume) for every breath delivered.

   There is one condition in which the ventilator will terminate the breath before the minimum volume being delivered. Should the high-pressure limit be met or exceeded before the minimum tidal volume being delivered, inspiration ends and the high-pressure limit alarm would activate.
3. The Inspiratory Rise (Insp Rise) control adjusts the rate at which pressure is delivered during inspiration during a mandatory pressure breath in the following modes: A/C-PV, SIMV-PC, TCPL-A/C, TCPL SIMV, and PRVC. It is similar to the rise time or sloping feature in other ventilators. A setting of 1 is the most rapid rise in pressure, whereas a setting of 9 is the slowest. A separate control is available for adjusting the rise in PSV ventilation. It is termed PSV Rise. It is adjusted in the same fashion as Insp Rise. (*Note*: Also see Vsync Rise in the following section.)
4. *Flow Cycle* allows adjustment of the percentage at which the ventilator will flow-cycle a breath during pressure-targeted ventilation (A/C and SIMV) and TCPS (A/C and SIMV). Thus, mandatory pressure breaths can be time- or flow-cycled (range 0 to 45%). (*Note*: Flow-cycling for PSV is adjusted using the PSV Cycle feature.)
5. PSV Tmax sets the maximum length of inspiratory time allowed during a PSV breath (range is 0.2 to 5.0 seconds [adult/ped] and 0.15 to 3.00 [neonates]).
6. The *Waveform* feature allows the operator to select either a square wave (constant flow) or a decelerating (descending) ramp flow pattern during volume ventilation. The default is a descending ramp. With this waveform selected the ventilator begins flow delivery at the set peak flow and decreases flow until 50% of the set peak flow is reached.
7. The Sigh control allows the ventilator to deliver a sigh breath at 1.5 times the set tidal volume, every 100 breaths for adult and pediatric patients.
8. Bias Flow is flow present in the patient circuit during the expiratory portion of a breath. This feature establishes the flow from which flow-triggering is accomplished (range 0.4 to 5.0 L/min, default 2 L/min.) (see Chapter 11 for an additional explanation of flow triggering).
9. Pressure-triggering is available in addition to flow-triggering on the AVEA. Both trigger mechanisms are always active (relative to their sensitivity setting). The ventilator will respond to whichever trigger threshold is reached first. The range of pressure-triggering is from –0.1 to –20 cm H_2O, whereas the range for flow triggering is 0.1 to 20 L/min.
10. Vsync can be activated in volume modes (Volume A/C and Volume SIMV). When selected, a single test breath is delivered to measure end-inspiratory pressure (plateau pressure). System compliance and resistance are measured to determine the initial pressure needed to deliver the set volume. Each subsequent breath will be delivered at a pressure sufficient to provide the volume. Should the volume be less than or more than the set volume, the inspiratory pressure is moved up or down in increments of no more than 3 cm H_2O on the next breath to ensure delivery of a set volume. (Note: Vsync is only available for adult and pediatric patients.)
11. Vsync Rise, which is only active when Vsync is enabled, functions similarly to the Inspiratory Rise feature in adjusting the slope of the inspiratory

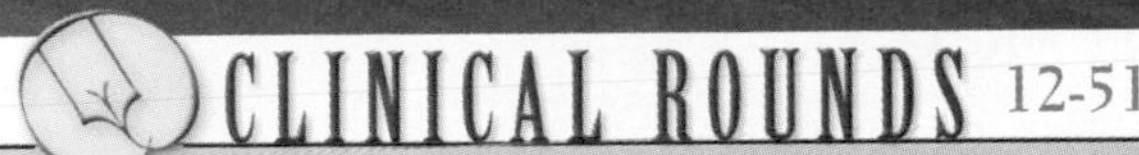

CLINICAL ROUNDS 12-51

A patient is receiving pressure-targeted SIMV ventilation on the AVEA ventilator at a rate of 6 breaths/min. Inspiratory pressure is set at 20 cm H_2O, PSV is 15 cm H_2O and CPAP/PEEP is 5 cm H_2O. The PSV Cycle is set at 20% and the Flow Cycle is set at 40%. T_I is set at 1.5 seconds. Peak inspiratory flow for a pressure supported breath is noted from the flow-time waveform to be about 50 L/min. The inspiratory flow curve for a mandatory breath does not reach zero before inspiration ends.

Question 1: What is the peak inspiratory pressure for a mandatory breath and for a pressure support breath?

Question 2: Is a mandatory breath time- or flow-cycled?

Question 3: At what flow will pressure supported breaths cycle out of inspiration?

See Appendix A for the answer.

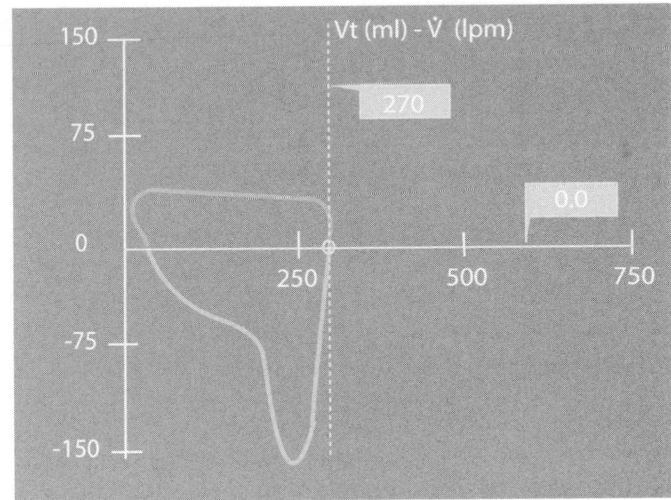

Figure 12-118 The graphic display shows a flow-volume loop in the freeze mode with the tidal volume (270 mL) and the flow (0.0 lpm) at the dotted line. The horizontal axis is volume, and the vertical axis is flow. (Courtesy VIASYS Healthcare, Critical Care Division, Palm Springs, Calif.)

pressure rise during breath delivery (range 1 to 9, with 9 the slowest). See Clinical Rounds 12-51 for a problem using advanced settings.

Monitors and Displays

The AVEA has both digital and graphic monitoring displays. The main screen continuously displays up to five monitored parameters (see Figure 12-116, left-hand column). The operator can customize these 5 main screen displays or an extended display of 15 on the monitor screen from a list of 32 items. The monitor screen is accessed by touching the Screen Indicator or by pressing the SCREEN button. Table 12-50 lists the monitored parameters.

A maximum of three waveform tracings can be displayed simultaneously on the main screen (see Figure 12-116). The operator can touch the waveform title bar and a menu will appear with choices for airway pressure, esophageal pressure, tracheal pressure, flow, volume, and two analog input signals. All waveforms are graphed against a horizontal time axis.

The Loop screen displays two real-time loops, flow-volume and pressure-volume. Up to four loops can be saved at a time using the Freeze function. Any saved loop can be selected as a reference loop for comparison to live loops (Figure 12-118).

The STANDBY mode is available for use when a patient is temporarily away from the ventilator. While in STANDBY, the ventilator supplies 2 L/min of gas continuously through the patient circuit to prevent damage to the circuit or overheating of the chamber water should the heated humidifier be left on. Ventilation will resume at the most recent control settings after the RESUME button on the STANDBY screen is pressed.

Alarms and Indicators

Alarms and Indicators are used to notify clinicians when automatic as well as adjustable alarm limits are violated or when conditions affecting ventilator function are detected. Visual displays exist for all types of alarms. Alarm messages appear in the Alarm Indicator at the upper right of the touch screen. When multiple alarms are present a white triangle appears to the right of the alarm message. This touch icon is used to open and close a drop-down display of up to nine alarm messages. The highest priority alarm is always displayed in the top position.

Alarm conditions result in visual and audible alarms at three different levels:

- High priority—five tones repeated with a flashing red alarm indicator
- Medium priority—three tones repeated with a flashing yellow alarm indicator
- Low priority—single tone with a solid yellow alarm indicator
- Normal status—solid green alarm indicator

Table 12-51 provides information on ventilator alarms. To set the limits for an alarm, the operator selects the Alarm Limits button and the ALARM LIMITS screen appears (Figure 12-119). The operator presses the touch screen immediately over the alarm control. The control highlights. The alarm value is adjusted by using the data dial until the control reaches the value required. Pressing the touch screen above

Table 12-50 The Monitor Screen Displayed Data—AVEA Ventilator

Displayed Data	Description
Vte	Exhaled tidal volume (mL)
Vte/Kg	mL of Vte per kg adjusted for patient weight
Vti	Inspired tidal volume (mL)
Spon V_T	Spontaneous Vt (mL)
Spon V_T/Kg	mL of Spon Vt per kg adjusted for patient weight
Mand V_T	Mandatory (mL)
Mand VT/Kg	Mand Vt per kg adjusted for patient weight
% Leak	Percent leakage. The difference between the inspiratory and expiratory volume in % difference
Ve	Calculated minute volume (L/min) based on set V_T and rate for volume breaths only
Spon Ve/kg	Spontaneous minute volume adjusted for patient weight
Rate	Respiratory rate (breaths/min)
Spon Rate	Spontaneous rate (breaths/min)
Ti	Inspiratory time (sec)
Te	Expiratory time (sec)
I:E	Calculated value for inspiratory-to-expiratory ratio, based on set rate, Vt, and peak flow for volume breaths, and rate, and inspiratory time for pressure, TCPL and PRVC breaths. Range 1:99.9 to 99.9:1
f/Vt	Rapid shallow breathing index (B/min/L), respiratory rate, divided by tidal volume
Ppeak	Peak inspiratory pressure (cm H_2O)
Pmean	Mean airway pressure (cm H_2O)
Pplat	Plateau pressure (cm H_2O) if available
PEEP	Positive end-expiratory pressure (cm H_2O)
Air inlet	Air inlet pressure (psig)
O_2 Inlet	Oxygen inlet pressure (psig)
F_IO_2	Percent of oxygen displayed as a whole number
Cdyn	Dynamic compliance (characteristic) (mL/cm H_2O)
Cs (Cstat)	Static compliance (mL/cm H_2O). Requires an inspiratory hold maneuver.
Rrs	Respiratory system resistance (cm H_2O/L/sec). This calculation is performed during an inspiratory hold maneuver.
PIFR	Peak inspiratory flow rate (L/min)
PEFR	Peak expiratory flow rate (L/min)

the control or pressing the ACCEPT button sets the new alarm limit.

Troubleshooting

Before using the ventilator on a new patient or when the patient circuit is changed, pretesting is performed using Operational Verification Testing. The first test reviewed is for general operations and the second for alarm function. These tests are performed to ensure the ventilator is performing safely and accurately. The Operator's Manual provides more information on how to perform testing for those individuals using the AVEA in the clinical setting.

Newport e500 Ventilator[1-3]

The Newport e500 (Newport Medical Instruments, Costa Mesa, Calif.) ventilator is intended for use with infants, pediatric, and adult patients requiring a tidal volume 20 mL or more. It can be used for noninvasive and invasive positive pressure ventilation (Figure 12-120).

Power Source

The Newport e500 requires an electrical and a high-pressure gas source for operation. The rear panel contains DISS connectors for high-pressure air and oxygen sources as well

Table 12-51 Alarms—AVEA Ventilator

Alarm	Description
Vent Inop	Ventilator failure. The safety valve opens (Safety Valve message appears). The spontaneously breathing patients can breath room air
Loss of Air	Wall or cylinder air below 18 psig. No compressor installed
Loss of O_2	O_2 supply below 18 psig
Loss of Gas Supply	All gas sources failed. Safety valve opens
Low P_{PEAK}	Peak inspiratory pressure less than the set Low P_{PEAK} value
High P_{PEAK}	Peak inspiratory pressure greater than High P_{PEAK} value. Inspiration ends
Ext High P_{PEAK}	Occurs when the High P_{PEAK} alarm is active for more than 5 seconds. The Safety Valve Opens. No breaths are delivered
Low PEEP	Baseline pressure drops below the set Low PEEP level
Low Minute Volume	Monitored exhaled Ve is less that the set value for the Low Ve alarm
High Minute Volume	Monitored exhaled Ve is greater than the set High Ve alarm
High V_T	Monitored exhaled V_T is greater than the High V_T alarm
Apnea	Apnea alarm occurs if the ventilator does not detect a breath during the set apnea interval
High rate	The monitored total breath rate exceeds the high rate value
I-Time Limit	Inspiratory time exceeds the set MAX I-time plus any set pause time (5.0 sec for adult/pediatric patients; 3.0 sec for neonatal patients)
I:E Limit	I:E ratio exceeds 4:1 for a mandatory breath. Inspiration ends
Low F_IO_2	Delivered O_2 falls below set F_IO_2 minus 6%, or falls below 18%
High F_IO_2	Delivered O_2 rises above the set F_IO_2 plus 6%

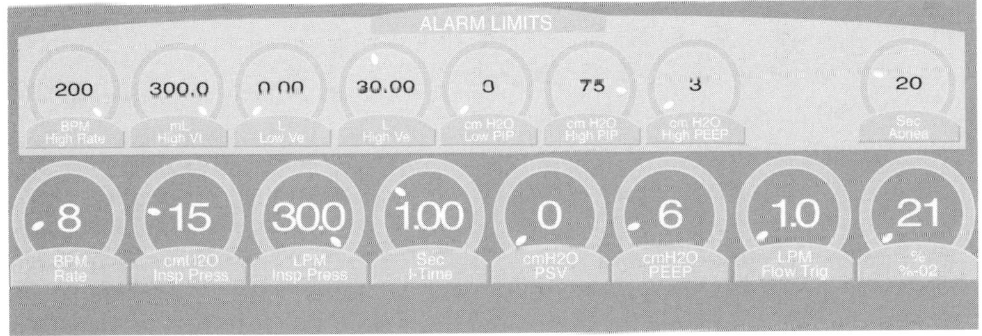

Figure 12-119 The Alarm Limits screen that appears above the screen display of ventilator parameters. This screen appears at the bottom of the touch screen. (Courtesy VIASYS Healthcare, Critical Care Division, Palm Springs, Calif.)

as an AC power cord connector, a DC power source input connector, and two electronic cable connectors that attach to the control panel and the graphics display module. Figure 12-121 shows a picture of the rear panel of the e500. Table 12-52 gives a description of each of the panel connectors and devices.

The internal battery can provide about 1.5 hours of backup power when fully charged and ventilation remains fully functional. The e500 can also use an external (DC) battery as a power source.

On the center left-hand side of the front panel is an indicator section, which provides information about the batteries and power sources. The word "charging" illuminates to show the internal battery is recharging and the ventilator is connected to an AC power source. (*Note*: The internal battery will charge whenever the ventilator is plugged into an AC source whether the unit is on or in the standby mode.) The INT BATTERY indicator illuminates and the ventilator beeps every 5 minutes when the e500 is operating off the internal battery and not an AC source. The battery

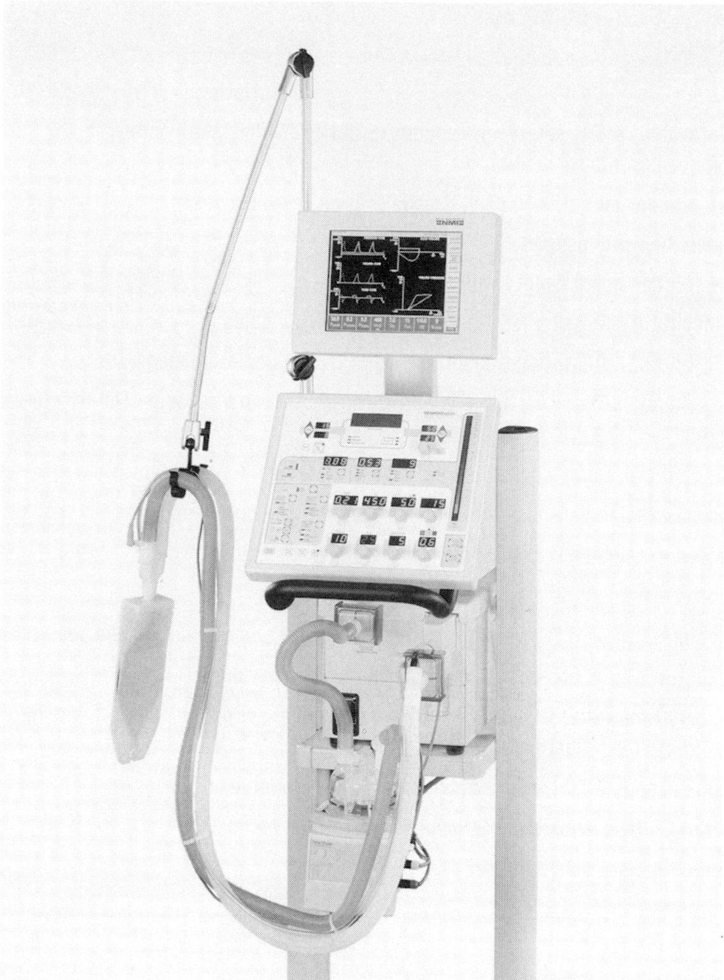

Figure 12-120 The Newport e500 ventilator including the Graphics Display Monitor and the patient circuit. (Courtesy Newport Medical Instruments, Costa Mesa, Calif.)

charge bar on the right of this section shows the relative charge remaining on the internal battery. The MAINS light illuminates when the ventilator is operating on AC power (*Note*: The charge light will also be illuminated.)

The EXT BATTERY lights when an external battery is in use. The amount of charge remaining is NOT indicated for the external battery.

On/Standby Control and Patient Circuit

The ON/STANDBY control switch is located on the left side of the front of the ventilator gas delivery unit (GDU) where the patient circuit connectors are located (Figure 12-122). The main inspiratory and expiratory lines of the patient circuit should have bacterial filters installed. A bacterial filter is placed between the inspiratory limb and the inspiratory port (TO PATIENT) to prevent contaminants from exhaled gases entering the inspiratory line in the event of a Device Alert shut down (Box 12-128).

A bacterial filter is used between the expiratory limb and the expiratory port (FROM PATIENT) to prevent exhaled gas contaminants from entering the exhalation system. The exhalation valve assembly is heated to prevent moisture in exhaled air from condensing on the expiratory flow sensor. The exhalation assembly has low resistance to allow for rapid return to baseline pressure after a positive pressure breath and reduce the potential for auto-PEEP resulting from expiratory resistance.

A proximal pressure connecter is located between the inspiratory and expiratory connectors on the front of the GDU. This connector is used to attach a line from the ventilator to the patient Y-connector for monitoring proximal airway pressure. A small amount of flow from the ventilator purges the proximal line to keep moisture from collecting.

Just below the main inspiratory line connector is an emergency air intake. This opening must be kept unobstructed. In the event of a Device Alert condition (see Alarm section), this opening allows the venting of patient circuit pressure.

The ventilator includes a built-in oxygen analyzer, which provides automatic high and low F_IO_2 alarms and is

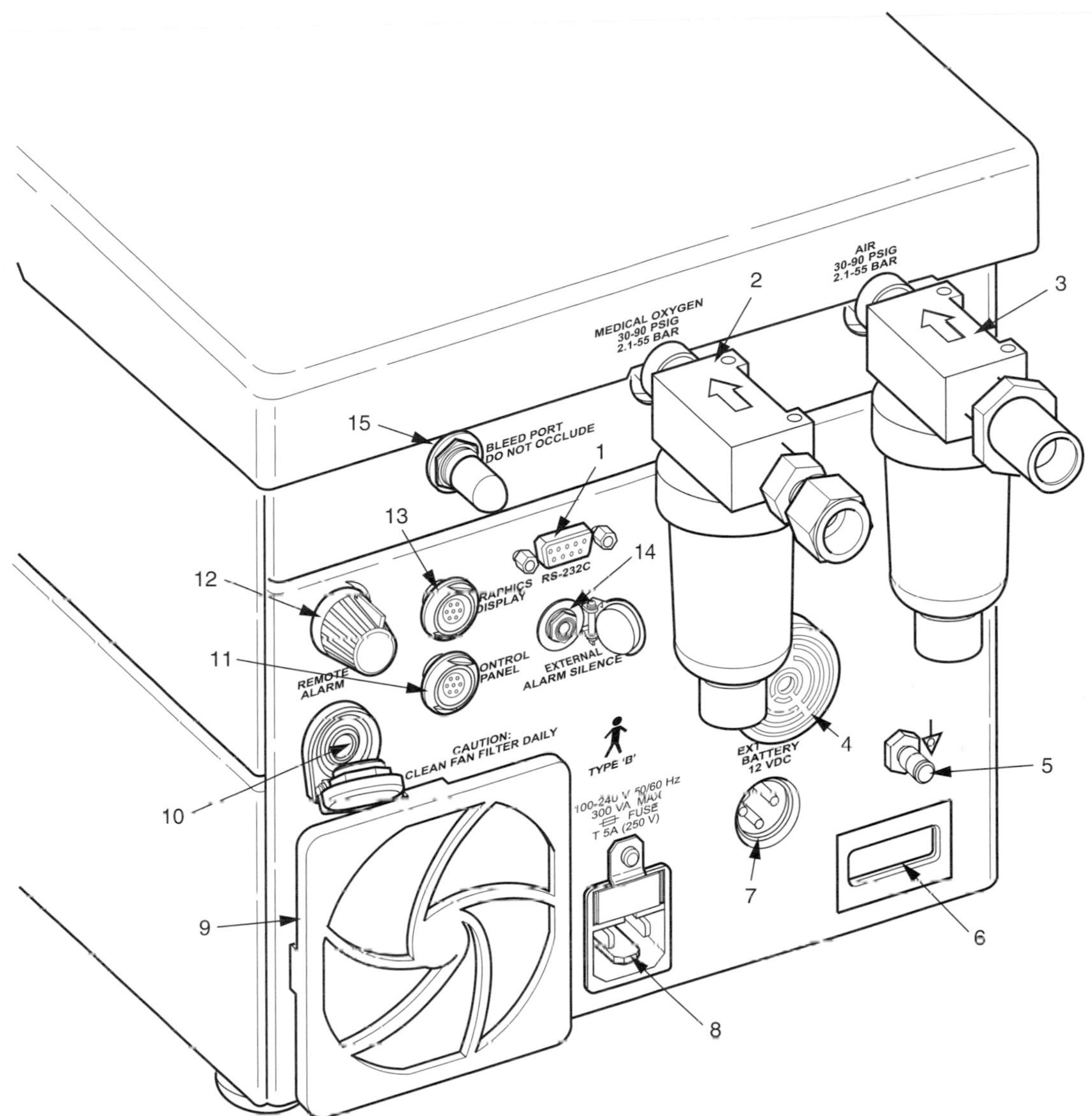

Figure 12-121 The rear panel of the e500 ventilator gas delivery unit (GDU). Table 12-52 describes each of the numbered components. (Courtesy Newport Medical Instruments, Costa Mesa, Calif.)

automatically calibrated when the e500 is turned on, recalibrated every 30 minutes for the following hour, and every 8 hours of operation thereafter.

Internal Drive Mechanism

The e500 features an electronically controlled inlet gas mixing system, which blends and delivers gas with sufficient flow to accommodate a high inspiratory flow demand from the patient (100 L/min ped/infant, 180 L/min adult). The gas mixing system allows a quick change of F_IO_2 (next breath) when the F_IO_2 control is adjusted or the 100% (3 min) button is pressed. When the F_IO_2 is set at 0.21, the e500 can operate with one gas supply (compressed air gas supply [>10 psig]).

When the ventilator is turned on, a power on self-test (POST) verifies the integrity of the software-controlled indicators, displays, audible alarm, and memory. Additional tests and calibrations are performed on an ongoing basis during operation. These include verification of software "watchdog" signals, flow and pressure transducer auto-zeroing, and oxygen analyzer calibration. The ventilator begins ventilation with the last set ventilator parameters that were used.

Ventilator User Set-Up Procedure

Before use, a few tests or calculations should be performed. Before running these, the operator must be sure the patient circuit and humidification system are attached. A test lung is placed at the patient Y-connector. While pressing the Preset Vent Settings button, the operator turns the power switch (front of the GDU) to the "On" position. This procedure allows entry to the User Set Up routine. (*Note*:

Table 12-52 Rear Panel of the Gas Delivery Unit (Figure 12-121)

Item No.	Description
1	Serial port for interface to central monitoring systems (RS-232C connector)
2	DISS high-pressure oxygen connector
3	DISS high-pressure air connector
4	Alarm beeper
5	Alternate site for electrical grounding equipment
6	Hour meter displays ventilator's operating hours (power on)
7	Connector for external battery
8	AC power module. Replaceable fuses located above connector port
9	Fan filter housing (with cover)
10	Remote alarm connector to interface to hospital nurse-call system
11	Connector for e500 Control Panel to GDU
12	Alarm loudness control
13	Connector for e500 Graphic Display Monitor to GDU
14	Connection for external alarm silence cable
15	Bleed port (diffuser head) for gas exhaust from the ventilator pneumatic system

Pressing and holding the Preset Vent Settings button while in User Set Up causes the e500 to enter normal ventilating conditions. To turn the Set Up routine off at this point, the operator must turn the power switch to the Standby position and press the Alarm Silence button.)

The Set-up procedure allows selection of any of the following:

- Language
- Pressure measurement units (cm H_2O or mbar)
- Perform a leak test on the patient circuit
- Calculate and enable circuit compliance compensation (volume ventilation)
- Enable a 90-second slow inflation
- Set time and date
- Adjust for operation at ambient altitude

When starting a new patient, the operator should be sure to use the Leak Test to ensure the integrity of the patient circuit and select the Compliance Compensation feature. (*Note*: Although some settings are automatically retained when the ventilator is turned off, the leak test and compliance compensation are not.)

To perform the leak test, the operator rotates the trigger knob until "**c1**" is displayed in the *trigger* window. The directions are followed as they appear in the message window. The operator will be required, for example, to occlude the patient Y-connector. The criteria for this leak test are based on a pressure drop during the test. The final message will be either "no leak" or "leak test failed." If the leak test is failed because of an excessive drop in pressure during the test, the operator must be sure to check the circuit and any attached accessories for potential leak sites and correct these before repeating the test.

In addition to the leak test, the e500 also features an automatic leak compensation to stabilize the baseline pressure when there is a small leak. The leak compensation during ventilation adjusts breath-by-breath with 8 L/min maximum for ped/infant patient selection and 15 L/min maximum for adult patient selection. The adjustment for leak compensation is based on flow measurement at end exhalation. Leak compensation helps to minimize the chance of auto-triggering.

As with the leak test, the compliance compensation calculation should be run whenever the patient circuit is changed. The patient cannot be connected during this procedure. (*Note*: Chapter 11 reviews volume loss associated with tubing compliance and its standard calculation.) To have the ventilator perform this calculation, the operator rotates the *trigger* knob to display **c2** in the trigger window. When the message window displays *Compliance Comp test Hit Exp Hold*, the operator presses EXP HOLD. The operator then follows the directions in the message window as they are displayed.

The breathing compensation factor may be viewed by selecting V_TE in the monitor section of the control panel and reading the digital information displayed in the adjacent window. If the circuit compliance is outside acceptable range, the message window will display CC TEST FAILED CC>10 mL/cm H_2O. This typically indicates a significant leak in the patient circuit. The operator should check the integrity of the exhalation system, breathing circuit and accessories before repeating the compliance test. After the test is passed, the ventilator will automatically compensate for losses of volume associated with tubing compressibility based on the new calculated value. The Ccomp indicator illuminates during the inspiratory phase of a volume controlled breath when this feature has been enabled.

The additional set up window features, such as Altitude compensation, can also be reviewed or checked while the User Set Up feature is in operation. The Newport e500 operating manual provides a detailed explanation of these items for users of the e500. As an example, Box 12-129 reviews the slow inflation technique, available in the User Set Up, which is used to obtain a pressure-volume loop and establish points on the loop where changes in lung compliance are occurring.

To start ventilation once the User Set Up has been completed, the Preset Vent Settings button is pressed and held. The next step is to select the appropriate patient category (adult or pediatric/infant) and then the breath type

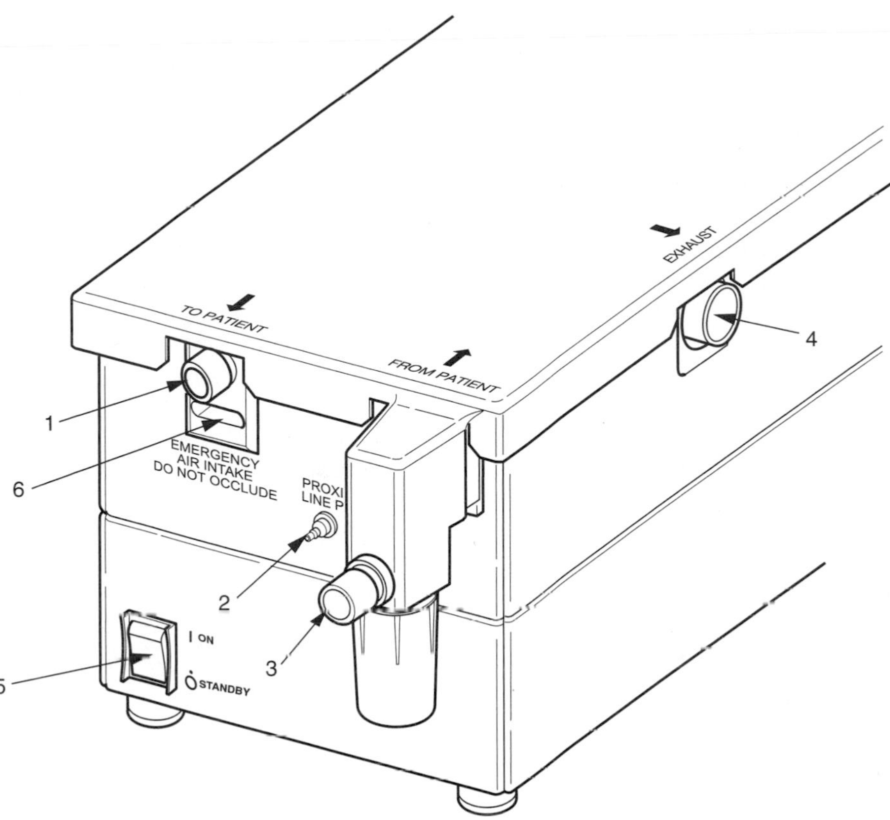

Figure 12-122 The front panel of the e500 ventilator showing the connections for the patient circuit and the on/off switch. *(1)* Inspiratory port, *(2)* Proximal pressure line port, *(3)* Expiratory port, *(4)* Exhaust outlet which allows exhaled gases to vent to room air, *(5)* ON/STANDBY switch, and *(6)* emergency air intake opening. (See text for further explanation.) (Courtesy Newport Medical Instruments, Costa Mesa, Calif.)

Box 12-128 Device Alert Alarms

If a Device Alert alarm occurs, a message will appear in the message window stating the problem. These alerts are related to battery problem or processor errors that may render the ventilator unable to adequately ventilate the patient. For example, a low battery power during battery operation or a component malfunction will result in a Device Alert. The emergency intake/relief and exhalation valves open. The ventilator supplies 8 L/min of air through the proximal pressure line if a supply is available. This allows a spontaneously breathing patient to obtain room air through the breathing circuit. The patient must be disconnected from the ventilator and provided with an alternative method of ventilation. The error message and the time it appeared are recorded in memory and can be reviewed in the user's set-up. Take the ventilator out of service until the problem can be corrected.

and mode, and adjust parameters as needed for the patient. Controls, breath-type modes, and alarms will all be reviewed.

Controls

The front control panel of the e500 contains three main areas: a control section, a monitored data section, and an alarm and message section (Figure 12-123). The control section is subdivided into a left-hand box with the mode keys and a few other controls. The right-hand section contains the commonly set ventilator parameters such as respiratory rate control.

Box 12-129 Slow Inflation Function

The Slow Inflation function is enabled and disabled under the User Set Up. When slow inflation is enabled and the ventilator is in Adult volume ventilation, with flow set at 1 to 2 L/min, pressing the "manual inflation" key delivers a slow manual inflation that can last up to 90 seconds as long as the airway pressure does not reach the high Paw limit or 60 cm H_2O. A slow inflation allows clinicians to view the upper and lower inflection points on the monitor for evaluation of an optimum PEEP setting and maximum safe distending pressure.

The mode control box includes a button for selecting patient size, either adult or pediatric/infant (Ped/Infant). An indicator light shows the selected category. Changing the patient size selection also governs the range of parameters. For example, the adult tidal volume range is 100 to 995 mL (5 mL resolution) or 1.00 to 3.00 L (0.01 resolution). The

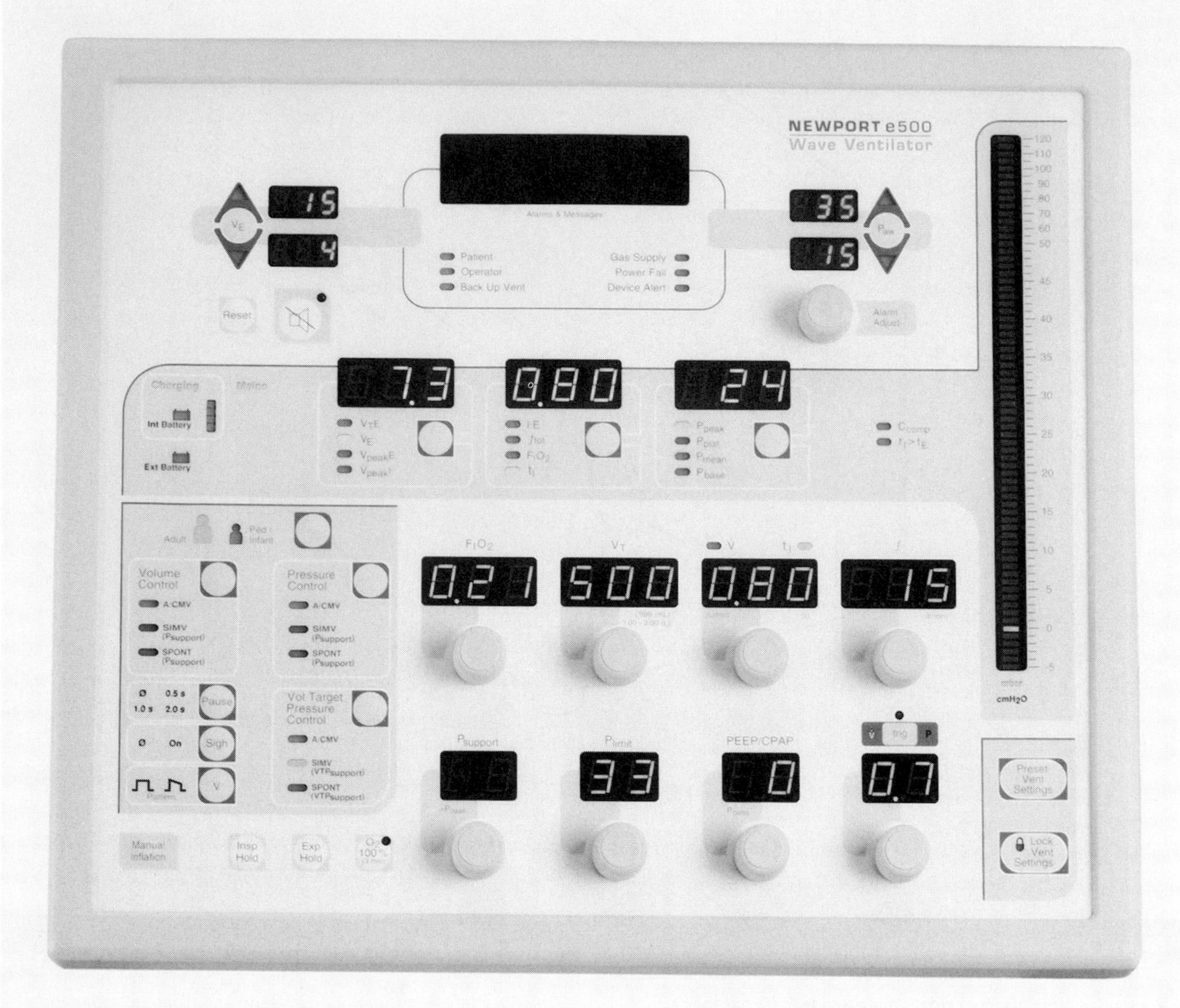

Figure 12-123 The front operating panel of the Newport e500 ventilator. (See text for further description.) (Courtesy Newport Medical Instruments, Costa Mesa, Calif.)

Ped/Infant range for tidal volume is 20 to 1000 mL (0.01 mL resolution).

The VOLUME CONTROL button is used to select volume-targeted breaths for assist/control (A/CMV), SIMV, or spontaneous (SPONT). An indicator illuminates to show the breath type and mode. To the right is the PRESSURE CONTROL button, which allows selection of pressure-targeted breaths in A/CMV, SIMV, or SPONT modes. Again, an indicator light illuminates to show the selected breath type and mode. The final mode and breath type panel is the VOLUME TARGETED PRESSURE CONTROL button. When this mode and breath type is selected, pressure ventilation is adjusted breath-by-breath to achieve the user set volume. These controls will be more extensively reviewed under the section on modes of ventilation and breath types.

The volume control section also includes a PAUSE control, a SIGH control and a FLOW WAVEFORM control. The PAUSE button is for setting an inspiratory pause during volume-targeted breaths (off, 0.5, 1.0 and 2.0 sec). The SIGH button activates sigh breath delivery with a sigh tidal volume equal to $1\frac{1}{2}$ times the set tidal volume. Sigh breaths occur every 100 breaths. The FLOW WAVEFORM control allows selection of either constant (square) or descending ramp flow waveforms during volume-targeted breath delivery.

Below the mode section are four additional controls: MANUAL INFLATION, INSPIRATORY HOLD, EXPIRATORY HOLD, and 100% OXYGEN DELIVERY (3 min). When pressed, the MANUAL INFLATION button delivers a manual inspiration that is up to 5 seconds long or ends when a high Paw alarm limit occurs. In pressure-controlled A/CMV and SIMV modes, MANUAL INFLATION is pressure-targeted at the set pressure limit. In SPONT mode (all breath types), as well as in VTPC, A/CMV, and SIMV modes, MANUAL INFLATION delivers a breath with a target pressure of PEEP/CPAP plus 15 cm H_2O. (*Note*: The maximum time for manual inflation is affected by the *slow inflation* control (see User Set Up Section).

When the INSPIRATORY HOLD button (INSP HOLD) is pressed, it starts an inspiratory hold at the end of inspiration for up to 5 seconds after a positive pressure breath. This allows the estimate of plateau pressure (P_{plat}). If INSPIRATORY HOLD is pressed during an exhalation, the hold takes place during the next positive pressure breath until the button is released or until 5 seconds elapses. The measured plateau pressure is displayed in the P_{plat} display until the end of the next inspiration. A reading of "- -" means the ventilator was unable to obtain a stable reading (usually resulting from a patient spontaneous breathing effort). P_{plat} is also displayed on the e500 GDM numeric screen with a time stamp indicating the time the measurement was made. The measurement of P_{plat} allows the e500 to calculate lung compliance and resistance when applicable. These are also displayed on the e500 GDM with time stamps.

Pressing the EXPIRATORY HOLD button (EXP HOLD) starts an expiratory hold maneuver at the end of the current exhalation for up to 20 seconds. This allows an estimated measurement of the auto-PEEP level. The ventilator displays this as P_{base}. If pressed during inspiration, the hold takes effect during the next exhalation until the button is released or 20 seconds has elapsed. Selecting EXP HOLD can be used to detect auto-PEEP as long as patient spontaneous breathing efforts are absent. If a stable reading is obtained, the total PEEP (auto-PEEP plus set PEEP) is shown in the P_{base} display. Otherwise, the display remains unchanged. "PEEPtotSTAT" is displayed on the e500 GDM along with a time stamp. This value is also used in the calculation of static compliance (Cstat), which is also time-stamped.

The O_2 100% (3 min) button delivers 100% O_2 for 3 minutes when activated. The indicator on the O_2 100% (3 min) button lights when 100% oxygen is delivered. Pressing the button again cancels 100% oxygen delivery.

Table 12-53 Ventilator Control Parameters

Control and Type	Description
F_IO_2 knob and display	Selects delivered oxygen concentration (0.21 to 1.0)
V_T knob and display	Selects delivered tidal volume for mandatory volume-targeted breaths and the target tidal volume for mandatory and spontaneous breaths in Volume Targeted Pressure Control ventilation
$\dot{V}/t_I$ indicator, knob and display	The knob selects the peak inspiratory flow for mandatory display breaths. If the $\dot{V}$ indicator is lit, the breath is volume-targeted and the display shows the flow setting. Flow range: adult, 1-180 L/min; pediatric/infant, 1-100 L/min. If the t_I indicator is lit, the breath is pressure-targeted and the display shows the inspiratory time setting. Inspiratory time range: adult, 0.1 to 5.0 sec; pediatric/infant, 0.1 to 3.0 sec
f knob and display	This knob controls the mandatory breath rate (f) and displays as breaths/min
Psupport knob and display	This knob controls the pressure support level (above PEEP/CPAP setting) for spontaneous breaths in SIMV or SPONT settings in either breath type (Volume Control or Pressure Control). The display is the set pressure level, which is added to the set PEEP/CPAP level. PS range: for adult, 0 to 60 cm H_2O; for pediatric/infants, 0 to 50 cm H_2O
P_{limit} knob and display	Target pressure is set with this knob and the value display. This is for Pressure Control mandatory breaths and both mandatory and spontaneous breaths in Volume Target Pressure Control mode. Pressure range: adult, 0 to 80 cm H_2O; pediatric/infant, 0 to 70 cm H_2O
PEEP/CPAP knob and display	This knob selects the baseline pressure for all breath types and modes and displays PEEP/CPAP. Range Adult 0 to 45 cm H_2O and ped/infant 0 to 30 cm H_2O
Trigger indicator, knob, and display	The trigger button selects either flow ($\dot{V}$) or pressure (P) triggering. The operator presses the button to highlight the trigger type desired. The knob adjusts the sensitivity value for either trigger variable. The display shows the selected setting. The *trig* indicator flashes when the ventilator recognizes a patient effort. During exhalation, the e500 uses a ventilator-set bias flow, which is functional during flow-triggering. The bias flow also functions to flush exhaled CO_2 and stabilize temperature, humidity and baseline pressure in the patient circuit. The bias flow is turned off during an expiratory hold maneuver

Using Ventilator Controls

Adjusting any of the ventilator parameter controls is basically the same for all variables. The adjacent knob for any parameter is adjusted until the display window above the knob shows the desired setting. The ventilator retains the settings in memory within 10 seconds of selection. If the ventilator is turned off (placed in Standby), these values are retained in memory and used when the unit is powered up again. Setting a parameter outside of the available range causes three things to happen. The Operator indicator blinks, an audible alarm sounds and the message window describes which parameter is out of range.

Ventilator Parameter Controls

The right hand area of the controls section contains the following: F_IO_2, V_T, $\dot{V}$, or T_I, frequency (f), Psupport, P_{limit}, PEEP/CPAP, and trigger: $\dot{V}$ or P trigger. Table 12-53 describes each of these controls.

Below the pressure manometer on the right side of the control panel are two additional controls: LOCK VENT SETTINGS and PRESET VENT SETTINGS.

The LOCK VENT SETTINGS button does just that; it locks and unlocks all the buttons and knobs in the control section except for the MANUAL INFLATION control and the O_2 100% (3 min) control. The lock indicator illuminates when the lock is in effect.

Pressing the PRESET VENT SETTINGS button simultaneously as the ventilator is turned "on" enters the *User Set Up* procedure and suspends ventilation. The PRESET VENT SETTINGS function can also be used during ventilation. Pressing the PRESET VENT SETTINGS button during ventilation allows selection of ventilation parameters for a different mode/breath type, without affecting current ventilator settings. The operator follows these steps:

- Presses Preset Vent Settings
- Selects the desired breath type/mode (*Note*: The preset breath type/mode indicator flashes, but the ventilator continues ventilation in the currently selected breath type and mode [current breath type/mode indicator remains steadily lit].)
- Sets the desired ventilator parameters
- To exit the Preset state, presses the PRESET VENT SETTINGS button again or waits 5 seconds after the last ventilator setting adjustment.
- The ventilator saves the settings selected during Preset as long as the ventilator is on.
- After the new breath type/mode is selected, the settings changed by the operator during Preset become effective.

Box 12-130 describes the safety benefit of setting parameters for ventilator modes not currently in use. (*Note*: If a new breath type/mode is not selected in the Preset state, or if a ventilator parameter change is made before selecting a new breath type/mode, the changes to settings become immediate for the current breath type and mode.) (See Clinical Rounds 12-52.)

Box 12-130 Patient Safety and Preset Vent Settings

To ensure patient safety, it is advisable to use the Preset Vent Settings button to set safe values for all parameters for the patient being ventilated. Should someone inadvertently change the ventilator to a different breath type or mode, the parameters for the new breath type or mode would still be appropriate for the patient. For example, if an adult patient is being pressure ventilated, a tidal volume is not set. Assume the ventilator holds in memory a V_T of 100 mL. If the mode were changed from pressure to volume A/C, the 100 mL V_T might not be appropriate for the patient currently being ventilated. It is advisable to adjust breath and mode type and their variables to guard against this type of problem.

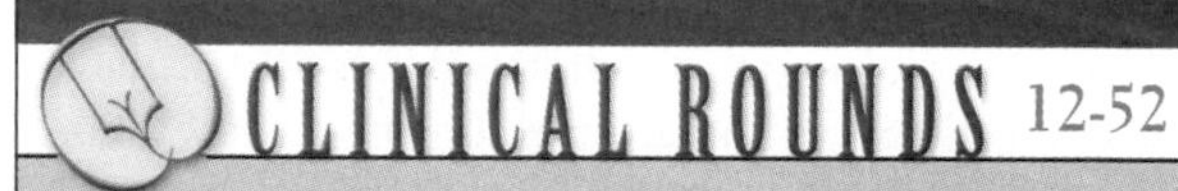

Making Parameter Changes with the e500.
A respiratory therapist is ventilating a patient with Pressure Control SIMV with the e500 at a mandatory rate of 6 breaths/min. The therapist presses the Preset Vent Settings button, selects Volume Control with SIMV as the breath type and mode and sets the respiratory rate to 2 breaths/min. How will the ventilator respond?

See Appendix A for the answer.

Sloping

Although many new ventilators have a separate sloping or rise time feature that adjusts the rate of pressure delivery during pressure ventilation, the e500 is programmed to adjust sloping based on the real-time response of the system. During pressure-targeted breaths of any type, the ventilator delivers a flow at a software-optimized rate to quickly achieve and maintain the set pressure until the end of inspiration. Flow is adjusted to provide automatic sloping (rise) for every breath. The program is designed to avoid overshooting the set pressure for the breath (see Chapter 11 for a description of sloping or rise time).

Monitored Data Section

The center portion of the front panel contains the monitored data section. On the far left are the battery and power indicators described earlier. The first data monitoring display is for volume and flow information. By pressing the button adjacent to the available list, any of the following can be displayed:

CLINICAL ROUNDS 12-53

A respiratory therapist presses the Insp. Hold button to obtain a plateau pressure reading for calculation of lung compliance. The Pplat display in the pressure section of the monitored data window reads "- -" and does not provide a value. What is the problem?

See Appendix A for the answer.

Box 12-131 Range of High and Low Minute Volume and Pressure Alarms

- High minute volume alarm range: adult 2 to 80 L/min, ped/infant 0.2 to 60 L/min.
- Low minute volume alarm range: adult 1 to 50 L/min, ped/infant 0.01 to 30 L/min.
- High peak airway pressure alarm range: adult 5 to 120 cm H_2O, ped/infant 5 to 100 cm H_2O.
- Low peak airway pressure alarm range: adult 3 to 95 cm H_2O cm H_2O, ped/infant 3 to 75 cm H_2O.

- V_{TE}—expiratory tidal volume (mL)
- $\dot{V}_E$—expiratory minute volume (L)
- $\dot{V}$peakE—peak expiratory flow (L/min)
- $\dot{V}$peakI—peak inspiratory flow (L/min)

An indicator lights to show which variable is being displayed.

The second set of data displayed is for timing and F_IO_2 data. Pressing the button displays any of the following:

- I:E ratio (inspiratory-to-expiratory ratio)—Displays 99:1 to 1:99. In SPONT mode, this display shows "- -".
- f_{tot}—the total breath rate in breaths/min.
- F_IO_2—displays the measured fractional inspired oxygen concentration. The display will show "- -" if the oxygen supply pressure is below minimum, or the ventilator is connected to air only and the F_IO_2 is set at 21%. It will also display "- -" if the oxygen sensor is disconnected, defective, or not calibrated since power up, or oxygen sensor calibration is in progress.
- t_I—measured inspiratory time displayed in seconds and updated following each spontaneous or mandatory breath.

An indicator light shows which variable is currently being displayed in this section.

The third section of the display data is for patient pressure information. Using the adjacent button allows display of one of the following:

- P_{peak}—peak airway pressure (cm H_2O) updated after each positive pressure inflation (range 1 to 120 cm H_2O).
- P_{plat}—plateau pressure (cm H_2O) displayed at the end of an inspiratory hold or pause (range 0 to 120 cm H_2O). The display shows "- -" if there is no Pause or Insp Hold or the ventilator cannot measure a stable plateau pressure.
- P_{mean}—mean airway pressure (cm H_2O), the average pressure in the patient circuit for the past 30 seconds (range 0 to 120 cm H_2O).
- P_{base}—baseline pressure (cm H_2O) (range 0 to 99 cm H_2O).

As with the other monitored variables, a light indicator shows the current parameter on display. See Clinical Rounds 12-53 for an exercise related to pressure monitoring.

Toward the right of the monitor displays are two light indicators. The C_{comp} indicator illuminates when the ventilator is correcting for patient circuit compliance. When C_{comp} is used, the ventilator adjusts volume delivery for volume controlled breaths to allow for the compliance of the patient circuit.

The t_I>t_E indicator illuminates when inverse I:E ratios are present (inspiratory time is longer than expiratory time). To the far right of the monitor data section is a pressure bar graph. This provides a continuous display of real-time pressure measured in the patient circuit in cm H_2O or mbar (millibars). The display range is –5 to 120 cm H_2O or 5 to 117 mbar. The desired units of measure are set using the User Set Up procedure.

Alarms

The alarm controls and indicators of the c500 are located in the upper section of the front panel. The alarm system can be divided into three basic sections: adjustable alarms, nonadjustable, and controls.

Adjustable Alarms

Adjustable alarms include the high and low minute volume and high and low peak airway pressure. The minute volume alarm control is located in the upper left section of the alarm area. Pressing the center $\dot{V}_E$ button selects between the high and low V_E alarm limit for adjustment of the high and low V_E values (Box 12-131 for alarm range). Pressing the button once selects the high alarm limit, twice selects the low alarm limit, and three times exits alarm setting conditions. The adjacent display for the selected alarm limit flashes and the message window describes the selected alarm. While the display is flashing, the operator rotates the Alarm Adjust knob located at the right hand side of the alarm section to set the desired value. The alarm limit is adjusted until the display shows the value wanted. Once adjusted, the adjacent display windows show the high and low V_E alarm limits setting. When a violation of these settings occurs, an indicator above or below the button blinks red and an audible alarm sounds.

Table 12-54 Non-Adjustable Alarms and Related Messages*

Message	Condition
Apnea	20 seconds have elapsed without a patient effort detected or a breath delivered
F_IO_2 High	Measured F_IO_2 >0.07 (7%) above set F_IO_2
F_IO_2 Low	Measured F_IO_2 > 0.07 (7%) below set F_IO_2
High Baseline Pressure	Monitored P_{base} > (set P_{base} + 5 cm H_2O) for 2 consecutive breaths
Low Baseline Pressure	Monitored P_{base} < set P_{base} by a software determined amount for more than 0.5 seconds for 2 consecutive breaths
Prox Line Disconnect	The outlet pressure from the ventilator is greater than the proximal pressure when proximal pressure is near zero
Sustained High Baseline	Monitored P_{base} has been ≥8 cm H_2O above set PEEP/CPAP for over 6 seconds for pediatric/infant patients or more than 10 seconds for adults

OPERATOR-RELATED ALARMS

Operator indicator blinks indicating an attempt to select an invalid setting when the Message window displays these:

Alarm	Description
Insp Time Too Long	Inspiratory time >5 seconds
Insp Time Too Short	Inspiratory time <0.1 seconds
I:E Ratio Inverse Violation	Inverse ratio >4:1
P_{limit} Below P_{base}	Current P_{limit} setting is lower than the P_{base} (PEEP/CPAP) setting
Low Paw Below P_{base}	Current low Paw alarm setting is lower than the P_{base} (PEEP/CPAP) setting
Vol Target Not Met	The set volume target is not met before the breath ends
Out of Range	An alarm or setting is out of range for the selected patient category
Back Up Ventilation	Back Up Vent indicator blinks and a message appears, "Back Up Ventilation" indicating that back-up ventilation is occurring in response to a Low $\dot{V}_E$ alarm
Gas Supply Alarms	Gas Supply indicator blinks and the message window displays an alarm message if one or both gas supplies are below the operational pressure level of 10 psig. (*Note*: If the F_IO_2 is set at 0.21, this alarm is only active if air is lost)
Power Fail Alarm	The Power Fail indicator blinks and the message window displays an alarm message in case of the loss of AC power or low internal battery power level
Device Alert	Device Alert blinks when the ventilator is inoperative or less than 10% of the internal battery charge remains when the ventilator is battery operated. The emergency intake/relief and exhalation valves open and a spontaneously breathing patient can receive room air. If available, 8 L/min of air is delivered through the proximal pressure tubing of the breathing circuit

*The *Patient* indicator blinks when the Message window displays any of these alarm messages and an audible alarm occurs.

The high and low airway pressure alarm indicators and control button are located on the right side of the alarm section. As with the minute volume alarm, the button is pressed to select between the high- and low-pressure alarm setting and set the pressure alarm limits in the same manner as the minute ventilation alarm limits are set. The display windows to the left show the value for the high and low peak airway pressure alarms (see Box 12-131 for alarm range). The indicator above or below the selector button blinks red and an audible alarm sounds to indicate a high or low airway pressure condition.

Nonadjustable Alarms

Table 12-54 lists the nonadjustable, patient-related alarms and the related message that appears in the Alarms and Message window at the top center portion of the front operating panel.

Alarm Controls

In addition to the high- and low-pressure and minute ventilation alarm controls described previously, there are four additional alarm controls.

- Alarm Silence—This button mutes audible alarms for one minute, including alarms that occur after the silent period begins. Pressing the Alarm Silence button again turns off the silence function. A *Device Alert* alarm cannot be silenced by this button unless the e500 is powered down first (see Box 12-128).
- Alarm Silence Suction/Disconnect Function—Holding down the Alarm Silence button for ≥1 second (a short audible beep will occur) enables a disconnection function. If the ventilator detects a circuit disconnection within 20 seconds, a suction disconnect function results. "Ventilation Suspended" appears in the message window. The automatic leak compensation is suspended and a bias flow of gas is delivered through the circuit (10 L/min adult, 5 L/min pediatric/infant). Ventilation only resumes when the breathing circuit is reconnected or when 3 minutes elapses, whichever occurs first.
- Alarm Reset Button—Pressing this button clears visual indicators and messages for alarms that are no longer active.
- Alarm Loudness Knob—This knob adjusts the audible alarm volume (located on the rear panel of the GDU).

Modes of Ventilation and Breath Types

The Newport e500 provides three breath types: volume, pressure, and volume-targeted pressure-control breaths (VTPC). These three breath types are available in A/CMV, SIMV, and SPONT modes of ventilation.

Breath Types

The e500 can provide volume- or pressure-targeted breaths as well as volume-targeted pressure-control breaths.

Volume Control

During volume ventilation, the ventilator delivers mandatory breaths based on the set tidal volume (V_T), flow ($\dot{V}$), frequency (f), PEEP/CPAP, oxygen concentration (F_IO_2), Pause, Sigh, and flow pattern setting. A constant (square) flow pattern and a descending ramp flow pattern are available for volume breaths. For a descending ramp, inspiration begins at the flow setting, decreases at a constant rate to 50% of the flow setting, and ends inspiration when the tidal volume has been delivered (volume-cycled) unless a pause is set. Patient demand cannot result in additional flow from the ventilator so the operator must set flow appropriate to the patient's needs.

Pressure Control

During pressure control ventilation, mandatory breaths are provided that are based on the set pressure (P_{limit}), inspiratory time (T_I), frequency (f), PEEP/CPAP, and F_IO_2 settings. The ventilator adjusts the flow during inspiration and the flow slope to best achieve an immediate rise in the pressure delivery to the set pressure (P_{limit}), without overshooting the pressure. During pressure control the ventilator adjusts flow in response to patient demand to maintain the set pressure. Inspiratory flow ends when the set inspiratory time has elapsed (time-cycled) or sooner if alveolar pressure reaches the target pressure.

Volume-Targeted Pressure Control (VTPC) Breaths

During VTPC ventilation, the e500 ventilator delivers mandatory breaths based on set values for pressure (P_{limit}), inspiratory time (t_I), V_T, f, PEEP/CPAP, and F_IO_2. This breath type is similar to pressure control, but unlike pressure control ventilation, the set pressure is the maximum allowable target pressure. The pressure varies to achieve a set V_T. Unlike volume ventilation, the V_T is a target and is not guaranteed for each breath. The ventilator determines the pressure needed to achieve the set V_T and increases or decreases the pressure by a maximum of 6 cm H_2O (up or down) per breath as needed. This is similar to pressure regulated volume control (PRVC) described in Chapter 11. Clinical Rounds 12-54 provides an example problem using VTPC.

The target pressure of the first breath is 40% of the set P_{limit} or P_{base} plus 5 cm H_2O, whichever is higher. The maximum pressure permitted during this mode is the P_{limit} value. The minimum pressure is P_{base} plus 5 cm H_2O.

If the set V_T is not achieved by the end of inspiration when the target pressure equals P_{limit}, an operator alarm occurs and the message window will display "Vol Target Not Met." The operator should investigate the cause of higher pressures being required and try to correct any problem that may have changed the patient's lung compliance or airway resistance. It is also possible that the V_T, P_{limit}, or T_I are set inappropriately.

Volume-Targeted Pressure

Control breath delivery is available in Volume Target Pressure Control A/CMV and SIMV modes. In the SIMV mode, the same target V_T and P_{limit} apply to both mandatory and

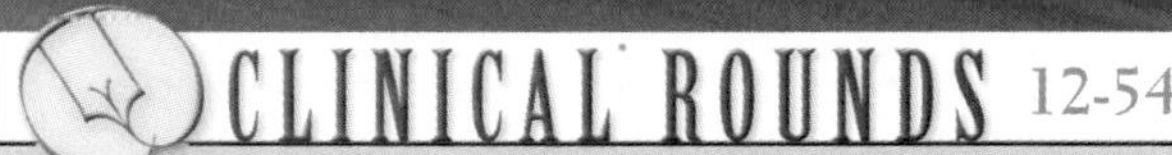

A patient is being ventilated with volume-targeted pressure control. The set tidal volume is 500 mL, the PEEP/CPAP is 10 cm H_2O and the P_{limit} is 35 cm H_2O with a rate of 10 mandatory breaths/minute. After the first few breaths, the peak pressure is 25 cm H_2O and the exhaled V_T is 460 cm H_2O.

Question 1: How will the ventilator respond to these measured values?

Question 2: What is the maximum pressure the ventilator will rise to?

See Appendix A for the answer.

spontaneous breaths. However, mandatory breaths are time-cycled and spontaneous breaths flow-cycled, based on the same flow-cycling threshold adjusting feature as standard pressure support described in the following section.

Volume Target Pressure Support Breaths

As with VTPC breaths, the e500 can also target a tidal volume during pressure support breaths. Because pressure support breaths are always spontaneous breaths, volume-targeted pressure support (VTPS) is available whenever the patient can receive spontaneous non-mandatory breaths. This includes volume-targeted pressure control SIMV and SPONT (spontaneous) modes.

As with VTPC, the target pressure in VTPS for the first breath is 40% of set P_{limit} or P_{base} plus 5 cm H_2O, whichever is highest. The ventilator delivers a flow to achieve and maintain the pressure. The lowest available pressure is the P_{base} setting plus 5 cm H_2O. The highest pressure is the set P_{limit}.

The e500 establishes a target pressure after each breath with the goal of meeting the set V_T. Pressure is adjusted up or down by a maximum of 6 cm H_2O breath by breath to achieve the set V_T. The set V_T may not be achieved with every breath, but is still targeted.

Three criteria end a VTPS breath:

- The patient stops demanding flow (flow decays to the flow-cycling off threshold).
- The pressure rises above the ventilator's current target level plus a small time-varied margin.
- Inspiratory time reaches a maximum value (2 sec adult, 1.2 sec pediatric/infant).

The standard cycling mechanism for VTPS and Psupport is flow-cycling. It is user adjustable from 5% to 55% of measured peak flow (Box 12-132) or the user may choose to have it automatically adjusted by the ventilator.

If the target pressure is equal to the P_{limit} (the maximum permitted pressure), and the target V_T is not reached by the end of a breath, an operator alarm will activate and the message window will display "Vol Target Not Met." The operator should determine the cause of higher pressures being required to deliver the volume, such as changes in the patient's lung compliance or airway resistance. The obvious advantage of this mode and VTPC is the use of pressure-targeted ventilation and the automatic adjustment of pressure target for the lowest level that accommodates volume delivery.

Box 12-132 Flexcycle

A flow-cycling feature called Flexcycle is being used for flow-cycling PS and VTPS breaths. Flexcycle uses pulmonary time constants calculated at end exhalation and the slope of the pressure waveform at end inspiration to automatically adjust the flow-cycling off threshold to specifically suit patient needs. It is adjusted on a breath-by-breath basis by the microprocessor.

Modes of Ventilation

Assist/Control (A/CMV) Ventilation

In A/CMV ventilation all breaths are mandatory. Triggering of inspiration is by time based on the machine rate or by the patient (flow or pressure-triggering). The set rate establishes the minimum breath rate. The breath can be volume- or pressure-targeted or VTPC. Inspiration normally ends as follows:

- Volume breaths are volume-cycled
- Pressure breaths are time-cycled
- VTPC breaths are time-cycled

Synchronized Intermittent Mandatory Ventilation (SIMV)

In SIMV the set breath rate establishes the mandatory breath rate. The patient can breathe spontaneously between mandatory breaths. Mandatory breaths can be volume- or pressure-targeted or VTPC. The mandatory breath trigger and cycling variables are the same as in A/CMV ventilation; that is, time- or patient-triggered and volume-cycled (volume-targeted breaths) or time-cycled (pressure-targeted breaths).

The baseline will be the set PEEP/CPAP level. Spontaneous breaths in volume or pressure-targeted SIMV can be supported with pressure support (Psupport) or set at zero Psupport. If zero is set, the ventilator actually delivers 1.5 cm H_2O of pressure above the set P_{base} during spontaneous inspiration.

If Psupport is set, the ventilator delivers the software-optimized flow (see Sloping, described earlier) to achieve the set pressure change. Inspiratory flow ends when one of three criteria occurs:

- The patient stops demanding flow (flow decays to the flow-cycling off threshold).
- The pressure rises above the PS target pressure level plus a small time-varied margin.
- Inspiratory time reaches a maximum value (2 sec adult, 1.2 sec pediatric/infant).

If VTPC is selected, spontaneous breaths are Volume Targeted Pressure Supported (VTPS), as described previously. In this case, the maximum target pressure is $\leq P_{limit}$ for both the VTPC mandatory breaths and the VTPS breaths. The distinguishing feature between these breaths is that VTPC breaths are time-cycled and VTPS breaths are flow-cycled. (*Note*: The nonsupported spontaneous breath type is not available when VTPC is selected. Only A/CMV, SIMV, and SPONT VTPS are available.)

Spontaneous (SPONT)

When SPONT is selected, the operator sets F_IO_2, PEEP/CPAP, Psupport or V_T, and P_{limit} (VTPS) and trigger sensitivity for patient-triggered breaths. The patient's spontaneous efforts determine the rate, flow, volume, and cycling of each breath, except for VTPS breaths. VTPS can be used in the SPONT mode (see VTPS above).

Back-Up Ventilation (BUV)

When the ventilator detects that the low minute ventilation alarm setting has been violated, BUV begins. The Back-up Vent indicator blinks and the message window displays "Back Up Ventilation." If the current mode is volume- or pressure-targeted A/CMV or SIMV, the ventilator employs the current control panel settings except for respiratory rate (f). The rate increases to 1.5 times the current setting or 15 breaths/min minimum and 100 breaths/min maximum.

For all modes in VTPC breath type or the SPONT mode in volume- or pressure-targeted breath type, the ventilator delivers pressure-targeted breaths with the following settings: P_{limit} (target pressure) 15 cm H_2O above the current PEEP/CPAP setting, inspiratory time (T_I) 0.6 second for pediatric/infant and 1.0 second for adult patients and respiratory rate 20 breaths/min for pediatric/infant and 12 breaths/min for adult patients.

BUV is suspended (disabled) for 1 minute in the following situations: suction disconnect function, changing a ventilator setting that affects mode, breath timing, flow/volume, pressure or trigger sensitivity. Pressing alarm silence, alarm reset, or adjusting alarm limit settings does not suspend the back-up ventilation nor cause normal ventilation to resume. The normal ventilation settings resume when the patient's minute ventilation rises to the low minute volume alarm setting plus 10%.

Special Features—Newport e500 Graphic Display Monitor (GDM)

The GDM is a monitor designed for use with the Newport e500 ventilator (Figures 12-120 and 12-124). The GDM connects to the ventilator via a serial communication interface. The GDM receives power from the ventilator when the e500 is connected to an AC power source. (*Note*: The GDM switches off during battery operation to conserve power.)

The GDM uses pressure and flow signals from the e500 to produce real time graphics of pressure, volume, and flow measured by the ventilator. The screen is touch-sensitive and allows the operator to select a waveform or loop to display in addition to offering freeze screen with cursor, scaling and auto-scaling, trends, and printing features (right column controls). In addition to the control features, a row of measured and calculated numeric data is displayed at the bottom of the screen (see Figure 12-124). Three predetermined sets of numeric data for display are available. The "basic set" is normally displayed on power-up. There is a separate screen that allows the viewing of all the numeric values on one screen (NUMERIC button).

GDM Setup

To set up the GDM, select the SETUP button. The following can be set: date, time, patient information, units of measure, units of weight, breath averaging, slope/rise, manual or automated (under extended functions menu),

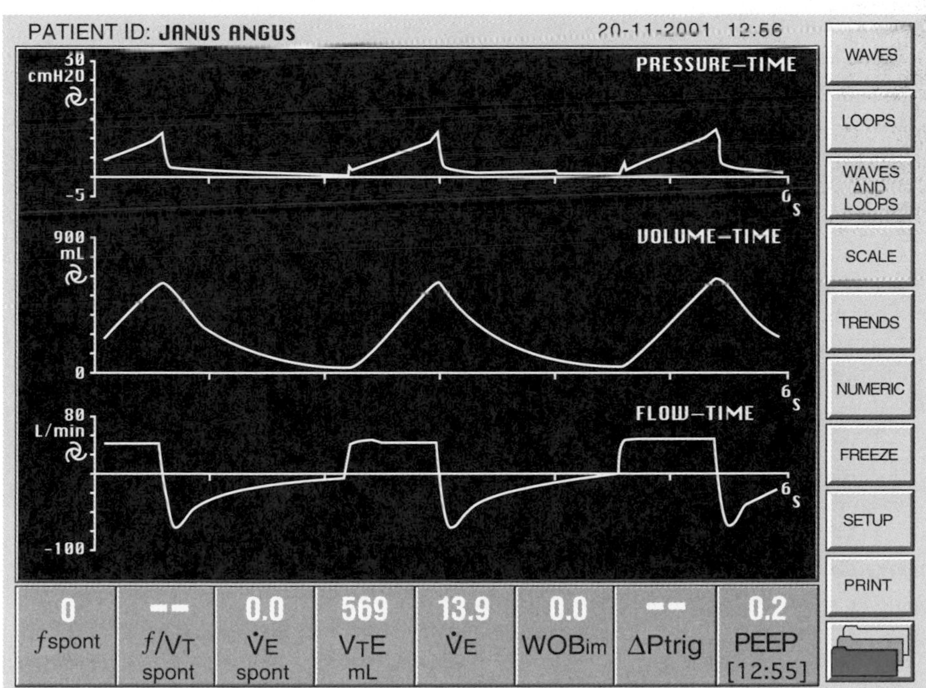

Figure 12-124 The Newport e500 Graphic Display Monitor Screen. (See text for further description.) (Courtesy Newport Medical Instruments, Costa Mesa, Calif.)

and expiratory threshold. To set any of these variables, the operator performs the following: touches the desired item to be set up, selects the value (keypad or alpha keys), and presses ENTER to update. To view the set-up parameters, the operator touches the SETUP button and the current settings are displayed. To exit without changing any date, the operator can press ENTER or touch any command button at the right edge of the screen.

Waveforms and Loops

Pressure, volume, and flow scalars and volume-pressure and flow-volume loops can be selected for display. The screen can feature three scalars and two loops simultaneously. The FREEZE function suspends current plotting of graphs and holds the current display for extended viewing (FREEZE/START button). When FREEZE is on, a green vertical dashed cursor appears in the center of the screen. Left and right touch-sensitive arrow buttons allows the cursor to be moved. Numeric values are displayed for each point on a waveform or loop intersected by the cursor.

In addition to freezing a screen for reviewing, the GDM also allows saving a reference loop. Touching LOOP and then REFERENCE LOOPS MENU access this function. A loop can be stored in memory and later used for comparison with other loops to evaluate changes in patient lung characteristics, for example, after bronchodilator therapy. Active loops can also be displayed overlaying previous loops. The One Touch™ feature automatically plots, and freezes a quasi-static, volume-pressure loop when the operator performs a manual slow inflation maneuver. The movable cursor allows for estimating lower and upper inflection points on the curve.

Trends functions can save up to 24 hours of selected trending parameters. The two trends screens can display the following:

TREND (SCREEN) 1

V_TE/flow, $\dot{V}_E$/time, f tot/time, %leak/time

TREND (SCREEN) 2

P_{peak}/time, P_{mean}/time, P_{base}/time, f/V_T spont/time

Troubleshooting

The alarms and indicators on the front panel help the operator solve the majority of problems that might occur during operation. In addition, the Operator's Manual provides regular users with a symptom driven table with common problems identified along with possible causes and solutions. For example, if a "Power Failure" alarm occurs, any of the following might be the problem: disconnected power cord, open fuse, loss of AC power, battery completely discharged, or a hardware failure. If checking the fuses and power sources does not correct the problem, the user should contact a qualified service technician.

A few troubleshooting situations are reviewed here.

1. If a Device Alert alarm occurs, the emergency intake/relief valve opens. If a bacterial filter is not in use, the inspiratory gas line of the patient circuit may be exposed to expiratory gas and its potential contaminants. Clean and sterilize the inspiratory gas delivery system after this event.
2. If monitored values for exhaled flows or volumes differ from set values, the flow sensor screen may be dirty or not calibrated correctly or a leak may be present in the circuit.
3. When monitored F_IO_2 values do not match set values, the oxygen or air pressure source(s) may be too low or a leak may be present in the pneumatic system for F_IO_2 monitoring.
4. If a High Baseline Pressure alarm message is present and the Patient indicator flashes, this means the measure baseline pressure has been ≥ 5 cm H_2O above the set PEEP/CPAP for two consecutive breaths. Check the breathing circuit for kinks or obstructions. Evaluate the ventilator settings and make any necessary adjustments.
5. An I:E Ratio Inverse Violation alarm occurs (Operator indicator flashes) when ventilator settings (t_I, f, flow, V_T) would result in an inverse I:E ratio greater than 4:1. The ventilator will not permit an I:E ratio > 4:1. The operator should be sure to check flow, T_I, frequency, and so on.
6. When an Insp Time Too Long alarm occurs and the Operator indicator flashes, the ventilator settings have resulted in an inspiratory time more than 5 seconds long. Check and correct the V_T, flow, f, T_I, and pause settings.
7. An inspiratory time less than 0.1 seconds, excluding any pause or inspiratory hold is not permitted. An Insp Time Too Short alarm indicates this condition. Evaluate and readjust V_T and flow settings as needed.
8. Prox Line Disconnect Alarm (Patient indicator flashing) occurs when the ventilator outlet pressure is higher than the measured proximal pressure when proximal pressure is near zero. Check the proximal pressure line connection and the patient to be sure the patient circuit is not disconnected or leaking. The ventilator will continue to ventilate the patient and monitors the ventilator via the ventilator outlet pressure rather than the proximal pressure line.
9. A Sustained High Baseline Pressure alarm (Patient indicator flashing) means an obstructed or kinked breathing circuit, a restricted or defective exhalation valve or a malfunctioning exhalation system. Monitored baseline pressure has been ≥ 8 cm H_2O above the set PEEP/CPAP for more than 6 seconds (pediatric) or 10 seconds (adult).

The ventilator opens the emergency intake/relief and exhalation valves. Provide alternative ventilation for the patient. Check the patient circuit for kinks or obstructions. Make sure the exhalation valve is functioning properly and replace the exhalation filter if necessary. Evaluate ventilator settings and make appropriate adjustments. If the alarm recurs, remove the ventilator from service and provide another means of ventilation to the patient. Contact a qualified service representative.

10. When the Ventilation Suspended message appears, and no alarm is heard, the ventilator detects a circuit disconnect and the Suction Disconnect Function is enabled. The ventilator will resume normal operation when it detects that the circuit is reconnected or when 3 minutes elapses, whichever happens first. The alarm will resume after one minute.

The e500 GDM monitor and the e500 ventilator are protected from common electromagnetic environments. However, e500s may be adversely affected by some high-frequency surgical devices or radiofrequency transmitting devices such as cell phones, cordless phones, and citizen band radios. Do not use the ventilator or monitor near magnetic resonance imaging equipment

SUMMARY

This chapter reviews a significant number of current and newly released mechanical ventilators. The text for each was reviewed by manufacturing representatives and clinicians using these units in intensive care areas whenever possible. Occasionally there are discrepancies between the operating manual material and the material in this chapter. Sometimes printed operating manuals lag behind the addition of new options and the updating of software. In such situations, information taken directly from manufacturer representatives took precedence over what had been printed. These individuals were invaluable resources in providing assistance in making this material as accurate as possible. When mechanical ventilators are operating in the clinical setting, users should always refer to the manufacturer's materials and resources and defer to these as accurate representations of current operating instructions.

The authors will be using the EVOLVE website for this text to provide updates and new features for the various ventilators and links to the manufacturers.

Review Questions

Bear 1000

1. The flow-control valve of the Bear 1000 is powered by which type of device so that rapid changes in flow are possible?
   a. An electronic flow transducer
   b. A linear drive, microprocessor-controlled piston
   c. A proportional rotary microswitch
   d. A stepper motor

2. To adjust the V_T setting on the Bear 1000, which of the following should be performed?
   a. Turn the tidal volume knob to the desired value
   b. Press tidal volume, key in the value on the numeric key pad, and press enter
   c. Press the tidal volume touch pad and rotate the control knob (at the far right on the second row of controls) until the desired value for V_T appears
   d. Reduce the $\dot{V}_E$ setting, then change the rate until the desired V_T appears in the message window

3. To set the high total $\dot{V}_E$ alarm on the Bear 1000, which of the following must be performed?
   I. Unlock the alarm panel
   II. Touch the left upward pointing triangle below the total $\dot{V}_E$ digital window
   III. Turn the alarm control knob until the desired value is displayed
   IV. Press the activated touch pad to the right of the alarm
   a. III only
   b. I and II only
   c. II and IV only
   d. I, II, and III only

4. An alarm sounds, and the respiratory therapist notes that the gas supply failure LED is illuminated. This indicates which of the following?
   a. One or more of the gas sources is <35 psig
   b. If one gas supply is still available, the ventilator will continue to operate
   c. Measured F_IO_2 has dropped below the set value
   d. Inspiratory pressure in the patient circuit is below the set value

5. True or False? The Bear 1000 requires both an air and an oxygen gas source and an electrical power source.

6. True or False? Both volume- and pressure-targeted mandatory breaths are available with the SIMV mode.

7. A nurse is trying to readjust the V_T on the Bear 1000 ventilator. Although the V_T reading is 0.5 L and the LED next to the V_T control is illuminated, turning the control has no effect. What could be the problem?

8. A physician is attempting to change the V_T setting during ventilation of a patient, but the digital display on the V_T control is blank and turning the control knob gets no response. What could be the problem?

9. The graphic display of pressure and time for a pressure-support breath shows the following:
   - a slight dip in the curve below baseline at the beginning of inspiration
   - a sharp rise in pressure to a peak, which falls to a plateau value during inspiration
   - a smooth drop in pressure to baseline at the end of inspiration

   Does this description fit an appropriate PSV breath delivery?

10. The COMPLIANCE COMP. control indicates a value of 3 cm H_2O. The set V_T is 0.7 L (700 mL); the PIP is 25 cm H_2O. The digital exhaled volume fluctuates from 0.68 to 0.71 L (680-710 mL). If a respirometer is placed in the main inspiratory side coming out of the ventilator and going to the patient, what would the volume read?

11. A patient is on pressure augmentation. The pressure-time graph shows a rapid rise to the set value, which is maintained constantly during inspiration. Flow rapidly rises to a peak, which progressively descends to 30% of peak flow and ends. Set volume is 0.5 L (500 mL), but delivered volume is 0.75 L (750 mL). Is the patient actively breathing? How do you know?

Bird 8400STi

1. The Bird 8400STi uses which of the following flow control valves?
   a. Variable-orifice solenoid
   b. Low resistance piston
   c. Electromechanical stepper valve
   d. Venturi injector

2. The PRES. CTRL key is used to set the:
   a. high-pressure limit
   b. pressure-support level
   c. pressure-control mode
   d. low-pressure alarm

3. Pressure reaches 30 cm H_2O, ending inspiration and causing an audio and visual alarm. This alarm is most likely the:
   a. high-pressure limit alarm
   b. low peak pressure alarm
   c. high PEEP/CPAP alarm
   d. VENT. INOP. alarm

4. A respiratory therapist is switching a patient from pressure-control ventilation to volume ventilation (A/C mode). Inspiratory pressure is set at 10 cm H_2O and PEEP is at 5 cm H_2O for a total PIP of 15 cm H_2O. Whenever the therapist presses the pressure-control pad to switch to volume ventilation, the unit will not do so. The most likely problem is:
   a. the mode must be SIMV
   b. the pressure-control setting must be reduced to 5 cm H_2O
   c. the ventilator cannot perform volume ventilation
   d. an alarm is active

5. "F 2" is shown in the sensitivity control display window. This indicates that the sensitivity is:
   a. set for flow trigger at 2 L/min below base flow
   b. set for pressure trigger at –2 cm H_2O, but is in fault (F)
   c. favorable (F) for the patient based on patient size
   d. set outside of available range

6. In which of the following conditions will the ventilator give a vent inop. alarm?
   I. Loss of electrical power
   II. Detection of an internal system problem
   III. Improper installation of the expiratory valve
   IV. Prolonged occurrence (>1 sec) of excessive high pressure (>24 psig)
   a. I only
   b. II and IV only
   c. I and III only
   d. I, II, and IV only

7. Following an interval of back-up ventilation, the 8400STi will resume normal ventilation when which of the following events occurs?
   I. Two consecutive spontaneous breaths occur with a $V_T \geq$ the set V_T for each breath during volume ventilation
   II. Two consecutive spontaneous breaths occur during pressure-targeted ventilation
   III. The operator presses the reset button and activates the control setting for breath rate
   IV. The alarm silence button is pressed
   a. IV only
   b. I and II only
   c. II and IV only
   d. I, II, and III only

8. True or False? On the Bird 8400STi, the control knob for V_T is also the control knob to set inspiratory pressure for pressure-targeted breaths.

9. True or False? All Bird 8400STi units can provide pressure-control ventilation.

10. The unit is operating in the VAPS mode and the pressure-time curve on the graphics display shows a slight dip in the curve just before inspiration begins, then a rapid rise in pressure during inspiration where it reaches and sustains a plateau. The pressure drops rapidly to baseline during exhalation. How would you describe the patient's breathing pattern? Is the breath volume- or flow-cycled?

Bird T-Bird AVS

1. The internal mechanism that establishes breath delivery to the patient on the T-Bird is called a(n):
   a. drag turbine
   b. air compressor
   c. rotary drive piston
   d. stepper motor

2. Flow waveforms available for volume ventilation on the T-Bird include which of the following?
   I. Descending ramp
   II. Ascending ramp
   III. Constant
   IV. Sine waveform

a. I and III only
b. II and IV only
c. I, III, and IV only
d. I, II, III, and IV

3. During patient transport, a respiratory therapist hears an alarm coming from the T-Bird ventilator. The external battery indicator is yellow, and the message window reads "EXT. BATTERY." Which action should be taken?
a. The alarm should be silenced, and no other action taken.
b. The ventilator should be immediately plugged into a grounded AC electrical outlet.
c. The ventilator should be manually switched from the external battery to the internal battery source.
d. The patient should be disconnected from the ventilator, and manual ventilation begun.

4. A respiratory therapist is trying to measure plateau pressure and have the T-Bird calculate a patient's static compliance, but after repeated attempts using the inspiratory hold control, the therapist cannot get a plateau pressure reading to appear in the message window. Which of the following are possible causes of this problem?
I. The patient is trying to breathe actively during the maneuver.
II. The therapist is holding down the inspiratory hold touch pad for too long.
III. Inflation hold is not the correct control to use.
IV. The internal computer is detecting a problem.
a. I only
b. I and III only
c. II and IV only
d. III and IV only

5. Which of the following is a reliable information source for reviewing the UVT for the T-Bird?
a. Operator's manual
b. Head nurse
c. Respiratory care clinical specialist
d. Pulmonologist

6. Which of the following modes are available on the T-Bird AVS III?
I. SIMV
II. PCV
III. PSV
IV. VAPS
a. I only
b. II and III only
c. I, II, III only
d. I, II, III, and IV

7. True or False? The T-Bird requires two high-pressure gas sources (air and oxygen) as part of its power source.

8. True or False? The exhalation valve is mounted within the unit and can be located in the lower central portion of the front.

9. True or False? Setting the value of a parameter requires the use of both the parameter's touch pad and the central control knob on the T-Bird.

10. Comparing pressure augment on the Bear 1000 with VAPS on the T-Bird, what is the difference in the cycling mechanism when the set V_T is met during inspiration without having to sustain flow?

Dräger Evita

1. Which of the following variables are functional during CMV ventilation on the Dräger Evita?
I. V_T
II. PRESS. CONTROL (PRESS. LIMIT)
III. f(SIMV) rate
IV. pressure-support rise time
a. I and II only
b. II and IV only
c. III and IV only
d. I, II, and III only

2. What mode touch pad is pressed to activate the PCV mode with the Evita?
a. PCV
b. CMV
c. Spont.
d. MMV

3. During PCV, the pressure set on the PRESS. CONTROL knob equilibrates with pressure in the lungs when which of the following conditions occurs?
a. The patient actively inspires and increases flow delivery above the set flow value.
b. The pressure limit is set below the current plateau pressure.
c. The flow-time curve shows flow returning to zero before the end of inspiration.
d. The flow is set at 60 L/min, and the I:E ratio is 1:3.

4. During PSV with the Evita, the low $\dot{V}_E$ alarm activates. The respiratory therapist notes that T_I is 4 seconds long on the pressure-time curve. The most likely cause of the problem is which of the following?
a. Patient's respiratory rate has dropped
b. Patient's lung compliance is reduced
c. Leak in the circuit
d. Trigger sensitivity is not sensitive to patient effort

5. Which of the following parameters can be used to assess a patient's neuromuscular drive?
a. Intrinsic PEEP
b. Plateau pressure
c. Occlusion pressure
d. Sensitivity setting

6. Which of the following procedures is used to begin the set-up of APRV ventilation in the Evita?

a. Press the APRV mode key until the LED remains lit.
b. Set the pressure limit at Pplateau 3 cm H_2O during CMV ventilation.
c. Activate the MMV mode touch pad and set the SIMV rate knob to the desired rate.
d. Select the F5 MENU SELECT function key and proceed with other function keys, depending on the menu provided.

7. Which of the following statements is (are) true about the measurement of occlusion pressure with the Evita?
   I. The procedure is first begun by selecting F5 to obtain a menu screen.
   II. The procedure is automatically performed after all the steps in its selection have been completed.
   III. The INSPIRATORY and EXPIRATORY HOLD touch pads are pressed when the message "measure P 0.1" appears at the top of the main screen.
   IV. The ventilator performs this measurement 0.1 seconds after inspiratory flow has started.
   a. I only
   b. IV only
   c. II and III only
   d. I, II, and IV only

8. True or False? Most of the controls on the Evita are rotary knobs and touch pads.

9. True or False? A patient can breathe spontaneously at any time during APRV.

10. Describe APRV ventilation.

Dräger E-4

1. Proportional pressure support (PPS) is similar to which one of the following modes of ventilation described in Chapter 11?
   a. Airway pressure-release ventilation
   b. Pressure-regulated volume control ventilation
   c. Pressure-support ventilation
   d. Proportional assist ventilation

2. AutoFlow on the E-4 is similar to which mode on the Servo 300?
   a. PRVC
   b. Pressure augment
   c. APRV
   d. VAPS

3. When the patient actively inspires during proportional pressure support, the E-4:
   a. increases its support
   b. maintains a constant pressure
   c. slows flow delivery
   d. allows the patient to breathe spontaneously from a steady baseline pressure

4. Which of the following are accurate descriptions of the function of AutoFlow?
   I. AutoFlow allows spontaneous inspiratory flows up to 180 L/min.
   II. AutoFlow regulates inspiratory pressure delivery to achieve the set V_T.
   III. AutoFlow fixes flow delivery at the set flow value.
   IV. It allows the patient to cough without significant build-up of pressure in the circuit.
   a. I only
   b. II only
   c. II and III only
   d. I, II, and IV only

5. True or False? During PCV ventilation with the E-4, the patient can breathe spontaneously at any time during a mandatory breath, even during the expiratory portion of the breath.

6. True or False? The Pmax pressure limit function of the E-4 is an upper airway pressure alarm.

7. True or False? The function of Neoflow on the E-4 is to provide flow triggering.

8. Describe the controls on the front panel of the Dräger E-4 ventilator.

9. Explain how to change the numerical value for a parameter, such as V_T, with the E-4.

10. An audible 5-tone alarm is heard, and a red area is present at the top right corner of the E-4 computer screen. Inside the red area is a message that reads "High frequency!!!" What priority level is this alarm, and what does it indicate?

Dräger Evita 2 Dura

1. Which of the following components are present on both the Evita 2 Dura and the E-4?
   I. A single-dial knob control
   II. A screen for viewing waveforms (graphics)
   III. Touch pads for selecting variables and alarms
   IV. Mode-selection touch pads
   a. I and III only
   b. II and IV only
   c. I, II, and III only
   d. I, II, III, and IV

2. The function of the control or dial knob is to:
   I. Change the numerical value of a selected parameter
   II. Activate new parameters
   III. Move the cursor (vertical line) on the screen
   IV. Turn the unit on and off
   a. I only
   b. II and IV only
   c. I, II, and III only
   d. II, III, and IV only

3. During patient ventilation, PIP is 20 cm H_2O and baseline pressure is 5 cm H_2O. What is the low airway pressure alarm value?
   a. 5 cm H_2O
   b. 10 cm H_2O
   c. 15 cm H_2O
   d. Cannot be determined from the information given

4. The nebulizer function during pediatric ventilation is only operational during:
   a. volume-targeted ventilation (Autoflow inactive)
   b. Neoflow function
   c. pressure-targeted modes of ventilation
   d. independent lung ventilation

5. An audible tone occurs and 3 exclamation points ("!!!") appear in the upper right corner of the Dura. Which of the following statements is true?
   I. This is a low priority alarm.
   II. A message will appear on the screen describing the alarm condition.
   III. This is a warning message (high-priority) that must be acknowledged by the operator.
   IV. This alarm will automatically reset once the problem has been corrected.
   a. I and II only
   b. II and III only
   c. III and IV only
   d. II, III, and IV

6. True or False? The exp. hold touch pad can prolong the expiratory phase up to 15 seconds.

7. True or False? As in the E-4 ventilator, the Evita 2 Dura requires you to select neonatal, pediatric, or adult patient before selecting additional parameters.

8. True or False? The LED on the V_T touch pad flashes, indicating that the value can be changed.

9. Describe what occurs during an alarm situation on the Evita 2 Dura.

10. Explain the function of the Pmax setting on the Evita 2 Dura compared with that on the E-4.

Hamilton VEOLAR^{FT}

1. The peak inspiratory flow is 60 L/min during delivery of a breath using a constant flow waveform. If the flow waveform is changed to a 50% descending ramp, what will be the peak flow?
   a. 60 L/min
   b. 80 L/min
   c. 90 L/min
   d. Cannot be determined from the information given

2. Which of the following controls has two functions (dual knobs)?
   I. Rate (breaths/min)
   II. Tidal volume
   III. Flow pattern
   IV. Minute ventilation alarm
   a. I only
   b. I and IV only
   c. II and III only
   d. III and IV only

3. During the initial setting of an SIMV rate of 5 breaths/min, appropriate CMV rate and % CYCLE TIME settings include:
   a. CMV = 15 breaths/min; % Cycle Time = 33%
   b. CMV = 10 breaths/min; % Cycle Time = 50%
   c. CMV = 8 breaths/min; % Cycle Time = 25%
   d. CMV = 5 breaths/min; % Cycle Time = 33%

4. A patient is being assisted with the spontaneous mode on the VEOLAR^{FT} with 5 cm H_2O of CPAP and PSV of 10 cm H_2O when the low internal pressure alarm activates. What is the most likely cause of this alarm?
   a. An endotracheal tube cuff leak
   b. An inappropriately set alarm limit
   c. A loss of high-pressure gas source
   d. A patient disconnection

5. When using the MMV or PCV modes of ventilation on the VEOLAR^{FT}, the operator must use which of the following?
   I. The message window in the alarm section
   II. The YES or NO touch pads
   III. The up and down arrows
   IV. The PCV inspiratory pressure knob
   a. I and II only
   b. II and IV only
   c. I, II, and III only
   d. I, II, III, and IV

6. True or False? The AMADEUS^{FT} flow sensor monitors flow and volume at the airway while the VEOLAR^{FT} monitors flow, volume, and pressure.

7. True or False? The function of the flush control on the VEOLAR^{FT} is to provide 100% oxygen to the patient circuit.

8. True or False? Using the nebulizer control affects the F_IO_2 and the V_T on the VEOLAR^{FT}.

9. The following settings are being used on the VEOLAR^{FT} rate = 15 breaths/min, the percent inspiratory time (I%) = 25%. Calculate the percent expiratory time (E%), TCT, T_I, T_E, and I:E.

10. How do you use the HOLD control to obtain a reading of end-expiratory pressure (auto-PEEP)?

Hamilton GALILEO

1. To select and set a specific ventilator control on the GALILEO, which of the following should be performed?
   I. Scroll through screen options or ventilator parameters using knob C.
   II. Select a highlighted option (parameter) by pressing knob C.
   III. After an icon is red, rotate knob C to change the numerical value.
   IV. Press knob C to select the newly set value.
   a. III only
   b. I and IV only
   c. II and III only
   d. I, II, III, and IV

2. Which of the following options can be configured as a cycling mechanism in volume ventilation?
   I. T_I
   II. Peak flow
   III. TCT
   IV. I:E
   a. I and IV only
   b. II and III only
   c. I, II, and IV only
   d. II, III, and IV only

3. A patient, who is not currently triggering breaths, is being ventilated with ASV on the GALILEO. Which of the following best describes the breath delivery in this situation?
   a. Time-triggered, pressure-targeted breaths that are volume guaranteed
   b. Flow- or pressure-triggered PS breaths that are volume guaranteed
   c. Pressure-triggered, volume-targeted breaths with a constant flow delivery
   d. Time-triggered, volume-targeted breaths with a constant flow delivery

4. Expiratory trigger sensitivity functions by which of the following?
   a. Flow-triggering inspiration
   b. Pressure-triggering the expiratory phase
   c. Flow-cycling PS breaths at a specified flow
   d. Limiting the maximum airway pressure during expiration

5. True or False? In PCV, the set pressure for breath delivery is also the maximum pressure that can be reached in the circuit.

6. True or False? After all desired parameters are set for a specific mode, you must select the CONFIRM icon to confirm and activate the new mode.

7. Explain how a ventilator parameter such as V_T is adjusted on the Hamilton GALILEO.

8. When the viewing screen is in the alarms menu, how do you determine the actual (current) value for airway pressure?

9. If the patient's IBW is entered as 50 kg and the $\dot{V}_E$ support is set at 100%, what will be the $\dot{V}_E$ delivery in an adult?

10. Compare the setting of PSV and PEEP levels during spontaneous ventilation on the VEOLAR^{FT} with that on the GALILEO.

Puritan Bennett 740

1. During ventilation of a patient with the 740, the message window reads "O_2% Low" and "Low O_2 Supply." The red alarm indicator is flashing, and an audible pattern of three beeps, then two beeps repeats. Which of the following statements about this situation is (are) true?
   I. The oxygen % setting is more than 21%.
   II. The oxygen sensor is malfunctioning.
   III. The measured O_2% is at least 10% less than the set O_2% for 30 seconds or more.
   IV. The high-pressure oxygen gas source is not providing adequate pressure.
   V. This is a medium-priority alarm message.
   a. I only
   b. III and V only
   c. II and IV only
   d. I, III, and IV only

2. After a POST, the 740 ventilator gives the message "PM due 24," indicating which of the following?
   a. It is midnight.
   b. A maintenance check is due in 24 hours.
   c. The patient's next treatment is in 24 minutes.
   d. The patient has been on the ventilator for 24 hours.

3. An SST should be run under which of the following conditions?
   I. Every 15 days
   II. When a new patient is to be started
   III. When the patient circuit is changed
   IV. After any alarm situation
   a. II only
   b. I and III only
   c. I, II, and III only
   d. I, II, III, and IV

4. Which of the following functions would the respiratory therapist activate before suctioning a patient?
   I. Standby mode
   II. Alarm silence
   III. 100% O_2
   IV. Clear
   a. I only
   b. II only
   c. III and IV only
   d. II and III only

5. The respiratory therapist returns to a patient's bedside that is being ventilated with a 740 and notices that the alarm indicator is illuminated steadily in red. The message window reads "HIGH PRESSURE," and no alarm is sounding. Which of the following statements is true?
   a. Inspiration has ended because high pressure was reached.
   b. The inspiratory line is occluded.
   c. An autoreset of the high-pressure alarm has occurred.
   d. The patient needs suctioning.

6. The modes of ventilation on the 740 include which of the following?
   I. PSV
   II. A/C volume ventilation
   III. PCV
   IV. SIMV volume ventilation
      a. II and III only
      b. III and IV only
      c. I, II, and IV only
      d. I, II, III, and IV

7. True or False? When the 740 is not in use, it should be kept plugged in and turned off.

8. True or False? Apnea ventilation works in all modes on the 740.

9. True or False? Flow triggering of all breath types is available on the 740.

10. A 20-second interval of apnea has occurred with a patient receiving three mandatory breaths/min in the SIMV mode on the 740. Will the apnea ventilation mode begin? If not, why not?

11. Which of the following power sources are required for the 740 to deliver a breath?
   I. AC electrical outlet
   II. High-pressure oxygen outlet
   III. High-pressure air outlet
   IV. Internal battery power
      a. I only
      b. I and II only
      c. II, III, and IV only
      d. I, II, III, and IV

12. After completing the mode set-up on a patient who is being switched from A/C to SIMV, the respiratory therapist notices the rate key flashing and the digital display is 10 breaths/min. Pressing "accept" does not initiate the settings she has selected and begin SIMV. The most likely cause of the problem is:
   a. The rate is set too low for the SIMV mode
   b. She should have pressed the "accept" key after each parameter setting change
   c. She must adjust all parameters in that mode before pressing "accept"
   d. SIMV is not an available mode on the 740 ventilator

Puritan Bennett 760

1. Which of the following controls adjusts the flow percent at which a pressure support breath ends on the 760 ventilator?
   a. Expiratory pause
   b. Exhalation sensitivity
   c. Rise Time Factor
   d. Inspiratory pause

2. Which of the following features is NOT available on the 740, but is on the 760?
   a. Pressure support
   b. Trigger sensitivity
   c. Volume bar graph
   d. I:E ratio display

3. What is the easiest way to determine the presence of auto-PEEP in a patient on the 760?
   a. Observe the end expiratory pressure
   b. Set the exhalation sensitivity to 100
   c. Check the flow/time curve on the graphic display
   d. Check the end expiratory flow in the message window

4. To set the T_I as the constant when PCV is activated, you must:
   a. set it on the control panel using the T_I/I:E control
   b. go to the user settings in the menu and select T_I/I:E
   c. keep the rate the same at all times
   d. use another ventilator because the 760 will not allow T_I as a constant

5. Setting the Rise Time Factor to 100 during PCV gives you:
   a. the most rapid rise to the set pressure
   b. a flow-cycle of 100% of peak flow measured
   c. an inspiratory pause that is 0.01 seconds long
   d. the slowest rise to the set pressure

Puritan Bennett 840

1. The function of the expiratory filter includes which of the following?
   I. Protect the ventilator from contamination with the patient's secretions.
   II. Filter exhaled air to protect clinicians from contamination.
   III. Protect the patient from potential contamination from the ventilator.
   IV. Measure expiratory gas flows for calculating flows and volumes.
      a. II only
      b. I and IV only
      c. I, II, and III only
      d. II, III, and IV only

2. The back-up power source will do which of the following, when electrical AC power is lost or drops below a minimum level?
   I. Illuminate the battery indicator in the status indicators area of the screen
   II. Provide power for about 30 minutes
   III. Not power the compressor
   IV. Not power the humidifier
   a. I only
   b. II and III only
   c. I and IV only
   d. I, II, III, and IV

3. Which of the following must the respiratory therapist perform to begin an SST?
   a. Disconnect the patient from the ventilator
   b. Turn the ventilator "on" from its off position
   c. Press the SST on the touch screen or the test button on the side of the ventilator
   d. All of the above

4. During PSV the E_{SENS} in the 840 is set at 20%. The respiratory therapist notices that inspiratory time is prolonged and appears to time-cycle rather than flow-cycle. What might be the problem?
   a. There may be a leak in the system and the inspiratory flow never drops to the 20% value.
   b. The patient is actively exhaling against the gas flow.
   c. The patient is making no spontaneous inspiratory effort to begin the next breath.
   d. The E_{SENS} may be set too high for the patient.

5. True or False? The main ventilator settings are always visible, even when the Apnea screen appears.

6. The upper screen of the GUI contains which of the following?
   a. Patient data
   b. Miscellaneous data
   c. Alarm status
   d. All of the above

7. An indicator, located in the 840's Status Indicator Panel, is blinking rapidly, suggesting a hazardous situation. Which indicator is being described?
   a. Low-priority alarm
   b. Medium-priority alarm
   c. High-priority alarm
   d. Battery low alarm

8. Which of the following tests is NOT available with the SST?
   a. Leak test
   b. Tubing compliance test
   c. Oxygen sensor calibration
   d. Expiratory filter resistance

9. The on/off power switch for the 840 is located on the:
   a. BDU
   b. GUI
   c. BPS
   d. Compressor

10. The freeze control on the ventilator graphic screen will allow freezing the last ______ seconds of data.
   a. 30
   b. 48
   c. 60
   d. 90

11. The control which adjusts the time scale on the graphics screen is the:
   a. horizontal control
   b. vertical control

12. True or False? A leak can cause an error in the respiratory mechanics measurements.

13. True or False? Rise time percentage allows you to adjust the inspiratory rise or slope in PC and PSV.

14. True or False? The mode that provides APRV is called BiLevel on the 840.

15. The speed by which inspiratory pressure rises to the set pressure value is determined by all EXCEPT which of the following?
   a. Percent setting on rise time percentage
   b. An active patient inspiration
   c. Compliance and resistance of the patient's lungs
   d. An active patient exhalation

Puritan Bennett 7200

1. A respiratory therapist accidentally unplugs the 7200 ventilator being used for a patient in the ICU. Besides activating alarms, the ventilator will:
   a. continue to ventilate the patient using the current settings and be powered by the internal battery
   b. stop functioning
   c. continue to ventilate the patient using the default ventilator settings in memory
   d. continue to ventilate the patient using disconnect parameters

2. A respiratory therapist changes the respiratory rate from 10 to 15 breaths during volume ventilation with the 7200. An error message appears in the display window: "DECR RESP RATE FIRST." How can the therapist maintain the new $\dot{V}_E$ and correct the error message?
   a. Increase the peak flow setting
   b. Decrease the set V_T
   c. Add a plateau time
   d. Change to pressure-control ventilation

3. A patient is switched from CMV to SIMV with a rate of 4 breaths/min. After about 30 seconds, an alarm sounds and apnea ventilation begins. Which of the following is (are) true?
   I. The patient did not trigger a mandatory breath.
   II. The apnea period is probably set at 30 seconds.

III. Switching from CMV to SIMV resulted in a delay in mandatory breath delivery.
IV. The respiratory therapist should have given a mandatory breath after the switch to avoid the alarm condition.
a. I only
b. II only
c. III and IV only
d. I, II, III, and IV

4. A respiratory therapist has set a peak flow of 80 L/min and selected the descending flow waveform. At the beginning inspiration, what will be the actual flow delivered to the patient?
a. 160 L/min
b. 120 L/min
c. 100 L/min
d. 80 L/min

5. When changing from a constant (rectangular) to a descending ramp waveform on the 7200, what happens to the T_I?
a. increases
b. decreases
c. stays the same

6. A patient is being ventilated with SIMV at a rate of 3 breaths/min. Set V_T is 0.75 L (750 mL), spontaneous V_T is 0.35 L (350 mL), and spontaneous rate is 10 breaths/min. Low V_T is set at 0.65 L (650 mL), and apnea time is 20 seconds. Based on this information, which alarm is likely to activate?
a. Apnea alarm
b. Low V_T alarm
c. Low-pressure alarm
d. Low rate alarm

7. A respiratory therapist wants to perform weaning measurements using the 7200 ventilator. Which of the following are available under the respiratory mechanics option (Options 30 and 40)?
I. Slow vital capacity
II. Maximum inspiratory pressure
III. Static compliance
IV. Rapid shallow breathing index
a. I and II only
b. II and III only
c. I, II, and III only
d. II, III, and IV only

8. The 7200 microprocessor detects inconsistencies in airway pressure, PEEP measurements, and the gas delivery in the pneumatic system. Which of the following will occur?
a. Apnea ventilation begins
b. Back-up ventilation begins
c. Disconnect ventilation begins
d. Alarms activate, but regular ventilation continues

9. During PCV, the following parameters are set: pressure = 20 cm H_2O; T_I = constant at 1.0 second; rate = 10 breaths/min; mode = CMV; and PEEP/CPAP = 0 cm H_2O. What will be the I:E ratio if the rate is decreased to 6 breaths/min and the patient does not trigger additional breaths?
a. 1:5
b. 1:6
c. 1:9
d. Cannot be determined from the information given

10. With the 7200, what flow-trigger and base flow would the therapist set for a 34 kg patient?

Newport Breeze E150

1. A respiratory therapist has initiated ventilation on a patient using the A/C mode on the Breeze E150. The patient appears to be struggling to get a breath. The therapist notes that the pressure gauge is indicating pressures of −10 cm H_2O and the effort indicator does not illuminate before mandatory breath delivery. What could be causing this condition?
a. Spontaneous flow is set too low.
b. The ventilator is in the control mode.
c. Trigger sensitivity is not set correctly.
d. Inspiratory flow is set too low.

2. The therapist is delivering aerosolized medications to a ventilated patient using the nebulizer control. Although the volume is set at 0.5 L (500 mL), she notes that the V_T display reads 0.53 L (530 mL). What is the most likely cause of this difference?
a. Use of the nebulizer function
b. A leak in the patient circuit
c. An error in the inspiratory flow transducer
d. An increase in the patient's spontaneous rate

3. The respiratory therapist has initiated volume ventilation on a patient using the E150 and notes that the pressure only rises to 10 cm H_2O. It then plateaus at this value for the length of inspiratory delivery. V_T is set at 0.8 L (800 mL). No alarm is sounding. What is the most likely cause of this problem?
a. The high pressure limit alarm is being reached and the alarm is silenced.
b. The ventilator is set for pressure-targeted—not volume-targeted—ventilation.
c. The pressure-relief valve is set at 10 cm H_2O and is limiting inspiratory pressure.
d. There is a large leak in the inspiratory line.

4. A patient is being supported in the spontaneous mode with 10 cm H_2O of CPAP at an F_IO_2 of 0.5. A low press alarm activates. The pressure gauge reads 3 cm H_2O. The low-pressure alarm is set at 5 cm H_2O. Which of the following is true about this situation?
I. Circuit pressure has been lower than the low CPAP pressure alarm setting for 4 seconds.
II. The apnea alarm is not available because a low CPAP alarm has been set.

III. There is a small leak in the circuit or around the patient airway.
IV. The gas sources have failed.
a. I and III only
b. I and IV only
c. II and IV only
d. I, II, and III only.

5. Which of the following modes of ventilation are available on the Breeze E150?
I. A/C volume-targeted
II. Pressure-control ventilation
III. Pressure-support ventilation
IV. Spontaneous
V. Mandatory minute ventilation
a. I and V only
b. II and III only
c. I, II, and IV only
d. I, II, IV, and V only

6. A plateau pressure during volume ventilation is achieved using what feature on the E150?
a. Inspiratory plateau time
b. Pressure-relief valve
c. PIP setting
d. High-pressure alarm limit

7. A high-pitched continuous reed alarm sounds during patient ventilation. This indicates which of the following?
a. The internal battery is charged and being used as a power source.
b. One of the high-pressure gas sources has lost pressure.
c. The measured F_IO_2 has exceeded the set F_IO_2 by 5% for 30 seconds.
d. The pressure-relief valve has been activated.

8. True or False? Use of the nebulizer feature on the E150 increases volume delivery during volume ventilation.

9. True or False? V_T delivery during volume ventilation is based on the V_T control setting.

10. A respiratory therapist observes a patient's chest wall movement and notes inspiratory efforts. However, the effort indicator does not illuminate. As a result, mandatory breaths are all time-triggered. How can the therapist change the ventilator settings to achieve better sensing of patient effort?

Newport Wave E200

1. The Wave E200 uses which internal flow delivery device?
a. An electromagnetic poppet valve
b. A stepper motor with a scissors valve
c. A linear drive piston
d. An internal bellows device

2. During volume ventilation of a patient with the E200, the airway pressure reaches the pressure limit set on the pressure-relief valve before it reaches the HIGH PRESSURE alarm. Which of the following statements about this situation is (are) true?
I. The operator should have set the pressure-relief valve higher than the high pressure alarm.
II. An audible alarm will sound and the high pressure alarm LED will illuminate.
III. Pressure will plateau, but inspiration will not end.
IV. Volume delivery will remain the same.
a. I and III only
b. II and IV only
c. I, III and IV only
d. I, II, III, and IV

3. During PCV using the E200, the respiratory therapist wants to give a nebulized medication treatment to a patient. What should she do?
a. Select an external flowmeter to power the nebulizer and (while it is on) set the pressure relief valve 1 cm H_2O above set pressure.
b. Until the treatment is finished, switch to a volume-targeted mode and use the pressure-relief valve to limit pressure.
c. Connect the nebulizer line to the device and press the nebulizer button on the lower panel of the ventilator.
d. Change the patient to another ventilator.

4. When the use of sigh is selected, which of the following is (are) true?
I. A sigh breath is delivered every 100 breaths.
II. This can only be used in volume-targeted A/C.
III. Sigh V_T is 1.5 times V_T set.
IV. Sigh T_I is 1.5 times T_I set.
a. I only
b. II only
c. III and IV only
d. I, III, and IV only

5. The operator sets the Wave E200 up for volume-targeted A/C ventilation. However, it is noted that the pressure only rises to 10 cm H_2O, and the desired volume is not achieved. No alarms are active. What could be the problem?
I. The pressure control knob is not in the off position.
II. There is water in the circuit.
III. The pressure is being released through the pressure-relief valve.
IV. The bias flow is set too low.
a. I only
b. III only
c. I and III only
d. II and IV only

6. The respiratory therapist wishes to use inverse ratio PCV on a patient being ventilated with the Wave. Rate is set at 12 breaths/min, and T_I is 2 seconds. T_I is increased to 3 seconds, and an audible alarm sounds. The IT TOO LONG LED illuminates. How can this problem be solved?

a. Reduce the flow instead of increasing T_I.
b. Change the setting of the I:E ratio switch on the back panel.
c. Increase the pressure setting for PCV.
d. Increase the bias flow to 10 L/min.

7. True or False? Either pressure- or volume-targeted SIMV can be set with the Wave E200.

8. True or False? The Wave E200 requires both an electric and pneumatic power source to operate.

9. The operator notices the set V_T in the upper panel reads 0.7 L (700 mL), and the inspired V_T in the monitor section reads 0.63 L (630 mL). What is a possible cause of this discrepancy?

10. To calculate a patient's lung compliance, the plateau is set at 20% on the back panel of the Wave. The peak pressure suddenly changes from 28 to 30 cm H_2O. What causes this change?

Pulmonetics LTV Series

1. Of the four ventilators available in the LTV series, which does not include flow-cycling?
a. LTV 1000
b. LTV 950
c. LTV 800
d. All include flow cycling

2. When the LTV ventilator is connected to a low pressure oxygen source, an example source might be:
a. an oxygen concentrator
b. an O_2 flowmeter attached to a wall oxygen outlet
c. an oxygen cylinder with a regulator and flowmeter attached
d. all of the above

3. All EXCEPT which of the following power sources can be used to power the LTV ventilator:
a. Two high pressure gas sources (40 to 70 psig)
b. External DC battery
c. Internal DC battery
d. Automobile lighter outlet with adapter

4. Which of the following statements is (are) true regarding PEEP and the LTV series?
I. When PC is used, the set pressure is added to the PEEP level selected.
II. PEEP is manually adjusted using the externally located exhalation valve.
III. The monitored PEEP value is shown in the display window along with other monitored data.
IV. The set PEEP value is the lowest pressure allowed for all modes and breath-types.
a. I and II only
b. II and IV only
c. II, III, and IV only
d. I, II, III, and IV

5. Immediately after the LTV is turned off using the power on/off control,
a. The InOP indicator illuminates
b. No audible alarm sounds
c. All indicators and displays are darkened
d. The standby mode indicator flashes

6. Which of the following features is available in the Extended Features menu?
I. Rise time
II. Flow termination
III. PC flow termination
IV. Inspiratory hold
a. III only
b. IV only
c. I and II only
d. I, II, and III only

7. Which of the following alarm conditions is set when "VC/PC Only" is selected using low peak pressure alarm in the extended features menu alarm operations?
a. All breaths in VC/PC including the SIMV settings have a low peak pressure alarm available.
b. Only mandatory breaths (pressure or volume) have the low peak pressure alarm active.
c. Only spontaneous breaths would have a LPP alarm in this setting.
d. There is no such alarm parameter available.

8. True or False? The sensitivity can be turned completely off on the LTV ventilator.

9. A Respiratory Therapist walks into the ICU room where a patient is being ventilated by the LTV 1000. All digital displays are blank. This would indicate:
a. The unit is operating on the internal battery.
b. The ventilator is not operational and the patient should be manually ventilated.
c. The visual dimmer has been turned all the way to low intensity
d. The ventilator has been turned off.

10. A Respiratory Therapist notices that a patient being ventilated with the LTV 1000 is having difficulty triggering a breath. The current sensitivity setting on the front panel is 9. The pressure manometer drops to −3 cm H_2O prior to inspiration being triggered. Which of the following statements is true regarding this situation?
a. The therapist should check for a leak in the system.
b. The 9 sensitivity setting represents cm H_2O of pressure.
c. The sensitivity should be changed to 2 or 3 and reevaluated.
d. The therapist should reduce the bias flow using the extended features menu.

11. The message LMV LPPS OFF appears in the display window. What does this indicate?

Respironics Esprit

1. The respiratory therapist assembles the Esprit for patient use and turns on the main power switch, but nothing happens. What could be the problem?
   a. It is not plugged into an AC outlet.
   b. The back-up battery is not charged.
   c. The main circuit breakers are not on.
   d. All of the above.

2. Which of the following statements about the high inspiratory pressure alarm is (are) true?
   I. When the pressure during inspiration reaches the high pressure alarm setting, inspiration ends.
   II. The high pressure alarm can only be adjusted using the alarm setting screen.
   III. During NPPV, the high pressure alarm is automatically set to 10 cm H_2O above IPAP.
   IV. High inspiratory pressure can be adjusted using the HIP icon next the pressure manometer on the touch-sensitive screen.
   a. I only
   b. II only
   c. II and III only
   d. I, III, and IV only

3. The 100% oxygen indicator above the screen will illuminate when:
   a. the alarm silence has been pressed
   b. 100% oxygen has been measured in the patient circuit by the O_2 sensor
   c. the 100% O_2 control button has been pressed
   d. the high-pressure oxygen source has been lost

4. During operation of the Esprit, an audible alarm sounds, the BATTERY LOW indicator is illuminated and the MAINS indicator is off. These conditions indicate:
   a. five minutes or less of battery power remains and the main AC power cord is not connected to an electrical source
   b. the external battery is low and it is being charged
   c. the unit is now on standby and the external battery is not available
   d. the unit is off and needs to be connected to a power source to recharge the battery

5. Which of the following statements about SST and EST is correct?
   a. These are self-tests used to verify system safety and correct operation.
   b. These tests can be run during ventilation of a patient.
   c. These functions are accessible through the normal ventilation screen.
   d. These are alarm conditions indicating that the safety valve is open.

6. Apnea ventilation in the Esprit:
   a. occurs when 20 seconds have passed without a breath being detected
   b. is not available on the ventilator
   c. cannot have an apnea rate set lower than the mandatory rate in A/C and SIMV
   d. has preset factory parameters for rate, volume, PEEP, flow and oxygen percent

7. Which of the following statements is true about the modes and breath types available on the Esprit?
   I. The available modes depend on the breath type selected.
   II. Breath types include VCV, PCV, and NPPV.
   III. A back-up breath rate is available in NPPV-Spont/T.
   IV. There is no PSV available for spontaneous breath support.
   a. I only
   b. II only
   c. III and IV only
   d. I, II, and III only

8. True or False? All pressure-targeted breaths, including PSV, PCV, and IPAP can have the rise time percent feature available to slope or taper the pressure delivery.

9. During NPPV–Spont/T:
   a. IPAP must be set equal to or higher than EPAP
   b. pressure support can be added to breath delivery
   c. only pressure-triggering is available
   d. all breaths must be patient-triggered

10. Expiratory trigger is best defined as:
    a. the variable that triggers inspiration
    b. the baseline pressure setting (PEEP/CPAP)
    c. the flow percentage at which inspiration ends during PSV
    d. the transition during NPPV between IPAP and EPAP

11. The actual breath rate is set at 8 breaths/min. The apnea rate is set at 6 breaths/min in the A/C mode. Which of the following is true?
    a. If apnea ventilation occurs, the rate will be 6 breaths/min.
    b. Apnea ventilation cannot occur because the rate is set at greater than 8 Breaths/min.
    c. A message will appear on the screen telling the operator the apnea rate must be $\geq$ the set rate (defaults to the set rate).
    d. Apnea ventilation is not available in the A/C mode.

12. During NPPV, the IPAP is set at 14 cm H_2O and EPAP at 4 cm H_2O. The high pressure limit is set:
    a. based on department policy
    b. 10 to 15 cm H_2O above IPAP
    c. between 4 and 14 cm H_2O
    d. automatically at 10 above IPAP

13. When setting flow trigger at 2 L/min, the bias flow will automatically be set at:
    a. 6 L/min
    b. 3 L/min above flow trigger
    c. 10 L/min
    d. twice the set flow

Siemens Servo 900C

1. Which type of internal drive mechanism is used in the Servo 900C?
   a. Linear drive piston
   b. Proportioning valve
   c. Spring-loaded bellows
   d. Rotary drive piston

2. To estimate the auto-PEEP level with the Servo 900C, which control is used?
   a. T_I%
   b. Pause time %
   c. Expiratory pause hold
   d. Gas change

3. The inspiratory servo valve consists of which components?
   I. A scissor-like valve controlled by a stepper motor
   II. A bacterial filter
   III. An inspiratory flow transducer
   IV. An electromagnetic solenoid
   a. I only
   b. I and III
   c. II and IV
   d. III and IV

4. At which level should the working pressure be set?
   a. 10 cm H_2O above PEEP
   b. 5 cm H_2O above the patient's plateau pressure
   c. 120 cm H_2O
   d. Above the peak pressure for the patient

5. During ventilation in the SIMV mode, the therapist has set the SIMV rate at 10 breaths/min, but notes that the patient is receiving 8 mandatory breaths/min. The most likely cause of this is:
   a. the patient is triggering additional mandatory breaths
   b. the SIMV-rate toggle switch is in the up position
   c. the breaths/min control set at 8 breaths/min
   d. the SIMV rate cannot go as high as 10 breaths/min

6. If the T_I% is set at 33%, the pause time is at 5%, and the rate is 10 breaths/min, what is the approximate T_I?
   a. 1.5 seconds
   b. 2.3 seconds
   c. 3.0 seconds
   d. 6.0 seconds

7. True or False? The 900C has a built-in oxygen analyzer.

8. True or False? If a patient becomes apneic during SIMV ventilation with a mandatory rate of 3 breaths/min, the apnea alarm is activated.

9. The $\dot{V}_E$ control is set at 12 L/min, the breaths/min at 12, flow is constant, and T_I% is 20% (inspiratory pause is 0%) during volume ventilation on the Servo 900C. What are the V_T, T_I, and inspiratory flow?

10. During pressure control ventilation with the Servo 900C, what control determines the inspiratory pressure, and does this value include the baseline pressure?

Siemens Servo 300

1. As air and oxygen high-pressure gases enter the Servo 300, they pass to a:
   a. large pressurized reservoir
   b. pair of servo-controlled stepper motors
   c. mixing chamber
   d. spring-loaded bellows

2. The Servo 300 can be pressure- or flow-triggered in which of the following modes of ventilation?
   I. Pressure control
   II. SIMV (vol. contr.)
   III. Pressure support
   IV. PRVC
   a. II only
   b. I and IV only
   c. II and III only
   d. I, II, III, and IV

3. A patient is switched from volume control ventilation to SIMV (VOL. CONT.). The SIMV frequency is set at 9 breaths/min, but only eight mandatory breaths are being delivered. The yellow indicator next to the CMV frequency control flashes. The most likely cause of this condition is that:
   a. the CMV rate control is set at 8 breaths/min
   b. mode change was not activated correctly
   c. the SIMV rate control is out of calibration
   d. patient has become apneic

4. Which of the following modes will guarantee volume delivery using pressure-targeted breaths and has a minimum set respiratory rate?
   a. Pressure-regulated volume control
   b. Volume support
   c. Automode
   d. SIMV (PRESS. CONTR.) + PS

5. An adult patient is being ventilated in volume support and becomes apneic. Which of the following will occur?
   I. The ventilator switches to PRVC.
   II. A light diode flashes next to the PRVC control.
   III. After 20 seconds, the apnea alarm activates.
   IV. The ventilator will begin to ventilate the patient at the set rate.
   a. I only
   b. III only
   c. II and IV only
   d. I, II, III, and IV

6. A patient is in the pressure-support mode. The rate is set at 12 breaths/min. The patient's endotracheal tube cuff becomes deflated, and a leak develops, preventing flow-cycling. In this situation, what will end inspiratory flow?

I. It will not end, but an apnea alarm will sound.
II. It will end after 4 seconds (80% of TCT).
III. It will switch to PRVC, and the apnea alarm will sound.
IV. The circuit pressure reaches the upper pressure limit.

a. II only
b. I and III only
c. II and III only
d. I, II, and IV only

7. True or False? Digital display of values is in red for measured values and in green for set values.

8. True or False? Similar to the Servo 900C, the Servo 300 uses a stepper motor for the inspiratory flow valve.

9. Explain how the Servo 300 establishes appropriate ventilating pressures during PRVC to achieve the desired volume?

10. During volume-support ventilation, the following parameters are noted: upper pressure limit setting = 35 cm H_2O, set V_T = 0.6 L, PEEP = 10 cm H_2O, CMV frequency = 10 breaths/min. The pressure required to deliver the V_T rises to 30 cm H_2O. How will the ventilator respond to this situation? How would you respond to this situation?

Dräger Savina

1. Which of the following statements about the power sources for the Savina ventilator is (are) true?

I. Two high-pressure gas sources are required to power the Savina.
II. An electrical power source is required to power the Savina.
III. Attaching the ventilator to a high pressure O_2 source allows for an adjustable F_IO_2.
IV. An internal DC battery is available to act as a back-up power supply.

a. I and II only
b. II and IV only
c. I, II, and IV only
d. II, III, and IV only

2. To set the sensitivity (trigger) on the Savina, the operator must access which of the following screens?
a. Settings
b. Configuration
c. Alarm limits
d. Waveforms (Main)

3. After selecting the "O_2 ↑suction" the respiratory therapist disconnects the patient for suctioning and then reconnects the patient. Following reconnection the ventilator will:
a. reset the F_IO_2 back to the original setting.
b. resume ventilation and provide 120 seconds of 100% O_2 to the patient.
c. give a low priority alarm to signify reconnection.
d. wait until Alarm Reset is pressed before beginning ventilation.

4. AutoFlow can be described as:
a. a method for providing flow to the patient on demand
b. pressure-targeted ventilation with a volume guarantee
c. a feature available for volume-targeted modes on the Savina
d. all of the above

5. The feature used to slope the beginning of the pressure curve by adjusting the rate of pressure and flow delivery is called:
a. inspiratory rise time percentage
b. sloping
c. ramping of inspiration
d. flow acceleration

6. When the sigh feature is activated on the Savina, the ventilator delivers a sigh breath equal to:
a. 1½ times the V_T setting every 100th breath
b. airway pressure that is set above the PEEP baseline pressure for two breaths every 3 minutes
c. the set sigh volume at the set sigh rate and frequency
d. a pressure breath with a peak inspiratory pressure 1½ times the normal Pinsp

7. Which of the following statements about CMV A/C is (are) true?

I. Breaths can be delivered as volume breaths with a maximum pressure depending on the features selected.
II. Volume-targeted breaths can be volume- or time-cycled.
III. Sensitivity can be turned "off" making the mode CMV (control ventilation).
IV. Patient-triggered breaths are flow-triggered.

a. I only
b. III only
c. II and IV only
d. I, II, III, and IV

Servo^i

1. The battery package in the Servo^i being used with a 68-year-old patient contains three fully charged batteries. The respiratory therapist must transport the patient still connected to the ventilator from the intensive care unit to the radiology department, which will take 20 to 30 minutes. How long will the available batteries last?
a. 30 minutes
b. 90 minutes
c. 3 hours
d. 6 hours

2. The on/off control for the Automode on the Servo[i] is located:
   a. in the top row of pads (top tool bar) on the main screen
   b. as a fixed key on the right side of the front panel
   c. under the list of available modes
   d. in mode screens where Automode is available

3. A patient in the radiology department is being ventilated with the Servo[i] and requires a stat aerosol treatment with bronchodilators. The respiratory therapist connects Servo[i] Ultra Nebulizer in-line with the patient circuit, but is unable to activate the nebulizer function. A possible cause of this is:
   a. there is no medicine in the cup of the nebulizer
   b. the patient circuit has a leak in it
   c. the ventilator is operating from battery power
   d. the Servo[i] does not have a built-in nebulizer function

4. A quick method for increasing the F_IO_2 delivery to a patient being ventilated using the Servo[i] is to use the:
   a. direct access knob adjacent to the F_IO_2 screen parameter
   b. main rotary dial to proceed through the necessary steps
   c. touch screen controls
   d. main menu

5. A respiratory therapist is changing the pressure limit for a patient on pressure control ventilation. As he decreases the "PC above PEEP" control, the screen area begins to illuminate with a red color and a low expiratory minute volume occurs. The most likely cause of this is:
   a. a low pressure alarm
   b. an apnea alarm
   c. the patient has triggered inspiration
   d. the therapist has set the pressure too low to maintain $\dot{V}_E$ above the alarm level

6. Which of the following controls sets the percent of peak inspiratory flow that cycles the ventilator out of inspiration?
   a. inspiratory rise time
   b. breath cycle time
   c. inspiratory cycle off
   d. trigger time-out

7. A patient being ventilated with the volume control mode is actively breathing and frequently inspires deeply during the inspiratory phase of the breath. This will result in:
   a. a concave dip in the inspiratory pressure curve to below baseline pressure
   b. no change in the constant (square) inspiratory flow waveform
   c. triggering of another breath
   d. an increase in flow and volume delivery

Viasys Avea

1. A 2-day-old infant is being ventilated with the AVEA at 35% oxygen. The respiratory therapist presses the INCREASE O_2 button before suctioning. The resulting oxygen delivery will be:
   a. 100% for 2 minutes
   b. 35% for 2 minutes
   c. 55% for 2 minutes
   d. 100% for 1 minute

2. The easiest way to determine if the ventilator is connected to an AC power source is to:
   a. check the on/off switch on the back panel
   b. check the Power On indicator for a green light
   c. see if the touch screen is on
   d. see if the AC Power indicator is illuminated green.

3. When "New Patient" status is accepted after the AVEA is turned on:
   a. the ventilator resets all settings to the default values
   b. the ventilator begins working at the most recently stored values
   c. you are required to enter all new parameters
   d. parameters are present based on the patient's body surface area

4. When volume-targeted breaths are activated, triggering is based on which of the following?
   a. time
   b. flow
   c. pressure
   d. all of the above

5. To set a descending flow waveform in volume A/C and volume SIMV:
   a. go to the Advanced Settings window and press peak flow control
   b. go to the Mode selection screen and pick waveform
   c. touch the waveform icon on the lower portion of the touch screen whenever volume-targeted ventilation is active
   d. do nothing, because the Avea only has a descending flow waveform

6. When the tidal volume is set at 500 mL and the Sigh control is enabled, which of the following statements is (are) true?
   I. A Sigh volume of 750 mL will be delivered
   II. The operator must also select sigh frequency
   III. A sigh breath occurs every 100 breaths
   IV. The sigh tidal volume is set at twice the tidal volume setting
   a. I only
   b. IV only
   c. I and III only
   d. II and IV only

7. Pressing the "Main" icon in the Screens selection window:

a. checks the main circuit breaker
b. displays the main screen
c. lists the main ventilator parameters
d. displays the main alarm limits

8. An alarm occurs accompanied by three audible tones and a yellow flashing bar in the upper right area of the touch screen. This indicates:
a. a high priority alarm
b. a medium priority alarm
c. a low priority alarm
d. a change in a ventilator parameter

9. The maximum available I:E ratio for a mandatory breath is:
a. 1:1
b. 2:1
c. 3:1
d. 4:1

Newport e500

1. Which of the following statements are true when an external battery is used for powering the Newport e500 ventilator?
a. The external battery charge remaining is displayed on the charge indicator bar.
b. The external battery icon illuminates.
c. The "Charging" indicator illuminates.
d. The e500 cannot use an external battery source.

2. The function of the Manual Inflation button is to delivery breath that, when pressed
a. is up to 5 seconds or when a high P_{aw} alarm limit occurs
b. will NOT deliver a breath in spontaneous mode
c. cannot provide slow inflation
d. delivers a breath at the set ventilator parameters

3. Which of the following statements is (are) true regarding flow delivery in the e500 ventilator?
I. During a pressure breath, flow delivery depends on patient demand.
II. Two flow waveform patterns are available with volume breaths, square and descending.
III. The available flow depends on the patient size selected.
IV. During pressure breaths, flow is determined by the value set on the flow control.
a. I only
b. II and IV only
c. I, II, and III only
d. II, III, and IV only

4. When the e500 ventilator is turned on:
a. the default values for ventilator parameters become active
b. the last ventilator parameters used are available in memory for use
c. the ventilator automatically goes into a new patient setup mode
d. all display windows read "- -" and require resetting

5. To provide sloping (ramping) of a pressure breath on the e500:
a. the operator uses the % rise time feature
b. a slope control is adjusted from 1 to 9 (no slope/ maximum slope)
c. flow is adjusted by the ventilated to provide automatic sloping (rise) for every breath
d. enter the Setup screen and select inspiratory ramp

6. The F_IO_2 display in the monitored data section of the e500 displays "- -" under which of the following circumstances?
a. If the oxygen supply pressure is below minimum
b. If the ventilator is connected to air only and the F_IO_2 is set at 21%
c. If the oxygen sensor is disconnected, defective, or not calibrated since power-up
d. If oxygen sensor calibration is in progress
e. All of the above

7. The Preset Vent Settings control on the e500:
a. can only be accessed when the ventilator is powered on.
b. is normally used to adjust current breath and mode parameters.
c. should be used to set breath type and mode parameters for patient safety.
d. is the first window to appear when the ventilator is turned on.

8. During VTPC assist/control ventilation, the message window displays the message "Vol Target Not Met," and an audible alarm sounds. What is one variable the respiratory therapist could increase to meet the set V_T?
a. The set V_T
b. The P_{limit}
c. The set pressure
d. The baseline pressure

9. An Insp Time Too Short alarm occurs during ventilation of a patient. The respiratory therapist should:
a. review and readjust V_T and flow settings as needed.
b. increase the upper pressure limit.
c. check for an obstruction in the circuit.
d. evaluate the patient for hiccups.

10. A "Sustained High Baseline Pressure" message appears, an audible alarm sounds, and the Patient indicator is flashing. A possible cause of this problem might be:
a. the set PEEP/CPAP is higher than the PEEP/CPAP upper pressure limit
b. the operator has tried to set the baseline pressure higher than the available range for the patient size
c. there is a kink in the patient circuit or a possible obstruction in the exhalation valve
d. the patient is having a sustained coughing episode

References

Bear 1000

1. Bear 1000 ventilator instruction manual, pub no 50-10613-00, Palm Springs, Calif, 1995 and L-1575, and 6/2001 version A, Viasys Healthcare, Critical Care Division.
2. Pilbeam SP: *Mechanical ventilation: physiological and clinical applications*, ed 3, St Louis, 1998, Mosby.
3. Greg Oliver, personal correspondence, Palm Springs, Calif, June, 2002, Viasys Healthcare, Critical Care Division.

Bird 8400STi

1. Bird 8400STi Ventilator operation manual and options L1297, Palm Springs, Calif, 1994, Viasys HealthCare, Critical Care Division.
2. Bird 8400STi Volume ventilator instruction manual L1141R2, Palm Springs, Calif, 1994, Viasys HealthCare, Critical Care Division.
3. Bird graphics monitor instruction and service manual L1282, Palm Springs, Calif, 1995, Viasys HealthCare, Critical Care Division.
4. Pilbeam S: *Mechanical ventilation: physiological and clinical applications*, ed 3, St Louis, 1998, Mosby.

Bird T-Bird

1. T-Bird: the seamless solution, T-Bird AVS, ventilator series, operator's manual L1331, Palm Springs, Calif, 1997; and L1580 revision B, 2001, Viasys HealthCare, Critical Care Division.

Dräger Evita

1. Dräger Evita: intensive care ventilator operator's manual, 90 28 225, Telford, Penn, 1993, Dräger, Inc.
2. GF Lear, personal communication, Telford, Penn, 1998, 2002, Dräger, Inc, Drägerwerk AG.

Drager E-4

1. Evita 4: Intensive care ventilation operating instructions 90 28 676-GA 5664.510, ed 1; and version 4.n, Telford, Penn, 1996, 2001, Dräger, Inc, Drägerwerk AG.
2. Pilbeam SP: *Mechanical ventilation: physiological and clinical applications*, ed 3, St Louis, 1998, Mosby.
3. GF Lear, personal communication, Telford, Penn, 1998, 2002, Dräger, Inc, Drägerwerk AG.
4. Breathing support package proportional pressure support PPS, tube compensation, ATC, supplement to the instructions for use of the Evita 4 as from software version 2.n 90 28 825-GA 5664.520 e, ed 1, Telford, Penn, 1996, and version 4.n, 2001, Dräger, Inc, Drägerwerk AG.
5. E-4 plus option NeoFlow NI 5664.515e/117D, Telford, Penn, 1997, Dräger, Inc.
6. NeoFlow: neonatal mode, supplement to the instructions for use of the Evita 4 as from software version 2.n ED 2077947.97, ed 2, Telford, Penn, 1997, and version 4.n, 2001, Dräger, Inc, Drägerwerk AG.

Dräger Evita 2 Dura

1. Evita 2 Dura intensive care ventilator operating instructions, software 3 n, 90 28 961, Telford, Penn, 1997, Dräger Inc.
2. Pilbeam SP: *Mechanical ventilation: physiological and clinical applications*, ed 3, St Louis, 1998, Mosby.

Hamilton Medical: VEOLAR^{FT}

1. Hamilton Medical: VEOLAR^{FT} operating manual, Reno, Nev, 1992, Hamilton Medical Inc.
2. Hamilton Medical, VEOLAR^{FT} study guide, part no 51061-SG, Reno, Nev, 1994, Hamilton Medical Inc.
3. Hamilton Medical, VEOLAR^{FT} users guide, part no 51061-UG, Reno, Nev, 1994, Hamilton Medical Corp.
4. Pilbeam SP: Mechanical ventilation. In Burton GG, Hodgkin JE, Ward JJ, editors: *Respiratory care: a guide to clinical practice*, ed 4, Philadelphia, 1997, Lippincott.

Hamilton GALILEO

1. Operating manual: GALILEO, 610 175/00, 1997 and Galileo Intensive Care Ventilator, 610862/00, (version 3) Switzerland, 2000, Hamilton Medical.
2. Branson RD, et al: Closed-loop mechanical ventilation, *Resp Care* 47:427, 2002.
3. Pilbeam SP: *Mechanical ventilation: physiological and clinical applications*, ed 3, St Louis, 1998, Mosby.
4. Radford EP, Ferris BG, Kriete BC: Clinical use of a nomogram to estimate proper ventilation during artificial respirations, *N Engl J Med* 251:877, 1954.
5. Iotti GA, et al: Respiratory mechanics by least squares fitting in mechanically ventilated patients: applications during paralysis and during pressure support ventilation, *Intensive Care Med* 21:406, 1995.
6. Otis AB, Fenn WO, Rahn H: Mechanics of breathing in man, *J Appl Physiol* 2:592, 1950.
7. Brunner JX , et al: Simple method to measure total expiratory time constant based on the passive expiratory flow-volume curve, *Crit Care Med* 23(6):1117, 1995.
8. Laubscher TP, et al: The automatic selection of ventilation parameters during the initial phase of mechanical ventilation, *Intensive Care Med* 22:199, 1996.
9. Laubscher TP, et al: Automatic selection of tidal volume, respiratory frequency and minute ventilation in intubated ICU patients as startup procedure for closed-loop controlled ventilation, *Int J Clin Monitoring Computing* 11:19, 1994.

Puritan Bennett 740

1. 740 Ventilator System operator's manual, G-060143-00 revision B 0697, Pleasanton, Calif, 1997, Puritan Bennett, a Division of Tyco Healthcare.
2. 740 Ventilator System pocket guide, A-AA2213-00 revision A (06/97), Pleasanton, Calif, 1997, Puritan Bennett, a Division of Tyco Healthcare.
3. Puritan-Bennett 700 Series Ventilator System—Operator's Manual, G-061874-00, revision D, Pleasanton, Calif, 2000, Puritan Bennett, a division of Tyco Healthcare.
4. David Hyde, RRT, Product Manager, personal communication, Pleasanton, Calif, 2000, Puritan Bennett, a division of Tyco Healthcare.

Puritan Bennett 760

1. Puritan-Bennett 700 Series Ventilator System—Operator's Manual, G-061874-00, revision D, Pleasanton, Calif, 2000, Puritan Bennett, a division of Tyco Healthcare.
2. David Hyde, RRT, Product Manager, personal communication, Pleasanton, Calif, 2000, Puritan Bennett, a division of Tyco Healthcare.

Puritan Bennett 840

1. Puritan Bennett Operator's and Technical Reference Manual, 840 Ventilator System, part no 4-070088-00, revision C, Pleasanton, Calif, Nov, 1998, Puritan Bennett, a division of Tyco Healthcare.
2. Puritan Bennett User's Pocket Guide, 840 Ventilator System, part no 4-076767-00, revision C, Pleasanton, Calif, Jan, 2000, Puritan Bennett, a division of Tyco Healthcare.
3. Puritan Bennett, Learning and mastering the Puritan-Bennett 840 ventilator system, Computer Based Training, part no A-AA2287-00 revision A, Pleasanton, Calif, 1999, Puritan Bennett, a division of Tyco Healthcare.
4. Dave Hyde, Product Manager, personal correspondence, Pleasanton, Calif, 2002, Puritan Bennett, a division of Tyco Healthcare.
5. Pilbeam SP: *Mechanical ventilation: physiological and clinical applications*, ed 3, St Louis, 1998.
6. Hess DR et al: *Respiratory care: principles & practice*, Philadelphia, 2002, WB Saunders.

Puritan Bennett 7200

1. Puritan Bennett Corp: 7200 series microprocessor ventilator operator's manual, Carlsbad, Calif, 1993, Puritan Bennett, a Division of Tyco Healthcare.
2. Pilbeam SP: Mechanical ventilation. In Burton GG, Hodgkin JE, Ward JJ: *Respiratory care: a guide to clinical practice*, ed 4, Philadelphia, 1997, Lippincott.

Newport Breeze E150

1. The Newport Breeze E150 ventilator: operating manual, OPR150, revision B, Newport Beach, Calif, 1993, Newport Medical, Inc.
2. Pilbeam SP, Payne FR: Mechanical ventilators. In Burton GG, Hodgkin JE, Ward JJ: *Respiratory care: a guide to clinical practice*, ed 4, Philadelphia, 1997, Lippincott.
3. Cyndy Miller, personal communication, Newport Beach, Calif, July, 2002. Newport Medical, Inc.

Newport Wave E200

1. Newport Wave ventilator operating manual model E200, version 1.5, 1993, Newport Beach, Calif, 1993, Newport Medical Instruments, Inc.
2. Pilbeam SP, Payne FR: Mechanical ventilators. In Burton GG, Hodgkin JE, Ward JJ: *Respiratory care: a guide to clinical practice*, ed 4, Philadelphia, 1997, Lippincott.
3. Cyndy Miller, personal communication, Newport Beach, Calif, July, 2002. Newport Medical, Inc.

Pulmonetics LTV 1000

1. LTV Series Ventilator Operator's Manual, part no 10664 revision J, Colton, Calif, 2000, Pulmonetic Systems, Inc.
2. LTV Series Caregiver Video, part no 11522 revision A, Colton, Calif, 2001, Pulmonetic Systems, Inc.
3. LTV Series In-Service Video, part no 11462 revision B, Colton, Calif, 2000, Pulmonetic Systems, Inc.
4. Produce Simulator for the LTV 1000 Ventilator, LTV 1000 Series Software CD, part no 11600, version 1.03, Colton, Calif, 2001, Pulmonetic Systems, Inc.
5. Angela King, personal communication, Colton, Calif, 2002, Pulmonetic Systems, Inc.

Respironics Esprit

1. Esprit Operator's Manual, Respironics, 580-1000-01F, Carlsbad, Calif, Aug 2001, Respironics, Inc.
2. Esprit Ventilator 4.0 software release notes, part no 1010639-05/22/02, Carlsbad, Calif, 2000, Respironics, Inc.
3. Barry Feldman, personal communication, Carlsbad, Calif, 4/2002, Respironics Corp.

Siemens Servo 900C

1. Mushin WW, et al: *Automatic ventilation of the lungs*, ed 3, Oxford, 1980, Mosby.
2. Siemens-Elema Servo Ventilator 900 operating manual, ME 461/5098.101,1974; and Servo Ventilator 900B preliminary supplement to operating manual, Solna, Sweden, 1974, Siemens-Elema AB, Siemens Medical Solutions.
3. Ingestedt S, et al: A servo-controlled ventilator measuring expired minute ventilation, airway flow and pressure, *Acta Anaesthesiol Scand Suppl* 47:9, 1972.
4. Mike MacGregor, personal communication, Siemens Servo, Danvers, Mass, March 2002, Siemens Medical Solutions.

Siemens Servo 300

1. Siemens Servo Ventilator 300, operating manual 6.0, s-171 95; part no 60 27 408 E313E, 1997, Solna, Sweden, Siemens, Elema AB, Siemens Medical Solutions.
2. Siemens Servo Ventilator 300A: Automode, order no 64 08 897 E315E, Solna, Sweden, 1997, Siemens Medical Solutions.
3. Mike MacGregor, personal communication, Danvers, Mass, April 2002, Siemens Servo, Siemens Medical Solutions.

Dräger Savina

1. Savina Intensive Care Ventilator, Operating Instructions, software 1.n, Dräger Medical, ed 2, July 2001, part no 90-37-22, Dräger, Inc, Drägerwerk AG.
2. Geof Lear, personal communication, Telford, Penn, June, 2002, Dräger Medical.

Servo^{i}

1. User's manual (U.S. edition), Servo^{i} Ventilator System, version 1.1, order no 66-00-261-E313E, Danvers, Mass, 2001, Siemens' Medical Systems, Inc.
2. Sara Corcoran, Clinical Product Manager, personal communication, Danvers, Mass, June 2002, Siemens Medical Systems, Inc.

Viasys AVEA

1. Avea Ventilator Systems, Operator's Manual, (revision A), L1523, Palm Springs, Calif March, 2002, VIASYS Healthcare, Critical Care Division.
2. Clinical Education Materials, Monographs and Presentations, L1490 revision A, software disc, Palm Springs, VIASYS Healthcare, Critical Care Division.
3. Christine Reilly, Clinical Marketing Manager, personal communication, Yorba Linda, Calif, June, 2002, VIASYS Healthcare, Critical Care Division.

Newport e500

1. Operating Manual, Newport e500 Wave Ventilator, OPR500 revision A, version 1.5, Costa Mesa, Calif, 2001, Newport Medical Instruments, Inc.

2. Operating/Service Manual, Newport e500 GDM Graphic Display Monitor, OPRGDM1900 revision B, Costa Mesa, Calif, 2001, Newport Medical Instruments, Inc.

3. Cyndy Miller, Director of Clinical Education, personal communication, Newport Beach, Calif, July 2002, Newport Medical, Inc.

Internet Resources

Amethyst Research: www.amethyst-research.com

Dräger, Inc: www.draeger.com

Hamilton Medical, Inc: www.hamilton-medical.com

Newport Medical Products, Inc: www.NewportNMI.com

Novametrics Medical Systems: www.novametrix.com

Pall Medical, Inc: www.pall.com

Puritan Bennett: www.puritanbennett.com and www.Mallinckrodt.com

Pulmonetics, Inc: www.pulmonetic.com

Sensormedics, Inc: www.sensormedics.com

Siemens Medical Systems, Inc: www.siemens.com

Ventilator website: www.VentWorld.com

Viasys Healthcare, Critical Care Division and the Viasys AVEA ventilator: www.ViasysCriticalCare.com

Bird and Bear Products Corp, www.birdprod.com and www.bearmedical.com

Chapter 13

Infant and Pediatric Ventilators

Kenneth F. Watson

Chapter Outline

**The general outline is an overview used for each of the CPAP units and ventilators and represents the sequence in which the material is presented. This outline varies slightly, reflecting the differences between the many types of devices.*

Chapter Learning Objectives

Upon completion of this chapter, the reader should be able to:

1. Systematically review continuous positive airway pressure delivery devices and infant and pediatric ventilators.
2. List the modes of ventilatory support provided by each ventilator.
3. When given flow and inspiratory time (T_I), calculate the approximate tidal volume (V_T) delivered by a typical infant ventilator.
4. Describe noteworthy internal functions of infant and pediatric ventilators.
5. Explain the location and function of the controls, monitors, alarm, and safety systems for each infant and pediatric ventilator.
6. Describe the precautions and key troubleshooting points for each ventilator.

Key Terms

Accumulator
Amplitude
Analog Pressure Output Cable Outlet
Aneroid Manometer
Assist Back-Up
Background Flow Control
Back-Pressure Switch
Bias Flow
Check Valve
Circuit PEEP
Control Circuit
Demand Flow System
Differential-Pressure Transducer
DIN Connector
Dump Valve
Electromagnetic
Electronic Pressure Switch
Exhalation Block
Expiratory Synchrony
Flow Interruption
Gel-Cell Battery
Hertz
High-Frequency Jet Ventilator
Hi-Lo Jet Tracheal Tube
Illuminated Bar Graph
Impedance
Infrared Sensor
Jet Solenoid
Leak Compensation
Leak Makeup
Mechanical Oscillator
Mechanical Stop
Message Log
Micro-Controller Unit (MCU)
NCPAP Generator
Nickel Cadmium (NiCD) Battery
On/Off Locking Toggle Switch
Oscillating Quartz Crystal
Oscillator Subsystem
Overpressure-Relief Valve
Piston Assembly
Piston Centering
Polarity Voltage
Positive/Negative Pressure-Relief Valve
Proportioning Valve
Pulsation Dampener
Purge Valve
Rotary Baffle
Serial Output Connector
Soft Key
Square-Wave Driver
Subambient Relief Valve
Termination Sensitivity
Tracking-Relief Pressure Valve
Variable Inspiratory Variable Expiratory (VIVE)
Volume Limit

The Infant Ventilator

For more than three decades, infants have been ventilated primarily in the time-triggered, pressure-limited, time-cycled ventilation (TPTV) mode. The reason for this probably relates to the historical evolution of infant ventilators. Although no scientific evidence supports TPTV as superior to volume control in infants, many clinicians have believed that this mode reduces the risk of barotrauma.[1] Therefore, until recently, infant ventilators were designed to provide TPTV and continuous positive airway pressure (CPAP) exclusively. These ventilators were simple in design and incorporated many similar features.

Today, however, more precise monitoring and patient sensing has made it possible to apply additional modes of ventilation in infants. These modes previously were associated only with adult and pediatric patients. Manufacturers have introduced more sophisticated models with unique features. Although these infant ventilators have retained the basic design that enables them to provide TPTV and CPAP, many now offer additional options. Volume limited ventilation and pressure support are available on many models, for example.

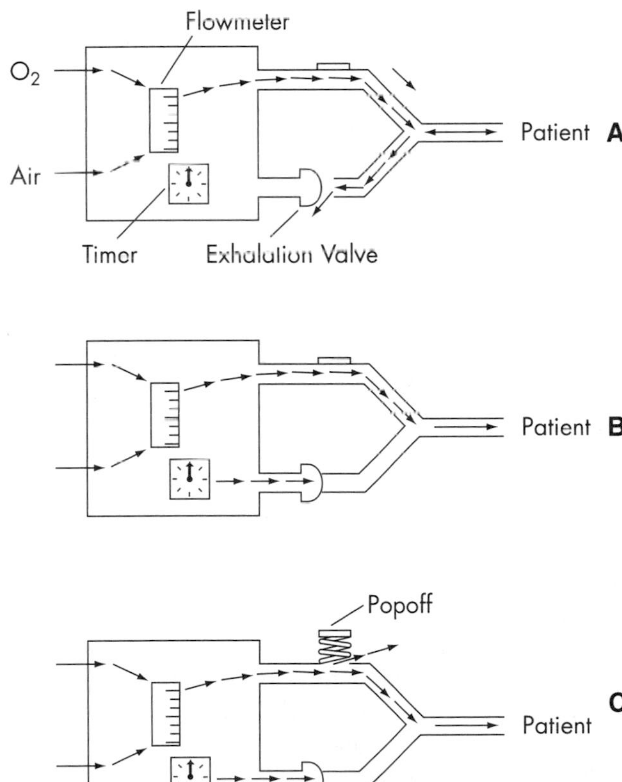

Figure 13-1 The typical continuous-flow ventilator circuit designed for time-triggered, pressure-limited, time-cycled ventilation (TPTV). **A,** spontaneous phase; **B,** inspiratory phase; **C,** pressure-limiting phase. (From Koff PB, Eitzman D, Neu J: *Neonatal and pediatric respiratory care*, ed 2, St Louis, 1993, Mosby.)

Most infant ventilators have been designed to provide a continuous flow of an air/oxygen mixture into the ventilator circuit (Figure 13-1, *A*).[2] In this design, a positive pressure breath results when the machine's exhalation valve closes, permitting the gas mixture to flow to the patient (Figure 13-1, *B*). During the inspiratory phase when a preset pressure limit is reached, pressure is maintained until the ventilator time-cycles into expiration (Figure 13-1, *C*). When the exhalation valve opens, the expiratory phase begins. As long as the exhalation valve remains open, a constant flow of the gas mixture passes by the patient's airway and is available for spontaneous breaths.

If the pressure limit is reached in this type of ventilator, tidal volume will depend on flow, pressure limit, and inspiratory time (see calculation, Box 13-1). However, alterations in the patient's compliance and airway resistance can affect the tidal volume. For example, consider the patient whose compliance improves over a few hours. If the ventilator settings are not modified, the patient's lungs will accommodate flow from the ventilator over a longer period during the inspiratory phase. Peak pressure will be reached later in the inspiratory phase. Therefore, a larger than desired tidal volume may be delivered by the ventilator. Inspiratory time and flow are set and digitally displayed on most TPTV ventilators. The calculation shown in Box 13-1 should be used to estimate the available tidal volume if the pressure limit is reached. If the pressure limit is reached early in the inspiratory phase, however, tidal volume could be substantially less than calculated.

Some ventilators use a **demand flow system** to provide inspiratory gas for spontaneous breaths. This type of system delivers flow at a variable rate proportional to patient inspiratory flow. The ventilator matches the patient's inspiratory flow. Demand flow is believed by some clinicians to be advantageous to operator selected continuous flow systems because continuous flow systems tend to produce resistance to expiration at the airway, commonly known as **circuit PEEP.** For patients whose ventilatory needs include high inspiratory flows but low end-expiratory pressure, the demand system eliminates the needs to set a high continuous flow. Some patients may present with highly variable ventilatory patterns. The use of a demand system may assure sufficient flow to meet transiently high inspiratory flow needs.

In a typical demand system, a minimal preset continuous flow is delivered by the ventilator. On spontaneous inspiration

Box 13-1 Calculation of Maximum Available Tidal Volume for TPTV

$$V_T = \frac{\text{Inspiratory time (seconds)} \times \text{Flow (L/min)}}{60}$$

this flow rate will increase to maintain the baseline pressure. When the ventilator delivers a mandatory breath, the flow rate increases to the value set with the FLOW RATE control knob.

With the development of improved flow-sensing capability, newer ventilator models can now distinguish between the patient's inspiratory flow and machine-generated flow. This allows the clinician to select the TPTV mode and adjust the ventilator to deliver patient-triggered mandatory breaths. This type of continuous flow SIMV is possible even with small endotracheal tube leaks. Technically, the addition of SIMV to this mode means that it is no longer purely TPTV because triggering is by the patient rather than by a time interval. However, default triggering is still according to a time interval. Flow-sensing capability has led to other advances, many of which are unique to a specific ventilator model. The ways in which flow-sensing applications have been developed will be discussed with each ventilator that uses this technology.

The same flow-sensing technology that provides better ventilator/patient synchrony has enabled clinicians to return to volume modes of ventilation in small infants. By closely monitoring inspired and expired tidal volume, ventilatory pressures, and waveforms, clinicians can better adjust ventilator settings according to physiologic changes. Compliance and airway resistance measurements are now possible. Providing the appropriate level of support, responding to physiologic changes more quickly, and weaning infants from the ventilator more effectively are greatly facilitated by some of the latest developments in infant ventilators.

As dual modes of ventilation have become widely used in adults, their application in infants and pediatric patients has been increasing as well. Clinicians working with adults have long recognized that pressure control and pressure support modes are desirable in many clinical situations primarily because of their decelerating waveforms. With the addition of a volume-targeting capability to these modes, a patient receives a more consistent tidal volume in spite of compliance or airway resistance changes. In infants, rapid and sometimes dramatic changes are often seen in an infant's compliance after surfactant replacement therapy. In many pediatric patients, marked compliance or airway resistance changes can occur very rapidly because of the progression of a disease process or after an intervention. Therefore, a ventilator that is capable of delivering consistent tidal volumes while providing decelerating flow can be very useful in the neonatal and pediatric setting.

With infants, many clinicians continue to prefer to use mechanical ventilators that were designed exclusively for infants and small children. However, manufacturers are beginning to design models that are suitable for any patient size. Features such as flow-triggering and cycling, short response times, volume monitoring, and low internal compressible volume are being incorporated into most new ventilator designs. Today, some hospitals have chosen to employ a single ventilator model that can be used with both adult and neonatal patients. Caution should be used, however, in employing these ventilators in very small patients, especially with uncuffed artificial airways. It is good practice to monitor tidal volume at the infant's airway when using these ventilators for a more precise determination. The use of calculations to correct for compressible volume does not take artificial airway leak into account. Moreover, in situations in which compliance is markedly low or airway resistance is markedly high, volume loss in the patient/circuit system can be greater than that calculated.

CPAP Systems

Traditionally, the use of CPAP in neonates has served as a bridge to extubation or a stepping stone from mechanical ventilation to normal breathing. Many low-weight infants who show an increased work of breathing after extubation can be managed on nasal CPAP systems rather than reintubating them and placing them back on the ventilator. Many clinicians prefer to construct their own CPAP systems using readily available blenders, humidifiers, adapters, tubings, and valves. Others prefer to deliver CPAP using an infant ventilator. Both of these types of CPAP delivery systems are often referred to as conventional CPAP systems. Both use continuous flow to either a nasal cannula or to prongs inserted into the nasopharynx.

Recent applications of CPAP in neonates have gone beyond traditional uses. In one study, infants who were treated with exogenous surfactant were subsequently placed on nasal CPAP. Although intubation was required to administer the surfactant, patients were duly extubated and maintained on nasal CPAP until their oxygen requirements and work of breathing decreased to acceptable levels. For most patients in this study, mechanical ventilation was avoided.[3]

Another less traditional use of CPAP has been its application after a period of high-frequency ventilation. Some neonates can be weaned from the high-frequency ventilator directly to a CPAP system. Conventional mechanical ventilation and prolonged endotracheal intubation can be avoided. One study suggests that the judicious use of CPAP facilitates early weaning from high-frequency ventilation and reduces the incidence of chronic lung disease.[4]

Experience and evaluation of conventional CPAP delivery systems has revealed the presence of mechanical impedance to exhalation resulting from turbulent flow. Some clinicians believe that this impedance, combined with flow starvation during the inspiratory phase, prevents the delivery of stable pressures to the infant's airway and produces an imposed work of breathing. That some infants do not tolerate CPAP could be because of these phenomena. To overcome these issues, new CPAP generators have been developed that tend to match inspiratory flow and to minimize expiratory flow impedance. Employing fluidic principles, these delivery devices reportedly accommodate the spontaneous ventilatory pattern of the infant by implementing a "fluidic flip" between inspiration and expiration. It has been observed that these devices are particularly effective in reducing work of breathing in very low birth weight infants, rendering CPAP better tolerated in this population and helping to avoid positive pressure ventilation.[5] These CPAP delivery systems represent the only freestanding CPAP devices available on the market today.

EME Infant Flow NCPAP System

The EME Infant Flow System (Electro Medical Equipment, East Sussex, England) is designed to provide nasal CPAP to infants. The system consists of a 12 V DC electrically powered driver, a humidifier/heated wire delivery circuit, an infant flow generator with prongs, and a cap for fitting and stabilizing the prongs in the nasal passages (Figure 13-2). A small nasal mask is also available and can be used in lieu of nasal prongs. The driver consists of a flowmeter, a blender with a fractional inspired oxygen (F_IO_2) control, a digital pressure bar graph, an alarm system, and a high-pressure relief system. Any humidifier that accommodates standard temperature sensors and heater wire connections can be used with this unit.[6]

Compressed air and oxygen from 50 psig sources are introduced into the back of the driver. A decrease in one source gas pressure to less than 30 psig will activate the SUPPLY GASES FAILURE alarm. Until the alarm condition is corrected, the gas at the higher pressure will be delivered to the patient. The supply gases failure alarm can only be silenced by correcting the pressure drop or disconnecting both gas sources. Blended gas at a constant flow exits the driver, passes through the humidifier, and is carried to the infant flow generator (Figure 13-3, *A*). The generator consists of two fluidic jets. The geometric design of the jet delivery ports facilitates the Coanda effect (Chapter 11). On inspiration, flow from the driver passes through the nasal prongs to the infant. However, if the infant's inspiratory flow is less than that delivered by the driver, excess flow is diverted away from the prongs. On expiration, expiratory flow pressure "flips" the direction of flow away from the prongs and through an expiratory port. Only a baseline amount of flow remains to maintain the set CPAP level. Diverting flow away from the nasal prongs enables the infant to exhale through a low resistance system.

Nasal prongs, made from a soft silicon-based elastomer, are available in three sizes. Nasal masks, also made from silicon elastomer, are available in two sizes. A mounting system incorporates a head cap, available in 10 sizes with each size color-coded, and two positioning straps (Figure 13-3, *B*). The straps attach to the two flanges of the nasal attachment and are inserted into slits along the edge of the head cap. The gas delivery tube and exhalation tubing are positioned above the patient's head and can be tied to the head cap. The infant can then be repositioned or held while the CPAP prongs remain in position.

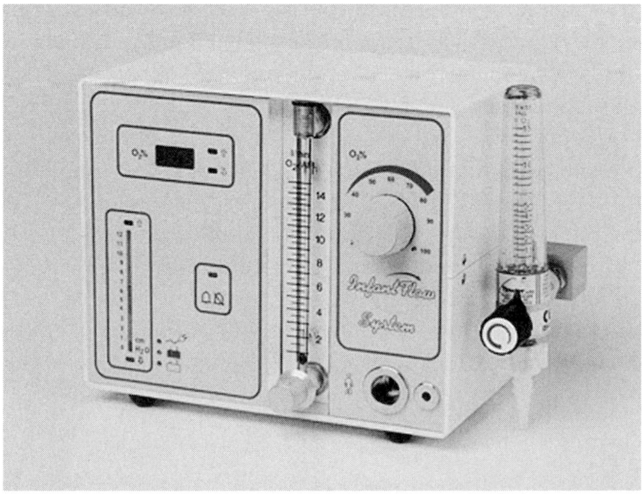

Figure 13-2 The EME Infant Flow System. (Courtesy Electro Medical Equipment, East Sussex, England.)

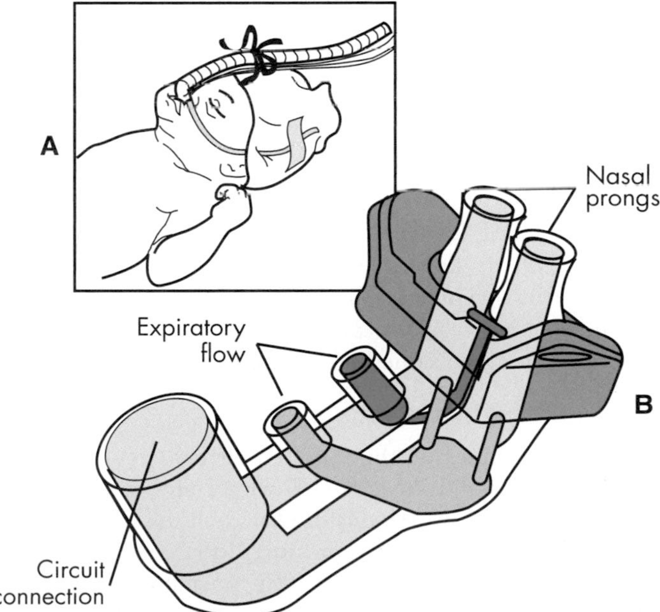

Figure 13-3 **A,** The infant flow generator used with the Alladin Infant Flow System. **B,** The infant flow generator mounting system.

Controls, Monitors, and Alarms

All controls are located on the driver. They include an ON/OFF SWITCH, FLOWMETER, an OXYGEN (%) control, and an ALARM MUTE button. A digital pressure manometer provides a dynamic display of airway pressure. Alarm conditions are audible and are visually displayed on the front panel.

Power Switch

An on/off power toggle switch is located on the driver's rear panel. Immediately after the power to the driver is turned on, the system's software version will be displayed in the oxygen (%) window for 2 seconds. The clinician should use the operator's manual specific to each driver's software version.

O_2%

F_IO_2 is variable from 0.21 to 1.0. The O_2% knob is calibrated in 10% increments but will allow adjustment in 1% increments. The set oxygen concentration is according to the knob's position. The digital display, also marked O_2%, is a reading from the unit's built-in oxygen analyzer. This analyzer is calibrated by the clinician before each use by adjusting two potentiometers on the driver's left side panel, one while the O_2% knob is set at 21 percent and the other at 100 percent.

An alarm system is incorporated into the analyzer's digital display. The microprocessor sets alarm limits either automatically within 2 minutes of a stable reading or when the alarm keypad is pressed and held for 3 seconds. When the monitored F_IO_2 falls outside of these limits, a red high or low light-emiting diode (LED) will light and an audible alarm will sound.

Flowmeters

A non-back pressure-compensated flowmeter, incorporated into the driver and adjustable to 15 L/min, sets the peak flow available to the patient. The flow setting also determines the CPAP level. A chart is available to guide the clinician in setting the flow for the desired CPAP level. Ideally, if prongs are sized and fitted correctly, a flow of 8 L/min should provide a CPAP level of 5 cm H_2O.

An auxilliary flowmeter is mounted to the side of the driver. This flowmeter, which is adjustable to 15 L/M, is intended to power accessory devices. Gas exiting this flowmeter is at the same F_IO_2 as the O_2% setting.

Pressure Manometer

The proximal pressure line of the delivery circuit attaches to a port on the front panel. Proximal airway pressure is measured in cm H_2O and is displayed on the multicolored bar graph. This graph reads pressures to 12 cm H_2O. Colors within the bar graph indicate the operational ranges as shown in Table 13-1.

Red LEDs above and below the bar graph will light when pressure alarm limits are manually set and when pressure alarm limits are violated. If alarm limits are not manually set by pressing the alarm keypad for 3 seconds, the driver's microprocessor will set them automatically within 2 minutes. See Clinical Rounds 13-1 for questions related to the EME.

Table 13-1 Colors within airway pressure bar graph indicating operational ranges for the EME Infant Flow System

Color	Pressure (cm H_2O)
Red	0
Yellow	1-3
Green	4-6
Yellow	7-12

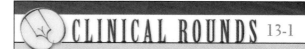

CLINICAL ROUNDS 13-1

A respiratory therapist notices the red LEDs illuminated above and below the pressure bar on the pressure manometer of the EME Infant Flow NCPAP System. What should she do?

See Appendix A for the answer.

Alarm Keypad/Alarm Limits

The alarm keypad serves two functions. During an alarm condition, the audible portion may be silenced for 30 seconds by touching the keypad briefly.

The keypad is also used to set alarm limits. After the infant is placed on the desired levels of CPAP and F_IO_2, pressing and holding the keypad for 3 seconds will set alarm limits. A green LED above the keypad will light when alarm limits have been set. Alarm conditions must persist for 15 seconds before alarms are activated.

When limits are set, audiovisual alarms activate when pressures rise more than 3 cm H_2O or fall below 2 cm H_2O from baseline CPAP level. Oxygen alarm limits are ± 5% of the digitally displayed oxygen concentration.

To protect against excessive system pressures, a solenoid control valve within the driver opens at a pressure of 11 cm H_2O and vents to ambient. An alarm also sounds. After 3 seconds, the driver will attempt to restore flow to the patient circuit.

Battery Power

A lead acid battery is contained within the driver. With a full charge, the driver unit will operate for four hours on battery power.

Troubleshooting

The prongs should be checked first for fit before adjusting the straps as this can result in the prongs moving towards the eyes. In general, the straps should not need adjustment if the fit is correct. Obviously some adjustment may be required as not all babies have the same shaped faces. Care should be taken not to pull too tightly on the straps and squash the infant's nose in an effort to get a good seal.

The most common problem seen in the EME is leaking at the nose. When leaks are present, the size of the prongs should be checked. Readjusting the straps also improves the fit. Care should be taken, however, not to adjust the straps too tightly to achieve a seal. Doing so will put too much pressure on the nose and will cause patient discomfort and skin breakdown. The prongs or mask should seal gently. Patient agitation occasionally presents a problem to keeping the system tight and delivering the desired level of CPAP.

In the case of oxygen alarms, recalibrating the oxygen analyzer usually resolves the problem. If frequent calibrations are necessary, the oxygen fuel cell may require replacing.

Hamilton Arabella System

The Hamilton Arabella (Hamilton Medical, Inc., Reno, NV) is an integrated noninvasive CPAP system similar in design to the EME Infant Flow. The Arabella system consists of a Universal Generator Set with interchangeable silicone nasal prongs, a heated wire delivery circuit, the Arabella Cap, and the Monitoring Gas Mixer.

Prongs for the Arabella come in four sizes. Choosing the appropriate size is facilitated by using the Knosmeter, which is a guide with printed silhouettes that can be matched to the infant's nares. Caps are available in five color-coded sizes.[7]

The major difference between the Arabella and the EME systems lies in the design of their flow generators. In the Arabella, the jets delivering expiratory flow extend part way into a single common chamber within the generator housing. In the EME the jet nozzles are positioned flush with the housing wall and each set serves a separate chamber. The cavity of the Arabella's generator is slightly larger and the geometric angles for guiding flows are arranged differently. Also, unlike the EME, the Arabella's jets protrude into a single common chamber. Because of the Arabella flow generator's design, the difference in functional characteristics is that the flow of gas from the jet is more stable than in the EME. A more stable jet flow seems to require a more substantial patient expiratory flow to cause the device to switch into expiration. The additional flow that is required implies that a higher work of breathing could result when using the Arabella system.

The Arabella's Monitoring Gas Mixer and the EME's Infant Flow Driver, although labeled differently, are essentially the same device. Both are set up and operated in exactly the same way. The Arabella device is not available with an internal battery.

Healthdyne 105 Infant Ventilator

The Healthdyne 105 Infant ventilator was presented in the sixth edition (1999) of this text. This material is now available on the EVOLVE website for this text.

Sechrist IV-100B Infant Ventilator

The Sechrist IV-100B Infant ventilator was presented in the sixth edition (1999) of this text. This material is now available on the EVOLVE website for this text.

Sechrist IV-200 Infant/Pediatric Ventilator and Savi Total Synchrony System

The Sechrist IV-200 Infant/Pediatric ventilator (Figure 13-4) is a pressure-limited, time-cycled, continuous flow ventilator. It is capable of providing time cycled pressure limited (TCPL) ventilation in either the CMV or IMV modes. This ventilator also can provide continuous flow CPAP.

Pneumatic requirements for this ventilator are medical grade air and oxygen 30 to 60 psig. A pressure differential of 20 psig can exist between the two gases without affecting the ventilator's operation.

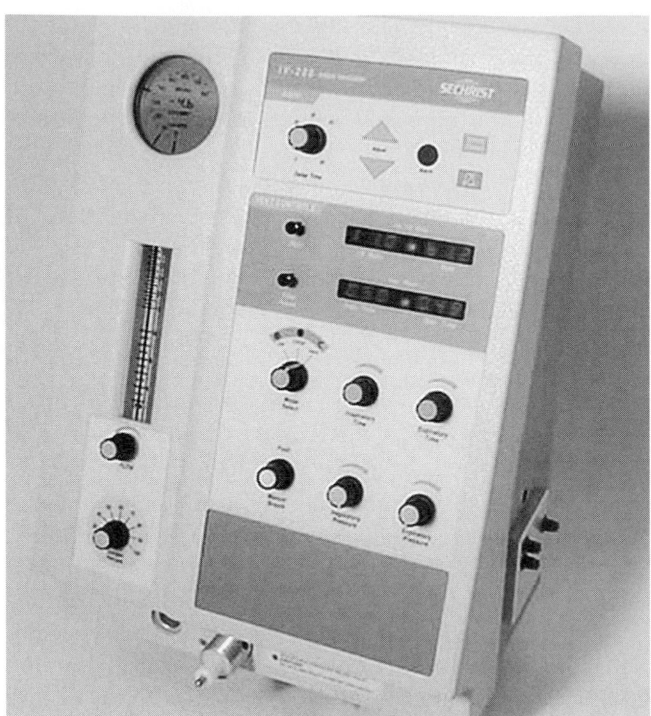

Figure 13-4 The Sechrist model IV-200 Infant/Pediatric Ventilator. (Courtesy Sechrist Industries, Inc, Anaheim, Calif.)

Table 13-2 Specifications for the Sechrist IV-200 Infant/Pediatric Ventilator

Flow	0 to 32 L/min; Flush 40 L/min
Oxygen Percentage	21-100%
Inspiratory Time	0.10 to 2.90 seconds
Expiratory Time	0.30 to 60.0 seconds
Inspiratory Pressure	5 to 70 cm H_2O
Expiratory Pressure (PEEP)	-2 to 20 cm H_2O
Safety Pressure Relief Valve	15 to 85 cm H_2O
ALARMS, DISPLAYS, AND SAFETY FEATURES	
Delay Time (Low pressure alarm)	3 to 60 seconds
Alarm Mute	30 ± 5 seconds
Alarms	High Pressure Limit, Peak Overpressure, Low Pressure Limit, Low Airway Pressure Leaks, Patient Disconnect, Fail-to-Cycle, Apnea, Prolonged Inspiration, Source Gas Failure, Power Failure (Battery Back-up)
Displays	Inspiratory Time, Expiratory Time, I:E Ratio, Rate, Airway Pressure, High Pressure Alarm, Low Pressure Alarm Mean Airway Pressure
Indicators	Inspiratory Phase, Inverse I:E Ratio, Mode Selection, Alarm, High and Low Pressure Alarm, Limit Set Points
Safety Auto Lock Out Circuit	Inspiratory phase is terminated at the 4 sec. point, even in the presence of microprocessor failure

The Sechrist IV-200's electronic components can be operated with 100-240 VAC, 50/60 Hz. The ventilator can also be operated from a 12 V DC power supply using an accessory power cable.[8]

Overview of Control and Alarm Panel

The three-position MODE SELECTOR CONTROL can be set to OFF, CPAP, or VENT. When set in the VENT mode, either intermittent mandatory ventilation (IMV) or controlled mandatory ventilation (CMV) can be delivered. A flowmeter can be adjusted to deliver the desired level of continuous flow. Below the flow setting is the F_IO_2 control.

The mandatory rate on the IV-200 is a function of the INSPIRATORY TIME and the EXPIRATORY TIME controls. A TIME PRESET control allows the clinician to preview and select the desired inspiratory and expiratory times while in the CPAP mode before switching to the VENT mode.

Ventilatory pressures are set by the Inspiratory Pressure control, which establishes the pressure limit of the inspiratory phase, and the EXPIRATORY PRESSURE control, which establishes the desired level of positive end expiratory pressure (PEEP). A SAFETY PRESSURE RELIEF VALVE is a safety feature to protect against excessive system pressures. A MANUAL BREATH button is also located on the front panel.

A WAVEFORM CONTROL allows the user to vary the inspiratory waveform. A TEST button is pressed to perform electronic checks of the microprocessor, display, and alarm functions.

The alarms on the Sechrist IV-200 are extensive (see Table 13-2). However, only two alarm limits are adjustable: the high inspiratory pressure and the low inspiratory pressure. These alarm limits are set by first pressing the SELECT (RESET) button to select either the high- or low-pressure alarm and then pressing and holding the upper or lower ALARM SET ARROWS and observing the visual display. The SELECT (RESET) is also pressed to cancel the high pressure alarm when it is activated.

The DELAY TIME alarm is used to establish a time delay before the low pressure alarm is audibly and visually activated. An ALARM MUTE button silences the audible alarm for 30 ± 5 seconds.

The alarms, displays, indicators, and safety features for the Sechrist IV-200 are listed in Table 13-2.

SAVI Total Synchrony System

The SAVI Total Synchrony System is an optional module that can be added to the Sechrist IV-200 ventilator (Figure 13-5). The purpose of the module is to allow the ventilator to be synchronized to the patient's ventilatory pattern through the application of impedance pneumography.[9]

The SAVI system is interfaced by a cable to the patient's electrocardiogram monitor, which measures changes in thoracic impedance. The monitor translates the impedance change into a voltage which is sent to the SAVI module. The output voltage signal is used by SAVI to trigger the ventilator as impedance changes during normal breathing. As the impedance waveform begins to rise, the ventilator immediately trigger into the inspiratory phase. When the waveform peaks and begins to fall, the ventilator will cycle to the expiratory phase. The ventilator's ability to cycle into expiration is referred to as "Exhalation-on-demand." Should the impedance monitoring system fail for any reason, the ventilator will automatically revert to back-up settings that the clinician enters at set-up.

The interfacing of impedance pneumography to control ventilator triggering and cycling represents an alternate approach to achieving ventilator synchrony. Whereas other infant/pediatric ventilators rely on flow and pressure changes at the airway to effect a synchronous ventilatory pattern, the SAVI Total Synchrony System can be employed without the use of an airway sensor. However, as is the case with flow synchrony, the use of any synchrony system renders it difficult for the clinician to sort out how much work is being done by the patient versus how much by the ventilator. Weaning and withdrawing the ventilator become more challenging. However, the goal in using a ventilator synchrony system is to shorten the duration of mechanical ventilation and limit the incidence of volutrauma. These desirable outcomes are more attainable when clinicians become fully aware of the strengths and limitations of these systems and become more skilled in using them.

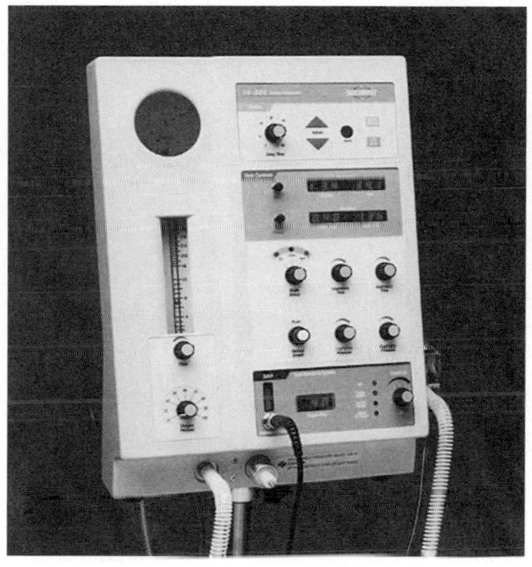

Figure 13-5 The Sechrist model IV-200 Infant/Pediatric Ventilator with SAVI system. (Courtesy Sechrist Industries, Inc, Anaheim, Calif.)

Bear Cub BP 200 and BP 2001 Infant Ventilators

The Bear Cub BP 200 and BP 2001 Infant Ventilators and the Bear CEM Controller and NVM Monitor were presented in the sixth edition of this text (1999). This material is now available on the EVOLVE website for this text.

Bear Cub 750vs Infant Ventilator

The Bear Cub 750vs (VIASYS Healthcare System, Critical Care Division, Palm Springs, CA) is a comprehensive redesign of the Bear infant ventilator intended to replace the Cub 2001 (Figure 13-6). Although this unit is designed for neonates, it can be used with pediatric patients weighing up to 30 kg. Like its predecessors, the 750vs is pneumatically and electrically powered and controlled. In this model, flow-triggering, spontaneous rate, and machine/patient tidal volume monitoring are fully integrated into the machine. Also new to this model are independent base and inspiratory flows, a volume limit feature, and an internal battery back-up.[10]

Two micro controller units, or MCUs, determine all of the ventilator's functions. One is designated the controller MCU and the other the monitor MCU. Each is assigned specific and duplicate tasks. The controller MCU receives information from the control settings as well as signals communicated from the flow sensor, pressure transducer, and monitor MCU. In turn, it signals the unit's components to operate. The monitor MCU reads information from all switches and potentiometers and monitors ventilator performance. It also receives data from the controller MCU. Each of the MCUs monitors the performance of the other. Each has the ability to shut down the ventilator and trigger alarms if software or hardware errors are detected.

A key component to the unit's features is the flow sensor, which is an anemometer consisting of two platinum hot wires. This sensor incorporates an electronic memory circuit

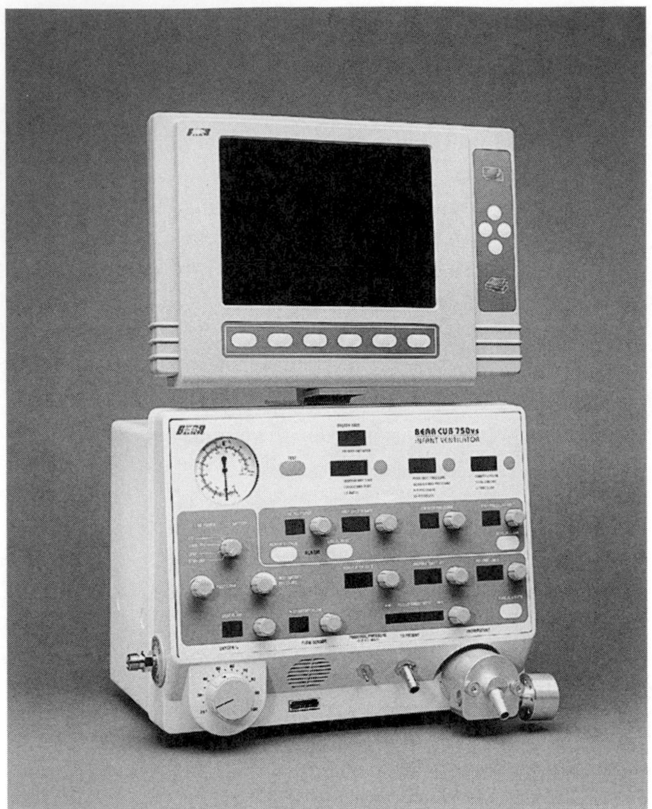

Figure 13-6 The Bear Cub 750vs Infant Ventilator. (Courtesy VIASYS Healthcare, Critical Care Division, Palm Springs, Calif.)

that eliminates the need for calibration. It is capable of determining flow in two directions. Designed to be placed at the patient airway, the sensor permits monitoring and display of patient tidal volume and respiratory rate. It also provides patient flow-triggering and enables the "Volume Limit," explained in a section following. The percentage of endotracheal tube leak is calculated using inspired and expired tidal volume measured by the flow sensor. The monitor MCU makes this calculation and displays it on the front panel. Use of the flow sensor is optional. If the clinician wishes to employ the ventilator without monitoring and synchronization functions, the sensor can be disabled.

Connections to both compressed air and oxygen are required for the ventilator to operate. An optional external air compressor, the model 3100, is provided by the manufacturer. If one of the two gas sources were to fail, a back-up system will assure continued operation using the remaining gas source. However, a source gas failure will alter the F_IO_2. When the ventilator is connected to compressed air and oxygen and is in STAND-BY, blended gas is available from the AUXILIARY GAS OUTLET. Gas flow to this outlet is set using the BASE FLOW control.

Patient circuits and humidification units are provided by the manufacturer. Commercially available infant/pediatric circuits and humidifiers may be used if they meet the manufacturer's specifications.

CLINICAL ROUNDS 13-2

A respiratory therapist is setting the PEEP/CPAP level of the Bear Cub 750vs and notices an audible alarm with a message "Pressure Setting Incompatible." What is one possible explanation for this alarm condition?

See Appendix A for the answer.

Controls and Monitors (Figure 13-7)

PEEP/CPAP and Inspiratory Pressure

PEEP/CPAP is adjustable from 0 to 30 cm H_2O. INSPIRATORY PRESSURE is adjustable to a maximum of 72 cm H_2O. Desired levels can be set by rotating each control knob clockwise and observing the pressure on the analog manometer at end expiration and peak inspiration. The desired peak inspiratory pressure (PIP) level can be set by rotating the control knob clockwise and observing the pressure on the analog manometer at peak inspiration.

The ventilator is designed for proximal airway pressure monitoring. A $\frac{1}{8}$-inch internal diameter tubing is required to connect the proximal airway to the PROXIMAL PRESSURE outlet of the ventilator. A flow of 100 mL/min continuously purges this tubing to prevent moisture accumulation and patient contamination of the ventilator.

The exhalation valve consists of a seated diaphragm that operates as a pneumatic servo-controlled regulator. Exhaled gas passes through the diaphragm and is vented to the atmosphere. PEEP/CPAP and PIP levels are regulated by a differential pressure transducer called the control transducer. This transducer is signaled electronically to reference one level of pressure during a mandatory breath and another during expiration. The control transducer is separated from the proximal airway transducer by the control diaphragm.

During inspiration, when the control pressure equals the set PIP, the control diaphragm opens. This in turn pressurizes the exhalation valve diaphragm to maintain the PIP level until the set inspiratory time lapses. During expiration, when the control pressure drops to the set PEEP, the control diaphragm closes and allows the exhalation valve to open until the PEEP level is reached. The control diaphragm opens sufficiently to maintain the PEEP level during the expiratory phase.

The exhalation valve assembly incorporates a jet venturi to eliminate or reduce circuit PEEP generated by the base flow. This venturi enables a PEEP/CPAP level of 0 cm H_2O at a base flow of 10 L/min and 4 cm H_2O at 20 L/min.

If PEEP/CPAP is set higher than the INSPIRATORY PRESSURE control, the PRESSURE SETTINGS INCOMPATIBLE alarm will activate. When this occurs, the set PEEP/CPAP will be maintained, but mandatory breaths will not be delivered (Clinical Rounds 13-2).

Rate

The VENTILATOR RATE control is adjustable from 0 to 150 breaths per minute. This control sets the number of mandatory breaths in the synchronized IMV (SIMV)/IMV mode or the minimum number of breaths to be delivered in the assist/control mode. The set number of breaths per minute is indicated by the LED to the left of the control.

Inspiratory Time

The INSPIRATORY TIME control is adjustable from 0.1 to 3.0 seconds. The set inspiratory time is indicated in seconds by the LED to the left of the control. If this control is set to deliver an inverse inspiratory-to-expiratory (I:E) ratio, the digital display will flash and the SETTINGS INCOMPATIBLE alarm will sound. During the alarm condition, the ventilator will limit the inspiratory time to provide an I:E ratio of 1:1 at the set ventilator rate. Adjusting the INSPIRATORY TIME control to an I:E ratio of 1:1 will correct the alarm condition.

Volume Limit

The VOLUME LIMIT control sets a ceiling for tidal volume delivered by mandatory breaths. This control is adjustable from 5 to 300 mL. If the set volume limit is reached, the ventilator will terminate inspiration before the set inspiratory time is delivered. The volume limit LED will illuminate and an audible alarm will sound to alert the clinician that the breath has volume-cycled rather than time-cycled. To correct this alarm condition, the clinician must either select a higher volume limit or decrease the inspiratory pressure. During the alarm condition, the set inspiratory time is not delivered. Also, the set inspiratory pressure may not be delivered (see Box 13-2).

Base Flow and Inspiratory Flow

The background flow available to the patient for spontaneous breathing is set using the BASE FLOW control. The flow delivered to the patient during mandatory breaths is set using the INSPIRATORY FLOW control. Each of these flows is adjustable from 1 to 30 L/min. Both the base flow and inspiratory flow are regulated by individual flow control valves. The two control valves are switched by a solenoid valve. Each is connected to a potentiometer which provides signals to the monitor MCU. The ventilator's internal barometer calculates the flow setting for the barometric pressure. The calculated flow is then displayed on the front panel.

Insufficient or excessive flow settings will result in an INCOMPATIBLE SETTINGS alarm. During this alarm condition, either the BASE FLOW or INSPIRATORY FLOW displays will flash, depending on which of the flows is inappropriately set. Adjusting the control(s) to a more appropriate flow will correct the alarm condition (see Box 13-3).

Assist Sensitivity

The amount of inspiratory effort the patient must exert to trigger a mandatory breath is determined by the ASSIST SENSITIVITY control. Adjustable from 0.2 to 5.0 L/min, this control sets the minimum flow the patient must generate to trigger assist/control or SIMV breaths. Also, in either the SIMV or CPAP modes, this control permits spontaneous breaths to be counted and displayed in the BREATH RATE window.

To the left of the ASSIST SENSITIVITY control is a flow indicator. During a mandatory breath, as flow delivered to the airway increases, the horizontal bar graph illuminating toward the right indicates an increasing flow. As flow diminishes at peak inspiratory pressure, the illuminating bar moves back to the left. If an artificial airway leak is present, more flow is directed toward the airway, and the horizontal flow graph will display the degree of baseline leak. The greater the baseline leak, the further to the right the bar graph will illuminate during the expiratory phase. Along the horizontal bar graph is another illuminated indicator that moves along the graph as the ASSIST SENSITIVITY control is adjusted. The flow at which a mandatory breath can be triggered is reflected by the location of the indicator. If the indicator is adjusted too far to the left so that it intersects with the baseline flow graph, the ventilator will auto-trigger. If the indicator is adjusted too far to the right of the baseline flow, triggering is more difficult. The appropriate position of the indicator is just to the right of the indicated baseline flow.

Box 13-2 Important Technical Note About the Volume Limit Setting

The ventilator's microprocessor is programmed with flow and pressure limits for each volume limit setting. If the inspiratory flow setting is too high, the volume limit LED will flash, alternating with the message "E.FL." If the inspiratory pressure setting is too high, the volume limit LED also will flash, alternating with the message "E.PL." If the flow sensor is disconnected or disabled, the volume limit LED will display dashes.

Box 13-3 Important Technical Note About Gas Flow

The total flow capability of the 750vs is 30 L/min. When the auxiliary gas outlet is used, flow coming from the outlet added to the base flow or inspiratory flow, whichever is higher, represents the total flow output of the ventilator. When total flow exceeds 25 L/min, the actual base flow or inspiratory flow may be less than set. Therefore, the clinician should be alerted to a potential decrease in base flow or inspiratory flow when high flows are used through the auxiliary gas outlet.

Essential to patient triggering and breath rate monitoring is the flow sensor. If the sensor is disconnected or disabled, no flow will be displayed on the Assist Sensitivity horizontal bar graph and the patient will be unable to trigger a breath. Along the horizontal bar graph is another illuminated indicator that moves along the graph as the ASSIST SENSITIVITY control is adjusted.

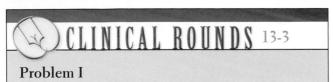

Problem I

While using the 750vs, the clinician has the auxiliary flow set at 5 L/min, the inspiratory flow at 10 L/min and the base flow set at 5 L/min. Total gas flow will be what?

Problem II

Inspiratory pressure is set at 15 cm H_2O and the high-pressure alarm at 20 cm H_2O. During inspiration, the pressure reaches 10 cm H_2O. What could cause this?

See Appendix A for the answer.

Manual Breath

The MANUAL BREATH button delivers a single mandatory breath when pressed. Each manual breath is delivered at the set inspiratory time, flow, and inspiratory pressure.

Auxiliary Gas Outlet

Located on the left side of the ventilator, the AUXILIARY GAS OUTLET provides an additional flow of blended gas. This port is a spring-loaded diameter index safety system (DISS) fitting to which a flowmeter may be added. Up to 8 L/min flow is available through this outlet. In the event of electric power disruption, this valve is still functional and can be used with a manual resuscitator.

Oxygen %

Delivered oxygen concentration is adjusted by the OXYGEN % control. The control knob regulates an internal air/oxygen blender.

Over Pressure Relief

An external mechanical OVER PRESSURE RELIEF valve is located on the ventilator's back panel. Adjustable from 15 to 75 cm H_2O, this valve relieves excessive pressure in the inspiratory limb of the ventilator circuit.

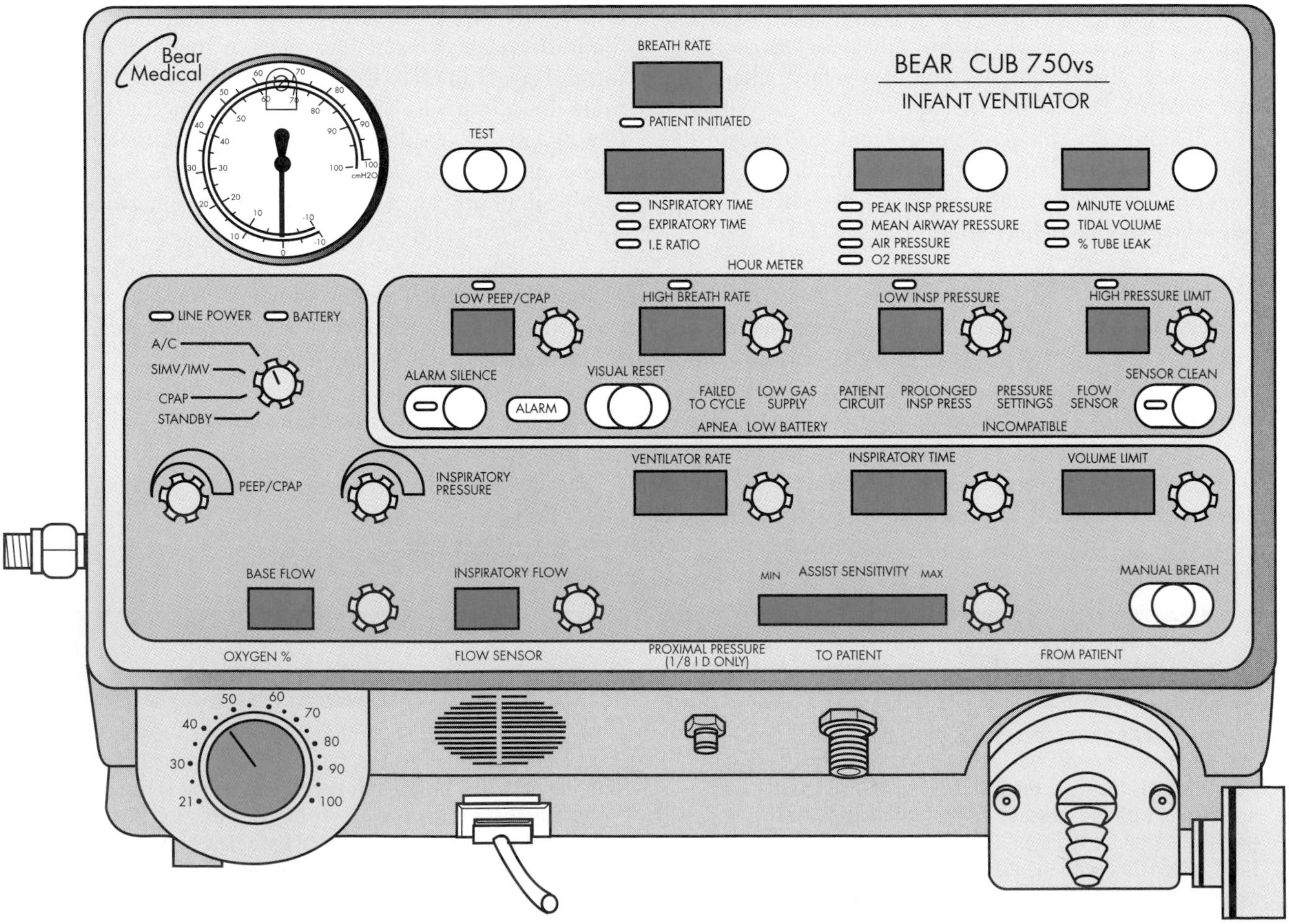

Figure 13-7 The Bear Cub 750vs Infant Ventilator control panel.

This valve is not intended to be used as the ventilator's primary peak inspiratory pressure control but rather a safety valve. If set lower than the INSPIRATORY PRESSURE control, the unit's audible and visual high pressure alarms will **NOT** alert the clinician to a high pressure situation (Clinical Rounds 13-3).

Table 13-3 Adjustable alarms on the Bear Cub 750vs Infant Ventilator

Alarm	Adjustable Range	Condition Triggering Alarm
Low PEEP/CPAP	-5 to 30 cm H_2O	Measured proximal airway pressure falls below the set value for at least 60 ms
High Breath Rate	3 to 255 bpm	Monitored value for breath rate exceeds alarm setting
Low Inspiratory Pressure	1 to 65 cm H_2O	Proximal airway pressure does not exceed set threshold during delivery of a mechanical breath
High Pressure Limit	10 to 75 cm H_2O	Proximal airway pressure exceeds set threshold

Alarms

Visual alarm indicators, all red LEDs, are grouped together in the mid-portion of the front panel (Figure 13-7). These include four adjustable alarms and nine fixed alarms. When an alarm condition occurs, both a visual and an audible alarm are activated. Although the audible portion is intended to alert the clinician to an alarm condition, the visual portion indicates the specific problem. When an alarm condition is corrected, the audible portion will stop automatically. The visual portion will continue to indicate the alarm condition until the VISUAL RESET button is pressed. With the exception of the FAILED TO CYCLE alarm, the audible portion of an alarm can be silenced by pressing the ALARM SILENCE button. The alarm will be silenced for 60 seconds unless the clinician cancels the silence period by pressing the button a second time. A control to adjust alarm loudness is located on the ventilator's rear panel. Adjustable alarms for the Bear Cub 750vs are described in Table 13-3. Fixed alarms are listed in Table 13-4.

Table 13-4 Fixed alarms on the Bear Cub 750vs Infant Ventilator

Alarm	Condition Triggering Alarm
Failed to Cycle	Microprocessor detects an internal or external malfunction; after alarm condition is corrected, Mode Select switch must be turned to the Standby position and then to the desired ventilation mode.
Low Gas Supply	Either air or oxygen inlet pressure or both inlet pressures decrease to below 24 ± 2 PSIG
Patient Circuit	Occlusion of inspiratory limb of breathing circuit; proximal sensing line disconnect
Prolonged Inspiratory Pressure	Proximal airway pressure remains above reference value (low PEEP/CPAP + 10 cm H_2O) for more than 3.5 seconds
Settings Incompatible	One or more of the following: Inspiratory time and ventilator rate settings incompatible (Inspiratory Time and Ventilator rate displays will flash) Base Flow is set higher than Inspiratory Flow (Base Flow and Inspiratory Flow displays will flash) Volume Limit setting is incompatible with Flow and Inspiratory Pressure settings (If Inspiratory Flow setting is too high, Volume Limit LED digits will flash, alternating with "E.FL." If Inspiratory Pressure setting is too high, Volume Limit LED digits will flash, alternating with "E.PL."
Pressure Settings Incompatible	Inspiratory Pressure Setting is greater than PEEP/CPAP setting or PEEP/CPAP setting is greater than Inspiratory Pressure setting.
Flow Sensor	Sensor malfunction or disconnect from ventilator.
Apnea	Lack of breath initiation within set period; apnea period can be adjusted with control located on the ventilator's rear panel. Apnea period is adjustable from 5 to 30 seconds in 5-second increments. When flow sensor is in use, apnea alarm is activated when no flow is detected within set time period. When flow sensor is disconnected or is disabled in the A/C or SIMV/IMV modes, the apnea alarm will activate if mechanical breaths fail to be delivered. When flow sensor is disconnected or is disabled in the CPAP mode, the apnea alarm becomes inactive.
Low Battery	Internal battery has approximately 5 minutes of power remaining before full discharge

Table 13-5 Specifications for the Bear Cub 750vs Infant Ventilator

Rate	1 to 150 breaths per minute
Inspiratory Time	0.1 to 3.0 seconds
Inspiratory Flow	1 to 30 L/min
Base Flow	1 to 30 L/min
Volume Limit	5 to 300 mL
Oxygen Concentration	21% to 100%
Pressure Limit	0 to 72 cm H_2O
PEEP/CPAP	0 to 30 cm H_2O
Audiovisual Alarms	Low PEEP/CPAP, High Breath Rate, Low Inspiratory Pressure, High Pressure Limit, Failed to Cycle, Low Gas Supply, Patient Circuit, Prolonged Inspiratory Pressure, Settings Incompatible, Pressure Settings Incompatible, Flow Sensor, Apnea, Low Battery
Monitors	Breath Rate, Breath Type (Patient Initiated), Minute Volume, Tidal Volume (Exhaled), % Tube Leak, Inspiratory Time, Expiratory Time, I:E Ratio, Peak Inspiratory Pressure, Mean Airway Pressure, Air Pressure, O_2 Pressure, Proximal Airway Pressure, Hourmeter, Test, Battery
Alarm Silence	60 seconds

*Volume Limit audible alarm can be disabled.

Special Features

A graphics display is available on the Bear Cub 750vs as an upgrade option. With the display, scalar pressure, flow, and volume waveforms can be simultaneously viewed. Loops and additional data can also be displayed. A computer interface also is available, allowing a computer to be used in lieu of the graphics monitor. Three analog signals are generated by the ventilator for connection to an oscilloscope or strip chart recorder. These signals represent pressure, flow, and breath phase.

Within the grouping of alarm indicators is a SENSOR CLEAN button (Figure 13-7). This feature provides a means to help free the sensor wires of organic contaminants. When the button is pressed, an instantaneous 1-second increase in the sensor wires' temperature will occur during the ventilator's next expiratory phase. Mucus and other debris clinging to the sensor wires will "burn off," reducing interference in the sensor's performance. This feature is useful in that the clinician can sometimes avoid having to remove and clean or exchange the sensor when erratic readings occur.

An internal battery will operate the ventilator when electrical power is interrupted. With a full charge, the battery will provide power for approximately 30 minutes.

Specifications for the Bear Cub 750vs are listed in Table 13-5.

Troubleshooting

An extensive troubleshooting guide can be found in the ventilator's instruction manual. Leaks in the patient circuit cause most problems. The ventilator's extensive alarm and diagnostic system facilitates resolving most troubleshooting issues.

Bear Cub 750psv

Overview

The Bear Cub 750psv (Figure 13-8) represents an update of the model 750vs. Some features have been added to this model, making it a more flexible ventilator for both neonatal and pediatric applications. Because this model is very similar to its predecessor, only its differences will be discussed here.[11]

Central to the updated design is an improved flow sensor, which provides a more accurate reading of tidal volume, both inspiratory and expiratory. The flow sensor remains an anemometer consisting of two platinum hot wires but its housing and cable are more durable. The sensor and cable are a single unit. On this new version of the Bear Cub, the sensor clean feature has been discontinued.

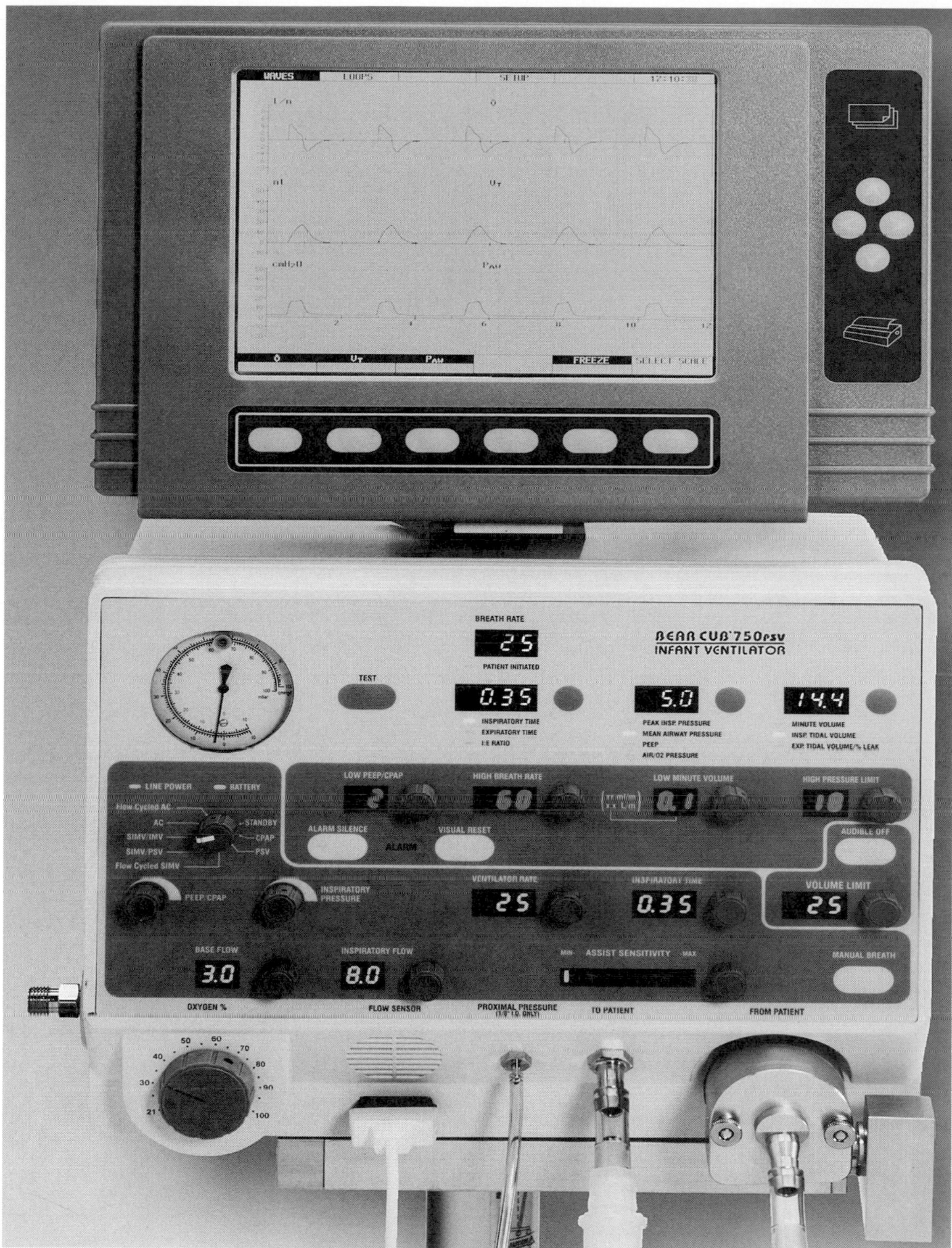

Figure 13-8 The Bear Cub 750psv Infant Ventilator with graphic monitor. (Courtesy VIASYS Healthcare, Critical Care Division, Palm Springs, Calif.)

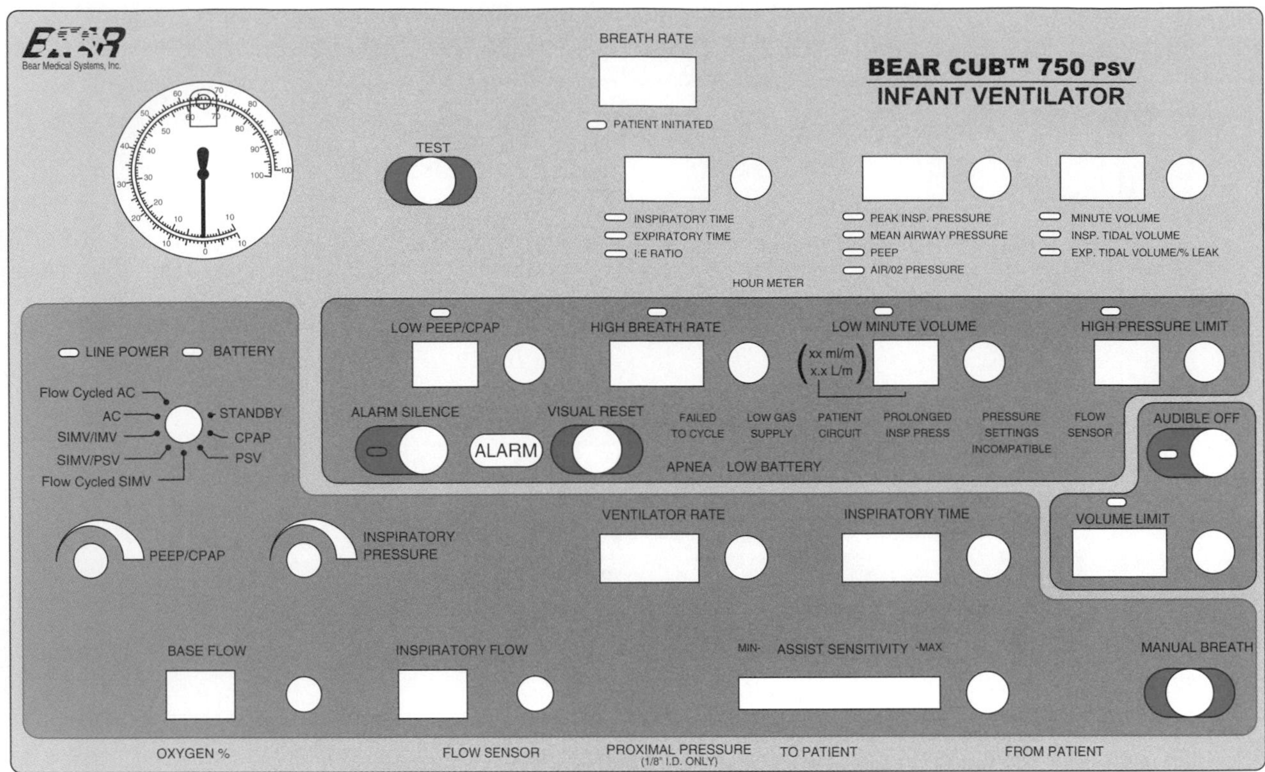

Figure 13-9 The Bear Cub 750psv Infant Ventilator control panel.

Table 13-6 Specifications for the Bear Cub 750psv Infant Ventilator

Rate	**1 to 150 breaths per minute**
Inspiratory Time	0.1 to 3.0 seconds
Inspiratory Flow	1 to 30 L/min
Assist Sensitivity	0.20 to 5.0 L/min
Over Pressure Relief	15 to 75 cm H_2O
Base Flow	1 to 30 L/min
Volume Limit	5 to 300 mL
O_2%	21% to 100%
Inspiratory Pressure	0 to 72 cm H_2O
PEEP/CPAP	0 to 30 cm H_2O
Manual Breath	×1
Apnea Alarm (selectable)	5, 10, 20, or 30 seconds
Audiovisual Alarms	Low PEEP/CPAP, High Breath Rate, Low Inspiratory Pressure, Low Minute Volume, Volume Limit*, High Pressure Limit, Failed to Cycle, Low Gas Supply, Patient Circuit, Prolonged Inspiratory Pressure, Settings Incompatible, Pressure Settings Incompatible, Flow Sensor, Apnea, Low Battery
Monitors	Breath Rate, Breath Type (Patient Initiated), Minute Volume, Tidal Volume (Inspired and Expired), % Tube Leak, Inspiratory Time, Expiratory Time, I:E Ratio, Peak Inspiratory Pressure, Mean Airway Pressure, PEEP, Air Pressure, O_2 Pressure, Proximal Airway Pressure (gauge), Hourmeter, Test, Battery
Alarm Silence	60 seconds

*Volume Limit audible alarm can be disabled.

The volume limit feature on the model 750psv is identical to the 750vs except that the audible high-volume limit alarm can be disabled. Disabling this alarm has no effect on the other alarm systems.

A low minute volume alarm has been added to the 750psv. Adjustable from 0 to 9.9 L, this alarm adds an important safety feature to the new model.

Additional Modes

Four additional modes have been added to this new model, bringing the total number of available modes to seven.[11] The multi-positional mode selector control (see Figure 13-9) has been redesigned to accommodate these additional modes. The new modes are flow-cycled assist-control, flow-cycled SIMV, flow-cycled SIMV plus pressure support ventilation (PSV), and PSV only. All of the new modes provide flow-triggered and flow-cycled breaths. With these additions, the clinician may elect to operate ventilator in assist-control or SIMV with or without breath termination by flow-cycling. When a flow-cycled mode is selected, the switchover from inspiration to expiration occurs at a fixed 10% of peak flow. The operator cannot alter the percentage of peak flow at which cycling occurs.

Pressure support ventilation is available on the model 750psv either combined with SIMV breaths or as a separate mode. When PSV and SIMV are used together, the inspiratory pressure cannot be set independently. Therefore the inspiratory pressure for both mandatory breaths and pressure support breaths are set by the single INSPIRATORY PRESSURE control.

Specifications for the Bear Cub 750psv are listed in Table 13-6.

Infrasonics Infant Star Ventilators

There are three versions of the Infrasonics Infant Star ventilator: the original version, the Infrasonics Infant Star 500, and the Infant Star 950. The original version was available as either a conventional ventilator or as a conventional ventilator with high-frequency ventilation. The Infant Star 500 is an updated version of the original but is available as a conventional ventilator only. The Infant Star 950 offers all of the features of the 500, but also incorporates high-frequency ventilation. All can be used with the optional Star Sync, which allows patient triggering of IMV breaths.

The Infrasonics Infant Star Neonatal Ventilator (Original Model)

Overview

The original Infant Star (Figure 13-10, A) is electrically and pneumatically powered and microprocessor controlled. It is time-triggered and time-cycled with pressure limiting. The ventilator is designed to provide either continuous flow or continuous plus demand flow.[12] The ventilator's pneumatic components are housed in a separate case making up the base of the unit. Sitting on top is the electrical module with all of the ventilator's electronic controls and indicators. This module rotates to permit it to be viewed from different angles.

Either AC power or an external battery can be used to power the ventilator. When the ventilator is connected to AC power, the battery is being recharged. A battery will be completely recharged in 1 to 1.5 hours. A fully charged battery will power the ventilator for approximately 30 minutes.

Compressed air and oxygen are required for the Infant Star's operation. These gases are blended and reduced to a 18 psig pressure source, which drives a series of solenoid valves to control gas flow to the patient. These solenoid valves work together to provide flow in 2 L/min increments from 2 to 16 L/min for spontaneous breathing and from 4 to 40 L/min for mandatory breaths. These flow limits allow the ventilator to be used in infants weighing up to 10 Kg.[13]

High-frequency ventilation is an optional feature on the original Infant Star ventilator. Those units fitted with this option operate similarly to the Infant Star 950 (described later in this section).

Controls

Mode Selector

Using the four-position MODE SELECTOR switch, the clinician can select IMV or CPAP with either continuous or demand flow. When selecting CONTINUOUS FLOW, the set flow is delivered through the circuit during both a mandatory breath and a spontaneous breath. During spontaneous breathing, if pressure within the patient circuit drops below 1 cm H_2O of the set PEEP/ CPAP level, flow is increased in 2 L/min increments. This enables the clinician to select low flows without limiting the patient's inspiratory flow demand. When selecting DEMAND FLOW, a background flow of 4 L/min is delivered continuously during spontaneous respiration. With DEMAND FLOW, if pressure within the patient circuit drops below 1 cm H_2O of the set PEEP/CPAP level during spontaneous breathing, flow will increase in 2 L/min increments. When set in the IMV mode with DEMAND FLOW, mandatory breaths are delivered at the set flow.

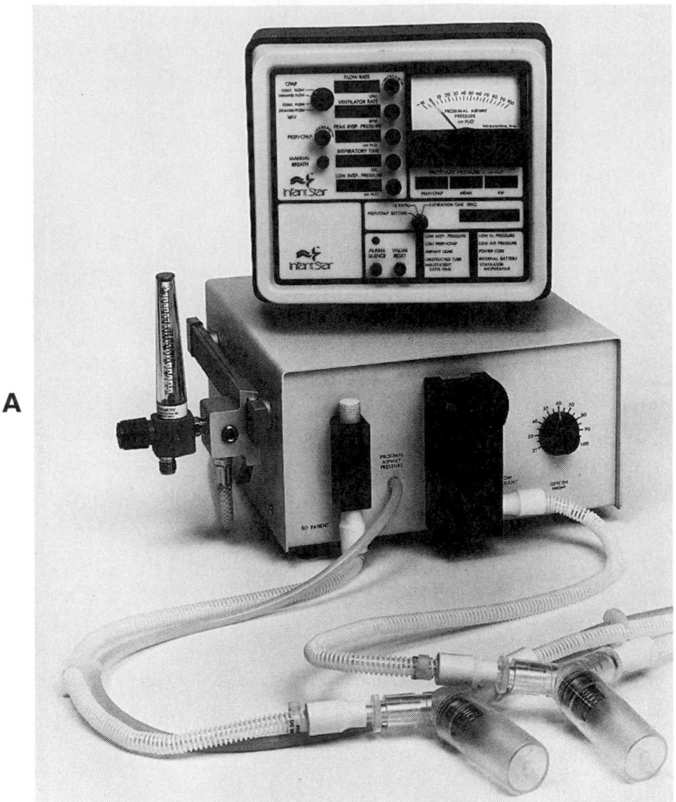

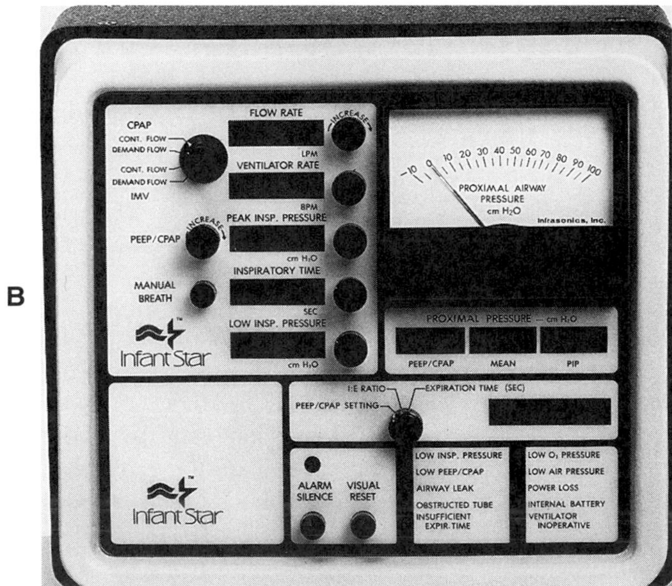

Figure 13-10 **A,** Infant Star Ventilator; **B,** control panel of an Infant Star Neonatal Ventilator. (Courtesy Puritan Bennett, a division of Tyco Medical, Pleasanton, Calif.)

PEEP/CPAP

PEEP/CPAP is adjustable from 0 to 24 cm H_2O. Turning this control knob clockwise increases the pressure within the exhalation valve diaphragm that opposes flow from the expiratory limb of the patient circuit. The set PEEP/CPAP level is read from the lower digital display with the knob on the left turned to PEEP/CPAP SETTING. Monitored PEEP/CPAP is displayed in the "PEEP/CPAP" monitoring window, in the SELECTED DATA window ("PEEP/CPAP" setting), and by the PROXIMAL AIRWAY PRESSURE analog meter.

Manual Breath

The MANUAL BREATH control knob is located beneath the PEEP/CPAP control. When depressed, this button delivers a single breath at the set PIP, flow, and inspiratory time.

Flow Rate

The FLOW RATE control knob is located at the top and to the left of the proximal airway pressure meter. Adjusting this knob clockwise increases flow from 4 to 40 L/min. Flow is digitally displayed in the window to the left of the control. During a mandatory breath, the ventilator delivers the set flow. However, during spontaneous breathing, a maximum flow of 16 L/min is available to the patient regardless of the flow setting. This is true even if the flow setting is greater than 16 L/min. When the ventilator is operating in the IMV mode with continuous flow, the set flow reflects the actual flow when set between 4 and 16 L/min. However, at any point during a mandatory breath, the patient can override the set flow to the maximum 16 L/min.

PIP and Mean Airway Pressure

PEAK INSPIRATORY PRESSURE (PIP) is adjustable from 8 to 90 cm H_2O by turning the control knob clockwise. The set PIP is displayed in the window to the left of the knob. Monitored PIP is displayed in both the PIP PRESSURE monitoring window and the PROXIMAL AIRWAY PRESSURE analog meter. Proximal airway pressure is monitored by an electrical pressure transducer that is connected by tubing directly to the patient Y connector.

At the beginning of a mandatory breath, the exhalation valve closes and the set flow is delivered. After proximal airway pressure almost reaches the set PIP, the ventilator's microprocessor begins to reduce flow. If PIP is reached, flow will stop completely and the exhalation valve will remain closed until the set inspiratory time lapses. If a leak is present, one or more solenoid valves will deliver a flow of gas sufficient to maintain the desired PIP for the full duration of the inspiratory time.

Mean airway pressure is displayed in the MEAN PRESSURE monitoring window. The microprocessor recalculates mean airway pressure every second and updates the visual display every five seconds.

Ventilator Rate, Inspiratory Time, and I:E Ratio

Adjusting the VENTILATOR RATE control knob clockwise increases the mandatory breath rate from 1 to 150 breaths/minute. The ventilator rate is digitally displayed in the window to the left of the control knob. Below this control is the INSPIRATORY TIME control. Adjusting this knob clockwise increases the inspiratory time from 0.1 to

3.0 seconds. The inspiratory time is digitally displayed in the window to the left of this knob. I:E ratio is determined by the ventilator rate and inspiratory time. Digital displays of I:E ratio and expiratory time can be monitored using the SELECTED DATA switch at the lower center of the control panel. Although inverse I:E ratios are attainable, the ventilator's microprocessor does not permit expiratory time to be less than 0.2 to 0.3 seconds, depending on the rate control setting (see the discussion of alarms).

Alarms

Alarm Silence/Visual Reset

The ALARM SILENCE button will silence the audible alarm for 60 seconds. Pressing the button a second time will cancel the silence period. An indicator light will illuminate during the silence period. After alarm conditions are corrected, the audible alarm will stop sounding. Visual alarms will continue to be displayed until the VISUAL RESET button is pressed.

Low Inspiratory Pressure

Adjustable from 0 to 60 cm H_2O, the LOW INSPIRATORY PRESSURE audible/visual alarm is set at or slightly below the PIP setting. Should a leak develop in the ventilator circuit or the ventilator fail to deliver the desired PIP, this alarm will be activated. Each breath not reaching this setting will trigger the alarm. When the alarm condition is corrected, the audible alarm will terminate.

Low PEEP/CPAP

The LOW PEEP/CPAP alarm is not adjustable by the operator, but rather is set automatically by the microprocessor. If the measured PEEP or CPAP is less than the set level for a 25-second period, this audible/visual alarm will be triggered. The difference between set and measured pressure that triggers the alarm varies with the PEEP/CPAP setting. Those pressure differences are listed in Table 13-7. It is important to note that the low PEEP/CPAP alarm may not be activated in the presence of an accidental extubation. This is because back pressure produced by endotracheal tube resistance may prevent a difference between measured and set PEEP/CPAP levels sufficient to trigger an alarm.

Table 13-7 Difference in Set/Measured Pressure Difference Triggering a Low PEEP/CPAP Alarm in the Infant Star Ventilator

PEEP/CPAP Setting (cm H_2O)	Set/Measured Pressure Difference That Triggers Low PEEP/CPAP Alarm (cm H_2O)
0-5	2
6-8	3
9-12	4
13-24	5

Airway Leak

A circuit leak that drops PEEP and activates demand flow may trigger the AIRWAY LEAK alarm. This alarm system can detect a leak smaller than one that would trigger the LOW PEEP/CPAP alarm. Specifically, the AIRWAY LEAK alarm is activated if the leak is large enough to decrease the PEEP by 1 cm H_2O and cause the demand flow to increase 8 L/min or more above background flow for 4 seconds or longer. Some ventilators automatically detect and compensate for sizeable leaks by increasing circuit flow. This feature is most useful in ventilator applications involving small, uncuffed artificial airways. Although the Infant Star compensates for leaks, it determines a large leak greater than 8 L/min as an alarm condition that must be corrected to eliminate the alarm condition.

Obstructed Tube Alarms

If obstructions occur in the inspiratory or expiratory limbs of the ventilator circuit, audible and visual alarms are triggered. Also, a message is displayed. For all of these alarms, the OBSTRUCTED TUBE LED will flash.

If proximal airway pressure rises to 5 cm H_2O above set PIP, inspiration will immediately terminate. An "AO1" visual alarm condition will occur. The message "HI-PP-AO1" will appear in the monitoring window, and the yellow OBSTRUCTED TUBE LED will flash. If proximal airway pressure rises to 10 cm H_2O above set PIP, inspiration will immediately terminate and an "AO2" alarm condition will occur. The exhalation valve and an internal safety valve will open allowing the patient to breathe from room air. A digital display "HI-PP-AO2" will appear in the monitoring window accompanied by an audible alarm.

If the expiratory tubing becomes blocked, an "AO3" alarm will result. Normally, when the exhalation valve opens, pressure must fall to one half the difference between PIP and PEEP settings within 200 milliseconds. If this does not occur, the flow solenoid valves will close and the internal safety valve will open. "HI-PP-AO3" will be displayed and an audible alarm will sound.

An "AO4" visual and audible alarm will occur if proximal airway pressure exceeds the set PEEP/CPAP level by ≥ 6 cm H_2O for 5 seconds. When this occurs, the flow solenoid valves will close and the internal safety valve will open. The message "HI-CP-AO4" will be displayed.

If pressure within the ventilator circuit rises to 15 cm H_2O above set PIP, an "AO5" audible/visual alarm results. This alarm condition is determined by the internal pressure transducer rather than the proximal airway pressure transducer. Therefore, it can occur even when the proximal airway pressure tubing is blocked or disconnected. The exhalation valve and the internal safety valve will open.

For all of the above alarm conditions, the visual or audio/visual alarms will continue until the next mandatory breath. If conditions causing the alarm are corrected, the ventilator will resume normal operation. The message display and the audible alarms will also terminate.

Insufficient Expiratory Time

An audible and visual alarm indicating insufficient expiratory time will be activated when combined ventilator settings prevent in expiratory time of 0.2 or 0.3 seconds. When the rate setting is greater than 100 breaths/min and the inspiratory time is set so that expiratory time is less than 0.2 seconds, the alarm will be activated. If the rate is set below 100 breaths/min but the inspiratory time is set so that expiratory time is less than 0.3 seconds, the alarm will also be activated. In this alarm condition, inspiration will terminate earlier than the set time. After the alarm condition is corrected, the ventilator will resume normal operation. The yellow INSUFFICIENT EXPIRATORY TIME indicator will flash until the VISUAL RESET button is pressed.

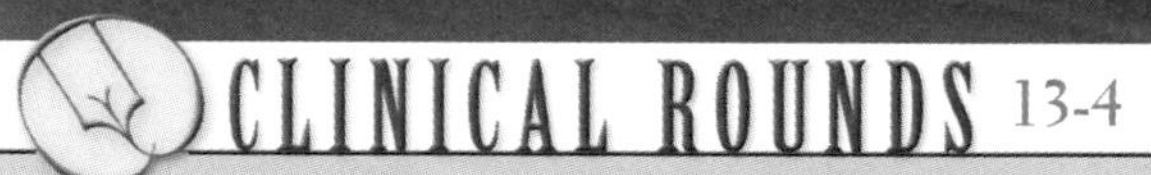

A spontaneously breathing infant is receiving assistance via the original Infant Star ventilator during transport from one unit to another. An audible ventilator alarm sounds. The Power Loss and Internal Battery LEDs are flashing. A few minutes later the ventilator stops operating.

I. What is the cause of the problem?

II. Can the infant breathe room air through the ventilator?

III. What should the therapist do immediately?

See Appendix A for the answer.

Box 13-4 Using the External Pressure Limit as the Primary Inspiratory Pressure, or PIP Control

Some clinicians advocate using the external pressure control limit on the Infant Star as the primary pressure control in certain situations. For example, when a small-volume nebulizer is placed in line, the additional flow can increase system pressure and activate an A04 alarm. Some clinicians also recommend setting the PIP with the external pressure limit in patients who cough frequently or may have a tendency to periodically fight the ventilator.

If the external pressure limit is used to establish the baseline PIP, the ventilator's inspiratory pressure control should be set 5 to 10 cm H_2O higher as a safety limit.

Low Oxygen Pressure or Low Air Pressure

If either compressed gas pressure drops below 40 psig, the LOW OXYGEN PRESSURE or LOW AIR PRESSURE alarm is activated. An audible alarm will sound and the yellow LOW OXYGEN PRESSURE or LOW AIR PRESSURE LED will flash. The ventilator will continue to operate if only one gas source pressure drops, but F_IO_2 will vary. However, if both pressures drop, the internal safety valve will open.

Power Loss

The ventilator can be operated by an internal battery that will last 30 minutes when fully charged. At 5 to 10 minutes before complete battery discharge, the POWER LOSS and INTERNAL BATTERY LEDs will begin flashing. The audible alarm will also sound. When the battery becomes fully discharged, the ventilator will stop operating and the exhalation valve and internal safety valve will open. Audible and visual alarms will continue (Clinical Rounds 13-4).

Table 13-8 Specifications for Infant Star Neonatal Ventilator

Control Setting	Range
Rate	1 to 150 breaths per minute
Flow Rate	4 to 40 L/min
Peak Inspiratory Pressure	8 to 90 cm H_2O
Inspiratory Time	0.1 to 3.0 seconds
PEEP/CPAP	0 to 24 cm H_2O
Oxygen Percent	21% to 100%
Monitors/Displays	I:E Ratio, Expiratory Time, Monitored PEEP/CPAP, Mean Airway Pressure, Measured Peak Inspiratory Pressure
ALARMS	
Airway Leak	
Low Inspiratory Pressure	0 to 60 cm H_2O
Low PEEP/CPAP	Varies with set PEEP/CPAP (see text)
Obstructed Tube Conditions	A01 to A05 (see text)
Insufficient Expiratory Time	<0.2 to 0.3 seconds
Low Oxygen Inlet Pressure	<40 psig
Low Air Inlet Pressure	<40 psig
Power Loss	5 to 10 minutes of battery use left
Ventilator Inoperative Conditions	Various causes (see text)
Alarm Intensity	Rotary baffle
Alarm Silence	60 seconds
Alarm Silence	60 seconds

Internal Battery

When the ventilator is turned on but not connected to an A/C power source, the internal battery will automatically power the ventilator for up to 30 minutes. The visual yellow LED will light up while the unit is operating on the internal battery. No audible alarm will sound until the battery approaches full discharge (Clinical Rounds 13-4).

Ventilator Inoperative

When the audible/visual VENTILATOR INOPERATIVE alarm is activated, flow through the solenoid valves will stop and the internal safety valve will open. This alarm condition will occur if at least one of the following is present:

1. The exhalation valve does not open for 3.5 seconds.
2. The exhalation valve does not close for 66 seconds in the IMV mode
3. The microprocessor fails

Safety Relief Valve

A spring-loaded PRESSURE RELIEF VALVE is located at the ventilator outlet. When the pressure set by this valve is reached, excess gas will be vented to the atmosphere. Turning the valve clockwise increases relief pressure. This valve is intended to be used as a back-up safety valve in case the primary PIP control and the high-pressure alarm system were to fail. Normally the SAFETY RELIEF VALVE is set to at least 13 cm H_2O above the desired PIP. Exceptions to the way the valve is normally used are discussed in Box 13-4.

Additional Features

The original Infant Star incorporates additional features to enhance its operation. Alarm loudness can be adjusted using a rotary baffle on the unit's back panel. Although the ventilator does not incorporate a graphics monitor, an analog pressure output cable outlet permits connection to an oscilloscope, or strip chart, recorder. A serial output connector enables connection to a computer or cardiac monitor.

Connections are also available to add an external DC power source, a remote alarm, and the Star Synch interface (described in a section below).

Table 13-8 lists specifications for the Infant Star.

Troubleshooting

The exhalation valve diaphragm on the Infant Star must be turned in the proper direction and seated properly. The housing must be properly assembled and tightened. Circuit leaks are also common. The ventilator can be tight tested according to the manufacturer's instructions. A "Quick Checkout" procedure is also outlined in the ventilator's instruction manual. This should be used before placing the ventilator back into service after cleaning or when optimum performance is questioned.

Infrasonics Infant Star 500 Ventilator

Overview

The Infant Star 500 (Figure 13-11) is electrically and pneumatically powered. All of the ventilator's functions are controlled by dual microprocessors. One controls all of the unit's operations and the other controls display information. Continuous operational checks between the two microprocessors assure more dependable operation.[13] As with the original model, the ventilator's pneumatic components are housed in an updated case making up the base of the unit. Sitting on top is the electrical component module with all of the ventilator's electronic controls and indicators. This module rotates to permit it to be viewed at different angles.

The model 500 is time-triggered and time-cycled with pressure limiting. The ventilator is designed to provide continuous background flow for spontaneous breathing. This background flow is supplemented by a demand system that will provide additional flow to the patient if required.

The ventilator's power switch is located on the rear panel. Either AC power or an external battery can be used to power the ventilator. A fully discharged external battery will be completely recharged in 1 hour if the ventilator is turned off but connected to electrical power. If the ventilator is turned on, a discharged battery will require 1-½ hours to fully be recharge.

Compressed air and oxygen are required for the Infant Star's operation. These gases are blended and reduced to an 18 psig pressure source, which drives a series of solenoid valves to control gas flow to the patient. These solenoid valves work together to provide flow in 2 L/min increments from 2 to 30 L/min for spontaneous breathing and from 4 to 40 L/min for mandatory breaths. These flow limit ranges differ slightly between software versions. The ventilator may be used in infants weighing up to 18 Kg.

A standard infant circuit and approved humidifier can be used with the Infant Star 500.

Controls

The front panel (see Figure 13-12) is organized into three sections from left to right: (1) the ALARM STATUS section, (2) the VENTILATOR SETTINGS section, and (3) the PATIENT MONITORING section. Each of these sections will be discussed.

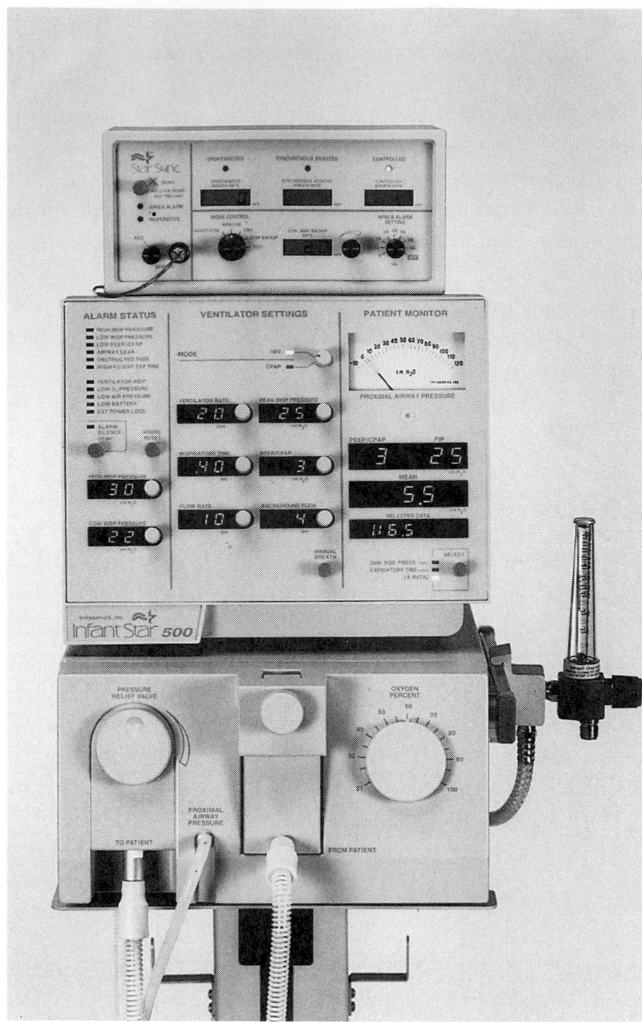

Figure 13-11 The Infrasonics Infant Star 500 Neonatal Ventilator. (Courtesy Puritan Bennett, a division of Tyco Medical, Pleasanton, Calif.)

Alarm Status Section

The ALARM STATUS section features visual LED indicators that illuminate in red when alarm conditions occur. An audible alarm is also activated for all alarm conditions with the exception "ext power loss." Because the battery automatically begins to power the unit when external power is lost, only a visual indicator is activated. If the battery were discharged, a visual and audible alarm would immediately activate.

The ALARM SILENCE button will silence the audible alarm for 60 seconds. Pressing the button a second time will cancel the silence period. The ALARM SILENCE indicator light will illuminate during the silence period. For certain alarm conditions, such as electrical and internal function failures, the audible alarm cannot be silenced.

After alarm conditions are corrected, the audible alarm will stop sounding. The LED corresponding to the alarm will continue to be lit after alarm conditions are corrected until the VISUAL RESET button is pressed.

High Inspiratory Pressure

The HIGH INSPIRATORY PRESSURE alarm is activated when the PIP exceeds a set limit. This limit can be adjusted from 5 to 105 cm H_2O using the HIGH INSPIRATORY PRESSURE control knob. The pressure limit is digitally displayed in the window to the left of the control.

The limit should not be adjusted more than 15 cm H_2O above the PIP set for ventilation. If a limit greater than 15 cm H_2O is selected, the HIGH INSPIRATORY PRESSURE LED will flash and the microprocessor will automatically set the pressure limit to 15 cm H_2O above the set PIP.

When the pressure limit is activated, the exhalation valve will open and the inspiratory phase is terminated (pressure cycled). The message "HI PIP, AO1" will appear in the PEEP/CPAP, PIP and selected data windows in the patient monitor section. The ventilator will attempt to deliver the next breath at the appropriate time interval. It will continue to sound the audible alarm and display the alarm message until the alarm condition is corrected.

Low Inspiratory Pressure

The LOW INSPIRATORY PRESSURE alarm is activated if a set minimum pressure is not reached during the inspiratory phase. This minimum pressure is selected using the LOW INSPIRATORY PRESSURE control. A digital display of the set low inspiratory pressure appears in the window to the left of the control.

Adjustable from 3 to 60 cm H_2O, the LOW INSPIRATORY PRESSURE setting must be less than the PIP setting. Should a large leak develop in the ventilator circuit or the ventilator fail to deliver the desired PIP, this alarm will be activated. This alarm will also be activated if the low inspiratory pressure control or the pressure relief valve is inappropriately set.

If the LOW INSPIRATORY PRESSURE control knob is turned fully counterclockwise to 3 cm H_2O and the PEEP/CPAP setting is higher, the ventilator will automatically track the PEEP/CPAP level as the minimum inspiratory pressure. The alarm will not be activated unless the PEEP level drops below 3 cm H_2O.

When the LOW INSPIRATORY PRESSURE alarm is activated, the ventilator will continue to deliver the next breath at the appropriate timed interval. Each breath not reaching the low inspiratory pressure setting will trigger the alarm (Clinical Rounds 13-5).

Low PEEP/CPAP

The LOW PEEP/CPAP alarm is not adjustable by the operator but is set automatically by the microprocessor. If the measured PEEP or CPAP is less than the set level for 25-second period, the alarm will be triggered. The difference between set and measured pressure that triggers the alarm varies with the PEEP/CPAP setting. Those pressure differences, which are shown in Table 13-7, are the same as in the original Infant Star.

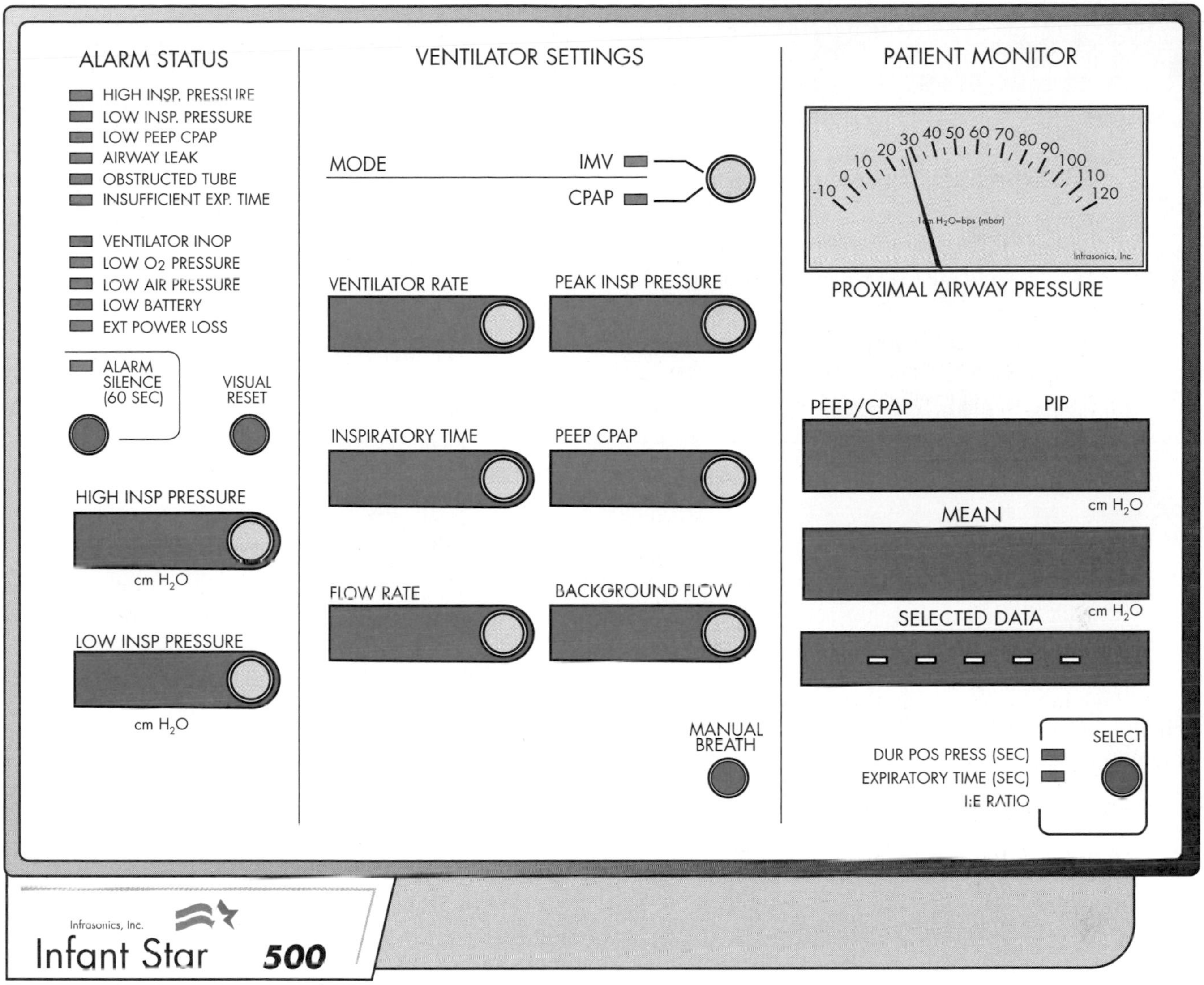

Figure 13-12 The Infrasonics Infant Star 500 Neonatal Ventilator control panel.

Airway Leak

The AIRWAY LEAK alarm is activated when large leaks are detected in the patient circuit when using 3 cm H_2O PEEP or CPAP or greater. Small circuit leaks are automatically compensated for by the ventilator's demand valve in order to maintain set PEEP/CPAP. The valve accomplishes this by adding a compensatory flow called "leak makeup." However, if this compensatory flow were to reach 13 L/min above the background flow setting for 4 seconds or longer, the AIRWAY LEAK alarm will be activated.

Obstructed Tube

If obstructions occur in the inspiratory or expiratory limbs of the ventilator circuit, the OBSTRUCTED TUBE alarm will be activated. Specifically, the alarm condition will be triggered if any of the following four conditions occur:

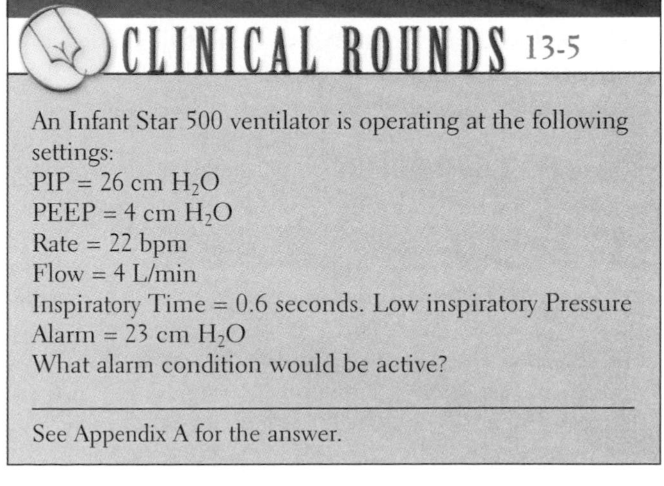

CLINICAL ROUNDS 13-5

An Infant Star 500 ventilator is operating at the following settings:

PIP = 26 cm H_2O
PEEP = 4 cm H_2O
Rate = 22 bpm
Flow = 4 L/min
Inspiratory Time = 0.6 seconds. Low inspiratory Pressure Alarm = 23 cm H_2O
What alarm condition would be active?

See Appendix A for the answer.

Table 13-9 Message Displayed for Obstructed Tube Alarm, Infant Star 500

Message	Problem
HI PIP, A02	Proximal airway pressure is 5 cm H_2O above high inspiratory pressure setting
HI PIP, A03	Less than 50% pressure drop from PIP to PEEP during expiration
HI CPP, A04	PEEP/CPAP is 6 cm H_2O higher than set for 5 seconds
HI PIP, A05	PIP at the outlet of the ventilator is 10 cm H_2O greater than high inspiratory pressure setting

1. Proximal airway pressure rises to 5 cm H_2O above the high inspiratory pressure setting
2. PEEP/CPAP rises above the set level
3. Partial or complete obstruction of the expiratory circuit
4. Internal pressure reading is 10 cm H_2O higher than high inspiratory pressure setting

When the OBSTRUCTED TUBE alarm is activated, one of four messages is displayed in the selected data window to alert the clinician to the reason for the alarm (Table 13-9).

For all of the OBSTRUCTED TUBE alarm conditions, either the exhalation valve or the internal safety valve will open. The audible alarm will continue until the next mandatory breath. If conditions causing the alarm are corrected, the ventilator will resume normal operation. The message display and the audible alarms will also stop.

Insufficient Expiratory Time

The INSUFFICIENT EXPIRATORY TIME alarm will be activated when combined ventilator settings prevent an expiratory time of 0.2 or 0.3 seconds. When the rate setting is greater than 100 breaths/min and the inspiratory time is set so that expiratory time is less than 0.2 seconds, the alarm will be activated. If the rate is set below 100 breaths/min but the inspiratory time is set so that expiratory time is less than 0.3 seconds, the alarm will also be activated. Until this alarm condition is corrected, the ventilator rate will decrease to permit sufficient expiratory time. The VENTILATOR RATE display will flash, indicating that the set rate is not the actual rate (Clinical Rounds 13-6).

Ventilator Inoperative

The VENTILATOR INOP alarm is activated when either microprocessor detects an electronics error. With this alarm condition, mandatory breath delivery stops, gas flow stops, and the internal safety valve opens. Spontaneous breathing of room air is possible through the internal safety valve. The audible portion of the alarm cannot be silenced.

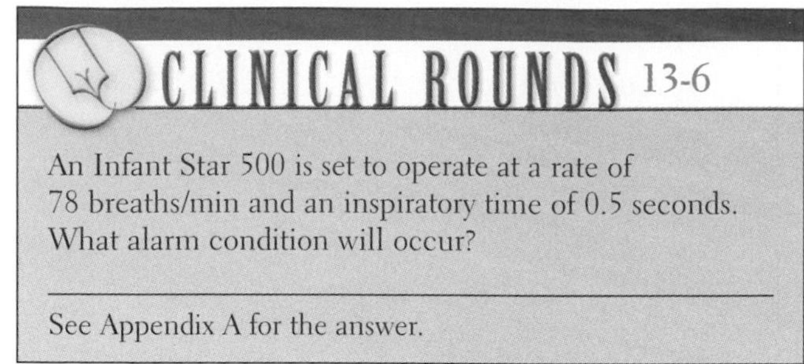

CLINICAL ROUNDS 13-6
An Infant Star 500 is set to operate at a rate of 78 breaths/min and an inspiratory time of 0.5 seconds. What alarm condition will occur?
See Appendix A for the answer.

When a VENTILATOR INOP alarm condition occurs, an error message will appear in the selected data window. The operator must be sure the patient has another means of ventilation. The message is a code that may be useful to service personnel. Before turning off the ventilator, the clinician should record this code.

Low O_2 Pressure

The LOW O_2 PRESSURE alarm will be activated if oxygen line pressure drops below 35 psig. When the alarm is activated, the ventilator will continue operating but will deliver 21% oxygen. However, if the oxygen concentration is set above 80%, ventilator performance may be impaired.

Low Air Pressure

The LOW AIR PRESSURE alarm will be activated if the compressed air line pressure drops below 35 psig. When the alarm is activated, the ventilator will continue operating but will deliver 100% oxygen. However, if the oxygen concentration is set below 30%, ventilator performance may be impaired.

Low Battery

When the ventilator is turned on but not connected to an A/C power source, the internal battery will automatically power the ventilator for at least 30 minutes. When the battery is 5 to 10 minutes from complete discharge, the low battery and external power loss indicators will begin to flash alternately. The audible alarm will sound, and it cannot be silenced.

When the battery completely discharges, the VENTILATOR INOP and LOW BATTERY indicators will light up and the audible alarm will sound. Once again, the audible alarm cannot be silenced. Mandatory breath and gas flow delivery will stop and the internal safety valve will open. Room air will be available to the patient for spontaneous breathing through the safety valve.

External Power Loss

If electrical power is interrupted, the EXT POWER LOSS LED will light up. However the ventilator will continue to be operated by the internal battery. No other alarms will be activated and no audible alarm will sound until the battery is almost discharged.

Ventilator Settings Section

The ventilator settings section includes all of the unit's operational controls. Each setting is digitally displayed using green LEDs in a window to the left of the control.

Mode Selector

Modes on the Infant Star 500 are set using the two position MODE SELECTOR switch. Either IMV or CPAP are available. Green LEDs indicate the mode selected.

When using the CPAP mode, only the BACKGROUND FLOW and PEEP/CPAP controls are operational. The other controls should be set to back-up settings in case manual breaths are given or ventilation in the IMV mode becomes necessary.

Ventilator Rate

Adjusting the VENTILATOR RATE control knob clockwise increases the mandatory breath rate from 1 to 150 breaths/min Adjustments can be made in increments of one breath to a rate of 60 breaths/min. From 60 to 130 breaths/min, adjustments can be made in two breath increments. For rates from 130 to 150, the maximum rate, only five breath increments are possible.

Inspiratory Time and Flow Rate

The INSPIRATORY TIME control knob, when turned clockwise, increases the inspiratory time from 0.1 to 3.0 seconds. The inspiratory time is adjustable in 0.01 second increments from 0.10 to 0.60 seconds. From 0.60 to 1.0 seconds, the control is adjustable in 0.02 second increments. For inspiratory times from 1.0 to 3.0 seconds, the control is adjustable in 0.1 second increments.

I:E ratio is determined by the ventilator rate and inspiratory time. Although inverse I:E ratios are attainable, the ventilator's microprocessor does not permit expiratory time to be less than 0.2 to 0.3 seconds (see alarm status section).

Adjusting the FLOW RATE control knob clockwise increases flow delivered during mandatory breaths from 4 to 40 L/min. This flow is adjustable in 2 L/min increments.

PIP

PEAK INSPIRATORY PRESSURE is adjustable from 5 to 90 cm H_2O by turning the control clockwise. If the control is not adjusted to at least 5 cm H_2O above the PEEP/CPAP setting, the PIP display to the left of the control will flash.

At the beginning of a mandatory inspiration, the exhalation valve closes and the set flow is delivered. When proximal airway pressure almost reaches the set PIP, the ventilator's microprocessor begins to reduce flow until it stops. If PIP is reached, flow will stop completely and the exhalation valve will remain closed until set inspiratory time lapses. If a leak or spontaneous breathing is present, one or more solenoid valves will deliver a flow of gas sufficient to maintain PIP over the inspiratory time.

PEEP/CPAP

PEEP/CPAP is adjustable from 0 to 24 cm H_2O. Turning this control knob clockwise increases the pressure within the exhalation valve diaphragm which opposes flow from the expiratory limb of the patient circuit.

After suctioning procedures or major changes in control settings, the measured PEEP/CPAP may be 2 to 3 cm H_2O above or below the set level. This also may occur after disconnecting and reconnecting the patient to the ventilator. Approximately 30 seconds is required for the pressure to stabilize.

Background Flow

The BACKGROUND FLOW control knob sets the flow available for spontaneous breathing in both CPAP and IMV modes. Turning this knob clockwise adjusts flow from 2 to 30 L/min in 2 L/min increments. If patient flow demand or a leak reduces PEEP/CPAP by 1 cm H_2O, the demand system will automatically provide additional flow up to 40 L/min.

The BACKGROUND FLOW control knob sets flow independently to that selected for the mandatory inspiratory phase. This control enables the clinician to minimize circuit PEEP, or the amount of back pressure that develops in the ventilator circuit because of gas flow. In many cases, flow sufficient for spontaneous breathing needs can be set significantly lower than the flow necessary for a mandatory breath.

Manual Breath

The MANUAL BREATH button delivers a single breath at the set PIP and inspiratory time. The button is operational in both IMV and CPAP modes.

Patient Monitor Section

The PATIENT MONITOR section of the Infant Star 500 front panel displays all monitored data in amber LEDs. A PROXIMAL AIRWAY PRESSURE manometer also displays dynamic airway pressures. Airway pressure is transmitted to the ventilator's pressure monitoring transducer by tubing connected directly to the patient Y connector. Fixed digital displays show monitored levels of PEEP/CPAP, PIP, and mean airway pressure. The PEEP/CPAP level is measured every 10 milliseconds and is updated every 200 milliseconds. The PIP is updated every breath. Mean airway pressure is measured every 5 milliseconds and is updated every 200 milliseconds.

A SELECTED DATA window digitally displays a choice of three additional data. By pushing the SELECT button, the clinician can toggle between the data choices, indicated by LEDs and displayed in the window. The DUR POS PRESS display indicates the amount of time the proximal airway pressure exceeds 1 cm H_2O during a mandatory breath. The EXPIRATION TIME display indicates the duration of the expiratory phase in seconds. The I:E RATIO display shows the relationship of the inspiratory phase to the expiratory phase. The inspiratory phase is always expressed

Table 13-10 Specifications for Infant Star 500 and 950 Infant Ventilators

Control Setting	Range
Rate	1 to 150 breaths per minute
Inspiratory Time	0.1 to 3.0 seconds
Inspiratory Flow	4 to 40 L/min
Background Flow	2 to 30 L/min
Rate	1 to 150 breaths per minute
Oxygen Concentration	21% to 100%
Pressure Limit	5 to 90 cm H_2O
PEEP/CPAP	0 to 24 cm H_2O
Alarms	High Inspiratory Pressure, Low Inspiratory Pressure, Low PEEP/CPAP, Airway Leak, Obstructed Tube Conditions (see text), Insufficient Expiratory Time, Ventilator Inoperative, Low O_2 Pressure, Low Air Pressure, Low Battery, External Power Loss
Monitors	I:E Ratio, Expiratory Time, Monitored PEEP/CPAP, Mean Airway Pressure, Measured Peak Inspiratory Pressure
Alarm Silence	60 seconds
Audiovisual Alarms	Low PEEP/CPAP, High Breath Rate, Low Inspiratory Pressure, High Pressure Limit, Failed to Cycle, Low Gas Supply, Patient Circuit, Prolonged Inspiratory Pressure, Settings Incompatible, Pressure Settings Incompatible, Flow Sensor, Apnea, Low Battery
Monitors	Breath Rate, Breath Type (Patient Initiated), Minute Volume, Tidal Volume (Exhaled), % Tube Leak, Inspiratory Time, Expiratory Time, I:E Ratio, Peak Inspiratory Pressure, Mean Airway Pressure, Air Pressure, O_2 Pressure, Proximal Airway Pressure, Hourmeter, Test, Battery
Alarm Silence	60 seconds
HIGH FREQUENCY VENTILATION (MODEL 950 ONLY)	
HFV Rate	2 to 22 Hertz
Amplitude (oscillatory pulse flow)	12 to 120 L/min

as 1, whereas the expiratory phase is expressed in whole numbers and/or decimals. The expiratory phase is expressed in tenths of seconds for inverse relationships.

Safety Relief Valve

A spring-load PRESSURE RELIEF VALVE is located at the ventilator outlet. When the pressure set by this valve is reached, excess gas will be vented to the atmosphere. Turning the valve clockwise increases relief pressure. Adjustable from 5 to 120 cm H_2O, this valve is intended to be used as a back-up safety valve in case the primary PIP control and the high pressure alarm system fail.

Additional Features

The Infant Star 500 incorporates an additional feature to enhance its operation. The unit's exhalation valve assembly, called the EXHALATION BLOCK, is heated to 60° C. This minimizes condensation.

Alarm loudness can be adjusted using a rotary baffle on the unit's back panel. Loudness can be regulated from approximately 72 to 88 decibels.

Although the model 500 does not incorporate a graphics monitor, an analog pressure output cable outlet permits connection to an oscilloscope or strip chart recorder. A serial output connector enables connection to a computer or cardiac monitor. Ventilator settings and pressures can then be displayed in a central location with other patient data.

Connections are also available to add an external DC power source, a remote alarm, and the Star Synch, explained in a section later in this chapter.

Specifications for the Infant Star 500 are included in Table 13-10.

Troubleshooting

To avoid system leaks, the exhalation valve must be assembled properly and tightened. Circuit leaks will trigger low PEEP/CPAP and AIRWAY LEAK alarms. More complex troubleshooting problems are addressed in the ventilator's instruction manual.

Infrasonics Infant Star 950 Ventilator

The Infrasonics Infant Star 950 ventilator (Figure 13-13) is almost identical in design to the model 500. However, this model incorporates high-frequency ventilation, which can be used with or without conventional ventilation. Internally the two models differ only in the high-frequency components. Because the model 950's alarms, controls, and monitors are

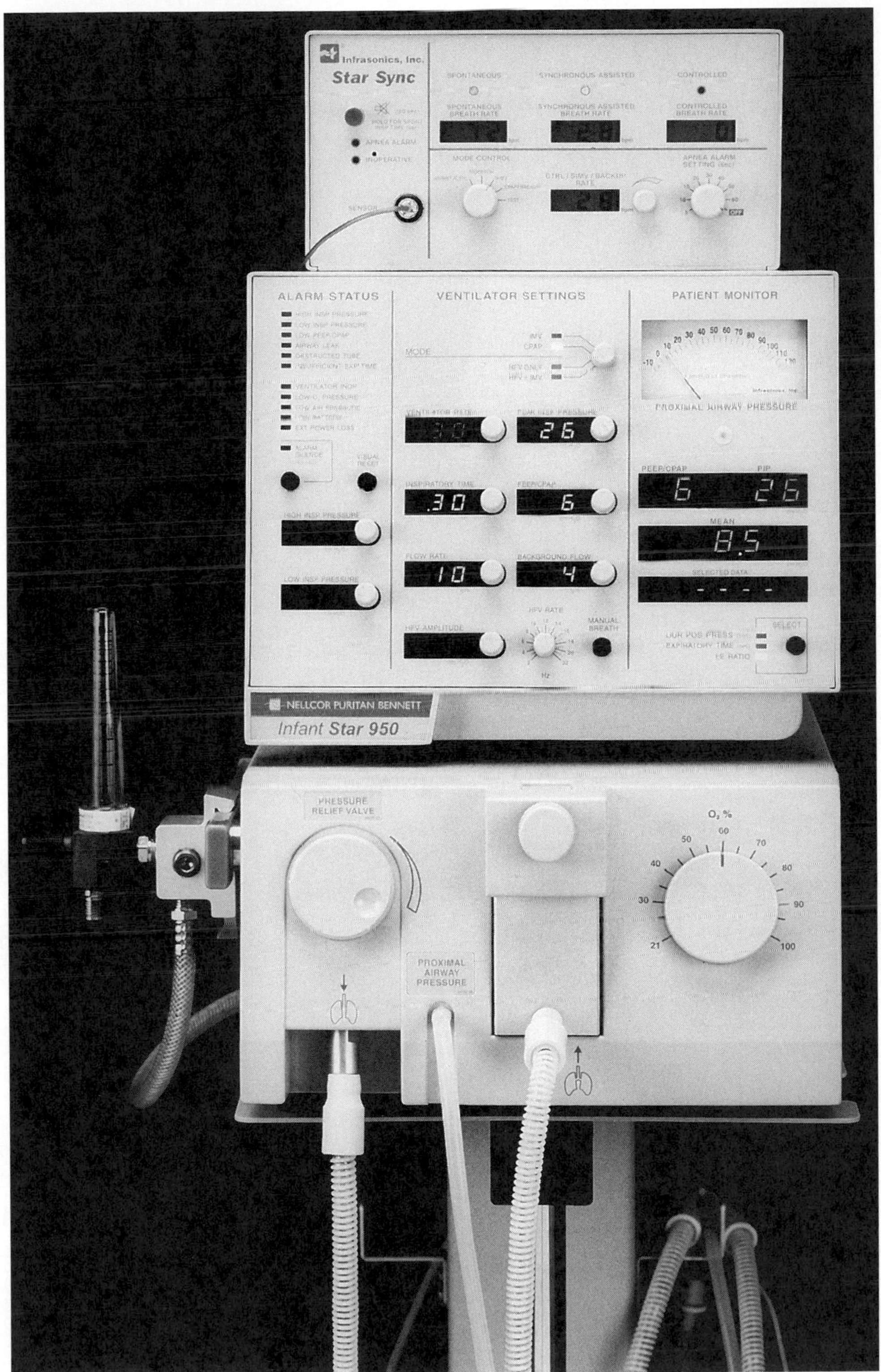

Figure 13-13 The Infrasonics Infant Star 950 Ventilator and Star Synch module. (Courtesy Nellcor Puritan Bennett, a division of Tyco Healthcare, Pleasanton, Calif.)

similar to those found on the model 500, only the differences between the two units will be discussed in this section.

Minimum compressed oxygen and air pressure for the Infant Star 950 is 45 psig rather than 35 psig for the model 500. Higher pressures are required to meet the additional gas flow demands of the high-frequency system.[14]

Standard infant ventilator circuits and humidifiers can be used with the model 950 to provide conventional ventilation. However, if high-frequency ventilation is employed, a reusable Tygon circuit specifically designed for the ventilator is recommended. This circuit minimizes compliance and provides greater **amplitude** to high frequency breaths. Also, a Fisher-Paykel humidifier with a low compressible chamber is recommended. If a continuous water feed system is not used, the chamber should be refilled hourly to its maximum water level mark.

The type of high frequency ventilation provided by the Infant Star 950 is comparable to a **mechanical oscillator,** a device that employs a diaphragm, piston, or plate to move gas bi-directionally. Although the Infant Star 950 also provides bi-directional flow, it is more accurately described as a flow interrupter, which is a type of pneumatic oscillator in which flow abruptly starts and stops at very high rates. The effect of **flow interruption** is the creation of pulses that have the ability to produce pressure swings at the patient's airway. These pressure swings provide the high-frequency amplitude.

Using proportioning valves, the Infant Star 950 delivers high, instantaneous pressure pulses to the inspiratory limb. A jet venturi positioned within the exhalation valve assembly creates a negative pressure. Between the positive pressure pulses and the negative flow from the expiratory limb, an

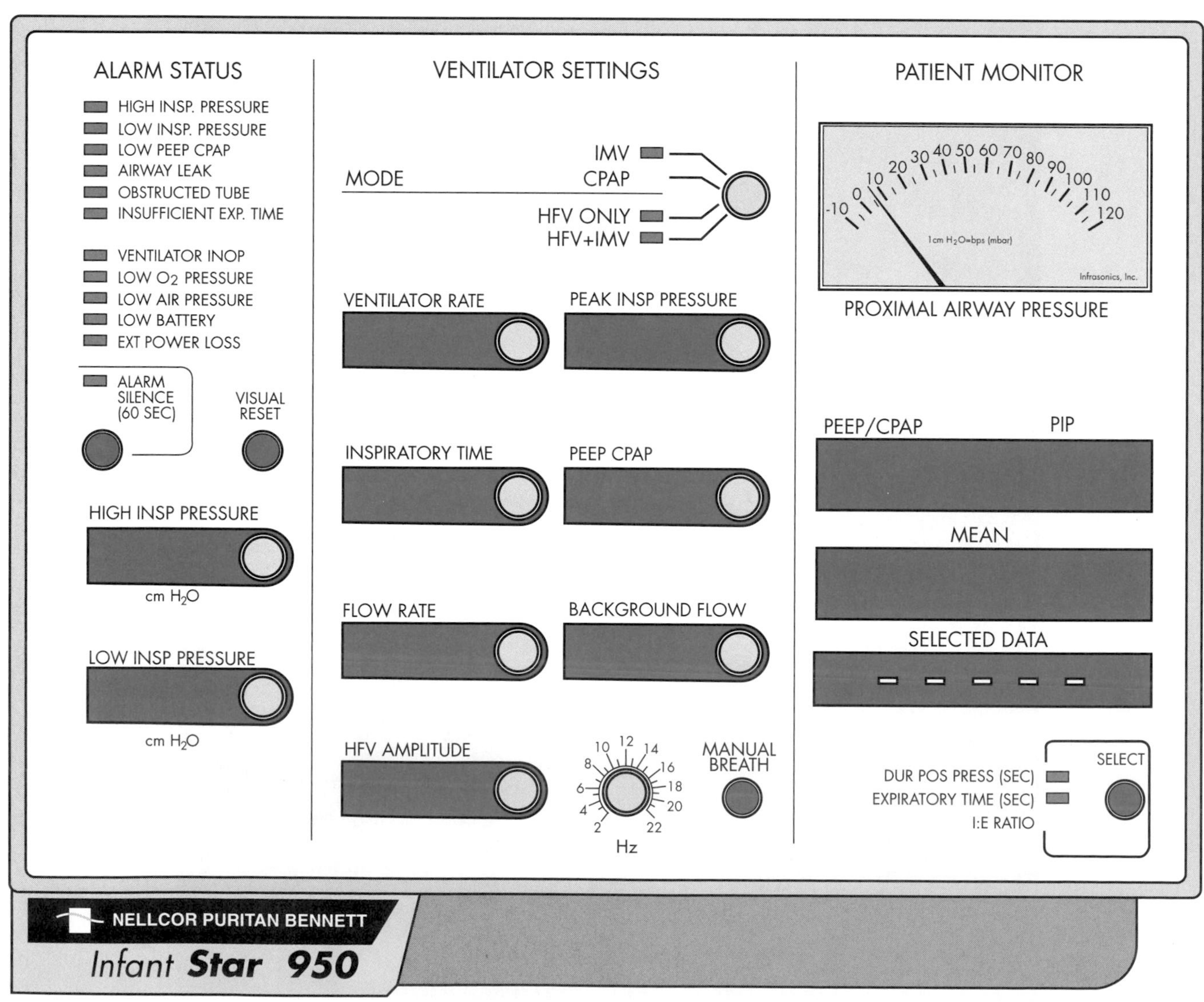

Figure 13-14 The Infrasonics Infant Star 950 Ventilator control panel. (Courtesy Puritan Bennett, a division of Tyco Medical, Pleasanton, Calif.)

"oscillator-like" bi-directional flow of gas is generated at the airway.

Controls

The front control panel (Figure 13-14) is almost identical to that of the Infant Star 500 except that two additional modes are available. Also, controls for AMPLITUDE and FREQUENCY are added. When using high-frequency modes, mean airway pressure is adjusted using the PEEP/CPAP control knob. There are no flow adjustments except for IMV breaths. Other aspects of the ventilator, including the rear panel, are identical to the model 500.

Mode

In addition to IMV and CPAP modes, high-frequency ventilation (HFV) ONLY or "HFV + IMV" can be selected. When in the HFV mode, conventional settings are dimly displayed and are non-functional. Only mean airway pressure (adjusted using the PEEP/CPAP control), F_IO_2, amplitude, and frequency can be adjusted. The MANUAL BREATH button is operational and will deliver a conventional breath at the set flow, inspiratory time, and PIP.

When in the "HFV + IMV" mode, all controls are operative except for BACKGROUND FLOW. The LED display for this control will remain dimly lit. In this mode, high-frequency oscillations will be momentarily interrupted and IMV breaths delivered at the set rate, flow, inspiratory time, and PIP.

HFV Rate and HFV Amplitude

The HFV RATE control knob adjusts the number of oscillations from 2 to 22 **Hertz.** One Hertz is equal to 60 cycles, or breaths, per minute. The HFV AMPLITUDE control varies the pressure of oscillatory pulses, also known as oscillatory pulse pressure, from 0 to 160 cm H_2O. Although this control is technically a flow control, adjusting it affects the intensity of the pulses. Therefore it alters the ΔP or the change from baseline pressure to peak pressure that occurs with every oscillation. As with other controls, green LED displays indicate control settings.

Specifications for the Infant Star 950 are included in Table 13-10.

Infant Star Synch

Patient triggering of SIMV or assist/control breaths is available through the Infant Star Synch interface, the top module seen in Figure 13-13. This unit, which can be attached to all Infant Star models, consists of the interface module, cable, and a disposable abdominal pillow. Using impedance detection of abdominal movements, the Star Sync system is designed to signal the ventilator to deliver a breath when the patient initiates an inspiratory effort. The module also provides digital display of spontaneous breaths, assisted breaths, unassisted breaths, and spontaneous inspiratory time. An optional time-adjustable alarm for apnea is also incorporated into the system.

Troubleshooting

In addition to the same troubleshooting issues that occur with the Infant Star 500, the clinician should be aware of the effect of water in the circuit when operating the ventilator in the high-frequency mode. Large collections of water affect gas movement and may dampen oscillations. Effects of water condensation of the ventilator are usually seen in undesirable changes in the amplitude reading. The circuit should be checked for condensation before readjusting the amplitude control knob.

Infant Star 100 Neonatal Ventilator

The Infant Star 100 Neonatal Ventilator (Infrasonics, Inc. San Diego, CA) (Figure 13-15) is a time-cycled, pressure-limited, continuous flow ventilator. It is designed for either in hospital or field transport of neonatal and pediatric patients. It is electrically powered with 120 volts AC and pneumatically powered by two external gas sources at 40 to 75 psig. It incorporates a low bleed flow to conserve gas during transport. It also includes an internal rechargeable gel-cell battery that can provide 6 to 8 hours of continuous operation.[15]

Control and Alarm Panel

Figure 13-15 shows a close-up of the control and alarm panel. The CPAP/IMV LOCKING TOGGLE SELECTOR SWITCH is located on the front bottom left panel. The control settings are: INSPIRATORY TIME (0.2 to 3.0 seconds), EXPIRATORY TIME (0.2 to 30 seconds), EXPIRATORY TIME X1/X10 (multiplies expiratory time setting by 1 or 10), FLOW (1 to 15 L/min), PEEP/CPAP (0 to 20 cm H_2O), and PIP (0 to 60 cm H_2O). A proximal airway pressure gauge has a range of –20 to 100 cm H_2O. The inspiratory indicator amber LED illuminates during mandatory inspirations. The MANUAL BREATH button

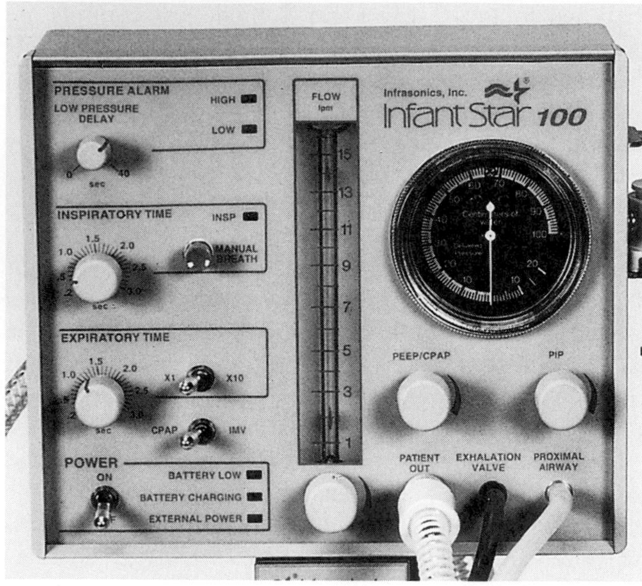

Figure 13-15 The Infant Star 100 Neonatal Ventilator control and alarm panel. (Courtesy Puritan Bennett, a division of Tyco Medical, Pleasanton, Calif.)

delivers a single mandatory breath in both modes. When the manual breath control is activated the breath is based on the peak inspiratory pressure, flow, and inspiratory time settings. Table 13-11 lists parameter specifications for the Infant Star 100 Infant Ventilator.

The locking toggle of the on/off Power switch prevents the unit from being accidentally turned on or off. Adjacent to the power switch are three power indictors. The BATTERY LOW indicator will illuminate and an alarm will sound when the internal battery does not have sufficient power to run the ventilator. The alarm remains active until the ventilator is connected to an external power source. The BATTERY CHARGING indicator lights up when the unit is plugged into an AC power source and remains lit until the battery is fully charged. The internal battery will recharge automatically as long as it is plugged into an AC outlet—even if the ventilator is off. A red EXTERNAL POWER LED indicator is illuminated when the ventilator is supplied with external power.

Alarms

The HIGH PRESSURE ALARM is a nonadjustable alarm with audible and visual indicators. It will activate when proximal airway pressure exceeds 72 to 92 cm H_2O. The LOW PRESSURE ALARM is also preset with audible and visual indicators when proximal airway pressure decreases below 2.5 cm H_2O. The LOW PRESSURE DELAY is adjustable from 0 to 40 seconds.

Table 13-11 Specifications for Infant Star 100 Neonatal Ventilator

Inspiratory time	0.2 to 3.0 seconds
Expiratory time	0.2 to 30 seconds
Flow	1 to 15 L/min
Peak inspiratory pressure	0 to 60 cm H_2O
PEEP/CPAP	0 to 20 cm H_2O
Rate (determined from Ti and Te settings)	2 to 150 bpm
Oxygen concentration	21 to 100%
Trigger mechanism	Time

Optional Low Air-Oxygen Blender

An optional low air-oxygen blender is supplied by external air and oxygen sources at 40 to 70 psig. The blender delivers oxygen concentrations through either the primary or auxiliary gas outlet. The primary gas outlet is the gas source for the ventilator. The auxiliary gas outlet supplies metered low flows (0 to 30 L/min) through a flowmeter. An audible alarm indicates a difference of 30 psig between the two gas sources.

Tracking Relief Pressure Valve

The TRACKING RELIEF PRESSURE VALVE automatically limits airway pressure and is located inside the ventilator. If the set PIP is greater than or equal to 10 cm H_2O, pressure release will occur at 10 to 15 cm H_2O above set PIP. If the set PIP is less than 10 cm H_2O, pressure release will occur at 15 to 20 cm H_2O above set PIP.

Infant Star 200 Neonatal-Pediatric Ventilator

The Infant Star 200 Neonatal-Pediatric Ventilator (Figure 13-16) (Puritan Bennett, a division of Tyco Medical, Pleasanton, CA) is a time-cycled, pressure-limited, continuous flow ventilator. It is electrically powered with 120 volts AC and pneumatically powered by two external gas sources at 40 to 75 psig. SIMV is made available with a 9 pin DIN connector providing communication between the Infant Star 200 and Star Sync Patient Triggered Interface.[16]

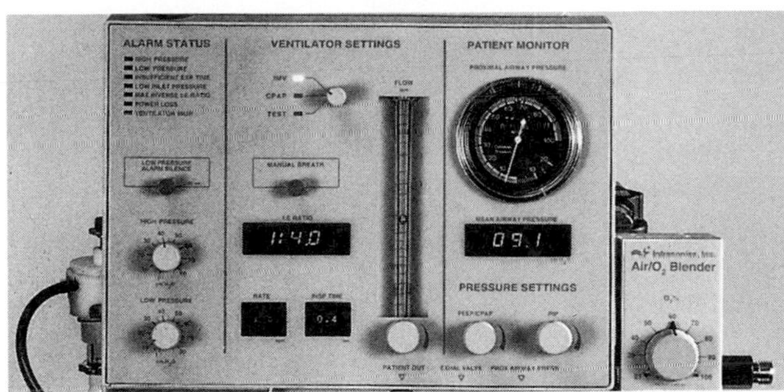

Figure 13-16 The Infant Star 200 Neonatal-Pediatric Ventilator control and alarm panel. (Courtesy Puritan Bennett, a division of Tyco Medical, Pleasanton, Calif.)

Table 13-12 Infant Star 200 Neonatal-Pediatric Ventilator

Inspiratory time	0.1 to 2.9 seconds
Rate	0 to 150 bpm
I:E Ratio	1:0.25 to 1:9.9
PEEP/CPAP	0 to 20 cm H_2O
Peak inspiratory pressure	0 to 70 cm H_2O
Flow	2 to 50 L/min
Trigger mechanism	Time

Control and Alarm Panel

The front panel is composed of three sections: alarm status, ventilator settings, and patient monitor (see Figure 13-16). The first section is the alarm status panel which is located on the left side of the ventilator. The HIGH PRESSURE ALARM has a range of 1 to 85 cm H_2O. The LOW PRESSURE ALARM has a range of 1 to 85 cm H_2O. The low pressure alarm silence is sixty seconds. The INSUFFICIENT EXPIRATORY TIME ALARM is activated when the inspiratory time and rate settings result in an expiratory time less than 0.2 seconds. The LOW INLET PRESSURE ALARM is activated when the gas source is below 40 psig. The MAX INVERSE I:E RATIO ALARM is activated when the ratio is greater than 4:1. The POWER LOSS ALARM is activated when insufficient power is present. When a malfunction is detected by the microprocessor the VENTILATOR INOP ALARM is then activated. The audible alarm intensity is adjusted by a rotary baffle which muffles alarm sound when rotated counterclockwise. A remote alarm output is available to connect to an external alarm system. Table 13-12 provides parameter specifications for the Infant Star 200 Neonatal/Pediatric Ventilator.

The middle section is the ventilator settings panel. The available modes of ventilation are IMV, CPAP, and TEST. The IMV and CPAP modes have continuous flow available for spontaneous respiratory efforts. The TEST mode verifies proper functioning of the monitoring LEDs and alarms and all mandatory breaths are ceased during this mode. The FLOW CONTROL range is 2 to 50 L/min. The flowmeter is calibrated in two ranges which are: 1 L/min increments from 2 to 12 L/min and 5 L/min increments from 15 to 50 L/min. The VENTILATOR RATE range is 1 to 150 breaths/minute in 1-breath increments. The INSPIRATORY TIME range is 0.1 to 2.9 seconds in 0.1 second increments. The MANUAL BREATH button delivers one mandatory breath in all modes. The tidal volume delivered depends on the set flow, inspiratory time, and peak inspiratory pressure. The I:E ratio range is 1:0.25 to 1:9.9.

The third section is the patient monitor panel. The pressure settings include PEEP/CPAP (0 to 20 cm H_2O) and PIP (0 to 70 cm H_2O). The monitored pressures are proximal airway pressure (–20 to 100 cm H_2O) and mean airway pressure (0 to 99.9 cm H_2O).

Optional Air-Oxygen Blender

The blender is supplied by external air and oxygen sources 40 to 70 psig. The blender delivers oxygen concentrations through either the primary or auxiliary gas outlet. The primary gas outlet is the gas source for the ventilator. The auxiliary gas outlet supplies metered low flows (2 to 90 L/min) through a flowmeter. An audible alarm indicates a difference of 30 psig between the two gas sources.

Tracking Relief Pressure Valve

The tracking relief pressure valve automatically limits airway pressure and is located inside the ventilator as in the 100 model, if the set PIP is greater than or equal to 10 cm H_2O, the pressure relief will occur at 10 to 15 cm H_2O above set PIP. If the set PIP is less than 10 cm H_2O, the pressure relief will occur at 15 to 20 cm H_2O above set PIP.

V.I.P. Bird Infant-Pediatric Ventilator

The V.I.P. Bird ventilator (VIASYS Healthcare – Critical Care Division, Palm Springs, CA) (Figure 13-17) mechanically supports neonatal, infant, and pediatric patients with the most common ventilator modes. It is electrically powered with 110 volts AC and pneumatically powered by external compressed air and oxygen at 40 to 75 psig. DC power operation from an external power source is possible. The V.I.P. Bird is microprocessor controlled by three processors. Flow-triggering and flow-cycling can be accomplished by using the Bird Partner IIi volume monitor and infant flow sensor. An oxygen blender auxiliary output flowmeter (0 to 15 L/min) is located on the side of the ventilator for use with a nebulizer or hand-held resuscitator.[17]

Noteworthy Internal Functions

The Microblender mixes the two gases according to the set oxygen percentage. The blended gas then enters the 1.1 liter accumulator (Figure 13-18). The accumulator reserves pressurized gas during the expiratory phase to meet high inspiratory flow demands of the patient with maximum flow capabilities up to 120 L/min. The gas exits from the accumulator and enters a pneumatic regulator that adjusts the flow control valve driving pressure to 25 psig (see Figure 13-18). A **pulsation dampener** is located between the regulator and flow control valve and is used to stabilize pressure and maintain driving pressure to the flow control valve. Gas flow is delivered to the patient by means of an electromechanical proportioning valve and an electromagnetic exhalation valve. The flow control valve shifts the rotary motion of a stepper motor to a linear motion of a plunger. Delivered flow rates are determined by the system driving pressure and the diameter of the valve opening. Flow rates are unaffected by downstream patient circuit pressures of up to a maximum level 350 cm H_2O using a system pressure of 25 psig.

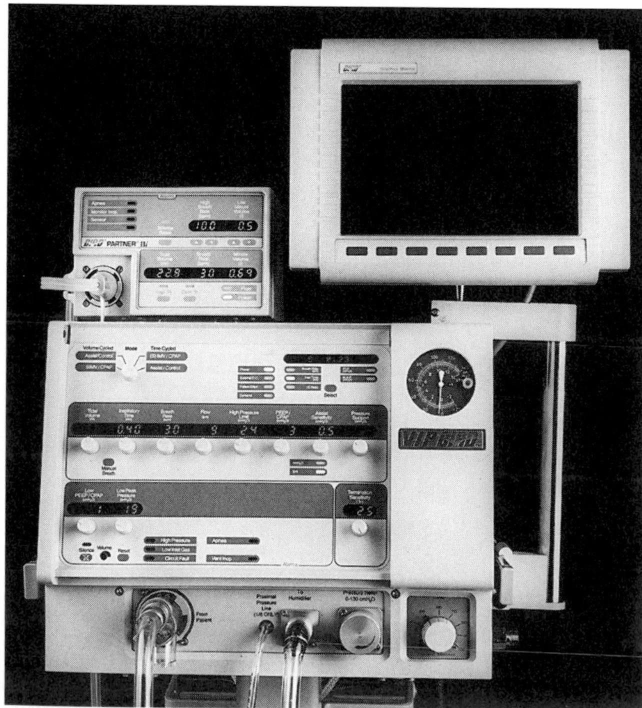

Figure 13-17 The V.I.P. Bird Ventilator. (Courtesy VIASYS Healthcare, Critical Care Division, Palm Springs, Calif.)

Because of the possibility of inadvertent PEEP developing from the continuous flow present in the expiratory limb of the patient circuit during time-cycled pressure-limited ventilation, a jet venturi is incorporated into the exhalation manifold. The jet solenoid controls the driving pressure to the exhalation valve jet venturi and is controlled by the microprocessor. It is active when the flow rate control is set at 5 L/min or greater with PEEP of 0 to 5 cm H_2O or when PEEP is set at zero and flow at any setting.

A pneumatically driven safety valve is activated when a ventilator inoperative event or electrical power failure occurs. This allows the patient to breath room air. For example, if a pressure difference of 20 psig occurs between the air and oxygen sources, the gas source with the highest pressure will be utilized by the ventilator. This will result in a delivered oxygen concentration of either 21% or 100%.

Control and Alarm Panel

Figure 13-19 provides a diagram of the control and alarm panel. The MODE SELECTOR knob is located on the front top left panel and has two groups of modes. The volume-cycled (VC) modes are Assist/Control and SIMV/CPAP. The TC modes are Assist/Control and (S)IMV/CPAP. The front panel control settings are: TIDAL VOLUME (20 to 995 mL), INSPIRATORY TIME (0.1 to 3.0 seconds), RATE (0 to 150 breaths/minute), FLOW (3 to 120 L/min for VC modes and 3 to 40 L/min for TC modes), HIGH PRESSURE (0 to 120 cm H_2O for VC modes and 0 to 80 cm H_2O for TC modes) (see Box 13-5), PEEP/CPAP (0 to 24 cm H_2O), ASSIST SENSITIVITY (off, 1 to 20 cm H_2O for VC modes and off, 0.1 to 5.0 L/min for TC modes with neonatal flow sensor in use only), and PRESSURE SUPPORT (0 to 50 cm H_2O). Table 13-13 lists parameter specifications for the V.I.P. Bird Infant-Pediatric Ventilator.

The MANUAL BREATH CONTROL is located in the control panel and is a single, operator-initiated controlled breath that is available in all modes. Illumination of displays highlights controls that are functional for that specific mode. Dimmed displays are controls that are not functional in a certain mode. For example, tidal volume will have a dimmed display when the ventilator is operating in a time-cycled pressure-limited mode. During CPAP the inspiratory

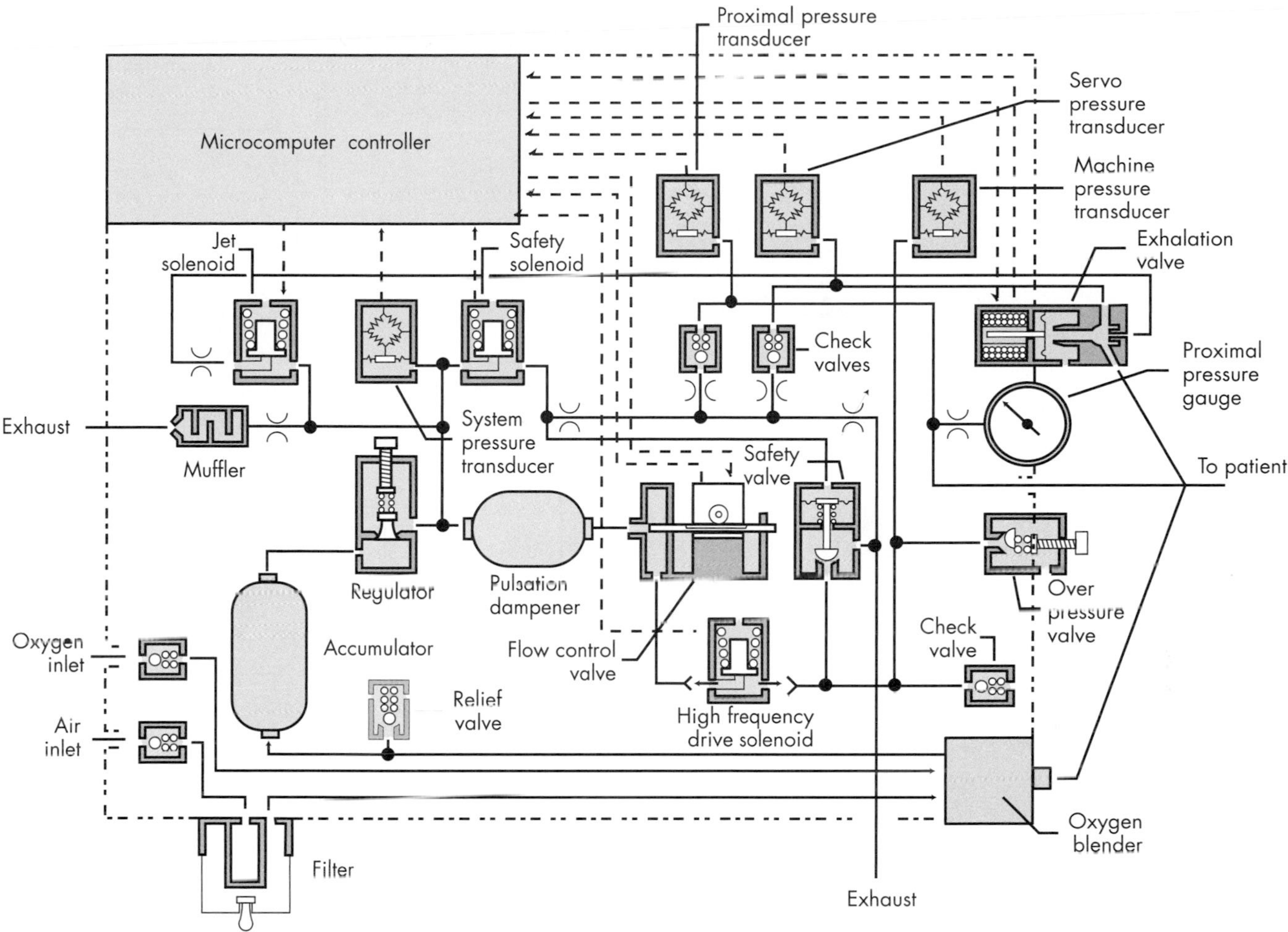

Figure 13-18 The V.I.P. Bird 1.1-L accumulator and internal circuit. (Courtesy VIASYS Healthcare, Critical Care Division, Palm Springs, Calif.)

time and peak inspiratory pressure displays remain illuminated and are functional during manual ventilation.

Directly below the control section is the alarm section which includes: LOW PEEP /CPAP (–9 to 24 cm H_2O), LOW PEAK PRESSURE (off, 3 to 120 cm H_2O), HIGH PRESSURE, LOW INLET GAS, CIRCUIT FAULT, APNEA (inactive with continuous flow), VENT INOP, ALARM SILENCE (60 seconds), and RESET. An additional safety feature is the MECHANICAL PRESSURE RELIEF knob which is located next to the oxygen concentration dial and can be adjusted between 0 and 130 cm H_2O in all modes. Turning the pressure relief knob clockwise increases the value and counterclockwise decreases the value. The high-pressure limit should be set below the over pressure relief valve setting for the high-pressure limit to be activated (Box 13-5).

When the power switch located on the rear top left panel is turned off, the ventilator inoperable alarm can be silenced by depressing the alarm silence button. The alarm silence is located on the front bottom left panel. It will silence the alarm for 60 seconds unless the RESET button located on the right is depressed.

Front panel digital displays include: BREATH RATE (0 to 250 breaths/minute), INSPIRATORY TIME (0.05 to 60 seconds), I:E RATIO (1:0.1 to 1:60), PIP (0 to 130 cm H_2O), MAP (0 to 120 cm H_2O), POWER (illuminates when power is on), EXTERNAL DC (illuminates when external DC power source is being used), PATIENT EFFORT (illuminates when assist sensitivity is met), and DEMAND (illuminates when demand system is triggered). The PATIENT EFFORT LED will flash when the patient's inspiratory effort exceeds the assist sensitivity setting. The DEMAND LED will flash when the demand flow system is triggered by spontaneous efforts decreasing airway pressure 1 cm H_2O below the baseline pressure during time-cycled IMV. Airway pressures are displayed on a pressure gauge. In the IMV mode only the mandatory breaths are displayed in the BREATH RATE display. The I:E RATIO LED flashes when inverse I:E ratio is present.

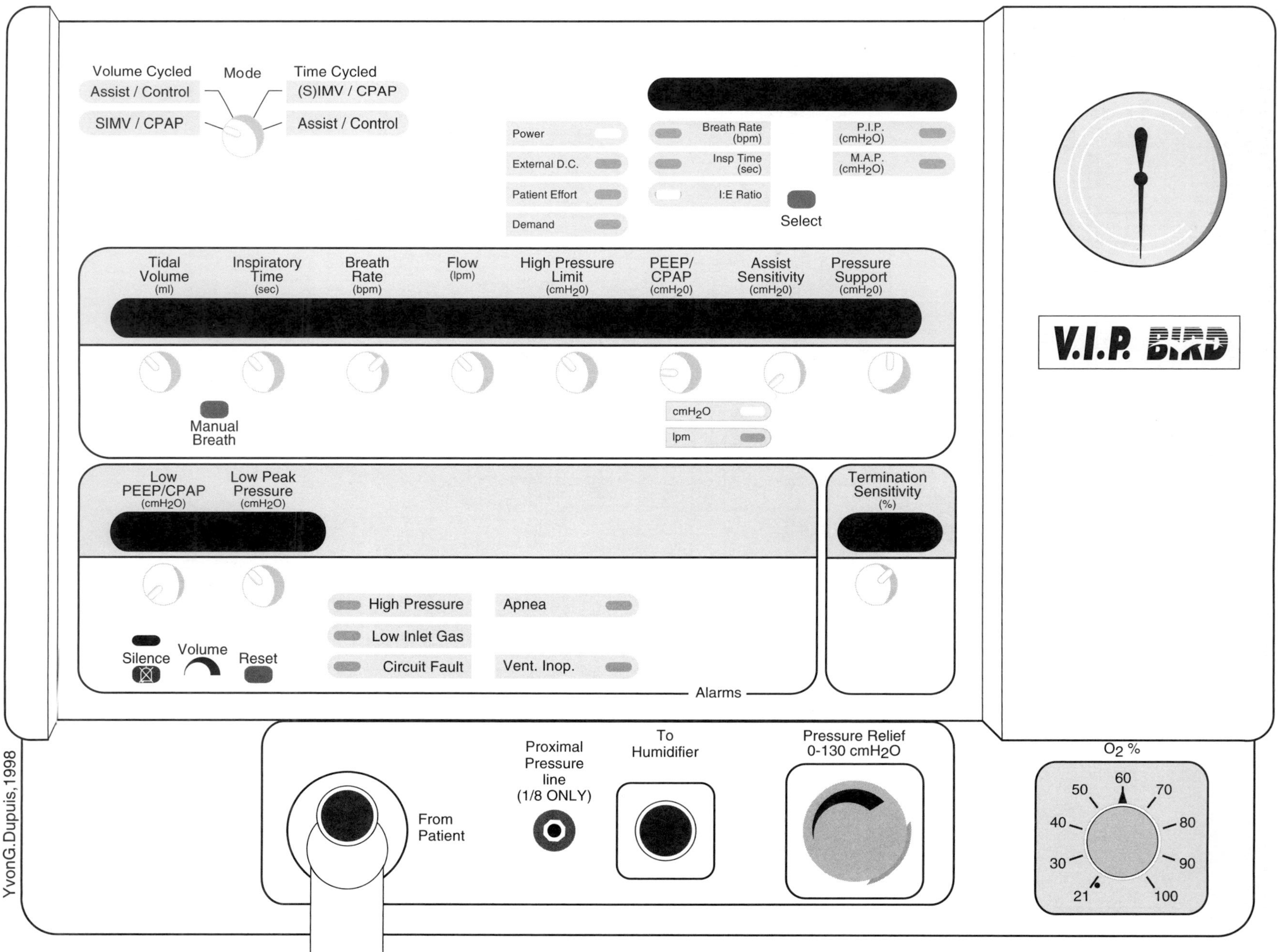

Figure 13-19 The V.I.P. Bird Ventilator control and alarm panel. (Courtesy Yvon Dupuis.)

Table 13-13 Specifications for V.I.P. Bird Infant-Pediatric Ventilator

Tidal volume	20 to 995 mL
Inspiratory time	0.1 to 3.0 seconds
Rate	0 to 150 bpm
Flow (TC modes)	3 to 40 L/min
Flow (VC modes)	3 to 120 L/min
Peak inspiratory pressure (TC modes)	0 to 80 cm H_2O
High pressure limit (VC modes)	0 to 120 cm H_2O
PEEP/CPAP	0 to 24 cm H_2O
Assist sensitivity (TC modes)	Off, 0.1 to 5.0 L/min
Assist sensitivity (VC modes)	Off, 1 to 20 cm H_2O
Pressure support	0 to 50 cm H_2O
Trigger mechanism	Pressure (VC)/Flow (TC)
Alarms	Low PEEP/CPAP Pressure, Low Peak Pressure, High Pressure, Low Inlet Pressure, Circuit Fault, Apnea, Ventilator Inoperative

Box 13-5 Function of the High Pressure Control

The high pressure limit controls the set peak inspiratory pressure in the time-cycled pressure limited modes. Its function in the volume-cycled modes is a high-pressure limit.

Box 13-6 Breath Termination Ranges According to Tidal Volume

5% peak flow for delivered V_T 0-50 mL, 5-25% peak flow for delivered V_T 50-200 mL, and 25% peak flow for delivered V_T > 200 mL

Modes of Ventilation

Volume-Cycled Modes

In the Assist/Control volume-cycled mode inspiration is volume-targeted, time- or pressure- triggered, flow-limited, and volume-cycled. Inspiration can be pressure-cycled if the airway pressure reaches the set high pressure alarm setting. The operator sets the following parameters: tidal volume, breath rate, flow, high pressure limit, PEEP/CPAP, and assist sensitivity.

In the SIMV/CPAP volume-cycled mode mandatory breaths are volume-targeted, time- or pressure-triggered, flow-limited, and volume-cycled. Inspiration can be pressure-cycled if the airway pressure reached the set high pressure alarm setting. Spontaneous respiratory efforts between mandatory breaths are pressure-targeted, pressure-triggered, pressure-limited, and pressure-cycled. Pressure support can be added to spontaneous efforts and are pressure-targeted, pressure-triggered, pressure-limited, and flow-cycled. The maximum demand flow available is 120 L/min for spontaneous and pressure supported breaths. The operator sets the following parameters: tidal volume, inspiratory time (pressure support time limit), breath rate, flow, high pressure limit, PEEP/CPAP, assist sensitivity, and pressure support (if desired).

Pressure support termination criteria are set up differently with the V.I.P. Bird ventilator because of the varied patient population that can be ventilated with this device. For example, if the unit fails to flow-cycle at 25% of peak flow due to an air leak around the artificial airway this may result in excessive inspiratory times (some units will time-cycle at 2 to 3 seconds). The termination criteria for the V.I.P. Bird are based on delivered tidal volume ranges (Box 13-6). The pressure support display will flash when the breath is time-cycled.

Time-Cycled Modes

In the IMV time-cycled mode mandatory breaths are pressure-targeted, time-triggered, pressure-limited, and time-cycled. In IMV the operator sets the following parameters: breath rate, inspiratory time, flow, high-pressure limit (PIP desired), and PEEP/CPAP. The continuous and demand flow systems support spontaneous efforts. Continuous flow is determined by the flow knob setting (range 0-15 L/min). Demand flow is available when spontaneous inspiration decreases the airway pressure 1 cm H_2O below the baseline pressure. The maximum level of demand flow is 120 L/min. Sensitivity is set at 1 cm H_2O below baseline pressure in the IMV/CPAP mode. CPAP is activated when the breath rate setting is zero.

In (S)IMV/CPAP (using Bird Partner IIi volume monitor and infant flow sensor) the mandatory breath is pressure-targeted, flow- or time-triggered, pressure-limited, and time-cycled. CPAP is activated when the breath rate setting is zero. In SIMV the operator sets the following parameters: breath rate, inspiratory time, flow, high pressure limit, PEEP/CPAP, and assist sensitivity (L/min).

In the Assist/Control mode inspiration is pressure-targeted, flow- or time-triggered, pressure-limited, and flow- or time-cycled. The patient receives the set pressure with every spontaneous respiratory effort. The breath rate setting acts as a back-up rate in the event of decreased respiratory effort. The operator sets the following parameters: BREATH RATE,

Box 13-7 Important Clinical Note About the Terminal Sensitivity and Mode

If the patient is unable to self-regulate ventilation (e.g., hiccups), the termination sensitivity should be turned off or change the mode of ventilation until the situation resolves.

INSPIRATORY TIME, FLOW, HIGH PRESSURE LIMIT, PEEP/CPAP, ASSIST SENSITIVITY, and **TERMINATION SENSITIVITY.**

The TERMINATION SENSITIVITY control is an additional feature that adjusts the flow termination point of the breath, preventing air trapping and inverse I:E ratio, therefore providing **expiratory synchrony.** It is only used in the assist/control time-cycled mode. TERMINATION SENSITIVITY ranges are off, and 5 to 25% of peak flow. For example, a setting of 25% means that the breath will be terminated when the flow (measured at the proximal airway) decreases to 25% of measured peak flow. If the flow fails to decrease to the % set, which might occur with lower % setting and presence of air leak around artificial airway, the breath is time-cycled. The termination % setting will flash to indicate that the breath is time-cycled. Airway graphics are helpful in evaluating patient/ventilator synchrony and their use is strongly recommended with this mode of ventilation (Box 13-7).

The ASSIST SENSITIVITY control is adjustable from 0.2 to 5 L/min with the use of the infant flow sensor. By pressing the CONTINUOUS FLOW button on the Bird Partner IIi monitor, the real time flow signal can be evaluated by observing the continuous flow readout at end exhalation. If the digital readout returns to zero the operator should set the ASSIST SENSITIVITY value at 0.2 L/min to provide optimal patient triggering capabilities. If there is a leak (flow readout does not return to zero), the ASSIST SENSITIVITY should be adjusted to 0.2 L/min above the digital readout. Adjusting the sensitivity above the leak avoids autocycling and requires the patient to generate only the flow difference between the leak and the ASSIST SENSITIVITY setting.

Graphics Displays

Airway graphics are an invaluable tool that allow the clinician to monitor and adjust ventilatory strategies for each patient. Graphical analysis also provides real-time and trend assessment of ventilator parameters and of patient/ventilator interactions. The Bird Graphics Monitor is designed for use with the V.I.P. Bird and Bird 8400 STi ventilators (Figure 13-17). It requires use of the Bird Partner or Bird Partner IIi monitor (see section below on Partner IIi monitor). The graphics monitor is portable and easily moved between ventilators. A communication port is available for a printer. Compatible printers include the HP ThinkJet and Epson FX-850.

The graphics monitor displays real time scalar waveforms for pressure, flow, and volume (vertical axis) plotted over time (horizontal axis). The waveform select screen allows the clinician to select two waveforms at a time. Positive values (above zero on the vertical axis) relate to the inspiratory phase and negative values to the expiratory phase of ventilation. Pressure/volume and flow/volume loops are also available, along with reference loop storage. The pressure/volume graphical loop displays tidal volume on the vertical axis and airway pressure on the horizontal axis. The flow/volume graphical loop displays flow on the vertical axis and tidal volume on the horizontal axis. The freeze screen provides movable target and reference cursors that allows the clinician to hold and evaluate significant events. The trend feature is provided with ten selectable parameters and can be set for 15 minutes or 1-, 2-, 4-, 8-, or 24-hour windows.[18]

Special Features of the V.I.P. Ventilator

Leak Compensation

Leak compensation is used to stabilize baseline pressure, prevent autocycling, and optimize assist sensitivity in the presence of leaks. It is only recommended for use with leaks around artificial airways. It is not recommended for those patients with minimal respiratory effort and no leak, because some patients are unable to trigger appropriately with the leak compensation active. Leak compensation is only functional in the volume-cycled modes.

When pressure decreases 0.25 cm H_2O below baseline pressure, the leak compensation feature introduces small amounts of flow into the circuit attempting to reestablish baseline pressure. The amount of leak compensation needed is learned by the exhalation valve pressure transducer so that the flow control valve returns to the determined value after each breath. The amount of flow is reevaluated every 8 milliseconds. The maximum amount of flow available is 5 L/min with assist sensitivity set at –1 cm H_2O and 10 L/min with assist sensitivity set at –2 to –5 cm H_2O. The default setting after any power-up is leak compensation on. The leak compensation is turned on or off by pressing the select button until the desired feature is displayed in the digital window (top left digital display).

Partner IIi Monitor

The Bird Partner IIi monitor is a microprocessor controlled volume monitor with a variable orifice differential pressure flow measuring device that is placed in the patient circuit near the upper airway. It measures effective inspiratory and expiratory volumes, displays digital measured values (tidal volume, breath rate, minute ventilation, and the real time flow signal-only with infant sensor), displays digital alarm parameters (high rate, low minute ventilation), and provides an adjustable apnea alarm (10 to 60 seconds in 5 second

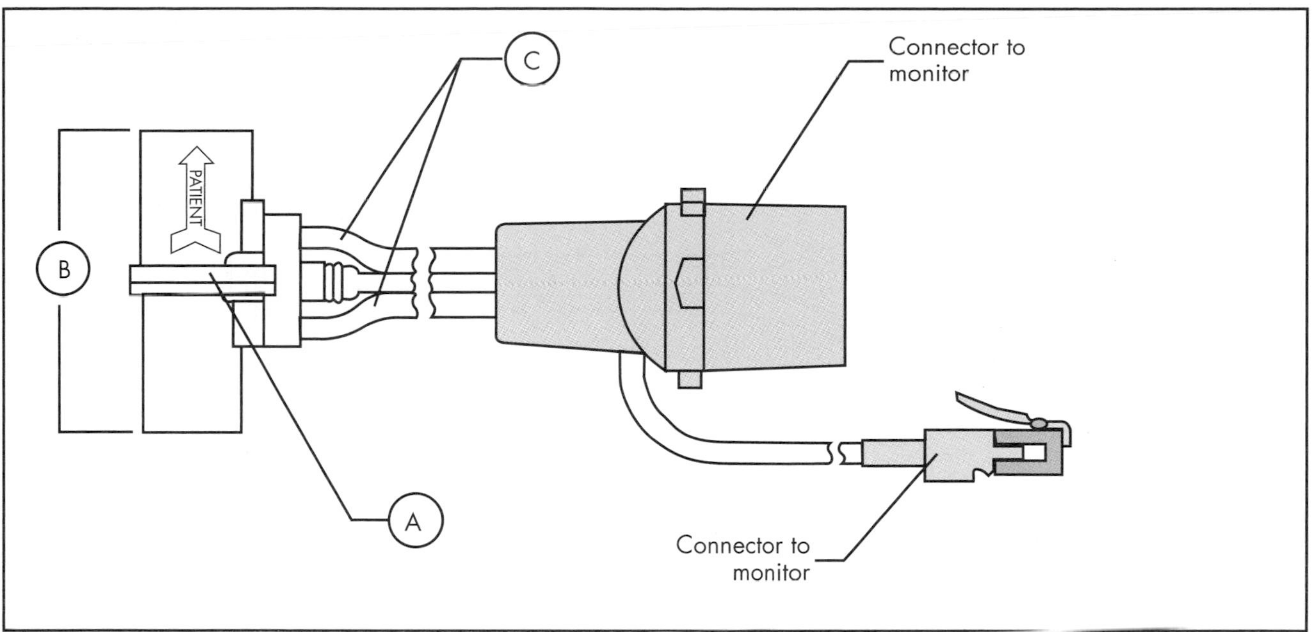

Figure 13-20 Infant sensor used with the Partner IIi monitor and the V.I.P. Bird. (Courtesy VIASYS Healthcare, Critical Care Division, Palm Springs, Calif.)

Box 13-8 Important Clinical Note Regarding the Flow Sensor

The infant flow sensor should be cleaned every 24 hours to maintain accurate tidal volume measurements and flow triggering capabilities. The sensor can be sterilized in a cold solution or gas sterilized. Steam autoclave or pasteurization cannot be used because the high temperatures will damage the flow element.

Box 13-9 Use of a Capnograph with an Inline Sensor

When using capnographic monitoring, place the end-tidal CO_2 sensor between the infant sensor and the patient circuit Y to provide optimal flow triggering capabilities. There are special connectors available to facilitate the additional monitoring. The infant sensor has less than 1 mm of dead space.

increments). Alarm limits can be set using the monitor's touch pad controls. The apnea button (red) is located on the rear panel of the monitor. The clinician can visualize the current apnea setting by depressing the red button and observing the displayed value in the tidal volume window. Repeated depression of the button will allow the clinician to adjust the apnea setting.

The monitor can be used with the infant or pediatric sensor. The infant sensor is placed at the proximal airway and circuit Y and can only be used with artificial airways with an internal diameter of 4.5 mm or less (Figure 13-20). The sensor *(B)* is placed with the arrow pointing towards the patient *(A)* and the monitoring tubes *(C)* facing upwards to prevent condensation or secretion accumulation within the lines (see Box 13-8 for important information about cleaning the infant sensor). The gas inlet on the back of the ventilator connects to a 50 psig source and is used to inject 12 mL/min of gas through the pressure line to prevent obstructions within the line and water from entering the differential pressure transducer. The gas flow is synchronized with the expiratory phase so no additional volume is delivered to the patient during inspiration. The tidal volume readout is the effective tidal volume since the sensor placement is at the patient airway. Box 13-9 explains the use of a capnograph with an infant flow sensor.

If a continuous artificial airway leak is present, the CONT V function can be used to determine the liter flow of the leak. By pressing and holding the CONT V touch pad, a real-time flow through the infant sensor is displayed. The clinician can use the baseline leak, or the flow displayed between breaths, to determine the best trigger sensitivity setting and avoid auto-triggering. Generally, trigger sensitivity is set 0.2-0.4 L/min above the baseline leak flow. Measurement of artificial airway leak is possible only while using the infant sensor.

The pediatric sensor (Figure 13-21, *B*) is placed just before the expiratory valve with the arrow pointing toward the direction of gas flow. The tidal volume readout includes

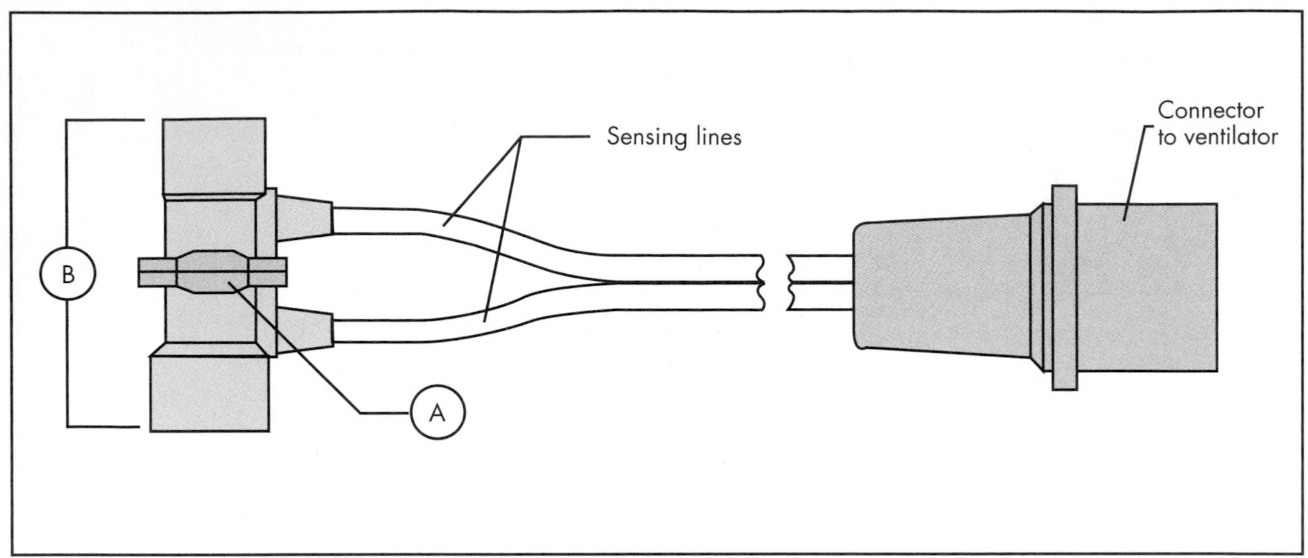

Figure 13-21 Pediatric sensor used with Partner IIi monitor and V.I.P. Bird. (Courtesy VIASYS Healthcare, Critical Care Division, Palm Springs, Calif.)

compressible volume and effective tidal volume. Tidal volume measurements are derived from the measurement of flow. As flow passes through the sensor and past the variable orifice flow element *(A)*, which is located between two chambers, the flow element bends in the direction of flow creating a small pressure difference between the two chambers. The differential pressure transducer measures the pressure differences between the two chambers, sends an analog signal that is read by the microprocessor, which compares the signal to a calibration curve and translates the value to a volume.[17]

V.I.P. Sterling and Gold Infant/Pediatric Ventilators

The V.I.P. Sterling and Gold Infant/Pediatric ventilators (VIASYS Healthcare – Critical Care Division, Palm Springs, CA) (Figure 13-22) are improved models of the original V.I.P. The internal design and most of the controls, alarms, and specifications are identical to the original. Therefore only the changes and new features will be presented here.

The most noteworthy changes are in two areas. First, both ventilators use redesigned flow sensors called the Infant "Smart" Flow Sensor and the Pediatric "Smart" Flow Sensor. The other major change is the incorporation of the functions of the Partner IIi Monitor into the main ventilator housing. Some expanded setting limits as well as some new features have been added. Volume assured pressure support (VAPS), a dual mode feature, is a key addition on the V.I.P. Gold. It is described later in this section.

The heart of the redesigned flow sensors for both the Sterling and the Gold is a stainless steel flap that replaces the former plastic design. A variable orifice differential pressure technology similar to the original sensors is employed to measure flow. With the new design, the Infant "Smart" Flow Sensor can be used with artificial airway sizes up to 5.5 mm I.D. For larger endotracheal tubes, the Pediatric "Smart" Flow Sensor is necessary. This sensor is placed at the exhalation valve rather than at the artificial airway.[19]

The ventilators' microprocessor is able to determine which flow sensor is in use. When using the Infant "Smart" Flow Sensor, a bias flow of 3 L/min is present unless the ventilator is operating in the TCPL mode. In the TCPL mode, flow is set by the operator. When using the Pediatric "Smart" Flow Sensor, bias flow can be turned on or off by pressing the Bias Flow control. Bias flow operates at a fixed 5 L/min with the pediatric sensor when turned on.

Changes in Controls/Alarms

Although many of the controls, indicators, and alarms on the Sterling and Gold models are identical to the original V.I.P., some additions and changes have been made. The front panel of the V.I.P. Gold is shown in Figure 13-23. The layout of controls and indicators is very similar to the original. As in the original model, push buttons are used to activate functions, visualize certain parameter settings, or turn functions on or off. A single selector switch is used to change modes. Dials are used to adjust parameters and alarm limits.

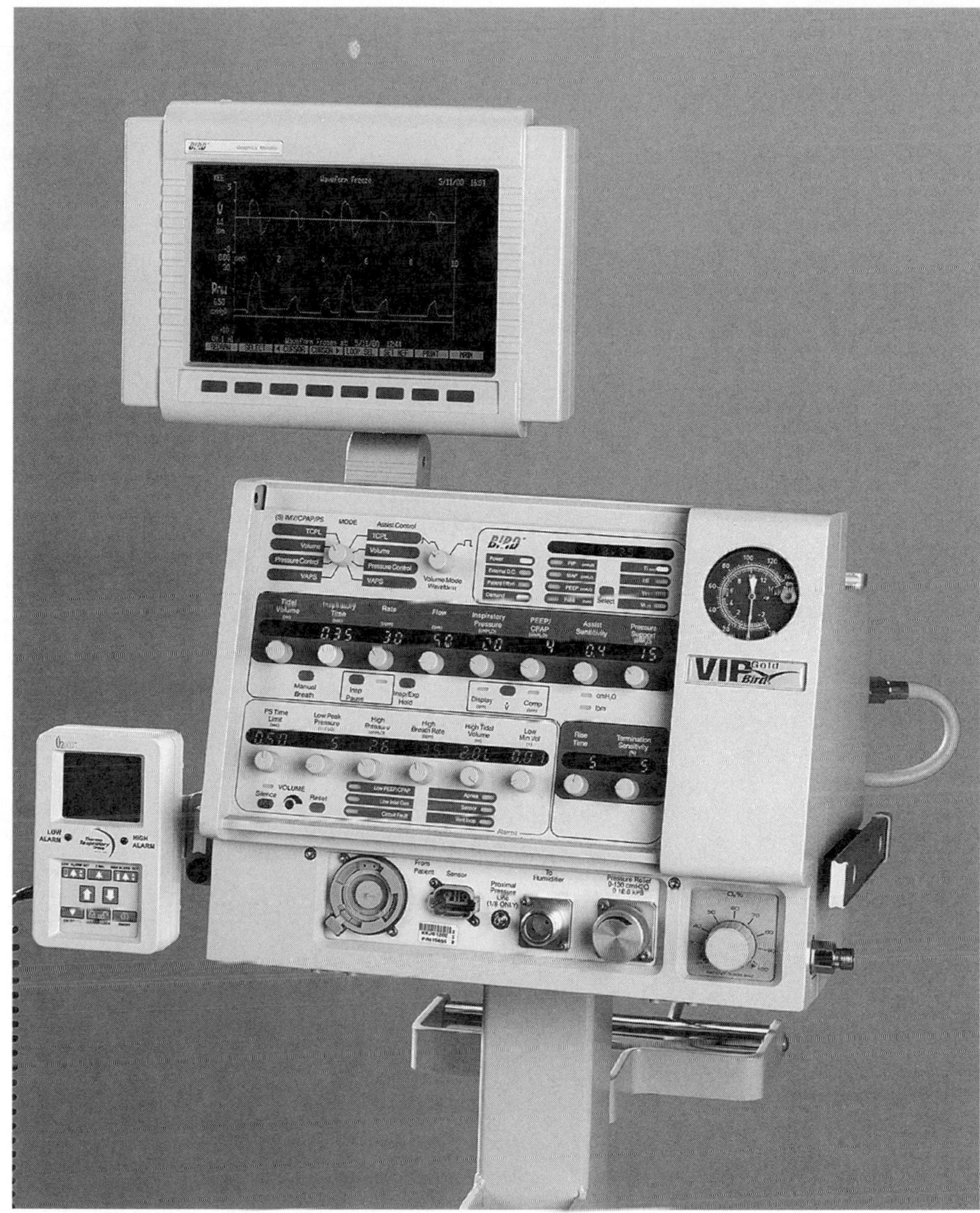

Figure 13-22 The Bird V.I.P. Gold Infant Ventilator. (Courtesy VIASYS Healthcare, Critical Care Division, Palm Springs, Calif.)

Ventilator Modes and the Mode Select Switch

The Mode Select Switch, located in the left upper portion of the front control panel, is a multiposition dial. The position of the switch sets either the mode or the breath type. As in the original V.I.P., some controls are deactivated when certain modes are selected. Displays for deactivated controls remain illuminated but dimmed.

The assist-control modes for both the Sterling and Gold models are grouped in a mode category column to the right of the control dial. Time-cycled, pressure-limited mode and volume-limited are the only assist-control modes available on the Sterling in this mode category. Two additional assist-control modes are available on the Gold model: Pressure Control and VAPS (described later). The left column of both models lists the (S)IMV/CPAP/PS modes. On the Sterling, only TCPL and Volume modes are available in this mode category. CPAP can be provided in either of these modes and pressure support can be added to nonmandatory breaths. In addition to the two (S)IMV/CPAP/PS modes on the Sterling, the Gold also provides Pressure Control and VAPS in this mode category. When adding pressure support to spontaneous breaths, the level can be adjusted with a separate control allowing separate inspiratory pressures for mandatory and pressure supported, spontaneous breaths.

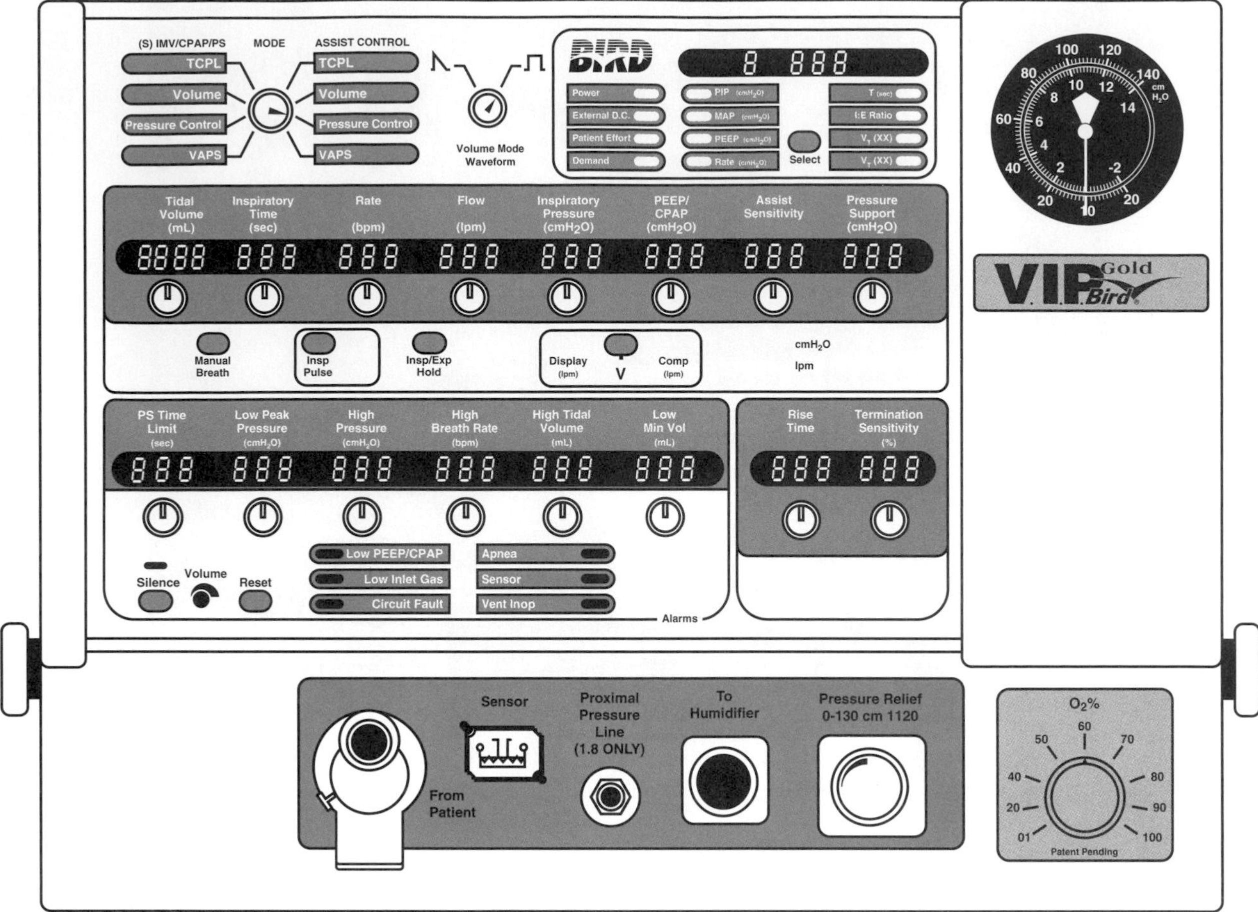

Figure 13-23 The Bird V.I.P. Gold Infant Ventilator. (Courtesy VIASYS Healthcare, Critical Care Division, Palm Springs, Calif.)

The VAPS mode is available only on the V.I.P. Gold model. It is a dual control mode that guarantees that a pressure control breath, a pressure supported breath, or a TCPL breath will reach a preset volume. During a VAPS breath, tidal volume may be augmented by extending the inspiratory phase at the set flow for a segment of time beyond the point that flow would otherwise terminate. An example of how the ventilator augments a breath is represented by waveforms in Figure 13-24. Breath A is a pressure supported breath that terminates at a set flow. In this breath, the desired tidal volume is reached within the set inspiratory time. In contrast, Breath B represents a breath in which delivery of the set tidal volume is not achieved during the allotted inspiratory time. When the ventilator determines that the delivered volume is too low, it allows flow to decelerate to its minimum set point. However, rather than terminating, the set flow continues over a slightly lengthened inspiratory time, causing the peak inspiratory pressure to rise. The breath is therefore augmented to the desired tidal volume. An augmented breath essentially transitions from a pressure control or TCPL breath to a volume control breath. With VAPS, electronic extension of the inspiratory phase only occurs if the microprocessor determines that the pressure settings alone cannot deliver the preset tidal volume (Clinical Rounds 13-7).

VAPS can be selected from either the (S)IMV/CPAP/PS column or the Assist/Control column of the Mode Select switch. When selected from the (S)IMV/CPAP/PS column, mandatory pressure control breaths are delivered at a guaranteed volume. The clinician must set TIDAL VOLUME, INSPIRATORY PRESSURE, RATE, and FLOW. Non-mandatory breaths in this form of VAPS will be unsupported if no pressure support level is present. When the clinician sets a PRESSURE SUPPORT level and a PRESSURE SUPPORT/VAPS TIME LIMIT (see below), pressure support breaths as well as mandatory pressure control breaths will be delivered at a guaranteed volume. The PRESSURE SUPPORT LEVEL and THE PRESSURE SUPPORT/VAPS TIME LIMIT controls must be set by the clinician.

When VAPS is selected from the Assist/Control column, breaths delivered to the patient are either patient-triggered or mandatory TCPL breaths. In this version of VAPS, the clinician sets INSPIRATORY PRESSURE as well as TIDAL VOLUME, FLOW, PRESSURE SUPPORT/VAPS TIME LIMIT, and RATE.

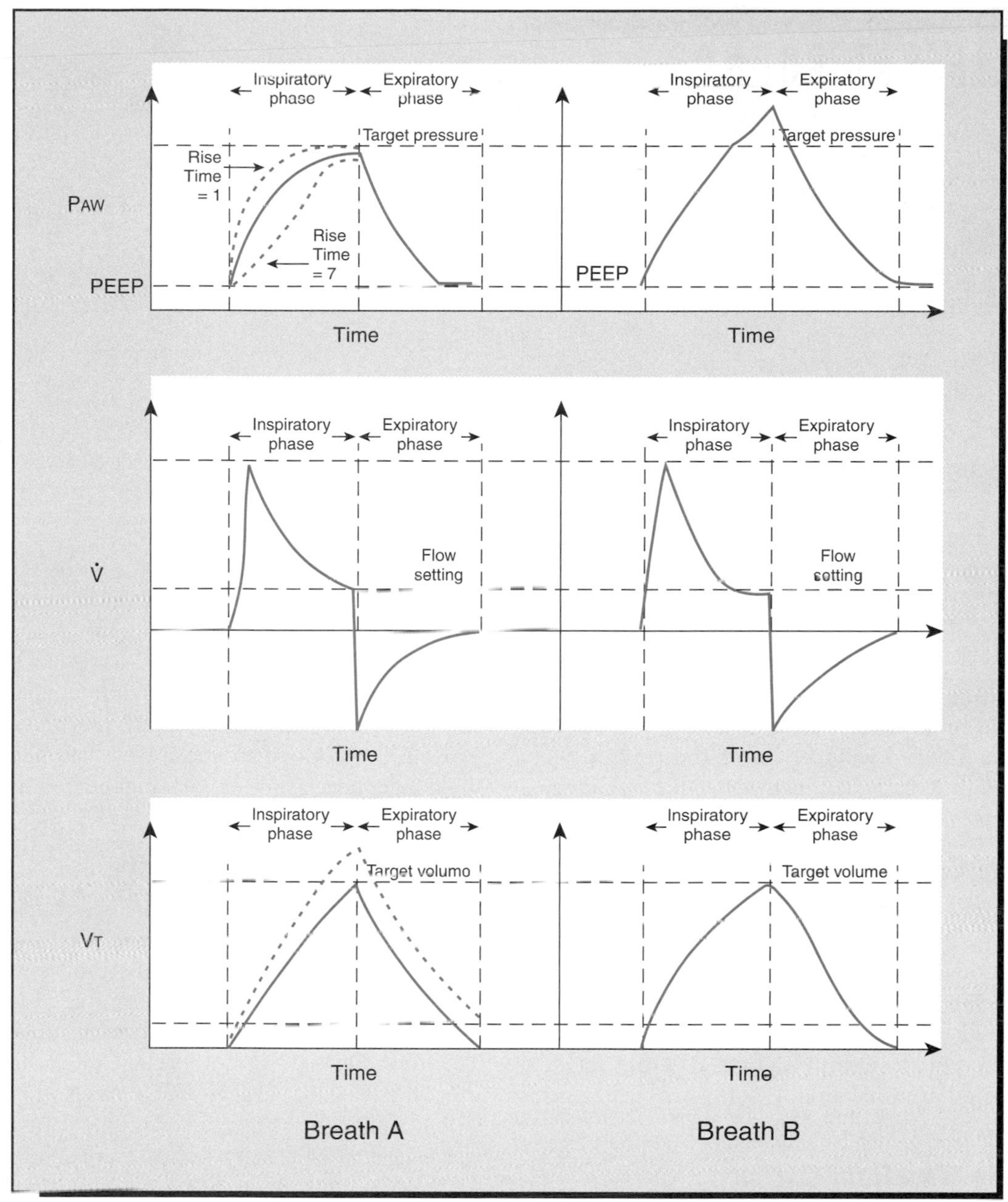

Figure 13-24 VAPS breath delivery with Bird V.I.P. Sterling and Gold Infant Ventilator. **Breath A** *(left column)* depicts breaths that flow-cycle at the set flow after the minimum tidal volume has been delivered. [*Note*: The target pressure is delivered. Flow decelerates to the flow setting. V_T has met or exceed the set V_T. The breath cycles out of inspiration at the set flow.] **Breath B** *(right column)* shows a transition from a PS breath to a volume-assured breath. Transition occurs when flow drops to the set peak flow and the set V_T has not been delivered. [*Note*: The target pressure is delivered. Flow decelerates to the flow setting. V_T has *not* met the set V_T. Flow remains constant at the set peak flow until the set V_T is achieved. Peak pressure continues to rise and T_I increases until V_T is delivered.] (Courtesy VIASYS Healthcare, Critical Care Division, Palm Springs, Calif.)

Pressure Support/VAPS Time Limit Control

This control is active only in the Pressure Support mode on both the Sterling and Gold and on the VAPS mode on the Gold. It is automatically activated when these modes are selected. This control sets a time limit for the inspiratory phase in case of a leak or any other condition in which inspiratory flow does not drop to the termination level. Adjustable from 0.1 to 3.0 seconds, the Pressure Support/VAPS Time Limit is displayed in a window above the control.

Rise Time Control

Available on the Gold model only, the Rise Time control allows the inspiratory pressure rise time to be adjusted. This control is active only in the Pressure Control, VAPS, and

CLINICAL ROUNDS 13-7

A respiratory therapist is setting VAPS on a patient who has spontaneous breathing efforts. The ventilator is in A/C volume ventilation with PEEP = 3 cm H_2O, flow = 15 L/min, V_T set at 50 mL, and a pressure limit of 20 cm H_2O. The therapist observes the flow-time curve rising rapidly at the beginning of inspiration and then tapering off until if finally reaches zero at the end of inspiration. Actual delivered V_T is 60 mL.

Question: What is the cycling variable that ends inspiration in this example?

See Appendix A for the answer.

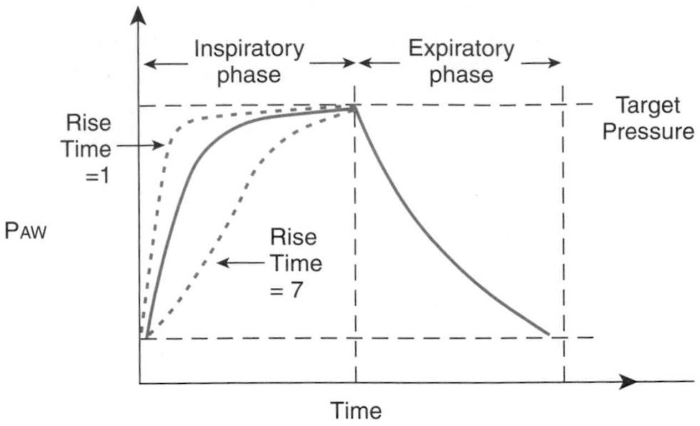

Figure 13-25 The RISE TIME control available on the Gold model tapers pressure delivery at the beginning of inspiration. See text for description. (Courtesy VIASYS Healthcare, Critical Care Division, Palm Springs, Calif.)

Pressure Support modes. The control is adjustable from a setting of 1 to 7. At a setting of 1, the fastest rise time, the set peak inspiratory pressure is reached quickly and is held for the duration of the set inspiratory time (Figure 13-25). At the slowest setting, 7, inspiratory flow is decreased to allow a gradual rise to set peak inspiratory pressure. The selected setting is displayed in a window above the control knob. The inspiratory time and the breath cycle are not affected by this control.

Tidal Volume Control

Tidal Volume for both the Sterling and Gold models is set and adjusted in the same way as for the original V.I.P. However, the tidal volume limit has been increased to 1200 mL. On the Gold model in the VAPS mode, the TIDAL VOLUME CONTROL setting establishes a target volume. This volume is not necessarily delivered if the set tidal volume, measured on exhalation, is achieved by the effects of inspiratory pressure settings alone.

Volume Mode Waveform Switch

The two-position VOLUME MODE WAVEFORM Switch is active only when volume controlled breaths are delivered. The left position sets a decelerating flow waveform during the inspiratory phase. The right position sets a square waveform.

Apnea Indicator and Apnea Interval Switch

A period of apnea equal to the set APNEA INTERVAL will trigger an audible alarm and a flashing visual indicator. The audible alarm can be silenced with the ALARM SILENCE button or it will silence itself once the alarm condition is corrected. The visual indicator will continue to flash until the RESET button is pressed.

The APNEA INTERVAL is set by the operator and is adjustable from ten to sixty seconds. The current APNEA INTERVAL can be determined by pressing and holding the SELECT button for two seconds. The interval will appear in the Monitor Display window. The APNEA INTERVAL is also displayed when the APNEA INTERVAL switch is pressed. This switch is a push button located on the rear panel of the ventilator. Upon pressing the button one time, the current apnea interval is displayed in the MONITOR DISPLAY window for 3 seconds. Each push of the button after the first time will increase the apnea interval by 5-second increments up to a maximum of 60 seconds. After the operator toggles to the 60-second maximum, pressing the button again returns the interval to 10 seconds.

Bias Flow, Assist Sensitivity, and Triggering

The purpose of bias flow within the patient circuit is to provide a reference flow for the sensors in order to effect flow-triggering. When the infant sensor is in use, the bias flow is automatically on and delivering 3 L/min. With the infant sensor, the bias flow status will not appear in the MONITOR DISPLAY window. When the pediatric sensor is used, the bias flow level runs at a preset 5 L/min. However, with the pediatric sensor, the bias flow status can be viewed in the MONITOR DISPLAY window by using the SELECT button. Repeatedly pressing the SELECT button scrolls through all monitored parameters. After the final parameter is scanned, the message "BF"ON or "BF"OFF will be displayed. At this point, the operator can turn the bias flow on or off by pressing and holding the SELECT button for 2 seconds. When no flow sensor is used, no bias flow is delivered.

Both the V.I.P. Sterling and Gold ventilators provide either flow- or pressure-triggering in all modes. The ASSIST SENSITIVITY control sets either the flow or pressure necessary to trigger the ventilator into inspiration, depending upon the type of triggering that is active. An indicator for each type of triggering illuminates when active. Triggering can be locked out completely by turning the ASSIST SENSITIVITY control to the off position. When using the infant flow sensor, only flow-triggering is active and is adjustable from 0.1 to 3.0 L/min using the ASSIST SENSITIVITY control. When using the pediatric flow sensor and Bias Flow is turned on, flow-triggering is active and is adjustable from 2.2 to

5.0 L/min. When the BIAS FLOW is turned on, pressure-triggering is active with the pediatric sensor and is adjustable from 1 to 20 cm H_2O. If no flow sensor is used, both models automatically default to pressure-triggering in all modes.

Flow Display/Comp

The FLOW DISPLAY COMP button on both the Sterling and Gold models replaces the CONT V on the original partner Iii Monitor. This control serves the same function as the CONT V button when the infant flow sensor is in use. When the FLOW DISPLAY COMP button is pressed, the "Display" indicator to the left will illuminate. Flow values will then be displayed in the ventilator's MONITOR DISPLAY window. The operator can then use the SELECT button to toggle between inspiratory and expiratory real time flows. This function is particularly useful in determining the amount of baseline leak at the artificial airway and adjusting the assist sensitivity to eliminate auto-triggering. The clinician can toggle to the inspiratory flow, note the amount of baseline leak, and set the ASSIST SENSITIVITY control at least 0.2 L/min above the detected leak.

When using the pediatric flow sensor, the FLOW DISPLAY COMP button serves another function. With this sensor, pressing the button establishes a zero point for the volume monitor based on the set level of continuous flow. This function is called flow compensation. To accurately monitor volumes, flow compensation should be activated each time the flow setting is changed. Upon pressing the FLOW DISPLAY COMP button with the pediatric sensor connected, the "Comp" indicator to the right will illuminate for 3 seconds and the level of flow compensation will appear in the MONITOR DISPLAY window. To disable flow compensation, the FLOW DISPLAY COMP function must be pressed and held for 2 seconds. The FLOW DISPLAY COMP function is not available when the ventilator is operated without either of the flow sensors.

Inspiratory/Expiratory Hold

An Inspiratory/Expiratory Hold function is available on the V.I.P. Gold model only. When the INSP/EXP HOLD button is pressed once, an "I/E Hold" prompt will appear in the MONITOR DISPLAY window. While this message is displayed, pressing the SELECT button once will toggle to the "I Hold" message. To attain an inspiratory hold for up to three seconds, the INSP/EXP HOLD button is pressed and held. When the button is released, the inspiratory plateau pressure appears in the MONITOR DISPLAY window.

An expiratory hold can be performed by first pressing the INSP/EXP HOLD button to bring up the "I/E Hold" prompt in the MONITOR DISPLAY window. The SELECT button is then pressed two times to display the "E Hold" message. To attain an expiratory hold for up to three seconds, the INSP/EXP HOLD button is pressed and held. When the button is released, an expiratory plateau pressure appears in the MONITOR DISPLAY window.

Inspiratory Pause

An INSPIRATORY PAUSE control is available only on the V.I.P. Gold. This control allows an inspiratory pause time to be set when operating the ventilator in either volume-targeted or VAPS modes. When the "INSP PAUSE" button is pressed once, the current setting, if any, is displayed in the DISPLAY MONITOR window. The window will first show IP followed by the current pause setting. While the pause time is being displayed, it can be changed by pressing the SELECT button. Each time the SELECT button is pressed, the inspiratory pause time will increase by 0.1 second up to a maximum of 2 seconds. Holding the button will also allow the pause time to increase. To reset the pause time to zero, the RESET button is pressed.

Leak Compensation Control

Leak compensation has been changed on the Sterling and Gold models. This function is no longer available when using the infant flow sensor. It can be activated only when using the pediatric sensor with the bias flow turned off or when using the ventilator without a flow sensor. Leak compensation can be activated on the V.I.P. Sterling only when in a volume mode or in the V.I.P Gold when in a volume mode or in pressure control or VAPS.

Leak compensation can be activated by scrolling through the displayed parameters using the SELECT button until the current leak compensation message appears in the Monitor Display window. This message will be either "LK ON" or "LK OFF." Pressing and holding the SELECT button will toggle between the "LK ON" and "LK OFF." settings.

Leak compensation is used when artificial airway leak prevents the ventilator from otherwise maintaining the PEEP level. Small increments of flow are introduced into the circuit to provide back pressure compensation for the leak. When using leak compensation, the patient's ability to trigger may be diminished. Careful attention to the assist sensitivity setting is necessary. In some cases, removing the source of the leak is preferable to using the leak compensation function (Clinical Rounds 13-8).

Specifications for the Bird V.I.P. Gold and Sterling ventilators are listed in Table 13-14.

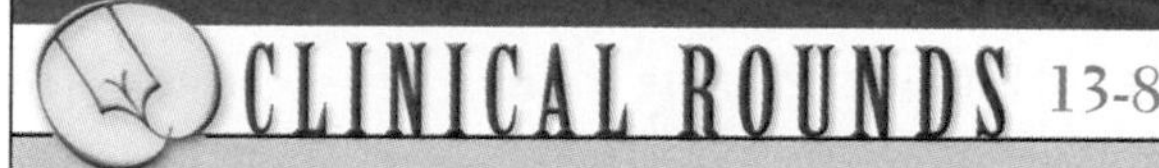

A respiratory therapist is assessing a patient being ventilated with the Infant Gold ventilator. The therapist notices the patient using accessory muscles to inspire. The patient's efforts do not trigger a ventilator breath even though the trigger sensitivity seems to be at an appropriate setting. What is a possible cause of the problem?

See Appendix A for the answer.

Table 13-14 Specifications for the V.I.P. Gold and Sterling Ventilators

CONTROLS	AVAILABLE SETTINGS AND RANGES
Mode Select	
Waveform Select	square wave/decelerating flow
Tidal Volume	10 to 1200 mL
Inspiratory Time	0.10 to 3.0 seconds
Breath Rate	0 to 150 bpm
Flow	3 to 120 L/min—Volume Modes and VAPS (Gold Only) 3 to 40 L/min—TCPL, Inspiratory Flow 3 to 15 L/min—TCPL, Expiratory Bias Flow
Inspiratory Pressure	3 to 80 cm H_2O
PEEP/CPAP	0 to 24 cm H_2O
Assist Sensitivity	Pressure-Triggered: 1 to 29 cm H_2O Flow-Triggered—Infant "Smart" Sensor: 0.02 to 3 L/M Flow-Triggered—Pediatric "Smart" Sensor: 1.0 to 5 L/M
Pressure Support	1 to 50 cm H_2O
Termination Sensitivity	5, 10, 15, 20, and 25 per cent of peak flow
Rise Time	1 to 7 (1 = fastest, 7 = slowest)
Manual Breath	
Inspiratory Pause	0 to 2 seconds
Inspiratory/Expiratory Hold	3 seconds maximum
Flow Display/Comp	
Alarm Silence	
Alarm Reset	
Monitor Display Select	
Apnea Switch	10 to 60 seconds
Alarm Intensity	Min. 66 dB
O_2 Concentration	21% to 100%
MONITORS AND INDICATORS	
Peak Inspiratory Pressure	0 to 130 cm H_2O
Airway Pressure Manometer	-20 to 140 cm H_2O
Inspiratory Time	0.05 to 60 seconds
Mean Airway Pressure	0 to 120 cm H_2O
I:E Ratio	1:0.1 to 1:60
Minute Volume	0.0 to 99.9 L (with flow sensor)
Positive End Expiratory Pressure (PEEP)	0 to 24 cm H_2O
Tidal Volume	0 to 9999 mL (with flow sensor)
Respiratory Rate	0 to 250

Continued

Table 13-14 Specifications for the V.I.P. Gold and Sterling Ventilators—cont'd

Alarms	Low Peak Pressure High Pressure Alarm Low PEEP/CPAP Pressure Alarm Pressure Support/VAPS Time Limit High Tidal Volume Alarm Low Minute Volume Alarm High Breath Rate Alarm High/Prolonged Pressure Alarm Low Inlet Gas Pressure Blender Input Gas Alarm Circuit Fault Alarm Apnea Sensor Alarm Ventilator Inoperative

Dräger Babylog 8000 Infant Ventilator

The Dräger Babylog 8000 Infant Ventilator (Dräger Inc. Critical Care Systems, Telford, PA) (Figure 13-26) is used to mechanically ventilate premature babies and infants. The weight limit use for the ventilator is 20 kilograms. It is electrically and pneumatically powered and microprocessor and pneumatically controlled. The incorporation of a hot wire anemometer placed at the patient Y connector allows the Babylog to monitor flow at the endotracheal tube level, thereby providing improved patient/ventilator synchrony.[20]

Noteworthy Internal Functions

The compressed air and oxygen sources pass through a filter and non-return valve before entering the pressure regulators (Figure 13-27). The two gas sources then enter the solenoid valves and flow adjusters, which blend and control the gas flowing through the inspiratory limb of the patient circuit. In the event of a gas supply or electrical failure, the patient can spontaneously breathe room air through a filter and non-return valve. Expiratory gas flow from the patient circuit is regulated by a pneumatic exhalation valve. The pneumatic safety valve directs excessive pressure build-up within the ventilator system through the exhalation valve.

Control and Alarm Panel

Figure 13-28 provides an illustration of the control and alarm panel of the Babylog 8000plus, which is almost identical to the 8000 (see section below on the 8000plus). In the 8000plus the CMV soft key pad of the 8000 is replaced with VENT.OPTIONS and the CPAP pad of the 8000 is replaced with VENT MODE.

The panel contains a rotary dial panel and a display/soft key panel. The dial panel contains buttons for the operating modes (CPAP and IPPV) and rotary dials for ventilator parameters. Activated modes are indicated by an illuminated LED located within the button. The button must be depressed until the green LED is continuously illuminated for the mode to be activated. This is a safety feature that is in place to prevent accidental mode changes. Illuminated green LEDs indicate mandatory parameters to be set for that particular mode of ventilation. If a parameter has been internally limited or needs attention the green LED will flash.

The rotary dial panel contains six dials. OXYGEN CONCENTRATION % (21 to 100%), INSPIRATORY TIME (0.1 to 2.0 seconds), EXPIRATORY TIME (0.2 to 30 seconds), INSPIRATORY FLOW (1 to 30 L/min), INSPIRATORY PRESSURE LIMIT (10 to 80 cm H_2O), and PEEP (0 to 15 cm H_2O). Table 13-15 provides parameter specifications for the Dräger Babylog 8000 Ventilator.

The screen and soft key panel that is located on the top of the ventilator serves various functions. The waveform display window displays either pressure or flow scalar waveforms over time. The measured values window digitally displays minute ventilation, oxygen concentration, peak inspiratory pressure, mean airway pressure, and PEEP. The current mode of ventilation and other pertinent information is displayed on the far right in the status window. The soft keys are used to select ventilation modes, ventilator functions, and access other windows. The menu keys are located on the bottom of the screen. The screen functions are selected from the monitoring and functions menu with their respective submenus. Green LED illuminating lights will indicate whether monitoring or functions has been selected. The MANUAL SOFT KEY is located above the monitoring LED and activates a manual breath or an extension of an existing breath in progress. The maximum

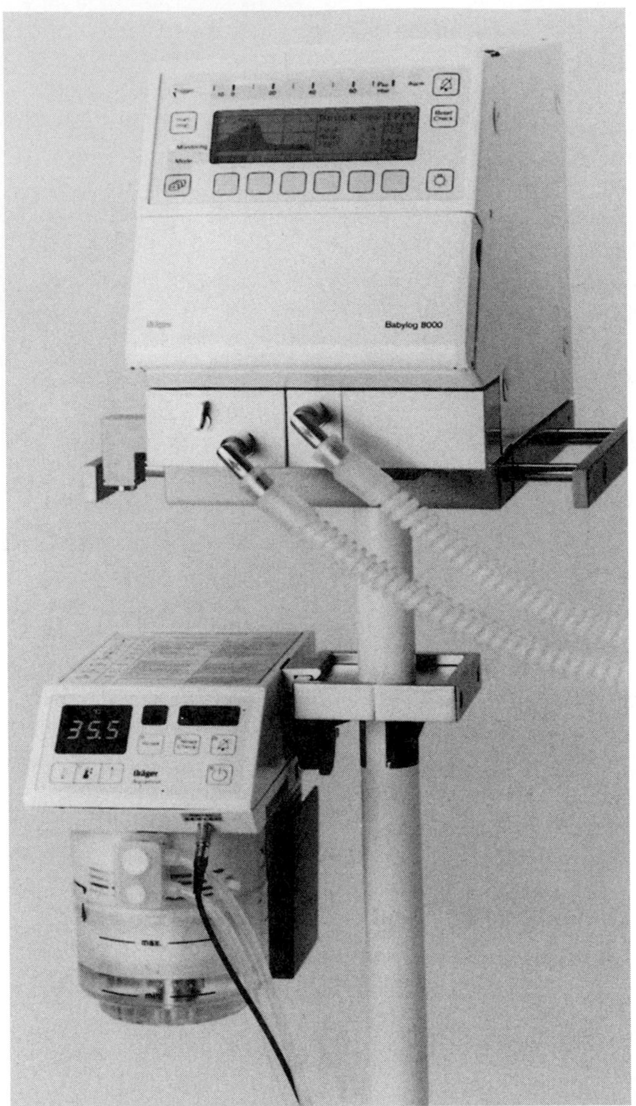

Figure 13-26 The Dräger Babylog 8000 Infant Ventilator. (Courtesy Dräger Corp, Telford, Penn.)

inspiratory time available is 5 seconds. Text messages are displayed as pop-up windows at the top of any current screen.

The ALARM SILENCE and RESET/CHECK soft keys are located on the top right panel. The ALARM SILENCE silences the alarm for 2 minutes, while the RESET/CHECK allows the clinician to recognize those messages and clear them from the screen. A red alarm light will flash when a warning or caution message is displayed on the screen.

Inspiratory and expiratory pressure sensors calculate the airway pressure, which is then displayed as real-time airway pressure measurements on an illuminating bar graph located on the top of the monitor. The yellow LED is illuminated when inspiration is triggered.

The OXYGEN CONCENTRATION ALARM limits are set internally at ±4%. The alarm limits for PEEP and PINSP are also set internally by the microprocessor. The LOSS OF PEEP/CPAP limit is –4 cm H_2O with a minimum of –2 cm H_2O. The HIGH PRESSURE ALARM is automatically set to PINSP +10 cm H_2O or PEEP/CPAP +4 cm H_2O. In the event of excessive pressure build up within the circuit, the exhalation valve opens allowing exhalation. Adjustable alarm limits include HIGH MINUTE VENTILATION, LOW MINUTE VENTILATION, MINUTE VENTILATION DELAY (0 to 30 seconds), and APNEA (5 to 20 seconds).

The ventilator alarms are arranged in order of importance. The alarms are grouped into advisory, warning, and alarm messages that are digitally displayed on the ventilator screen eliminating the guesswork of troubleshooting alarm conditions. Incidents such as obstructed endotracheal tube, kinked circuit, and apnea are clearly identified on the ventilator screen. Each alarm level has a distinctive audible tone that indicates its level of importance. Every message is recorded in the message log, which is capable of storing the most recent 100 entries. The log records the time of occurrence, displayed text, and information on the response.

Modes of Ventilation

The mandatory breaths in Assist Control and SIMV are time or patient-triggered, pressure-targeted, and time-cycled. The operator sets the following parameters: inspiratory time, expiratory time, inspiratory flow, inspiratory pressure, PEEP, and trigger sensitivity. Mandatory breaths are volume triggered when a patient's spontaneous inspiratory volume is equal to or greater than the set trigger volume (set value of 2 or greater), otherwise the mandatory breath is time triggered.

Continuous flow supports spontaneous respiratory efforts between the mandatory breaths in the CPAP mode. The amount of continuous flow available is determined by either the inspiratory flow control or the VIVE (Variable Inspiratory Variable Expiratory) flow option.

The VIVE operating mode allows the clinician to adjust the flow during the expiratory phase to match the patient's needs during mandatory and spontaneous breaths. The inspiratory flow rate is displayed on the left bar graph and adjustments can be made with the rotary dial. The expiratory flow rate is displayed on the right bar graph and can be adjusted with the up and down menu buttons.

Trigger sensitivity is set by accessing the main menu function and selecting the trigger button. The trigger sensitivity range is 1 to 10 with 1 (minimum) representing a more sensitive trigger sensitivity and 10 (maximum) representing the least sensitive trigger. The trigger threshold of 1 to 10 corresponds with a volume of 0 to 3 milliliters. The recommended setting is minimum; a yellow trigger LED is illuminated with each triggered breath. A setting of one indicates that when the Babylog measures a flow change of 0.25 L/min (straight flow-trigger), the mandatory breath is then synchronized with the patient effort. Settings above 1 indicate that the Babylog is evaluating the system

1. Sintered filter
2. Non-return valve
3. Pressure regulator
4. Absolute pressure sensor
5. Solenoid valve of mixer and flow unit
6. Flow adjuster for blender and flow unit
7. Solenoid switching valve
8. Solenoid valve
9. Solenoid valve
10. Non-return valve
11. Filter
12. Pneumatic control valve
13. Flow adjuster
14. O_2 measuring system
15. Pneumatic control valve
16. Pneumatic safety valve
17. Relative pressure sensor
18. Electrical PEEP control valve
19. Safety valve
20. Expiration valve
21. Bactericidal labyrinth
22. Relative pressure sensor
23. Solenoid valve
24. Ejector

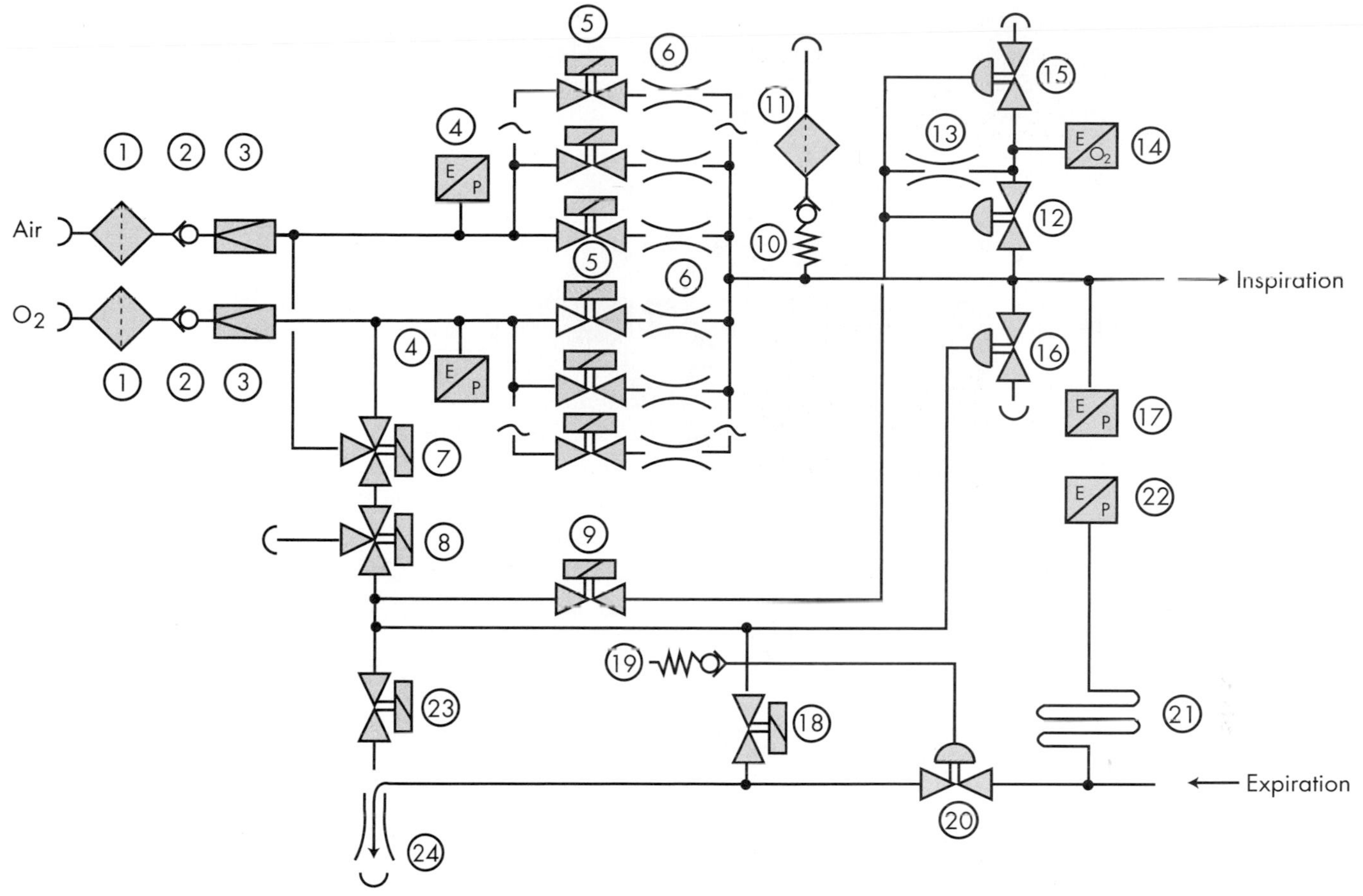

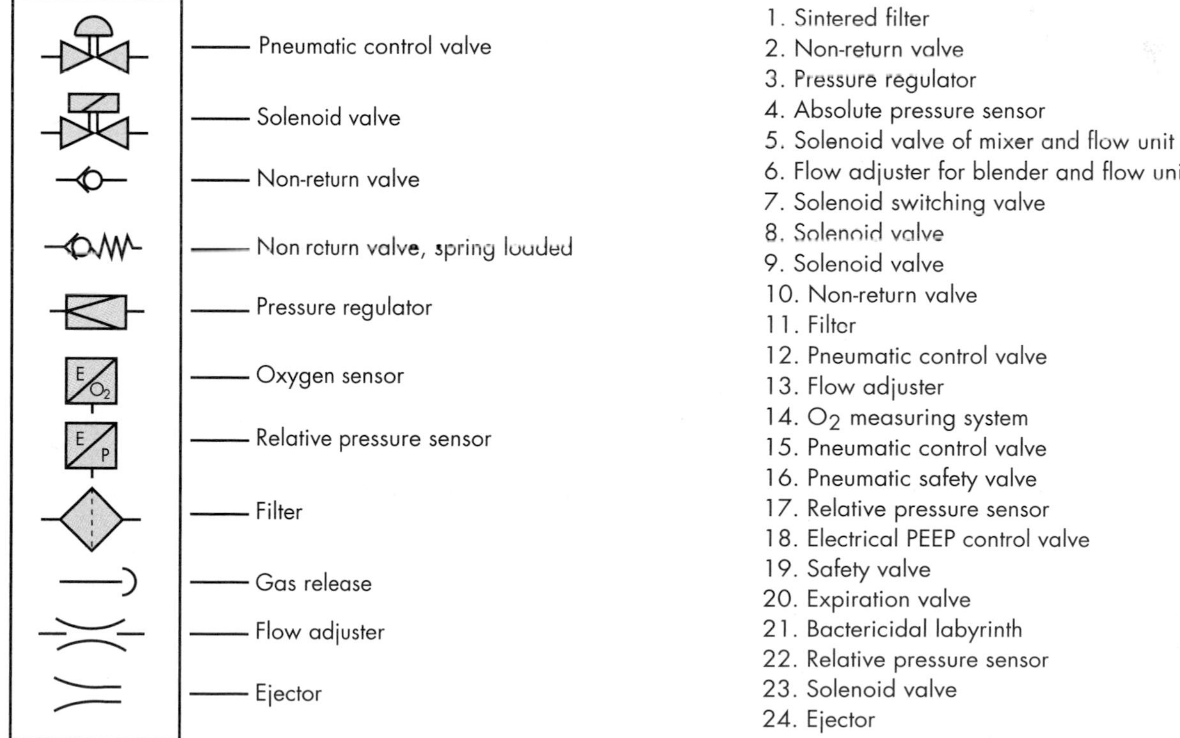

Figure 13-27 The internal pneumatic circuit of the Dräger Babylog 8000 Infant Ventilator. (Courtesy Dräger Corp, Telford, Penn.)

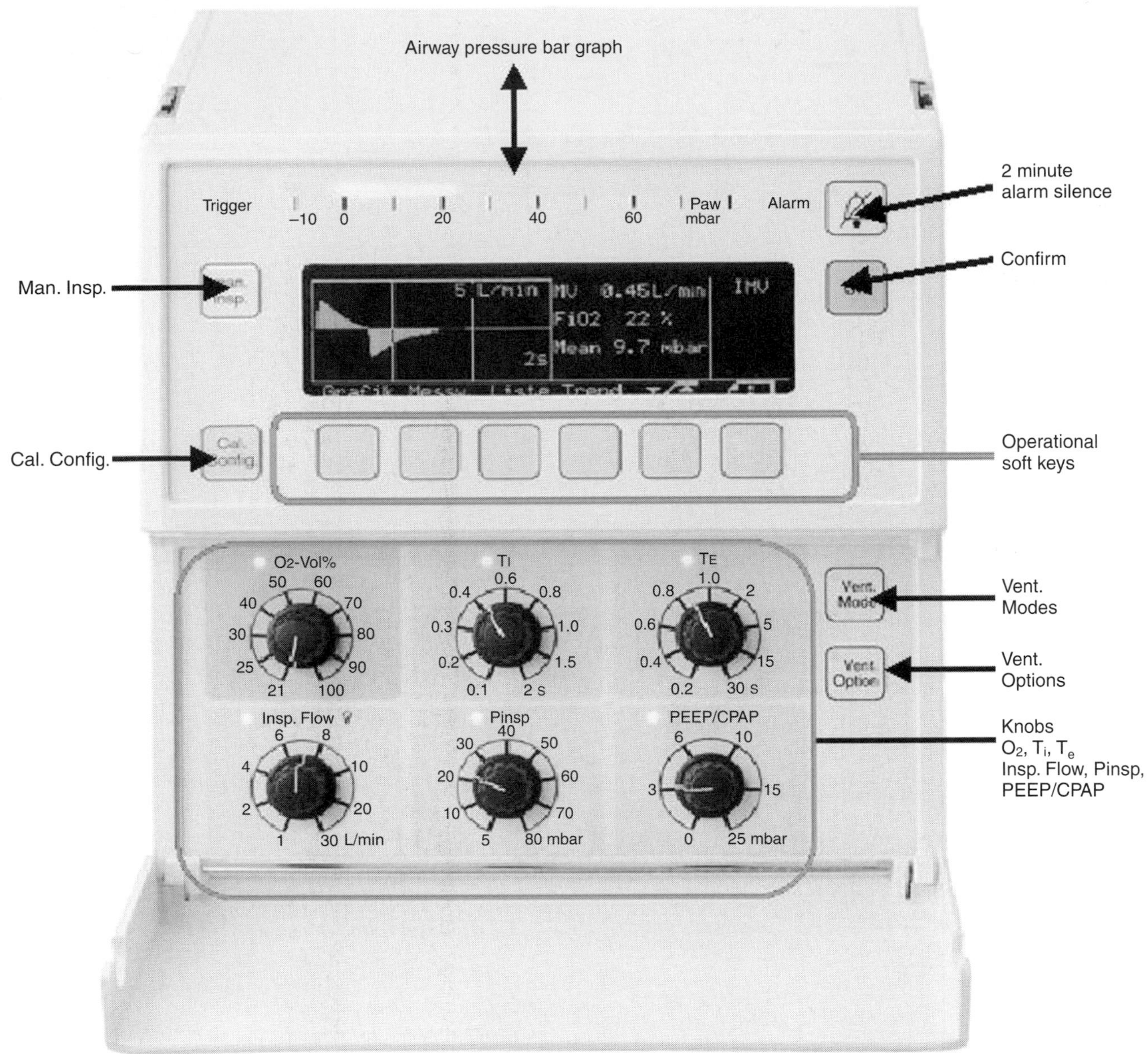

Figure 13-28 The control and alarm panel of the Babylog 8000plus Infant Ventilator (see text for description). (Courtesy Dräger Corp, Telford, Penn.)

for flow changes but waits until a particular volume moves across the flow sensor, then synchronizing the breath with the patient's negative effort (Figure 13-29).

The IMV breath is pressure-targeted, time-triggered, pressure- or flow-limited, and time- or pressure-cycled. The operator sets the following parameters: oxygen concentration, inspiratory time, expiratory time, inspiratory flow, inspiratory pressure, and PEEP. The mandatory rate is calculated by adding the inspiratory time and expiratory time that are set and dividing the sum into 60 seconds. The mandatory breath is time-triggered based on the rate calculation.

The application of nasal CPAP can be used but the flow measurement has to be disabled by disconnecting the connector from the flow sensor and pressing the reset/check button. The operator sets the following parameters: oxygen concentration, inspiratory flow, and PEEP.

Graphics Displays

Real-time pressure and flow scalar waveforms are displayed on the monitoring screen. The waveforms are accessed through the monitoring main menu and selecting the graph submenu and pressing either the $\overline{P}$aw or FLOW button. The waveform scale is automatically set by the ventilator. The displayed flow scalar waveform indicates the inspiratory flow pattern above the baseline and expiratory flow below. Freeze and trend options are also available if desired. The trend feature stores a 24-hour window.

Table 13-15 Specifications for Babylog 8000 Infant Ventilator

Inspiratory time	0.1 to 2.0 seconds
Expiratory time	0.2 to 30 seconds
Inspiratory flow	1 to 30 L/min
Expiratory flow	1 to 30 L/min
Peak inspiratory pressure	10 to 80 cm H_2O
PEEP/CPAP	0 to 15 cm H_2O
Oxygen concentration	21% to 100%
Rate	2 to 150 breaths/min
Trigger mechanism	Flow/volume trigger
Alarms	Loss of PEEP/CPAP; high pressure; high minute ventilation; low minute ventilation; minute-ventilation delay; and apnea

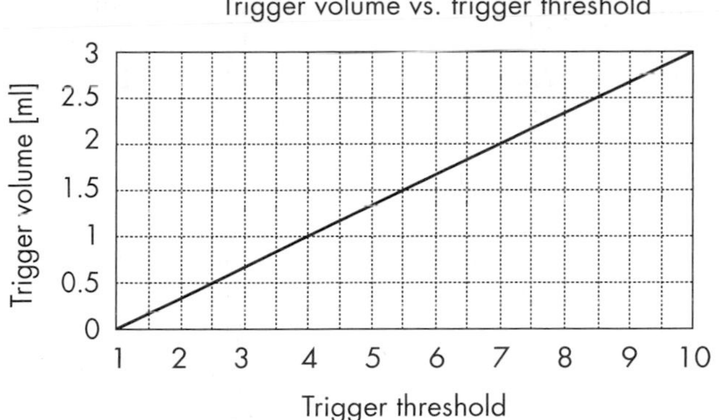

Figure 13-29 The trigger sensitivity setting on the Babylog 8000 Infant Ventilator (see text for further information).

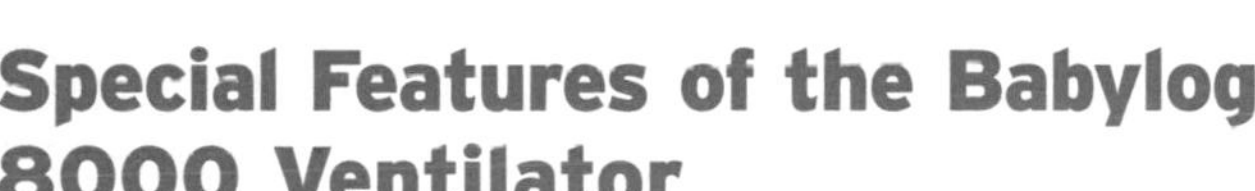

Special Features of the Babylog 8000 Ventilator

The ventilator performs an automatic calibration of the oxygen analyzer every 24 hours. Calibration can also be done manually under the "function menu" and "cal submenu." The calibration takes approximately 5 minutes to complete. The flow sensor calibration is accessed through the function menu and calibration submenu. To calibrate the flow sensor, the operator simply follows the instructions given on the screen. The monitoring of minute ventilation and apnea are only made possible with a calibrated flow sensor. Flow sensor calibration should be performed every time the ventilator is turned on, after sensor assembly, and after sensor replacement.

Dräger Babylog 8000plus Infant Ventilator

The Dräger Babylog 8000 has had several upgrades. Software version 4 is the original. The next two upgrades were version 5 and 6. The company then added "plus" to the unit, which is probably best defined as (1) extra monitoring; (2) pressure support, and (3) the addition of Volume Guarantee. [Note: Some individuals do not consider pressure support part of the plus package.]

The Drager Babylog 8000plus is an updated version of the original model 8000. In this newer model, additional monitoring parameters have been added. A pressure support ventilation mode and VOLUME GUARANTEE are available as options. A high-frequency feature capable of rates from 5 to 20 Hz is another option with this model, but is not available in the United States.

Additional monitoring includes measurement of lung mechanics. These parameters are accessible from the monitoring menu and include airway resistance, dynamic compliance, time constant, C20/C, and r, which is the correlation coefficient of linear regression. A low tidal volume alarm is also available.

The pressure support ventilation mode is provided as a spontaneous-only mode. It cannot be combined with other modes or used with mandatory breaths. However, if apnea is detected, the ventilator will begin delivering mandatory breaths according to the set pressure and inspiratory and expiratory times. Pressure support breaths are flow-triggered and either flow- or time-cycled. When inspiratory flow drops to a fixed 15% of peak flow, inspiration terminates. Flow termination is not adjustable. Time cycling will occur if the set Tin is reached.

VOLUME GUARANTEE is a dual mode feature that can be used in all patient-triggered modes. As its name implies, a tidal volume can be set by the clinician. However, the ventilator will continue to provide characteristic waveforms of pressure-targeted ventilation. In other words, VOLUME GUARANTEE is pressure-limited ventilation with a volume target. The clinician continues to have control over the delivered peak pressure but also can select a tidal volume target. The VOLUME GUARANTEE feature can only be employed when the airway flow sensor is in use.

When VOLUME GUARANTEE is activated, the ventilator software continuously measures and compares inspired and expired tidal volume. Each breath uses these comparisons from the previous breath to make adjustments to the peak inspiratory pressure to deliver a tidal volume as close as possible to the preset value. The lowest inspiratory pressure is administered that can result in delivery of the target tidal volume.

When activating VOLUME GUARANTEE, the clinician sets the maximum peak inspiratory pressure. This setting becomes an inspiratory pressure limit. Over the next six to eight breaths, the ventilator determines the appropriate inspiratory pressure and begins to achieve and maintain the target tidal volume. If the patient's inspiratory effort adds to the tidal volume, the ventilator PIP will immediately decrease. If the total inspiratory tidal volume exceeds the set target volume by 130%, the expiratory valve will open and no additional ventilator-driven gas will be delivered to the patient.

The clinician should exercise care when using VOLUME GUARANTEE to carefully monitor patient-ventilator interaction. An appropriate target tidal volume should be selected based on patient weight. A clinically safe peak inspiratory pressure should be set as well as an appropriate value for the low V_T alarm.

Bunnell Life Pulse High-Frequency Jet Ventilator

The Bunnell Life Pulse High-Frequency Jet ventilator (HFJV) (Bunnell Incorporated, Salt Lake City, Utah) (Figure 13-30) is indicated for patients with severe respiratory distress syndrome complicated by pulmonary air leak failing conventional mechanical ventilation strategies. The Bunnell HFJV is a microprocessor controlled, pressure-limited, time-cycled, constant flow high-frequency jet ventilator that works in parallel with a conventional ventilator. The conventional ventilator provides background conventional ventilation (if desired), supplies entrained gas, and regulates the PEEP level.[21]

Control and Alarm Panel

The ON/OFF switch is located midway on the front left panel. Pressing the button once powers the ventilator on (displays green light) and pressing the button again turns the ventilator off (no light). Figure 13-31 provides a diagram of the seven components of the ventilator which include the following sections: monitoring, alarms, controls, patient box, disposable cartridge/circuit, rear panel, and humidifier monitor, alarms, and controls.

The ventilator monitoring displays provide pertinent patient information and ventilator performance and are located on the front top left panel of the control panel. These displays are PIP, delta P (PIP-PEEP), PEEP, SERVO PRESSURE, and $\overline{P}$aw. The four patient pressures are sensed at the distal end of the Hi-Lo jet tube (if used) and measured by the transducer in the patient box. The displays are averages calculated over a short period and are not reflective of alveolar pressures. Mean airway pressure can be increased by increasing peak inspiratory pressure, increasing PEEP, and increasing the rate and tidal volume of the sigh breaths. The PEEP level is controlled by the conventional ventilator.

The SERVO PRESSURE measurement (0-20 psig) is the amount of internal pressure required to generate the PIP displayed in the NOW (current requirement) display and is a clinical indicator of improved lung status or acute changes (i.e., tension pneumothorax, endotracheal tube leak, atelectasis). For example, a decrease in lung compliance may result in a decrease in servo pressure because less gas is required to meet the set PIP. Increases in lung compliance or the development of a pneumothorax may result in elevated servo pressures (Clinical Rounds 13-9).

The pinch valve ON/OFF lights located on the front top left panel (monitor panel) indicate the communication between the ventilator and pinch valve (located on patient box). The illuminated on light indicates the valve is signaled to open for inspiration. The illuminated OFF light indicates the valve is signaled to close for expiration. The light will alternate rapidly between the ON and OFF displays.

The ventilator alarm displays are located on the front top right panel and include the following: SERVO PRESSURE (+1 cm H_2O present value), $\overline{P}$aw (+1.5 cm H_2O), HIGH (>5 cm H_2O PIP for 2 seconds or >10 cm H_2O for 30 seconds), and LOSS OF PIP (<25% PIP). The mean

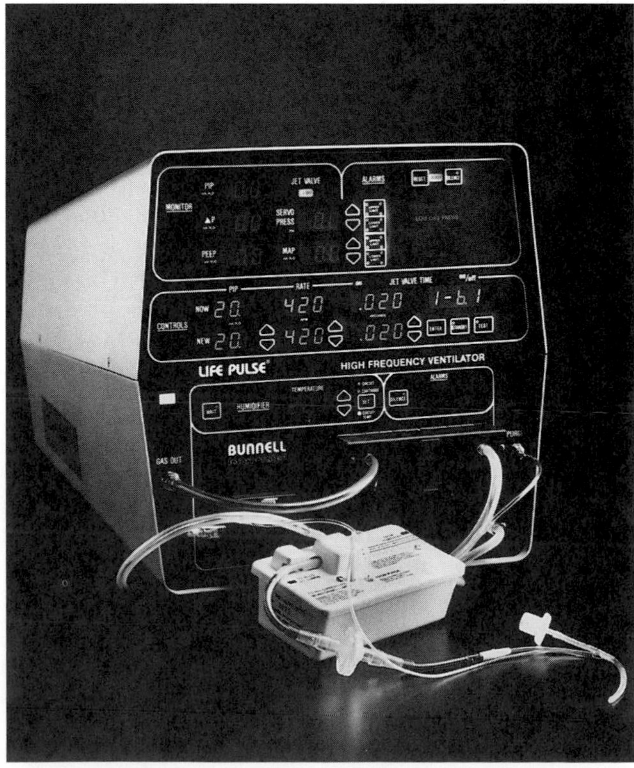

Figure 13-30 The Bunnell Life Pulse High-Frequency Jet Ventilator. (Courtesy Bunnell, Inc, Salt Lake City, Utah.)

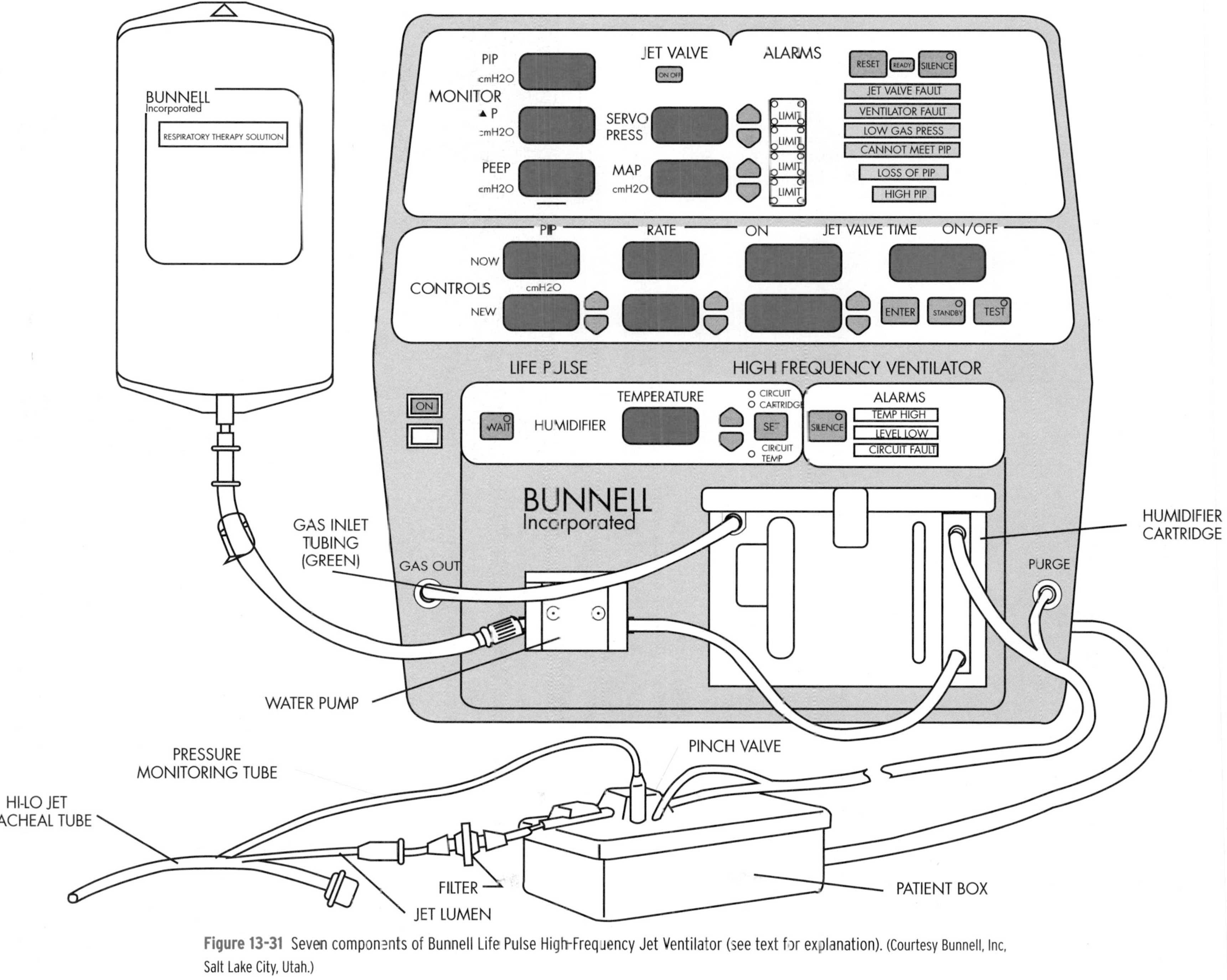

Figure 13-31 Seven components of Bunnell Life Pulse High-Frequency Jet Ventilator (see text for explanation). (Courtesy Bunnell, Inc, Salt Lake City, Utah.)

> **CLINICAL ROUNDS 13-9**
>
> An infant with acute respiratory distress syndrome is receiving high-frequency ventilation with the Bunnell Jet ventilator. Breath sounds and arterial blood gases have been improving over the past 24 hours. The servo pressure has been slowly increasing over several hours. The change in servo pressure might indicate what change in the patient?
>
> See Appendix A for the answer.

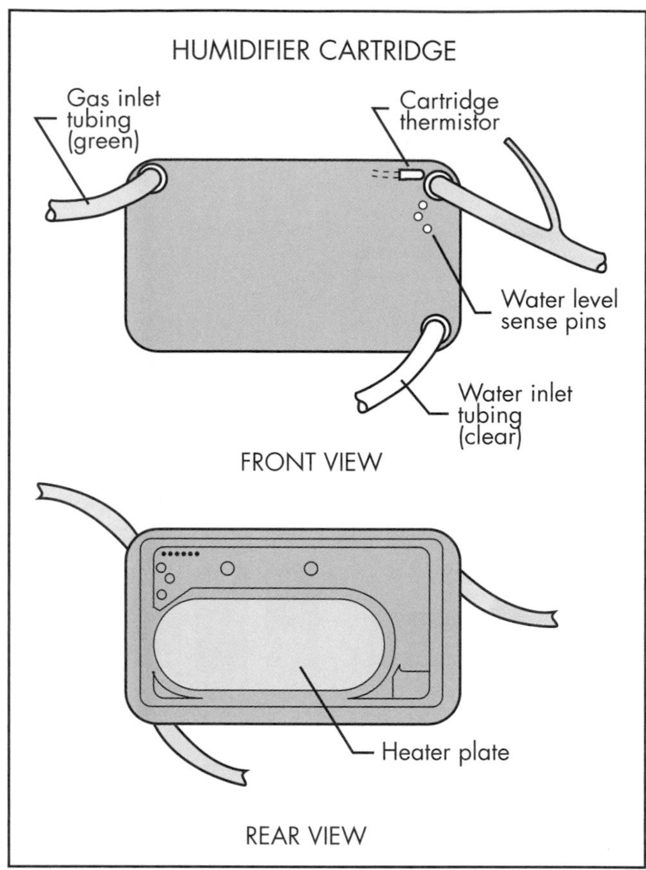

Figure 13-32 The humidifier cartridge/patient breathing circuit of the Bunnell Life Pulse High-Frequency Jet Ventilator.

airway pressure and servo pressure upper and lower limits can be adjusted manually. The HIGH PIP, JET VALVE FAULT, VENTILATOR FAULT, LOW GAS PRESSURE, CANNOT MEET PIP, and LOSS OF PIP alarms are back-lighted displays. The JET VALVE FAULT alarm alerts the clinician that the pinch valve in the patient box is not functioning appropriately. The microprocessor is continuously monitoring the pinch valve and activates the alarm when malfunctions are detected. The Life Pulse continues to operate even if the pinch valve is not cycling. The ventilator fault alarm alerts the clinician that a problem is present within the Life Pulse electronics or valves. A numerical code will be displayed in the jet valve on/off time window to indicate the type of failure.

The LOW GAS PRESSURE alarm alerts the clinician that the gas supply is less than 30 psig. The CANNOT MEET PIP alarm alerts the clinician that the ventilator is unable to deliver the pressures within a set range while the servo pressure has increased to the maximum level available. The alarm can be a result of a leak in the humidifier cartridge/patient circuit, incomplete connection of the circuit to the jet tube, defective or damaged jet tube (kinked tube, improper positioning, occlusion, or leak), present settings unable to ventilate larger patient, patient fighting the Life Pulse, or the pinch valve opening action is not effective resulting in higher servo pressures to meet current settings.

The RESET, READY light, and ALARM SILENCE (60 seconds) buttons are located above the ventilator alarm displays. The RESET button has the machine recalculate automatic upper and lower limits for the servo pressure, PIP, and mean airway pressure ($\overline{P}aw$) parameters. It is recommended for use when changes are made on the conventional side of ventilation and manual adjustments are not made. When the RESET button is pressed, the READY light turns off and alarm indicators are inactive. The Life Pulse calculates new alarm limits; after this is accomplished, the READY light will illuminate and all alarms are reactivated. The READY light indicates when the machine has stabilized after start-up or reset, calculated alarm limits, and is ready for operation. The SILENCE button will silence audible alarms for 60 seconds. The alarm will resume after this period of time if the condition has not resolved. A red light will illuminate in the corner of the silence button when the silence function is in effect.

The ventilator control parameters and displays are located on the front middle panel and include: PIP (8 to 50 cm H_2O), RATE (240 to 660 insufflations/minute), JET ON TIME (inspiratory time) (.02 to 0.034 seconds), and ON/OFF RATIO (1:1.2 to 1:12). The NOW displays indicate current operating settings. The NEW display and control area allows the operator to adjust set parameters and visualize the change prior to entering new parameters. Some hospitals interrupt HFJV by setting the sigh breath peak pressure (on conventional ventilator) higher than HFJV, whereas others adjust the sigh breath peak pressure (on conventional ventilator) equal or less than the HFJV PIP setting (HFJV breaths are not interrupted).

The operating mode selection buttons are ENTER, STANDBY, and TEST. Pressing the ENTER button changes the now parameters to the new parameters. Inappropriately high servo pressure may occur if the ENTER button is pressed before connecting the patient circuit to the patient, possibly resulting in high pressures and delivery of excessively high tidal volumes. The STANDBY mode is used when the operator wants to interrupt HFJV temporarily (i.e., suctioning or to monitor the effectiveness of conventional ventilation). Alarms are inactive while in the STANDBY mode. The functioning STANDBY mode is indicated by red lights and a 5-second audible alarm and is automatically set up with ventilator power-up. The TEST mode is an automatic test that checks the ventilator systems and circuitry for proper function and should not be performed with a patient connected to the jet ventilator.

The disposable humidifier cartridge/patient breathing circuit is a closed system that provides humidity, heating, and monitoring of the gas exiting the ventilator (Figure 13-32). The humidifier cartridge heats and humidifies the gas before patient delivery. The cartridge receptacle holds the humidifier cartridge in place by securing the latch into place. The water in the cartridge is warmed by the anodized aluminum heater plate.

The gas out and purge pneumatic connectors located on the front panel are of different sizes in order to prevent improper connections. The short green gas-inlet tube connects the gas flow from the ventilator to the cartridge. The clear water-inlet tube transfers water from the pump when the water level sensors detect a decrease in the water level, thus filling the humidifier cartridge. Water is transferred from a non-pressurized source (i.e., solution bag or bottle) to the pressurized humidifier cartridge by the water pump. The water level is regulated by the water level sensor pins in the cartridge. The purge port supplies gas to the **purge valve**, which is located in the patient box. The gas is used to provide a moisture free environment in the monitoring line of the Hi-Lo jet tube. The small, clear, second lumen of the patient circuit connects to this port.

The HUMIDIFIER WAIT button turns off the heater and water pump, allowing easy removal and replacement of the cartridge/circuit. A red light in the corner of the button will flash to indicate activation of the wait feature. To resume normal function, simply depress the button again.

A thermistor is located at the patient breathing circuit and cartridge connection to assure adequate gas temperature delivery to the patient. The available temperature range is 32° to 42° C.

The temperature is displayed in three separate windows, which are labeled CIRCUIT (desired), CARTRIDGE (desired), and CIRCUIT TEMPERATURE (actual temperature). The set button selects the temperature setting/measurement to be displayed. The window display will automatically return to the circuit temperature display reading. The humidifier system has a separate SILENCE button (separate from ventilator ALARM SILENCE) and various back-lighted alarm messages. The messages alert the clinician of any temperature/water level changes and/or electrical problems within the cartridge/circuit.

The PATIENT BOX is a satellite component that contains the pinch valve, purge valve, and pressure transducer (Figure 13-33). It is designed for placement near the patient's head for accurate pressure monitoring and delivery of jet bursts. The PATIENT BOX electrical cable connects to the rear panel of the ventilator. An **electromagnetic** solenoid activates the pinch valve. The pinch valve breaks the flow of pressurized gas into small bursts with the pinch and release action on the silicone tube of the patient breathing circuit. The PUSH TO LOAD button opens the valve to allow correct placement of the silicone tube within the PATIENT BOX and to allow repositioning of the silicone tube. The silicone tube should be moved 2 millimeter every 8 hours to prevent areas of wear and avoid tearing.

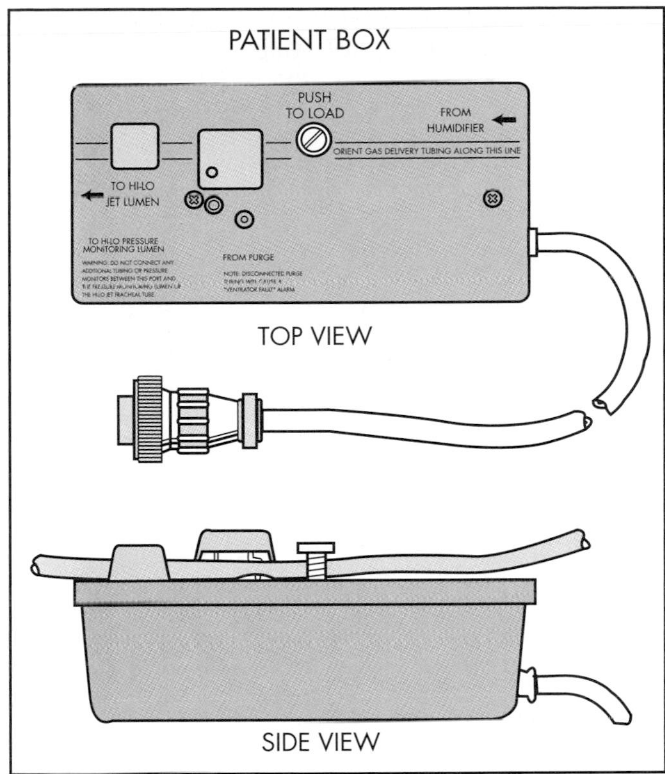

Figure 13-33 The PATIENT BOX on the Bunnell Life Pulse High-Frequency Jet Ventilator.

A bacterial filter is present downstream from the pinch valve to provide particle filtration. A millimeter measuring guide is printed on the PATIENT BOX for visual use. The purge valve maintains a moisture-free pressure monitoring line of the endotracheal tube by allowing pressurized gas from the ventilator to pass through the line. A 10-millisecond burst of gas is introduced through the monitoring line. The pressure transducer measures tracheal pressure and sends the information to the microprocessor.

The rear panel contains the mixed gas input connection, oxygen sensor connection, hour meter, circuit breaker, alarm volume control, PATIENT BOX connector, analog output, and dump valve outlet. The gas input fitting connects the ventilator to an oxygen blender in order to provide varied oxygen concentrations. A 30-100 psig supply source is required. The oxygen sensor connection allows continuous

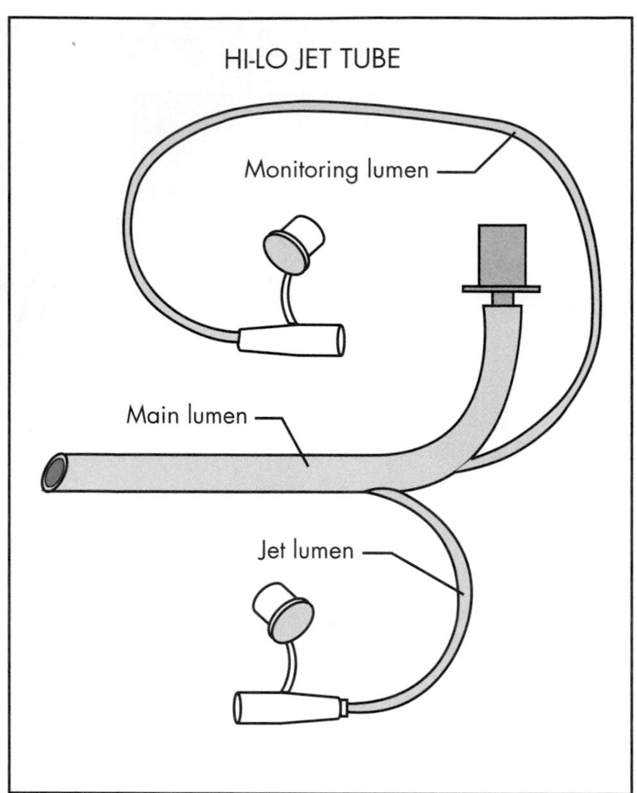

Figure 13-34 Triple-lumen Hi-lo Jet tracheal tubes for use in high-frequency jet ventilation. (Courtesy Puritan Bennett, a division of Tyco Medical, Pleasanton, Calif.)

monitoring of F_IO_2. The **dump valve** is a safety valve that releases internal pressure.

Special Features

Hi-Lo Jet Endotracheal Tube

The triple lumen Hi-Lo Jet tracheal tubes (Figure 13-34) are uncuffed and range in size from 2.5 to 6.0 mm inner diameter (ID) in 0.5 mm increments. The external diameter is approximately equal to the external diameter of a half-size larger standard endotracheal tube. For example, a 3.0 mm ID Hi-Lo Jet tube has an external diameter that is approximately equal to a 3.5 mm ID standard endotracheal tube.[21]

The three lumens of the Hi-Lo Jet tube serve various functions. The main lumen contains a 15 mm connector that provides the connection point for the conventional ventilator circuit Y connector. The jet lumen provides the connection to the patient breathing circuit from the patient box. The jet bursts are delivered through this lumen. The monitoring lumen is used to monitor pressures at the distal end of the Hi-Lo Jet tube. This lumen is connected to the TO HI-LO PRESSURE MONITORING LUMEN connection on the patient box.

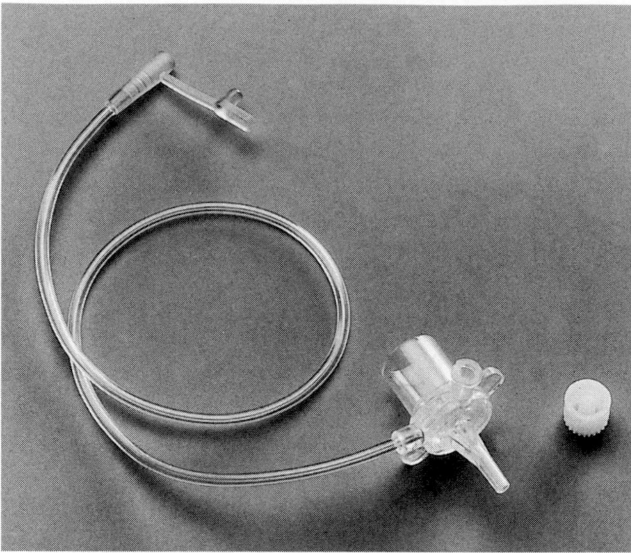

Figure 13-35 Bunnell Life Port Endotracheal Tube Adaptor for use in high-frequency jet ventilation. (Courtesy Bunnell, Inc, Salt Lake City, Utah.)

LifePort Endotracheal Tube Adaptor

The development of the LifePort Endotracheal Tube Adaptor (Figure 13-35) has alleviated the requirement of intubating/reintubating patients with the specialized jet tube prior to initiation of HFJV. With the use of the double-port endotracheal tube adapter and a conventional single-lumen endotracheal tube, HFJV can be implemented easily and quickly. The adaptors are available in sizes 2.5 mm ID, 3.5 mm ID, and 4.5 mm ID. To initiate HFJV, simply replace the 15 mm standard endotracheal tube adaptor with the 15 mm connection of the jet tube adaptor. The jet port provides entry of gas from the jet ventilator. The inspired gas is redirected through a nozzle, which increases the gas velocity. The momentum of the gas is converted to pressure as the gas exits from the nozzle.

Bunnell Incorporated suggests adjusting the HFJV PIP to equal the conventional PIP when utilizing the 2.5 mm ID LifePort adaptor. When using the larger adapters, set up the initial HFJV PIP at 90% of the conventional PIP.

Sensormedics 3100 and 3100A High-Frequency Oscillatory Ventilators

The model 3100 was the first of the two high-frequency oscillators originally introduced by the SensorMedics Corporation of Yorba Linda, CA (now VIASYS Healthcare systems, Palm Springs, CA) for use with neonates. An improved model, the 3100A, followed and replaced the 3100 (Figure 13-36, A). Both of these models have been used extensively in the treatment of acute respiratory failure in infants. The 3100A is also being used in older pediatric patients and adults.

Noteworthy Internal Functions

The heart of the SensorMedics models is the **oscillator subsystem,** or the **piston assembly** (Figure 13-37). The system incorporates an electronic control circuit, or **square-wave driver,** which powers a linear drive motor. The motor consists of an electrical coil within a magnet, similar to a permanent magnet speaker. When a positive polarity is applied to the square wave driver, the coil is driven forward. The coil is attached to a rubber bellows, or diaphragm to create a piston. When the coil moves forward, the piston moves toward the patient airway, creating the inspiratory phase. When the polarity changes to negative, the electrical coil and the attached piston are driven away from the patient, creating an active expiration.[22]

The amount of **polarity voltage** applied to the electrical coil determines the distance that the piston will be driven toward and away from the patient airway. Therefore, increasing the polarity voltage increases piston movement, or amplitude. Piston excursion is limited, however, by resistance from the pressure within the patient circuit. The oscillator subsystem also limits the piston stroke to 365 mL. The total time for a piston stroke is a few milliseconds. When oscillations are at low frequencies, the piston has sufficient time to travel the available excursion length during either the inspiratory or expiratory phase and remain at maximum position until it begins its movement in the opposite direction. Conversely, as oscillating frequency is increased, the excursion time of the piston becomes a larger percentage of the breath phase. The percentage of time the piston remains completely forward or backward decreases. At very high frequencies, the polarity to the coil changes so rapidly that the piston does not have time for a complete excursion and arrival to its maximum position. In fact, it may only travel a fraction of its potential distance before changing direction. Therefore, volume delivered by the piston is decreased as oscillatory frequency is increased.

Although the piston subsystem is designed to produce as little friction as possible, the rapid movement of the piston generates some heat. Therefore, a venturi-type air amplifier is used on the 3100A to introduce cooling air around the electrical coil. A separate compressed air source of at least 30 psig serves this system, which consists of a regulator and venturi. The regulator reduces air flow to 15 L/min, and the venturi entrains 45 L/min room air. This provides 60 L/min of cooling air for the subsystem.

Circuit Design

Figure 13-38 shows the basic circuit of the 3100A. After exiting the back panel of the ventilator and passing through a humidifier, blended gas enters the patient circuit at the **bias flow** inlet. Flow is set using the bias flow control on the front panel (Figure 13-36, *B*). The gas mixture fills the space in front of the piston, flows past the limit valve and on to the endotracheal tube connection. Gas then passes the dump valve, and exits through either the control valve or a small restricted orifice next to the control valve housing. The oscillating piston moves the circuit gas in a forward and backward direction toward the airway. The rate of bias flow, the pressure maintained at the airway, and the speed and excursion of the piston are all set by the clinician.

Any standard humidifier can be used with the 3100 and 3100A. Circuits are designed to accommodate heater sensors to provide servo controlled temperature at the airway. Heated wire circuits are available to reduce water condensation. All circuits incorporate a water outlet, tubing, and water trap that permits water condensate to drain away from the piston.

Controls (Figure 13-36, *B*)

On/Off

The ventilator's ON/OFF SWITCH is located on the front of the unit below the piston and to the right (Figure 13-36, *A*). If power to the unit is turned off or electrical power is interrupted while the ventilator is in operation, an audible alarm will sound and the red POWER FAILURE LED on the front control panel is illuminated. This alarm can only be silenced by depressing the RESET button on the front panel. With any interruption in ventilator operation, pressurization of the circuit's three mushroom valves stops immediately, allowing the circuit to vent to the atmosphere. This venting allows the patient to breathe room air. The proximity of the vented DUMP VALVE close to the airway enables the patient to breathe room air with minimal resistance from the ventilator circuit.

Piston Centering

The piston's forward and backward excursions are limited by two **mechanical stops.** If time and amplitude allow the piston to encounter one of the stops, it will remain stationary

A

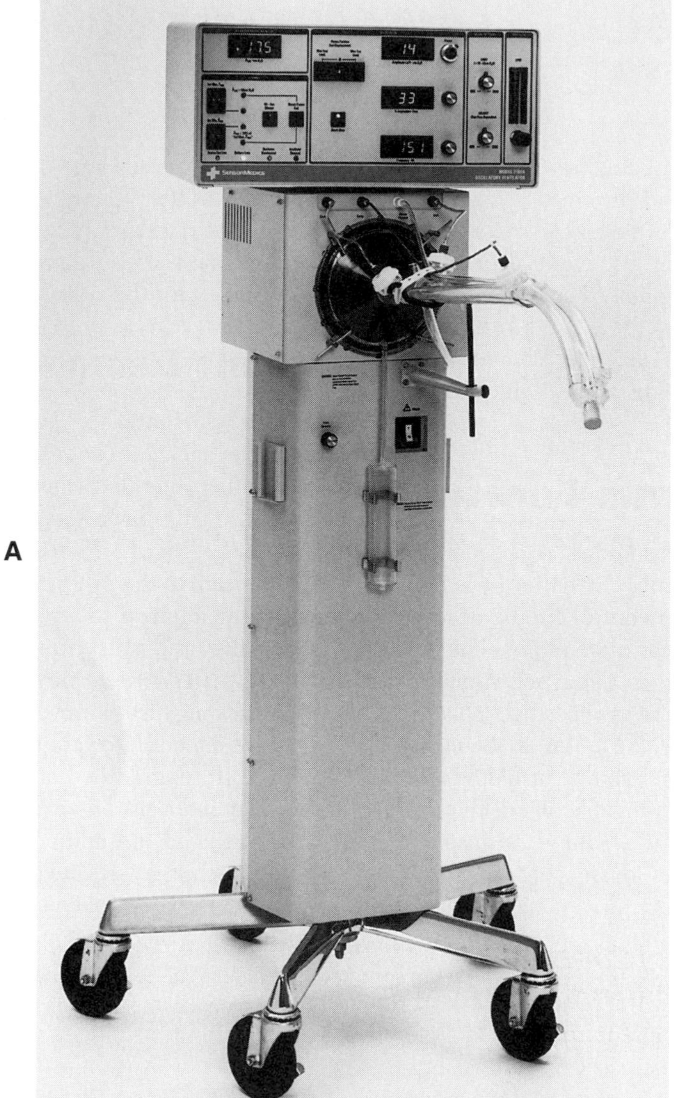

B

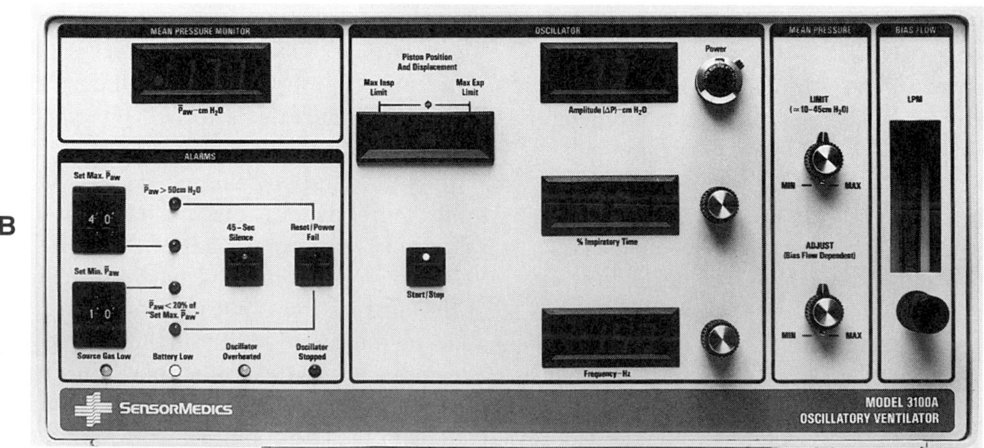

Figure 13-36 **A,** SensorMedics Model 3100A High-Frequency Oscillator. **B,** Control panel of the 3100A. (Courtesy VIASYS Healthcare, Critical Care Division, Palm Springs, Calif.)

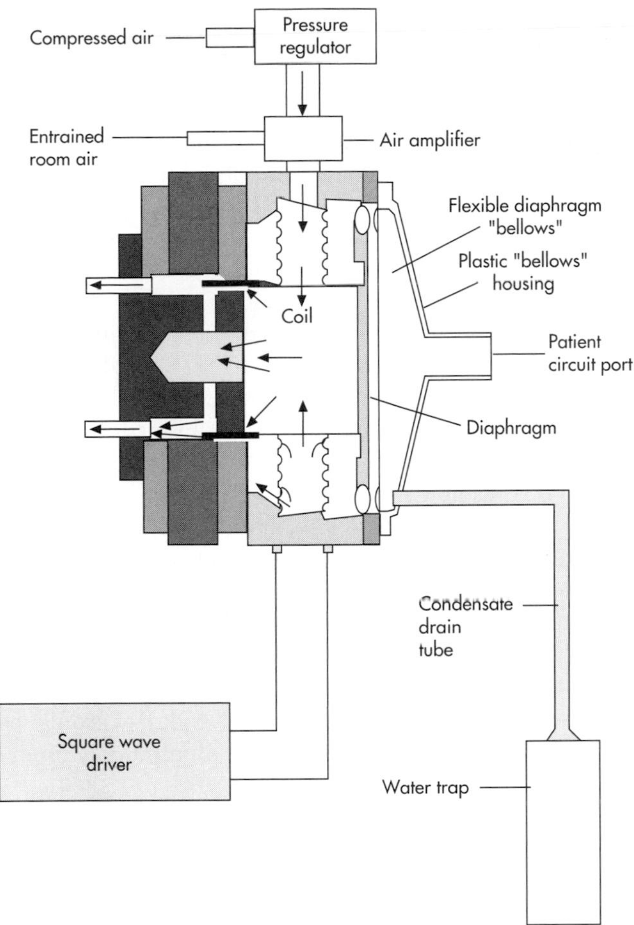

Figure 13-37 The piston assembly of the SensorMedics Model 3100A High-Frequency Oscillator. (Courtesy VIASYS Healthcare, Critical Care Division, Palm Springs, Calif.)

for the duration of the inspiratory or expiratory time and then change direction. An infrared sensor is used to track the movement of the piston between the mechanical stops. Piston movement is displayed by a bar graph on the control panel. The left end of the bar graph is labeled MIN INSP LIMIT and the right MAX INSP LIMIT. The dot represents the piston's center position.

The PISTON CENTERING control knob (Figure 13-36 A, beneath and to the left of the diaphragm) adjusts an electrical counter force to the piston. This counter force acts in opposition to the Paw on the front side of the piston. The result of this opposing counter force is a centering effect on the piston. At a constant Paw, as the PISTON CENTERING control knob is turned clockwise, the piston will move toward the MAX INSP LIMIT, one of the mechanical stops. The oscillator should not be operated so that the piston is driven against a mechanical stop for an extended period of time. The piston should be maintained in the center of the bar graph to maintain piston efficiency and to maximize the life of the oscillator mechanism.

Adjusting other controls, such as the MEAN PRESSURE ADJUST control or the POWER control, will change the piston position. The clinician should check and adjust piston centering after making changes in other settings.

Bias Flow

The BIAS FLOW control sets the rate of continuous flow through the patient circuit. Adjusting this control counter-clockwise increases flow to an internal limit of 40 L/min. Gas flow is indicated by a ball float which is located within a glass tube. The tube is graduated in 5 L/min increments.

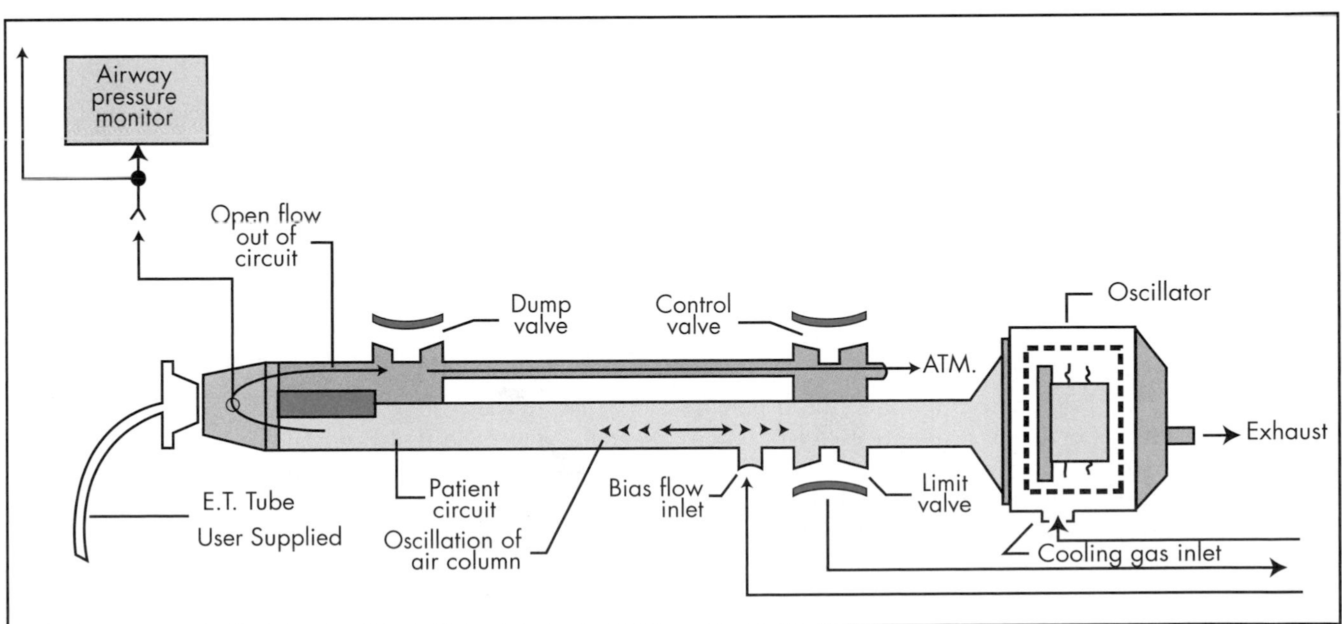

Figure 13-38 The basic breathing circuit of the SensorMedics Model 3100A High-Frequency Oscillator. (Courtesy VIASYS Healthcare, Critical Care Division, Palm Springs, Calif.)

F_IO_2

A standard air/oxygen blender is used to provide blended gas to the ventilator. A minimum pressure of 30 psig is required. The gas mixture is adjusted to the desired F_IO_2 before entering the ventilator.

Mean Pressure Adjust

The MEAN PRESSURE ADJUST control knob adjusts the $\bar{P}$aw. This control varies the resistance placed on the CONTROL VALVE, the mushroom valve in the patient circuit at the end of the expiratory limb. $\bar{P}$aw is digitally displayed in the MEAN PRESSURE MONITOR window. Although the MEAN PRESSURE ADJUST control is the primary determinant of $\bar{P}$aw, other controls will also affect it. For example, increasing bias flow will increase $\bar{P}$aw. Changes to the POWER, FREQUENCY, INSPIRATORY TIME, and PISTON CENTERING controls will also change the $\bar{P}$aw. Therefore, if a change in $\bar{P}$aw occurs because another control has been adjusted, the MEAN PRESSURE ADJUST control knob should be used to return the $\bar{P}$aw to the desired level.

Mean Pressure Limit

The MEAN PRESSURE LIMIT control knob is normally used to set a limit above which the $\bar{P}$aw cannot be exceeded. Adjustable to a maximum of 45 cm H_2O, this control can be used to protect the patient from an inadvertent rise in mean airway pressure. This control sets a pressure in the LIMIT VALVE, a mushroom valve located close to the bias flow inlet of the patient circuit. If the pressure within the circuit were to exceed this pressure, the LIMIT VALVE would open to permit excess pressure to be vented to the atmosphere.

An alternative use of the MEAN PRESSURE LIMIT control is to set it above the mean airway pressure that would otherwise exist using only the MEAN PRESSURE ADJUST control. Using the control in this way assures the clinician that $\bar{P}$aw will not exceed that prescribed, regardless of changes made in bias flow, percent inspiratory time, or frequency. However, the clinician should be aware that changes made to controls which result in an uncentered piston can still change $\bar{P}$aw, regardless of where the MEAN PRESSURE LIMIT control is set. Increasing the power, or amplitude, also can increase $\bar{P}$aw.

Power/ΔP

The POWER control determines the amount of polarity voltage applied to the oscillator's subsystem electrical coil. Adjusting this control clockwise increases the forward and backward displacement of the piston, therefore increasing oscillatory pressure (ΔP), or amplitude, and delivered volume. Pressure is adjustable from approximately 7 to 90 cm H_2O. Another term for ΔP is amplitude.

The extent to which the ΔP increases depends on the resistance the piston encounters to forward movement. For example, when the oscillator is used with a patient with extremely low pulmonary or chest wall compliance, the piston will meet a high resistance in the inspiratory phase. Increasing the POWER setting will increase ΔP but not in the same proportion as according to the amount of resistance the piston encounters from the $\bar{P}$aw. Therefore, if a low level of $\bar{P}$aw is present, ΔP adjustments for the same change in power would be greater than if a high level of $\bar{P}$aw is present.

% Inspiratory Time

The fraction of time that the piston is in the inspiratory position is determined by the % INSPIRATORY TIME control. For example, if the control is set at 33%, the piston will spend 33% of the breath cycle in the inspiratory position and the remaining 67% in the expiratory position. The control is adjustable from 30 to 50%. The setting is digitally displayed in the window to the left of the control knob.

Changing the inspiratory time affects the symmetry of the oscillator waveform. If, for example, the clinician decreases the % INSPIRATORY TIME control from 50 to 33%, the amount of time for the piston to travel during the inspiratory phase may be limited. This is especially true at high frequencies. Therefore, the ΔP and $\bar{P}$aw could be affected by changes in the percentage of inspiratory time.

Frequency

The FREQUENCY control sets the oscillatory frequency, or breaths per minute, in Hertz. One Hertz is equal to 60 cycles, or 60 breaths per minute. The control is adjustable from 3 to 15 Hz, and the setting is digitally displayed in the window to the left of the control.

As frequency is increased, excursion of the piston will be limited by the time allotted for each breath cycle. Therefore, changes in the frequency will affect mean airway pressure and ΔP (Boxes 13-10 and 13-11).

Start/Stop

The START/STOP control button either enables or disables oscillator operation. Pressing this START/STOP button will light the green LED labeled OSCILLATOR STOPPED if the ventilator's microprocessor determines that the unit is safe to operate. This control only allows the oscillator to begin operation if the start-up procedure was properly performed.

Reset

The RESET button sets or resets the unit's safety alarms and the power failure alarm. Conditions triggering an alarm must be corrected before resetting can occur. This button does not function unless the ventilator has been activated with the START/STOP button.

Certain alarm conditions, such as the PAW $<20\%$ SET MAX PAW alarm, cause the circuit dump valve to immediately deflate. When the clinician depresses the RESET button, the DUMP VALVE will reinflate. It is necessary to hold the RESET button in until the airway

Box 13-10 Clinical Example of Changing Frequency with the 3100A

A patient is on the SensorMedics 3100A at a frequency of 15 Hz. The clinician decides to lower the frequency to 10 Hz. Doing so allows the piston more travel time. This results in greater piston displacement, or more delivered volume to the patient. The exact amount of the volume increase is unknown. In some patients, an inadvertent (and unknown) increase in tidal volume may contribute to volutrauma. Therefore, the clinician should always use caution when lowering the oscillatory frequency.

Box 13-11 Effect of Control Changes on Mean Airway Pressure

Many of the controls on the 3100 affect more than one parameter. For example, when adjusting the amplitude with the power control, the change in piston thrust will change the level of mean airway pressure. When adjusting the frequency, changes in amplitude, piston position, and mean airway pressure will occur. Therefore, the clinician should use caution when making a setting change and carefully readjust other settings that might also change.

pressure exceeds 20% of that on the SET MAX PAW thumb wheel. Otherwise reset may not occur.

The RESET button also is used to silence the ventilator's battery powered audible POWER FAILURE alarm when the unit is turned off or if electrical power is interrupted.

Alarms

45 Second Silence

For most alarm conditions, the audible portion can be silenced for 45 seconds by pressing the 45-SEC SILENCE button. When activated, the button's yellow LED will light until the silence period lapses.

When the oscillator is turned off at the POWER switch or stops because of a power interruption, the audible alarm can only be silenced by pressing the RESET button.

Set Maximum and Minimum Paw

The SET MAX PAW and SET MIN PAW thumb wheel switches enable the clinician to set maximum and minimum limits for $\bar{P}$aw. Because some drifting of $\bar{P}$aw may occur because of endotracheal tube leaks or spontaneous breathing, a safety range should be set. When either limit is reached, a red LED next to the corresponding thumb wheel will light and an audible alarm will sound. The ventilator will continue to operate, but the alarm condition will persist until the MEAN PRESSURE ADJUST control is readjusted or new alarm limits set.

PAW <20% SET MAX PAW

Conditions causing a sharp drop in $\bar{P}$aw to a level less than 20% of the value set on the SET MAX PAW. The thumb wheel will trigger a PAW <20% SET MAX PAW alarm. When this alarm is triggered, the oscillator stops, the red LED lights indicating this alarm condition, and the audible alarm sounds. Bias flow will continue to be delivered to permit spontaneous ventilation.

PAW >50 cm H_2O

The "Paw >50 cm H_2O" alarm is activated if mean airway pressure rises above 50 cm H_2O for any reason. When this alarm is activated, the DUMP VALVE opens, causing the oscillator to stop. The red LED lights up indicating this alarm condition, and an audible alarm sounds. Although the audible alarm can be silenced with the 45-SEC SILENCE button, the oscillator will not resume operating until the RESET button is pressed and held until mean airway pressure exceeds 20% of that set with the SET MAX PAW thumb wheel.

Power Failure

The battery powered POWER FAILURE alarm is activated if the POWER switch to the ventilator is turned off or if electrical power is interrupted. If the unit's main circuit breaker is tripped or the main power supply were to fail, this alarm condition would also occur. The POWER FAILURE LED will light up and the audible alarm will sound. Both can be extinguished by pressing the RESET button.

When power is restored to the ventilator, the circuit must be occluded and the RESET button pressed and held until mean airway pressure exceeds 20% of that set with the SET MAX PAW thumb wheel. Only then will oscillations resume (Box 13-12).

Box 13-12 Returning the Oscillator to Operation after Disconnect

When alarm conditions occur, especially those which shut down the oscillator, the clinician should immediately remove the patient from the circuit and provide manual ventilation. After the cause of the alarm condition is corrected, the airway connector should be plugged and oscillations restarted using the RESET button. Plugging the circuit and restarting oscillations is necessary to confirm safe operation. When that is done, the plug is then removed and the connection is immediately hand occluded. Next, the circuit is quickly reconnected to the patient's airway.

Battery Low

The yellow BATTERY LOW LED lights up when the battery serving the power failure alarm is low. No audible alarm is activated.

Source Gas Low

The yellow SOURCE GAS LOW LED lights up whenever gas pressure from the blender falls below 30 psig. This LED also lights up if the pressure drops below 30 psig in the separate compressed air source for cooling the piston subsystem. The most common cause of this alarm condition is obstruction of the Inlet Filter Cartridge with dirt. If this problem is not corrected, the piston subsystem is likely to overheat resulting in piston failure.

Oscillator Overheated

The yellow OSCILLATOR OVERHEATED LED will light when the oscillator coil temperature reaches 175° C. No audible alarm will sound. Failure to correct this problem can result in piston failure.

Troubleshooting

The array of visual and audible alarms assists the clinician in troubleshooting specific problems with the Sensormedics oscillator. The instruction manual also provides a troubleshooting guide.

Circuit leaks are most likely to occur at the many connection points. For example, the pressure line going from the airway Y connector to the front of the unit could be loose. Lines going from the front to each of the mushroom valves can be the source of leaks. All of these lines have Luer connections that should be tight. Although it occurs rarely, any of the mushroom valves can rupture, which would cause the unit to stop oscillating and activate the alarm.

When using a circuit not equipped with heater wires, pooling of water can occur at any low point in the circuit. If the patient is positioned lower than the circuit, excessive condensate can run into the patient airway. Care should be taken to keep water drained from the circuit. The clinician should note any unusual knocking coming from the piston. If the Sensormedics is operated for long periods of time at very low frequencies, the piston can begin to fail. If the piston housing is not connected to a compressed air source or if the unit is operated without sufficient piston centering, the piston will wear out more rapidly than normal. Usually piston failure can be detected by a knocking sound and by drifting in the mean airway pressure and amplitude levels.

Every clinician who uses the Sensormedics oscillators should be capable of performing a system calibration and check. An outline of this procedure is printed on the left side and top of the unit. If problems are noted in maintaining desired settings, the patient should be removed from the ventilator and this procedure performed. Doing so often reveals the source of the problem.

Sensormedics 3100B High-Frequency Oscillatory Ventilator

The Sensormedics 3100B High-Frequency Oscillatory Ventilator, a newer version of the model 3100A, is intended to be used with adult patients. Appropriate for the patient with a weight greater than 35 Kg., the model 3100B (Figure 13-39, *A*) is designed with greater power, flow and pressure capabilities than its predecessor. Because the design and controls of the two models are very similar, only the differences between the two will be discussed here.

Overview of Differences Between 3100A and 3100B Models

Power and mean airway pressure controls for the 3100B are identical to the 3100A. Although the power control remains at graduated 10-turn locking dial, the ΔP is adjustable to greater than 90 cm H_2O of the maximum amplitude of the proximal airway pressure. Mean airway pressure is adjustable to approximately 55 cm H_2O. Piston centering is performed automatically by updated electronic sensors. Therefore, the Center Piston control has been eliminated from this model.[23]

The MEAN PRESSURE LIMIT control has also been eliminated. The SET MAX PAW is the only adjustable control to prevent inadvertent increases in mean airway pressure. The limit controls are discussed below.

The bias flow capability of the 3100B has been expanded to an internal limit of 60 L/min. The rotameter glass tube, which indicates flow, is graduated from 0 to 60 L/min in 5 L/min increments (Figure 13-39, *B*).

The FREQUENCY control and digital display, which operate identically to the 3100A, permit the operator to adjust frequency from 3 to 15 Hertz. These are the same limits as on the 3100A. The INSPIRATORY TIME control is also identical with limits from 30 to 50 per cent.

The ALARMS panel on the model 3100B is arranged identically to the 3100A. However, there are several differences in alarm limits and function. A major difference is in the SET MAX PAW control. The maximum setting for this control is 59 cm H_2O. When the ventilator is operating and the set pressure limit is reached or exceeded by the proximal pressure, the unit no longer shuts down entirely. The audible and visual alarm will activate, but instead of shutting down, the ventilator will depressurize the Limit Valve seat until the mean airway pressure falls to a level of 12 (±3) cm H_2O below the set mean. After the pressure drops to this point, the Limit Valve will allow the circuit to re-pressurize and rise again and the audible and visual

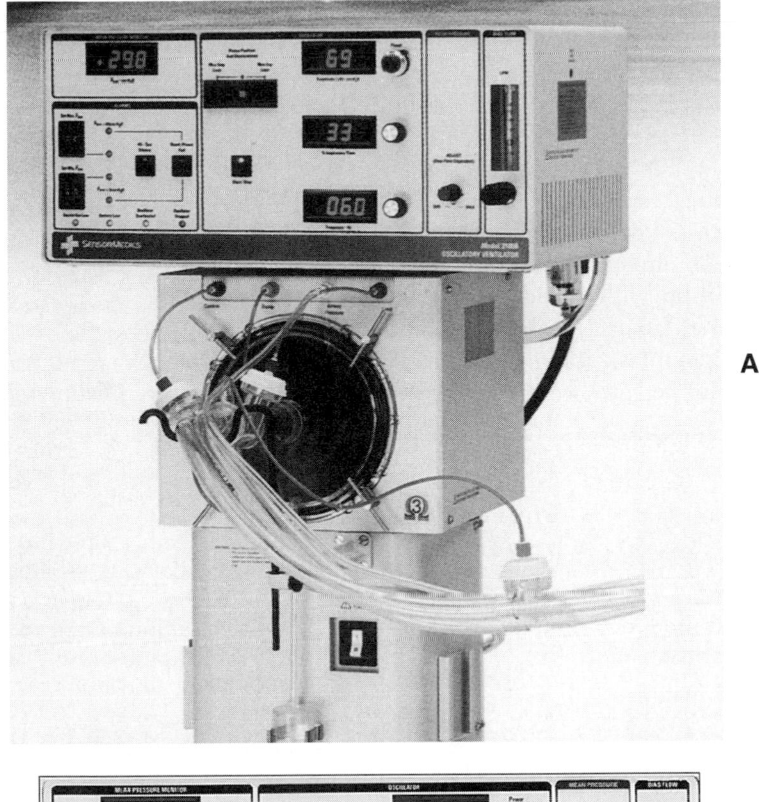

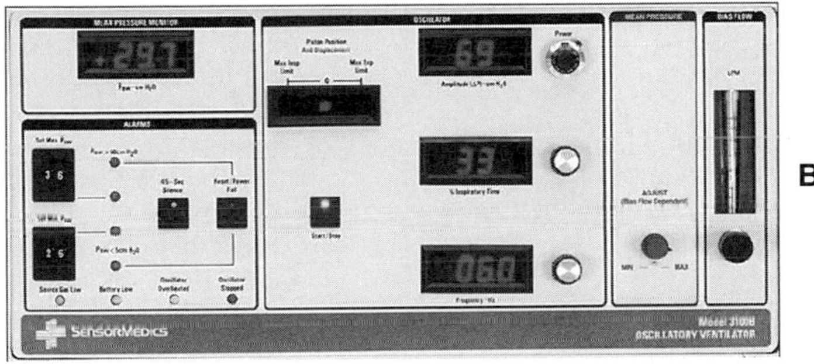

Figure 13-39 **A,** The SensorMedics Model 3100B High-Frequency Oscillator. **B,** The control panel of the 3100B. (Courtesy VIASYS Healthcare, Critical Care Division, Palm Springs, Calif.)

alarms will be deactivated. If the proximal pressure rises again to meet or exceed the limit setting, the same cycle of events will repeat until the alarm condition is resolved.

The "PAW>60 CMH_2O" red LED and audible alarm operate the same as the "PAW>50 CMH_2O" on the 3100A, with the only difference being the higher pressure required to trigger the alarm condition. The "PAW<5 CMH_2O" red LED and alarm operate identically to the "PAW<20% OF SET MAX PAW," except that a mean airway pressure less than 5 cmH_2O will trigger the alarm.

Chapter Summary

The ventilators discussed in this chapter represent those that are widely and exclusively used in pediatric settings. Some models covered elsewhere in this text are equipped to effectively monitor and ventilate the largest adults down to the smallest infants. In fact, this capability is a trend in newer ventilator designs.

Many ventilators that were originally designed to be used with adults have been found to be easily adapted to pediatric applications and, in some cases, to neonatal applications. In many clinical settings mechanical ventilation is provided to patients of all ages and sizes using a staff that also works with this wide range of patients. In such settings, a ventilator that is easily adapted to fit any need presents a cost savings and saves time in staff technical training.

Infant and pediatric ventilators will continue to be developed, particularly to provide better monitoring capabilities. Additional developments in specialized applications unique to the neonatal/pediatric population are certain, including ventilatory support to spontaneously breathing patients and high frequency technology. Recently clinicians have shown interest in ventilators capable of delivering subambient oxygen concentrations. Others have envisioned systems capable of providing specialty gases such as nitric oxide and heliox. Units providing liquid ventilation may some day see their way into the market. In the planning stages for years, prototype closed loop systems that monitor arterial blood and expired gases and adjust their own ventilator settings are being tested.

As with all technology, necessity drives the scope and the direction of advancement. As clinical problems present themselves, technical innovation will provide ever more sophisticated solutions. Other factors, such as medical advances, economics, demographics, and even ideology will continue to affect the infant/pediatric ventilator market.

Review Questions

See Appendix A for answers.

1. One of the most common modes of ventilation that has been used in infants for more than 30 years is:
   a. Volume ventilation
   b. SIMV with pressure support
   c. Time-triggered, pressure-limited, time-cycled ventilation
   d. Volume assured pressure support

2. Better ventilator-to-patient synchrony has been developed in infant ventilation because of the technological advancement of which of the following devices?
   a. Floating expiratory valves
   b. Flow sensing devices
   c. Volume measuring devices
   d. Rapid response pressure monitors

3. The Aladdin Infant Flow System incorporates an alarm system for which of the following conditions?
   a. Spontaneous respiratory rate falling outside of set parameters
   b. F_IO_2 reading different from set F_IO_2
   c. Apnea
   d. Spontaneous minute volume falling outside of set parameters

4. Which of the following best describes the volume limit feature of the Bear Cub 750vs ventilator?
   a. Activates an alarm if tidal volume decreases to a preset level
   b. Phases out mandatory breaths from the ventilator when spontaneous breaths fall within certain parameters
   c. Allows the PIP to adjust itself upward or downward to maintain the patient's tidal volume within set parameters
   d. Sets a ceiling for volume delivered by mechanical breaths

5. Which of the following ventilators uses an anemometer with two platinum hot wires for bidirectional flow measurement?
   a. Bear Cub 750vs infant ventilator
   b. VIP Bird Gold version
   c. Hamilton Arabella CPAP system
   d. Sechrist IV 200 infant ventilator

6. A respiratory therapist is ventilating an infant using the Bear Cub 750vs. The horizontal bar graph indicating flow shows that the indicator is adjusted too far to the left and intersects the baseline flow graph. The most likely problem to result from this is:
   a. increased ventilating pressures
   b. a reduced inspiratory time
   c. inadequate flow to the patient
   d. auto-triggering of the ventilator

7. The Bear Cub 750psv has which additional features when compared to the Bear Cub 750vs?
   a. An improved flow sensor
   b. The addition of four more modes of ventilation
   c. A low minute volume alarm
   d. All of the above

8. A respiratory therapist increases the PEEP from 3 to 5 cm H_2O on a patient being ventilated with the original Infant Star. To readjust the low PEEP/CPAP alarm the therapist is required to:
   a. take no action because the alarm is automatically reset by the microprocessor
   b. use the interlocking low/high PEEP alarm control
   c. press the low PEEP alarm touch pad, use the dial control to adjust the value and press the dial control to confirm the setting
   d. take no action because there is no low PEEP alarm control

9. A respiratory therapist uses an external flowmeter to power an inline nebulizer being used to give an aerosol treatment to an infant who is receiving ventilator support with the original Infant Star. The added flow increases the system pressure and activates an AO4 alarm. To correct this situation, the therapist should
   a. reduce the flowmeter setting
   b. set the EXTERNAL PRESSURE LIMIT and the primary inspiratory pressure control
   c. discontinue the treatment
   d. increase the peak pressure alarm during the treatment

10. The peak inspiratory pressure (PIP) on the Infant Star 500 is set at 13 cm H_2O. The therapist adjusts the high pressure limit alarm to 30 cm H_2O. Which of the following will occur as a result of this action?
   a. The ventilator high pressure alarm will activate if the pressure reaches 30 cm H_2O and end inspiration
   b. 30 cm H_2O is beyond the available range and an out of range alarm will occur

c. The ventilator high pressure alarm will activate if the pressure reaches 30 cm H_2O but inspiration will continue until T_I ends
d. The high inspiratory pressure LED will flash and the microprocessor will automatically set the Plimit 15 cm H_2O above PIP

11. During operation of the Infant Star 500 the PEEP/CPAP control is set at 5 cm H_2O and the PIP at 9 cm H_2O. The respiratory therapist notes that the PIP indicator flashes. This means which of the following?
a. Inspiratory time is too short to reach the PIP
b. The flow is inadequate to reach PIP during the set inspiratory time
c. PIP is <5 cm H_2O above the PEEP value
d. There is a leak in the circuit

12. The purpose of the background flow feature on the Infant Star 500 and 950 ventilators is to:
a. maintain a minimum gas flow past humidifier temperature probes to prevent inspiratory gas from overheating
b. compensate for leaks around the endotracheal tube
c. maintain a gas flow sufficient for spontaneous inspiratory demands but low enough to minimize circuit PEEP
d. provide a back-up flow of blended gas to the patient in case the demand valve fails

13. The Infant Star 950 ventilator differs from the Sensormedics 3100A in which of the following ways?
a. The Infant Star creates gas pulses rather than piston-generated mechanical oscillations
b. The Infant Star can provide both conventional and high-frequency ventilation
c. When operating in one of its high-frequency modes, the Infant Star can provide greater flows, mean airway pressures, and oscillatory frequencies
d. Both A and B

14. The tracking relief pressure valve on the Infant Star 100 and 200 ventilators serves which of the following functions?
a. Automatically sets a high-pressure safety limit
b. Prevents the operator from setting the safety pressure-relief valve too high
c. Automatically sets an appropriate PIP level
d. Prevents the operator from setting the minimum inspiratory pressure alarm too low

15. Termination sensitivity is an added feature on the VIP Bird ventilator that:
a. allows the clinician to adjust the flow termination point of the breath
b. operates in all modes
c. can be adjusted from 0 to 25% in increments of 5%
d. A and C

16. On the VIP Bird, the termination sensitivity setting flashes when the:
a. breath is terminated at the set value
b. breath is time-cycled
c. breath is both flow-triggered and flow-cycled
d. expiratory time is deemed too short by the ventilator's microprocessor

17. On the VIP Bird, leak compensation is:
a. available in all modes
b. only available in volume-cycled modes
c. used to stabilize baseline pressure in the presence of leaks
d. B and C

18. The flow sensor in the Sterling and Gold versions of the VIP Bird differ from the original because it:
a. incorporates a heated wired anemometer
b. contains a stainless steel flap in the variable orifice differential pressure transducer
c. uses an ultrasonic wave detection monitor
d. incorporates a laser beam splitter

19. In the Dräger Babylog 8000 infant ventilator, all EXCEPT which of the following are automatically set by the microprocessor?
a. Oxygen concentration alarms
b. PEEP alarm limits
c. Low V_T alarm
d. Inspiratory pressure alarm

20. When the VIP Gold ventilator Rise Time control is set at 1:
a. a rapid rise to set pressure occurs
b. only volume breaths are affected
c. the inspiratory time increases
d. the respiratory rate increases

21. When the VIP Bird mode switch is set at time-cycled SIMV, what are the breath variables for mandatory breaths?
I. Time- or patient-triggering
II. Volume-targeted breaths
III. Pressure-targeted breaths
IV. Time-cycled
a. III only
b. I and II only
c. I, III, and IV only
d. I, II, and IV only

22. The Bunnell Jet Ventilator:
a. operates in tandem with a conventional ventilator
b. requires the use of the Hi-Lo Jet tube
c. delivers rates of 240 to 660 insufflations/minute
d. A and C

23. The triple lumen Hi-Lo Jet tube:
a. is the type of only endotracheal tube that can be used with the Bunnell Jet ventilator
b. ranges in size from 2.5 to 6.0 mm ID
c. must be replaced with a standard endotracheal tube when the patient is switched to conventional ventilation
d. all of the above

24. The Dräger Babylog 8000 Infant Ventilator:
    a. is used to ventilate premature and term infants
    b. has a weight limit of 10 kilograms
    c. has a built-in battery
    d. all of the above

25. The power control on the Sensormedics 3100A is primarily used to change the:
    a. mean airway pressure
    b. frequency
    c. bias flow
    d. amplitude

26. If the frequency on the Sensormedics 3100A is increased from 10 to 15 Hertz and no other settings are changed, which of the following will occur?
    a. Inspiratory time will increase
    b. Volume delivered by the piston will decrease
    c. Amplitude will increase
    d. None of the above

27. Mean airway pressure in the SensorMedics 3100A high frequency oscillator can be affected by which of the following?
    I. Bias flow
    II. Frequency setting
    III. % Ti
    IV. Piston-centering
    V. Mean airway adjustment control
    a. V only
    b. I and III only
    c. II, IV, and V only
    d. I, II, III, IV, and V

28. A new feature of the SensorMedics 3100B oscillator compared to the 3100A is the:
    a. frequency control
    b. inspiratory time control
    c. automatic piston centering
    d. mean airway pressure control

References

1. Chatburn RL: Principles and practices of neonatal and pediatric ventilation, *Respir Care* 36:573, 1991.
2. Betit P, Thompson JE, Benjamin PK: Mechanical ventilation. In Koff PB, Eitzman D, Neu J, editors: *Neonatal and pediatric respiratory care,* ed 2, St Louis, 1993, Mosby.
3. Thompson MA: *Early nasal CPAP and prophylactic surfactant for neonates at risk of RDS: the IFDAS trial,* presented at the European Society for Paediatric Research, annual meeting, Helsinki, Finland, August 2001.
4. Claris O, Bassir M, Verellen G, Debauch C, Lapillonne A, Salle BL: *Nasal CPAP as a weaning tool after ventilation by oscillation,* abstract presented at ReaSoN Meeting, Leeds, UK, 1996.
5. Klausner JF, Lee AY, Hutchinson, AA: Decreased imposed work of breathing with a new nasal continuous positive pressure device, *Pediatr Pulmonol* 22:188-194, 1996.
6. Instruction manual, EME Infant Flow System, Brighton, East Sussex, England, 2000, Electro Medical Equipment, Ltd.
7. Instruction manual, Arabella System, Reno, Nev, 2001, Hamilton Medical, Inc.
8. Operator's manual: Sechrist Model IV-200 Infant Ventilator, Anaheim, Calif, 2000, Sechrist Industries, Inc.
9. Operator's manual: SAVI Total Synchrony System, Anaheim, Calif, 2000, Sechrist Industries, Inc.
10. Instruction manual, Bear Cub 750vs Infant Ventilator, form P/N 51-10641-00, Palm Springs, Calif, 1996, VIASYS Healthcare Systems, Critical Care Division.
11. Instruction manual, Bear Cub 750psv Infant Ventilator, form P/N 51-10697-00, Palm Springs, Calif, 1999, VIASYS Healthcare Systems, Critical Care Division.
12. Operating instructions: Infant Star Neonatal Ventilator, form P/N 9910005, Pleasanton Calif, 1986, Puritan Bennett, a division of Tyco Healthcare.
13. Operating instructions: Infant Star 500 Ventilator, Pleasanton Calif, 1996, Puritan Bennett, a division of Tyco Healthcare.
14. Operating instructions: Infant Star 950 Ventilator, Pleasanton Calif, 1996, Puritan Bennett, a division of Tyco Healthcare.
15. Operating instructions: Infant Star 100 Neonatal Ventilator, Pleasanton Calif, 1995, Puritan Bennett, a division of Tyco Healthcare.
16. Operating instructions: Infant Star 200 Neonatal-Pediatric Ventilator, Pleasanton, Calif, 1995, Puritan Bennett, a division of Tyco Healthcare.
17. Instruction manual: V.I.P. Bird Infant-Pediatric Ventilator, Palm Springs, Calif, 1991, VIASYS Healthcare Systems, Critical Care Division.
18. Instruction manual: V.I.P. Graphics instruction manual, Palm Springs, Calif, 1991, VIASYS Healthcare Systems, Critical Care Division.
19. Operator's manual: V.I.P. Bird Gold and Sterling Ventilator Systems, Palm Springs, Calif, 2000, VIASYS Healthcare Systems, Critical Care Division.
20. Operator's manual: Dräger Babylog 8000, 1st U.S. edition, Telford, Penn, 1993, Dräger Inc.
21. Operator's manual: Life Pulse High Frequency Jet Ventilator, Salt Lake City, Utah, 1991, Bunnell Incorporated.
22. Operator's manual: 3100A High Frequency Oscillatory Ventilator, form P/N 767124, Palm Springs, Calif, 1991, VIASYS Healthcare Systems, Critical Care Division.
23. Operator's manual: 3100B High Frequency Oscillatory Ventilator, form P/N 767164, rev. J, Palm Springs, Calif, 2001, VIASYS Healthcare Systems, Critical Care Division.

Internet Resources

Dräger Inc: www.draeger.com

Puritan Bennett, a division of Tyco Medical: www.puritanbennett.com

Sechrist Respiratory Products: www.sechristind.com

Ventilator Website: www.VentWorld.com

Viasys Healthcare, Critical Care Division-Bear and Bird products: www.ViasysCriticalCare.com, www.birdprod.com, and www.bearmedical.com

Hamilton Medical: www.Hamilton-Medical.com

Chapter 14

Transport, Home-Care, and Alternative Ventilatory Devices

Kevin Lord
Susan P. Pilbeam

Chapter Outline

Chapter Learning Objectives

Upon completion of this chapter, the reader should be able to:

1. Compare the ventilators described and provide a list of their common characteristics.
2. Explain the factors that determine tidal volume (V_T), rate, and flow for each ventilator described.
3. Discuss the desirable characteristics of a transport ventilator, a home-care ventilator, and a noninvasive positive pressure ventilator.
4. Explain how PEEP is applied and used for each ventilator.
5. Describe the oxygen system for each ventilator and how it regulates and monitors the fraction of inspired oxygen (F_IO_2).
6. Identify an alarm situation with any of the ventilators discussed.
7. Explain the flow of the gas source through the internal mechanisms of each ventilator.
8. Describe what type of clients would be best suited for home-care ventilation.
9. Compare and contrast the differences between positive- and negative-pressure ventilators.
10. Describe the benefits of noninvasive positive pressure ventilation (NPPV) over traditional ventilation.
11. Describe the various NPPV interfaces and the proper procedure for their attachment.

Key Terms

Antisuffocation Valve
Caudal
Cephalad
Chest Cuirass
External PEEP Valve
Internal Regulator
Iron Lung
Microprocessor
Pneumatic System
Pneumobelt
Poppet Valve
Potentiometer
Pressure-Relief Valve
Rocking Bed
Solenoid Valve
Transport Ventilator

TRANSPORT VENTILATORS

There are few other procedures that require greater care and skill than the transportation of a critically ill patient. Advancements in technology and the ability of diagnostic tests to render information critical to treatment of the patient have created a gray area between risk and benefit. The current literature suggests that physiologic changes that occur during transport are in fact not a result of the transport but of the gravity of the patient's condition.[1] The statement can then be made that likelihood of changes in heart rate, respiratory rate, blood pressure, and oxygen saturation developing on transport is no different than if the patient remained in the intensive care unit (ICU). However, transport of a patient is not without the risk of complications. Loss of an intravenous line, changes in body temperature, hyper- or hypoventilation, which can perpetuate arrhythmias, and equipment malfunction are all perceivable problems resulting from the relocation of the patient. Therefore, every attempt should be made to ensure that monitoring, ventilation, oxygenation, and patient care remain constant during movement and that protocols and policies are put in place to guide the decision to transport and serve as a checklist for the transport team. The movement of a patient from one location to another should never be considered routine. Preparation and communication are vital components to a successful transport.

Ventilators are designed and developed to meet the specific needs of the patient. The attributes commonly shared among transport ventilators include a compact, lightweight unit (compared with the traditional ICU ventilators) that can be maintained by a reliable power source. The power source must allow the ventilator to operate from an internal battery or a gas source to permit mobility. Durability and ease of use are two added features that compose a good transport ventilator.

The device must be capable of working in extreme conditions that include temperature, vibration, and altitude and should contain sufficient shielding to protect its internal mechanisms from electromagnetic energy. In addition to durability, the control panel should remain simplistic. This does not infer that the machine should be basic in operation, only that the front panel controls are easily recognized and easy to adjust. The volume, rate, and pressure controls should be large and easy to find and all displays should be clearly visible in the daytime as well as night time to reduce the chance of mistakes due to missed information. Today's transport ventilator has become very sophisticated and reliable, but nothing should be overlooked or assumed when transporting a critically ill patient.

The American Association for Respiratory Care (AARC) has developed a clinical practice guideline specifically

Clinical Practice Guidelines 14-1

In-Hospital Transport of the Mechanically Ventilated Patient

Definition/Description

Transportation of the mechanically ventilated patients for diagnostic or therapeutic procedures is always associated with a degree of risk. Every attempt should be made to assure monitoring, ventilation, oxygenation and patient care remain constant during movement. Patient transport includes preparation, movement to and from, and time spent at destination.

Indications

Transportation of mechanically ventilated patients should only be undertaken following a careful evaluation of risk-to-benefit ratio.

Contraindications

Contraindications include the inability to maintain an airway, provide adequate oxygenation and ventilation, maintain acceptable hemodynamic performance and adequately monitor cardiopulmonary during transport.

Precautions and Complications

Hazard and complications of transport include the following:

- Hyperventilation, during manual ventilation, resulting in respiratory alkalosis, cardiac dysrhythmias and hypotension
- Loss of PEEP/CPAP resulting in hypoxemia
- Position changes that result in hypotension, hypercarbia, and hypoxemia
- Dysrhythmias resulting from the transport
- Equipment failure resulting in inaccurate data or loss of monitoring capabilities.
- Inadvertent disconnection of intravenous pharmacologic agents resulting in hemodynamic instability
- Accidental extubation
- Accidental removal of vascular access
- Loss of oxygen supply resulting in hypoxemia

Limitations

The literature suggests that nearly two thirds of all transports for diagnostic studies fail to yield results that affect patient care.

Monitoring

Monitoring provided during transport should be maintained at the level of stationary care.

For complete guidelines see AARC clinical practice guidelines: In-hospital transport of the mechanically ventilated patient, *Resp Care* 47(6):721, 2002.

addressing the purpose, indications, methods of providing, and complications associated with transporting mechanically ventilated patients, which is a valuable resource to practitioners interested in transport ventilation (Clinical Practice Guideline 14-1).

In addition to transport ventilators, this chapter also includes home-care ventilators used with noninvasive and invasive patient interfaces, and adjunct ventilating devices such as negative pressure ventilators.

Achieva, Achieva PS, and Achieva PSO_2 Ventilators

The Achieva (Figure 14-1, A) is a transport ventilator that comes in three models. A list of the differences between the models is presented in Table 14-1. The following discussion will focus on the Achieva PSO_2 (Puritan Bennett, Pleasanton, Ca, a division of Tyco Healthcare).

The Achieva PSO_2 is a flow- or pressure-triggered, volume-, or pressure-targeted, pressure-, flow-, or time-cycled ventilator that is gas powered and electronically controlled. It is used for pediatric patients as well as adults and is capable of functioning in assist/control (A/C), synchronized intermittent mandatory ventilation (SIMV), or spontaneous modes. It weighs less than 32 lb and is 10.75″ × 13.30″ × 15.6″ in size.

Power Source

The Achieva PSO_2 requires an electrical power source to function properly. The electronic system can use any of the following three separate power sources:

- An alternating current (AC) outlet
- An external 24- or 12-volt DC battery (24 volt is always preferred)
- An internal 24-volt DC battery

The ventilator, when plugged into an outlet, will automatically choose the AC power. If an AC power failure occurs, the ventilator switches to the next available power source. When an external battery is employed, the manufacturer recommends using their connecting cables and a 24-volt DC battery (a 12-volt DC battery may also be used) for optimum performance. When the ventilator is in operation, the External Battery light is illuminated.

The internal battery is intended only as a backup when all other sources have failed. The battery is able to support the ventilator for about four hours under normal working

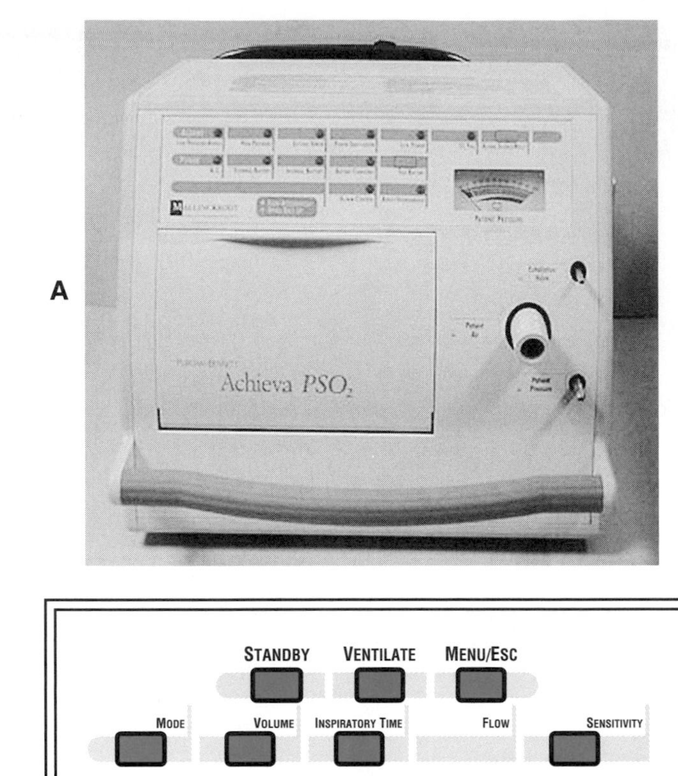

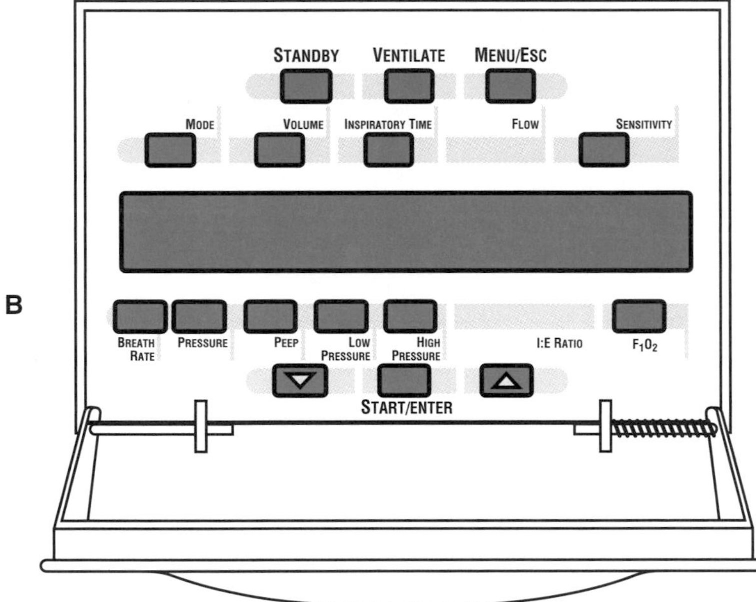

Figure 14-1 **A,** The Achieva Ventilator. **B,** The front panel controls on the Achieva. (Courtesy Puritan-Bennett, a division of Tyco Medical, Pleasanton, Calif.)

conditions and about 1 hour under stressful conditions of large tidal volumes and high respiratory rates. When the ventilator is in operation, the Internal Battery light is illuminated. The internal battery is charged whenever the ventilator is in the STANDBY mode and plugged into an AC outlet.

There are three alarms that work to alert the clinician when the internal battery is getting low. These include the LOW INTERNAL BATTERY alarm (about 45 minutes of power remaining), the EXTREMELY LOW INTERNAL BATTERY alarm (about 10 minutes of power remaining), and the BATTERY CHARGE DEPLETED alarm. When the latter occurs, another method of ventilating the patient must be found and used immediately.

Internal Mechanism

The internal compressor of the Achieva draws air through an inlet filter at the rear of the machine and directs the air through the internal pneumatic circuit. When a 50-psig O_2 source (45 to 80 psig) is connected to the ventilator, the air can be mixed with oxygen using the internal oxygen blender. From the blender the gas flow passes a check valve and is then directed to the patient outlet tube.

Table 14-1 Differences among Achieva models

Modes of Ventilation	Achieva	Achieva PS	Achieva PSO_2
Assist/control	Yes	Yes	Yes
with pressure control capability	Yes	Yes	Yes
SIMV	Yes	Yes	Yes
with CPAP	Yes	Yes	Yes
with pressure support	No	Yes	Yes
Spontaneous (pressure support)	No	Yes	Yes
with CPAP	No	Yes	Yes
Apnea back up rate (in spontaneous mode)	No	Yes	Yes
Dial in PEEP (3-20 cm H_2O)	Yes	Yes	Yes
Flow triggering	Yes	Yes	Yes
Internal O_2 blender	No	No	Yes
Internal modem	No	Yes*	Yes*
Access to stored events with the Achieva Report Generator software	Yes	Yes	Yes
Pediatric capability	Yes	Yes	Yes
Internal battery	Yes	Yes	Yes
External battery capability	Yes	Yes	Yes
Portability	Yes	Yes	Yes

Courtesy Puritan-Bennett, a division of Tyco Healthcare, Pleasanton, Calif.
*Available only in the United States and Canada.

During spontaneous breathing, a parallel pathway exits from the inlet filter, which connects directly to the patient outlet tube. This allows the patient to spontaneous breath room air after opening a demand valve (2 cm H_2O effort required). If the ventilator fails, a spontaneously breathing patient can obtain air through this route.

Although the ventilator does have an internal blender it does not come equipped with an oxygen analyzer, so it is important to periodically check the oxygen concentration in the circuit to confirm the F_IO_2 being delivered to the patient.

Ventilator Setup

The Achieva PSO_2 uses a patient circuit with an exterior exhalation manifold. The exhalation manifold serves the purpose of directing the inspiratory and expiratory gas flows as well as providing the desired positive end expiratory pressure (PEEP) to the system. The PEEP is actually controlled by a voltage sensitive orifice inside of the machine that monitors the client's airway pressure and restricts the degree of opening of the mushroom valve inside of the exhalation manifold. The PEEP range is 0 and 3 to 20 cm H_2O.

Before attaching the ventilator to the client, a USER SELF-TEST should be performed in addition to verifying alarm functions. To execute the USER SELF-TEST the ventilator should be placed in the STANDBY mode and the Menu/ESC key activated. The test is the first option on the menu. The clinician must then press "ENTER" and follow the remaining instructions.

To validate the alarms functions, each alarm should be checked individually.

Operations of the Ventilator

Pressing the START/ENTER switch located on the bottom front panel of the ventilator turns powers on the machine. The current settings are displayed on the front panel and the clinician is able to make changes to these settings while the machine is in the STANDBY mode. This allows for the correct settings to be entered before the patient is connected. After the ventilator has been checked and the correct settings entered, the clinician activates the ventilator by depressing the VENTILATE key.

Control and Alarms (see Figure 14-1, *B*)

Parameters

The main control parameters include tidal volume, rate, pressure, inspiratory time, and sensitivity. Depressing the VOLUME key in the center left of the control panel determines the tidal volume. This control will only function when the pressure value is 0. The tidal volume range is 50 to 2200 mL for A/C and 50 to 1750 mL in SIMV.

The RESPIRATORY RATE function is located on the bottom left of the control panel and functions in A/C and SIMV modes. It has a range of 1 to 80 breaths per minute.

The PRESSURE control is used in pressure-targeted ventilation. It is located on the bottom left of the control panel. When this value is set to zero (0) cm H_2O, the machine operates as a volume-targeted ventilator.

The INSPIRATORY TIME control is located in the middle of the control panel. It is utilized in A/C and SIMV modes of ventilation (range 0.2 to 5.0 seconds).

The SENSITIVITY key is located at the top right of the control panel. The Achieva PSO_2 is able to be flow- or pressure-triggered. The default setting is flow-triggered; however, it is possible to use both flow and pressure simultaneously. Whichever threshold is reached first (pressure or flow) activates the ventilator. To set the trigger parameter the clinician must first go to the MENU/ESC switch and scroll down the menu to the desired trigger parameter selection. If flow-triggered is preferred, the clinician can then choose the minimum flow setting required to activate inspiration. The set flow trigger range is 3 to 25 L/min. Inspiration is activated when the change in flow through the circuit is within ±0.5 L/min of the set value. If pressure-triggering is desired, the operator selects the MENU/ESC key and scrolls down to the pressure-trigger selection. The pressure sensitivity range is 1 to 15 cm H_2O below the baseline pressure.

Additional Controls

Additional controls and features include FLOW ACCELERATION, PRESSURE SUPPORT, PEEP, and ALTITUDE SETTING. The flow acceleration is only active when using pressure-targeted ventilation with pressure-supported breaths. This feature is designed to limit the flow at the beginning of inspiration thereby controlling the rate of rise in pressure within the system. When flow acceleration is activated, the maximum flow rate that can be delivered is 180 L/min.

Pressure support ventilation is available in the SIMV and spontaneous modes. Pressure support (PS) breaths are patient-triggered, pressure-limited, and flow-cycled. When the patient triggers a PS breath, the delivered inspiratory flow will be the maximum amount available from the ventilator unless FLOW ACCELERATION is on; in which case, the inspiratory flow will be determined by the FLOW ACCELERATION, which is set by the clinician.

PS stops when the inspiratory flow drops below 15% to 55% of the peak flow. The EXPIRATORY SENSITIVITY setting controls the termination of pressure support.

PEEP can be used in any of the modes of ventilation. The Achieva contains an external exhalation PEEP valve that is capable of maintaining a maximum of 20 cm H_2O of pressure in the circuit. As a safety feature the PEEP valve remains in the open position during ventilator failure. This allows the patient to exhale through the exhalation valve.

CLINICAL ROUNDS 14-1

A 7-year-old patient is being air transported from Vail, Colo., (10,000 feet), to a Denver hospital (altitude 5,000 feet) after a skiing accident. She required ventilatory support during the transport. The respiratory therapist noted after landing that the measured F_IO_2 was not the same as the set F_IO_2. What should the therapist do?

See Appendix A for the answer.

To ensure the ventilator's oxygen blender performs properly at high altitude, the Achieva can be adjusted to accommodate a high-altitude environment. The operator depresses the MENU/ESC button and scrolls to the altitude selection. Activation of the altitude selection automatically adjusts the internal barometric pressure (Clinical Rounds 14-1).

Alarms

Alarms include LOW PRESSURE/APNEA, HIGH PRESSURE, SETTING ERROR, POWER SWITCH OVER, LOW POWER and O_2 FAIL (only available on the Achieva PSO_2 model). The LOW PRESSURE alarm sounds when the pressure in the ventilator circuit fails to reach a minimal set value for two consecutive cycles. There is an exception to this. When operating in the SIMV mode, the LOW PRESSURE alarm will not sound if it is set above the pressure in the circuit during spontaneous breathing (above the pressure support). Therefore, the ventilator monitors the peak pressure in the ventilator circuit for the last two consecutive mandatory breaths. If this pressure fails to achieve the set low pressure limit, the LOW PRESSURE alarm will sound.

The APNEA alarm visual indicator is the same indicator as the LOW PRESSURE alarm. The apnea alarm sounds when the machine fails to cycle for 10 seconds in A/C or 20 seconds in SIMV or spontaneous modes.

The HIGH PRESSURE alarm establishes the maximum pressure allowed in the patient circuit during all breaths. This alarm is at the top left part of the control panel and cannot be set below the PEEP setting. When the set HIGH PRESSURE level is exceeded, inspiration stops and the machine cycles into exhalation, venting the remaining volume and pressure to room air.

The SETTING ERROR alarm is located in the middle top portion of the control panel and is a function of the inspiratory to expiratory (I:E) ratio. The Achieva allows the clinician to set the inspiratory time from 0.2 seconds to 5.0 seconds. If the expiratory time was to exceed the inspiratory time (inverse I:E ratio) the SETTING ERROR alarm would be activated.

The POWER SWITCH OVER alarm located in the top middle of the control panel warns the clinician when the power source operating the ventilator is changed. This alarm sounds when the operator changes from an AC source to an external or internal battery and when the ventilator is operating on an external battery and it is changed to an internal battery.

The LOW POWER alarm sounds first when the internal battery has less than 45 minutes left of operating power. A single beep occurs every 5 seconds and the visual indicator in the top right portion of the control panel flashes. When the battery power of the internal battery can no longer provide 10 minutes of operation the low battery alarm sounds with three pulsating bursts. The visual alarm will continue to be activated.

The O_2 fail alarm, found only on the Achieva PSO_2 model, provides a visual and an audible alarm when the oxygen concentrator fails to detect a source flow. The cause of such a problem may be the result of inadequate pressure from the oxygen source or from a leak between the oxygen high-pressure source and the oxygen blender.

Modes

The Achieva PSO_2 can provide volume- or pressure-targeted, time-cycled ventilation in A/C or SIMV modes. When operating in A/C volume ventilation, the clinician sets the tidal volume, inspiratory time, sensitivity, breath rate, and PEEP, if desired. The pressure control is set to zero. A backup rate is also available as part of the apnea alarm feature. When working in A/C with a breath rate of less than 6 breaths/minute, if the ventilator fails to cycle into inspiration within 10 ± 1 seconds, an apnea alarm will sound and the ventilator will deliver the set tidal volume at a rate of 10 times a minute until the patient initiates a spontaneous breath. This feature is present in all modes but the apnea delay may vary.

To change from volume- to pressure-targeted ventilation the clinician must set an inspiratory time, breath rate, sensitivity, PEEP, and a pressure value greater than zero. When the pressure setting is greater than zero, the tidal volume is not displayed.

When operating in SIMV, the same rules apply for volume- or pressure-targeted mandatory breaths as does in A/C. Spontaneous breaths are allowed between mandatory breaths. When the mandatory breath rate is set less than 6 breaths/min and the patient fails to trigger a breath in 20 ± 1 seconds, the apnea alarm sounds and a backup rate is initiated until the patient's next spontaneous breath. The same time delay of 20 ± 1 also holds true when the patient is being ventilated using the spontaneous mode of ventilation (see below). The SIMV mode also allows for the clinician to use continuous positive airway pressure (CPAP) or PS during the spontaneous breathing phase.

The SPONTANEOUS mode in the Achieva PSO_2 allows for the setting of pressure support and PEEP/CPAP. When CPAP is selected, the pressure control (touch pad) must be set to zero. The PEEP control (touch pad) is used to adjust the baseline pressure. Since all breaths are patient dependent in the spontaneous mode, the Achieva allows the clinician to activate an optional backup rate. The optional backup rate becomes active when no patient inspiratory effort has been detected for a time period of 20 ± 1 seconds. (*Note:* This may be the same time interval to initiate the apnea alarm; however, apnea ventilation is not activated when the back rate has been selected.) The ventilator will deliver a set tidal volume at a rate of 10 breaths/min and an I:E ratio of 1:2 until the patient triggers a spontaneous breath.

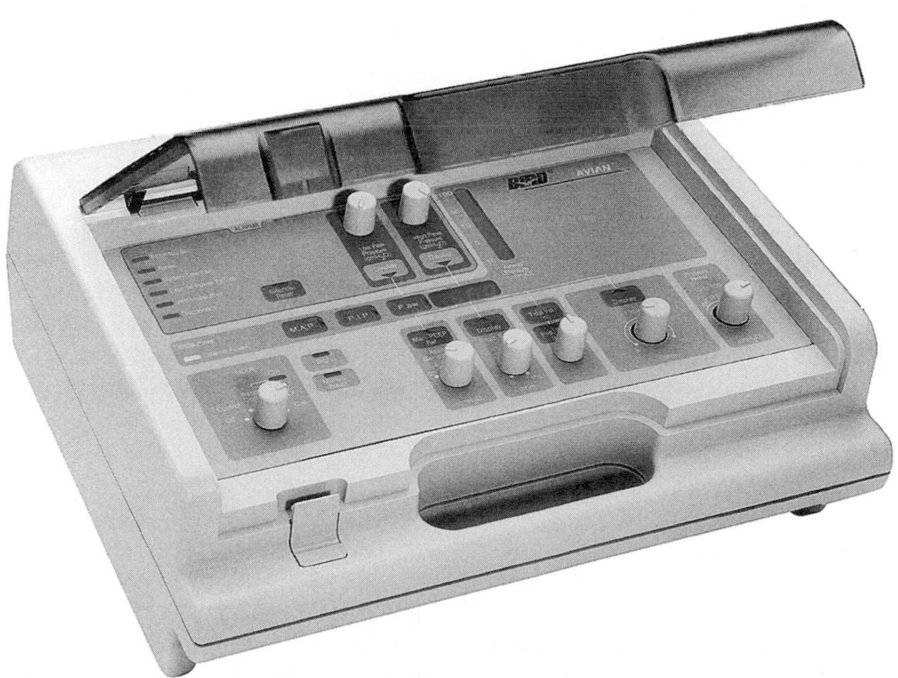

Figure 14-2 The Avian Ventilator. (Courtesy VIASYS Healthcare, Critical Care Division, Palm Springs, Calif.)

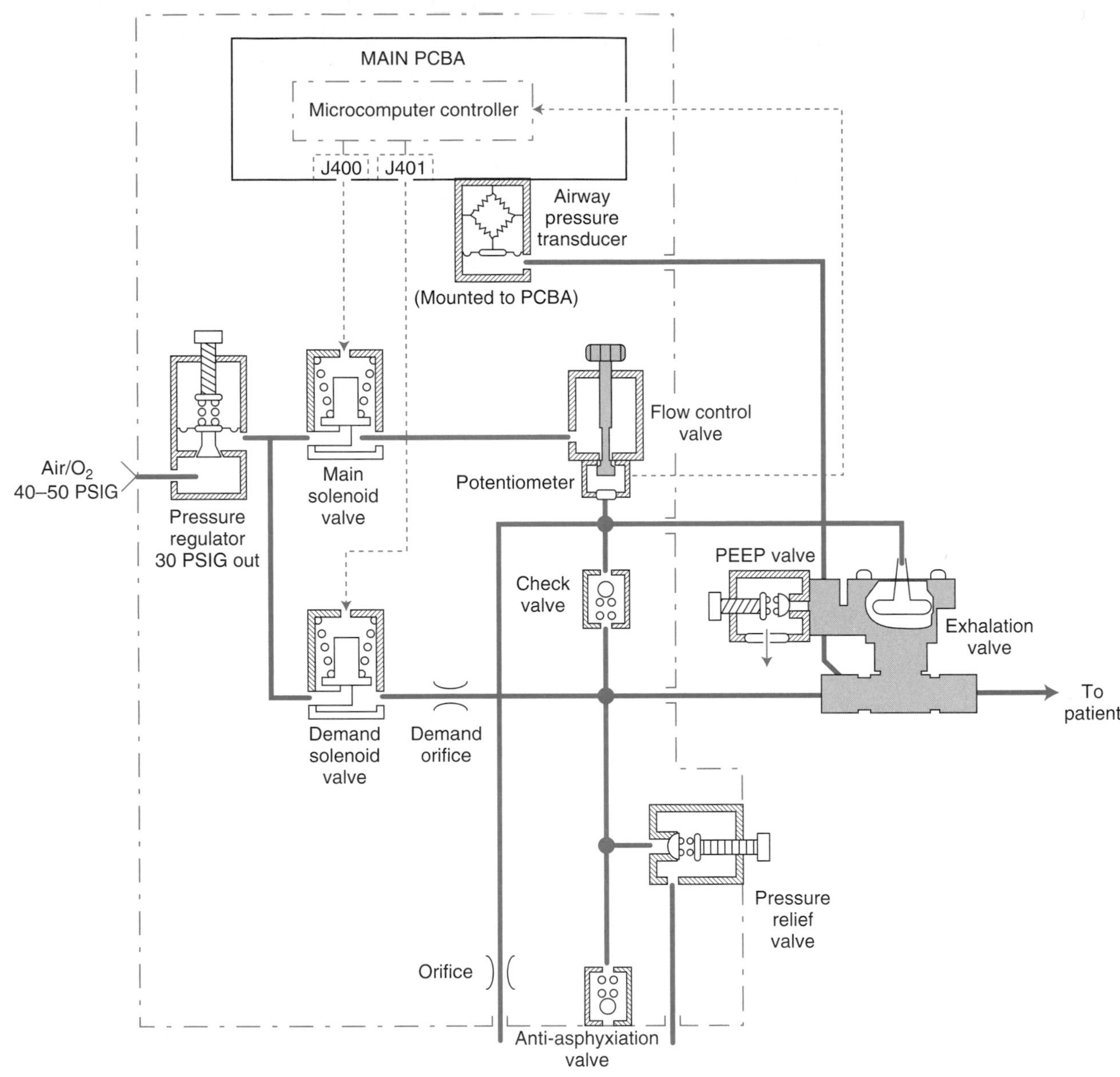

Figure 14-3 The internal pneumatic circuit of the Bird Avian. (Courtesy VIASYS Healthcare, Critical Care Division, Palm Springs, Calif.)

Bird Avian

The Bird Avian transport ventilator (Figure 14-2) is available through VIASYS Healthcare, Critical Care Division, Palm Springs, Calif. It is a microprocessor-controlled ventilator primarily used for transporting pediatric and adult patients. It can function in four modes: control, A/C, SIMV, and CPAP ventilation. It is lightweight (11 lb) and portable (10″ × 12″ × 5″).

Power Source

The Avian is electrically and pneumatically powered and requires both sources to properly perform all of its operations. The electronic system can use three possible power sources:

- An internal 6-volt DC battery
- An external 12-volt DC battery
- A standard AC outlet

The internal battery can sustain ventilator operation for about 11 hours and requires about 18 hours to be fully recharged. The external DC battery must be able to maintain an output of 11 to 30 volts to sustain ventilator operation, and the AC power option requires an adapter to properly function.

The pneumatic system requires a medical-grade, high-pressure source gas that can deliver 40 to 60 psig and has minimum flow-rate capabilities of 100 L/min. The source may be a cylinder, wall outlet, or oxygen/air blender with a DISS connector.

Internal Mechanism (Figure 14-3)

Source gas enters through a gas inlet port at the top of the ventilator. The gas pressure is reduced by a regulator to a constant working pressure of 30 spsig. This pressure ensures optimal machine function. When a mandatory breath is delivered, the gas moves from the regulator to a main solenoid valve, which controls inspiratory flow. Gas flows from the main solenoid valve to a flow-control poppet valve, which has two functions. First, it regulates and maintains gas flow to the patient based on the desired control settings. Second, a potentiometer valve attached to the flow-control poppet valve measures changes in valve position, and relays this information to the microprocessor. This information allows tidal volume (V_T) to be calculated during mandatory breath delivery.

Before the gas leaves the internal circuit for the patient circuit, it passes through a one-way check valve, a pressure-relief valve, and a proximal airway pressure line. The pressure-relief valve is a safety feature that prevents airway pressure from exceeding a set value. If a high-pressure situation occurs, the excess pressure and volume are vented to room air. The proximal airway line allows for communication with the airway pressure transducer and monitors the airway pressure and pressure alarms.

A demand valve provides flow for spontaneous breaths that may be initiated by a patient during SIMV or CPAP modes. The patient effort required to open the demand valve is determined by the sensitivity setting. (*Note*: Mandatory breath triggering is determined by the sensitivity setting as well.) Once triggered, gas flows through the demand orifice and through a fixed resistor that regulates flow to 60 L/min. Because the check valve is bypassed, the exhalation valve stays open, allowing any excess flow to be vented to the atmosphere.

A removable PEEP valve can be attached to the outlet port of the exhalation valve. The Avian automatically compensates the sensitivity or the trigger mechanism for any changes in the PEEP level, so that work of breathing does not increase.

The Avian operates from a 100% gas source (air or oxygen); therefore, the oxygen percentage depends upon the gas powering the ventilator. To accurately adjust the F_IO_2, the unit requires an air/oxygen blender for its gas power.

Controls and Alarms

The front panel of the Avian contains several controls for setting ventilator parameters and for monitoring patient data and alarms.

Mode Control Knob

The mode selector has five possible settings: OFF, CONTROL, ASSIST/CONTROL, SIMV/CPAP, and CAL. The OFF setting turns the ventilator off and triggers the VENT INOP. alarm, which can be silenced by the ALARM SILENCE/RESET button. The visual alarm, however, continues to flash for 30 minutes. The CAL setting lets the operator calibrate the airway pressure transducer to properly read "O" at ambient pressure. The other modes are presented in the section on modes of ventilation later in this chapter.

Control Parameters

The control parameters include the following functions:

- TIDAL VOLUME
- INSPIRATORY TIME
- RATE
- FLOW
- PEEP

The TIDAL VOLUME function is active when the machine is operating in volume-targeted ventilation. It allows the operator to set a range of 50 to 2000 mL for a mandatory breath. When the machine is initially turned on, the unit defaults to volume-targeted ventilation with volume-cycling, which requires a V_T setting in all modes except CPAP.

Mandatory breaths can be changed from volume- to time-cycling by using the tidal volume/inspiratory time (T_V/T_I) control button. To activate time-cycled ventilation, the T_V/T_I button is pressed and the T_I set. The new selection is displayed in the monitor window. To activate the new setting, the operator presses the T_V/T_I button a second time. If the operator wants to change T_I, the new setting is entered and then the display button is pressed. (*Note*: Because volume-cycled ventilation is the default setting when the ventilator is switched on, when time-cycled ventilation is desired, this change must be made when the power is turned on.)

The RESPIRATORY RATE control in the center of the panel allows for time-triggering of a mandatory breath (0 to 150 breaths/min). The flow control on the bottom right regulates the maximum flow delivered to the patient for all mandatory breaths (5 to 100 L/min).

The PEEP valve is a separate attachment to the exhalation valve. To access this function, the operator presses the MANUAL PEEP reference button on the front panel and holds it for 3 seconds until the "A" in the display window disappears. This allows manual setting of PEEP from 0 to 20 cm H_2O. If the PEEP value deviates by more than 5 cm H_2O from the desired value, an audible alarm activates, and the display window reads "PEEP Not Set," to alter the operator to the problem.

The ASSIST SENSITIVITY control allows the operator to set the trigger sensitivity for all breath types (–2 to –8 cm H_2O). The sensitivity is automatically PEEP compensated. For example, if PEEP is 5 cm H_2O and the sensitivity is –2 cm H_2O, the breath triggers when an inspiratory effort drops the baseline pressure to 3 cm H_2O.

The PRESSURE-RELIEF control is in the middle, right part of the control panel. It is designed to allow the operator to set the maximum acceptable pressure in the circuit during a mandatory breath. The PRESSURE-RELIEF control serves one of two purposes. First, it is a safety feature, and is normally set 5 to 15 cm H_2O above the HIGH PEAK PRESSURE alarm in case the HIGH PEAK PRESSURE alarm fails. Second,

CLINICAL ROUNDS 14-2

A patient is being ventilated with the Bird Avian in the A/C mode. V_T is 0.6 L; rate is 10 breaths/min; PIP is 25 cm H_2O; and the high peak pressure alarm is set at 35 cm H_2O. A decision is made to switch to pressure-limited ventilation. Where should the respiratory therapist set the high peak pressure alarm and the pressure-relief control to still achieve approximately the same V_T?

See Appendix A for the answer.

the PRESSURE-RELIEF control also functions as a pressure-limiting device when set to the desired limit. In the latter use, the HIGH PEAK PRESSURE alarm is set at 5 to 15 cm H_2O above the PRESSURE-RELIEF setting. The PRESSURE-RELIEF control has an adjustable range from 10 to 100 cm H_2O. It is a spring-loaded valve with no electronic input, so it can act as a secondary safety backup for situations of high circuit pressures if there is an electronic failure (Clinical Rounds 14-2).

The SIGH function is on the front left part of the control panel. When activated, it delivers a breath 1.5 times the V_T or T_I setting, depending on which is active. The maximum limits are 3 seconds for T_I and 2000 mL for V_T. The frequency is one sigh every 100 breaths or one every 7 minutes, whichever comes first.

The MANUAL breath control allows the operator to deliver a mandatory breath at the current ventilator settings. When activated, the breath rate timer is reset so that a time-triggered breath will not occur until the next full cycle.

Airway Pressure Alarms

The operator can set and monitor high and low airway pressures. The HIGH PEAK PRESSURE alarm establishes the maximum pressure allowed in the patient circuit during all breaths. This alarm is at the top central part of the control panel, has an allowable range of 1 to 100 cm H_2O, and cannot be set below the PEEP setting. When the set alarm level is exceeded, inspiration stops and the machine cycles into exhalation, venting the remaining volume and pressure to room air.

The LOW PEAK PRESSURE alarm is only active during mandatory breaths in the control, A/C, and SIMV modes. It is located in the central top section of the control panel (range of 2 to 50 cm H_2O). The LOW PEAK PRESSURE alarm is activated when a patient does not exceed the alarm setting during the inspiratory phase of each breath.

Box 14-1 Recoverable Alarms on the Avian

- Loss of electrical power
- Mode switch momentarily turned off
- Power voltage out of range

Additional Alarms

Additional alarms that are monitored include the following:

- DISCONNECT
- VENTILATOR INOPERATIVE
- EXTERNAL POWER LOW/FAIL
- BATTERY LOW/FAIL
- ALARM/SILENCE RESET
- I:E RATIO
- APNEA

The DISCONNECT alarm is at the bottom of the alarm section on the control panel. It monitors the airway pressure in the patient circuit and is activated if the pressure does not exceed 2 cm H_2O above the baseline pressure during a mandatory breath.

The VENTILATOR INOPERATIVE alarm is in the alarms section of the control panel and has two conditions: recoverable and nonrecoverable. The nonrecoverable alarm is usually the result of a software problem or central processing unit (CPU) malfunction. In this case, the machine must be turned off, and the ALARM/SILENCE button pressed to silence the alarm. The patient must be disconnected and manually ventilated until the problem is resolved. For a list of the recoverable problems, see Box 14-1. When any one of the recoverable problems occurs, the machine returns to normal working function after the condition has been corrected.

The EXTERNAL LOW/FAIL alarm is activated when the external power supply connected to the ventilator is operating outside of the acceptable range (11 to 30 DC for an external battery). The machine automatically switches to the internal battery. When the internal battery voltage falls below 5.6 ± 0.2 volts and no external supply is connected, the BATTERY LOW/FAIL alarm is activated. The battery life remaining depends on the machine settings.

The ALARM/SILENCE RESET button is in the alarm section on the control panel. When it is activated, this control silences the alarm for a certain time (depending on the problem) and resets the visual alarm in the display window.

The Avian does not allow I:E ratios greater than 1:1 to occur. If any combination of T_I or V_T, flow, and breath rate creates a T_I >50% of the TCT, the ventilator generates an audiovisual alarm. This alarm cannot be reset until the problem is alleviated. In the meantime, the ventilator continues to function with a T_I of 50% of the TCT.

The APNEA alarm is also in the alarm section of the control panel and is activated when 20 seconds elapse with no breath detected (spontaneous or mandatory). The audiovisual alarms are activated, and the ventilator resorts to a backup rate of 12 breaths/min in the A/C mode, using the set parameter. The backup ventilation can be terminated by pressing the ALARM/RESET button.

Modes of Ventilation

The Bird Avian can provide control, A/C, SIMV, or CPAP ventilation. As previously mentioned, the machine may be set to volume- or time-cycled ventilation, but the default setting is volume-cycled. Therefore, when operating in any modes but CPAP, the operator must be aware of how the machine is cycling. In the control mode, T_I or V_T, flow and breath rate are all active, offering a time- or volume-cycled, volume-targeted breath. The ASSIST SENSITIVITY setting is not functional in this mode.

The A/C mode allows the patient to initiate mandatory breaths, and thus control the total breath rate of the ventilator. All other functions set in the control mode are still active in this mode except for ASSIST/SENSITIVITY. When operating in A/C, the patient must generate an inspiratory effort greater than the set sensitivity to initiate a breath.

The SIMV mode allows for spontaneous breathing between the volume-targeted mandatory breaths. All previous functions are still active, and PEEP and sigh operations are added.

When operating in the CPAP mode, the control function is turned to SIMV, the rate is set to "0," and the PEEP valve is adjusted to the desired setting. All breaths are spontaneous and completely controlled by the patient. If the patient fails to trigger the ventilator within 20 seconds (not an adjustable time period), the APNEA alarm is activated, and the ventilator reverts to back-up ventilation. Back up ventilation consists of 12 breaths/min with all set controls operational in the A/C mode. To terminate this function, the ALARM SILENCE/RESET button must be pressed.

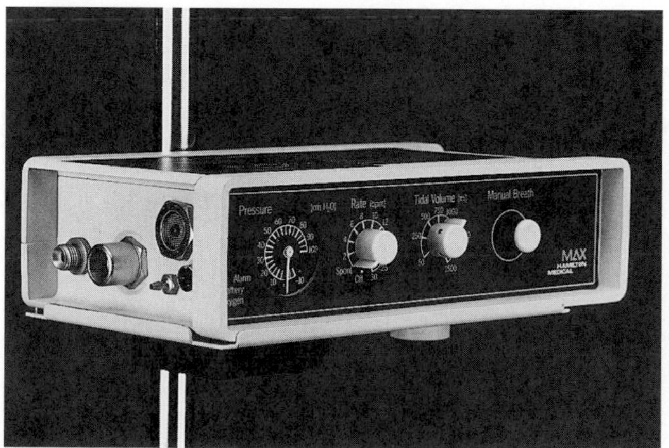

Figure 14-4 The Hamilton MAX Ventilator. (Courtesy Hamilton Medical, Reno, Nev.)

Hamilton Medical MAX

The Hamilton Medical, Inc., MAX (Figure 14-4) is used to ventilate pediatric or adult patients during transport. It uses intermittent mandatory ventilation (IMV) to provide time-triggered, volume-targeted, and time-cycled mandatory breaths that are delivered with a constant flow. Spontaneous breaths are pressure-triggered and pressure-limited. The device is lightweight (~5 lb) and compact (11.5″ × 6″ × 3″).

Power Source

The MAX is electrically controlled and pneumatically powered, and requires energy supplies for both systems to properly operate. The electronic system normally uses four 1.5-volt AA batteries to power the control panel and solenoid valve. As an alternate electrical power source, an external DC battery source with an input range of 12 to 28 volts and a minimum of 150 mA can be used. The MAX can also be connected to a standard 120-volt AC outlet with a 12-volt converter.

The pneumatic system is designed to use 100% medical-grade oxygen as its primary source gas. For proper operation, it requires a pressure of 50 to 90 psig from a cylinder, wall outlet, or oxygen/air blender. If compressed gas is used instead of oxygen, there can be an increase in V_T by as much as 10% because of the difference in densities between the gases.

Because the MAX operates from a high-pressure gas source, oxygen delivery depends on the gas powering the ventilator. When oxygen is the source gas, F_IO_2 is 1.0. When air is used, it is 0.21. To provide variable oxygen concentrations, the unit must be connected to an external air/oxygen blender.

The internal components of the ventilator do not consume any gas during operation, allowing the operator greater accuracy in predicting the length of time a cylinder will last during transport (Clinical Rounds 14-3).

Internal Mechanism

The source gas enters through a connection on the side panel (Figure 14-5) and is routed through an internal regulator that precisely adjusts the pressures to 50 psig. After

CLINICAL ROUNDS 14-3

A respiratory therapist is asked to transport a ventilated patient from the ICU to x-ray using the MAX ventilator. The respiratory rate is 15 breaths/min with no additional spontaneous breaths, and the V_T is 500 mL. The oxygen E cylinder has 1200 psi available, and the estimated time of the trip (one-way) is 30 minutes. Does the therapist have to change to a full cylinder to make the round trip?

See Appendix A for the answer.

passing through the regulator, the flow is guided to an electronically controlled solenoid valve. During mandatory breaths, this valve opens for a set period of 1 second, thus fixing the T_I. Next the source gas branches, directing flow to a second flow-control valve and pressure regulator. The flow-control valve regulates the flow/V_T that is to be delivered to the patient. The pressure regulator functions as a pressure-relief valve, limiting the maximum allowable pressure in the patient circuit. The pressure relief is factory-set at 45 cm H_2O, but can be manually changed from 10 to 100 cm H_2O inside the machine.

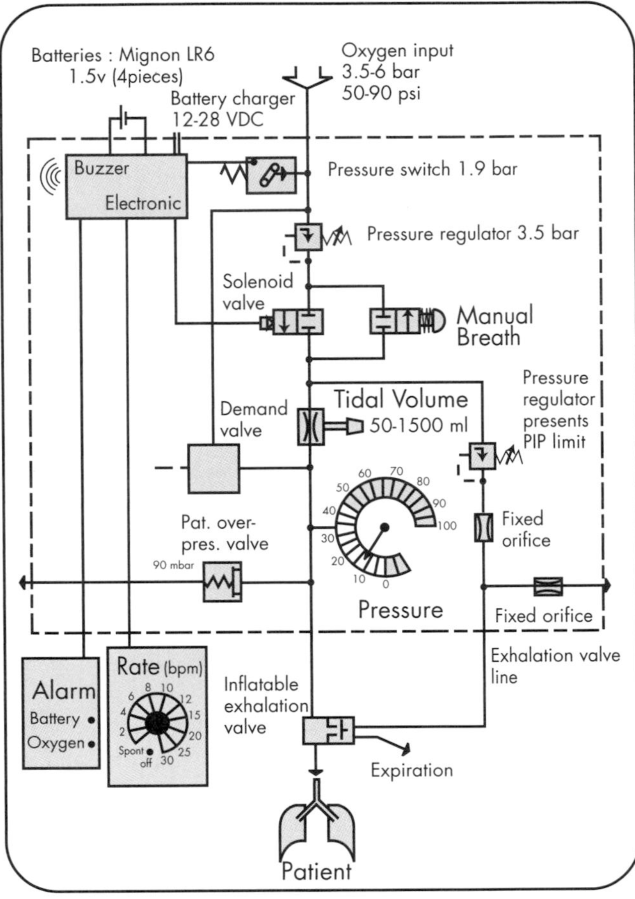

Figure 14-5 The MAX internal pneumatic diagram. (Courtesy Hamilton Medical, Reno, Nev.)

When spontaneous breaths are initiated, the patient must open the pneumatically controlled demand valve. This differs from mandatory breaths in the following two ways:

1. It requires the patient to provide an inspiratory effort sufficient to drop circuit pressure 1 to 2 cm H_2O below ambient pressure to generate inspiratory flow. When PEEP is required, it becomes increasingly difficult for the patient to trigger a spontaneous breath because the ventilator does not compensate for PEEP.
2. The demand valve is powered by the source gas and can provide flows up to 145 L/min.

When a manual breath is delivered, the electronically powered solenoid valve is bypassed and gas enters directly into the circuit (see description of manual breath in the following section on controls).

Controls

Figure 14-6 provides a view of the front panel controls. The three primary controls are the rate, tidal volume, and manual breath control.

Rate

The RATE control allows mandatory breaths to be set from 2 to 30 breaths/min. It also has a spontaneous setting in which mandatory breaths stop and all breaths are spontaneously triggered breaths (preset sensitivity of –1 to –2 cm H_2O). Under these conditions, the patient determines the rate and V_T of each breath. (*Note*: This setting provides no back-up mandatory rate.) The OFF position of this control stops mandatory and patient-triggered breaths and inactivates the alarm system (see the discussion of alarms at the end of this section).

Tidal Volume

The MAX is a flow-controller, so V_T delivery is a function of flow and T_I. Thus when the V_T is adjusted, it is the flow rate (variable from 0 to 90 L/min) that is actually being

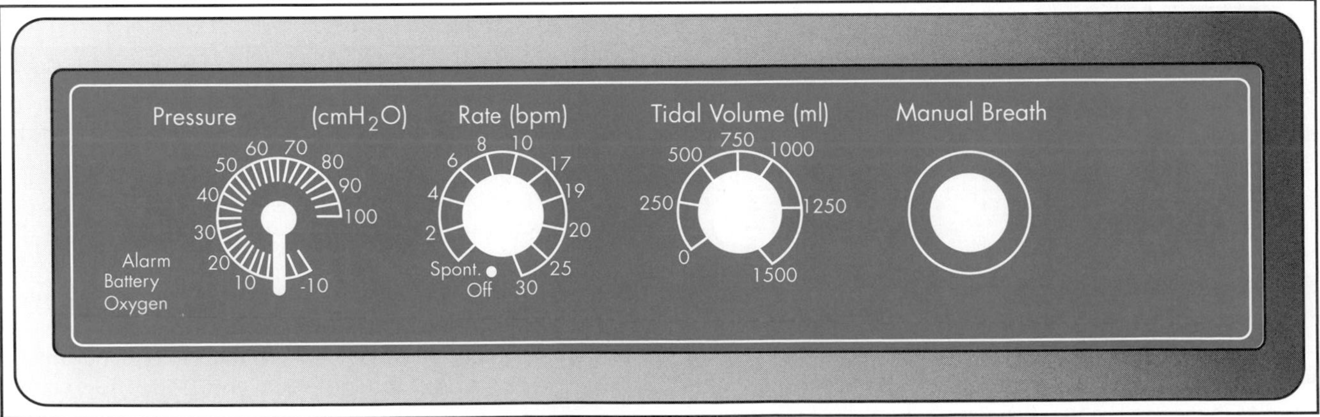

Figure 14-6 The front control panel of the Hamilton MAX ventilator.

Box 14-2 Manual Inhalation Button

There is no maximum length of time that the MANUAL INHALATION button can be pressed, but the patient is protected from overinflation by the internal safety pop-off valve (set at 45 cm H_2O).

If there is an electrical power failure, the transport team can ventilate a patient with manual breaths because pneumatic power can still provide flow delivery. The manual breath control does not require electricity to work. It diverts the gas around the electronically controlled solenoid valve (see Figure 14-5).

adjusted. The front panel, however, displays incremental changes in adjustable volumes of 50 to 1500 mL for mandatory breaths.

Manual Breath

By depressing the MANUAL BREATH button, a positive-pressure breath can be delivered at any time. Volume delivery depends on how long the button is pressed. After the button is released, inspiration ends. For example, if it is pressed for 1 second, the set V_T will be delivered because the normal T_I is fixed at 1 second (Box 14-2).

Pressure Gauge

The pressure gauge on the left side of the front panel is calibrated in cm H_2O (10 to 100 cm H_2O) and allows the operator to view the active pressure in the circuit, the PEEP level or baseline, and the maximum pressure change from baseline.

Alarms

The MAX has two alarms (LOW BATTERY and LOW OXYGEN) and a pressure-limit feature. If there is a low battery condition, a constant visual indicator is illuminated and a pulsating tone sounds simultaneously. The LOW BATTERY alarm indicator is activated when the rechargeable batteries have less than 10 minutes of power left or the alkaline batteries have less than 30 minutes left.

The low oxygen indicator also has audiovisual indicators that are activated when the input pressure source falls below 27 psig and alert the operator to the insufficient pressure from the source gas. (*Note*: There is no built-in O_2 analyzer.) The low oxygen light indicates the pressure level at the gas source inlet.

There is no low pressure alarm for circuit leaks, but there is an audible alarm for excessive high pressures. Excessive pressures are limited by the internal pressure alarm system that is part of the exhalation valve circuit assembly. This internal pressure system acts as a pressure relief, venting excessive flow through the exhalation valve to room air when circuit pressure exceeds the set value producing a noise as it does so. The pressure relief limits pressure delivery but does not end inspiration. As previously mentioned, the pressure relief limit is preset by the manufacturer at 45 cm H_2O and can be internally adjusted from 10 to 100 cm H_2O.

CLINICAL ROUNDS 14-4

A patient is being transported with the MAX ventilator. The rate is set at 10 breaths/min, and the V_T is at 500 mL. An expiratory CPAP valve has been added to the exhalation valve outlet; the CPAP is set at 7 cm H_2O. The respiratory therapist observes the pressure manometer and notices that the pressure drops to $^-1$ to $^-2$ cm H_2O at the beginning of inspiration, peaks at 25 cm H_2O, and then goes to 7 cm H_2O during exhalation. What accounts for the observed pressure changes, and what can be done to correct them?

See Appendix A for the answer.

Modes of Ventilation

The design of the Hamilton MAX provides only one mode of ventilation: IMV; but the unit is set up to allow for control, and spontaneous (CPAP) ventilation as well. When the patient does not trigger any additional breaths above the set minimum set rate, the ventilator operates in a control mode with the V_T and breath rate controlled by the ventilator.

When the RATE control is set to SPONTANEOUS, there is no set mandatory breath rate. All spontaneous breaths are pressure-triggered, pressure-limited, and pressure-cycled. The ventilator provides inspiratory flow when the patient generates sufficient pressure to open the demand valve (1 to 2 cm H_2O). Inspiration ends when the circuit pressure rises above the required pressure to maintain an open demand valve. This setting in spontaneous ventilation can act as CPAP, or rather as EPAP (expiratory airway pressure), when an external PEEP valve is added to the expiratory valve outlet. The MAX does not have an internal mechanism for PEEP compensation. Any additional rise in baseline pressure will require the patient to generate a negative pressure of 1 to 2 plus the additional baseline pressure. If high PEEP levels are used, this could increase the patient's work of breathing (Clinical Rounds 14-4).

During ventilation, mandatory breaths are delivered minimally at the rate set on the RATE control.

When the MAX is used in the IMV mode, mandatory breaths are time-triggered, volume-targeted, and time-cycled. Adequate spontaneous inspiratory efforts that occur between the mandatory breaths are delivered as spontaneous breaths. (*Note*: If the patient is in the middle of a spontaneous inspiration and the ventilator determines it is time for

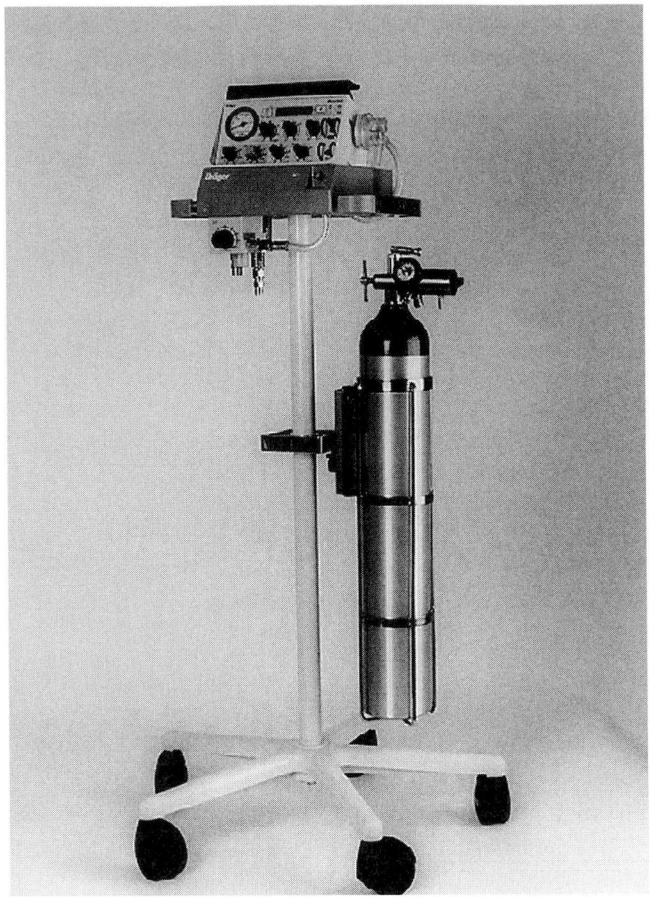

Figure 14-7 The Dräger Microvent Ventilator. (Courtesy Dräger Medical, Telford, Pa.)

Box 14-3 Calculation of Cylinder Duration for the Microvent

For the estimated cylinder duration for the Microvent in the control mode, use the following formula:

$$\text{Expected time of operation} = \frac{\text{pressure of gas supply (liters)}}{\text{minute ventilation} + 1\ \text{(liters/min)}}$$

Pressure of gas supply = tank pressure $\times$ conversion factor

For example:

2200 psig = tank pressure

0.28 = conversion factor for an E cylinder

volume of gas supply = (2200 psig) (0.28) = 622 L

The reason that 1 is added to the minute ventilation is to account for the consumption of 1 L of gas/min. Suppose an E cylinder has a pressure reading of 1800 psig. The patient is breathing 10 times per minute at a set V_T of 0.5 L. How long will is take for the tank to be completely empty?

volume of gas supply = (1800 psig) (0.28) = 504 L

minute ventilation = rate $\times$ V_T

= (10 breaths/min) (0.5 L) = 5 L

$$\text{expected time of operation} = \frac{(504\ \text{L})}{(5 + 1)\ \text{liters/minute}}$$

= 84 min

another mandatory breath, the mandatory breath is delivered on top of the spontaneous breath.) The mandatory breaths are not synchronized with the patient's spontaneous efforts. If breaths are not synchronous and breath stacking ensues, the operator can increase the mandatory breath rate to override the spontaneous rate and reduce the chance of any additional breath stacking. The pressure relief valve prevents excessive airway pressure if breath stacking does occur.

Dräger Microvent

The Dräger Microvent (Figure 14-7) is a time- or patient-triggered, volume-targeted ventilator primarily used for transporting adult patients. It may also be used on pediatric patients weighing more than 33 lb (Dräger Medical, Telford, Pa). The Microvent can function in four modes: control, A/C, SIMV, PSV, and CPAP. It is lightweight (9.5 lb) and portable (8.5″ × 4.7″ × 8.1″).

Power Source

The Dräger Microvent requires an electrical and a pneumatic power source to properly operate. The electronic system can use the following three separate power sources:

- An AC outlet
- An external, 12-volt battery
- An internal, rechargeable or non-rechargeable battery

The internal battery has a lifespan of about 2 hours when fully charged and requires about 5 hours for recharging. When approximately 10 minutes of operating time is left, the message "CHARGE NiCd" is illuminated in the display window. When the ventilator is connected to one of the two external power sources, the green power connected status indicator lights up and the internal battery pack begins charging. This occurs regardless of whether the ventilator is on or off. The internal battery is essential to the operation of the machine; without it the ventilator cannot function.

The pneumatic component requires medical-grade gases (air and oxygen), at 38 to 84 psig. The sources may be cylinder gas, wall outlets, or an oxygen/air blender, as long as a DISS connector is provided.

When the Microvent is operating with an air and oxygen blender, the oxygen percentage depends upon the F_IO_2 setting on the external blender. There is no entrainment feature. (*Note:* To ensure accurate F_IO_2s, the operator should monitor the patient's inspiratory gas flow with an oxygen analyzer.)

The ventilator consumes 1 L/min of gas for its pneumatic functions. When estimating the amount of oxygen available from a cylinder for patient transport, the operator must include this factor in the calculations (Box 14-3).

Internal Mechanism

The source gas enters through the inlet filter at the rear of the machine (Figure 14-8) and is immediately reduced by the internal regulator to a constant working pressure. From the regulator, flow is diverted to the PEEP and exhalation valves to be primed and also to the INSPIRATORY/EXPIRATORY (I/E) valve. The gas is then routed to the electronically-controlled pressure regulator, which governs the rate and pattern of gas flow to the patient. From this pressure regulator, gas passes a one-way check valve and is then sent to the patient circuit. A flow sensor at the Y-connector of the patient circuit monitors inspiratory and expiratory minute ventilation and patient airway pressures.

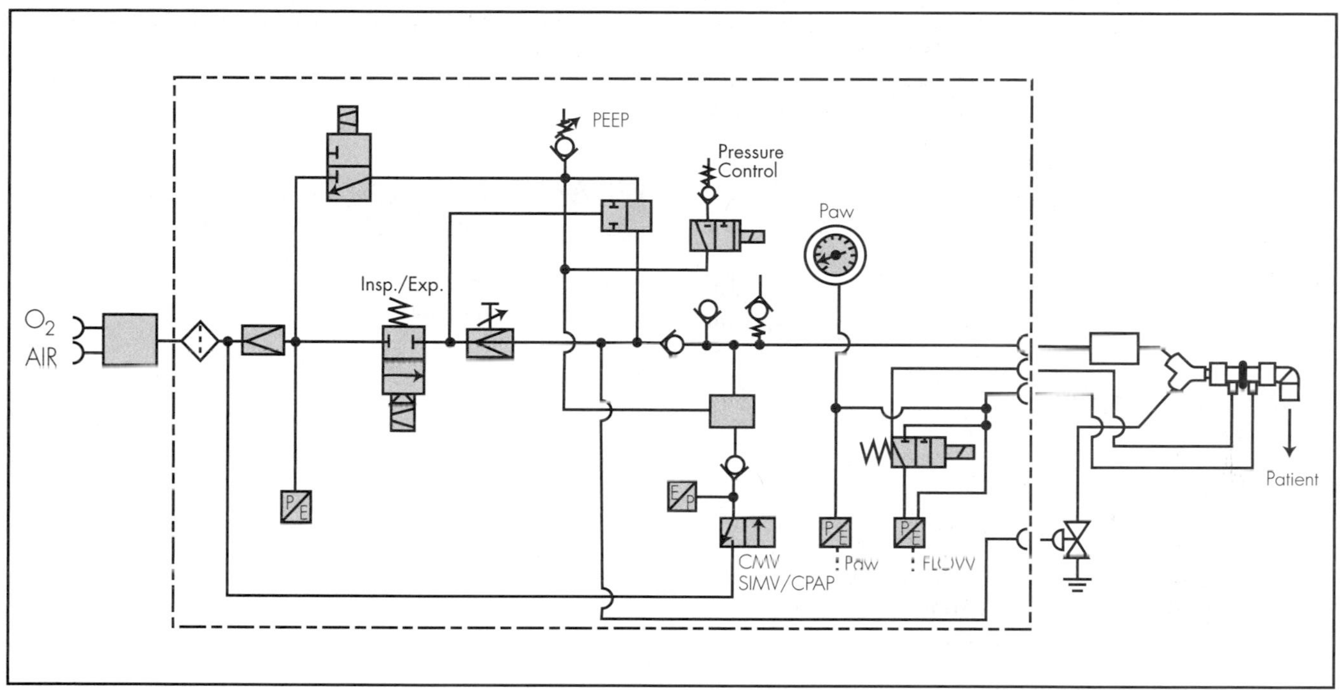

Figure 14-8 The Microvent internal pneumatic circuit. (Courtesy Dräger Medical, Telford, Pa.)

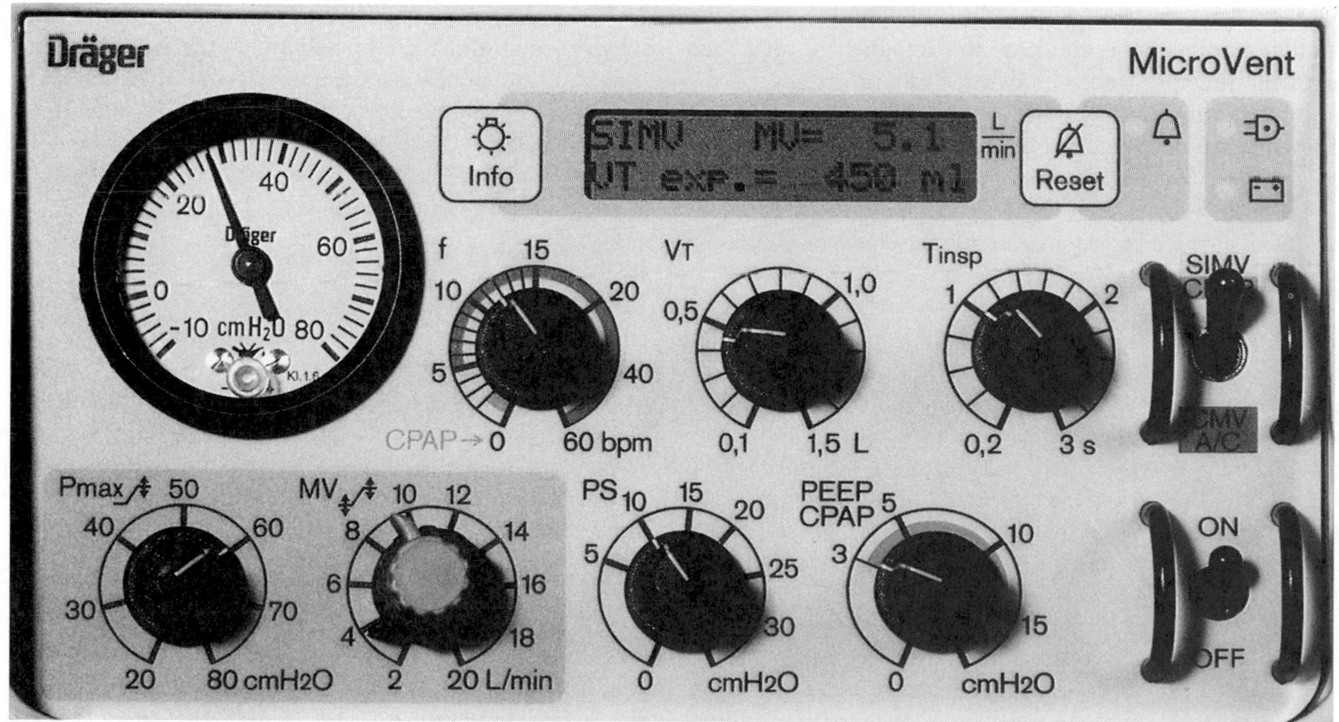

Figure 14-9 The Microvent control panel. (Courtesy Dräger Medical, Telford, Pa.)

The Microvent provides a continuous, 10 L/min flow of gas through the patient circuit (bias flow). This flow is controlled by the demand valve and is intended to help reduce the patient's work of breathing for spontaneously-triggered breaths. If the patient requires a flow above 10 L/min, the demand valve can provide flows up to 120 L/min.

If the gas supplies fail, ambient air can be drawn in through an antisuffocation valve.

Controls

The front panel of the Microvent is easy to operate and contains a pressure monitor, liquid crystal display (LCD), alarm controls and indicators, and the basic unit controls (Figure 14-9).

Pressure Gauge

The pressure manometer is on the top left section of the control panel and continuously monitors airway pressure (10 to 80 cm H_2O).

Liquid Crystal Display

An LCD at the top center part of the panel shows the measured parameters, alarms, and advisory messages that are monitored and detected by the unit.

The three controls in the middle of the front panel are the VENTILATOR RATE, V_T, and T_I. The ventilator rate is active in control, A/C, and SIMV modes. The knob is to the left of the three controls. It sets the number of mandatory breaths in the control mode, the minimum number of mandatory breaths in the A/C mode, and the maximum mandatory breaths in SIMV. The adjustable range is 0 to 60 breaths/min.

The V_T control is in the middle of the three controls and regulates the volume delivered to the patient during each mandatory breath (range of 100 to 1500 mL).

The T_I control is on the far right of the three controls and regulates the length of time spent in inspiration (range of 0.2 to 3 seconds). The V_T and the T_I settings are responsible for the delivered flow for mandatory breaths. To the right of the T_I control is the mode selection switch.

Pressure Support and PEEP

PRESSURE SUPPORT and PEEP/CPAP controls are located on the lower part of the front panel. The PS control has an operational range of 0 to 35 cm H_2O. It only functions during spontaneous breaths and must be set higher than the CPAP/PEEP level or it will not function. The level of PS provided to the patient during each breath is determined by the difference between the pressure support and the PEEP settings (Clinical Rounds 14-5). The on/off switch is to the right of the PEEP/CPAP control.

The PEEP/CPAP control has an operational range of 0 to 18 cm H_2O and functions in all modes of ventilation. To use the CPAP mode, the operator must place the mode selector in SIMV and turn the RATE setting to "0" breaths/min.

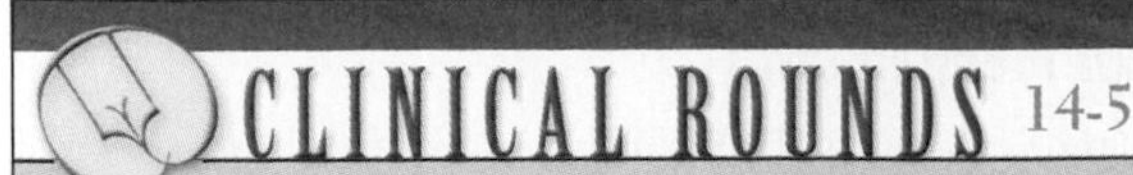

CLINICAL ROUNDS 14-5

In the CPAP mode, the PEEP is set at 5 cm H_2O, and the pressure support is at 15 cm H_2O. What is the actual amount of pressure support that the patient receives with each spontaneous breath?

See Appendix A for the answer.

Box 14-4 Microvent Alarms

- High peak pressure (Pmax)
- Low airway pressure
- High PEEP
- Apnea
- High and low minute ventilation
- Power system alarms (O_2 pressure low, power failure, charge NiCd)

Alarms

The Microvent can monitor several parameters and alert the operator to fluctuations that exceed set alarm limits (Box 14-4).

High Peak Pressure Alarm and Pmax

The PMAX control is on the bottom left section of the panel and limits upper airway pressure (20 to 80 cm H_2O). When circuit pressure exceeds the set PMAX level, the HIGH PEAK PRESSURE alarm (audiovisual) is activated. The I/E solenoid valve closes, which stops inspiration and allows the remainder of the breath to be vented to room air.

Low Airway Pressure and High PEEP Alarms

The LOW AIRWAY PRESSURE and HIGH PEEP alarms (audiovisual) are set by the manufacturer and alert the operator when exceeded. The LOW AIRWAY PRESSURE alarm is activated when the pressure in the patient circuit fails to reach 5 cm H_2O within 15 seconds of the previous mandatory breath. The high PEEP alarm is activated when airway pressure fails to drop below 22 cm H_2O during exhalation.

Apnea Alarm

The apnea alarm is only functional during CPAP (SIMV rate = 0 breaths/min). When the patient fails to make a sufficient effort to trigger the ventilator within 15 seconds, the alarm is activated. It does not have an adjustable range.

High and Low Minute Ventilation Alarms

HIGH and LOW MINUTE VENTILATION settings are adjustable from 2 to 20 L/min and alert the operator when the patient exceeds the set parameters.

Power System Alarms

The power system alarms include O_2 PRESSURE LOW, POWER FAILURE, and CHARGE NiCd. The O_2 PRESSURE LOW alarm activates when the gas inlet pressure falls below 22 psig, indicating that the gas source is not providing enough pressure to the ventilator for proper function. The POWER FAILURE and CHARGE NiCd alarms are activated when the external power supply fails or the internal battery has less than 10 minutes of operational power left.

Reset Button

The RESET button at the top right part of the front panel can be used to silence alarms for 2 minutes when pressed.

Modes of Operation

The Microvent offers the following modes of ventilation:

- CMV
- A/C
- SIMV
- CPAP
- PSV

In CMV, rate, V_T, and T_I are all active, offering time-triggered, volume-targeted, and time-cycled breaths. All breaths are ventilator-controlled.

When in the A/C mode, the mode selector switch remains in CMV. To access the A/C function, the operator must press the INFO key until the display message reads "CMV—A/C." In this mode, the rate, V_T, and T_I controls are all functioning. The A/C mode allows mandatory breaths to be patient-triggered (flow), and there is no adjustable sensitivity control to set. The ventilator responds to a 4 L/min decrease in baseline flow to trigger a mandatory breath.

When the Microvent is in the SIMV mode, mandatory breath delivery is the same as that in A/C with one exception. In A/C, every patient effort that exceeds the trigger sensitivity level (4 L/min) results in a mandatory breath. In SIMV, the maximum mandatory breath rate is limited to the rate control setting. An asterisk appears in the display window with the delivery of every triggered mandatory breath. The patient may breathe spontaneously between these breaths.

To use CPAP with the Microvent, the mode switch remains in the SIMV setting, but the rate is adjusted to "0." When in CPAP, all breaths are spontaneous, requiring the patient to generate a –1 cm H_2O pressure to trigger the ventilator. (*Note*: Mandatory breaths are flow-triggered, and spontaneous breaths are pressure-triggered.) PEEP and pressure support are active controls in CPAP. The pressure support setting must always be greater than PEEP to operate. If there is an apneic period longer than 15 seconds, the ventilator initiates a backup rate of 8 breaths/min at the set V_T and T_I. It is important to set these controls even when the rate is set to 0 because of their use in an apneic event.

Dräger Oxylog 2000

The Oxylog 2000 (Figure 14-10) is a time- or patient-triggered, volume-targeted ventilator used primarily for emergencies and transporting adults, or pediatric patients weighing at least 33 lb. The Oxylog can function in three modes: control, SIMV, and CPAP. It is lightweight (9.5 lb) and portable (8.5″ × 4.7″ × 8.1″) (Dräger Medical, Telford, Pa).

Power Source

The Dräger Oxylog requires an electrical and a pneumatic source to properly function. The electronic system can use the following three separate power sources:

- An AC outlet
- An external 12-volt battery
- An internal rechargeable or non-rechargeable battery

When the ventilator is connected to one of the two external power sources, the green POWER CONNECTED status light goes on and the rechargeable internal battery pack starts charging regardless of whether the ventilator is on or off. This internal battery is essential to the operations of the machine. It has a functional lifespan of about 6 hours when fully charged and requires about 8 hours to recharge to maximum capacity. When approximately 10 minutes of

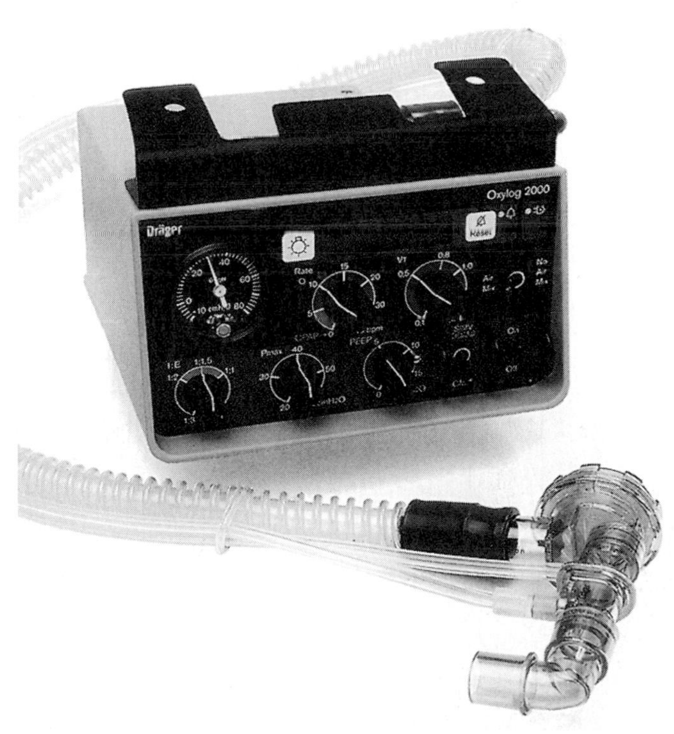

Figure 14-10 The Dräger Oxylog 2000 ventilator. (Courtesy Dräger Medical, Telford, Pa.)

operation is left, a message in the display window reads: "CHARGE NiCd."

The pneumatic component requires a high-pressure medical-grade gas (oxygen or air) supplied in a range of 38 to 84 psi. The source may be a cylinder, wall outlet, or oxygen/air blender with a DISS connector.

In the Oxylog the F_IO_2 delivery is not only dependent on the gas source being used, but also on the AIR/MIX switch and the mode selected for use. The AIR/MIX switch allows the operator to choose from 1.0 to 0.60 F_IO_2 when oxygen is the gas source. The AIR/MIX function is only operational for mandatory breaths. All spontaneous breaths receive 100% of the source gas. Attaching an air/oxygen blender to regulate F_IO_2 gives the operator more control over oxygen delivery.

Box 14-5 The Oxylog 2000 Air/Mix Injector

When the AIR/MIX switch is on, the gas source passes through the internal injector, which draws ambient air from the room to dilute the mixture to 60%. This conserves gas use by 50% and allows for prolonged transport when a limited source gas is used.

The internal pneumatic components of the ventilator consume 1 L/min of gas to support their functions. It is necessary to include this factor in the calculation for cylinder duration when a cylinder is used to power the unit during transport. The Oxylog is also equipped with an oxygen-conserving device, an AIR/MIX injector (Box 14-5).

Internal Mechanism

The gas source enters through the inlet port at the rear of the machine (Figure 14-11) and is immediately filtered and reduced to a constant working pressure by a regulator. From the regulator, the flow is diverted to the PEEP and exhalation valves to be primed and then to the inspiratory/expiratory (I/E) valve. The I/E valve regulates the release of inspiratory flow in a time-cycled fashion. Next, the gas source passes an electronically controlled pressure regulator, which governs the rate and pattern of flow before it passes through one of the following two valves:

1. A pneumatic control valve that supplies the patient with a 100% gas source.
2. An injector that supplies the patient with a 60% gas source.

The route is determined by the position of the AIR/MIX switch (see Box 14-5). After its route through the pneumatic valve or the injector, the gas flows to the patient circuit.

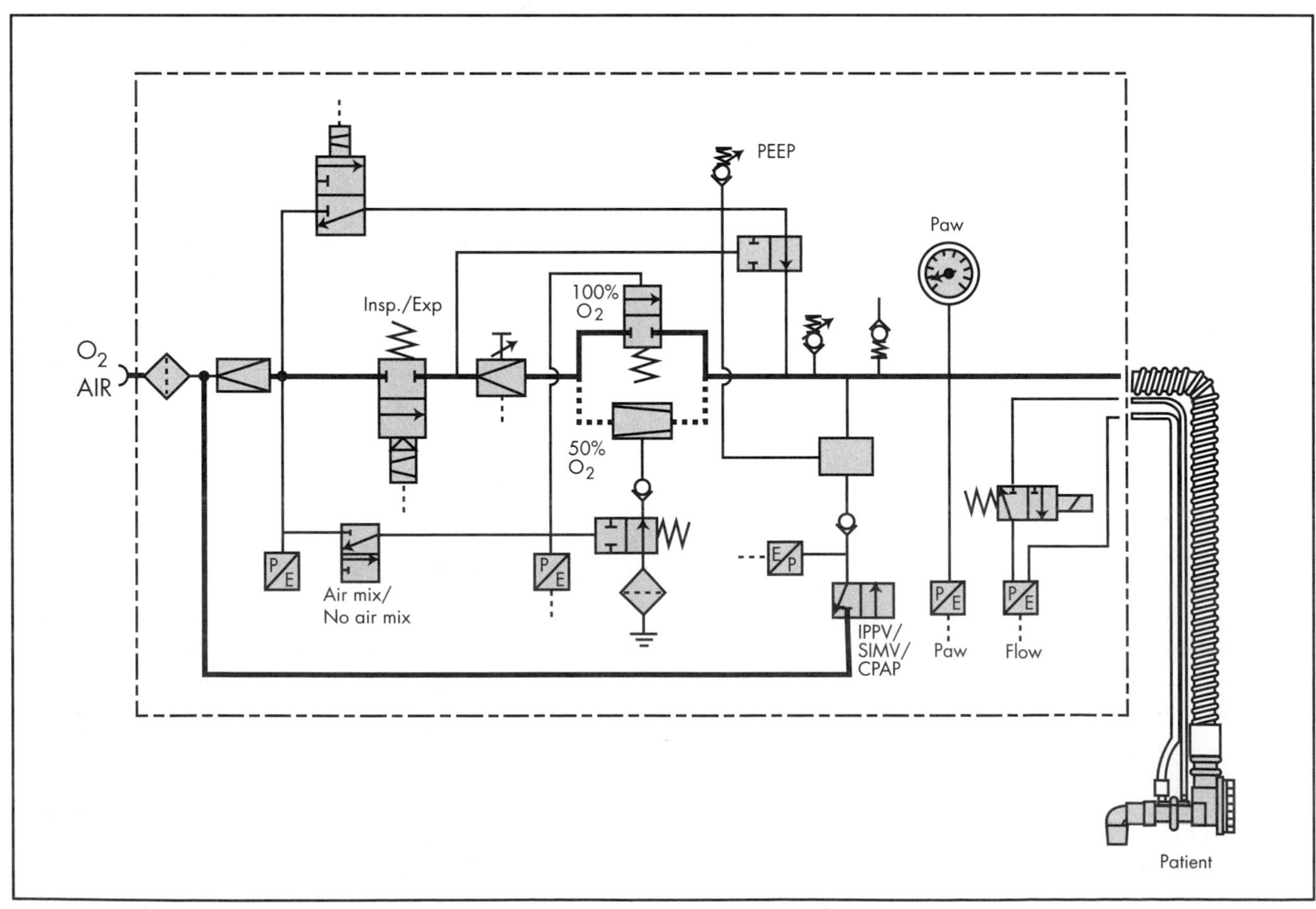

Figure 14-11 An internal pneumatic diagram of the Dräger Oxylog 2000 ventilator. (Courtesy Dräger Medical, Telford, Pa.)

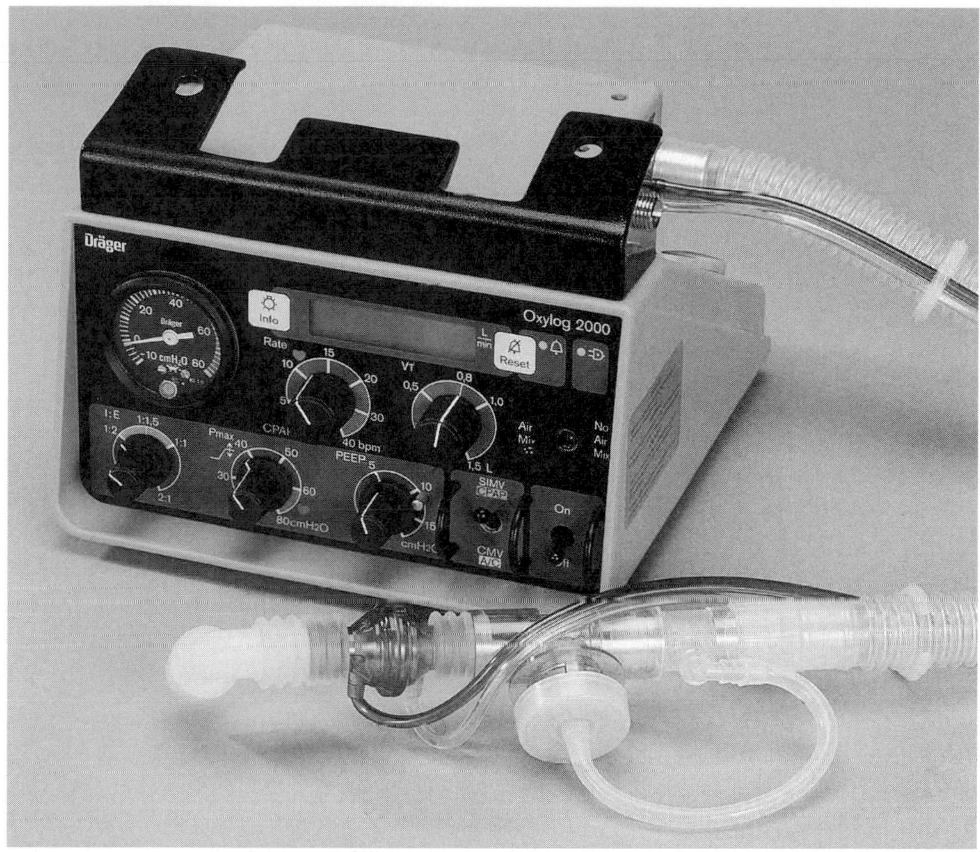

Figure 14-12 Dräger Oxylog 2000 control panel and patient circuit. (Courtesy Dräger Medical, Telford, Pa.)

Table 14-2 The Oxylog 2000 color-coded settings

	Range (kg)	Minute Ventilation	Ventilator Rate
Green (infants)	10 to 20 kg	0.1 to 0.3 L	30 to 40 breaths/min
Blue (children)	20 to 40 kg	0.3 to 0.8 L	20 to 30 breaths/min
Brown (adults)	above 40 kg	0.8 to 1.5 L	5 to 20 breaths/min

Courtesy Dräger, Inc, Telford, Pa.

To initiate a spontaneous breath, the patient must open the demand valve by generating a minimum pressure change of –1 cm H_2O. During a spontaneous breath, gas from the demand valve bypasses the injector that is regulated by the AIR/MIX switch. As a result, all spontaneous breaths are provided at 100% source gas. The maximum flow for a spontaneous breath is 120 L/min.

Controls and Alarms

The controls and alarms on the Oxylog 2000 are simple and easy to operate (Figure 14-12).

Pressure Monitoring Gauge

The pressure gauge is on the top left part of the control panel and provides continuous measurements of airway pressure in centimeters of water.

Control Parameters

The control parameters include the following: V_T, RATE, I:E RATIO, and PEEP. The V_T knob regulates the volume delivered to the patient during each mandatory breath (100 to 1500 mL). The V_T is also color-coded for quick setting (see the discussion of additional features in this section or Table 14-2 for a complete explanation).

Table 14-3 I:E Ratio in the SIMV mode for the Oxylog 2000

Frequency Setting	Effect
0	No ventilator breaths (CPAP)
5 to 12 breaths/min	Fixed T_I (2 seconds)
12 to 40 breaths/min	Fixed T_I (1:1.5)
	I:E = 1:1.5 seconds

Courtesy Dräger, Inc, Telford, Pa.

The RATE knob is to the left of the volume setting and functions to regulate the set number of mandatory breaths in the control mode and the minimum number of mandatory breaths in SIMV. The ventilator has an adjustable range of 5 to 60 breaths/min in the control and SIMV modes. When the mode selector is placed in SIMV and the rate is less than 5 breaths/min, the ventilator switches to CPAP.

The I:E knob is at the bottom-left of the control panel and has an operational range of 1:3 to 2:1 (±5%.) The Oxylog allows for inverse ratio ventilation in the control mode, which is not a common feature in transport ventilators. In the SIMV mode, the I:E ratio is determined by the rate setting (see Table 14-3 for complete details).

The PEEP control is located on the lower middle part of the control panel and has an operational range of 0 to 15 cm H_2O. The PEEP control is functional in all modes.

Alarms and Alarm Reset

The Oxylog provides HIGH and LOW AIRWAY PRESSURE ALARMS, HIGH and LOW MINUTE VENTILATION ALARMS, and POWER SOURCE alarms.

High-Pressure Alarm

The high-pressure alarm labeled PMAX is on the lower left section of the control panel and has an adjustable range of 20 to 60 cm H_2O. When airway pressures exceed the PMAX setting, a red alarm status light starts blinking and an intermittent audible alarm is triggered. Simultaneously, the inspiratory flow stops, and the exhalation valve opens. When the problem is corrected, the audible alarm is silenced, but the visual display must be manually reset with the ALARM RESET button at the top right of the control panel. The ALARM RESET can also be used to silence audible alarms for 2 minutes. If the problem is corrected, the ALARM RESET button clears the display screen.

Low-Pressure Alarms

The LOW-PRESSURE alarm does not have a control knob. It is activated when the pressure in the patient circuit does not reach at least 10 cm H_2O pressure in 20 seconds after the previous mandatory breath. An audiovisual alarm is activated that is not functional in the CPAP mode.

High and Low Minute Ventilation Alarms

Minute ventilation is an additional parameter that is monitored by the Oxylog. The Oxylog monitors expired minute ventilation through the flow sensor near the expiratory valve and ensures that the patient is being properly ventilated. The current reading is shown in the display window. A fluctuation outside of set parameters may activate the audiovisual alarm. If the expiratory minute volume falls below 40% of the inspiratory minute volume, the alarm is activated. Tubing and connections should be checked for any possible problems because a leak is suggested.

Apnea Alarm

The apnea alarm is only functional in the CPAP mode. When the patient does not make sufficient effort to open the demand valve within 15 seconds, an audiovisual alarm is activated.

Power System Alarm

The pneumatic system has an O_2 PRESSURE LOW alarm that is activated when the gas inlet pressure falls below 28 psig. This indicates that the gas source is not providing sufficient pressure for proper ventilator function. The electronic system has a power failure and a CHARGE NiCd alarm that are activated when the external power supply fails or the internal battery has less than 10 minutes of power left.

Modes of Ventilation

The Dräger Oxylog offers control, SIMV, and CPAP modes. In the control mode, the ventilator requires that the V_T, rate and I:E ratio be set. The unit is then time-triggered. To trigger a mandatory breath, the machine requires the patient to initiate a 4-L/min change in flow. To receive gas flow for a spontaneous breath in the SIMV mode, the patient must generate a pressure change of –2 cm H_2O below baseline to open the demand valve. As in the control mode, V_T and rate are set and active in SIMV, but the I:E ratio is not; it is determined by the rate setting (see Table 14-3).

The third option of ventilation is CPAP. In CPAP, only the PEEP control is set. As with spontaneous breaths in SIMV, to trigger gas flow in this mode, the patient must generate a pressure change of –2 cm H_2O below baseline. The AIR/MIX switch is nonfunctional because all breaths come from the demand valve, which bypasses the AIR/MIX injector.

Newport Medical Instruments E100i

The Newport E100i was originally presented in the sixth edition (1999) of this text. The material for that ventilator has been moved to the Evolve website for the text (Newport Medical Instruments, Newport Beach, Calif).

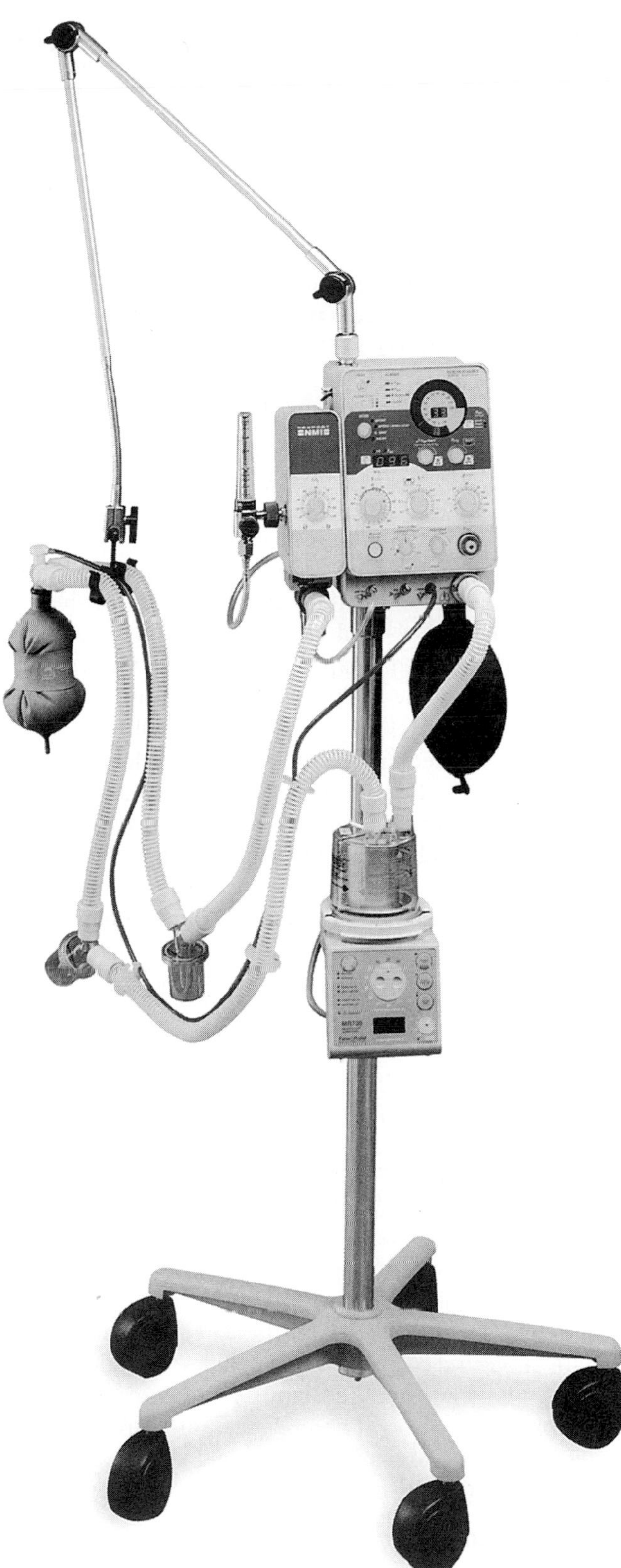

Figure 14-13 The Newport E100M ventilator. (Courtesy Newport Medical Instruments, Newport Beach, Calif.)

Newport Medical Instruments E100M

The Newport E100M (Figure 14-13) is a pressure- or time-triggered, volume- or pressure-targeted, and time-cycled ventilator that is pneumatically powered and electronically controlled. It is used for infant, pediatric, and adult patients and can operate in assist/control volume ventilation (A/CMV), SIMV, spontaneous and "SPONT + APNEA A/CMV" modes. The E100M is lightweight (18 lb) and compact (10.5″ × 9.5″ × 6.5″) and able to be used as a transport ventilator.

Power Source

The E100M requires both an electrical and a pneumatic power source to properly function. The electronic system integrates two microprocessors that control all mechanical components and visual displays. The system requires an AC power source (110 or 220 volts) or power supplied by the internal back-up battery. The back-up battery on the E100M has an operational time of 6 to 8 hours and a "Battery in Use" alert is displayed in the monitor window when it is active. To allow for optimal charging time, the battery pack is recharged whenever the ventilator is connected to an AC power source, regardless of whether the ventilator power switch is on or off. A convenient "% CHARGE" indicator approximates the total charge of the battery for the clinician.

The pneumatic system requires two medical-grade gases supplied to an air/oxygen mixer at 35 to 90 psi (50 psig is nominal). The air and oxygen sources may be cylinders or wall outlets. (*Note*: If one gas sources runs out before the other, an automatic crossover valve in the air/oxygen mixer allows the ventilator to continue operating on the remaining gas source. If this occurs, the F_IO_2 may be altered.)

Internal Mechanism

The source gases enter an air/oxygen mixer and where pressure is immediately reduced to a constant working pressure. From the mixer, the gas splits into three channels, two mixed gas sources for patient breathing and one 50 psi air control line. One source of mixed gas goes to the mandatory (main flow) breath flow system and the other goes to the spontaneous breathing flow systems. The 50 psi air control line is used for control systems, one of which is the solenoid that controls the spontaneous (normally open) and main flow (normally closed) pneumatic interface valves. The microprocessor signal for the mandatory breath or Time Limited Demand Flow breath timing goes to the solenoid. While the signal is present, the solenoid sends control gas to the normally open Spontaneous pneumatic interface valve, signaling it to close, and to the normally closed main flow pneumatic interface valve, signaling it to open. When the signal stops, the valves return to their respective resting positions. The solenoid valve signal is based on the set respiratory rate, set inspiratory time (T_I), and set Time Limited Demand Flow on the front panel.

Box 14-6 Time Limited Demand Flow

Time limited demand flow works by allowing the operator to deliver a mandatory flow rate (set by the operator) at the onset of a spontaneous breath for a set time (determined by the operator). The operator should set the Time Limited Demand Flow to provide the higher, mandatory flow for the larger part of the spontaneous breath (exhalation valve remains at the PEEP setting during this time), allowing the patient to finish inhaling from the SPONT flow system. Using Time Limited Demand Flow allows the SPONT flow to be set at a lower value since it is no longer needed to meet the patient's peak flow needs. The higher Time Limited Demand Flow can aid in overcoming the resistance of the circuit and reduce the work of breathing of the patient while the lower SPONT flow can minimize expiratory resistance and minimize the chance for auto-PEEP.

The flow ($\dot{V}$) control determines the flow rate delivered to the patient during a mandatory or Time Limited Demand Flow spontaneous breath.

The E100M provides the operator with three means of delivering gas flow to the patient during spontaneous breathing, Time Limited Demand Flow, which uses the mandatory flow setting, the constant flow switch (V_1) and the auxiliary flow meter (V_2). Both SPONT (V_1) and SPONT (V_2) flow sources are connected to the reservoir bag and the patient circuit. When V_1 is turned on, the ventilator delivers 8 L/min to the reservoir bag (located on the right side of the machine) and into the patient breathing circuit between mandatory, Time Limited Demand Flow or manual breaths. (*Note*: The F_IO_2 of this gas is set by the clinician on the control panel.)

The auxiliary flow meter, V_2, attached to the side of the air/oxygen mixer (see Figure 14-13) can be turned on independent of V_1 or in combination with V_1, which would allow a flow rate for spontaneous breaths above 8 L/min to the patient. (*Note*: When set to flush, the flow is 36 L/min.) V_2 thus serves a dual purpose. When spontaneous flows of less than 8 L/min are required for the patient, V_2 can be activated alone and the flow can be adjusted appropriately (pediatric patients). If an adult patient requires higher flows, V_1 can be turned on with a constant flow of 8 L/min, and V_2 can be adjusted to add additional flow up to a total flow of 44 L/min (8 L/min from V_1 + 36 L/min from V_2).

When ventilating pediatric and adult patients, the user may observe the reservoir bag to ensure proper adjustment of flow from the flow meter and continuous flow switch. This bag should not completely deflate at any time during periods of spontaneous breathing nor should it remain fully inflated. (*Note*: Using excessive flows during spontaneous breathing may contribute to an increase in expiratory resistance, and thereby increase the potential for auto-PEEP.)

An additional feature of the E100M is the Duoflow system. The Duoflow system allows the clinician to control mandatory and spontaneous breaths separately. The gas flow for mandatory breaths can be adjusted by the mandatory flow control ($\dot{V}$ [L/min]) on the front panel.

The inspiratory flow available for spontaneous breaths is determined by the V_1 and V_2 as described earlier. V_1 and V_2 can be used in combination with time-limited demand flow described under Control Parameter below. Box 14-6 also provides a detailed description of time-limited demand flow. (*Note*: The reservoir bag provides for an additional gas source if the client's need were to exceed the preset flow rate.) If all electrical and pneumatic systems fail, the patient may draw ambient air through an emergency intake valve. The patient effort required to open this valve is approximately 2.0 cm H_2O.

Controls

The rear panel of the E100M contains the power (on/off) switch, alarm loudness control, internal battery test button, which displays the percent charge in the display window, and the remote alarm output. The remote alarm output connection allows the E100M to interface with most nurse call systems. In the event of an alarm or malfunction the call station is alerted to the problem immediately.

The front panel controls and alarms are divided into several sections. The first is the air/oxygen mixer, which is mounted on the left side of the ventilator and controls the F_IO_2 delivery. The other sections are located on the main panel of the ventilator. At the very bottom are connectors for the following:

- The exhalation valve assembly
- A nebulizer line
- The proximal airway line
- The main inspiratory line connector

The ventilator front panel above this section includes controls for ventilator parameters, and alarms, as well as monitors and indicators.

The bottom row of the front panel contains the controls for MANUAL INFLATION, TIME-LIMITED DEMAND FLOW, PEEP/CPAP (PBASE) and pressure limit (PLIMIT). The next section up contains the breath control parameters: FLOW ($\dot{V}$), t_I, and RESPIRATORY RATE (f). The third up section contains mode indicators—a display window and adjustments for high and low pressure alarms and a pressure-trigger (SENSITIVITY) control. The top section displays alarm indicators and controls. These controls will be described beginning with breath control parameters.

Control Parameters–Middle Section (see Figure 14-14)

The breath control parameters include a mandatory FLOW control ($\dot{V}$ [L/min]), inspiratory time control (t_I, seconds) and respiratory rate (f, breaths/min). (*Note*: When the E100M is set up to deliver volume-targeted mandatory breaths, V_T delivery is determined by the set mandatory flow [range 1-100 L/min] and the set t_I [range 0.1 to 3.0 seconds]. Recall from Chapter 11 that V_T = flow (L/sec) × T_I (sec).

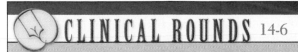

CLINICAL ROUNDS 14-6

Tidal Volume Delivery and Limiting Inverse Ratios With the Newport E100M

Problem 1

During A/CMV ventilation the respiratory rate is set at 30 breaths/min, flow is 60 L/min, and T_I is set at 1 second. What is the tidal volume? What is the I:E ratio?

Problem 2

Assume the rate is 20 breaths/min, flow is 6 L/min (0.1 L/sec), and the T_I is 2.5 seconds. Calculate the tidal volume, total cycle time (TCT), expiratory time T_E, and I:E ratio.

If the I:E is greater than 4:1, what will the resulting V_T delivery be when the ventilator reduces the ratio to 4:1? (*Note:* Although this situation might not occur clinically, it provides a simple example for calculating T_E, T_I, TCT, and I:E [see Chapter 11 for a further explanation of calculating these values].)

See Appendix A for the answer.

The mandatory FLOW control ($\dot{V}$ [L/min]), as described previously, lets the operator adjust the flow delivery during a mandatory breath and during Time Limited Demand Flow. It is not delivered by way of the reservoir bag as it is with a spontaneous breath but directly to the patient.

The t_I control (0.1 to 3.0 seconds) determines the length of time mandatory flow is delivered for either time- or pressure-triggered mandatory breaths in A/CMV or SIMV. The Time Limited Demand Flow determines the length of time mandatory flow is delivered at the onset of spontaneous breaths. The Newport E100M allows for inverse I:E ratios up to 4:1. If the t_I and rate settings result in an inverse I:E ratio of greater than 4:1, the I:E ratio display adjacent to the t_I control flashes. t_I is then shortened by the ventilator to provide a I:E ratio of no more than 4:1. This results in a reduced tidal volume delivery. To reestablish the desired V_T, the operator can either increase the mandatory flow or reduce the set t_I (Clinical Rounds 14-6).

The respiratory rate control (f, B/MIN; range 1 to 120 breaths/min) is operational in A/CMV, SIMV and "SPONT + APNEA A/CMV." This control regulates the time-triggered activation of the electronic solenoid valve described earlier (see Internal Mechanism).

Lower Front Panel Controls

The MANUAL breaths button on the lower left section of the front panel is pneumatically controlled; therefore, it can be used even if there is an electric power failure. This control by-passes the electronic solenoid valve and delivers the flow determined by the $\dot{V}$ setting. The breath is terminated when the clinician stops pressing the control, the set pressure limit is reached, or after four seconds have elapsed.

Next, the TIME-LIMITED DEMAND FLOW control is designed to decrease the work of breathing for spontaneous breaths by delivering a set flow rate, determined by the mandatory flow setting, for a predetermined amount of time at the beginning of inspiration. The adjustable time range is 0 to 1.0 seconds. Because of the added flow from the ventilator at the beginning of the breath, less flow is required for the reservoir bag. This feature is designed to be used for the larger portion of the breath. The SPONT flow and reservoir bag are intended to provide the patient with the remaining flow/volume for the spontaneous breath.

The PEEP/CPAP control regulates the internal PEEP valve on the Newport E100M and allows for an adjustable range of 0 to 25 cm H_2O in all modes. When PEEP is used during transport, a small amount of additional flow is required to maintain airway pressure. This flow should be considered when the operational time of the cylinder is assessed.

When PEEP/CPAP is increased, the trigger sensitivity is adjusted relative to the new baseline pressure so that the patient incurs no additional work of breathing. (*Note:* Trigger sensitivity is also automatically optimized when the advanced trigger control is set [see below].)

The pressure-limit (PLIMIT) control can be set in all modes of ventilation to limit the maximum pressure in the patient circuit from 0 to 100 cm H_2O. It is important to set the pressure-limit control above the HIGH PRESSURE ALARM setting when using volume control ventilation. This is because the pressure limit feature does not end inspiration, but merely holds the pressure in the circuit at the set value until the end of inspiration.

The PLIMIT is also used to set the maximum pressure during pressure-targeted ventilation. Again, exceeding the PLIMIT value does not end inspiration, but vents excess flow and pressure from the patient circuit to room air (see the modes of ventilation section). The HIGH PRESSURE alarm should be set 5 to 10 cm H_2O above the PLIMIT setting as an additional safety feature.

The constant flow switch is located on the right side of the machine. When it is activated, it delivers 8 L/min of mixed gas flow to the patient circuit between mandatory breaths (see Internal Mechanism).

Top Front Panel Controls

The MODE control switch is located in the top section of the front panel and allows for changing the ventilating mode (see modes of ventilation). Just below the MODE control this is a window that displays total respiratory rate (f_{TOT}) tidal volume (V_T) or I:E ratio. To the right of the window is the control for the LOW and HIGH AIRWAY PRESSURE alarm (see Top Front Panel Alarms and Indicators).

The trigger sensitivity control (P_{TRIG}) determines the pressure change required to trigger a mandatory or Time

Limited Demand Flow breath. When the E100M is first turned on, the P_{TRIG} default setting of -5 cm H_2O becomes effective. The operator should readjust the trigger to the patient's effort (range -10 to $+25$ cm H_2O). The trigger sensitivity control automatically adjusts to changes in the baseline pressure. If PEEP/CPAP is changed, P_{TRIG} is also changed. If advanced trigger control (ATC) has been activated, the trigger setting is also optimized. (When ATC is active, optimization occurs regularly, not just with a PEEP change.)

When activated, ATC automatically adjusts the trigger sensitivity to keep it as sensitive as possible without auto-triggering. The change in sensitivity is based on a predetermined algorithm. (*Note*: P_{TRIG} must always be set lower than baseline pressure to prevent auto-triggering and must also be set for breath detection in spontaneous and "SPONT + APNEA A/CMV" modes. This is to allow the TIME-LIMITED DEMAND FLOW feature to be activated.)

Front Panel Alarms and Indicators

The knob for the airway pressure alarms (P_{AW} ALARM control) is located adjacent to the display window. This single knob is used to set both the LOW and HIGH-PRESSURE alarm settings. When the knob is rotated, both alarm values change proportionally. To independently adjust the HIGH-PRESSURE alarm setting, the operator must pull out the control knob before rotating it. As the P_{AW} ALARM control is adjusted, the selected alarm limit value is displayed on the pressure gauge (nonblinking bars) (see Figure 14-14).

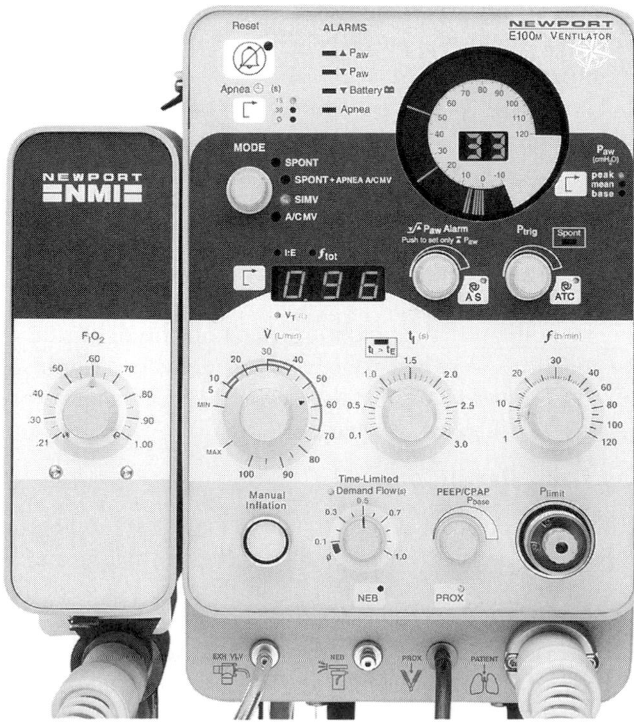

Figure 14-14 The Newport E100M ventilator control panel. (Courtesy Newport Medical Instruments, Newport Beach, Calif.)

The AS (Auto-Set Alarm) button next to the P_{AW} ALARM control automatically selects high and low pressure alarm settings based on current ventilator settings when it is activated. The alarm settings are determined by the current peak pressure for a mandatory breath. These are specific settings established by the manufacturer. (*Note*: Users of the E100M should refer to the operator's manual for more extensive information on alarm settings at specific peak pressures.)

The HIGH PRESSURE alarm is active in all modes. When the HIGH PRESSURE alarm setting (5 to 120 cm H_2O) is reached, the inspiratory phase of a time- or patient-triggered mandatory breath or manual inflation ends.

The LOW PRESSURE alarm is only active in the A/CMV and SIMV modes. It is activated if the airway pressure does not exceed the LOW PRESSURE alarm setting during a time- or pressure-triggered mandatory breath.

The APNEA alarm control (spontaneous alarm) is found at the top left portion of the ventilator just below the alarm silence/reset button. The APNEA alarm is functional in all modes. The operator sets the desired apnea time period by depressing the APNEA button until the appropriate time select indicator is illuminated. There are three available time settings for this alarm: Off (0), 15, or 30 seconds. The Off setting disables the APNEA (spontaneous) alarm. If the set apnea time elapses without a spontaneous effort being detected, an audible and visual alarm occurs. The alarm remains illuminated until one breath is recognized in the spontaneous mode or until four consecutive breaths have been initiated in the "SPONT + APNEA A/CMV" mode.

The alarm indicators to the right of the apnea alarm provide a visual alert the operator when certain alarm limits have been violated. They include:

- High and low pressure alarm violations
- Low battery charge, and
- Apnea (called "spontaneous alarm")

All of the visual alarms are accompanied by audible alarms. The pressure and battery charge alarms have been reviewed.

The top right section of the front panel is occupied by an electronic pressure gauge (range $^{-}10$ to 120 cm H_2O). The center provides digital numeric displays of peak, mean and base pressures. The outer band provides a visual display of real-time measured airway pressure. The continuously lit segments indicate the high and low pressure alarm limits. The blinking segment indicates the trigger level setting.

Additional Alarms

The E100M offers additional audible-only alarms including AC and DC power failure, air/O_2 low source gas pressure, and low battery. The power failure alarm is a continuous pulsating alarm that is activated when there is a loss of electric power. The air/O_2 low source gas pressure alarm is also a continuous alarm that is activated when the air or oxygen source gas pressure falls below 35 psig. The low battery alarm is activated when about 20 minutes of normal battery backup power remains. It is also a continuous alarm that cannot be silenced and can only be terminated when the problem is resolved.

Modes of Ventilation

The Newport E100M offers A/CMV, SIMV, and spontaneous modes, and a backup mode called "SPONT + APNEA A/CMV." The MODE control button is located in the top left section of the front panel.

In both A/CMV and SIMV, mandatory breaths may be volume- or pressure-targeted. When using volume-targeted A/CMV, the operator must set the trigger (sensitivity) FLOW, flow, t_I, and RATE (f). Mandatory breaths are either time- or pressure-triggered, and the set V_T is determined by the FLOW and t_I settings.

When the E100M is in the volume-targeted SIMV mode, mandatory breath delivery is the same as in A/CMV with one exception. In A/CMV, every patient effort that exceeds the trigger sensitivity level results in a mandatory breath. In SIMV, the mandatory breath rate is limited to the rate control setting. The patient can take additional breaths between mandatory breaths, without receiving a mandatory breath. The flow for a spontaneous breath is obtained from Time Limited Demand Flow (mandatory flow without pressurization) and then finished from the SPONT flow 1 and/or 2 or it may be obtained from the SPONT flows alone if Time Limited Demand Flow is not activated by the user (see spontaneous mode). The spontaneous V_T completely depends on patient effort and patient lung characteristics.

The E100M lets the operator pressure-target mandatory breaths in both A/CMV and SIMV (see Chapter 11 for further description pressure-targeted ventilation). When the parameters for pressure ventilation are set, the pressure relief control is set at the desired pressure limit and the high-pressure alarm is fixed at a value above the pressure-relief setting by about 10 cm H_2O. This prevents the high-pressure alarm from ending inspiration prior to achieving the set t_I.

After the pressure in the patient circuit reaches the pressure-relief (PLIMIT) setting, the excess flow is vented to room air maintaining the set pressure plateau until the set t_I has ended. Recall that changes in patient compliance or resistance can affect the V_T delivered during pressure ventilation (Chapter 11).

In the spontaneous mode no mandatory breaths are delivered. The flow to the patient for spontaneous breaths are determined by Time Limited Demand Flow (mandatory flow without pressurization) and the V_1 switch or V_2 flow meter setting located on the right side of the control panel (refer to internal mechanisms). Although the patient is not required to trigger a spontaneous breath, it is important that the trigger level to be set appropriately or ATC activated. This allows the ventilator to detect all spontaneous breaths and reset the APNEA delay alarm. If the E100M does not detect a patient inspiratory effort within the set apnea time, the spontaneous alarm is activated. When operating in the "SPONT + APNEA A/CMV" mode a backup rate is initiated until four consecutive spontaneous breaths are detected. The settings for the backup mode feature are the same parameters that are set in the A/CMV mode.

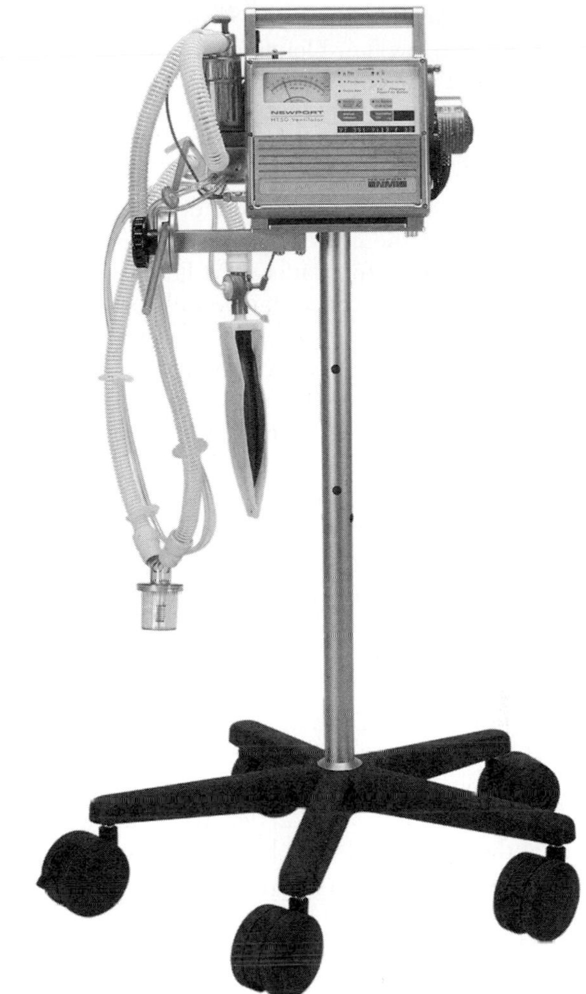

Figure 14-15 The Newport HT50 ventilator. (Courtesy Newport Medical Instruments, Newport Beach, Calif.)

Newport HT50

The Newport HT50 (Newport Medical Instruments, Newport Beach, CA) is a portable ventilator designed for homecare, subacute, transport and hospital use (Figure 14-15). It is a microprocessor-controlled ventilator that may be used for adult or pediatric patients (≥10 kg). The device functions in three modes: assist/control (A/CMV), SIMV, and spontaneous ventilation (SPONT). It is lightweight (15 lb without a humidifier) and compact (10.6″ × 7.87″ × 10.24″).

Power Source

The HT50 is electrically powered and requires no gas sources to properly perform all of its operations. Oxygen enrichment is available through a 50 psi entrainment (zero bleed) mixer or a low flow blending bag kit. The electronic system can use three possible power sources:

- A standard AC outlet (100-240V)
- An external DC battery (12-30V)
- An internal DC battery

Indicators on the top right section of the front provide information about the current power source (Ext. Power/ Charging Int. Battery, Int. Battery (Push to Test).

The internal battery can sustain ventilator operation for about 10 hours and requires 8 hours to fully recharge from any AC or DC power source, even while the ventilation is in operation. Newport recommends charging the battery for a minimum of 5 hours after the battery has been completely depleted (approximately 80% of a full charge).

The HT50 has a universal power entry module. This module allows the clinician to use the same port for connecting the plug for an AC current as it does for an external DC current. To use an external DC current the source must be capable of delivering a minimum of 12 volts and a maximum of 30 volts to be compatible with the ventilator. The auto DC power connector allows for powering the HT50 from the cigarette lighter in an automobile.

The HT50 comes equipped with several battery indicators and alarms that monitor the status of the power supply to the ventilator. The indicators are located in the upper right section of the front panel. The button, labeled "Int Battery (Push to Test)," allows you to read the battery charge level in the pressure gauge window when operating from the internal battery. When the light-emitting diode (LED) adjacent to this control is amber, the internal battery is medium-to-fully charged. When red, the battery is low.

The Message Display Window in the center of the front panel will provide written messages of battery conditions. They include: BATTERY LOW alarm, BATTERY EMPTY alarm, and NO EXT. POWER (a POWER SWITCH OVER alarm). When the BATTERY LOW message appears in the Message Display Window, an audible, intermittent three-pulse cautionary beep sounds and a visible alert (LED blinks red adjacent to "Int. Battery") is activated. This alarm indicates that the internal battery is in use and less than 2 hours of battery charge remain. Pressing the SILENCE/RESET button can silence the audible alarm, but the visual alarm will remain illuminated until the ventilator is plugged into an AC outlet or an external battery is connected.

The BATTERY EMPTY message is activated when less than 30 minutes of power remains in the internal battery. It is accompanied by an audible, intermittent three-pulse cautionary alarm and a visible alert (LED blinks red adjacent to "Int. Battery").

The POWER SWITCH OVER alarm notifies the clinician that the external power source has failed and the internal battery is now in use. It occurs when a switch from an external battery to the internal battery has occurred because of disconnection from the power cord or a power interruption. The message "No ext. power" appears in the message window, the LED next to the "Int Battery" blinks red and the red LED next the "Ext.Power/Charging Int. Battery" is constantly lit. This alarm can be silenced by pressing the SILENCE/RESET button or by plugging the ventilator into a working outlet.

The internal pneumatic circuit does not require external compressed air but does require a medical-grade high-pressure oxygen gas source capable of delivering 35 to 90 psi or low flow oxygen. The 35 to 90 psi oxygen source may be a cylinder or wall outlet. The low flow source may be a flowmeter from a cylinder, wall outlet, liquid system or concentrator.

Internal Mechanism

All gas enters the HT50 through an opening in the filter cover located on the right side of the machine. If neither oxygen accessory is connected, the ventilator delivers room air to the patient. For oxygen enrichment, either the air-oxygen entrainment mixer or oxygen blending bag kit is inserted into the opening. This ventilator uses a dual micro-piston delivery system that allows the ventilator to operate without an external air compressor. The respiratory rate, trigger sensitivity, pressure control or tidal volume, PEEP, and pressure support set by the clinician determine the stroke rate and stroke speed of the pistons.

Oxygen Source and Humidifier

The HT50 comes with two oxygen delivery options: (1) an optional air oxygen entrainment mixer or (2) an oxygen-blending bag kit. The air oxygen entrainment mixer attaches to the fresh gas intake valve on the right side of the ventilator and allows for the attachment of a high pressure oxygen gas source. This device allows the clinician to control the oxygen percentage delivered to the patient from 21% to 100% oxygen with a knob located on the blender itself. It is a unique high pressure-ambient mixing system that uses no bleed.

The oxygen-blending bag kit also attaches to the fresh gas intake valve on the right side of the ventilator and allows for the attachment of a low-flow oxygen gas source. This device allows the clinician to control the oxygen percentage delivered to the patient by varying the flow rate set on a flowmeter attached to the blending bag kit. Two charts (one for use with PEEP and one for use without PEEP) assist the clinician in setting proper flow rates to achieve a given F_IO_2.

The HT50 offers a humidifier option. When the optional humidifier is attached (left side of machine), it is only functional if the ventilator is powered by an external AC power source. The humidifier is activated by a button located on the front right of the control panel, which allows the clinician to activate the humidifier and set a temperature ranging from 19° to 39° C. The operator presses the humidifier button to adjust the temperature and uses the up and down arrows in the center of the front panel to increase or decrease the temperature setting. During ventilation, the displayed temperature is measured at the patient connector.

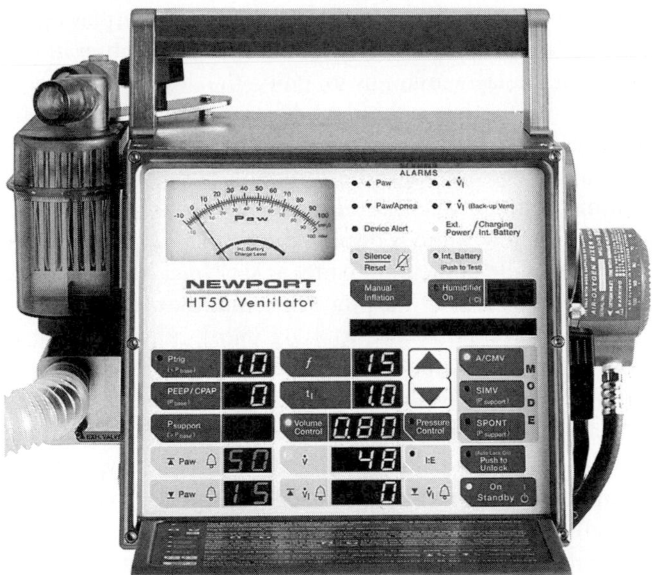

Figure 14-16 The Newport HT50 control panel (see text for further description) (Courtesy Newport Medical Instruments, Newport Beach, Calif.)

Box 14-7 Setting Ventilator Parameters in the SETTINGS Position and in the ON Position

In the SETTINGS position, if the mode is changed or breath control switched from volume control to pressure control and vise versa, the change is implemented without further action on the part of the user. On the other hand, if the ventilator had been in the ON position, the clinician would have had to confirm the mode or breath control change by depressing the button for the newly selected parameter a second time. If the parameter change is not confirmed when the ventilator is in the ON position then it will return to the previous setting.

In the setting condition, the displayed temperature is measured at the humidifier bottle outlet. To turn off the humidifier, the operator presses and holds the button for 3 seconds.

If the message "Check Humidifier" appears in the Message Display Window and the LED adjacent to the humidifier control blinks red, a malfunction has been detected. The humidifier shuts down. One of five possible messages is displayed. The user is advised to see the operating manual for instructions.

Patient Circuit

The connections for the patient circuit are located on the left side of the ventilator. They include a temperature plug when the humidifier is attached, a proximal pressure line with filter, a drive line for the externally mounted exhalation valve and the main inspiratory line.

Control Panel and Alarms

The front panel of The HT50 contains several controls for setting parameters, monitoring patient data and alarms, as well as powering up the ventilator (Figure 14-16). The ON/STANDBY selector is located at the bottom right of the front panel. It allows the user to select one of three operating conditions by pressing the ON/STANDBY button. In the first condition, the ventilator is off/standby. Standby means that the ventilator is plugged into an external power supply and therefore the internal battery is charging. The second condition (button pressed once) is the SETTINGS feature. The SETTINGS feature allows the clinician to program the ventilator settings prior to turning the machine on and connecting it to a patient. It is also the condition during which an exhalation valve calibration is performed. This simple procedure (occlude circuit and press MANUAL INFLATION twice) performs a leak check on the breathing circuit and also provides a linearization curve for the ventilator pressure management in conjunction with the exhalation valve in use. When operating in SETTINGS, the parameter values that are entered (e.g., tidal volume, respiratory rate) do not have to be confirmed by pressing the key a second time, as they do during as they normal do during operation (Box 14-7). The third condition (button pressed again) begins ventilation.

Two safety features help prevent any accidental changes in the set parameters from occurring. The first is a panel cover, which blocks the control settings from view and must be opened to gain front panel access. The second is the PANEL LOCK feature located at the bottom right of the ventilator, just above the ON/STANDBY selector. When activated, it locks all settings on the ventilator and prevents someone from inadvertently changing the parameters.

Control Parameters

The front panel is divided roughly into three sections: the central panel containing parameter controls and modes, the bottom section of alarms and the top section of monitored data and alarm indicators (see Figure 14-16).

As a general rule, when changing parameter values, the operator first presses the desired parameter button, uses the up or down arrow to change the displayed setting and then presses the parameter button again to confirm and activate the change. Alarms are set in the same way. A setting limitation message will appear in the message display window when the operator adjusts a parameter to its limits. Table 14-4 lists setting limitation messages.

The first control parameter displayed is trigger sensitivity (PTRIG; 0 to –9.9 cm H_2O). The sensitivity is automatically PEEP compensated. For example, if PEEP is 5 cm H_2O and the sensitivity is –0.5 cm H_2O, the breath triggers when an inspiratory effort drops the airway pressure to 4.5 cm H_2O. The PTRIG LED indicator light illuminates every time a spontaneous breath is detected allowing the clinician to tract the patient's breathing pattern.

Table 14-4 Setting limitation messages on the HT50

Message	Meaning
REACHED MAX $\dot{V}$	Maximum flow setting reached
REACHED MIN $\dot{V}$	Minimum flow setting reached
INVERSE I:E	An inverse I:E ratio has been set
REACHED MAX I:E	The maximum inverse ratio of 3:1 has been reached
$\dot{V}$ UNAVAILABLE	Flow value cannot be displayed during pressure ventilation
PEEP + PS TOO HIGH	Maximum limit of PEEP + PS is 60 cm H_2O
PC − PEEP TOO LOW	PC − PEEP is <5 cm H_2O
↑− PEEP TOO LOW	High P_{limit} − PEEP is <5 cm H_2O
REMINDER MESSAGES	
PANEL LOCK	Operator has tried to change a parameter with the panel lock activated
PRESS AGAIN	Pressing on the same button is required to confirm and activate the parameter change requested

The PEEP/CPAP (0 to 30 cm H_2O) control governs the baseline pressure. PEEP/CPAP cannot be set higher than the pressure control target setting minus 5 cm H_2O. This is to ensure that the ventilator is able to deliver a breathe during pressure ventilation, even it is just 5 cm H_2O, i.e., the difference between set pressure target and PEEP.

Pressure support (Psupport) has an available range of 0 to 60 cm H_2O. The ventilator will not allow the combined value of PEEP/CPAP plus pressure support to be greater than 60 cm H_2O.

The available mandatory respiratory rate (f) range is 1 to 99 breaths/min. Inspiratory time (t_I) is adjustable from 0.1 to 3.0 sec. The next control is the VOLUME CONTROL (100 to 2200 mL)/PRESSURE CONTROL (5 to 60 cm H_2O). This allows the operator to select either volume-targeted or pressure-targeted breaths and set the desired parameter value, that is, volume in liters or pressure in cm H_2O.

Mode controls include assist control (A/CMV), SIMV, and SPONT (see section on Modes of Ventilation). To activate the mode the operator presses the desired mode once and then a second time to activate it. However, before confirming a mode, all the appropriate parameter settings for that mode should be set and checked.

The lower section of the panel includes the high and low pressure alarm controls (P_{AW}), inspiratory flow display, and I:E ratio display, minute volume display and the high and low minute volume alarm controls ($\dot{V}_I$). The alarms will be reviewed later in this section.

The inspiratory flow ($\dot{V}$) and I:E ratio LCD display allow the clinician to select viewing either one or the other in the adjacent display window by touching the desired parameter control. To the left is the flow display. When operating in volume control ventilation, the flow rate delivered to the patient is determined by the inspiratory time and the tidal volume setting: V_T (L) = T_I (sec) × Flow (L/sec). The calculated flow value is displayed in an LCD panel in the bottom middle of the front panel as $\dot{V}$. (*Note:* If the t_I allows the flow to reach a maximum or minimum range level [available flow range is 6 to 100 L/min], adjustment of t_I stops and a beep sounds. A setting limitation message appears in the Message Display Window.) The flow display is not available during pressure control or spontaneous ventilation.

The I:E ratio is determined by the frequency and the inspiratory time settings (range 1:99 up to 3:1). When the entered parameters generate an inverse I:E ratio, the ventilator briefly alarms making the clinician aware of the changes but continues with ventilation. The I:E ratio cannot exceed 3:1.

The upper portion of the control panel contains a pressure gauge (−10 to 100 cm H_2O or mBar) that monitors real-time airway pressure. This section of the front panel also includes a manual inflation control (3 sec. maximum) and the humidifier control described previously. The manual inflation feature is only active in the A/CMV and SIMV modes. It allows the clinician to control the size of the tidal volume for the manual breath by controlling the inspiratory time. The flow rate is determined by the variables of V_T and t set for in volume-targeted A/CMV and SIMV. In pressure control, the set pressure is delivered. The breath is terminated when the clinician stops pressing the control, the set high pressure alarm limit is reached, or three seconds have elapsed. A backup safety feature will not allow the clinician to deliver a manual breath while the patient is in inspiration or if the airway pressure is >5 cm H_2O above PEEP.

Just below the Manual Inflation control is the Message Display Window discussed previously. When the display is blank, the operator can view monitored parameters by using the up and down arrows on the front panel. Monitored values that appear include V_T, $\dot{V}_I$, f, or Paw (peak, mean and base). These are updated every 10 seconds or at the end of each breath, allowing the operator to record current values.

Airway Pressure and Minute Ventilation Alarms

The high airway pressure alarm control is located on the lower left portion of the control panel and has an adjustable range of 4 to 99 cm H_2O. When the set high-pressure level is reached, audiovisual alarms are activated, and the machine cycles into exhalation. The visual indicator is in the top section of the front panel. (*Note*: The high peak pressure alarm cannot be set below the PEEP setting.)

The low airway pressure alarm control is below the high airway pressure alarm control. Its operating range is 3 to

98 cm H_2O. The low airway pressure alarm is only active during mandatory breaths in the A/CMV and SIMV modes. It is activated when the rise in pressure does not exceed the alarm setting during the inspiratory phase of two consecutive patient- or time-triggered mandatory breaths. The visual indicator is in the top section of the front panel.

The high and low minute ventilation alarm controls are also located on the lower panel. The high $\dot{V}_I$ (high inspiratory minute volume) alarm has a setting range of 2 to 50 L. The low $\dot{V}_I$ (low inspiratory minute volume) has a setting range of 0.3 to 49 L. If the measured minute volume falls outside of the set limits, the appropriate alarm becomes active producing both an audible and visible alert. The visual indicator is in the upper section of the front panel. (*Note*: The alarm measures the volume delivered from the ventilator and not what is exhaled by the patient.) If at any time the minute ventilation falls below the "low minute ventilation" alarm value, the backup ventilation (BUV) feature is activated and the $\dot{V}_I$ (Back-up Vent.) indicator illuminates. This feature is active in all modes and is described in the section on modes of ventilation.

Additional Alarms

Additional alarms that are monitored and have messages that appear in the Message Display Window include the following: high baseline pressure, occlusion, low baseline pressure, check proximal line, apnea, PC cannot be reached and device alerts.

The high baseline pressure alarm occurs when the baseline pressure is greater than the low airway pressure alarm setting at the beginning of a time-triggered, mandatory breath. The message reads "HIGH Pbase." The alarm resets when airway pressure drops to within 5 cm H_2O of the set PEEP/CPAP.

The occlusion alarm ("OCCLUSION") is activated when the airway pressure remains +15 cm H_2O above the PEEP setting for 3 seconds after beginning exhalation or at end exhalation, whichever comes first. It is corrected if airway pressure falls to within 5 cm H_2O of baseline. If this alarm occurs, no additional mandatory breaths are delivered until it is corrected. The Device Alert indicator blinks and the ventilator attempts to release pressure through the redundant safety system. The safety system allows the patient to draw ambient air into the breathing circuit through an emergency intake valve when no other flow is available. The patient effort required to open this valve is approximately 2 cm H_2O.

The low baseline pressure alarm ("LOW Pbase") indicates an unstable baseline. For example, this could occur with a large leak in the patient circuit ($P \geq 2$ cm H_2O below baseline for three seconds). In addition to the message displayed, the low P_{AW} indicator blinks. The alarm resets when the baseline pressure difference is less than 2 cm H_2O.

The check proximal line ("CHECK PROX LINE") alarm occurs when, during inspiration, the proximal pressure measured is significantly different from the internal back-up pressure sensor measurement taken inside the ventilator. In addition to the message, the low P_{AW}/Apnea indicator blinks red. Causes include disconnections, kinking of the circuit, and a water-filled proximal sensor line. Ventilation continues during this condition using the pressure monitored by the internal pressure transducer.

When a patient breath goes undetected for 30 sections, an apnea alarm occurs ("APNEA").

"PCV not reached" signals to the operator that the maximum inspiratory pressure measured is less than 50% of the set pressure during pressure control ventilation. The operator should check the patient to be sure they are being adequately ventilated and check the circuit for leaks.

When the Device Alert LED illuminates a steady red and an internal beep occurs, the ventilator has detected one of four message conditions: OCCL Shutdown, Motor Fault, 10V SHUTDOWN, or SYSTEM ERROR. With the exception of an occlusion alert, the ventilator will stop ventilating. Another means must be found to ventilate the patient and the HT50 should be taken out of service and not used on patients until check by a qualified technician.

The ALARM/SILENCE-RESET button is in the upper alarm indicator section on the control panel. When it is activated, this control silences the alarm for 60 seconds. It is also used to clear "latched" alarms that are no longer active, including alarm messages in the message window.

Modes of Ventilation

The mode settings located on the right front panel the HT50 include control-assist/control (A/CMV), SIMV and SPONT. (*Note:* When selecting a mode after the ventilator has been turned on, the operator must press the button twice to confirm the selection. If the button is not pressed a second time within 5 seconds, the selection is cancelled.)

When operating in the A/CMV or SIMV mode the ventilator can be programmed for either volume control (VC) or pressure control (PC) ventilation for the mandatory breaths. This control was described previously. When choosing volume control, the LED display allows the clinician to determine the tidal volume delivered. If pressure control is the desired option, then the LED display allows the clinician to determine the pressure target delivered to the patient.

In A/CMV VC mode, the clinician sets the V_T, frequency (minimum respiratory rate), inspiratory time, and trigger sensitivity. PEEP can also be set. All breaths have the same V_T delivered, regardless of whether they are patient-triggered or time-triggered.

The SIMV VC mode lets the patient breath spontaneously between mandatory breaths without receiving the set V_T. The operator sets V_T, breath rate, t_I, pressure support for spontaneous breaths, PEEP, and trigger sensitivity.

For PC mandatory breaths, the operator selects the pressure control option and adjusts the pressure to the desired target value. Mandatory breaths in either A/CMV or SIMV then become pressure-targeted rather than volume-targeted.

When using the spontaneous mode to ventilate, all breaths become patient-triggered and pressure-targeted. Pressure support may be utilized as well as PEEP/CPAP to aid the spontaneous breaths. (*Note*: When a patient circuit is disconnected during pressure control or pressure support, flow may increase through the circuit to compensate for the low pressure. After reconnecting the patient circuit, the operator should press the pressure control or pressure support button twice to quickly readjust the flow to a lower level.)

BUV is a safety feature that becomes active, as noted, when the low $\dot{V}_I$ alarm is violated. It is available in all modes. During BUV the message "Low $\dot{V}_I$ (BUV)" is displayed. When the HT50 is operating in the spontaneous mode and BUV becomes active, the ventilator delivers a pressure-targeted breath. The pressure delivered to the patient is 15 cm H_2O above the PEEP setting and it is maintained for 1 second at a respiratory rate of 15 breath/min. The BUV feature is deactivated if there is a recorded rise in minute ventilation to 10% above the set low $\dot{V}_I$ alarm value. It is important to note that the "low minute ventilation" alarm responds to the volume delivered from the ventilator, not the volume exhaled from the patient. If there is a leak or the circuit becomes disconnected, the alarm will not sound and backup ventilation will not be activated. In fact a high minute volume is usually the indicator of an increase in leak or disconnection.

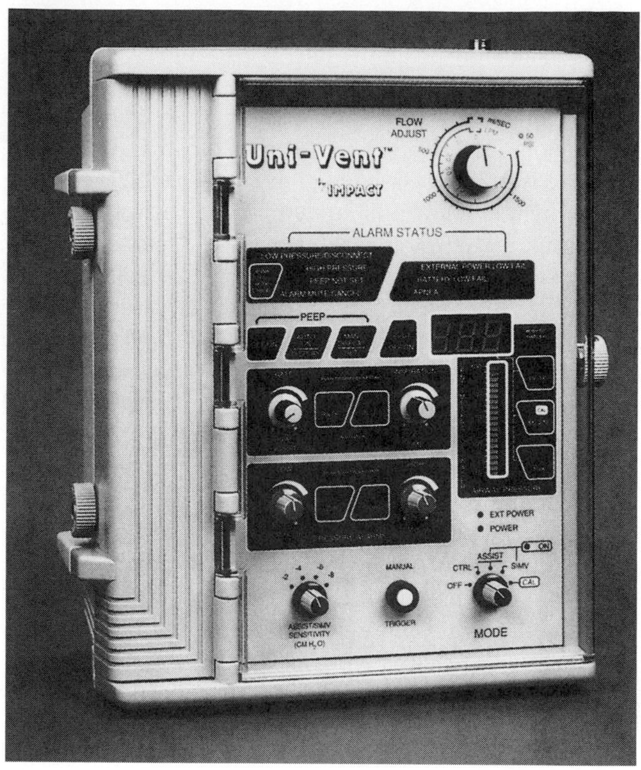

Figure 14-17 The Impact Uni-Vent 750 Ventilator. (Courtesy Impact Instrumentation, Inc, West Caldwell, NJ.)

Impact Uni-Vent 750

The Uni-Vent 750 (Figure 14-17) is a pressure- or time-triggered, volume-targeted, pressure- or time-cycled microprocessor-controlled ventilator used primarily for patient transport. It is 9″ × 11.5″ × 4.5″ and weighs about 12.5 lb. This ventilator can provide control, A/C, and SIMV modes of ventilation (Impact Instrumentation, Inc., West Caldwell, NJ).

Power Source

The Uni-Vent 750 requires pneumatic and electric power supplies to perform properly. The electronic system requires one of the following three sources to power the microprocessor and its electrical components:

- An internal DC battery
- An external DC battery
- A 120-volt AC outlet (with a converter)

The internal battery has an estimated life of 9 hours.

The pneumatic system requires a high-pressure source gas at 50 to 100 psig to properly perform. The source may be a cylinder, wall outlet, or oxygen/air blender. Because the Uni-Vent operates exclusively from one gas source, the oxygen percentage depends on the gas powering the ventilator. To precisely regulate the F_IO_2, the operator should connect the unit to an air/oxygen blender. There is no entrainment feature on this ventilator.

Internal Mechanism

The internal elements (Figure 14-18) of the pneumatic system receive the source gas from the oxygen inlet on the rear panel and route the gas through an internal regulator that precisely adjusts the pressure to 50 psig. After passing the regulator, the gas flow is guided through two parallel circuits. The first circuit, which contains two main inspiratory flow valves, is used during control and A/C modes. If one valve does not close when the machine cycles into expiration, the second valve stops gas flow to the patient and prevents over inflation. This is a safety feature of the system. During a patient- or time-triggered breath, the inspiratory flow solenoid opens and gas passes the flow-control valve and is directed to the patient. The Uni-Vent has no V_T setting. The volume delivered to the patient depends on the set T_I and flow.

When spontaneous breaths are initiated, the flow through the system is directed to the pneumatically controlled demand valve. The demand valve has an opening pressure of −1 cm H_2O below baseline. After the demand valve is opened, the gas source passes through a fixed orifice, which limits the peak flow to the patient to 60 L/min for spontaneous breaths.

When using disposable patient circuits, a separate anti-asphyxia valve must be attached at the patient connection to allow for spontaneous breaths in case of valve failure.

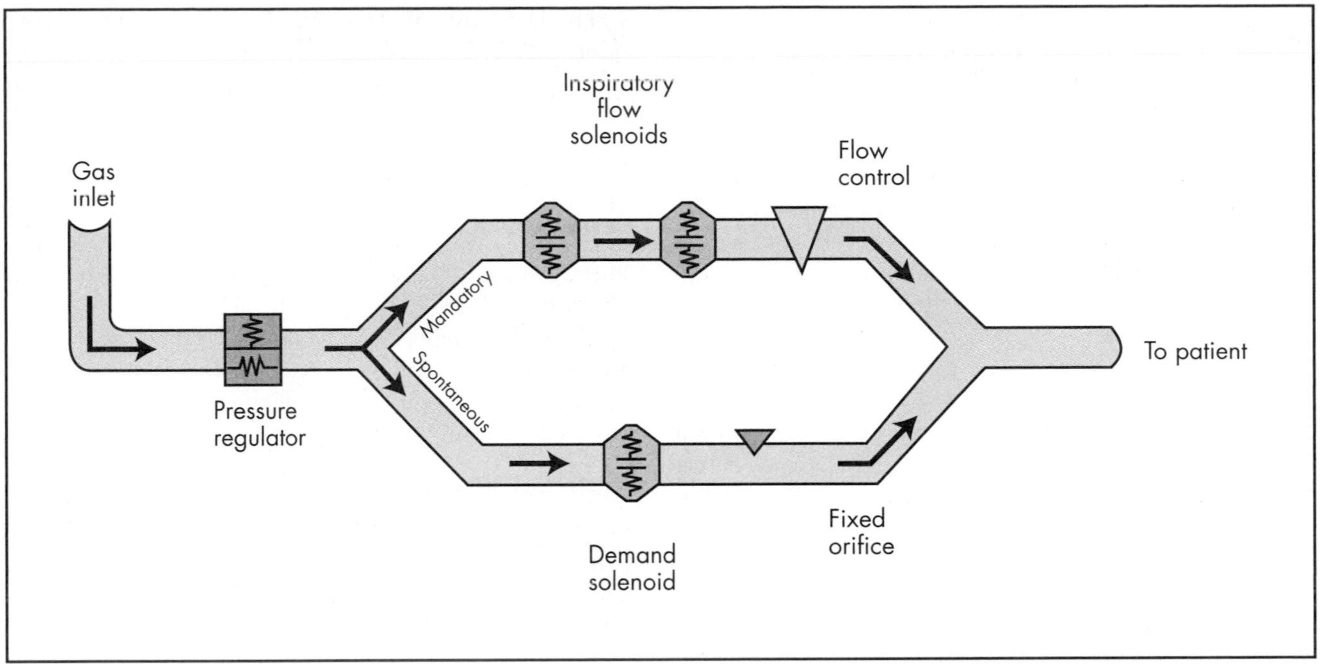

Figure 14-18 The Impact Uni-Vent 750 internal pneumatic circuit (see text for explanation).

The nondisposable circuits have a patient valve instead of an exhalation valve (Figure 14-19). The patient valves in the nondisposable units serve the purpose of the exhalation valve and also contain the anti-asphyxia valve.

The Uni-Vent 750 requires that an external PEEP valve be attached to the exhalation valve. The ventilator compensates for added PEEP with one of two mechanisms: automatic or manual. In the automatic mode, the microprocessor analyzes the patient circuit's pressure waveforms over three consecutive breaths to determine the level of PEEP. This process of updating the PEEP in the patient circuit is a continuous one. The manual process requires the operator to enter the PEEP value directly into the microprocessor using the keypad. When the operator chooses to use the manual method, the PEEP NOT SET alarm is inactivated.

Controls and Alarms

The Uni-Vent contains several controls for setting and monitoring parameters and alarms.

Rate

The respiratory rate control is active in control, A/C, and SIMV modes of ventilation and time-triggers a mandatory breath in each of these modes. It has an adjustable range of 1 to 150 breaths/min. The set rate, in combination with the set T_I, controls the I:E ratio of the ventilator.

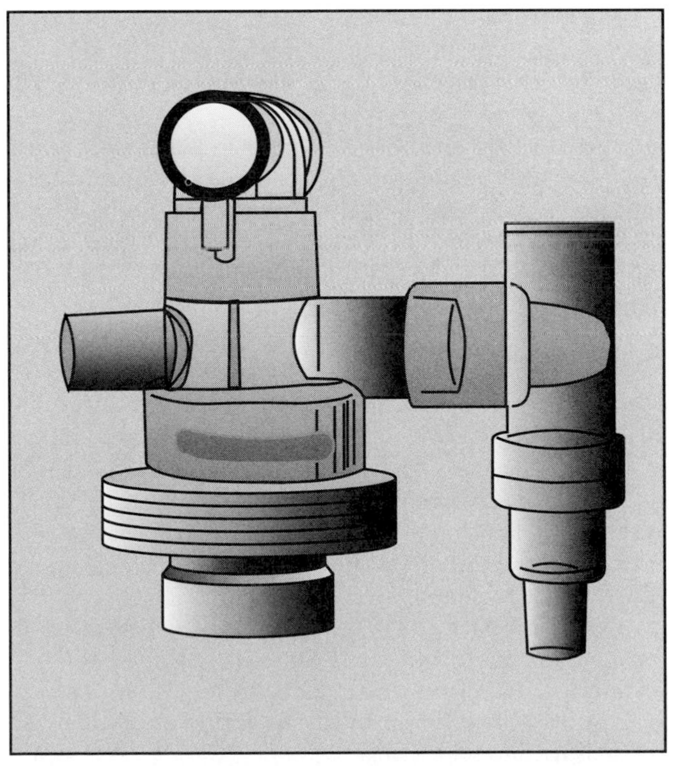

Figure 14-19 The Uni-Vent 750 patient valve. (Courtesy Impact Instrumentation, Inc, West Caldwell, NJ.)

Flow Adjust

The flow adjust control allows for adjustable flow rates from 50 to 1500 mL/sec (3 to 90 L/min). If the flow setting is insufficient for the inspiratory demands of the patient, then the anti-asphyxia valve allows room air to be entrained for additional flow. When air entrainment occurs, the valve creates a whistling sound, alerting the operator to the problem. (*Note:* Opening of the anti-asphyxia valve and entrainment of room air can alter the F_IO_2 delivered to the patient.)

Manual Breath

The MANUAL BREATH button can be used to deliver a positive pressure breath whenever the operator considers it appropriate. The MANUAL BREATH function is operational in all modes. When activated, the ventilator delivers a breath at the set flow for as long as the operator holds the button. This control is designed to be operational if there is a CPU or electronics failure. The breath timer is reset after a full exhalation period elapses, thereby preventing the stacking of a time-delivered breath.

Airway Pressure Alarms

There are two airway pressure alarms on the 750 that can be adjusted and monitored. They are the HIGH PRESSURE and the LOW PRESSURE/DISCONNECT alarms. The HIGH PRESSURE alarm is activated when the airway pressure exceeds the set HIGH PRESSURE alarm for 2 seconds during a single breath. It also acts as a pressure relief for the ventilator. If the HIGH PRESSURE setting is surpassed, the ventilator vents the excess flow to the atmosphere and allows the set T_I to complete its cycle. The adjustable range of this function is 15 to 100 cm H_2O.

The LOW PRESSURE/DISCONNECT alarm detects leaks and disconnections in the patient circuit and has an adjustable range of 0 to 50 cm H_2O. If the patient fails to meet the low-pressure setting, or if the airway pressure fails to reach +1 cm H_2O at the time of the next mandatory breath, the alarm is activated.

Additional Alarms

Three additional alarms on the Uni-Vent are the APNEA, the PEEP NOT SET, and the INVERSE I:E alarms. The APNEA alarm is activated when the patient fails to trigger a spontaneous or mandatory breath in 19 seconds (nonadjustable). The ventilator defaults to a back-up rate of 12 breaths/min and uses the currently set V_T. The APNEA alarm is only operational in the assist and SIMV modes.

The PEEP NOT SET alarm is activated when the end-expiratory pressure fails to return to the set value by +2 to −1 cm H_2O for three consecutive breaths. This alarm is inactivated when the manual instead of the automatic mode is used to set PEEP.

The Uni-Vent 750 does not allow for inverse ratio ventilation (IRV). Any combination of rate and T_I that creates a longer inspiratory than expiratory period activates the INVERSE I:E alarm. The ventilator defaults to exhalation and elicits an audiovisual alarm that cannot be deactivated until the problem is corrected.

Power Alarms

The Uni-Vent 750 has two power alarms: EXTERNAL POWER LOW/FAIL and BATTERY LOW/FAIL. The EXTERNAL POWER LOW/FAIL alerts the operator when the external power source is disconnected or fails. The BATTERY LOW/FAIL alarm is set off when the internal battery voltage falls below 11 V or is defective and will not recharge.

Modes of Ventilation

The Uni-Vent 750 offers three modes of ventilation: control, assist (A/C), and SIMV. In the control mode, the machine delivers time-triggered, volume-targeted breaths based on the set rate, T_I, and flow. If necessary, the patient can breathe spontaneously between the mandatory breaths through the anti-asphyxia valve (see Figure 14-19). In a sense, this is like an IMV mode.

The A/C mode lets the patient initiate mandatory breaths and ultimately control the total rate of the ventilator (time-triggered + patient-triggered). All other functions that were set in the control mode are still active in A/C mode with the addition of assist sensitivity. Breaths are patient- or time-triggered, volume-targeted, and time-cycled.

When the SIMV mode is used, the patient can breathe spontaneously through the internal demand valve and receive mandatory breaths through the main inspiratory valve. All controls set in the A/C mode are set for the mandatory breaths in SIMV. The patient's spontaneous efforts must generate a pressure change of at least −1 cm H_2O to open the internal demand valve and obtain flow (Box 14-8).

Box 14-8 CONTROL and SIMV Modes on the Uni-Vent 750

In the CONTROL mode, the patient receives time-triggered mandatory breaths from the machine. Between these breaths, the patient can breathe spontaneously from the anti-asphyxia valve in the patient circuit.

In the SIMV mode, the mandatory breaths are patient- or time-triggered. Between mandatory breaths, the patient breathes spontaneously from the internal demand valve.

In the CONTROL mode, spontaneous breaths are at room air (F_IO_2 = 0.21). In the SIMV mode, spontaneous breaths receive the F_IO_2 provided by the gas source.

Impact Uni-Vent Eagle 755

The Eagle 755 (Figure 14-20) is an upgraded version of Impact's Uni-Vent 750. (Impact Instrumentation, Inc., West Caldwell, NJ.) Additions include a direct V_T setting and an alarm package that features scroll knobs that allow high- and low-pressure alarms to be set directly on the digital bar graph. The 755 also includes a backup ventilation mode that is activated during apneic periods.

In addition, the Eagle 755 allows the operator the option of pressure plateau ventilation. In this mode, the ventilator limits the pressure allowed in the circuit and airways, but does not end inspiration until the desired V_T is delivered. If the pressure in the airways reaches the set pressure limit before the entire V_T is delivered, a pressure plateau occurs, venting the excess flow until the ventilator delivers the entire V_T.

The Eagle 755 also has an LCD display that lets the operator view all settings continuously along with real-time pressure waveforms, a built-in compressor with a blender, an F_IO_2 display, an interactive operator demonstration mode, and an internally calibrated and adjustable PEEP control.

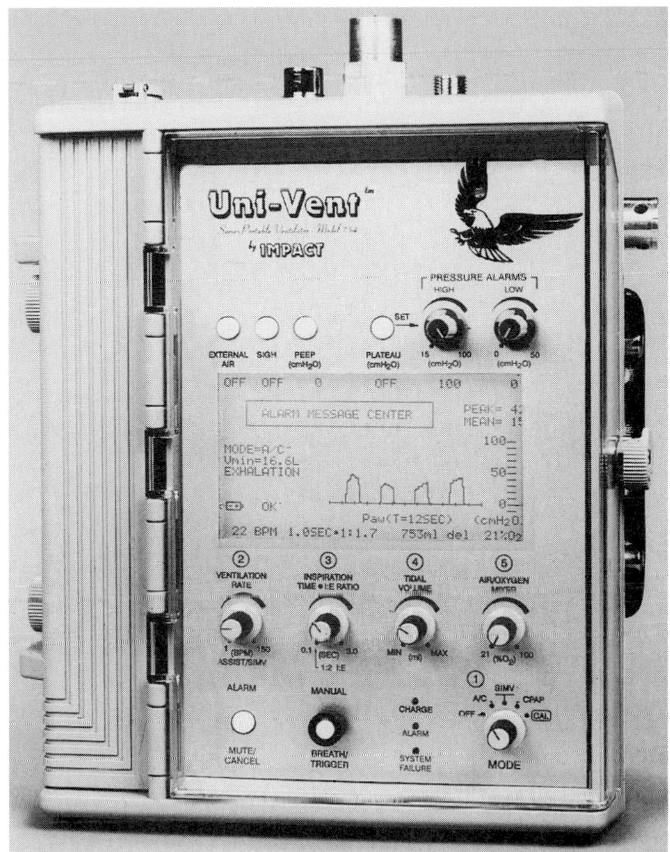

Figure 14-20 The Uni-Vent 755 Eagle ventilator. (Courtesy Impact Instrumentation, Inc, West Caldwell, NJ.)

Summary of Transport Ventilators

When transporting patients, particular care must be taken to ensure optimal monitoring of patient status, ventilation, oxygenation, and patient safety. Choosing and using the right equipment are part of the respiratory therapist's responsibilities. The ideal transport ventilator is small, lightweight, and able to withstand the rigors of transport while providing adequate ventilation at all times.

HOME-CARE VENTILATORS

Home care began in the United States more than 100 years ago.[2] Individuals discharged from the hospital that still required routine care were the primary candidates for this emerging sector of medicine. Today it is one of the fastest growing areas of health care. With the continued rise in the cost of caring for patients in the acute or extended care environment, home care is a realistic alternative for individuals battling primarily chronic diseases.

The following section focuses on the technical aspects of the equipment available for home-care ventilation. The supportive measures include primarily positive-pressure ventilators, which are the most commonly used, and noninvasive positive-pressure ventilators.[3]

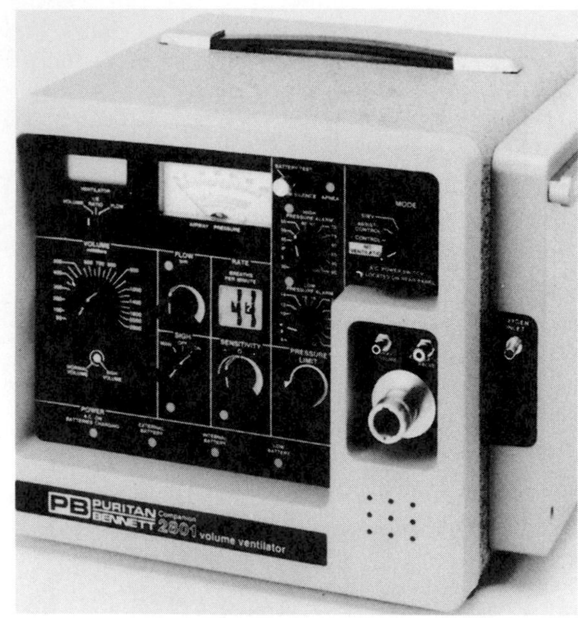

Figure 14-21 The Puritan Bennett Companion 2801 ventilator. (Courtesy Puritan-Bennett, a division of Tyco Medical, Pleasanton, Calif.)

Puritan Bennett Companion 2801

The Puritan Bennett Companion 2801 (Figure 14-21) is an updated model of the 2800 with a new front panel and several upgrades. (Puritan Bennett, Pleansanton, Calif). The airway pressure and exhalation valve connections are of different sizes, and the high and low airway pressures are calibrated with an increase in accuracy and ease in use. Additional upgrades include increases in the range settings for peak flow, peak inspiratory pressure, low inspiratory pressure, apnea alarm, and sensitivity.

The Companion 2801 is an electronically powered, rotary-piston–driven, microprocessor-controlled ventilator that is primarily used in home care (for a review of rotary-driven pistons see Chapter 11). Its dimensions are $12\frac{3}{4}'' \times 10\frac{5}{8}'' \times 13\frac{1}{4}''$ and it weighs about 31 lb. The 2801 produces a sinusoidal flow waveform for any mandatory breath in any of its working modes: control, A/C, and SIMV.

Power Source

The Companion 2801 can prioritize and then choose from the following three power sources:

- A standard AC outlet
- An external DC battery
- An internal DC battery

A standard electrical AC outlet is the primary energy source for routine daily operations. An external DC source is what the machine automatically switches to if there is a power failure. If neither AC nor external DC power is available, then the ventilator uses the internal battery. It is of the lowest priority because it has a maximum working capacity of only about 30 to 60 minutes, depending on ventilator settings. As soon as an AC outlet is available or an external battery is attached, the ventilator automatically switches to the available source with the highest priority rating.

During use, the 2801 is continuously recharging the internal battery. When the ventilator is not in use, it must be connected to an external power source and the mode switched to NO VENTILATION for the internal battery to be charged. It takes about 4 hours to recharge a totally depleted battery.

Internal Mechanism

The Companion 2801 delivers a breath by drawing in room air through the intake filter and check valve at the rear of the machine. The gas then enters into the piston chamber during the exhalation phase of the respiratory cycle. When the piston begins the forward stroke (inspiration), the gas moves from the piston chamber past a second check valve, an adjustable relief valve, and the exhalation manifold before entering the patient circuit. The adjustable relief valve monitors the internal pressure and does not allow it to increase above the set value. When pressures exceed this setting, the excess pressure is vented to room air (see the discussion of pressure limit ventilation in the section on modes of ventilation). If the clinician wishes to deliver an F_IO_2 greater than 0.21, an oxygen accumulator can be added to the rear of the machine (*Note*: an accumulator is a mixing chamber that provides a reservoir of mixed gas and lets the operator increase the delivered F_IO_2). The accumulator is not a calibrated device and an O_2 analyzer should be used.

The exhalation valve line attaches between the ventilator housing and the external valve. The line regulates the direction of flow during inspiration and expiration. The exhalation valve line is primed for operation by a branch of the main internal circuit before passing the second check valve. The expiration valve closes during inspiration, directing gas flow to the patient, and opens during expiration to allow the exhaled breath to be released.

Control Panel and Alarms

The front panel of the Companion 2801 (Figure 14-22) is divided into several sections and includes the mode switch, a monitor section, parameter controls, and an alarm section.

Mode Control

The mode selector is at the top right corner of the control panel. The 2801 allows the operator to select control, A/C, or SIMV. These settings are described further in the discussion of modes of ventilation.

Display Features

The Companion 2801 has two display capabilities: the airway pressure manometer (10 to 80 cm H_2O), which lets the operator view the measured pressure, and the LCD, which displays one of three possible parameters. A switch just beneath the LCD allows the operator to choose between volume, I:E ratio, and flow.

Control Parameters

The main control parameters include V_T, RATE, FLOW, and SENSITIVITY. The V_T control is on the middle left part of the control panel and sets the delivered V_T to the patient during a mandatory breath (50 to 2500 mL).

The respiratory RATE function on the middle of the control panel uses a two-digit rotary thumb wheel (see Figure 14-22) that lets the operator select a range from 1 to 69 breaths/min.

The FLOW function is in the middle of the control panel and regulates peak flow to the patient (20 to 120 L/min).

The SENSITIVITY setting is on the bottom center of the control panel and is active in the A/C and SIMV modes. This control allows the patient to pressure-trigger a mandatory or spontaneous breath (−10 to +10 cm H_2O).

Additional Controls

Additional controls include PRESSURE LIMIT and SIGH.

The PRESSURE LIMIT control is at the bottom right of the control panel and limits the maximum amount of pressure in the airway. The machine allows for an adjustable range of 10 to 100 cm H_2O.

The SIGH volume setting is an additional knob on the V_T control. When the SIGH function is switched to on, the ventilator delivers three consecutive sigh breaths every 10 minutes. The sigh volume cannot be set below the V_T or two times more than the V_T.

PEEP

There is no PEEP control on the Companion 2801. If the operator wants to provide PEEP to the patient, an external

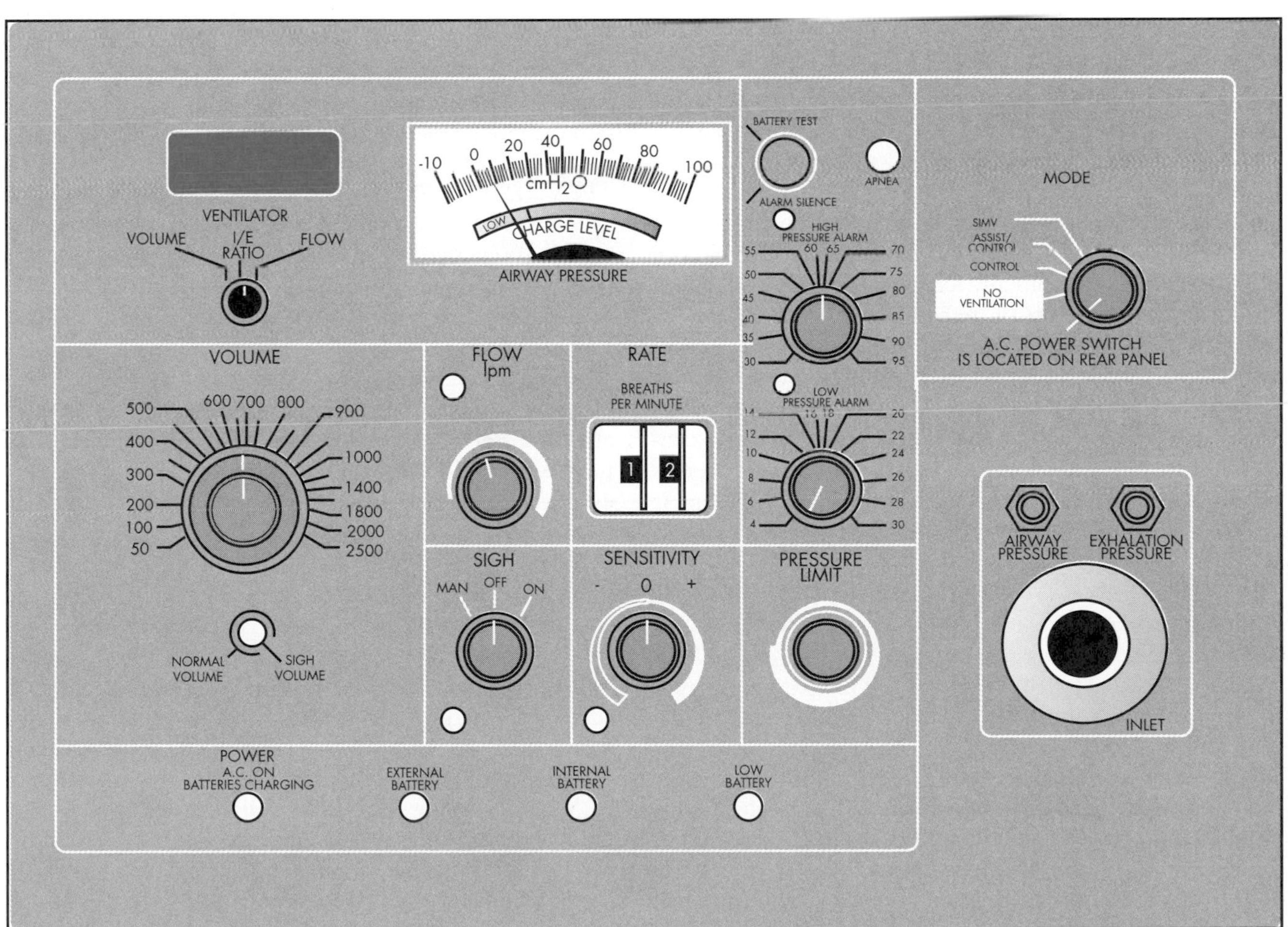

Figure 14-22 The front panel of the Puritan Bennett Companion 2801 ventilator.

CLINICAL ROUNDS 14-7

A respiratory therapist is called by the wife of a patient who is using the Companion 2801. The patient has recently resumed spontaneous breathing (A/C mode, $V_T = 0.5$, rate = 9 breaths/min, PEEP = 5 cm H_2O).

The wife states, "My husband seems to have trouble getting a breath started from the machine. When he breathes in, the pressure gauge goes to −1 cm H_2O, then it goes up to 20 cm H_2O, and then back down to 5 cm H_2O when he breathes out."

What do you think is the problem?

See Appendix A for the answer.

PEEP valve must be attached to the exhalation manifold. When using PEEP, the sensitivity must be adjusted to account for the increase in baseline pressure. The ventilator does not compensate for PEEP (Clinical Rounds 14-7).

Airway Pressure Alarms

The Companion 2801 lets the operator control settings that regulate and monitor airway pressure, including the HIGH PRESSURE alarm and the LOW PRESSURE alarm. The HIGH PRESSURE alarm is a separate control setting that allows for an adjustable range of 25 to 100 cm H_2O. When the setting is exceeded, an audiovisual alarm is activated, and inspiration stops. Any remaining volume is vented through the exhalation valve to room air. A continuous pulsating alarm sounds until the problem is resolved.

The LOW PRESSURE alarm is in the middle right part of the control panel and has an adjustable range of 2 to 32 cm H_2O. This alarm is activated if the pressure in the circuit does not achieve the desired setting for two consecutive breaths or for 15 seconds, whichever comes first. A continuous pulsating alarm sounds until the problem is resolved.

Additional Alarms

Additional alarms include APNEA, LOW BATTERY, POWER SWITCHOVER, and FLOW.

The APNEA alarm LED illuminates if the patient does not trigger a breath within 15 seconds (nonadjustable) while the SIMV mode is used. If the rate is set below 8 breaths/min and an apneic period is detected (15 seconds), then an alarm sounds. A back-up rate of 12 breaths/min is initiated if the apnea persists for longer than 30 seconds. For the ventilator to return to the original settings, the patient must trigger two breaths within 10 seconds. The visual alarm stays lit until the alarm silence/battery test button is pressed.

The LOW BATTERY alarm is activated when the power source in use falls below 11.9 volts of DC current. A pulsating alarm continues until the problem is resolved or the ALARM SILENCE/BATTERY TEST button is pressed. This alarm is also triggered when the internal battery falls below the set voltage of 11.9 volts. Every 15 minutes the ventilator tests the internal battery. If it does not meet the minimum standard of 11.9 volts, an alarm sounds for 5 seconds. The visual alarm is also activated and remains lit until the ALARM SILENCE/BATTERY TEST button is pushed.

The POWER SWITCHOVER alarm activates when the ventilator automatically switches from a higher priority power source to a lower one. The pulsating alarm continues to sound until the ALARM SILENCE/BATTERY TEST button is pressed. There is no alarm activated when the ventilator switches from a lower to a higher priority power source.

The FLOW alarm is an audiovisual alarm that is activated when the I:E ratio is more than 1:0.8 or the ventilator fails to deliver the set number of breaths.

Modes of Ventilation

The Companion 2801 can provide volume- or pressure-targeted ventilation in control, A/C, or SIMV modes. In volume-targeted control ventilation, the operator sets V_T, flow, and respiratory rate. Because this mode does not allow any patient interaction, the SENSITIVITY control is not functional, and the ventilator operates with time-triggering.

The A/C mode lets the patient initiate volume-targeted mandatory breaths as well as set a minimum back-up rate. The V_T, FLOW, RATE, and SENSITIVITY controls are all active.

When operating in SIMV, all controls used with the A/C mode are active. The patient is allowed to breathe spontaneously between mandatory volume-targeted breaths with triggering of a mandatory breath.

Pressure-targeted ventilation operates during a mandatory breath in any of the previously mentioned modes. Pressure-targeted ventilation is activated by setting the PRESSURE LIMIT control. It is recommended that the initial pressure limit be set at the current plateau pressure during a volume controlled breath. The V_T control is set slightly higher than normal requirements.

When a pressure-targeted breath is delivered, the set pressure is reached and an inspiratory pressure plateau occurs. The breath ends when the ventilator determines the set V_T has been delivered from the machine (volume-cycled). However, after the plateau pressure is reached, all additional pressure and volume are vented to room air. The higher than normal set V_T is actually not all delivered to the patient. This mode functions similarly to, but not exactly as PCV. The factor that differentiates this mode from traditional PCV is that the ventilator is volume-, not time-cycled. The machine remains in inspiration until the full V_T is delivered, regardless of whether it is to the patient or to room air. Fluctuations in V_T delivery to the patient are expected.

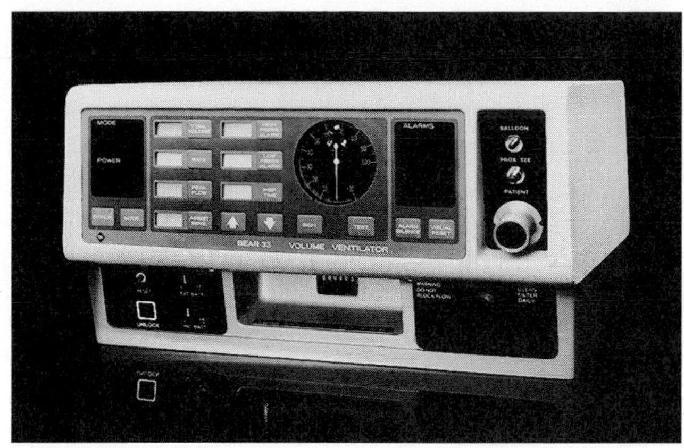

Figure 14-23 The Bear 33 ventilator. (Courtesy VIASYS Health Care, Critical Care Division, Palm Springs, Calif.)

Intermed Bear 33

The Bear 33 (Figure 14-23) is a microprocessor-controlled volume ventilator used primarily for home-care support. It is 7.5″ × 14″ × 12.8″, weighs 32 lb, and offers control, A/C, and SIMV modes (Viasys Healthcare, Critical Care Division, Palm Springs, Calif).

Power Source

The Bear 33 is an electrically powered ventilator. When the power switch on the front panel is turned on, the machine automatically selects from the following three power sources:

- An AC outlet
- An external DC battery
- An internal DC battery

The AC outlet, which has top priority, is a standard 110- or 220-volt AC outlet. The external DC battery gets second priority, and the internal DC battery is ranked third. (*Note*: When the internal battery is in use, it can provide power for about 1 hour, so that it should only be used as a back-up power source in case of emergencies.) As soon as an AC outlet becomes available or an external battery is attached, the ventilator automatically switches to the available source with the highest priority.

Internal Mechanism

Room air is drawn into the ventilator through the gas inlet filter (Figure 14-24). It then passes through the one-way check valve and enters into the cylinder assembly during the backstroke (expiration phase) of the piston. After the piston begins the upstroke (inspiration), the air passes through the output check valve en route to the patient circuit. This check valve is a one-way valve that prevents air from reentering the cylinder assembly. Before the gas source enters the patient circuit, it passes the set pressure-relief valve and the bypass check valve. The set pressure-relief valve limits the maximum pressure the ventilator can generate. When the pressure in the patient circuit exceeds the high-pressure setting, a solenoid valve is activated, and the exhalation valve vents the remaining breath to room air. All mandatory breaths are delivered in a characteristic sine-wave pattern.

For spontaneous breaths, the bypass check valve lets the patient draw in room air through the inlet port while the piston is positioning for the next mandatory breath. The patient must overcome the resistance of the circuit, including PEEP, and generate pressures more negative than 0.2 cm H_2O to open this valve. An additional gas source for spontaneous breaths is room air drawn past the deflated exhalation balloon in the exhalation valve assembly. This additional source becomes unavailable when an external PEEP valve is added to the port.

The PEEP valve on the Bear 33 is not part of the ventilator's internal mechanism. An external valve must be attached to the patient manifold if PEEP is to be applied, and can cause an increase in the patient's work of breathing. The Bear 33 does not offer any compensatory mechanism for spontaneous breaths when PEEP is applied. The higher the PEEP level, the more difficult it is for the patient to trigger a spontaneous breath. (*Note*: This is not the case for mandatory breaths because the assist sensitivity can be adjusted to compensate for the additional PEEP when the patient triggers a mandatory breath [Clinical Rounds 14-8]).[4]

The Bear 33 does offer the ability to deliver an oxygen concentration above 0.21; however, an oxygen accumulator must be attached. The accumulator is a mixing chamber that provides a reservoir of mixed gas and lets the operator increase the delivered F_IO_2. The accumulator is not a calibrated device, so that periodic checks with an O_2 analyzer are important.

Control Panel and Alarms

The Bear 33 has a simple control panel (Figure 14-25) that allows the operator access to parameters and alarm settings.

Control Parameters

The control parameters for the Bear 33 include V_T, RATE, PEAK FLOW, and ASSIST SENSITIVITY. The V_T control is at the top left part of the control panel and has an adjustable range of 100 to 2200 mL. To change the setting, the operator uses the up and down arrow keys. If an inappropriate V_T is set, the display blinks until an acceptable setting is chosen.

The RATE control is on the middle left part of the control panel and has an adjustable range of 2 to 40 breaths/minute. It is functional in all modes of ventilation.

The PEAK FLOW control is in the middle left part of the control panel and regulates the maximum flow delivered to the patient (20 to 120 L/min). This function is only active during mandatory breaths. If the set peak flow limit is reached, the display flashes until the selection is within an acceptable range.

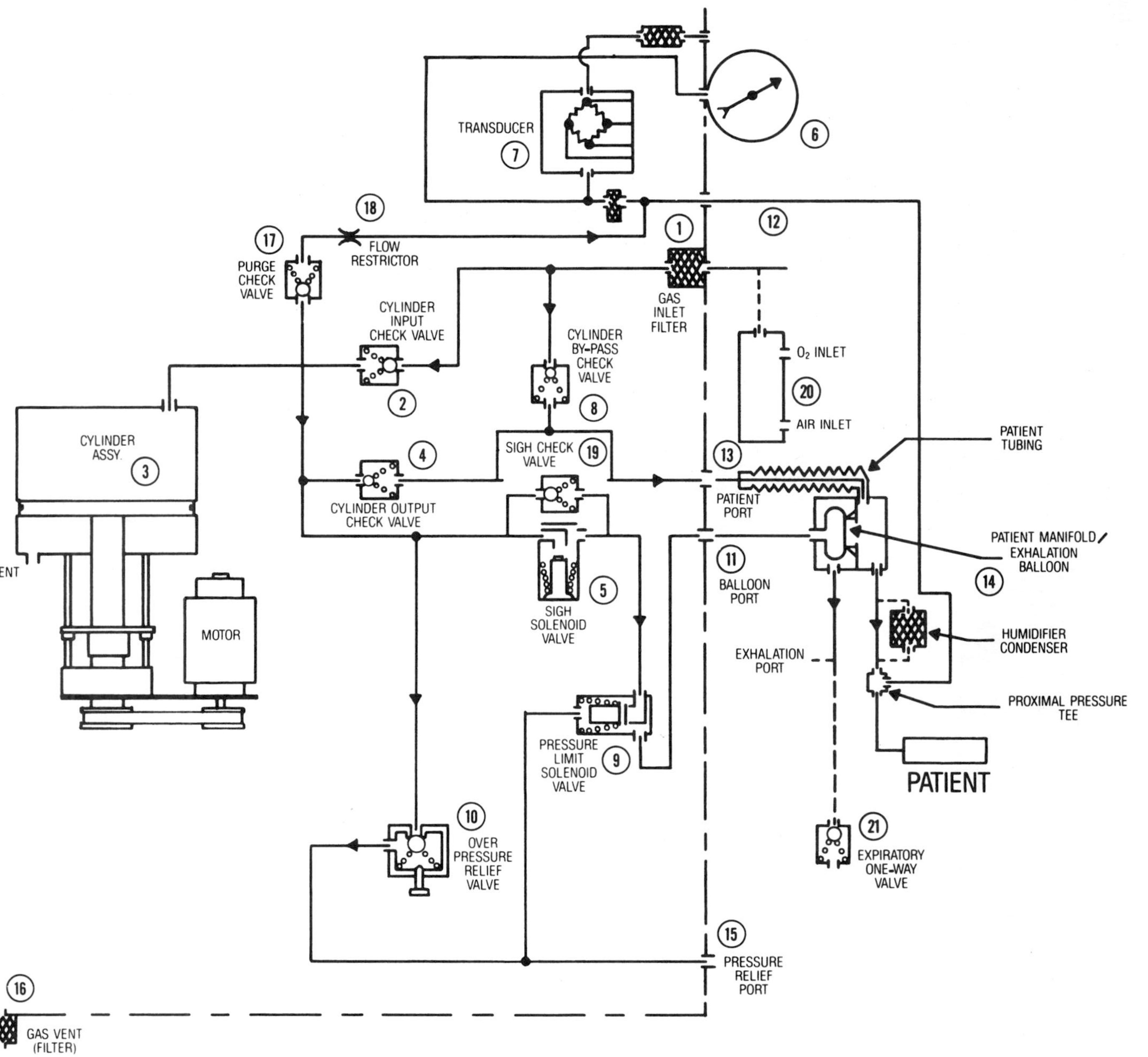

Figure 14-24 The pneumatic schematic of the Bear 33. (Courtesy VIASYS Healthcare, Critical Care Division, Palm Springs, Calif.)

The ASSIST SENSITIVITY control regulates the patient effort required to initiate a mandatory breath and is adjustable from −9 to +19 cm H_2O. When the patient initiates a spontaneous breath, the demand valve is bypassed, thereby negating the function of assist sensitivity (see Clinical Rounds 14-8).

Additional Control Parameters

The PEEP control is an additional attachment to the expiratory valve with an operational range of 0 to 20 cm H_2O. There is no control on the ventilator that allows the operator to adjust the setting; it must be done manually at the exhalation valve. (*Note*: The assist sensitivity must be adjusted when PEEP is added; however, the patient must be able to generate enough negative pressure on spontaneous breaths to return the airway pressure to baseline plus 0.2 cm H_2O.)

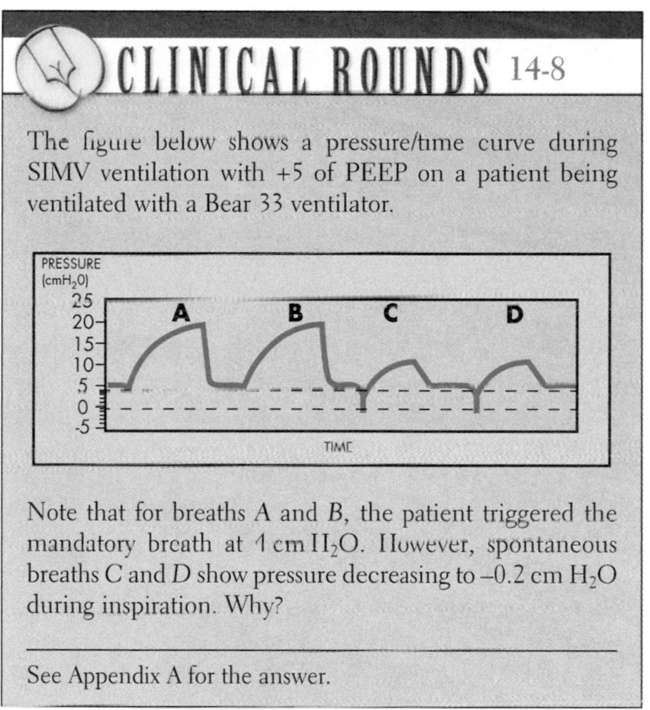
CLINICAL ROUNDS 14-8

The figure below shows a pressure/time curve during SIMV ventilation with +5 of PEEP on a patient being ventilated with a Bear 33 ventilator.

Note that for breaths A and B, the patient triggered the mandatory breath at 4 cm H_2O. However, spontaneous breaths C and D show pressure decreasing to −0.2 cm H_2O during inspiration. Why?

See Appendix A for the answer.

The SIGH function at the bottom right of the control panel delivers a breath 1.5 times the V_T to a maximum of 3300 mL. When activated, it delivers 6 sighs/hour. The Bear 33 also lets the operator deliver a manual sigh at any time.

Airway Pressures

The Bear 33 has two separate pressure alarms and an apnea alarm. The HIGH PRESSURE alarm is in the center of the top of the control panel and adjustable from 10 to 80 cm H_2O. If the patient exceeds this setting on any given breath, a visual indicator is activated. An audio alarm is only triggered if the setting is exceeded for two consecutive breaths. When the high pressure setting is reached, inspiration ends. If at any time the airway pressure exceeds 80 cm H_2O, the audible and visual alarms are activated immediately. This is a nonadjustable alarm limit.

The LOW PRESSURE alarm is at the center of the top of the control panel and has an operable range of 3 to 70 cm H_2O. The visual alarm is activated when the inspiratory pressure fails to reach the desired setting. If the patient does not attain the low pressure setting on two consecutive breaths, the visual indicator stays lit and the audible alarm sounds. The visual alarm remains illuminated until manually reset, even if the patient generates a sufficient pressure on following breaths.

Operational Alarms

The following alarms monitor the ventilator's function and electronic power supply: VENT INOPERATIVE, LOW INTERNAL BATTERY, POWER CHANGE, and APNEA alarms. The VENT INOPERATIVE alarm is audiovisual and is activated when one of the conditions presented in Box 14-9 occurs.

The LOW INTERNAL BATTERY is activated when the internal battery has about 25% or less of operating power remaining.

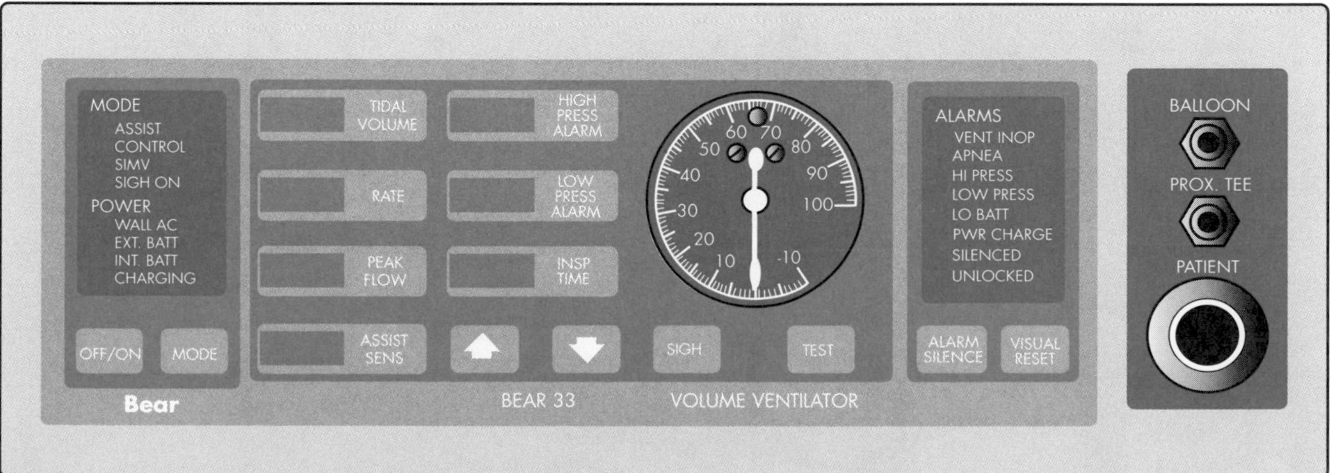

Figure 14-25 The front control panel of the Bear 33.

It can be silenced for 60 seconds with the alarm silence button or deactivated by changing to another power source.

The POWER CHANGE alarm is activated when the power supply has been switched to a lower priority source, for example from AC to internal battery. The audible alarm automatically resets when the power supply is reinstated. If this is not done, the operator must manually reset the alarm with the ALARM RESET button.

The APNEA alarm is not an adjustable control and is not on the front panel. It has a fixed setting of 20 seconds. If no spontaneous or mandatory breaths are detected within this time, the audiovisual alarm activates. Detection of spontaneous breaths is irregardless of the sensitivity setting (see the discussion on the internal mechanism).

Modes of Ventilation

The Bear 33 offers the control, A/C, and SIMV modes.

Box 14-9 Causes of the VENTILATOR INOPERATIVE Alarm

1. Failure to cycle.
2. High or low T_I. The ventilator does not allow for inverse I:E ratios. This alarm is activated when the T_I is less than 0.25 seconds or greater than 4.99 seconds. The I:E ratio is calculated based on the V_T, flow, and rate settings.
3. Timing circuit failure.
4. Internal power supply failure.
5. Internal battery supply insufficient to drive ventilator.

When in the control mode, the V_T, rate, and peak flow controls are set. The ventilator is time-triggered and does not use the assist sensitivity feature. Unlike traditional ventilators, however, the Bear 33 allows for spontaneous breathing that is not synchronized to occur between mandatory breaths (i.e., IMV). This is made possible by the bypass check valve (see Figure 14-24 or refer to the discussion of the internal mechanism in this section).

The A/C mode lets the patient initiate mandatory breaths. V_T and flow are both active in this mode, in addition to trigger sensitivity. When the ventilator "assists" the patient's breath, an "A" appears on the sensitivity display. The ventilator does not cycle into inspiration if triggered in the first 750 milliseconds from the beginning of expiration of the previous mandatory breath.

When operating in the SIMV mode, the patient is able to breathe spontaneously between mandatory breaths. The mode operates by generating an "assist window" that remains open until a patient-initiated, mandatory breath occurs. While the window is open, any effort sufficient to overcome the sensitivity setting triggers a mandatory breath. After a mandatory breath has been given, the window closes for a time to allow for spontaneous breaths by the patient. The rate setting is the factor that influences the time period available for mandatory and spontaneous breaths.

Lifecare PLV-100 and PLV-102

The Lifecare PLV-100 (Figure 14-26) and PLV-102 (Figure 14-27) volume ventilators are lightweight microprocessor-based units ideally suited for long-term home use (Respironics, Pittsburg, Pa). Their compact size and variable

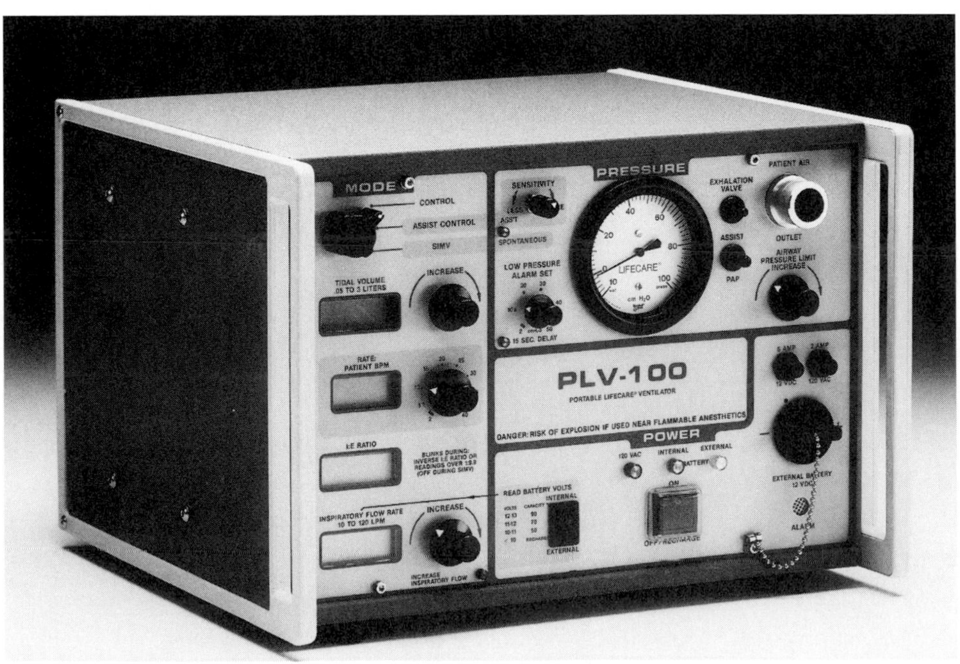

Figure 14-26 The Lifecare PLV-100 ventilator. (Courtesy Respironics, Inc, Pittsburgh, Pa.)

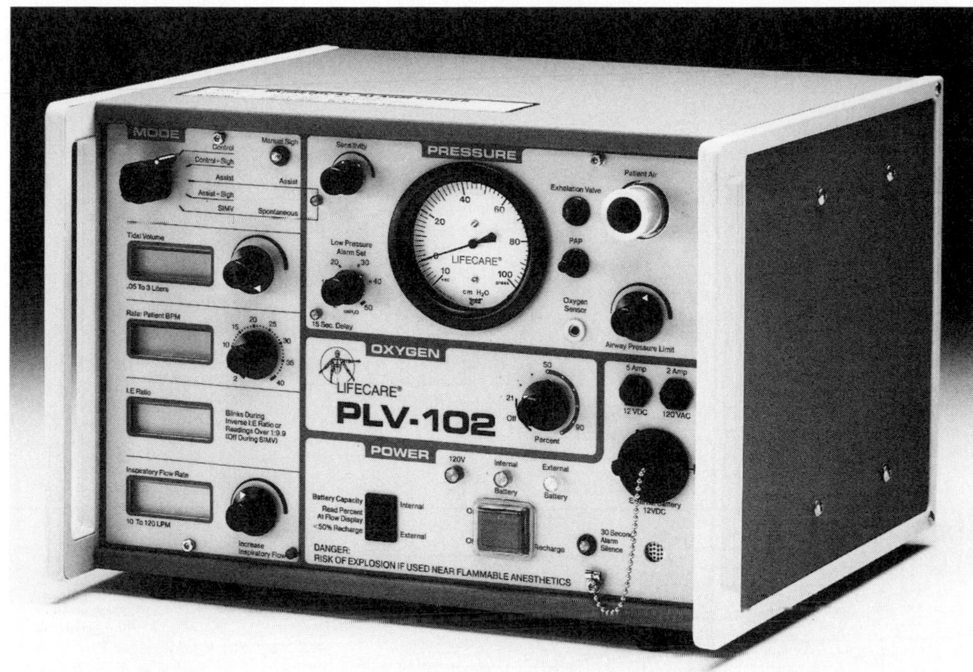

Figure 14-27 The Lifecare PLV-102 ventilator. (Courtesy Respironics, Inc, Pittsburgh, Pa.)

power sources make them highly portable, thus giving the advantage of mobility to the patient and caregiver.

Power Source

Both the PLV-100 and PLV-102 are designed to operate on the most practical power source available. The preferred power source is a 120-volt AC electrical current, but if there is a power failure, both ventilators automatically select a 12-volt DC external battery if connected. This external battery can power the ventilator for up to 24 hours depending on the ventilator's rate, volume, and pressure settings. The higher these settings, the shorter the time provided by the battery.

If the external power source is not connected, these units use a 12-volt DC internal battery. This internal battery is intended for emergency use only because it can only provide about 1 hour of power, depending on the ventilator's rate, volume, and pressure settings. The internal battery is automatically recharged whenever the ventilator is operating on a 120-volt AC power source. Each time the external or internal DC power source is selected, the ventilator sounds a 3-second alarm to alert the operator to verify the DC battery voltage level to ensure that safe operating time remains. This voltage level can be easily observed by reading the READ BATTERY VOLTS indicator on the front panel of both machines.

Both ventilators are programmed to provide a complete check of the microprocessor system, front panel digital displays, LEDs, audible alarms, and pressure transducer operation. This is a 5-second diagnostic sequence of checks that takes place each time the ventilators are turned on.

Internal Mechanism

The delivery of gas flow to the patient is provided by a rotary piston driven by a brushed motor and controlled by a microprocessor (Figure 14-28). The piston draws gas into the housing on the down stroke through a check valve and an air intake filter on the back of the machine. On the upstroke, the piston compresses the gas and pushes it out to the patient circuit and exhalation valve. The gas also passes a safety pressure-relief valve and a pressure transducer. Pressure is monitored by the proximal airway pressure line, which provides feedback to the microprocessor system. Because the drive mechanism is a rotary piston, gas is delivered in a characteristic sine-wave flow pattern with a sigmoidal pressure curve.

Oxygen Source

Administering oxygen with the PLV-100 ventilator may be accomplished by bleeding in oxygen through an inlet adapter attached to the patient circuit, or through an accumulator placed at the gas intake port. The addition of oxygen through an inlet adapter increases delivered V_T, and F_IO_2 varies depending on the delivered minute volume. In addition, extra flow into the circuit from the oxygen flow meter may necessitate adjustment of the machine's sensitivity in order for the patient to trigger assisted breaths.

The oxygen percent can be set by turning the OXYGEN % knob on the front of the PLV-102. Oxygen-enriched gas can be obtained on the PLV-102 by attaching a high-pressure oxygen hose to the DISS inlet on the back panel of the

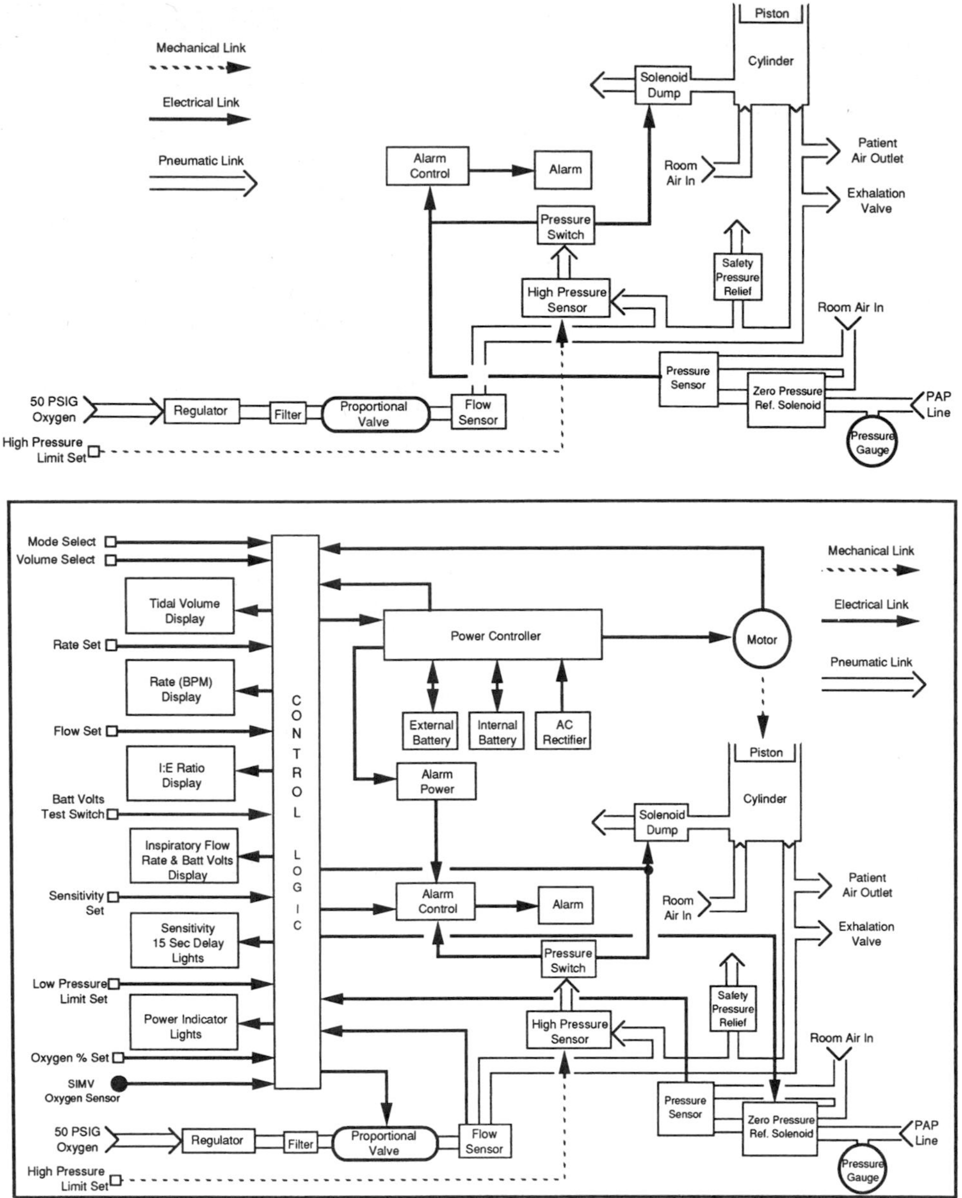

Figure 14-28 The pneumatic schematic of the Lifecare PLV-102 ventilator. See text for details. (Courtesy Respironics, Inc, Pittsburgh, Pa.)

machine. As oxygen enters, it passes through a proportional valve and flow sensor before going to the internal inspiratory circuit. Based on the set V_T and set oxygen percentage, the microprocessor system controls the proportional valve to deliver the desired F_IO_2. When using low V_T (<300 mL) and high oxygen percentage (>50%) settings, the accuracy of oxygen delivery cannot be guaranteed.

In the SIMV mode, the use of an oxygen sensor is recommended for more precise control of oxygen levels during spontaneous breathing. The sensor provides feedback to the ventilator's microprocessor system, allowing oxygen to be titrated into the circuit during inspiration of a spontaneous breath. This sensor should be placed inline with the ventilator circuit, between the humidifier and at least 18 inches from the H-valve or patient outlet. Regardless of mode, oxygen is only delivered during inspiration.

Controls

Both the PLV-100 and PVL-102 are volume-targeted ventilators. Actual volume delivery to the patient is determined by the backward and forward stroke of the rotary piston. By adjusting the TIDAL VOLUME control knob on the front panel of the machine, the operator is actually setting the length of the piston's backward stroke. As the piston's forward stroke occurs, the set V_T is delivered to the patient. The set V_T is shown on a LCD display adjacent to the V_T control knob. The V_T is adjustable from 0.05 to 3.0 liters.

The inspiratory phase of both ventilators is either pressure- or time-triggered, volume-targeted, or time-cycled. A sensitivity control determines the amount of patient inspiratory effort relative to patient airway pressure required to trigger an "assisted" breath. This control is adjustable from –6 to +3 cm H_2O on the PLV-100 and from –5 to +18 cm H_2O on the PLV-102. If the patient makes no spontaneous effort, inspiration begins as a result of the elapsed time between the set number of breaths. The rate range for both ventilators is 2 to 40 breaths per minute.

The AIRWAY PRESSURE LIMIT control establishes the maximal airway pressure allowed during the inspiratory phase. When the set pressure limit is reached, excess pressure is vented to the atmosphere through the piston safety valve as the motion of the piston continues. Thus the set pressure limit is not exceeded and T_I remains constant. The airway pressure limit is adjustable from 5 to 100 cm H_2O on the PLV-100 and from 10 to 100 cm H_2O on the PLV-102.

PEEP/CPAP

If the operator wants PEEP/CPAP on either the PLV-100 or PLV-102, an external threshold resistor valve can be added to the patient circuit (see Chapter 11 for a description of a threshold resistor). This valve should be placed proximal to the exhalation valve if a disposable circuit with an exhalation valve diaphragm is in use.[3] Placing the PEEP valve distal to this type of exhalation valve can cause incomplete sealing of the exhalation diaphragm, which results in a significant loss of delivered V_T. The application of PEEP/CPAP may also require readjustment of the machine sensitivity so that the patient can assist without significantly increasing his/her work of breathing (Clinical Rounds 14-9).

Alarms

Both the PLV-100 and PLV-102 have audio and/or visual alarms for low pressure, apnea, high pressure, inverse I:E ratios, increased inspiratory flow, switch to battery, low external battery, low internal battery, power failure, microprocessor failure, and ventilator malfunction.

Low-Pressure Alarm

This alarm is activated when a patient's proximal airway pressure falls below the set low airway pressure level. An LED on the front panel lights immediately after pressure drops below this set level, but the audible alarm only sounds when the pressure drop lasts more than 15 seconds. This alarm is adjustable from 2 to 40 cm H_2O.

Apnea Alarm

This alarm is incorporated in the LOW PRESSURE alarm and occurs only in the SIMV mode. It is activated if the machine does not sense a spontaneous breath from the patient within 15 seconds, or if proximal airway pressure falls below the set low airway pressure level for more than 15 seconds.

CLINICAL ROUNDS 14-9

A patient is being ventilated in the hospital with a PLV-102 ventilator in preparation for home-care ventilation. The patient has a threshold-resistor PEEP valve attached distal to the exhalation valve on a disposable circuit. The PEEP setting is 7 cm H_2O.

The respiratory therapist measures exhaled V_Ts at 0.5 mL when the set V_T is 0.7 mL. What is the possible cause of this problem?

See Appendix A for the answer.

High Pressure Alarm

This alarm is activated anytime ventilating pressure exceeds the set high pressure limit. As mentioned previously, excess pressure is vented to the atmosphere through the piston chamber. When ventilating pressure falls below the set high pressure limit, the alarm resets itself. This alarm is adjustable from 5 to 100 cm H_2O on the PLV-100 and from 10 to 100 cm H_2O on the PLV-102.

Inverse I:E Ratio Alert

This alarm is only a visual alarm and is activated whenever T_I exceeds T_E, or whenever the I:E ratio is $<$1:9.9. It is inactivated during the SIMV mode because of the patient's spontaneous breaths between mandatory breaths.

Increase Inspiratory Flow Alert

This alarm is also only a visual alarm and is activated if the set inspiratory flow rate is not sufficient to meet the other set parameters of V_T and respiratory rate. Under these conditions, the inspiratory flow is automatically increased.

Switch to Battery Alert

This is a 3-second audible alarm that sounds whenever the ventilator switches to internal or external DC power from an AC power source. This way, the operator is alerted that limited operation time remains.

Low External Battery Alarm

This alarm is an audiovisual alarm that is activated when the external battery voltage falls below 9.5 volts when in use.

Low Internal Battery Alarm

This is an audiovisual alarm that is activated when the internal battery voltage falls below 9.5 volts when in use.

Power Failure Alert

This is an audible alarm that is activated whenever the ventilator is turned on and all power sources are exhausted or disconnected. A source of power must be found immediately or an alternative form of ventilation must be provided to the patient.

Microprocessor Failure Alarm

This is a continuous audible alarm that is activated when the ventilator fails to pass its diagnostic self-test on start-up. When this alarm is activated, the piston motor is locked out to prevent uncontrolled piston motion.

Ventilator Malfunction

This is an audible "fast beep" alarm that is activated whenever the ventilator's pressure transducer or piston system fails.

In addition to these standard alarms, the PLV-102 has an OXYGEN SYSTEM alarm. This visual alarm is activated whenever the oxygen flow is inadequate or the source pressure falls below 35 psi. This alarm is also activated if oxygen flow is detected during the exhalation phase of a breath because this indicates either a defective flow sensor or oxygen flow at an inappropriate time.

Modes of Ventilation

Control, A/C, and SIMV modes are available on both the PLV-100 and PLV-102. In the control mode, all patient breaths are delivered by the ventilator at a preset V_T, rate, and inspiratory flow. Based on these settings, the T_I is determined and the I:E ratio is displayed on the front panel of the machine. In the A/C mode, the patient's spontaneous efforts may pressure-trigger the ventilator to deliver assisted breaths above the minimal rate setting, but the V_T and inspiratory flow rate remain constant at preset values. The I:E ratio display varies depending on the rate the patient is assisting.

In the SIMV mode, the ventilators deliver breaths according to a set respiratory rate, V_T, and inspiratory flow rate; however, the patient may breathe spontaneously between these mandatory machine breaths. The patient's spontaneous breaths may come through the air intake valve (on the back panel of the machines), or through a continuous flow H-valve assembly added to the ventilator circuit. The ventilator synchronizes the delivery of mandatory machine breaths with the patient's trigger efforts by allowing a 6-second window of time before mandatory breath delivery. If the patient makes an assist effort during this time window, the ventilator's microprocessor responds to this effort and delivers a mandatory breath.

In addition to the control, A/C, and SIMV modes, two additional modes have been added to the PLV-102 ventilator: Control + Sigh and A/C + Sigh. In either of these modes, a sigh breath at 150% of the set V_T is delivered every 100 breaths.

Aequitron LP6 Plus and LP10

The LP6 Plus (Figure 14-29) is an identical machine to the LP10 except for the PRESSURE LIMIT control, which gives the operator the option of PCV with the LP10.

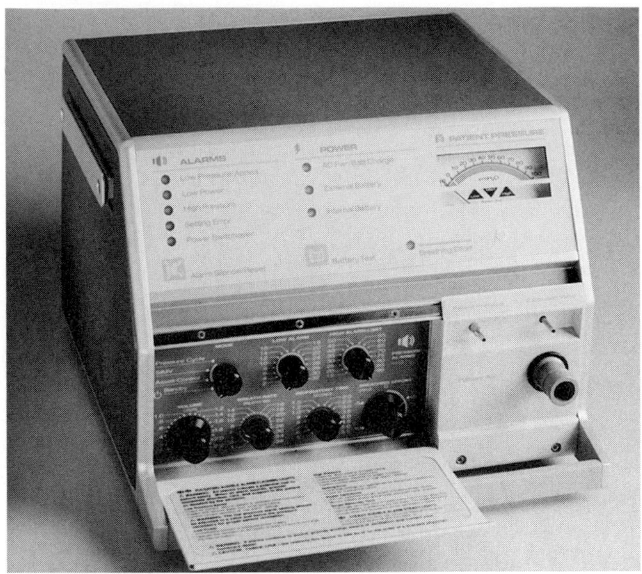

Figure 14-29 The LP6 Plus ventilator. (Courtesy Puritan Bennett, a division of Tyco Healthcare, Pleasanton, Calif.)

The Aequitron LP6 Plus and LP10 are microprocessor-controlled, volume-targeted ventilators primarily used for home-care ventilation (Puritan Bennett, Pleasanton, Calif). They are compact (9.25″ × 13.5″ × 12.5″ and lightweight (33 lb) and they can be used for pediatric and adult patients (Figure 14-30).

Power Source

Both machines operate on a standard 110- or 220-volt electrical outlet. If there is a power failure or an inability to use an AC outlet, the following alternative power sources are available:

- An external 12-volt battery
- An internal 12-volt battery

The internal 12-volt battery is intended as an emergency back-up only and is able to supply power for 30 to 60 minutes when fully charged. A power light display on the front panel enables the operator to see which power source is currently in use. When the AC light is green, the ventilator is using an AC outlet while charging the internal battery. A constant amber light indicates that an external power source in use, and a flashing amber light signifies that the internal battery is in use. When the internal battery is in use, and audible alarm sounds every 5 minutes to remind the operator that the battery is in use. When approximately 5 minutes of energy are left, the LOW POWER alarm rings continuously, signaling the need to change power sources. After using the internal battery, it is imperative to recharge it for at least 3 hours.

Internal Mechanism

The LP10 uses a rotary drive piston, which delivers a sinusoidal flow waveform to the patient (Figure 14-31). The

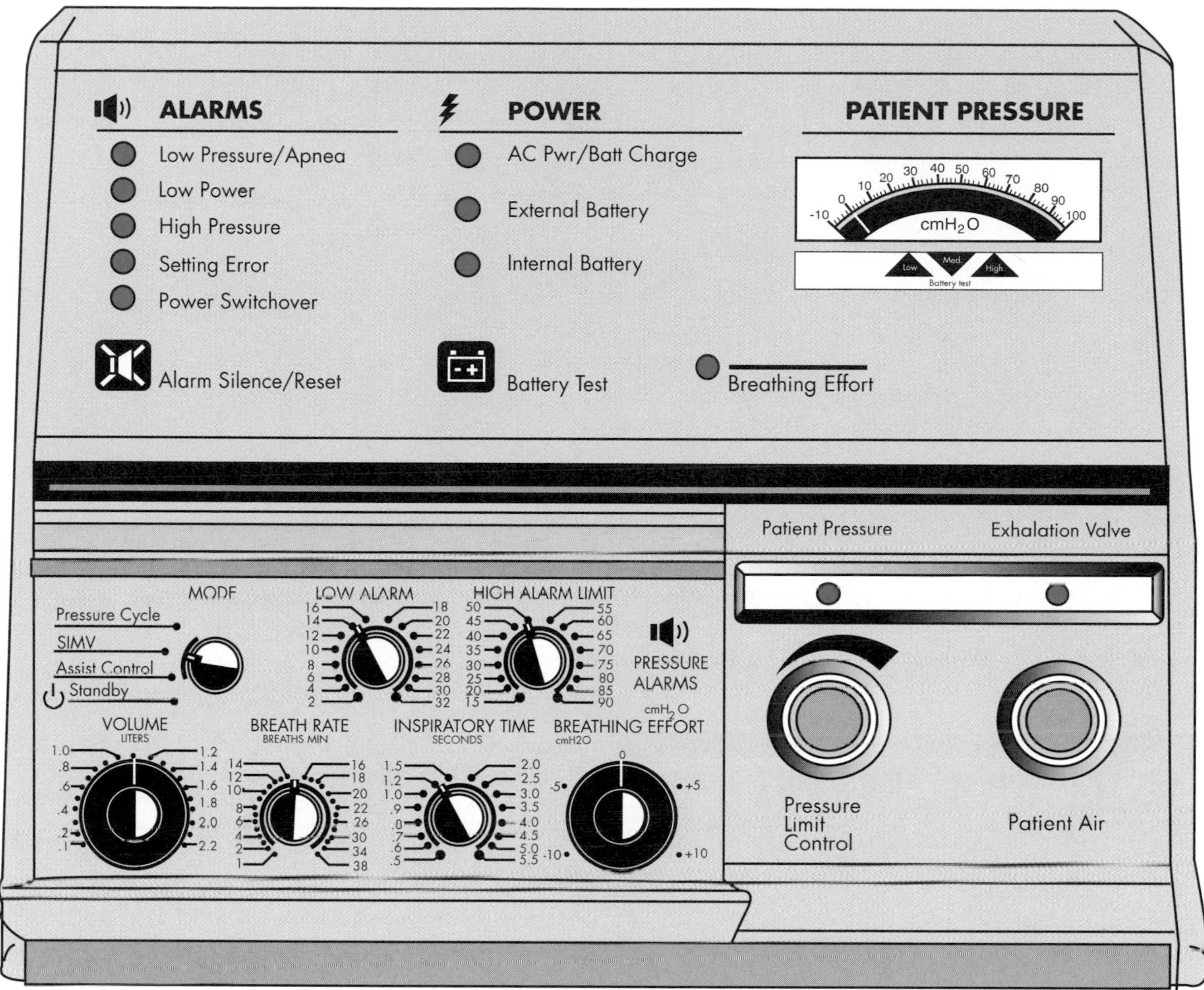

Figure 14-30 The LP10 front control panel. (See text for description.) (Courtesy Puritan Bennett, a division of Tyco Healthcare, Pleasanton, Calif.)

piston draws gas into the housing through the inlet filter port during a downward stroke of the piston. The gas passes a one-way check valve before entering the piston chamber. On the upstroke, the compressed gas moves through another one-way valve and out to the patient circuit and exhalation valve, passing the pressure transducer. The pressure transducer monitors airway pressures and relays the information to the microprocessor.

Oxygen Source

The LP10 can deliver oxygen concentrations greater than 21% by two methods. It bleeds oxygen directly into the patient circuit and can deliver F_IO_2s up to 0.4 with this method, but it is important to remember that additional volume is being added to the circuit as well. Be sure to consider this when setting the volume control. The second method of increasing F_IO_2 is by delivering oxygen directly into the rear panel air inlet port. This method can provide an F_IO_2 of 1.0. When delivering additional oxygen to the LP10, the F_IO_2 must be measured as close to the patient as possible with an oxygen analyzer. The machine does not provide a means of measuring F_IO_2.

Control Panel and Alarms

The front panel of the LP10 (see Figure 14-30) contains several controls for setting parameters and monitoring patient data and alarms.

Tidal Volume

The TIDAL VOLUME control is on the bottom left of the control panel. It has an operational range of 100 to 2200 mL that is adjustable in 100-mL increments.

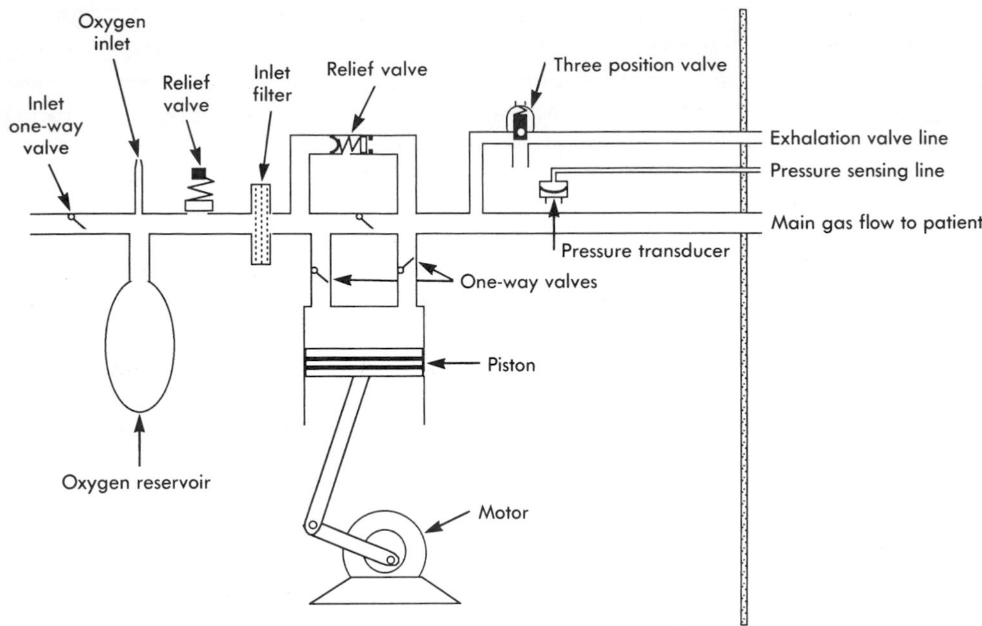

Figure 14-31 A functional diagram of the LP10 ventilator internal circuit. (Courtesy Puritan Bennett, a division of Tyco Healthcare, Pleasanton, Calif.)

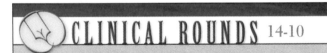

The respiratory therapist is using an LP10 to ventilate a home-care patient. The set rate is 15 breaths/min; the T_I is 2.5 seconds; and the V_T is 700 mL. Will the patient receive the full 2.5 seconds of inspiration?

See Appendix A for the answer.

Rate

The RATE control is on the bottom left part of the control panel (1 to 38 breaths/min) and sets the minimum number of mandatory breaths in A/C and the maximum number of mandatory breaths in SIMV.

Inspiratory Time

The inspiratory time control is at the bottom middle of the control panel (0.5 to 5.5 seconds).[3] The T_I and rate are responsible for the T_E and the I:E ratio. The machine does not allow an inverse I:E ratio to be set. If the operator uses inappropriate settings that create an inverse I:E ratio, an alarm sounds and the ventilator delivers the set number of breaths at an I:E ratio of 1:1 (Clinical Rounds 14-10).

Breathing Effort (Trigger Sensitivity)

The function of this control is to set the threshold pressure required for the patient to trigger a mandatory breath. It has an operational range of –10 to +10 cm H_2O. The breathing effort should be adjusted for increased levels of PEEP to prevent any unnecessary increase in the patient's work of breathing because the sensitivity is not PEEP compensated.

PEEP

The LP10 does not have an internal PEEP control, but an external valve can be attached to the exhalation manifold. The ventilator allows for PEEP compensation for mandatory breaths by adjusting the trigger sensitivity up to +10 cm H_2O. If the trigger sensitivity is set above the PEEP setting, auto cycling may occur. For example, if PEEP is +6 cm H_2O, and sensitivity is +7 cm H_2O, the unit may auto cycle.

Alarms

The LP10 monitors several parameters. When the parameters fall outside their acceptable ranges, the ventilator alarms to alert the operator to the specific problem. The first of these alarms is the HIGH ALARM/LIMIT, which is only active when the ventilator is working in a volume-targeted mode without the PRESSURE LIMIT control function. When the ventilator is using the PRESSURE LIMIT control, the alarm only sounds if the PRESSURE LIMIT valve fails to open. During pressure-targeted ventilation, the HIGH ALARM/LIMIT is used to determine the desired pressure level. It only alarms if the set pressure level is exceeded by 10 cm H_2O or more in this mode.

The LOW PRESSURE control is at the top middle of the control panel and has an adjustable range of 2 to 32 cm H_2O. When this alarm is activated, the LOW PRESSURE/APNEA light illuminates. The problems most commonly associated with this alarm are leaks in the circuit and lack of patient spontaneous breathing efforts. If the set rate is less than 6 breaths/min and the patient fails to trigger a breath within 10 seconds, the LOW PRESSURE/APNEA alarm sounds, and a back-up rate of 10 breaths/min starts. The delivered V_T is the same as that set on the control panel.

There are two basic alarms that monitor the LP10 power sources: the LOW POWER alarm and the POWER SWITCHOVER alarm. The LOW POWER alarm, which is a continuous audible alarm, is activated when approximately 5 minutes of power are left in the internal battery. The POWER SWITCHOVER alarm is activated when the ventilator switches from an AC outlet or an external DC source to the internal battery. Both features are in the alarms section of the control panel.

Modes of Ventilation

When using the A/C mode, the operator sets V_T, breath rate, T_I, and trigger sensitivity. In this mode, the patient can initiate mandatory breaths at or above the set rate, but every breath is at the set V_T.

The A/C mode also offers the ability of pressure-targeted, time-cycled breaths (PCV). When the PRESSURE LIMIT control function is active, it alters the pressure waveform of the ventilator, allowing for a plateau to occur during inspiration when the set pressure level is achieved. The ventilator vents the excess pressure for the remainder of the inspiratory cycle. The PRESSURE LIMIT control is not calibrated. It uses a spring-loaded valve for its operation.

Before the parameters are set, the patient should be disconnected. The operator then occludes the patient Y-connector, and rotates the dial until the desired pressure is achieved. After the patient has been reconnected, it is important to closely monitor the pressure because there may be a fall in the set pressure. Further adjustment of the PRESSURE LIMIT control may be necessary if this occurs.

The volume-targeted SIMV mode lets the patient breathe spontaneously between mandatory breaths. The operator sets V_T, breath rate, T_I, and breathing effort (trigger sensitivity). When operating in the SIMV mode, the operator can also use the PRESSURE LIMIT control, which operates the same in SIMV as in A/C.

The pressure-cycled mode operates by limiting the maximum pressure allowed in the patient circuit during inspiration. The ventilator assists or controls the patient- or time-triggered breaths. When the set pressure determined by the HIGH ALARM LIMIT is achieved, inspiration stops. There is no plateau phase. A high-pressure alarm only sounds if the pressure in the airway exceeds the pressure setting by more than 10 cm H_2O.

NONINVASIVE VENTILATION

The first successful use of noninvasive positive pressure ventilation (NPPV) was recorded as early as the mid-eighteenth century. The following 200 years involved improvements in the equipment used and the testing of this mode of ventilation as a possible form of treatment. During this period there were a number of pioneers. Dräger, one of the earliest supporters of NPPV, used a mask and a compressed gas source to manage the airway of drowning victims as early as 1911.[5] The experiments with positive pressure ventilation continued in the late 1930s when Barach and colleagues used intermittent positive pressure ventilation (IPPV) to treat pulmonary edema patients and in the 1950s with Motely and colleagues for the treatment of acute respiratory failure.[5,6] However, the mainstay of ventilatory support in the United States until the 1960s was the iron lung, with IPPB being relegated mainly for the administration of aerosolized medication. Improved patient interfaces and success for the treatment of obstructive sleep apnea in the 1980's led to noninvasive ventilation being reconsidered as a possible alternative to traditional ventilation.[7]

In the last 15 years NPPV has gained widespread approval for use in the hospital and home-care environment. The increased interest can be attributed to many factors (Box 14-10), with the most recent being the advent of portable and safe ventilators, user-friendly interfaces and a better understanding of respiratory muscle function. Physicians and clinicians are beginning to aggressively use NPPV for a variety of disease states that were previously managed with conventional mechanical ventilation. Currently, there are ongoing clinical trials evaluating the effectiveness of NPPV for neuromuscular disease patients, chronic obstructive pulmonary disease patients requiring nighttime respiratory muscle rest, acute respiratory failure, postoperative support, and facilitation of weaning. The remainder of this chapter will focus on the various patient interfaces and a description of many of the noninvasive positive pressure ventilators that are available.

Box 14-10 Factors Contributing to NPPV Interest

- Success in obstructive sleep apnea[2]
- Improved patient interfaces[2]
- Does not inhibit natural pulmonary defense mechanisms
- Allows the patient to eat, drink, and verbalize
- Allows the patient to expectorate secretions
- Less costly than conventional mechanical ventilation
- Possibility of use in acute and chronic ventilatory failure
- Avoidance of complications of intubation and tracheostomy[2]
- Ability to be used when patients refuse intubation[2]

A

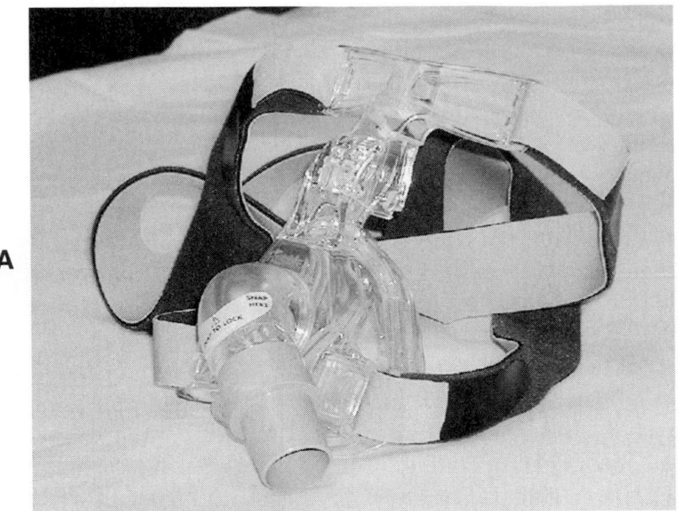

B

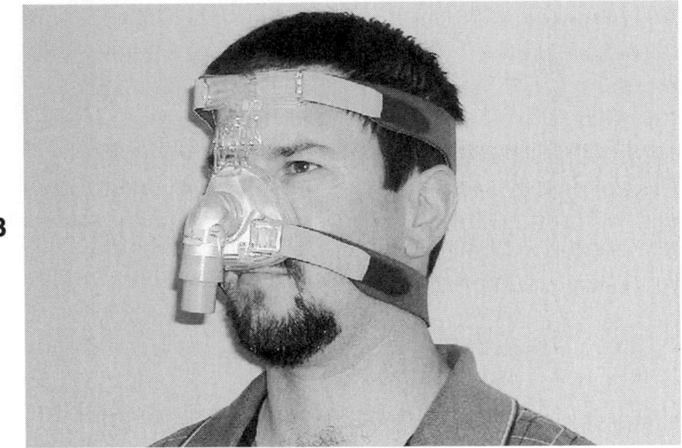

Figure 14-32 **A,** An example of a nasal mask with head gear. **B,** The nasal mask in place on a user.

A

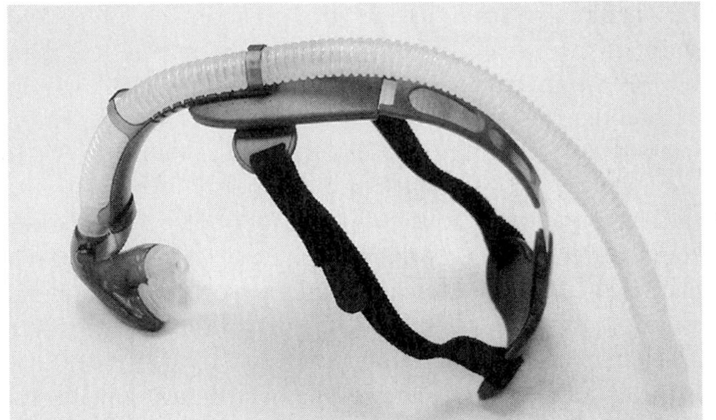

B

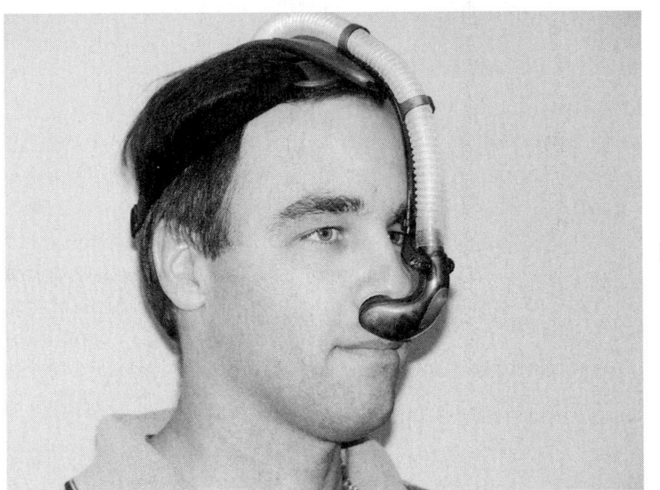

Figure 14-33 **A,** An example of nasal pillows attached to the inspiratory flow line and attached to the head gear. **B,** Nasal pillows in place on a user.

The Patient Interface[8]

When applying NPPV it is critical to use a properly fitting mask that combines minimal air leakage with maximum comfort. It does not matter how successful the device may be at alleviating the medical problem if the client is not comfortable. Poor comfort leads to poor compliance resulting in less use and a deterioration of the condition. The interfaces that are presently being used include: nasal mask, nasal pillows, oronasal mask, and a mouthpiece.

Selecting the correct mask size, particularly nasal mask size, may be the most challenging job for the respiratory therapist. The nasal mask is the most commonly used mask and often the most difficult to properly apply to the patient (Figure 14-32, *A* and *B*). The most common mistake associated with the device is using a larger than necessary mask. It is the patient's nose, not the face that needs to be covered. The top of the mask should lie at the junction of the nasal bone and the frontal bone and be fitted to cover the nares snuggly. The most frequent sizes used for the adult clients are small and medium. It is not uncommon for the maker of a nasal mask to provide a gauging device that guides the clinician in estimating the proper size. However, these devices are manufactured specifically for the home ventilator or CPAP device in use and should not be used with other equipment.

Nasal pillows are a second form of nasal NPPV and are often used as an alternative to the nasal mask (Figure 14-33, *A* and *B*). The interface consists of two cushions that are inserted into the nares of the patient that allow for ventilation. There is no pressure applied to the bridge of the nose as with the nasal mask, thereby reducing the risk of pressure sores. It is not uncommon to alternate between the nasal mask and nasal pillow interfaces to reduce the risk of developing pressure sores.

The oronasal mask is slightly larger than the nasal mask (Figure 14-34, *A* and *B*). Fitting the mask starts with placement above the junction of the nasal bone and frontal bone and includes the mouth as well as the nose. The bottom of the mask should rest just under the bottom lip. When first fitting the mask it is not unusual to have large air leaks around the mouth. A period of adjustment is usually required that allows the patient to acclimate to the oronasal mask. This adjustment generally results in a reduction in the

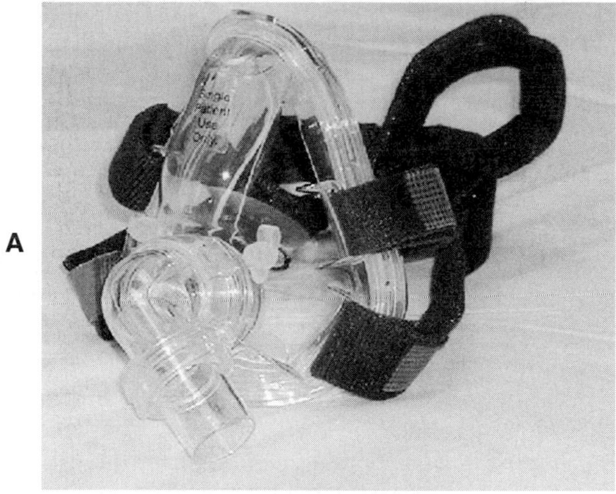

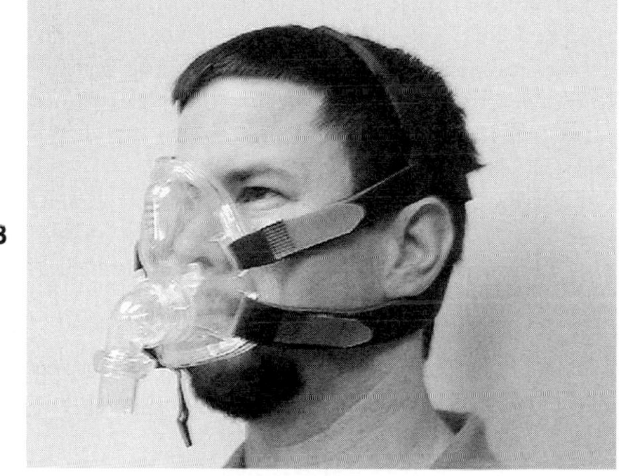

Figure 14-34 **A,** An example of an oronasal mask and the head gear. **B,** An oronasal mask in place on a user showing placement of the head gear.

amount of leak. None the less, leaks are inevitable. The NPPV machines that are used with these devices are designed to compensate for leaks and the subsequent loss of volume. A large uncontrolled leak, however, is not acceptable. A chinstrap may be effective at alleviating the problem, if an excessive leak persists. If a mask fits so tightly that no volume is lost, the pressure generated from the mask may cause the client to be uncomfortable and place the person at increased risk for pressure necrosis.

The final type of interface that can be used for NPPV is the mouthpiece or lip seal. Bennett developed the lip seal in 1972 for the purpose of allowing intermittent positive pressure ventilation when patients had trouble creating a tight seal around an ordinary mouthpiece. The actual device is a soft, oblong mask that fits around the patient's mouth. Depending on the needs of the patient, the device can be secured behind the patient's head, or if that is not possible, an impression of the patient's mouth can be made to custom fit the lip seal that can aid in securing the mouthpiece. The benefit of the mouth seal is that it rarely contributes to the development of pressure sores. In addition, it is easy to use.

The equipment used to attach the masks to the client is often overlooked. Securing the various interfaces is just as important as selecting the appropriate size. The apparatus most commonly used consists of cloth straps and Velcro headgear (see Figure 14-32). It is customary to have three points of attachment (prongs) on the oronasal and nasal mask that allow the straps to fasten to the headgear. These prongs are often found on the outer edge of the mask and allow the clinician to evenly distribute the pressure on the face, thereby reducing leaks. The prongs are positioned at the top of the nose and at the side of each nare. It is easiest if the clinician makes all strap attachments prior to placing the mask on the client. (*Note*: Although prongs are common on oronasal masks, they are rare on nasal masks. Instead nasal masks are generally fitted with hooks or loops that allow for an optimal seal.)

Ventilators

Home-care ventilators and other home-care ventilatory support devices may have any of the following features:

- The ability to provide full ventilatory support
- The ability to ventilate at night only
- Bilevel positive airway pressure support, or CPAP
- Low pressure or disconnect alarms

Controls that are common to noninvasive positive pressure ventilators include: A/C, SIMV, PSV, bilevel pressure ventilation modes, volume ventilation, respiratory rate, inspiratory time, PEEP, F_IO_2, and humidification. The following are several NPPV that are commonly used today.

Respironics BiPAP S/T[9]

The Respironics BiPAP (Respironics, Inc, Pittsburgh, Pa.) was the first to provide bilevel positive airway pressure, hence the acronym BiPAP. The unit currently has four models: S, S/T, S/T-D, and S/T-D30. The S model was the original BiPAP model, offering bilevel support only in the spontaneous mode. The next ventilator, the S/T, offered spontaneous and timed ventilation, providing the clinician with the ability to use time-triggered and time-cycled breaths. All other basic functions stayed the same as on the S model. The S/T-D and S/T-D30 improved upon the machine's diagnostic abilities and allowed the unit to interface with a recorder to log parameters. The underlying distinction between the S/T-D30 and S/T-D model is the maximum airway pressure the device is able to deliver. The S/T-D30 allows for a maximum pressure of 30 cm H_2O, compared with 20 cm H_2O for the S/T-D model. All discussion of the BiPAP unit here is limited to the S/T version.

The machine is a low-pressure, electrically driven, electrically controlled device. It is $7\frac{3}{4}'' \times 9'' \times 12\frac{3}{16}''$, weighs 9.5 lb, and can work in the IPAP (inspiratory positive airway pressure), EPAP, spontaneous (S), spontaneous/timed

(S/T), and timed (T) modes of ventilation. It has traits that make it useful in the hospital and home settings.

This ventilator is unique in its delivery of V_T and flow, and in its internal mechanics. Breaths are flow- or time-triggered, pressure-limited, and flow- or time-cycled and can deliver a square or a decelerating waveform. Because it is used with a mask for its patient interface, it uses a flow transducer in series with the patient air outlet to continuously adjust the instantaneous flows to account for leaks (see the discussion of controls in this section).

Power Source

The BiPAP has two potential power sources: AC current or an external DC battery. It neither contains an internal battery nor requires a pneumatic source.

Internal Mechanisms

The internal workings of the BiPAP are governed by a blower, which is controlled by the microprocessor. Room air is drawn into the unit through the filter on the front panel of the machine and is then directed to the pressure-controlling valve. This electronically controlled valve has two regulating factors: an electric current and a magnetic field. They both function in combination with the microprocessor and flow transducer to react to and compensate for changes in flow and pressure to maintain the desired settings. After the source gas leaves the pressure-controlling valve, it passes through the flow transducer and then to the patient.

The BiPAP uses a single-circuit patient circuit with an exhaust port and a pressure line to monitor patient flows and pressure changes (see Chapter 11 for a discussion on single and double circuits). The exhaust port may be one of several different types: the Whisper Swivel (most common), Castle Port, or NRV valve. The purpose of these ports is to exhaust CO_2 to room air. Under *no circumstance* should they be occluded. The occlusion could cause rebreathing of dead space air and improper ventilation of the patient. The proximal pressure line relays information to the microprocessor on the status of flow and volume changes within the patient circuit.

Leak Compensation

Because the BiPAP is flow-triggered for spontaneous breaths, there is a mechanism in place to compensate for the variations in the amount of air leak around the airway interface. There are three mechanisms that continuously monitor and adjust the baseline flow: total flow rate adjustment, expiratory flow rate adjustment, and tidal volume adjustment. Total flow rate adjustment is used when the operator first turns the machine on, or when gross leaks may occur. It establishes a baseline flow as quickly and as accurately as possible so that the flow transducer recognizes spontaneous efforts (i.e., a decrease in baseline flow by 40 mL/sec for 30 msec). The expiratory flow rate and tidal volume adjustments monitor additional parameters, such as no flow conditions and inspiratory and expiratory tidal volumes, to fine-tune flow on a breath-to-breath basis.

Oxygen Source

The Respironics BiPAP machine uses room air under normal conditions, but can be modified to increase F_IO_2 delivery. Oxygen may be bled directly into the patient's mask or into an oxygen-enrichment attachment that can be purchased from Respironics. The oxygen-enrichment device is attached to the tubing connector, allowing increased F_IO_2 delivery.

Control Panel

The BiPAP front panel (Figure 14-35) consists of an ON/OFF switch *(top right)* and a tubing connector for the patient circuit and the proximal pressure line. The remaining functions can be found on the back panel unless the unit is a S/T-D or S/T-D30 model with the detachable control panel (see the discussion of additional features in this section).

The rear control panel contains the airway pressure monitor (APM) and the detachable control panel (DCP) (Figure 14-36).

Behind the front panel door are the IPAP and EPAP settings, the FUNCTION SELECTOR knob, the RATE control knob (BPM), and the % IPAP control knob (Figure 14-37).

IPAP

The IPAP control knob lets the operator set the inspiratory positive airway pressure and is operational in all modes. It can deliver pressures of 4 to 20 cm H_2O.

EPAP

The EPAP control knob lets the operator set the expiratory positive airway pressure. The machine does not allow the

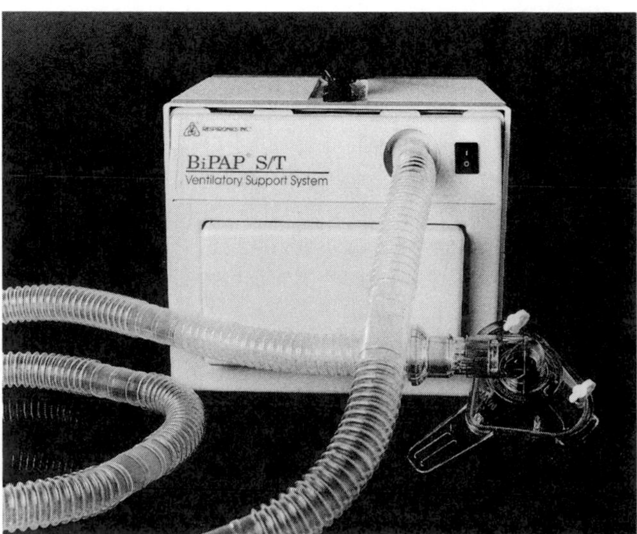

Figure 14-35 The front of the Respironics BiPAP S/ST-D. (Courtesy Respironics, Inc, Pittsburgh, Pa.)

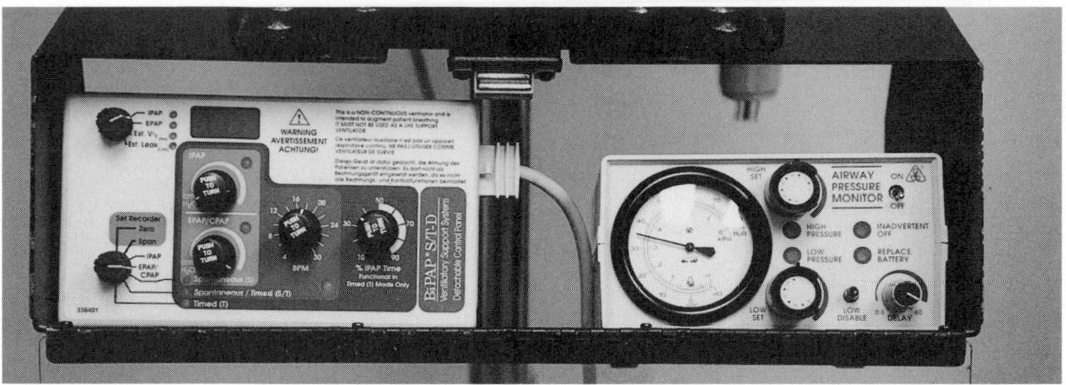

Figure 14-36 The rear panel of the Respironics BiPAP S/ST-D. See text for explanation. (Courtesy Respironics, Inc, Pittsburgh, Pa.)

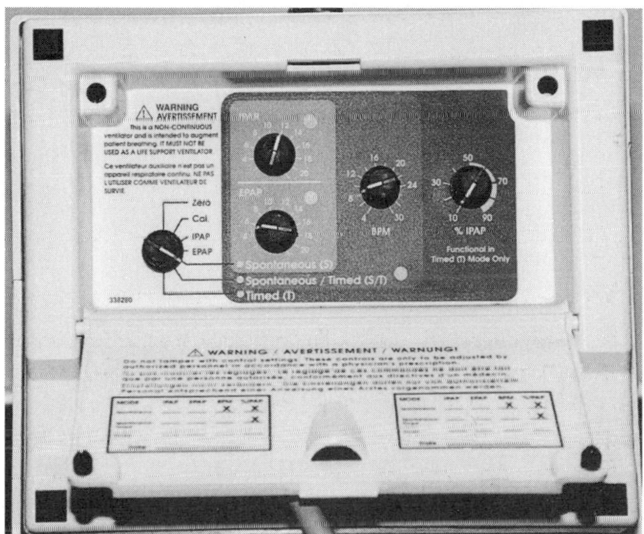

Figure 14-37 The front of the Respironics BiPAP S/ST-D with the door panel open showing the controls. (Courtesy Respironics, Inc, Pittsburgh, Pa.)

EPAP pressures to be set higher than the IPAP pressures. If this happens, IPAP levels are delivered throughout inspiration and expiration until proper adjustments are made (CPAP). This function is operational in all modes and has an adjustable range of 4 to 20 cm H_2O (Clinical Rounds 14-11).

BPM Control (Breaths per Minute)

The BPM control knob lets the operator set the minimal respiratory rate (4 to 30 breaths/min) and is functional in the S/T and T modes. When a timed breath is delivered, the LED under the BPM control is illuminated.

% IPAP Control

This control lets the operator control the fraction of time spent in inspiration during the respiratory cycle. It is only active in the T mode, can be set from 10% to 90%, and is capable of inverse I:E ratios.

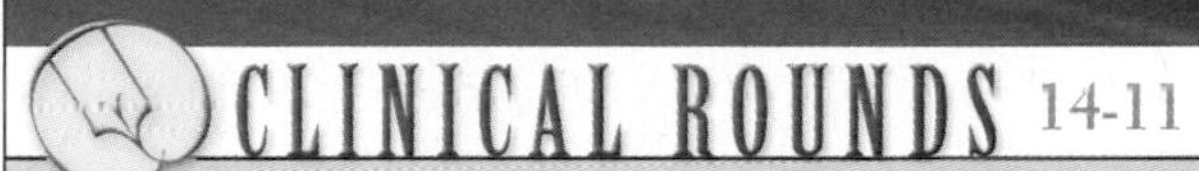

CLINICAL ROUNDS 14-11

The respiratory therapist notices that the ventilator is not cycling from IPAP to EPAP. The current settings are IPAP = 8 cm H_2O; EPAP = 8 cm H_2O; rate = 10 breaths/min; $\%T_I$ = 25%; mode = S/T. What is the problem?

See Appendix A for the answer.

Modes of Ventilation

The MODE selection knob sets the ventilator's mode: timed, spontaneous/timed, spontaneous, or CPAP (IPAP or EPAP).

When the MODE knob is set to the timed position, IPAP, EPAP, RATE, and % IPAP are activated. The mandatory breaths are time-cycled from inspiration to expiration. The patient may take additional spontaneous breaths over the set rate, but the ventilator does not cycle to the IPAP pressure level, but maintains flow to maintain the EPAP setting.

In the spontaneous/timed (S/T) mode, IPAP, EPAP, and RATE are set. The machine is flow-triggered by the patient or time-triggered based on the rate setting and the rate of the patient's spontaneous efforts. If the patient's spontaneous rate is equal to or greater than the set rate, all breaths are patient-triggered. If the patient fails to trigger a breath within the determined time interval, a time-triggered breath is delivered. In S/T, the RATE control does not guarantee a set number of mandatory breaths, but a set number of breath periods—regardless of whether they are patient- or machine-triggered (Clinical Rounds 14-12).

The spontaneous mode requires IPAP and EPAP pressures to be set; all breaths are flow-triggered and flow-limited by the patient. In this mode, the unit functions like

CLINICAL ROUNDS 14-12

A patient is being supported by the BiPAP in the S/T mode with a rate setting of 6 breaths/min. The spontaneous respiratory rate of the patient is 20 breaths/min. How many time-triggered breaths are delivered to the patient?

See Appendix A for the answer.

PEEP with pressure support. Every breath depends on patient effort, and pressure is maintained in both the inspiratory and expiratory phases of the respiratory cycle.

Although there is no CPAP position on the MODE selector knob, the machine functions as such when in either the IPAP or EPAP position. When the MODE selector is set to IPAP, the ventilator maintains the pressure set at the IPAP control throughout inspiration and expiration. When the selector is in the EPAP position, the ventilator performs similarly, using the EPAP control setting versus the IPAP setting. Because pressure is maintained at one pressure level throughout the respiratory cycle, the unit functions as if in a CPAP mode, regardless of the control setting used.

Additional Features

Additional features include the detachable control panel (DCP) and the airway pressure monitor, which are both available on the S/T-D and S/T-D30 models (see Figure 14-36).[3] The DCP lets the operator control all functions on the rear panel and also includes a selectable display feature. This display feature is an LCD that can provide IPAP or EPAP pressure readings, estimates of exhaled V_T, and estimated circuit leak information to the clinician.

The airway pressure monitor (APM) can continuously monitor circuit pressure. It contains an alarm package that alerts the operator when high and low pressure limits are exceeded, the battery power is low, or the machine is inadvertently turned off. The APM and the DCP enhance BiPAP's patient monitoring ability.

Respironics BiPAP Vision

The BiPAP Vision is a microprocessor-controlled ventilator that is capable of operating in CPAP mode or pressure support (S/T) mode (Figure 14-38) (Respironic Inc., Pittsburgh,Pa). The BiPAP Vision is generally thought of as a noninvasive system; however, it may be used to provide bilevel positive pressure ventilation to intubated patients. The specific guidelines set forth by the manufacture in the operating manual should be closely adhered to.

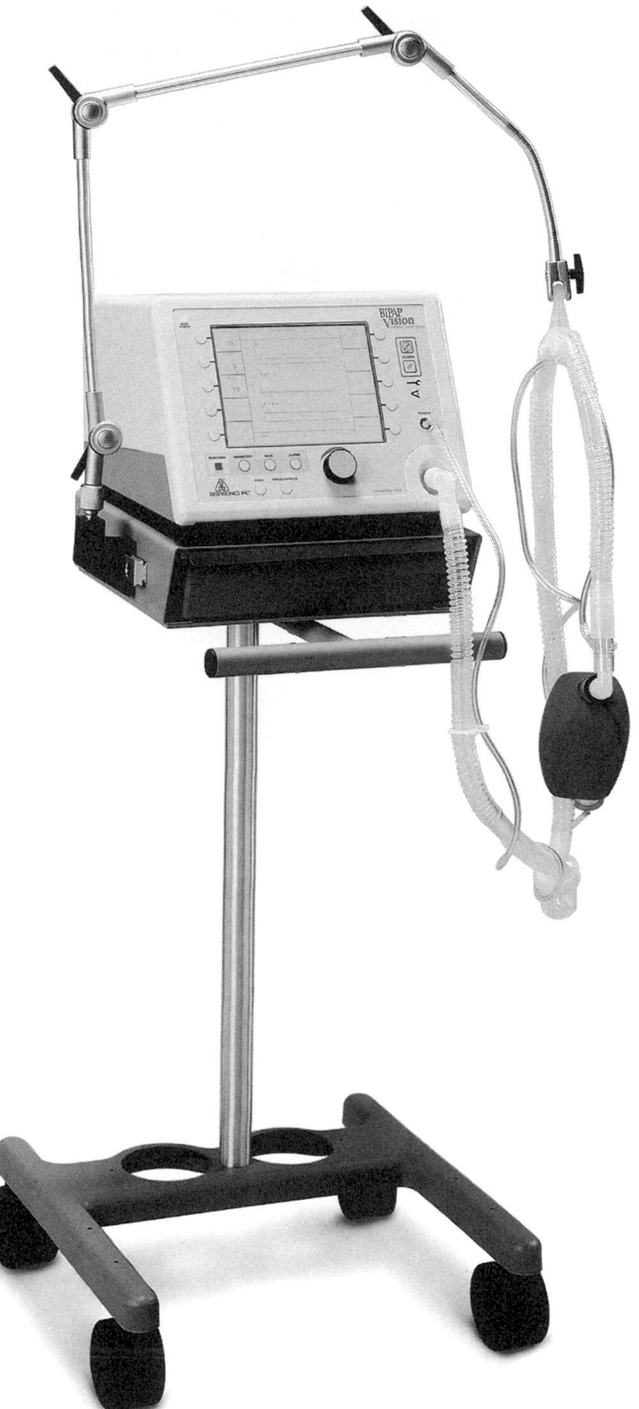

Figure 14-38 The Respironics BiPAP Vision ventilatory support system.

Power Source

A standard 120-volt AC electrical outlet powers the main operations of the BiPAP Vision in combination with a rechargeable NiCAD (nickel-cadmium) battery that drives the audible alarm system and a lithium cell that maintains the data retention functions. If at any time the system was to be disconnected from the electrical outlet the ventilator would cease to function. The NiCAD or lithium battery would not be able to support the operations of the machine; their purpose is strictly for adjunct functions. For example, the NiCAD battery powers the audible VENT INOP. alarm and the lithium battery maintains the internal clock.

Internal Mechanism

The ventilator uses a blower-driven, dual-valve-controlled system that is able to deliver and maintain pressures from 0 to 40 cm H_2O. The delivery of a breath begins with room air that is entrained through an inlet filter at the rear of the ventilator and then pressurized by the internal blower.

The entrained air moves from the blower to the pressure valve assembly (PVA), which regulates the desired inspiratory, expiratory or continuous pressures that are selected for the patient. The first valve in the PVA adjusts for the IPAP pressure to be delivered and a second valve works as an exhaust, modifying the pressure during the transition from IPAP to EPAP.

In line after the PVA and just prior to the machine outlet is the airflow module. This device monitors total gas flow and pressure being delivered to the patient and the pressure at the proximal pressure line. This information is sent to the main control system of the Vision where it is processed and used to maintain set pressure levels, trigger and cycle thresholds.

Oxygen Source

The BiPAP Vision allows the clinician to deliver an F_IO_2 greater than 0.21 (range 0.21 to 1.0) to the patient by attaching a high pressure gas source to the oxygen module found at the rear of the machine (Figure 14-39). The oxygen control located on the front control panel allows the clinician to regulate the amount of oxygen delivered to the blower. (*Note*: The accuracy of this device is ±3% at concentrations of 30% or less and may vary by as much as ±10% as the F_IO_2 approaches 100%.)

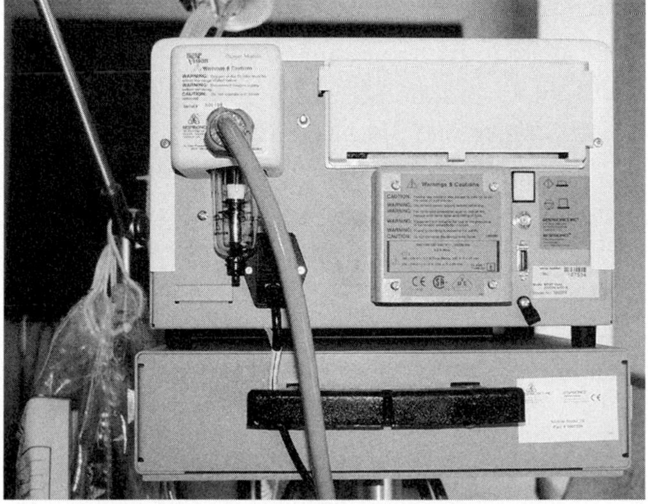

Figure 14-39 The rear panel of the Respironics BiPAP Vision.

Leak Compensation

Leaks are inherent to user interfaces and patient circuits in NPPV machines. Therefore, monitoring and compensating for changes in unintentional leaks are critical for maintaining the appropriate trigger and cycle levels for the ventilator. The BiPAP Vision uses a system called AUTO-TRACK SENSITIVITY that employs a combination of two mechanisms to identify and modify baseline values in response to leaks. These are expiratory flow rate and tidal volume adjustments.

The expiratory flow rate adjustment primarily works to make course adjustments in baseline values. When the ventilator is initially turned on it measures the total flow through the circuit before it is connected to the patient. This includes the intentional leak created by the exhalation port. The BiPAP Vision is then attached to the patient and the expiratory flow through the circuit is measured after the machine has cycled into expiration for 5 seconds. Through measurement and calculation, the ventilator is able to determine the intentional and unintentional leak of the system. This allows the ventilator to establish and monitor the baseline pressure, which allows the trigger and cycle values to be set.

The tidal volume adjustment is used for fine tuning of the baseline pressure on a breath-to-breath basis. Although the BiPAP Vision does not directly measure volume, it is able to estimate inspiratory and expiratory tidal volumes based on the patient flow and the time spent in inspiration and expiration. Differences that occur between the inspiratory and expiratory tidal volumes are then assumed to be the result of a change in the amount of intentional leak and are accounted for by an adjustment in baseline for the next breath. This feature allows the ventilator to adjust the baseline on a breath-to-breath basis thereby reducing large corrections.

Controls and Displays

The control panel of the BiPAP Vision contains eight hard keys or controls, soft keys and an adjustment knob, used to set ventilator parameters (Figure 14-40). The hard keys include: MONITORING, PARAMETERS, MODE, ALARMS, SCALE, FREEZE/UNFREEZE, ALARM SILENCE, and ALARM RESET. The soft keys are located to the left and right of the display panel. Soft keys change in accordance with the hard key activated. For example, if the hard key "PARAMETERS" was activated, the soft key options along the right and left side of the display panel would be IPAP, EPAP, RATE, TIME INSPIRATION, $\%O_2$ and IPAP RISE TIME. Depressing the soft key of choice and using the adjustment knob allows the clinician to change the value of the selected parameter.

Monitoring

The monitoring screen is also called the home screen. This screen displays graphic waveforms, calculated parameters and measured parameters and is the default screen when the machine is in operation. However, none of the displayed values can be changed. This screen is strictly for viewing the patient's current conditions. Information that can be

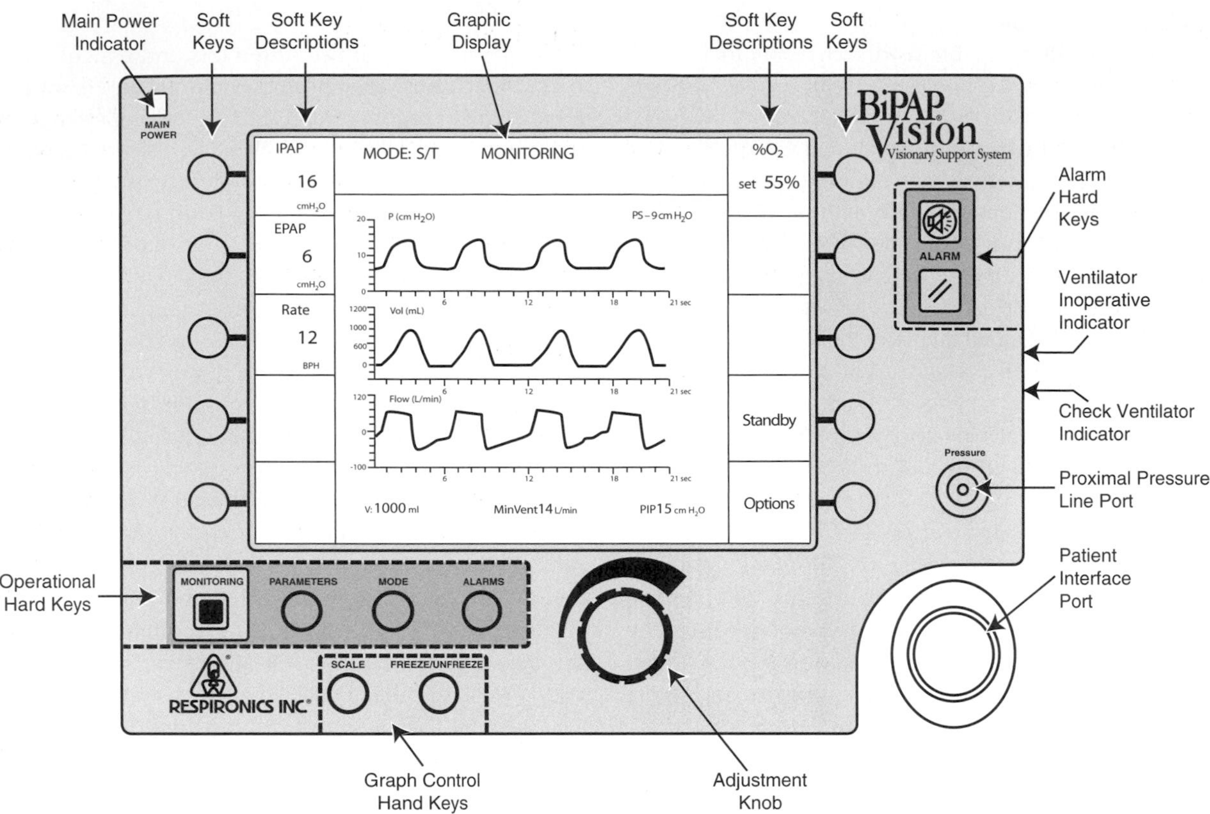

Figure 14-40 The control panel of the Respironics BiPAP Vision. (Courtesy Respironics, Inc, Pittsburgh, Pa.)

found on the home screen includes: CPAP or IPAP, EPAP, RATE (this is the total respiratory rate) V_T, minute ventilation, and peak inspiratory pressure.

Parameters

The PARAMETERS key displays the settings that are able to be modified in the current operating mode. These settings include: IPAP, EPAP, F_IO_2, INSPIRATORY TIME and RATE (if in the S/T mode). Additional information is displayed on the PARAMETERS screen that cannot be changed, but may be useful to the clinician. This includes: PATIENT LEAK (UNINTENTIONAL LEAK), INSPIRATORY TIME/TOTAL CYCLE TIME, and % OF PATIENT TRIGGERED BREATHS.

Mode Key

The MODE key displays the mode screen. This allows the clinician to view the current mode or change to a new operating mode. Whenever the clinician changes the mode of ventilation or any parameters within that mode, it is important that he/she confirms the new changes by depressing the soft key a second time. If the new settings are not confirmed, the ventilator will return to the previous values.

The BiPAP Vision operates in two modes: Continuous Positive Airway Pressure (CPAP) or Pressure Support mode (S/T). (Refer to the modes of ventilation section for additional details.)

Alarms

The ALARM hard key allows the clinician to view all current alarm settings and make any changes if necessary (see the alarms section for details).

Scale and Freeze/Unfreeze

The SCALE and FREEZE/UNFREEZE hard keys are self-explanatory. SCALE, allows the operator to increase or decrease the graph scales. The FREEZE/UNFREEZE key allows the operator to freeze and unfreeze the real time graphic display on the front panel.

Alarm Silence and Alarm Reset

The ALARM SILENCE key, when activated, turns off all audible alarms for two minutes. However, this does not prevent the ventilator from displaying a visual alarm. If an alarm limit is violated, a visual alarm will appear in the message box on the front panel. Once the two minutes has expired, any additional violations will result in an audible as well as a visual alarm.

The ALARM RESET function cancels the alarm silence and any alarm message displayed on the front panel. If another parameter were to exceed its alarm limits, the ventilator would display a visual and audible alarm.

Sensitivity

Because of the constant fluctuations in the amount of unintentional leak, the BiPAP Vision uses a series of algorithms to minimize the work to cycle the ventilator form IPAP to EPAP. The Vision uses specific threshold values above and below the base flow to determine when the patient is initiating inspiration and then beginning expiration. The clinician does not set the sensitivity. (*Note*: For information on how baseline values are obtained refer to the discussion on leak compensation.)

Alarms Controls

With the option of the newer generation noninvasive ventilators to ventilate intubated patients, it has become increasing important for the manufacturer to provide an extensive alarm system. The BiPAP Vision does just that. The available alarms include: HIGH PRESSURE, LOW PRESSURE, and LOW PRESSURE DELAY, APNEA, LOW MINUTE VOLUME, LOW RATE and HIGH RATE ALARMS, and a VENT INOP alarm.

High Pressure

The HIGH PRESSURE alarm (range 5 to 50 cm H_2O) is set above the IPAP value. An audiovisual alarm is activated when the airway pressure exceeds the HIGH PRESSURE alarm limit for more than 0.5 seconds. When this occurs, the machine immediately cycles from IPAP to EPAP.

Low Pressure and Low Pressure Delay

The LOW PRESSURE alarm (range 0 to 40 cm H_2O) and LOW PRESSURE DELAY alarm work together as a unit. The LOW PRESSURE alarm is set below the IPAP value and above the EPAP value. The LOW PRESSURE DELAY is set for the maximum amount of time that the patient is allowed between breaths. If a breath is not triggered in this time frame, then the airway pressure does not rise above the low-pressure alarm value. The LOW PRESSURE alarm activates indicating the ventilator or the patient has failed to cycle into inspiration. This alarm is active in both modes of ventilation. This may be indicative of a leak, insufficient rise time for the patient, or apnea.

Apnea

The APNEA alarm only monitors spontaneous breaths. It is an adjustable alarm that can be turned off or set at 20-, 30-, or 40-second intervals. If a spontaneous breath is not triggered within the set time frame, an audio and visual alarm will be activated.

Low Minute Volume

The LOW MINUTE VOLUME alarm (range 0 to 99 L/min) monitors the patient's exhaled volumes, calculated from patient flow and inspiratory time. The alarm activates if the measured minute volume does not meet the minimum setting.

Low Rate/High Rate

The BiPAP Vision is equipped with two alarm features that continuously compare the total respiratory rate of the patient with an adjustable maximal and minimal respiratory rate. If at any time the total respiratory rate goes above the HIGH RATE alarm or below the LOW RATE alarm, an audible and a visual indicator are activated. The alarms automatically reset when the total respiratory rate returns to acceptable limits.

Vent Inop

If at anytime the internal mechanisms of the machine were to fail or the AC power source were to fail, a red wrench icon would appear in the display window and it would be accompanied by a continuous audible alarm that can not be silenced. These conditions indicate a VENT INOP alarm. Box 14-11 lists causes of Vent Inop. As a safety feature, all system valves would open and the patient would be able to breathe room air. However, depending on the patient's respiratory pattern, it is very possible that he or she may experience rebreathing of exhaled gases due to the length of the circuit. In the event this alarm is activated the clinician should disconnect the patient from the machine and provide another means of ventilation.

Modes of Ventilation

As previously mentioned in the Controls and Display section, the BiPAP Vision offers two modes of ventilation: CPAP and the S/T mode. The CPAP mode delivers continuous positive airway pressure to the patient circuit and requires that the patient trigger each breath. If the patient is not breathing spontaneously than it is recommended that the clinician immediately change to the S/T mode.

During operation the monitoring screen displays the respiratory rate of the patient, the CPAP pressure that is delivered and the F_IO_2. At the bottom of the screen the ventilator also tracks estimated exhaled tidal volume, minute ventilation and peak inspiratory pressure (PIP). When operating in CPAP mode all alarms can be set to function.

The active S/T mode allows the clinician to set an IPAP (4 to 40 cm H_2O), EPAP (4 to 20 cm H_2O), respiratory rate (4 to 40 breaths/min), inspiratory time (0.5 to 3.0 sec) and IPAP rise time (Box 14-11). The S/T mode, unlike the

Box 14-11 IPAP Rise Time

The IPAP rise time is not a hard key, but it is an important soft key parameter in the mode display. It functions to adjust the rate of pressure change when the machine cycles from the EPAP to the IPAP. This value can be adjusted in increments of 0.05, 0.1, 0.2, and 0.4 seconds. The purpose of IPAP rise time is to gradually deliver the higher IPAP pressure to the patient to provide more comfortable breath delivery and improve patient-ventilator synchrony.

CPAP guarantees that the ventilator will cycle into IPAP a set number of times a minute based on the T_I setting. The rate setting and the inspiratory time setting are coupled so that the ventilator never allows an inverse in the I:E ratio. If at anytime this were to occur the ventilator would reduce the inspiratory time to ensure a 1:1 ratio. The pressure settings and rate setting would be unaffected.

There are two important points to note in regards to the IPAP and EPAP values. The EPAP setting can never be set higher than the IPAP value. If this were to occur, the ventilator would alarm and prevent any further increase in the pressure. If the EPAP is equal to the IPAP then the mode has essentially been changed to CPAP. Also, at very low EPAP values, the flow through the exhalation port may be insufficient to clear the expired tidal volume, which could result in a rise in the CO_2 levels of the patient. Clinical Rounds 14-13 provides some examples of these potential situations.

To reduce the sudden pressure change from EPAP to IPAP the BiPAP Vision allows the clinician to set an IPAP rise time when working in the active S/T mode. The ventilator allows the clinician to select a set amount of time that this pressure change is to occur: 0.05, 0.1, 0.2, or 0.4 seconds.

CLINICAL ROUNDS 14-13

IPAP and EPAP setting with the Vision

A respiratory therapist, who is used to using the Respironics BiPAP S/T, is adjusting the pressure levels for a patient during NPPV. The mode is set at S/T. IPAP is set at $^+10$ cm H_2O and EPAP at $^+12$ cm H_2O. Suddenly an alarm occurs. Pressures do not go to the $^+12$ cm H_2O setting. What should the respiratory therapist do to correct this situation?

See Appendix A for the answer.

Healthdyne Quantum PSV

The Quantum PSV (Figure 14-41) is a blower-driven ventilator capable of working in the CPAP, spontaneous, and spontaneous/timed modes.[10] Because of its size (8″ × 2.75″ × 3″) and weight (6.7 lb), it is commonly used in both the hospital and home settings.

Power Source

Unlike many home ventilators, the Quantum PSV only uses one power source, a standard 120-volt AC electrical outlet.

Internal Mechanisms

The Quantum PSV uses a blower-driven, valve-controlled system (Figure 14-42) that can provide various pressure levels to the patient to facilitate airway patency. The machine is flow- or time-triggered, pressure-limited, and flow- or time-cycled. It uses a flow transducer to continuously adjust the flow output to account for leaks around the patient's mask.

Air is entrained through the inlet filter and passes by the flow sensor, which relays information to the microprocessor that indicates the current status of flow moving to the patient circuit. Next air flows through the controlling valve, which regulates flows and pressures. The controlling valve is electronically governed based on the IPAP, EPAP, RISE TIME, RATE, and % I TIME settings. (*Note*: See the discussion of the control panel in this section for information on specific settings.)

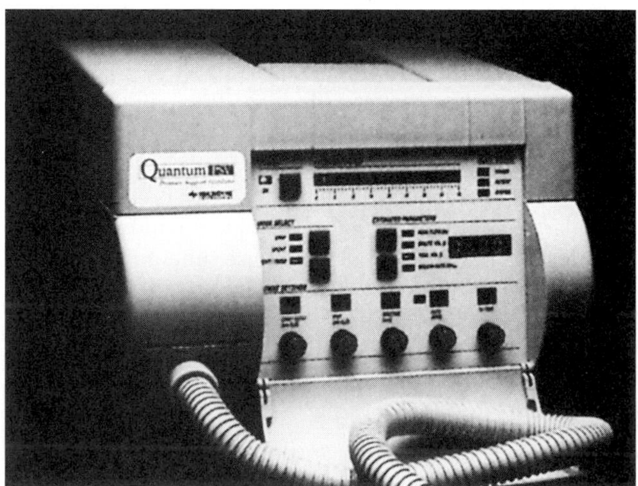

Figure 14-41 The Healthdyne Quantum PSV Ventilator. (Courtesy Respironics, Inc, Pittsburgh, Pa.)

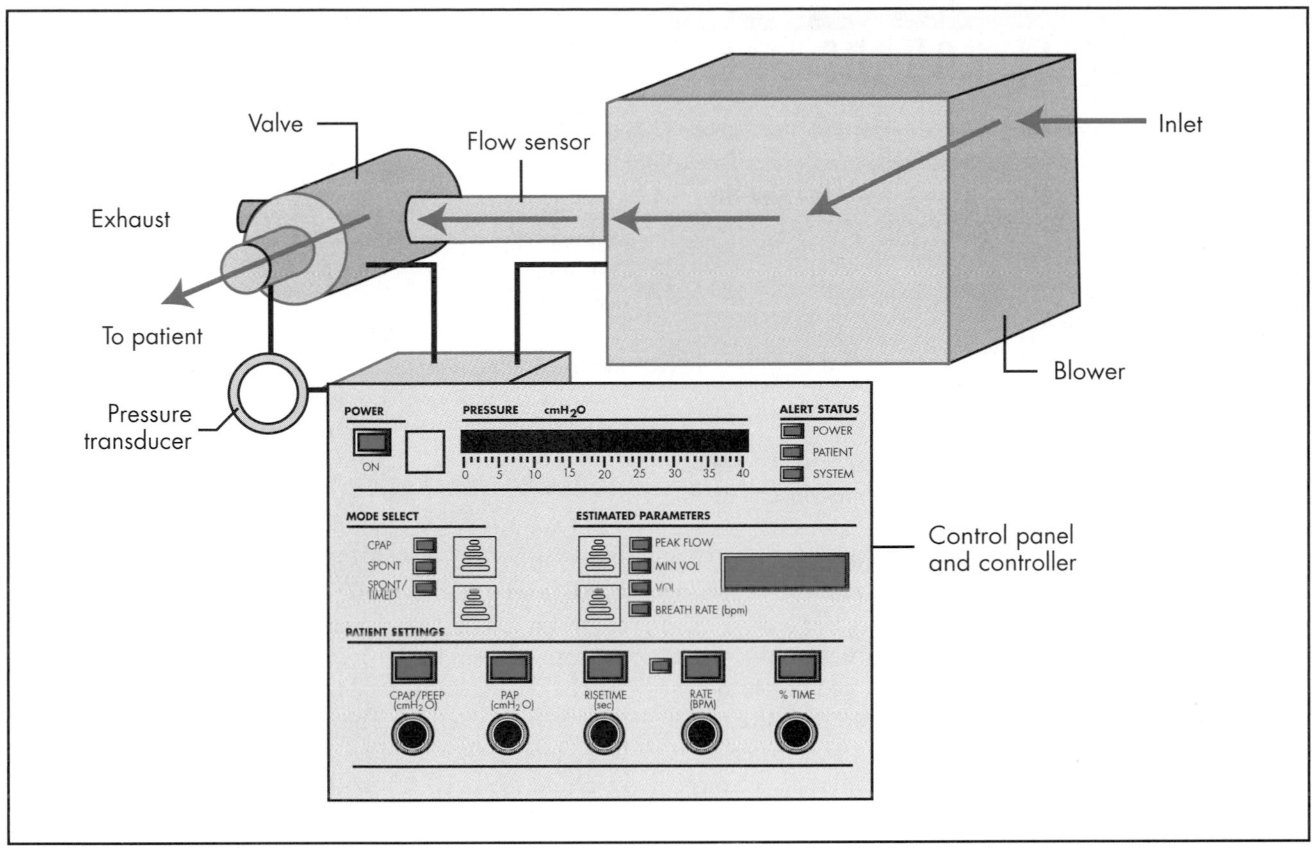

Figure 14-42 A flow diagram and the front control panel of the Quantum ventilator.

To flow-trigger a breath, the patient only needs to generate a flow change of 0.25 L/sec. After it is in inspiration, the unit measures the peak inspiratory flow and determines 75% of that value. Then it uses this measurement (75%) to determine the flow rate at which to cycle into exhalation. The flow sensor's continuous feedback of information to the microprocessor allows the Quantum PSV to adapt to small or large patient demand changes.

Oxygen Source

The Quantum delivers room air under normal conditions, but can be modified to increase the F_IO_2. A T-adaptor can be placed between the mask and the hose to bleed oxygen into the mask. There is no F_IO_2 adjuster, so periodic checks with an O_2 analyzer are required to monitor the delivered oxygen.

Control Panel

The Quantum PSV allows for a variety of functions, all of which can be managed with the control panel (see Figure 14-42). The controls that maybe adjusted to accommodate the patient needs are:

1. CPAP/EPAP
2. IPAP
3. RISE TIME
4. RATE
5. % I TIME

The CPAP/EPAP setting is at the lower left of the control panel (2 to 25 cm H_2O). The machine does not let the operator set the EPAP pressures higher than the IPAP pressures. For example, if the IPAP level is 5 cm H_2O and the EPAP level is 7 cm H_2O, then the EPAP level is automatically reduced to 5 cm H_2O and a state of CPAP exists. If this happens, the CPAP mode indicator light flashes.

The IPAP control sets the IPAP (2 to 30 cm H_2O) and should always be set above the EPAP setting, unless in the CPAP mode.

The RISE TIME lets the operator control the rate at which pressure change occurs between IPAP and EPAP, which ultimately affects the pressure curve. It has an operational range of 0.1 to 0.9 seconds and maximizes patient comfort by easing from one phase of the breath cycle into the other. The % I TIME must be set higher than the RISE TIME, or the RISE TIME control flashes, limiting the RISE TIME to maintain the desired T_I. The RISE TIME setting is reduced to the lowest possible setting, but always remains below the % I TIME (Clinical Rounds 14-14).

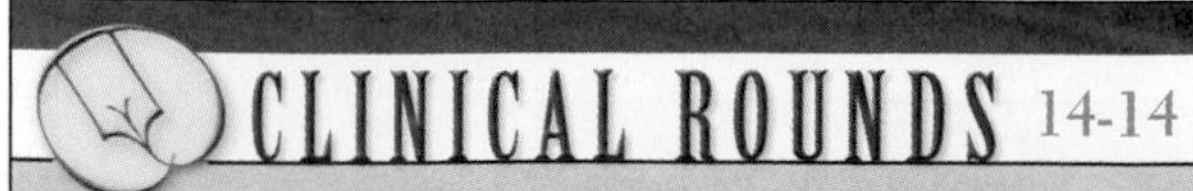

The respiratory rate on the Quantum PSV is set at 30 breaths/min; the $\%T_I$ is at 0.8 seconds; and the rise time is 0.9 seconds. The therapist notices that the rise time control light is flashing. What is wrong with the current settings?

See Appendix A for the answer.

The RATE control (4 to 40 breaths/min) is at the bottom right of the control panel and is only operational in the spontaneous/timed mode. When the operator changes the ventilator setting to the spontaneous/timed mode, there is a default setting of 10 breaths/min that automatically appears. Other desired rates have to be entered.

The % I TIME control is only functional in the spontaneous/timed mode. It allows the operator to determine the amount of time spent in inspiration relative to the TCT (10% to 90%). The Quantum allows for inverse I:E ratio ventilation. When the ventilator is initially changed from CPAP or spontaneous to spontaneous/timed, the % I TIME defaults to a setting of 33% until the operator enters the desired setting.

Estimated Parameters

The Quantum estimates the following parameters and presents them in the display window: PEAK FLOW, TIDAL VOLUME, MINUTE VOLUME, and BREATH RATE (all measured on inspiration). The PEAK FLOW parameter has a measurable range of 0 to 4.99 L/sec and is determined after the baseline flow and leaks have been measured. Any value above 4.99 L/sec causes the peak flow display to flash.

The TIDAL VOLUME (0 to 4.99 L) is calculated based on inspiratory flow and T_I. Any value above 4.99 L causes the TIDAL VOLUME display to flash.

The breath rate parameter is an estimate of the spontaneous breath rate plus the timed breath rate (0 to 99 breaths/min) that takes the average of the last four breaths. Any measurement greater than 99 breaths/min causes the display to flash.

The MINUTE VOLUME (0 to 99.99 L/min) is calculated by multiplying total respiratory rate by V_T (both estimated).

If the patient does not trigger a breath for more than 20 seconds, all estimated parameter windows show "________."

Modes of Ventilation

The Quantum PSV offers three modes: CPAP, spontaneous, and spontaneous/timed. CPAP is established by setting the EPAP level to the desired pressure setting. The blower and controlling valve work together to sustain the flow and pressure selected by the operator to maintain patient comfort.

The spontaneous mode requires an IPAP setting greater than the EPAP setting. The patient flow-triggers the ventilator by reducing the baseline flow by 0.25 L/sec to cycle the machine from EPAP to IPAP. The BREATH RATE and % I TIME settings determine the time spent in IPAP and EPAP. The V_T depends on patient effort.

When operating in the spontaneous/timed mode, the following controls must be set: EPAP, IPAP, RATE, RISE TIME, and % I TIME. The ventilator guarantees that a minimum number of breaths are delivered to the patient, and the RISE TIME and % I TIME can be adjusted to improve patient comfort. This mode lets the patient initiate and take spontaneous breaths. If the patient does not meet the number of set breaths, the ventilator initiates and delivers a breath.

OTHER NONINVASIVE SUPPORT DEVICES*

Negative-Pressure Ventilators

The following discussion focuses on two main types of negative-pressure ventilators: the iron lung and the chest cuirass. Negative pressure ventilation (NPV) attempt to mimic normal respiratory mechanics. During inspiration, negative pressure is applied outside of the chest cavity, creating a pressure gradient that allows air to flow into the lungs. The greater this pressure gradient, the greater the V_T delivered.

Although NPV reduces the side effects of positive-pressure ventilation, it is not without its own problems. NPV has been found to increase the risk of gastric reflux, induce obstructive sleep apnea, and cause rib fractures and hypotension. In addition, it is noisy; it is hard to ensure a proper seal around the patient's body or neck; patient care is hampered; and it creates a feeling of uneasiness in the patient.

NPV has the following three basic modes, depending on the generator's capabilities:

1. Inspiratory negative pressure only
2. Inspiratory negative pressure/positive expiratory pressure
3. Continuous negative pressure

The mode using inspiratory negative pressure only is the most common. Negative pressure only is generated on inspiration to assist or deliver a breath, and exhalation is allowed to occur passively via elastic recoil of the lung.

The next mode, negative inspiratory pressure/positive expiratory pressure, uses positive expiratory pressure

The previous edition of this text (edition 6, 1999) included the Rocking Bed and Pneumobelt as optional noninvasive respiratory support devices. This material has been moved to the EVOLVE website for this text.

similarly to PEEP on traditional positive-pressure ventilators. This mode is not commonly used and has been found to contribute to patient discomfort.

The third available option is continuous negative pressure. Negative pressure applied during end-expiration is referred to as NEEP. In addition to aiding in inspiration, NEEP applied to the upper airway facilitates expiration while allowing for increased respiratory rates and venous return. Its side effects additionally include the risk of airway collapse and ensuing increases in FRC. For these reasons, this later mode of ventilation is not often used. The following devices are machines that use negative pressure to ventilate the patient.

Body Respirator

The body respirator, or the iron lung (Figure 14-43), is a long cylinder that encases the patient from neck to toe, only exposing the head to ambient pressure. The airtight seal created at the neck allows the device to generate subatmospheric pressure around the thorax. The pressure gradient that develops is what lets the body respirator aid or deliver a negative-pressure breath to the patient.

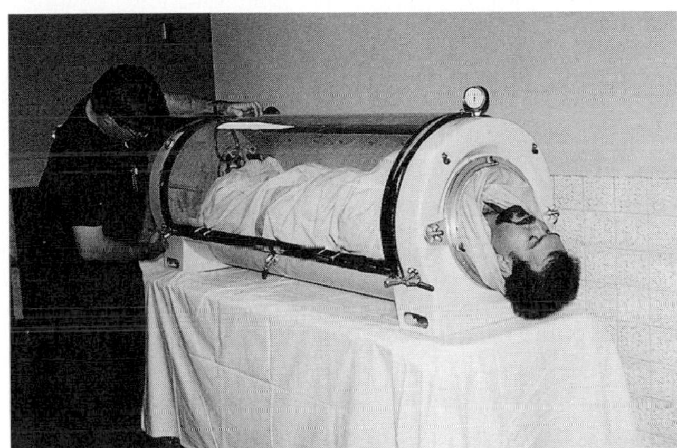

Figure 14-43 A body respiratory (iron lung).

Chest Cuirass

The chest cuirass (Figure 14-44) was developed to replace the body respirator; it is smaller and less cumbersome. The cuirass is a rigid shell that covers the thorax and abdomen and is secured to the patient with abdominal straps. A 2- to 3-inch barrier is used between the chest wall and the actual cuirass so that there is no restriction during inspiration. A tight seal is essential for the device to function properly. Therefore, for optimal performance, a custom shell should be made for the patient. A shell that conforms to the patient will have fewer leak problems. This device works with any negative-pressure pump.

Additional NPVs

Additional NPVs are the poncho, the raincoat, and the pneumosuit (Figure 14-45), which use NPV while aiding in patient comfort. The pneumosuit uses a negative-pressure generator and an iron-mesh cage that encapsulates the chest cavity in addition to the suit. The cage allows for a 2- to 3-inch barrier between the chest wall and the suit to prevent negative pressure from being directly applied to the thorax. A seal is made at the neck and extremities (which extremities is determined by the type of suit used), and maintaining these seals is the most common problem associated with this device.

Summary of Home-Care Equipment

With increasing life expectancy and our ability to support diseases once thought to be untreatable, home care is a viable alternative to hospital care. Indihar[11] did a cost-based

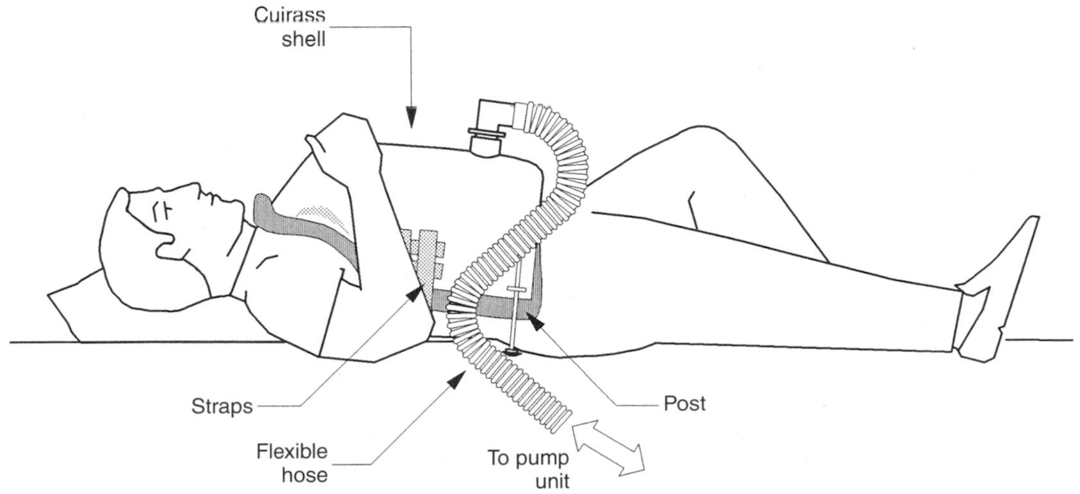

Figure 14-44 A cuirass shell used for negative-pressure ventilation. The patient is placed in the supine position, and the cuirass is stabilized with straps and posts. The method of ventilation is identical to that of the chest shell unit. (Redrawn from Dupuis Y: *Ventilators: theory and clinical application*, ed 2, St Louis, 1992, Mosby.)

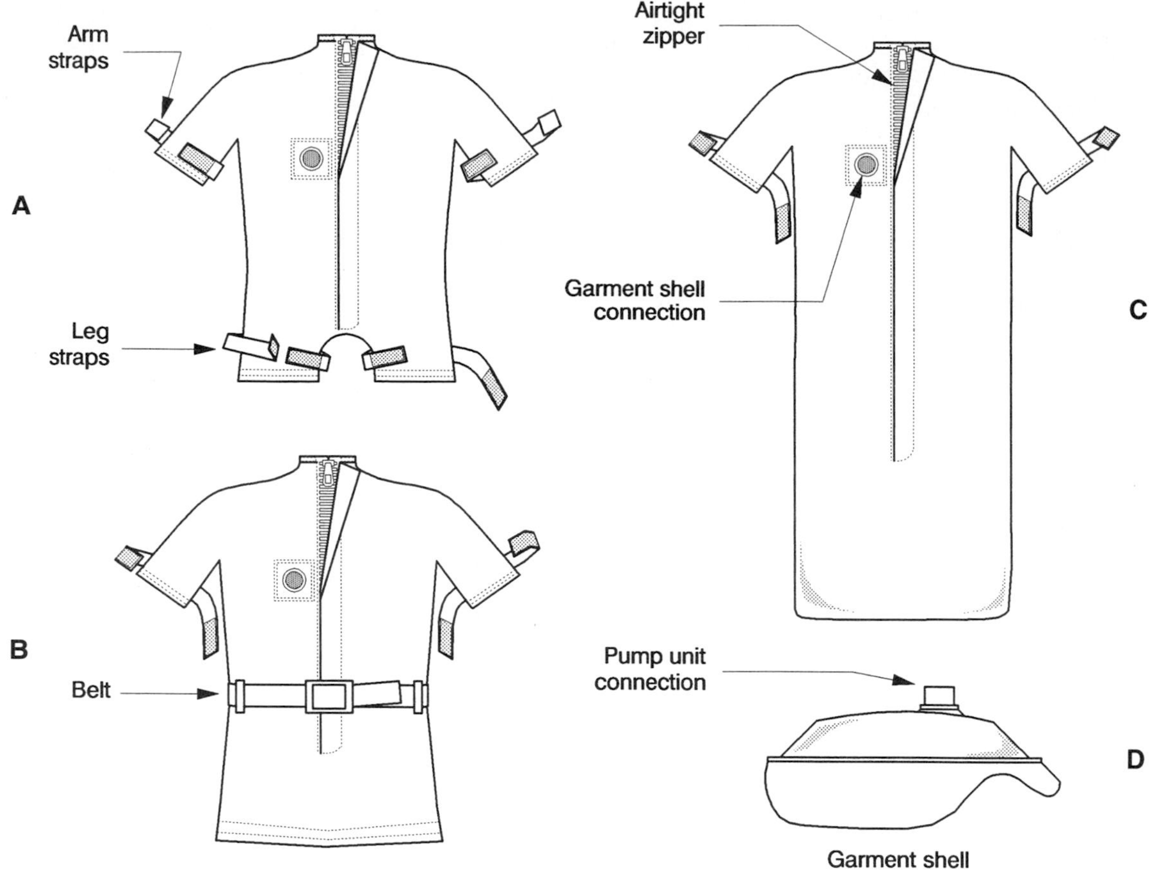

Figure 14-45 Airtight garments used for negative-pressure ventilation. **A,** Garment is sealed at neck, arms, and legs. **B,** Garment is sealed at neck, arms, and waist. **C,** Patient is placed in bag, sealed at neck and arms. **D,** Shell, fitted with pump connection extending through garment opening, is used to keep the garment off the patient's chest and enhance ventilation. (Redrawn from Dupuis Y: *Ventilators: theory and clinical application*, ed 2, St Louis, 1992, Mosby.)

study comparing five different sites of chronic ventilator care. When comparing the step-down unit in a hospital with home care supported by the family, the costs were reduced by approximately one third. Cost is not the only reason for home-care ventilation, but it is a major reason why it is being so aggressively pursued.

When choosing positive-pressure ventilators, invasive or noninvasive techniques, negative-pressure ventilators, or supportive aids, it is important that the patient and family are well educated about the operations of the equipment. They should be aware of the possible problems that might arise and how to identify them. When looking at supportive devices for the home, the clinician should choose one that is simple and operator-friendly with clear alarms to alert the user of any malfunctions. It is important to remember that the primary operators of home-care devices are non-medical personnel. Operators should refer to manufacturer's instructions to accomplish correct operation of any life-support device.

Review Questions

1. Which of the following alarms will occur when 10 minutes of internal battery power remains on the Achieva ventilator?
   a. Internal battery light illuminates
   b. Low battery alarm activates
   c. Extremely low battery alarm activates
   d. Battery charge depleted alarm activates

2. Which of the following statement(s) is (are) true in regard to the Achieva ventilator?
   I. The default sensitivity setting is flow-trigger
   II. The pressure-trigger is set by going under the Menu/ESC switch
   III. The flow-trigger value is set using the flow-trigger knob on the front panel
   IV. The Achieva is either pressure- or flow-triggered depending upon which threshold is reached first.

a. I only
b. II and IV only
c. I, II, and III only
d. I, II and IV only

3. Which of the following statements is (are) true about spontaneous breaths in the SIMV and CPAP modes with the Bird Avian?
   I. Flow for breaths is provided by the demand valve
   II. The effort required to trigger spontaneous breaths is determined by the sensitivity setting
   III. An H-valve assembly with reservoir bag is added to the patient circuit for spontaneous breaths
   IV. Spontaneous breaths can receive a flow of up to 60 L/min
   a. III only
   b. I and II only
   c. II, III, and IV
   d. I, II, and IV only

4. The PEEP not set indicator illuminates on the Bird Avian, indicating which of the following?
   a. PEEP is not in use on this patient
   b. The PEEP value deviates from the actual PEEP by more than 5 cm H_2O
   c. PEEP is not available on this ventilator
   d. The sensitivity needs readjusting because the PEEP has been changed

5. Which of the following statements is (are) true about the Hamilton MAX?
   I. The sensitivity is PEEP-compensated
   II. There is a low inspiratory pressure alarm available
   III. The sensitivity is not adjustable
   IV. The F_IO_2 is adjustable
   a. III only
   b. I and IV only
   c. I, II, and III only
   d. I, II, III, and IV

6. When using the Dräger Microvent, the high PEEP alarm might be activated with which of the following circumstances?
   a. PEEP > Pmax
   b. There is a leak in the circuit, and PEEP is in use
   c. There is a kink in the expiratory line
   d. There is water in the expiratory line

7. The apnea alarm on the Oxylog 2000 is:
   a. adjustable from 10 to 30 seconds
   b. constant at 15 seconds
   c. constant at 20 seconds
   d. based on the rate setting

8. The Newport E100M is set up for pressure-targeted ventilation. The pressure limit is set at 30 cm H_2O and the high pressure alarm at 35 cm H_2O. The patient coughs forcefully. This will result in:
   a. the pressure will peak at 30 cm H_2O and the inspiration will end
   b. the pressure will peak at 35 cm H_2O, but the breath continues until the set T_I is reached
   c. the pressure peaks at 30 cm H_2O, excessive pressures are vented to the room and the breath continues until the set T_I is reached
   d. the high pressure alarm will activate, pressure will peak at 35 cm H_2O and inspiration ends

9. During ventilation of a patient with the E100M, the PEEP is increased from 3 to 7 cm H_2O. The patient suddenly shows increased use of the sternocleidomastoid muscles. The pressure manometer shows the PEEP drop from 7 to 3 cm H_2O but no breath is triggered. The most likely cause of this problem is:
   a. ATC is not set
   b. sensitivity was not readjusted after increasing the PEEP
   c. the sensitivity needs to be changed to approximately 6 cm H_2O
   d. all of the above

10. The Newport HT50 can provide an enriched oxygen delivery by which of the following methods?
   I. An optional oxygen blender through a high pressure oxygen gas source
   II. An oxygen-blending bag for providing additional oxygen for spontaneous breaths
   III. By using the two high pressure gas sources required for powering the device
   IV. By bleeding oxygen into the patient circuit
   a. III only
   b. IV only
   c. I and II
   d. I and IV only

11. A respiratory therapist is increasing the PEEP/CPAP control on the HT50 from 5 to 10 cm H_2O. The patient's pressure setting is 10 cm H_2O. The ventilator does not allow the increase in PEEP. The most likely reason is:
   a. the therapist must toggle past a safety switch to increase PEEP above 9 cm H_2O
   b. the high pressure alarm is set at 20 cm H_2O and the settings would cause this alarm to activate
   c. the PEEP/CPAP level cannot be set higher than the pressure setting minus 5 cm H_2O
   d. the low pressure alarm must be readjusted before the change in PEEP can occur

12. The apnea alarm on the Uni-Vent 750 is activated; which of the following is (are) true?
   I. An apnea period of 15 seconds has been detected
   II. The ventilator is either in the A/C or SIMV mode
   III. A back-up rate of 12 breaths/min at the current settings for V_T delivery starts
   IV. The anti-asphyxia valve opens, letting the patient breathe spontaneously from room air
   a. IV only
   b. I and IV only
   c. II and III only
   d. I, II, and IV

13. The power switchover alarm on the Companion 2801 activates when the:
    a. ventilator switches to a lower priority source
    b. unit goes from battery to AC power
    c. internal battery has <11 volts left
    d. operator turns the ventilator off

14. During ventilation with the Bear 33, a patient's peak inspiratory pressure exceeds the high-pressure alarm setting. Which of the following will occur?
    a. The excess pressure vents into the room
    b. An alarm sounds
    c. Inspiration ends
    d. A plateau pressure is sustained until the percentage of T_I is reached

15. The INCREASE INSPIR FLOW light on the Lifecare PLV 102 is on. Which of the following statements is (are) true?
    a. The patient's inspiratory flow demand exceeds the set flow
    b. The operator tried to set a flow lower than the available flow range
    c. The machine detects airtrapping (auto-PEEP)
    d. Flow is not sufficient to meet the set parameters of V_T, f, and I:E limitations

16. A constant amber light is illuminated on the front panel of the LP10, indicating:
    a. an external power source is in use
    b. PEEP is active
    c. the sensitivity is turned off
    d. the internal battery voltage is adequate

17. The BiPAP Vision is connected to an oxygen source. The F_IO_2 is set at 0.8 on a patient in the ICU. The respiratory therapist measures the F_IO_2 as 0.9. A possible cause of this discrepancy is:
    a. the internal concentrator is out of calibration
    b. the setting control for O_2 is out of calibration
    c. the Vision has a ±10% error range for oxygen values approaching 100%
    d. the air source has failed

18. The CPAP light on the Quantum PSV is flashing, indicating:
    a. the unit is in the CPAP mode
    b. a high CPAP alarm is active
    c. EPAP is set higher than IPAP
    d. the CPAP level must be set

19. All spontaneous breaths on the Respironics BiPAP S/T are flow-triggered—true or false?

20. The range for the PEEP control on the Companion 2801 is 0 to 30 cm H_2O—true or false?

21. The Bird Avian can be time- or volume-cycled—true or false?

22. The Newport E100M can provide either volume- or pressure-targeted mandatory breaths—true or false?

23. When an apnea alarm activates on the Bear 33, backup ventilation begins at 12 breaths/min at the set V_T—true or false?

24. You can check the battery voltage on the Lifecare PLV 102 by using the read battery volts indicator—true or false?

References

1. Austin NP, Johannignan AJ: Transport of the mechanically ventilated patient, *Respir Care Clin North Am: Noninvasive Mechanical Ventilation* 8:1, 2002.
2. Pierson JD: Noninvasive positive pressure ventilation: history and terminology, *Respir Care* 42(4):370, 1996.
3. Dunne PJ, McInturff SL: *Respiratory home care: the essentials*, Philadelphia, 1998, FA Davis.
4. Gietzen JW, Lund JA, Swegarden JL: Effect of PEEP placement on function of home-care ventilators, *Respir Care* 36:1093, 1991.
5. Bach RJ: A historical perspective on the use of noninvasive ventilatory support alternatives, *Respir Care Clin North Am: Noninvasive Mechanical Ventilation* 2(2):161, 1996.
6. Mehta S, Hill SN: Noninvasive ventilation in acute respiratory failure, *Respir Care Clin North Am: Noninvasive Mechanical Ventilation* 2(2):267, 1996.
7. Sullivan CE, Berthon-Jones M, Issa FG: Reversal of obstructive sleep apnea by continuous positive airway pressure applied through the nose, *Lancet* 1:862, 1981.
8. Tobin MJ: *Principles and practice of mechanical ventilation*, New York, 1994, McGraw-Hill.
9. BiPAP clinical manual, S/T and S/T-D, Murrysville, Pa, 1990, Respironics, Inc.
10. Quantum PSV operator's manual, Marietta, Ga, 1997, Healthdyne Technologies.
11. Indihar SF: Cost of comparison care for chronic ventilator patients, *Chest* 99:260, 1991.

Bibliography

American Association for Respiratory Care: Clinical practice guideline: transport of the mechanically ventilated patient, *Resp Care* 38:1169, 1993.

Avian operators manual 4 248C, Palm Springs, Calif, 1995, VIASYS Healthcare, Critical Care Division.

Achieva operator's manual, Pleasanton, Calif, 2000, Puritan-Bennett, a division of Tyco Medical.

Bach JR: The prevention of ventilatory failure due to inadequate pump function, Resp Care 42:403, 1997.

Branson RD, Hess DR, Chatburn RL: *Respiratory care equipment*, Philadelphia, 1995, JB Lippincott.

Companion 2801 operator's instructing manual, Marietta, Ga, 1997, Healthdyne Technologies.

Dupuis YG: *Ventilators: theory and clinical application*, St Louis, 1986, Mosby.

Emerson Negative-Pressure Ventilator, Cambridge, Mass, 1961, JH Emerson Co.

Intermed Bear 33 clinical instruction manual 50000-10133, Palm Springs, Calif, 1987, VIASYS Healthcare, Critical Care Division.

Kacmarek RM, et al: Imposed work of breathing during synchronized intermittent mandatory ventilation provided by five home care ventilators, *Respir Care* 36:1093, 1991.

Kacmarek RM, Spearman CB: Equipment used for ventilatory support in the home, *Respir Care* 31:311, 1986.

MAX operator's manual 610253, Reno, Nev, 1991, Hamilton Medical.

Micovent operator's manual, Telford, Pa, 1995, Dräger Medical Inc.

Newport E100M operator's manual, Newport Beach, Calif, 2002, Newport Medical Instruments.

Newport NMI. HT50 and E100M ventilator presentation, 2002, Newport Beach, Calif, Newport Medical Instruments.

Oxylog Operator's Instruction Manual, Telford, Pa, 1995, Dräger Medical Inc.

Pilbeam SP: *Mechanical ventilation: physiological and clinical applications*, ed 3, St Louis, 1998, Mosby.

PLV-100 operating manual, Westminster, Co, 1990, Lifecare Inc.

PLV-102 operating manual, Westminster, Co, 1990, Lifecare Inc.

Uni-Vent 750/750M operator's manual, Rev B, West Caldwell, NJ, 1991, Impact Instrumentation Inc.

Internet Resources

Dräger Inc: http://www.draeger.com

Hamilton Medical Inc: http://www.hamilton-medical.ch/

Puritan Bennett: http://www.mallinckrodt.com/respiratory/resp/index.html

Sensormedics, Inc: http://www.sensormedics.com

Siemens Medical Systems, Inc: http://www.siemens.com/index.jsp

Newport Medical, Inc: http://www.newportnmi.com

Respironics, Inc: http://www.respironics.com

Ventilators: http://www.ventworld.com

Viasys Healthcare: http://www.ViasysCriticalCare.com

Chapter 15

Sleep Diagnostics

J.M. Cairo

Chapter Outline

Chapter Learning Objectives

Upon completion of this chapter, the reader should be able to:

1. Describe the various stages of sleep in adults and children.
2. Discuss the physiologic effects of sleep on cardiopulmonary function in healthy individuals.
3. List the most common measurements recorded during polysomnography.
4. Summarize the clinical and laboratory criteria used to diagnose obstructive, central, and mixed apnea.
5. Describe various strategies that can be used to monitor arterial oxygen saturation, nasal-oral airflow, and respiratory effort of patients with obstructive sleep apnea syndrome.
6. Explain the physiologic consequences of obstructive sleep apnea.
7. Name several common diseases associated with central sleep apnea.

Key Terms

Alpha Waves
Apnea/Hypopnea Index (AHI)
Apnea Index
Arousal Response
Beta Waves
Central Sleep Apnea
Cheyne-Stokes Respiration
Circadian Cycle
Collodion
Delta Waves
Holter Monitoring
International 10-20 EEG System
K-Complexes
Mixed Sleep Apnea
Non-REM Sleep
Obstructive Sleep Apnea (OSA)
Polysomnography
Relatively Low-Voltage, Mixed-Frequency (RLVMF) Waves
REM Sleep
Sleep Spindles
Theta Waves

The effect of sleep on breathing has received considerable attention in the past 30 years. Much of this attention relates to an increased awareness of sleep-related disorders and improved technology for assessing neurologic and cardiopulmonary functions during sleep. The physiologic effect of sleep on breathing is normally of little consequence in healthy individuals. Its effect on patients with altered respiratory function (i.e., those afflicted with chronic pulmonary diseases) can be profound, however, and lead to significant consequences.

Physiology of Sleep

Sleep is part of a cyclical phenomenon (i.e., **circadian cycle**) controlled by an endogenous pacemaker that remains active even in an isolated environment free of time cues.[1] Sleep in itself is a nonhomogenous phenomenon comprising two distinct states: non-rapid eye movement (non-REM) sleep and rapid eye movement (REM) sleep. As seen in Table 15-1, these states can be defined by electrographic and behavioral criteria, such as brain-wave activity, oculomotor activity, responsiveness to external stimuli, and muscle tone.[2,3]

Non-REM sleep, or quiet sleep, consists of four stages, which are thought to represent progressively deeper levels of sleep. At sleep onset (non-REM Stage 1), normal sleepers can be easily aroused because they alternate between wakefulness and sleep. The electroencephalogram (EEG) shows **alpha** and **beta waves,** which are present during wakefulness, diminishing as the sleeper's EEG converts to **relatively low-voltage, mixed-frequency (RLVMF) waves** (Figure 15-1, *A*). (Note that alpha waves are rhythmical waves that occur at a frequency of 8 to 13 cycles per second, whereas beta waves occur at frequencies of 14 to 80 cycles per second.[4]) Skeletal muscle tone changes only slightly from waking levels; eye movements throughout non-REM sleep are slow, rolling, pendulous, and disconjugate.[5]

Stage 1 sleep lasts for only a brief time and is followed by a transition to Stage 2 non-REM sleep, which is identified by the appearance of **sleep spindles** and **K-complexes** on the sleeper's EEG (Figure 15-1, *B*). Sleep spindles are waveforms with waxing and waning amplitude that occur at a frequency of 9 to 13 cycles per second. K-complexes are large, vertical, slow waves that have an amplitude of at least 75 microvolts with an initial negative deflection.[5] Arousal thresholds (i.e., the level of stimuli required to change to a "lighter" stage of sleep or wakefulness) are higher in Stage 2 than those in Stage 1.

The deepest stages of non-REM sleep (Stages 3 and 4) are referred to as slow-wave sleep because of the presence of large **delta waves** that appear when the sleeper enters these stages (Figure 15-1, *C*). Delta waves include all EEG waves with a frequency less than 3.5 cycles per second.[5] It is important to recognize that the distinction between Stage 3 and Stage 4 is somewhat arbitrary because both appear almost identical on EEGs. For example, most clinicians define the beginning of Stage 3 as that period when slow

Table 15-1 Behavioral and electrographic characteristics of sleep-wake states

Characteristic	Wake	Sleep: Non-REM	Sleep: REM
Eye lids	Open or closed	Closed	Closed
Eye movements	Slow or rapid	Slow or absent	Rapid
Responsiveness to external stimuli	Simple or complex	Simple	Often absent
Electroencephalogram	Low-voltage, high-frequency	High-voltage, low-frequency	Low-voltage, high-frequency
Electromyogram	High-level tonic activity	Lower-level tonic activity	Absence of tonic activity
Electrooculogram	Slow or rapid movements	Slow or rapid movements	Rapid movements

From Phillipson EA: Sleep disorders. In Murray JF, Nadel JE: *Textbook of respiratory medicine*, Philadelphia, 1997, WB Saunders.

waves constitute from 20% to 50% of the EEG recording. Stage 4, on the other hand, is identified by the presence of slow waves for at least 50% of the EEG recording.[2,5] The arousal threshold during Stages 3 and 4 is considerably higher than during Stages 1 and 2 of non-REM sleep.

After about 70 to 100 minutes of non-REM sleep, the normal sleeper enters **REM sleep.** During this phase of sleep, there is an increase in cerebral activity, as evidenced by the presence of a RLVMF pattern on EEG with a burst of **theta waves** (see Figure 15-1, *D*). Theta waves have a sawtooth appearance and occur at a frequency of 4 to 7 cycles per second.[4,5] It is generally accepted that dreaming occurs during REM sleep because sleepers who awaken after dreaming during REM sleep can recall their dreams. Although dreaming does occur during non-REM sleep, those dreams are usually not remembered. Eye movements during REM sleep are rapid, and conjugate eye movements are present. The arousal threshold (i.e., skeletal muscle tone) during REM sleep varies and may actually be absent. (It is interesting that if the arousal stimulus is incorporated into the dream content, arousal is less likely.[5])

During a typical night of sleep, a normal adult sleeper cycles between non-REM sleep and REM sleep about every 90 to 120 minutes.[1] Slow-wave sleep (non-REM Stages 3 and 4) is most prominent during the first half of the night and decreases as the night progresses. REM sleep, on the other hand, becomes longer and more intense throughout the sleep period, with the longest and most intense REM sleep occurring in the early morning hours.

Figure 15-2 illustrates the average amount of time that a healthy adult spends in each sleep state. Normally 4 to 6 cycles of sleep stages occur per night. Although there are variations between sleepers, these averages are a good approximation of the time distribution of non-REM sleep, REM sleep, and wakefulness during a typical night of sleep (Box 15-1).

The classic states of non-REM and REM sleep are not easily identified at birth with standard EEG, electromyographic (EMG), and electrooculographic (EOG) analysis. Although similarities exist between the sleep states that occur in newborns and adults, sleep stages during the neonatal period are generally categorized as active sleep, quiet sleep, and intermediate sleep. Active sleep is comparable to REM sleep; quiet and intermediate sleep states have many of the same characteristics of non-REM. It is worth noting that infants enter active sleep first instead of entering into quiet sleep as adults do. Between 6 to 8 weeks of age, infant sleep becomes more predictable; and by 12 weeks of age, the various stages of non-REM sleep and REM sleep are recognizable. By 12 months of age, infants exhibit the classic sleep stages seen in adults. As mentioned previously, sleep-state distribution for healthy adult sleepers during a typical 8-hour period of sleep usually involves non-REM and REM sleep states alternating cyclically every 90 to 120 minutes, with periods of REM sleep lasting from 10 to 30 minutes. In contrast, infants spend considerably more time in REM sleep than adult sleepers (i.e., during various stages in development, infants may spend as much as 75% of their sleep in REM).[1,5]

Effect of Sleep on Breathing

The effects of sleep on breathing are summarized in Table 15-2. As the sleeper passes through the various stages of non-REM sleep, there is a progressive reduction in chemosensitivity and respiratory drive. The reduction in respiratory drive that occurs during the early stages of non-REM sleep (Stages 1 and 2) predisposes the person to apneic periods (i.e., **Cheyne-Stokes respiration**) when fluctuating between being awake and asleep. With the establishment of non-REM slow-wave sleep (Stages 3 and 4), nonrespiratory inputs are minimized, and minute ventilation is regulated by metabolic control. Minute ventilation decreases by 1 to 2 L/min when compared with wakefulness. As a consequence, the partial pressure of arterial carbon dioxide ($PaCO_2$) rises by 2 to 8 mm Hg, and the partial pressure of oxygen in the arteries (PaO_2) decreases by 5 to 10 mm Hg.

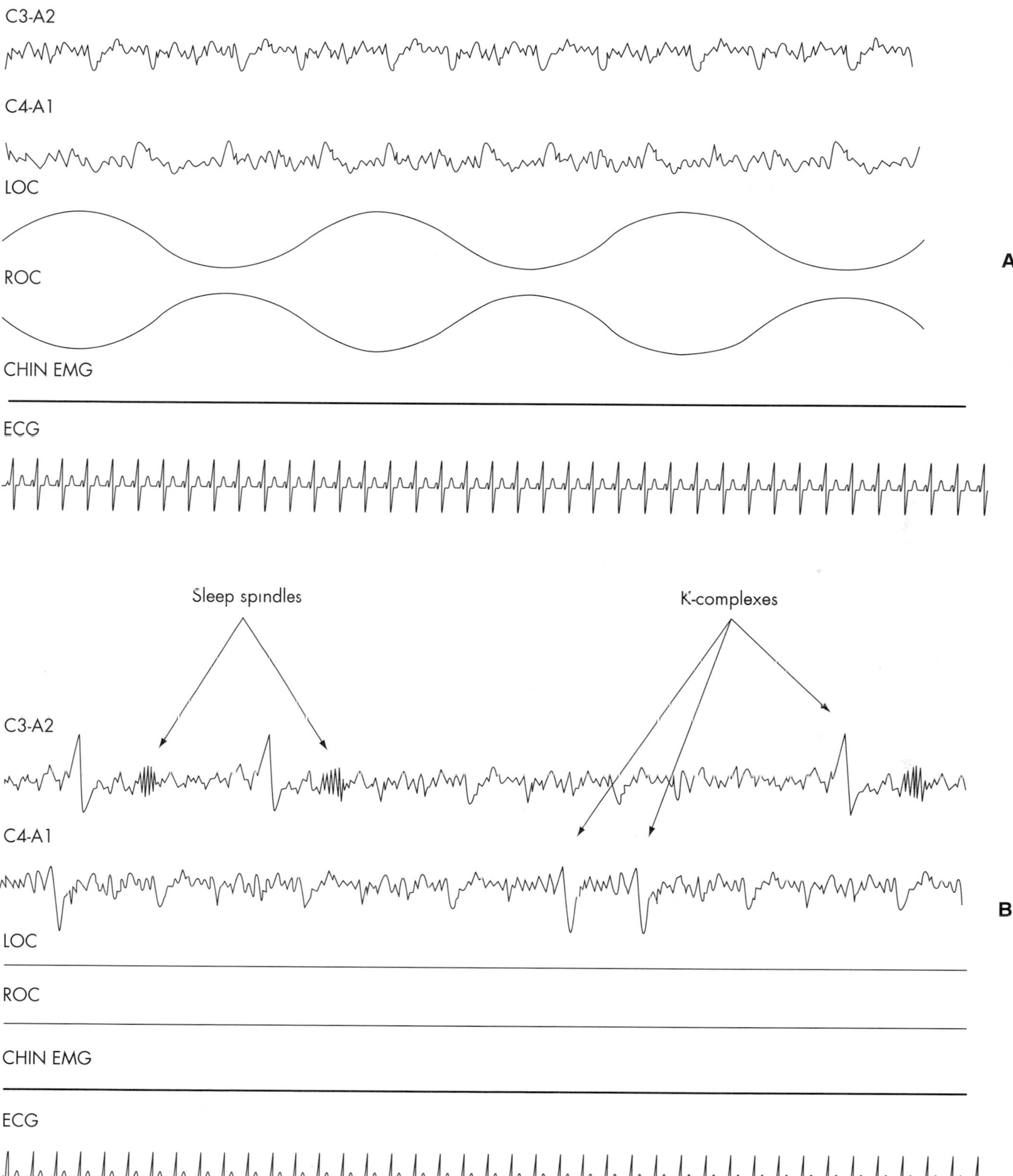

Figure 15-1 **A,** Stage 1 sleep. Stage 1 is characterized by a relatively low-voltage, mixed frequency EEG; slow, rolling eye movements (*LOC* and *ROC* relate to eye movements that are left of center and right of center, respectively); and tonic EMG activity. **B,** Stage 2 sleep. Stage 2 is characterized by relatively low-voltage background EEG activity; sleep spindles and K-complexes; absence of eye movements; and tonic EMG activity.

Continued

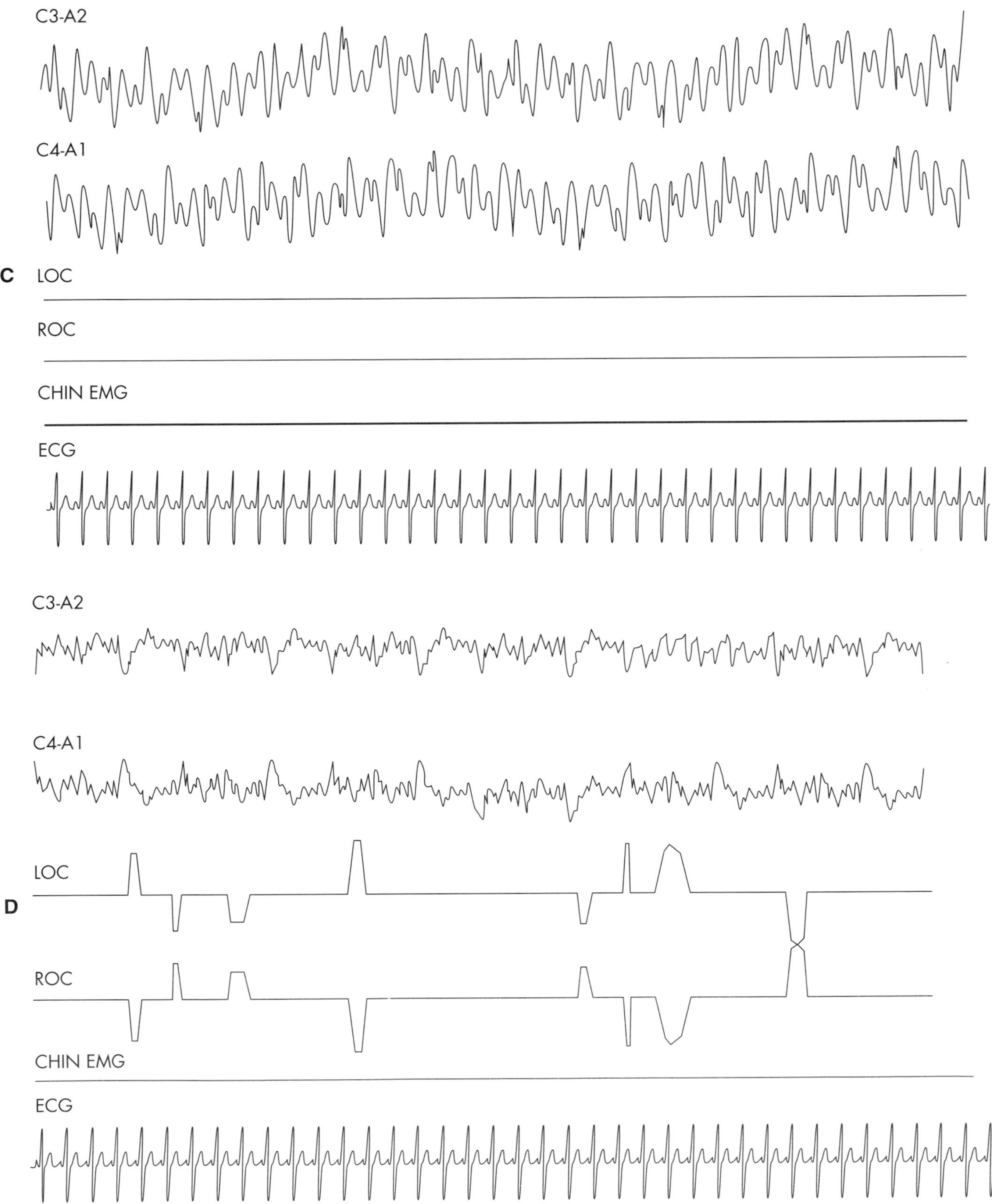

Figure 15-1 cont'd **C,** Stage 4 sleep. Stage 4 is characterized by high-voltage, slow-wave EEG activity; absence of eye movements; and tonic EMG activity. **D,** REM sleep. REM sleep is characterized by relatively low-voltage, mixed frequency background EEG activity, with a burst of notched theta waves; rapid, saccadic, conjugate eye movements; and chin muscle tone significantly decreased from waking and non–rapid-eye-movement (NREM) sleep level. (Redrawn from Sheldon SH, Spire JP, Levy HB: *Pediatric sleep medicine*, Philadelphia, 1992, WB Saunders.)

As the sleeper enters into REM sleep, breathing becomes irregular as the ventilatory response to chemical and mechanical respiratory stimuli is further reduced and even transiently abolished. Skeletal muscle activity, along with the intercostal and accessory muscles of respiration, is decreased, and the upper airway muscles are inhibited. This inhibition leads to an increase in upper airway resistance, whereas inhibition of the intercostal and accessory muscles is associated with diminished thoracoabdominal coupling and short periods of central apnea for durations of 10 to 20 seconds. $PaCO_2$ and PaO_2 levels are variable, but are generally similar to those in the latter stages of non-REM sleep.

Effect of Sleep on Cardiovascular Function

The effects of sleep on cardiovascular function are shown in Figure 15-3. In most individuals, both heart rate and blood pressure are generally reduced during sleep. Reductions in heart rate average about 5 to 10 beats/minute during non-REM sleep and up to 15 beats/minute during REM sleep.

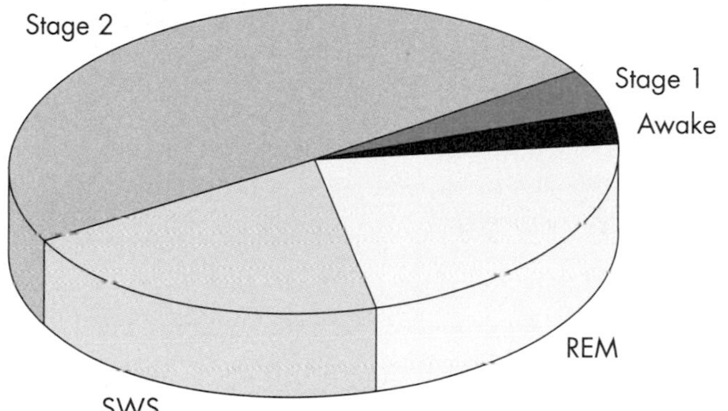

Stage	Percent of Total Recording Time
Wake after sleep onset	Less than 5%
Stage-1	2% to 5%
Stage-2	45% to 55%
Slow-wave sleep	13% to 23%
REM	20% to 25%

Figure 15-2 Sleep stage distribution in normal healthy adults. (Redrawn from Sheldon SH, Spire JP, Levy HB: *Pediatric sleep medicine*, Philadelphia, 1992, WB Saunders.)

Box 15-1 How Much Sleep Do We Need?

It is generally accepted that the amount of sleep that an individual requires is influenced by their age. Infants typically require about 16 hours per day, and teenagers need 8 or 9 hours per night on average. For most adults, 7 to 8 hours per night seems to be sufficient, although some people only require about 5 hours per day, and others require as many as 10 hours of sleep each day. As they get older (>60 years of age), people tend to sleep more lightly and for shorter periods. What may not be obvious is that we continue to need about the same amount of sleep that we require in early adulthood.

Certain conditions can also influence the amount of sleep that we require. That is, we have an increased need for sleep while recovering from an acute illness, such as a cold or the flu. Women in their first trimester of pregnancy often need several more hours of sleep than usual. The amount of sleep a person needs also increases when there has been a deprival of sleep in previous days. Getting too little sleep creates a "sleep debt," which ultimately must be repaid. Although we may think that we can adapt to getting less sleep than we need, sleep deprivation can severely alter our judgment, reaction time, and other neurologic functions.

See the National Institute of Neurological Disorders and Stroke website: *www.ninds.nih.gov* for more details.

Table 15-2 Physiologic effect of sleep on respiration

Feature	Sleep Stages 1 and 2	Sleep Stages 3 and 4	REM sleep
Pattern of breathing	Periodic	Stable	Irregular
Apneas	Short, central	Rare	Short, central
$PaCO_2$	Variable	↑ 2-8 mm Hg above wakefulness	Variable, similar to Stages 3, 4
Ribcage muscles	Active	Active	Inhibited
Diaphragm	Active	Active	Active
Upper airway muscles	Active	Active	Inhibited
Chemoresponsiveness	↓ Compared with wakefulness	↓ compared with Stages 1, 2	↓ compared with Stages 3, 4
Arousability to respiratory stimuli	Low thresholds	Low thresholds	High thresholds

From Phillipson EA: Sleep disorders. In Murray JF, Nadel JE: *Textbook of respiratory medicine*, Philadelphia, 1997, WB Saunders.

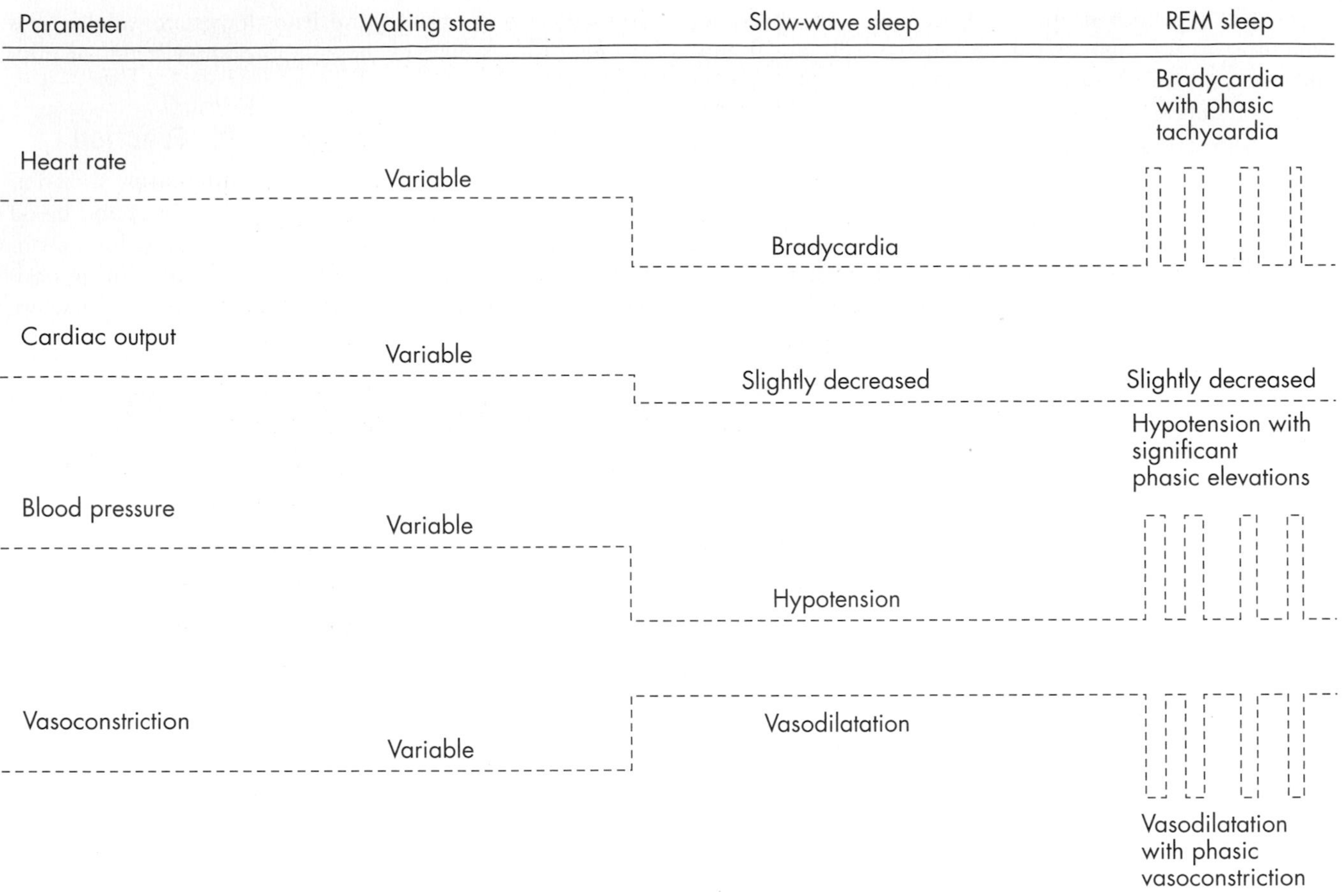

Parameter
Waking state
Slow-wave sleep
REM sleep
Heart rate
Variable
Bradycardia
Bradycardia with phasic tachycardia
Cardiac output
Variable
Slightly decreased
Slightly decreased
Blood pressure
Variable
Hypotension
Hypotension with significant phasic elevations
Vasoconstriction
Variable
Vasodilatation
Vasodilatation with phasic vasoconstriction

Figure 15-3 The effect of sleep on cardiovascular function in awake and sleep states. (Redrawn from Sheldon SH, Spire JP, Levy HB: *Pediatric sleep medicine*, Philadelphia, 1992, WB Saunders.)

Blood pressure shows a moderate decrease of 10 to 15 mm Hg during non-REM sleep and up to 25 mm Hg during REM sleep. Alterations in heart rate seen during sleep seem to parallel sleep-related alterations in blood pressure. These variations are especially evident during REM sleep, when arterial blood pressure varies to a greater extent than during non-REM sleep.[5] Changes in blood pressure during REM sleep are characterized as sharp increases in mean arterial pressure, which are superimposed on a relatively hypotensive state.

Cardiac output is usually only slightly reduced during non-REM sleep when compared with the waking state. The reduction in cardiac output, however, is more pronounced during REM sleep (e.g., approximately a 10% reduction).[5] Changes in cardiac output that are seen during sleep are not accompanied by changes in stroke volume, which tend to remain similar to values measured while the person is in a quiet, awake state.[5]

Diagnosis of Sleep Apnea

The ability to wake from sleep or to rouse to a lighter stage of sleep requires activation of higher neurologic centers (i.e., the reticular activating system and cortex).[2] Such activation results in an immediate increase in respiratory drive, activation of the upper airway muscles, stimulation of the cough reflex, and initiation of behavioral responses, specifically increases in skeletal muscle tone.[2,4] If these **arousal responses** do not occur, sleep apnea or alveolar hypoventilation can result.

Diagnosis of sleep apnea is based on information derived from patient history and physical examination and from laboratory studies that focus on sleep structure and cardiorespiratory function. The medical history and physical examination provide information that can be used to determine whether patients are at risk for sleep apnea and if they demonstrate the common symptoms and signs associated with various sleep-related disorders. Laboratory studies range from simple overnight monitoring of arterial blood gases with pulse oximetry and transcutaneous monitoring to analyzing cardiopulmonary and neuromuscular function with **polysomnography.**

Polysomnography

Although patient history and physical examination can provide evidence that a patient may be afflicted with sleep apnea, the data may be equivocal and thus lead the clinician to under- or overestimate the severity of the patient's sleep-

Table 15-3 Laboratory investigation of respiratory disturbances during sleep

Type of Test	Variable Measured	Technique
Screening	SaO_2	Ear oximeter
	PCO_2	Transcutaneous sensor
	Heart rate, rhythm	Holter monitoring
Standard polysomnography	EEG	Surface electrodes
	EOG	Surface electrodes
	Submental EMG	Surface electrodes
	Tibialis EMG	Surface electrodes
	Breathing pattern	Surface electrodes
	SaO_2, PCO_2	Ear oximeter, transcutaneous sensor
	Electrocardiogram	Standard electrodes
Special procedures	Intrapleural pressure	Esophageal catheter
	Diaphragm EMG	Esophageal or surface electrodes
	Esophageal pH	Esophageal electrodes
	Arterial blood gases	Arterial catheter
	Pulmonary arterial pressure	Swan-Ganz catheter
	Systemic blood pressure	Arterial catheter

From Phillipson EA: Sleep disorders. In Murray JF, Nadel JE: *Textbook of respiratory medicine*, Philadelphia, 1997, WB Saunders.

disordered breathing. For this reason, laboratory assessment of patients suspected to have sleep apnea should be performed to ensure a definitive diagnosis.

Table 15-3 summarizes the various laboratory procedures that can be used to investigate physiologic function during sleep. Although screening tests can provide valuable information about cardiopulmonary function during sleep, they do not allow for sleep staging and quantification of patient arousal or awakening during the course of the study. It is generally accepted that polysomnography is the gold standard for identifying the type and severity of sleep apnea. Polysomnography usually includes all-night audio/video monitoring of the patient, as well as recordings of ECGs, respiratory activity, EEGs, EOGs, and EMGs.[6] (Clinical Practice Guideline 15-1 summarizes the American Association for Respiratory Care (AARC) Clinical Practice Guideline for Polysomnography.) Besides being used to determine whether a patient demonstrates sleep apnea or hypopnea, polysomnography can also provide valuable information about the most effective means of treating these patients.

Electrocardiography

Cardiac activity, including heart rate and rhythm, is usually monitored with at least two ECG leads (e.g., lead II and a modified chest lead). It is important to recognize that monitoring two ECG leads can only provide limited information about the electrical activity of the heart. If more information about the patient's ECG is required, a 12-lead ECG or **Holter monitoring** may be indicated.

Electroencephalography

An EEG is a recording of fluctuations in the electric potentials of cortical neurons. These electric potentials are transmitted from the cortex through the coverings of the brain to the scalp, where electrodes placed at various points on the scalp are used to sense the sum of the potentials in the underlying cortex. EEGs provide valuable information on the integrity of the central nervous system and form the basis for identifying the various sleep stages that the patient enters during the sleep study.

To ensure that the information is meaningful and can be compared with that of different laboratories, a standardized system for electrode placement is used to record EEGs during sleep studies. The standard EEG montage used for polysomnography is based on the **International 10-20 EEG system** (Figure 15-4).[5,7] Note that modified EEG recordings that are typically used to stage sleep may not identify seizure disorders; therefore, in cases where seizures are suspected, more elaborate EEG recordings, as well as a neurologic consultation, may be necessary.

To place electrodes properly, one should first mark where they will be placed on the scalp. It is important to recognize that improper placement of these electrodes can severely affect the validity of the sleep study and lead to erroneous data. The scalp should be cleaned with alcohol to minimize

Clinical Practice Guidelines 15-1

Polysomnography

Indications

Polysomnography may be indicated for patients demonstrating any of the following conditions:

- Chronic obstructive pulmonary disease with an awake PaO_2 >55 mm Hg whose illness is complicated by pulmonary hypertension, right heart failure, polycythemia, or excessive daytime sleepiness
- Restrictive ventilatory impairment secondary to chest-wall and neuromuscular disturbances whose illness is complicated by chronic hypoventilation, polycythemia, pulmonary hypertension, disturbed sleep, morning headaches, or daytime somnolence and fatigue
- Disturbances of respiratory control with an awake $PaCO_2$ >45 torr, or patients whose illness is complicated by pulmonary hypertension, polycythemia, disturbed sleep, morning headaches, or daytime somnolence and fatigue
- Nocturnal cyclic bradyarrhythmias or tachyarrhythmias, nocturnal abnormalities of atrioventricular conduction, or ventricular ectopy that appears to increase in frequency during sleep
- Excessive daytime sleepiness or insomnia
- Snoring, which is associated with observed apneas or excessive daytime sleepiness

Contraindications

There are no absolute contraindications to polysomnography when indications are clearly established. Risk:benefit ratios should be assessed, however, if medically unstable inpatients are to be transferred from the clinical setting to a sleep laboratory for overnight polysomnography.

Precautions/Complications:

- Skin irritation may occur as a result of the adhesive used to attach electrodes to the patient
- At the conclusion of the study, adhesive remover is used to dissolve adhesive on the patient's skin. Adhesive removers (e.g., acetone) should only be used in well-ventilated areas.
- Engineering (or qualified biomedical personnel) must certify the integrity of the polysomnographic equipment's electrical isolation.
- The adhesive used to attach EEG electrodes, (e.g., collodion) should not be used to attach electrodes near the patient's eyes and should always be used in well-ventilated areas.
- Because of the high flammability of collodion and acetone, they should be used with caution, especially with patients requiring supplemental oxygen.
- Collodion should be used with caution in small infants and patients with reactive airway disease.
- Patients with parasomnias or seizures may be at risk for injury related to movements during sleep. Institution-specific policies and guidelines describing personnel responsibilities and appropriate responses should be developed.

Assessment of Need

Polysomnography should be used to assess oxygenation, cardiac status, and sleep continuity in those patients who are suspected of having sleep-related respiratory disturbances, periodic limb-movement disorders, or any of the sleep disorders described in the Internal Classification of Sleep Disorders Diagnostic and Coding Manual.

Assessment of Test Quality

- Polysomnography should either confirm or eliminate a diagnosis of a sleep-related respiratory disturbance.
- Documentation of findings, suggested therapeutic intervention, or other clinical decisions resulting from polysomnography should be noted on the patient's chart.
- Each laboratory should devise and implement indicators of quality assurance for equipment calibration and maintenance, patient preparation and monitoring, scoring methodology, and scoring variances between technicians.

For a complete copy of this guideline, see American Association for Respiratory Care: Clinical practice guideline: polysomnography, *Respir Care* 40(12):1236, 1995.

electrical impedance. The cup-shaped electrodes are filled with conductive paste or jelly and affixed to the scalp with cotton or gauze. The electrodes can be affixed to the scalp with tape or glue, or they can be anchored to the scalp by placing a piece of gauze soaked in collodion over the electrode (notice that the gauze can be dried with compressed air after it has been positioned over the electrode). After the electrodes are affixed to the patient, the electrode wires are then plugged into a junction box, which is coupled to the polygraph recorder.

Respiratory Activity

Assessment of respiratory activity during sleep usually involves measuring oxygen saturation, nasal-oral airflow, and respiratory effort. Oxygen saturation can be easily assessed using pulse oximetry or transcutaneous monitoring. (See Chapter 10 for a detailed discussion of noninvasive blood gas monitoring.) The pulse oximeter probe is placed on an earlobe, finger, or toe. Although transcutaneous monitoring can be used to assess oxygenation during sleep, the transcutaneous probe must be repositioned intermittently (every 2 to 4 hours), and may therefore interfere with the patient's sleep and lead to inadvertent arousal during the study. Indwelling arterial catheters can also be used to assess arterial blood gases, but the risks outweigh the benefits of using this approach and may lead to unnecessary complications.

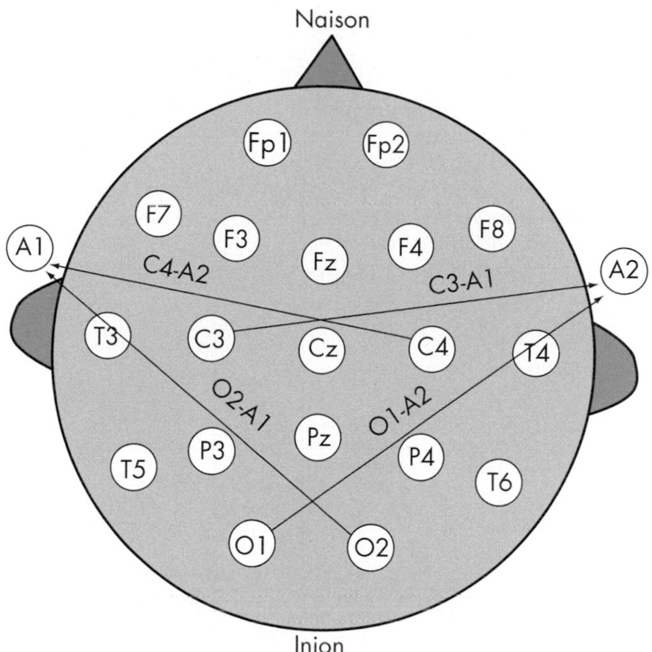

Figure 15-4 A standard polysomnographic EEG montage. (Redrawn from Sheldon SH, Spire JP, Levy HB: *Pediatric sleep medicine*, Philadelphia, 1992, WB Saunders.)

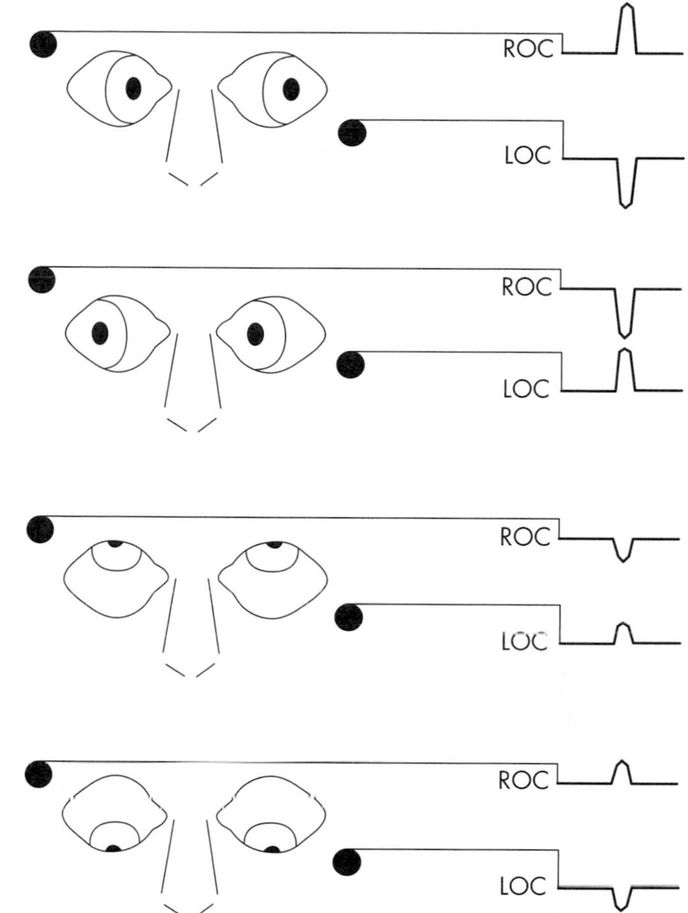

Figure 15-5 Electrooculogram electrode placement. ROC indicates eye movement to the right of center; LOC indicates eye movement to the left of center. (Redrawn from Sheldon SH, Spire JP, Levy HB: Pediatric sleep medicine, Philadelphia, 1992, WB Saunders.)

Nasal-oral airflow is typically measured by a thermistor or thermocouple device at the airway opening. The most common problems with these devices relate to probe position (i.e., the technician may have to reposition the probe frequently and adjust the amplifier sensitivity, thus disturbing the patient's sleep and reducing the validity of the study).

Respiratory effort can be measured by recording rib cage and abdominal movements, measuring intrapleural pressure changes, or measuring airflow at the airway opening with a pneumotachograph. A variety of devices are available for measuring rib cage and abdominal movements, including strain gauge or piezoelectric belts placed around the chest or abdomen, respiratory inductance plethysmography, and impedance pneumography. Intrapleural pressure changes can be measured with an esophageal balloon catheter positioned in the upper third of the esophagus that is connected to a standard strain-gauge pressure transducer.

Remember that, although all of these techniques can provide measurements of respiratory effort, techniques that restrict patient movement can compromise test results. Techniques that make the patient uncomfortable can ultimately decrease patient compliance during the study.

Electromyography

Electromyographic recording of various skeletal muscles can be accomplished during sleep using surface electrodes similar to those used for ECGs. Monitoring EMG signals can provide information about the patient's sleep-wake behavior and also allows arousal responses and sleep movements to be quantified. EMG signals recorded from the intercostal muscles can also be used to assess respiratory movements, which is a rather cumbersome technique considering the alternative methods of measuring respiratory activity that were discussed in the previous section.

Three electrodes are typically affixed to the chin with tape. Two of these electrodes are placed between the tip of the chin and the hyoid bone, lateral to each other and 2 cm apart; a third electrode is placed in the center of the chin. The submental EMG signal recorded from these electrodes is used to detect activation of the muscles that expand the upper airways (e.g., the genioglossus and the geniohyoid).[8] When leg movements are to be assessed, two surface electrodes are taped about 3 to 5 cm apart on each leg over the tibialis anterior muscle.

Electrooculography

Recording eye movements during sleep allows the non-REM and REM sleep states to be identified. Electrodes are placed on the skin surface in the periorbital region, specifically about 1 cm lateral to the outer canthi of the eyes and offset from the horizontal plane (i.e., 1 cm above the horizontal plane on one side and 1 cm below the horizontal plane on the other side). With this configuration, horizontal, vertical, and oblique eye movements can be detected. Figure 15-5 shows how these movements are recorded. Note that the height or depth of the deflection depends on the movement of the eyes relative to the fixed electrodes and is described as being either right-of-center (ROC) or left-of-center (LOC).[5]

Calibration of Polysomnography Signals

Calibration of the polysomnography equipment should be performed before the electrodes are placed on the patient using manufacturer's recommendations (check the user's manual for details on calibrating various channels). After the electrodes and sensors are affixed to the patient, a presleep calibration should be performed. This calibration lets the technician determine if all of the electrodes and sensors are positioned properly, if the amplifier settings are appropriate for retrieving meaningful data, and if there are any recording device malfunctions (i.e., chart recorder is functioning improperly). It also provides a series of baseline references for awake measurements. Documenting all calibrations is essential because if calibration is performed inadequately, the test results are ultimately invalid.

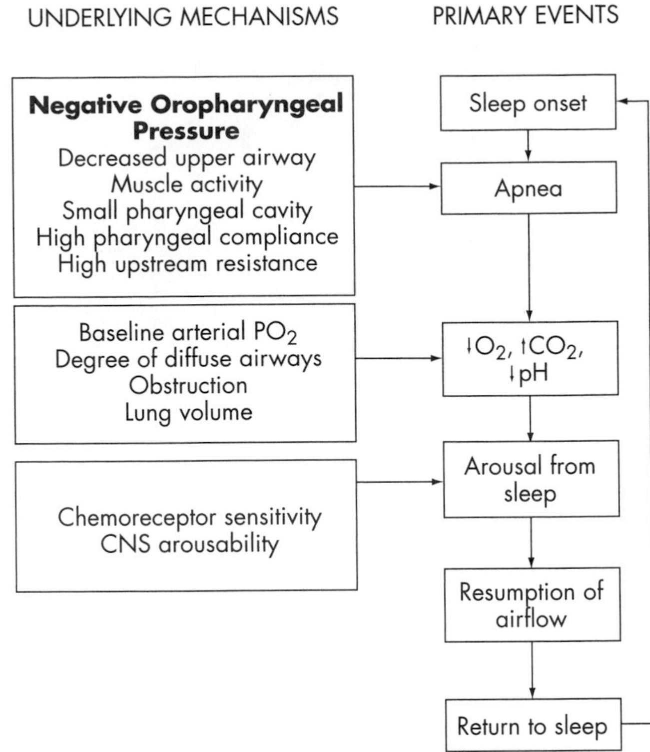

Figure 15-6 The primary sequence of events in OSA, along with the pathogenic mechanisms that contribute to these events. (Redrawn from Bradley TD, Phillipson EA: Pathogenesis and pathophysiology of the obstructive sleep apnea syndrome, *Med Clin North Am* 69:1169, 1985.)

Pathophysiology of Sleep Apnea

Sleep apnea is defined as repeated episodes of complete airflow cessation for longer than 10 seconds.[9] Hypopnea, in contrast, is usually defined as a reduction in airflow by 50% or more for 10 seconds, with some residual airflow and a physiologic consequence (i.e., arterial oxygen desaturation).[10,11] To compare the frequency of apnea with that of hypopnea during a sleep study, an **apnea index (AI)** or an **apnea/hypopnea index (AHI)** is usually calculated. The AI is the number of apneic periods observed divided by the total number of hours of sleep; the AHI includes both apneic and hypopneic episodes for the total number of hours of sleep. Normative data of asymptomatic individuals from Guilleminault and Dement[12] suggest that males average about seven apneic episodes per 8 hours of sleep, and females only average about two episodes per 8 hours of sleep.

Sleep apnea syndrome is considered to be present if apnea occurs in excess of five times per hour of sleep.[10,11] As such, three types of sleep apnea are generally described: obstructive sleep apnea (OSA), central sleep apnea, and mixed sleep apnea. OSA is characterized by the lack of airflow resulting from occlusion of the upper airways despite continued respiratory efforts. Central sleep apnea is characterized by the absence of airflow and respiratory efforts. Mixed sleep apnea has characteristics of both central and obstructive sleep apnea, with the central event usually preceding the obstructive event.

Obstructive Sleep Apnea

In OSA, airflow at the airway opening ceases because of complete occlusion of the upper airway. Occlusion of the upper airway may occur with posterior movements of the tongue and palate. As these structures move posteriorly, they come into apposition with the posterior pharyngeal wall, resulting in occlusion of the nasopharynx and the oropharynx.[2] Figure 15-6 shows the sequence of events that typically occur in OSA. Notice that obstruction of the upper airways initiates the primary sequence of events. Then apnea and progressive asphyxia develop until there is arousal from sleep, restoration of upper airway patency, and resumption of airflow. With relief of asphyxia, the person quickly returns to sleep—only to have the sequence of events repeat itself over and over. In fact, the sequence can repeat itself several hundred times per night.[13]

As seen in Figure 15-7, OSA is associated with several physiologic consequences and clinical features.[14] The physiologic consequences of OSA include the development of cardiac arrhythmias, pulmonary and systemic hypertension, acute hypercapnia, cerebral dysfunction, loss of deep sleep and sleep fragmentation, and excessive motor activity. These physiologic alterations can result in turn in restless sleep, excessive daytime sleepiness, personality and behavioral

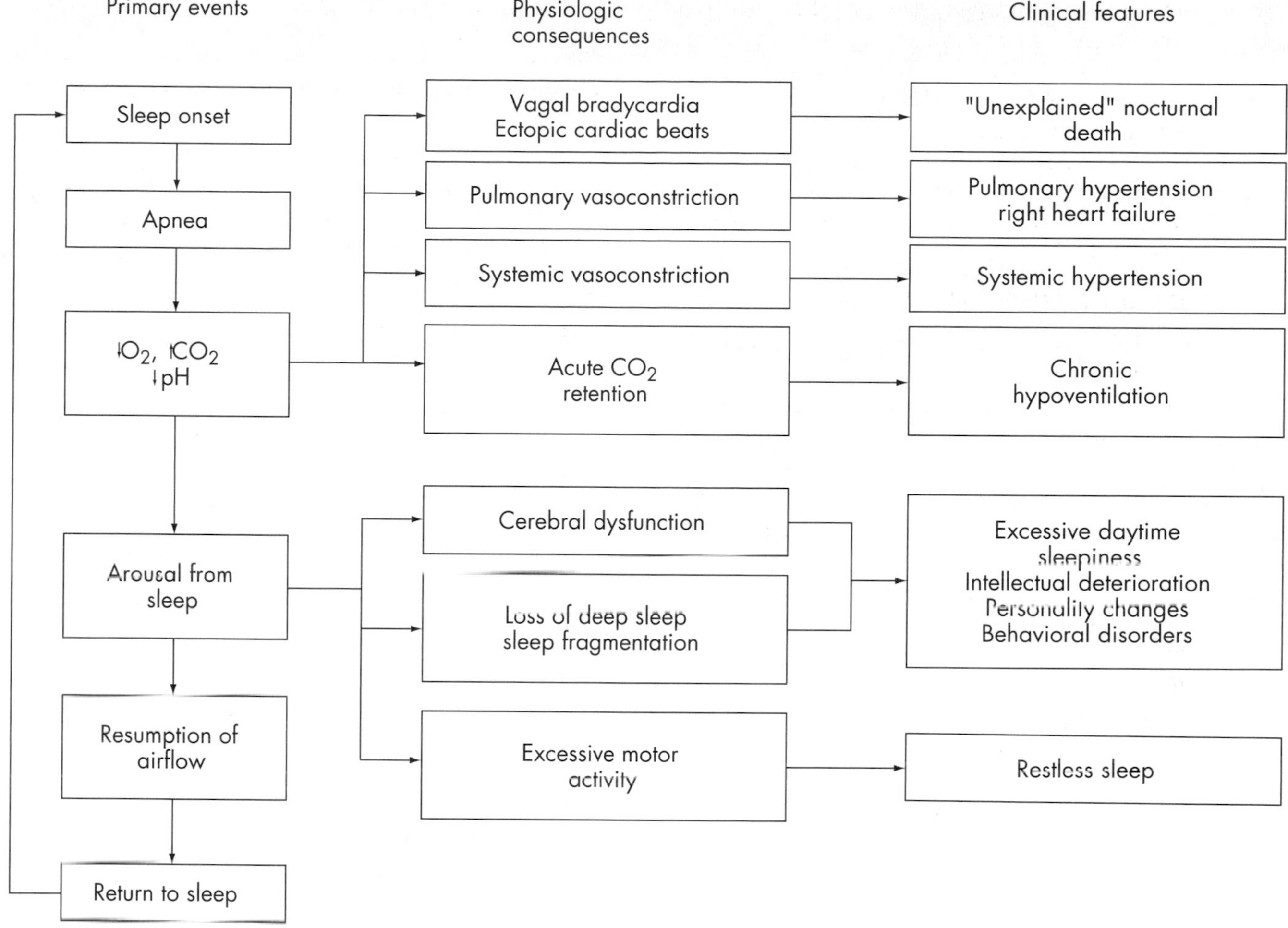

Figure 15-7 The physiologic response and clinical features that result from sleep apnea. (Redrawn from Bradley TD, Phillipson EA: Sleep apnea, *Med Clin North Am* 23:2314-2323, 1982.)

changes, intellectual deterioration, right-heart failure, and unexplained nocturnal death.[2]

The most common symptoms associated with OSA in adult patients include chronic loud snoring, gasping or choking episodes during sleep, excessive daytime sleepiness, morning headaches, and personality and cognitive deterioration related to fatigue from lack of sleep. Box 15-2 contains the standard definition of OSA, which was published by the American Sleep Disorders Association.[15] Patients at the greatest risk of developing OSA are those who are obese (particularly those demonstrating nuchal obesity [i.e., neck size >17 inches for men and >16 inches for women] and nasopharyngeal narrowing). Systemic hypertension also adds to the risk of OSA. The symptoms of OSA may be worse when patients ingest central nervous system depressants (e.g., sedatives, hypnotics) or consume alcohol, especially when it is ingested close to bedtime. Partial sleep deprivation, such as occurs with shift work, may also affect patients with moderate OSA symptoms. Respiratory allergies and environmental factors, such as smoking and ascent to altitude, can augment the symptoms of patients with mild OSA.

Figure 15-8 shows the key polysomnographic events that occur during the apneic episode of a patient with OSA. Although there is a cessation of airflow, respiratory efforts continue, as evidenced by movement of the rib cage and the abdomen. During the apneic episode, there is a fall in oxygen saturation. Clinical Rounds 15-1 presents the case of a patient with OSA.

The criteria for defining OSA in children are not as well-established as those for adults.[10] In children, OSA is best identified by combining phasic oxygen desaturation, hypercarbia, and intermittent paradoxical respiratory efforts. (Note that oxygen desaturation of less than 92% is generally considered abnormal in children, depending on their baseline oxygen saturation. Brief oxygen desaturations of >4% occur infrequently in children, and thus should be considered abnormal. Measurements of end-tidal partial pressure of carbon dioxide [$PetCO_2$] can also provide evidence of sleep-disordered breathing in children. It has

Box 15-2 Standard Definition of Obstructive Sleep Apnea

1. Patient complains of excessive sleepiness or insomnia. Occasionally, patients are unaware of the clinical features observed by others.
2. Patient experiences frequent episodes of obstructed breathing during sleep.
3. Associated features include loud snoring, morning headaches, a dry mouth upon awakening, and chest retraction during sleep in younger children.
4. Polysomnographic monitoring demonstrates more than five obstructive apneas >10 seconds each in duration per hour of sleep, and one or more of the following:
   - Frequent arousal from sleep associated with apneas
   - Bradytachycardia
   - Arterial oxygen desaturation in association with the apneic episode—with or without a multi-sleep latency of less than 10 minutes
5. OSA can be associated with other medical disorders (e.g., tonsillar enlargement).
6. Other sleep disorders can be present (e.g., periodic limb movement disorder or narcolepsy).

From Diagnostic Steering Committee: *The international classification of sleep disorders: diagnostic and coding manual,* ed 2, Lawrence, Kan, 1997, Allen Press.

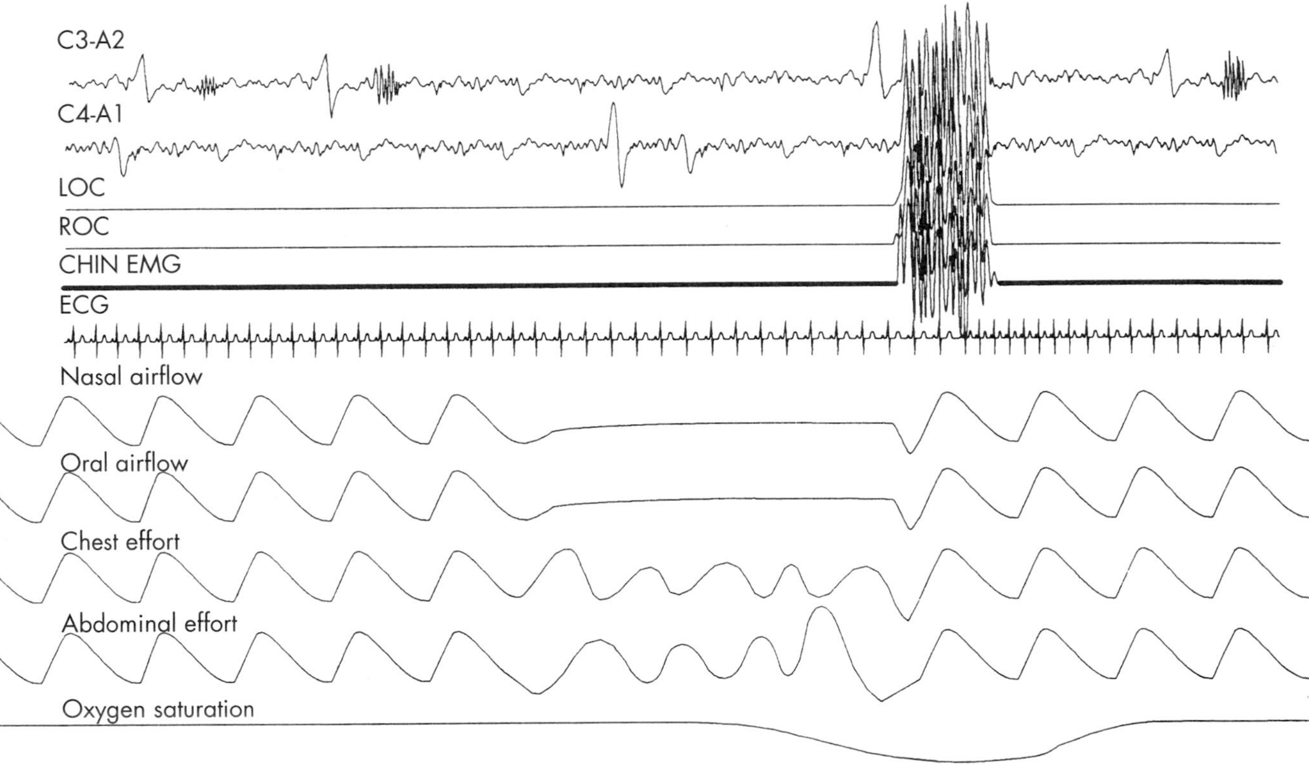

Figure 15-8 Polysomnographic tracings of a patient demonstrating OSA during REM sleep. The patient exhibited constant loud snoring, paradoxical movement of the chest and abdomen, and recurrent complete airway obstructions, leading to oxygen desaturation. (Redrawn from Sheldon SH, Spire JP, Levy HB: *Pediatric sleep medicine,* Philadelphia, 1992, WB Saunders.)

been suggested that $PetCO_2$ values of >45 torr for at least 60% of the total sleep time or $PetCO_2$ values >13 torr above baseline values indicate sleep-disordered breathing.)[10] Other criteria that should be noted when diagnosing sleep apnea in children include snoring, frequent arousal, and difficulty breathing while asleep, as well as failure to thrive, cor pulmonale, or neurobehavioral disturbances.[16]

Central Sleep Apnea

Central sleep apnea includes several disorders associated with cessation of respiratory drive and a complete loss of EMG activity of the respiratory muscles. Several mechanisms that have been proposed to account for these alterations involve defects in respiratory control or muscle function,

CLINICAL ROUNDS 15-1

Mr. H. is a 62-year-old automobile mechanic with a 60-pack-per-year history of smoking cigarettes. He was referred to the sleep laboratory after he was involved in an automobile accident when he reportedly fell asleep while driving home from work. He is unaware of any chronic abnormalities with his sleep pattern, but he does acknowledge that he has experienced excessive daytime sleepiness. His wife reports that she has noticed that he snores throughout the night and his sleep has become increasingly restless during the past 6 months. In fact, his wife reports that his snoring has become loud enough to disturb her sleep, and jokes that if his snoring gets any louder the neighbor may begin to complain. She also reports that his snoring episodes are more frequent and considerably louder if he has a nightcap (i.e., consumes an alcoholic drink) before going to sleep.

Does this patient demonstrate any history and physical findings that suggest the presence of OSA? Briefly describe a diagnostic strategy to properly diagnose his condition.

See Appendix A for the answer.

transient fluctuation in respiratory drive, and reflex inhibition of central respiratory drive.[2] Central sleep apnea is associated with central alveolar hypoventilation, neuromuscular diseases involving the respiratory muscles, and central nervous system diseases, but it can occur secondary to hyperventilation, such as occurs when a person ascends to high altitudes. Central sleep apnea is also a common finding in patients who experience esophageal reflux or upper airway collapse. It is important to mention that only about 10% of apneic patients seen in most sleep laboratories have central sleep apnea, thus our knowledge of this disorder is somewhat limited when compared with the information available about OSA.[17]

Patients with central sleep apnea typically report gasping for air and shortness of breath upon awakening from a central sleep apneic episode. Depression, as assessed both subjectively and by formal testing, is a common finding among patients with central sleep apnea. It is interesting to note that patients with central sleep apnea do not normally report insomnia and hypersomnolence as do those with OSA. Patients with central sleep apnea typically have a normal body habitus, although obese patients may also demonstrate this form of sleep apnea.

Figure 15-9 shows an example of a polysomnographic tracing for a patient with central sleep apnea. As with OSA, there is a complete cessation of airflow that lasts for

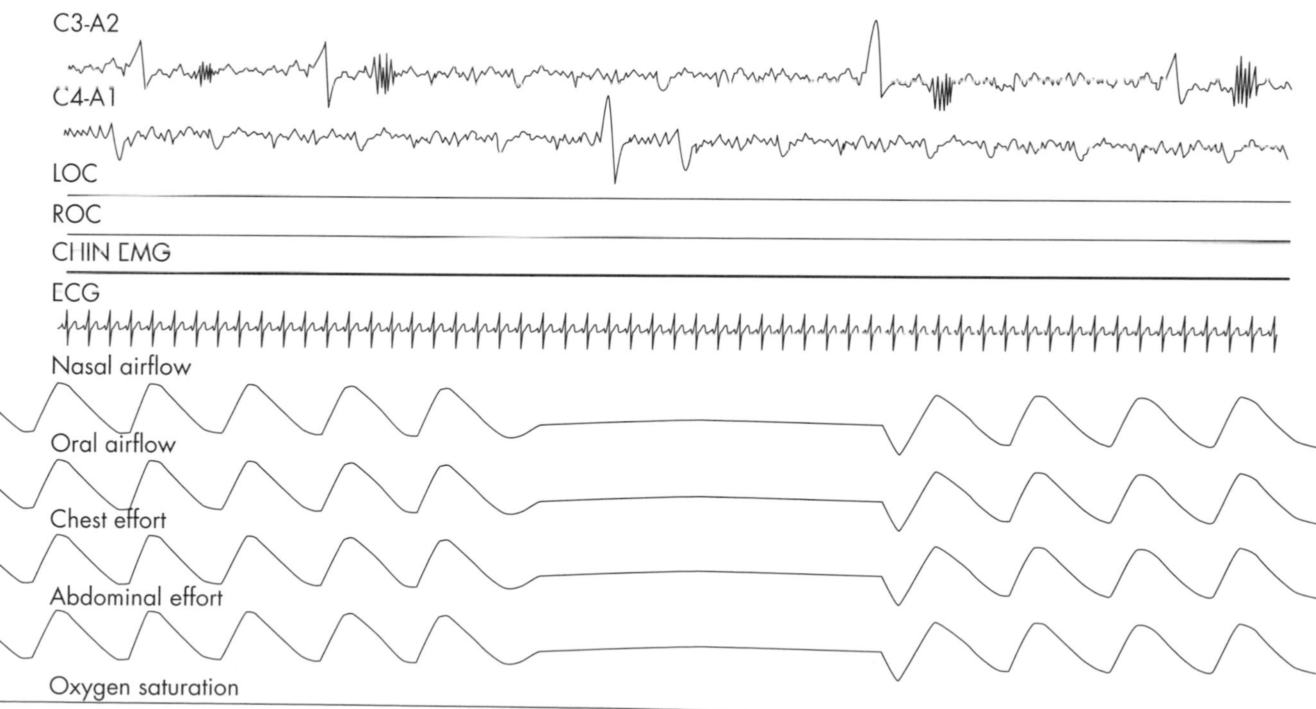

Figure 15-9 Polysomnographic tracings of a patient with central sleep apnea. Note that during the apneic episode there is complete cessation of nasal and oral airflow with concomitant absence of respiratory effort (i.e., no movements of chest or abdomen). (Redrawn from Sheldon SH, Spire JP, Levy HB: *Pediatric sleep medicine*, Philadelphia, 1992, WB Saunders.)

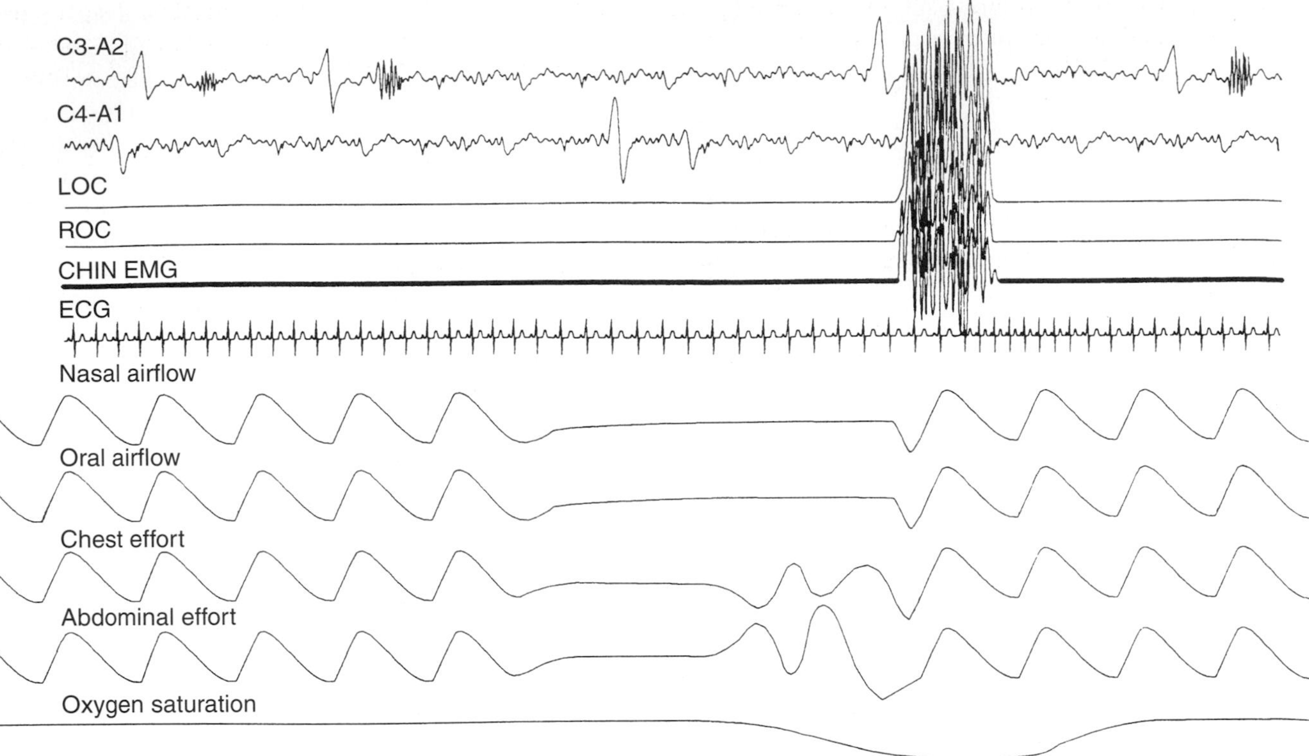

Figure 15-10 Polysomnographic tracings from a patient with mixed apnea. There is cessation of airflow at the nose and mouth. Initially, there is an absence of respiratory effort (central component), followed by at least two cycles of respiratory effort with continued absence of airflow (obstructive component). Significant oxygen desaturation is also present. Note that the EEG, EOG, and EMG signals are obscured by motion artifacts. (Redrawn from Sheldon SH, Spire JP, Levy HB: *Pediatric sleep medicine*, Philadelphia, 1992, WB Saunders.)

10 seconds or longer. In contrast to OSA, airflow cessation is associated with a cessation in respiratory effort, and thus no movement of the rib cage or abdomen.

Mixed Sleep Apnea

Most patients who experience central sleep apnea also demonstrate evidence of OSA. In fact, because these two types of apnea typically coexist, most authors define central sleep apnea as occurring in individuals in whom more than 55% of the apneic episodes are central in origin. The exact cause of mixed apnea is unclear at this time; but it has been suggested that the mechanisms responsible for central and obstructive sleep apnea may be related because several studies have shown that the upper airway muscles behave like respiratory muscles. That is, the upper airway muscles contract and dilate the pharynx when the diaphragm is stimulated.[18,19]

Polysomnography provides clear evidence of the presence of mixed apnea. As Figure 15-10 shows, airflow cessation is preceded by a central apneic event (i.e., no movement of the rib cage or abdomen). The obstructive component can be ascertained by observing that there is a resumption of respiratory effort, although there is still a

CLINICAL ROUNDS 15-2

The following polysomnogram was obtained from a 45-year-old post-polio patient who was referred to the sleep laboratory for diagnosis of sleep apnea. She complains of restless sleep, morning headaches, chronic fatigue, and daytime sleepiness.

Interpret these findings.

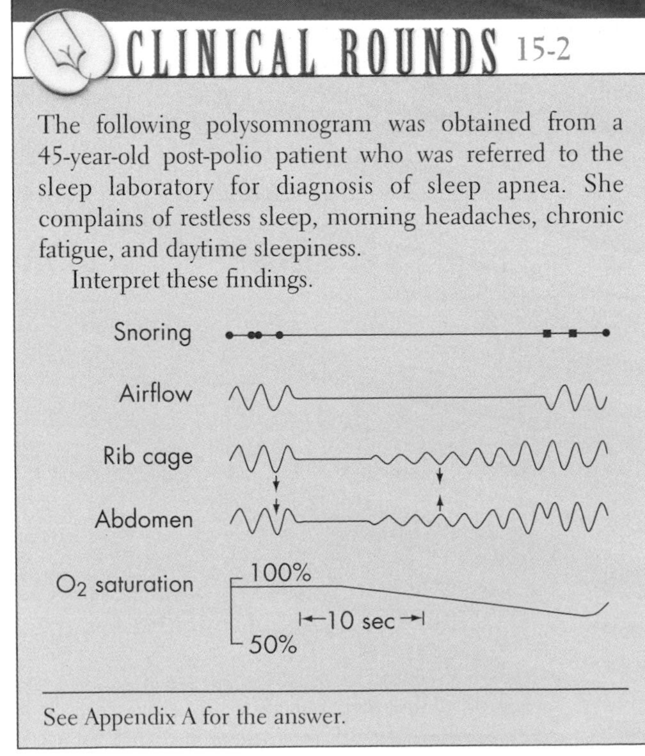

See Appendix A for the answer.

cessation of airflow. With arousal from sleep, the apneic event ends and airflow resumes as the airway opens (Clinical Rounds 15-2).

Summary

The physiologic effects of sleep on breathing are normally of little consequence in healthy individuals. In patients with altered respiratory function, however, sleep can have profound effects on physiologic function, which—if left untreated—can lead to dire consequences. Recent advances in our understanding of sleep structure and ability to assess cardiopulmonary and neuromuscular function during sleep have greatly improved our ability to recognize and treat sleep-related disorders.

Three types of sleep apnea are described: obstructive, central, and mixed. OSA is characterized by airflow cessation at the airway opening, even though the patient continues to make respiratory efforts. Central sleep apnea involves a complete cessation of respiratory efforts and airflow, and mixed apnea includes characteristics of both obstructive and central apnea. In patients with mixed apnea, the central apneic component typically precedes the obstructive event.

Diagnosis of sleep apnea is based on clinical findings, including patient history and physical examination, along with laboratory studies. Obtaining a complete history and physical examination is the first step of identifying if an individual is at risk for sleep apnea. Overnight monitoring of arterial blood gases with pulse oximetry or transcutaneous electrodes or polysomnography is then performed to make a definitive diagnosis of sleep apnea.

Although there is some controversy about the best strategy to use when attempting to diagnose sleep apnea, it is generally agreed that polysomnography is the gold standard for evaluating the presence and severity of sleep apnea. Polysomnography, which involves recording various electrogenic potentials (e.g., ECGs, EEGs, respiratory activity, and EOGs) can also be used to select the most effective management strategy after sleep apnea is identified in a patient.

Review Questions

See Appendix A for the answers.

1. Which of the following are characteristic findings of Stage 2 of non-REM sleep?
   I. Sleep spindles and K-complexes on EEG
   II. Slow pendulous and disconjugate movements of the eyes
   III. A relatively low threshold for arousal from sleep
   IV. Adult patients typically enter this stage of sleep after about 90 minutes of non-REM sleep
   a. I and II only
   b. II and IV only
   c. I, II, and III only
   d. II, III, and IV only

2. The classic states of non-REM and REM sleep are not easily identified at birth using standard polysomnography. Briefly describe the structure of sleep for a 2-week-old neonate.

3. Describe the impact of sleep on breathing in a healthy adult.

4. Which of the following changes in cardiovascular function occurs during sleep?
   a. Heart rate increases by about 5 to 10 beats/min during non-REM sleep
   b. Blood pressure decreases by as much as 25 mm Hg during REM sleep
   c. Cardiac output increases only slightly during non-REM sleep
   d. Stroke volume remains constant during non-REM and REM sleep

5. When performing polysomnography, it is suggested that the technician monitor a minimum of at least two modified ECG leads—true or false?

6. Sleep apnea is present if the person experiences at least ______ apneic events per hour of sleep.
   a. 3
   b. 5
   c. 8
   d. 10

7. List three variables that should be monitored to assess respiratory activity during polysomnography.

8. Which of the following are typical history and physical findings in patients with OSA?
   I. Chronic loud snoring
   II. Excessive daytime sleepiness
   III. Personality changes
   IV. Obesity
   a. I and III only
   b. II and IV only
   c. I, II, and III only
   d. I, II, III, and IV

9. Describe the physiologic consequences of OSA.

10. Which of the following are associated with central sleep apnea?
    I. Alveolar hypoventilation
    II. Myasthenia gravis
    III. Stroke
    IV. Angina pectoris
    a. I and II only
    b. II and III only
    c. I, II, and III only
    d. I, III, and IV only

11. Which of the following findings will a patient demonstrate during periods of mixed apnea with hypoxemia?

a. Systemic hypotension
b. Increased cardiac output
c. Decreased heart rate
d. Pulmonary hypertension

12. Which of the following are characteristic findings in children with obstructive sleep apnea?
I. Phasic oxygen desaturation
II. Hypercarbia
III. Intermittent paradoxical respiratory efforts
IV. Sinus tachycardia
a. I and III only
b. II and IV only
c. I, II, and III only
d. I, II, III, and IV

13. Which of the following are typical findings for patients with central sleep apnea?
I. These patients rarely reports insomnia.
II. The patient reports gasping for air upon awakening after an apneic event
III. Depression is a common finding in these patients
IV. Most patients with central sleep apnea are grossly overweight
a. I and II only
b. II and III only
c. I, II, and III only
d. II, III, and IV only

14. Define apnea/hypopnea index and describe how normative data for males differs from female subjects.

15. Which of the following drugs increase the incidence of obstructive sleep apnea?
I. Ethanol
II. Sedatives
III. Tricyclic antidepressants
IV. Hypnotics
a. II and III only
b. I, II, and III only
c. I, II, and IV only
d. I, III, and IV only

References

1. Guilleminault C, Dement WC: General physiology of sleep. In Crystal RG, West JB, editors: *The lung: scientific foundations*, New York, 1991, Raven Press, Ltd.
2. Bradley TD, Phillipson EA: Sleep disorders. In Murray JF, Nadel JA, editors: *Respiratory medicine*, ed 3, Philadelphia, 1994, WB Saunders.
3. Aserinsky E, Kleitman N: Regularly occurring periods of eye motility and concomitant phenomena during sleep, *Science* 118:273, 1953.
4. Guyton AC, Hall JE: *Human physiology and mechanisms of disease*, ed 6, Philadelphia, 1996, WB Saunders.
5. Sheldon SH, Spire JP, Levy HB: *Pediatric sleep medicine*, Philadelphia, 1992, WB Saunders.
6. American Association for Respiratory Care: Clinical practice guideline: polysomnography, *Respir Care* 40(12):1236, 1995.
7. Jasper HH: The ten-twenty system of the International Federation, *Electroencephalogr Clin Neurophysiol* 10:371, 1958.
8. Funsten AW, Suratt PM: Evaluation of respiratory disorders during sleep, *Clin Chest Medicine* 10:2, 1989.
9. Strollo PJ, Fernandez KS: Disorders of sleep. In Scanlan CL, Wilkins RL, Stoller JK, editors: *Egan's fundamentals of respiratory care*, ed 7, St Louis, 1998, Mosby.
10. Phillips BA, Anstead MI, Gottlieb DL: Monitoring sleep and breathing: methodology, *Clin Chest Med* 19(1):203, 1998.
11. Arand DL, Bonnet MH: Sleep-disordered breathing. In Burton GC, Hodgkin JE, Ward JJ: *Respiratory care: a guide to clinical practice*, ed 4, Philadelphia, 1997.
12. Guilleminault C, Dement WC: Sleep apnea syndromes and related sleep disorders. In Williams RL, Karacan I, editors: *Sleep disorders: diagnosis and treatment*, New York, 1978, Wiley & Sons.
13. McNicholas WT, Phillipson EA: *Breathing disorders in sleep*, Philadelphia, 2002, WB Saunders.
14. Phillipson EA: Sleep apnea, *Med Clin North Am* 23:2314, 1982.
15. Diagnostic Steering Committee: *The international classification of sleep disorders: diagnostic and coding manual*, ed 2, Lawrence, Kan, 1997, Allen Press.
16. Dyson M, Beckerman RC, Brouillette RT: Obstructive sleep apnea syndrome. In Beckerman RC, Brouillette RT, Hunt CE, editors: *Respiratory control disorders in infants and children*, Baltimore, 1992, Williams & Wilkins.
17. Guilleminault C, Van den Hoed J, Mitler M: Clinical overview of the sleep apnea syndrome. In Guilleminault C, Dement WC, editors: *Sleep apnea syndromes*, New York, 1978, Alan R. Liss.
18. Onal E, Lopata M, O'Connor T: Pathogenesis of apnea in hypersomnia-sleep apnea syndrome, *Am Rev Respir Dis* 125:167, 1982.
19. Dement, WC: *The promise of sleep*, New York, 1999, Random House.

Internet Resources

American Association for Respiratory Care: http://www.aarc.org

American Sleep Apnea Association: http://www.sleepapnea.org

American Thoracic Society: http://www.thoracic.org

The Association of Polysomnographic Technologists: http://www.aptweb.org

National Heart Lung and Blood Institute: http://www.nhlbi.nih.gov/

National Institute of Neurological Disorders and Stroke: http://www.ninds.nih.gov

National Jewish Medical and Research Center: http://www.njc.org

Sleep Net: http://www.sleepnet.com

Appendix A

Answers to Clinical Rounds and Review Questions

Author's Note

Decisions made in the clinical setting vary considerably among individuals and hospitals. There is usually more than one acceptable solution to a problem in patient care. The answers provided here represent only one or two possible choices of treatment. Readers are encouraged to talk these cases over with instructors, mentors, and colleagues.

Chapter 1

Clinical Rounds Exercises

Clinical Rounds 1-1

You can calculate the volume of gas in his lungs as he descends the pond by applying Boyle's law. We know that at sea level, where pressure surrounding the diver equals 1 atm (atmospheric pressure), the volume in his lungs equals 3000 mL. As the diver descends, the pressure surrounding him increases by 1 atm for every 33 feet. Thus, at 33 feet, the pressure exerted on the diver equals 2 atm. We can calculate the volume of gas in his lungs using the following variation of Boyle's law:

$V_2 = V_1P_1/P_2$
$V_2 = (3000\text{ mL})\ (1\text{ atm})/(2\text{ atm})$
$V_2 = 1500\text{ mL}$

At a depth of 66 feet, the pressure exerted on the diver equals 3 atm and his volume is calculated as

$V_2 = V_1P_1/P_2$
$V_2 = (3000\text{ mL})\ (1\text{ atm})/(3\text{ atm})$
$V_2 = 1000\text{ mL}$

Thus at 33 feet below the surface of the pond, the pressure to which the diver is exposed equals 2 atm, causing the diver's lung volume to decrease to one half (1500 mL) of the original volume at 33 feet and one third (1000 mL) of the original volume at 66 feet.

Clinical Rounds 1-2

According to Gay-Lussac's law, the pressure of a gas within a cylinder is directly related to the temperature at which the cylinder is exposed. Increasing this temperature therefore causes a proportional increase in the pressure of the gas within the cylinder. Thus, in this example, if the fire is not controlled and the temperature in the basement rises, the pressure within the cylinders can increase, creating an explosive hazard. Moving the cylinders therefore removes the hazardous condition.

Clinical Rounds 1-3

In this problem, $P_1 = 760$ mm Hg; $V_1 = 6L$; $T_1 = 273K$; $T_2 = 37°\ C$ (310 K); $P_2 = 3$ atm or 2280 mm Hg; V_2 = unknown. Thus,

$$P_1V_1/T_1 = P_2V_2/T_2\quad V_2 = P_1V_1T_2/P_2T_1$$
$$V_2 = [(760\text{ mm Hg})(6\text{ L})(310\text{ K})]/[(2280\text{ mm Hg})(273\text{ K})]$$
$$V_2 = 2.27\text{ L}$$

Clinical Rounds 1-4

Various conditions can cause a reduction in the rate of oxygen diffusion across the alveolar-capillary membrane. Decreasing the surface area of the membrane (e.g., resection of a lobe of the lung), increasing the thickness of the alveolar-capillary membrane (e.g., pulmonary fibrosis or the presence of pulmonary edema), and reducing the partial pressure gradient for oxygen between the alveoli and the blood flowing through the pulmonary capillary (e.g., reducing the partial pressure of inspired oxygen, such as when one ascends to high altitude) will reduce the rate at which oxygen crosses the alveolar-capillary membrane.

Review Questions

1. (a) 98.6° F; (b) 12° C; (c) 310 K; (d) 298 K
2. (a) 2.94 kPa; (b) 1034 cm H_2O; (c) 33 cm H_2O; (d) 3 atm
3. PO_2 = 158 mm Hg; PN_2 = 585 mm Hg; PCO_2 = 0.22 mm Hg
4. c
5. 793.15 mm Hg
6. 2.4 L
7. The density of oxygen = 32/22.4 = 1.43 g/L. The density of carbon dioxide = 44/22.4 = 1.973 g/L.
8. b
9. a
10. d
11. 2 A
12. (1) Ensuring that all devices attached to patients are electrically grounded; (2) ensuring that equipment circuit interrupters are functioning; (3) ensuring that all electrical devices used with a microshock-sensitive patient are well insulated and connected to outlets with a common, low-resistance ground.

13. A 1000-watt air compressor used for 24 hours would require 24 kilowatt-hours of energy (1000 W × 24 hrs = 24000 watts/24 hrs or 24 killowatts/24 hrs). If the cost of 1 kilowatt-hour is $0.10 then the total cost to operate the air compressor for 24 hrs would be $2.40 (24 hrs × 0.10 = $2.40).
14. d
15. b

Chapter 2

Clinical Rounds Exercises

Clinical Rounds 2-1

(1) Frozen carbon dioxide (dry ice); (2) Heliox; (3) Oxygen; (4) Nitric oxide.

Clinical Rounds 2-2

There is an apparent leak at the connection. The valve stem should first be closed, then the connection between the cylinder outlet and the regulator tightened.

Clinical Rounds 2-3

Turn off the zone valve that controls oxygen flow from the main oxygen supply to the affected area (in this case, the fifth floor of the north wing). Call for assistance to provide E cylinders of oxygen for patients requiring oxygen therapy.

Review Questions

1. b
2. d
3. c
4. d
5. d
6. c
7. a
8. b
9. b
10. d
11. a
12. b
13. c
14. a
15. False. The compressor will draw air in from the local environment and therefore will contain pollutants that may contaminate the local environment.

Chapter 3

Clinical Rounds Exercises

Clinical Rounds 3-1

The flow rate of oxygen is 6 L/min or 100 mL/sec (6000mL/60 sec). If the expired gas is exhaled in the first 1.5 sec of expiration, then 0.5 sec is available for filling the anatomic reservoir, which is approximately 50 mL for this patient. The anatomic reservoir includes the nose, nasopharynx, and oropharynx, which is about one third of the patient's deadspace, or 150 mL (1 mL for every pound is a good estimate of the amount of deadspace in a normal subject). The patient's inspiration lasts 1 sec, so he will inspire 100 mL of 100% oxygen. Therefore the anatomical reservoir and the inspiratory flow deliver 150 mL of 100% oxygen to the patient. The remaining 350 mL of tidal volume will be entrained room air, which has an F_IO_2 of about 0.20. This 350 mL of room air contains 70 mL of 100% oxygen (350 mL × 0.20 = 70 mL).

The delivered F_IO_2 can now be estimated:
50 mL of 100% oxygen from the anatomical reservoir.
100 mL of 100% oxygen (O_2 flow = 100 mL/sec).
350 mL of 21% oxygen (350 mL × 0.20 = 70 mL).
220 mL of 100% oxygen/500 mL tidal volume.
Estimated delivered F_IO_2 = 0.44.

Clinical Rounds 3-2

These are common complaints of patients who use nasal cannulas for long-term oxygen therapy. You could suggest that he consider using a transtracheal oxygen (TTO) device. These devices are more comfortable for patients requiring long-term oxygen therapy and are generally well tolerated by patients. Just as important, they are cosmetically more pleasing to most patients than are nasal cannulas. If the patient agrees to try the TTO device, you must teach him how to properly care for it. Adequate education is an essential part of ensuring patient compliance with any type of long-term oxygen therapy device.

Clinical Rounds 3-3

You should remove the helium-oxygen mixture, switch the patient to 100% oxygen (i.e., non-rebreathing mask), and immediately notify the physician of the patient's condition. You should recheck the concentration of oxygen delivered from the cylinder. It is possible that the contents of the cylinder were "unmixed," and thus the F_IO_2 delivered to the patient was actually much less than expected.

Review Questions

1. The easiest way to determine the number of stages in a regulator is to count the number of pressure-relief valves. Each chamber should have its own pressure-relief valve.
2. c
3. False
4. c
5. d
6. c
7. b
8. See Boxes 3-1 and 3-2.
9. d
10. d
11. c

12. The actual flow delivered to the patient is 18 L/min because you must multiply the indicated flow by the correction factor of 1.8. Thus 1.8 × 10 L/min = 18 L/min.
13. d
14. (1) Flushed skin; (2) full and bounding pulse; (3) the presence of premature ventricular contractions (PVCs); (4) hypertension; (5) muscle twitching.

Chapter 4

Clinical Rounds Exercises

Clinical Rounds 4-1

The most appropriate device for a 4-year-old child is a small-volume nebulizer. If possible, the aerosol should be administered through a mouthpiece to provide improved deposition of the medication. Although an MDI treatment could be suggested, this type of device may not be the most effective means of delivering aerosols to younger pediatric patients.

Clinical Rounds 4-2

Sample devices might include the Circulaire, RespirGard II, or Pari IS2. MMAD should be in the 1 to 3 micron range.

Clinical Rounds 4-3

A heated bland aerosol device with a MMAD of 1 to 5 microns, or a heated-wick device.

Clinical Rounds 4-4

The problem is that the device is unable to meet the inspiratory flow needs of the patient. As a consequence, he must entrain room air, which reduces the F_IO_2 that is being delivered. You can correct this situation by choosing a high-flow aerosol generator, such as a Misty-Ox device. Alternatively, you could connect two low-flow aerosol nebulizers together with a Brigg's adapter to increase flow. The key point is to choose an aerosol delivery device that can provide an inspiratory flow that will exceed the patient's inspiratory flow needs.

Clinical Rounds 4-5

A fitted respirator mask, gloves, and goggles probably will be adequate. A gown is also useful protection, but may not be practical in the home-care setting.

Review Questions

1. a
2. a
3. c
4. a
5. b
6. c
7. a
8. d
9. (1) Simple HMEs; (2) heat and moisture exchanging filters; (3) hygroscopic condenser humidifiers; (4) hygroscopic condenser humidifiers with filters.
10. b
11. b
12. b
13. b
14. b
15. c

Chapter 5

Clinical Rounds Exercises

Clinical Rounds 5-1

The clinical manifestations described point to a diagnosis of pneumonia. The laboratory findings suggest a bacterial pneumonia; *Streptococcus pneumoniae* sp. are most commonly associated with bacterial pneumonia.

Clinical Rounds 5-2

(1) *Pseudomonas aeruginosa* is a highly motile, gram-negative bacillus found in the human gastrointestinal tract. It is a contaminant in many aqueous solutions (vehicle route).
(2) Human immunodeficiency virus is transmitted through the exchange of body fluids (e.g., sexual contact) with an HIV-infected individual.
(3) Tuberculosis is a chronic bacterial infection that is almost exclusively transmitted within aerosol droplets produced by the coughing or sneezing of an individual with active tuberculosis.
(4) *Rickettsiae* spp are small pleomorphic coccobacilli. *Rickettsia* spp. are responsible for diseases that are transmitted by lice, fleas, ticks, and mites.

Clinical Rounds 5-3

First, determine if the device is contaminated. Microbiological identification requires that the hospital's clinical laboratory staff work with the staff of the respiratory care department to determine if infectious organisms are in the devices in question. The clinical microbiologist can provide information about nosocomial infections from direct smears and stains, cultures, serological tests, and antibiotic susceptibility testing.

Ongoing surveillance is required to ensure that an infection control program is adequately protecting patients and health care providers. Surveillance typically consists of the following: equipment processing quality control, routine sampling of in-use equipment, and microbiological identification. Equipment processing is monitored with chemical and biological indicators. Routine sampling of inuse equipment can be done with sterile cotton swabs, liquid broth, and aerosol impaction. Aerosol impaction is an effective method for sampling the particulate output of nebulizers.

Clinical Rounds 5-4

Most major burn wounds become infected during the first 48 to 72 hours after the incident. Care should therefore be directed to minimizing situations in which wound colonization can occur. For this reason, the most effective strategy is to use strict contact isolation procedures.

Review Questions

1. a
2. c
3. d
4. The Centers for Disease Control and Prevention updated its recommendations for hand washing technique on October 25, 2002. These updated guidelines specify that alcohol-based hand rubs should be used in conjunction with traditional soap and water to protect patients in health care settings.
5. c
6. (a) Semicritical; (b) critical; (c) noncritical; (d) semicritical; (e) semicritical
7. b
8. b
9. b
10. c
11. d
12. d
13. (1) A source of pathogens; (2) a mode of transmission of the infectious agent; (3) a susceptible host
14. (1) Monitoring equipment processing; (2) sampling in-use equipment routinely; (3) microbiologically identifying suspected pathogens
15. (a) semicritical; (b) critical; (c) semicritical; (d) semicritical
16. Standard Precautions: Hands should be washed between tasks and procedures on the same patient to prevent cross contamination of different body sites. Gloves, masks, protective eyewear and gowns should be worn when there is a chance of contacting blood. Needles and other sharp objects should be handled with care to prevent injuries. Needles should be recapped after use. Used needles and other sharps should be disposed in specially marked containers.
17. (1) e; (2) a; (3) c; (4) d; (5) b
18. See Table 5-3.

Chapter 6

Clinical Rounds Exercises

Clinical Rounds 6-1

Two devices that can be used in this emergency situation are laryngeal mask airways (LMA) and the Combitube.

Clinical Rounds 6-2

There are several possibilities. The tube could be in the esophagus, the patient's cardiac output could be low, or there could be no perfusion of blood through the lungs, as might occur as a result of a massive pulmonary embolus.

Clinical Rounds 6-3

First, the airway should be clear of any excessive secretions. The cuff is then deflated, which may necessitate suctioning the patient if secretions that were above the cuff become dislodged. The inner cannula is then removed, and the tracheostomy tube opening is occluded. The patient is evaluated to determine upper airway function.

Review Questions

1. a
2. c
3. c
4. b
5. b
6. a
7. d
8. a
9. d
10. a
11. (1) Detection of CO_2 with a capnograph; (2) auscultation of bilateral breath sounds and no audible sounds over the gastric region when the patient is artificially ventilated; (3) lateral chest radiograph
12. b
13. d
14. d
15. b
16. c
17. c
18. c
19. b

Chapter 7

Clinical Rounds Exercises

Clinical Rounds 7-1

This is a fairly common problem encountered by respiratory therapists. Most patients who have undergone abdominal surgical procedures avoid taking deep breaths because of the intense pain that occurs when the diaphragm pushes on the abdominal contents. This patient should be started on an aggressive plan that includes bronchial hygiene and lung expansion therapy to prevent postoperative atelectasis and pneumonia. The plan could include incentive spirometry, cough training (with instructions on splinting), aerosol therapy, and possibly chest physiotherapy and postural drainage.

Clinical Rounds 7-2

Although the patient is a candidate for antibiotic therapy as a medical treatment, respiratory care is needed to help clear secretions and re-expand lung bases that seem to be either secretion filled and/or atelectatic. Because the patient is unable to cooperate to perform therapies such as incentive spirometry and/or coughing and deep breathing, IPPB is an appropriate form of therapy in this case. This therapy might be accompanied by a beta adrenergic agent and a mucolytic to help mobilize secretions so that they can be cleared with suctioning. Postural draining and percussion might also be beneficial, particularly because this patient is not mobile.

Clinical Rounds 7-3

This is a primary indication for using IPV. Although it is a relatively new lung expansion technique, early studies indicate that IPV can be a useful bronchial hygiene technique for treating cystic fibrosis patients. Because of the acute nature of the patient's present illness, it is reasonable to give an initial IPV treatment and then reassess the patient in 1 to 2 hours. If the treatment improves gas exchange, as evidenced by physical assessment and pulse oximetry, further treatments would be indicated, thus preventing impending respiratory failure, which would require endotracheal intubation and mechanical ventilation. Other therapeutic modalities that might be considered would include aerosol therapy, chest physiotherapy and postural drainage, and PEP therapy.

Review Questions

1. a
2. (1) Upper abdominal surgery; (2) thoracic surgery; (3) presence of a restrictive lung defect associated with quadraplegia or a dysfunctional diaphragm; (4) to prevent atelectasis in patients with COPD who are scheduled for surgery
3. The most common problem encountered involves a leak in the system caused by a crack in the device, defective tubing, or failure of the patient to maintain a tight seal around the mouthpiece.
4. b
5. This patient is a good candidate for incentive spirometry; he is alert and cooperative. Although he does experience some pain when he takes deep breaths, he should be able to take deep breaths (vital capacity >10 mL/kg).
6. d
7. d
8. c
9. 100%
10. b
11. (1) Underwater seals, (2) weighted ball resistors, (3) spring-loaded valve resistors, and (4) magnetic valve resistors.
12. d
13. d
14. c

Chapter 8

Clinical Rounds Exercises

Clinical Rounds 8-1

There are several things that could interfere with the operation of the device: (1) The mouthpiece is connected to the wrong side of the device, and thus the exhaled gas cannot be measured. (2) The patient did not perform the test properly because either the technique was not clearly explained to him or he did not give a good effort. (3) The device was not plugged into the electrical outlet. (4) The patient's exhaled gas is leaking around the mouthpiece.

Clinical Rounds 8-2

Lung volume measurements by body plethysmography are an application of Boyle's law (i.e., when temperature is constant, volume and pressure are inversely related: $P_1V_1 = P_2V_2$).

Clinical Rounds 8-3

The FVC, $FEV_{1.0}$, and FEF_{25-75} are considerably reduced. The $FEV_{1.0}/VC$ is also reduced. The RV and FRC are elevated, indicating the presence of airtrapping. These findings are consistent with an individual with moderate to severe COPD.

Clinical Rounds 8-4

One possible explanation for this type of problem is that there is a leak in the sampling line. This problem can also occur when moisture builds up in the sampling line.

Review Questions

1. a
2. c
3. c
4. b
5. b
6. b
7. c
8. a
9. c
10. d
11. Inert gas techniques measure communicating lung volumes; body plethysmographs measure thoracic gas volumes (including gas trapped behind closed airways). For patients with airtrapping, the N_2 washout techniques underestimate the true FRC by the amount of trapped air present.
12. d
13. c
14. d
15. b

Chapter 9

Clinical Rounds Exercises

Clinical Rounds 9-1

The ventricular rate is 187 bpm. The rate can be calculated by using the formula, effective ventricular rate = 1500 ÷ (R-R interval); thus 1500 ÷ 8 = 187 bpm

Clinical Rounds 9-2

This ECG demonstrates elevated P waves in lead II (2.5 mm), suggesting right atrial enlargement. There are QS complexes throughout the precordial leads, suggesting the presence of a transmural infarction. The presence of peaked T waves also suggests this diagnosis. Note the presence of a prominent Q wave in lead I and aVL, suggesting an anterior lateral MI. The prominent Q waves seen in the inferior leads (II, III, and aVF) and the T wave changes seen in these leads also suggest an inferior infarct.

Clinical Rounds 9-3

(1) Measurements obtained from hypovolemic patients ventilated with PEEP will typically show exaggerated variations in pressure. This is particularly evident in patients ventilated with high inspiratory pressures, such as those patients with asthma or ARDS. (2) This problem can occur if the catheter is too proximal or if the balloon ruptures. (3) Excessive noise on the pressure tracing is usually associated with catheter whip or the catheter tip being located too close to the pulmonary valve.

Clinical Rounds 9-4

The cardiac output can be calculated using the Fick equation, or $\dot{V}O_2 = \dot{Q} \times (CaO_2 - C\bar{v}O_2)$. The steps for making this calculation follow:

$CaO_2 = (Hb \times 1.34)\ SaO_2 + (PaO_2 \times 0.003)$

$CaO_2 = (12\ gm\% \times 1.34)\ 0.92 + (60\ mm\ Hg \times 0.003)$

$CaO_2 = 14.97\ vol\ \%$

$C\bar{v}O_2 = (Hb \times 1.34)\ S\bar{v}O_2 + (P\bar{v}O_2 \times 0.003)$

$C\bar{v}O_2 = (12\ gm\% \times 1.34)\ 0.60 + (30\ mm\ Hg \times 0.003)$

$CvO_2 = 9.74\ vol\ \%$

$\dot{Q} = \dot{V}O_2 \div (CaO_2 \times C\bar{v}O_2)\ 10$

$\dot{Q} = 200\ mL/min \div (14.97\ mL/100\ mL - 9.74\ mL/100\ mL)\ 10$

$\dot{Q} = 3.82\ L/min$

Review Questions

1. a
2. d
3. d
4. c
5. c
6. d
7. b
8. d
9. c
10. c
11. c
12. c
13. b
14. b
15. d

Chapter 10

Clinical Rounds Exercises

Clinical Rounds 10-1

The presence of an air bubble will cause the PCO_2 to be lower than normal and the PO_2 to be higher than normal. The reason for this discrepancy is that room air has a PCO_2 of about 0.3 mm Hg and a PO_2 of approximately 150 mm Hg (see Chapter 3 for a full discussion of partial pressures of gases in room air).

Clinical Rounds 10-2

The interpretation of respiratory alkalosis is probably correct. The PO_2 results, however, need to be evaluated by another method because capillary PO_2 does not always correlate well with PaO_2

Clinical Rounds 10-3

Neither the SpO_2 nor the calculated SaO_2 accurately reflect the true oxygen saturation when CO poisoning is suspected. SpO_2 can be falsely high. SaO_2 is calculated by the ABG analyzer's microprocessor; PaO_2 is a measure of dissolved (not bound) O_2. The patient's blood sample should be run on a CO-Oximeter, which directly measures the oxyhemoglobin saturation and carboxyhemoglobin levels. For example, suppose that the CO-Oximeter measured the following: O_2 Hb = 83%; COHb = 15%; and thus HHb = 2%. Assume that the total hemoglobin equals 15 gm%. Then 83% of 15 gm% of Hb = 12.45 gm%; 15% of 15 gm% = 2.25 gm%; 2% of 15 gm% = 0.3 gm%. Notice that the pulse oximeter only detects the levels of O_2Hb and HHb. That is, the pulse oximeter reading suggests that only 2% of the hemoglobin is unsaturated and that 98% is saturated with oxygen. So 98% of the 15 gm% of Hb represents 14.7 gm% O_2Hb. Therefore the pulse oximeter overestimates the true level of oxyhemoglobin by about 2.25 gm%.

Review Questions

1. a
2. b
3. c
4. c
5. a
6. a
7. d

8. a
9. b
10. b
11. d
12. a
13. *Quality control* may be defined as a system that includes analyzing control samples (with known values of pH, PCO_2, and PO_2), assessing the results of these measurements against defined limits, identifying problems, and specifying corrective actions.

    Quality assurance involves proficiency testing, which provides a dynamic process of identification, evaluation, and resolution of problems that affect blood gas measurements.
14. a
15. a
16. c

Chapter 11

Clinical Rounds Exercises

Clinical Rounds 11-1

Part I: An open-loop system. The ventilator was told to deliver 650 mL and it did, but it did not make any adjustments when the exhaled volume was less than the set volume.
Part II: A closed-loop system. The ventilator has compared the exhaled volume to the set volume and progressively increased the peak pressure to achieve the set tidal volume.

Clinical Rounds 11-2

Problem 1: It seems that inspiratory flow is inadequate because pressures are dropping so low during inspiration. The patient may be opening the safety pop-in valve. Check the gas source to be sure it is on and connected and that the flow is adequate.
Problem 2: There is probably a leak in the system and pressure in the system cannot be maintained.

Clinical Rounds 11-3

The pressure must drop to +10 cm H_2O minus the sensitivity setting (i.e., 10 − 1 = +9 cm H_2O). Inspiration starts when the pressure drops to +9 cm H_2O or 1 cm H_2O below baseline pressure. This answer assumes that the ventilator is PEEP compensated, which most are.

Clinical Rounds 11-4

Base flow = 6 L/min − trigger flow. Measured flow must drop to 4 L/min.

Clinical Rounds 11-5

The trigger variable is pressure, the limit variable is pressure, and the cycling variable is time.

Clinical Rounds 11-6

Technically, referring to the variable as volume-cycled is incorrect, if volume-cycling is defined as the measurement of volume and the ending of inspiratory flow when the volume was achieved. A classic example of this cycling mechanism is the MA-1. In the MA-1, the rising of the bellows and the contact of a switch near the top of the bellows ends inspiration (i.e., until the volume leaves the bellows [a volume device] inspiration does not end). The MA-1 ventilator provides an example of true volume cycling.

One could argue, however, that the measurement of flow over time is a volume measurement because volume = time/flow. Modern flow-controlling valves are very accurate in their flow delivery. Should we split hairs over this issue? What is most important in the clinical setting? We're interested in volume ventilation or delivery of a tidal volume. We would want to know that the volume left the ventilator at the end of inspiratory flow. This is the case.

Both are correct. One is technically correct by very strict standards and definition. The other is correct based on common clinical usage and an acceptance that flow/T_I − volume.

Clinical Rounds 11-7

Part I: C_T = volume/PIP, C_T = 90 mL/45 cm H_2O = 2 mL/cm H_2O;

Volume lost = PIP × C_T = 20 cm H_2O × 2 mL/cm H_2O = 40 mL

Set tidal volume was 300 mL minus 40 mL lost to the circuit. The patient will receive 260 mL.

Part II: 3 ml/cm H_2O × 28 cm H_2O = 84 mL will be lost to the circuit. 640 mL × 84 mL = 556 mL will reach the patient.

Clinical Rounds 11-8

We know that PSV is patient-triggered, and that patients determine their own tidal volume based on their lung characteristics and their inspiratory effort, as well as by the set pressure. The ventilator algorithm that ends the breath does so when a predetermined flow that is a percentage of peak flow is reached. It can be argued that the programmer designed the algorithm so that the ventilator knows the patient's inspiration is ending (i.e., flow is declining). Therefore the programming is based on what the patient's breath is doing. So you could argue that it really is the patient's breathing pattern that determines all phases of a pressure-supported breath.

Clinical Rounds 11-9

No, the ventilator will measure a minute ventilation of 7.5 L/min (25 breaths/min × V_T of 0.3 = 7.5 L/min), which is well above the set minimum of 4.0 L/min. The patient has an increased work of breathing. Unless the high rate alarm is set, the operator will be unaware of the patient's problem.

Review Questions

1. Pneumatic and electric
2. This is a closed-loop or intelligent system.
3. b

4. Pressure-limited ventilation, pressure-controlled ventilation, and pressure-targeted ventilation
5. c
6. False
7. Controlled volume ventilation is time-triggered, volume targeted (limited), and time or volume cycled. The flow curve is constant (rectangular), and the volume and pressure curves are ascending ramps.
8. Patient-triggering; pressure or flow are the most common variables in patient triggering.
9. There is a leak in the circuit.
10. There seems to be an increase in Raw.
11. CPAP is only for spontaneously breathing patients. The term *PEEP* implies that mechanical ventilation also is in use.
12. d
13. b
14. High-frequency oscillatory ventilation
15. c
16. b
17. b
18. The four phases of a breath during mechanical ventilation and their phase variable include the following: (1) end of expiration and beginning of inspiration, (2) delivery of inspiration, (3) end of inspiration and beginning of expiration, and (4) expiratory pause. The variables are (1) trigger variable: begins inspiration, (2) control variable: remains constant during inspiration, e.g., volume or pressure, (3) limit variable: places a maximum value on a variable (pressure, volume, flow, or time) during delivery of a breath, and (4) cycle variable: ends inspiration.
19. The ventilator will trigger when the expiratory flow drops from 10 L/min to 7 L/min—a trigger of 3 L/min. To make the ventilator more sensitive, lower the trigger flow. For example, 1 L/min trigger flow will result in the ventilator beginning inspiration when the base flow drops to just 9 L/min.
20. No, downward deflection suggests that the patient is not triggering the breath, so it is time-triggered.

    Since inspiratory time is constant at 1 second, then the breath is time-cycled. Inspiratory flow is constant even though pressure has changed slightly, which is probably due to a change in the patient's lung conditions. A constant flow over a constant time delivers a constant volume. This mode is volume-targeted ventilation and the pressure is variable.
21. c
22. b
23. a
24. d
25. b
26. c
27. b
28. (1) High-frequency positive-pressure ventilation (HFPPV); (2) High-frequency jet ventilation (HFJV); (3) High-frequency oscillatory ventilation (HFOV); (4) High-frequency flow interruption (HFFI); (5) High-frequency percussive ventilation (HFPV)
29. d
30. A system leak causes the volume-time curve to remain above baseline during exhalation. To confirm, check the ventilator's inspiratory and expiratory volume measurements and the peak inspiratory pressure. Expiratory volumes will be lower than inspiratory volumes. The peak inspiratory pressure will be lower than previous readings. Leaks most commonly occur in the patient circuit or around the endotracheal tube cuff.

Chapter 12

Clinical Rounds Exercises

Clinical Rounds 12-1

With a constant flow of 1 L/sec and a V_T of 0.5 L, the inspiratory time is 0.5 seconds (T_I = flow/V_T). T_I will increase if the curve is changed to a descending ramp. With a descending ramp, the peak flow of 60 L/min is delivered only at the beginning of the breath and gradually slows to 50% of its value. The easiest way to determine the new T_I is to check the digital readout on the monitoring screen for T_I.

Clinical Rounds 12-2

The Insp/Exp Hold pad is pressed twice until "E HLD" is displayed in the monitor window. Next, the select key is pressed and held. The expiratory pressure (auto-PEEP) will be displayed in the window.

Clinical Rounds 12-3

The ventilator will switch to the A/C mode if apnea ventilation is activated. The rate will become whatever rate is set on the apnea back-up rate control. The tidal volume will become whatever is set on the tidal volume control. Normal operation can be resumed if the patient begins to spontaneously breathe again (two consecutive breaths with V_T >50% of set) or the operator presses the alarm reset button and activates the control setting for breath rate.

Clinical Rounds 12-4

Author's Note: These settings are pretty absurd for any patient and are only given here to demonstrate a point.

The "limited" alert tells the therapist that an incompatible settings condition exists. Check the T_I, V_T, and flow to see if the V_T can be delivered in the T_I determined by the set variables. TCT = 60/20 = 3 sec. Flow = 20 L/min, or 0.33 L/sec. T_I = V_T/flow plus inspiratory pause = 0.7 L/(0.33 L/sec) plus 1.2 sec = 3.32 sec. This means that the T_I would exceed TCT, which is an impossible condition.

The inspiratory flow definitely needs to be increased, and the use of a 1.2-second inspiratory pause should be questioned.

Clinical Rounds 12-5

The breath was flow-cycled. The breath ended when flow dropped to the set peak flow value of 60 L/min. Tidal volume delivery was about 0.8 L (800 mL), which was higher than the set value of 0.65 L (650 mL).

Clinical Rounds 12-6

(1) PCV is active in the CMV mode. The operator only has to set the pressure limit using the PRESS. CONTROL knob to establish the desired ventilating pressure. To check this setting, press the Paw touch pad below the measured values window and read the P_{peak} value.

(2) The manufacturer recommends using the plateau pressure from a volume-targeted breath and adding 3 cm H_2O. In this case, $P_{plateau}$ was 16 cm H_2O. A starting pressure would be about 19 cm H_2O.

(3) The $\dot{V}_E$ in volume ventilation was 6.5 L/min (0.65 L × 10 breaths/min = 6.5 L). You could start at a liter above and below the previous target, using 5.5 L/min (low alarm) and 7.5 L/min (high alarm). Then see how much the patient's $\dot{V}_E$ fluctuates once PCV is initiated. The exact amount for setting high and low $\dot{V}_E$ alarms is strictly up to clinicians and the institutions in which they practice.

(4) Tidal volume delivery can be checked by pressing the touch pad marked with a "T,V_T,f,R,C" below the measured values window. The measured expired V_T ("VTe") will appear in the window.

Clinical Rounds 12-7

(1) The flow waveform is constant because the ventilator is in volume-targeted ventilation.

(2) The inspiratory time of a mandatory breath is calculated as follows:

CMV rate = 15 breaths/min
60 sec ÷ 15 breaths/min = 4 sec is the mandatory breath cycle time. TCT/(sum of I:E) = inspiratory time
I:E is 1:3. I + E = 4
4 seconds/4 = 1 second; inspiratory time is 1 second

(3) Flow is 60 L/min, or 60 L/(60 sec) = 1 L/sec. V_T = 0.5 L. Time for delivery of volume = V_T/flow = 0.5 ÷ (1 L/sec).
Time for delivery of volume = 0.5 sec.
T_I = 1 second.
Pause time will be T_I – time for volume delivery, or 1.0 sec – 0.5 sec = 0.5 sec pause time.

(4) The time interval between mandatory breaths will be 60 sec ÷ 4 breaths/min, or 15 seconds.

Clinical Rounds 12-8

(1)

T_I = 2 sec
TCT = 6 sec (60sec/10 breaths per min)
T_E = TCT – T_I = 6 sec – 2 sec = 4 sec
I:E = 2:4 or 1:2

(2) At a flow of 60 L/min (1 L/sec), the ventilator can deliver 0.5 L in 0.5 sec. (T_I = V_T/flow in seconds.)

(3) Set T_I is 2 sec. V_T is delivered in 0.5 sec. The Dräger will time cycle the breath. An inspiratory pause will occur after a V_T delivery equal to 1.5 sec.

Clinical Rounds 12-9

Within only 4 hours, the ventilator is unable to deliver the set V_T using the previously set pressure. This suggests a change in patient lung characteristics. The respiratory therapist should evaluate the patient to determine the cause. Does the patient have a pneumothorax? Is the endotracheal tube becoming occluded? It is more appropriate here to further assess the patient and find out what is wrong than to make an immediate ventilator change.

Clinical Rounds 12-10

Disconnecting the patient may increase the risk of infection, which is one reason closed suction catheters are used.

Clinical Rounds 12-11

To complete the setting of an alarm value, you must press the dial knob to activate the new setting.

Clinical Rounds 12-12

In APRV, both pressure and time levels are treated as straight CPAP. In PCV + you have the option of adding PS to the expiratory phase of the breaths. Conceptually, you should not need PS during the release phase of APRV because you are not in that phase long enough to use it. T_{low} is a very short time period.

Clinical Rounds 12-13

Inspiratory pause is 15% of TCT (45% – 30% = 15%).
Expiratory time is 55% (30% + 15% + 55% = 100%).

Clinical Rounds 12-14

The % cycle time is based on 100%. By adding inspiration and expiration from the desired I:E ratio, you get a value of 5. This is divided into 100%:100% ÷ 5 = 20%. The I portion is 1 unit, or 20%. The E portion is 4 units, or 4 × 20% = 80%. With the T_I control (dark blue) set at 20%, and the T_E control (light blue) set right next to it, the result is 20% T_I and 80% T_E:20%:80% = 1:4.

Clinical Rounds 12-15

The ventilator will increase the pressure support level in 1 cm H_2O increments until the exhaled $\dot{V}_E$ equals or exceeds the MMV setting.

In this example, both $\dot{V}_E$ and $\dot{V}_A$ decreased. The patient's respiratory rate increased, perhaps in the patient's effort to maintain $\dot{V}_E$. This increased the work of breathing (WOB) for the patient. To alert the clinician that rate is increasing, it is important to set the high rate alarm. It should be placed at a value that the clinician deems appropriate for the patient and the situation.

Clinical Rounds 12-16

The therapist should check the option or DIP switches at the back of the ventilator. The number 3 switch should be in the on position.

Clinical Rounds 12-17

(1) TCT = 60 sec ÷ (10 breaths/min) = 6 sec.

$$T_I = 25\% \text{ of 6 sec, or 1.5 sec.}$$
$$\text{Flow} = V_T/T_I = 0.5 \text{ L}/1.5 \text{ sec} = 0.33 \text{ L/sec, or about 20 L/min.}$$

(2) If the rate is turned to 12 breaths/min, the new TCT will be 5 sec. 25% of 5 sec = 1.25 sec. With the same tidal volume, the new flow will be 0.4 L/sec, or 24 L/min. It makes sense that the flow would need to be faster to get the same V_T delivered in a shorter time.

(3) a. $T_I = V_T$/flow. (Convert flow to liters/second.) $T_I = 0.8 \div (1 \text{ L/sec}) = 0.8$ sec for inspiration.
b. When P-SIMV is selected, the ventilator is in a pressure-targeted mode. When configured for peak flow, this function only works in volume ventilation. T_I depends at what level the respiratory therapist sets that control.

(4) a. Because these configurations do not apply in PCV, we will assume volume ventilation. TCT = 4 sec. I:E is 1:3 and consists of 4 parts (1 + 3); inspiration is 1 part. Each part is 1 second long (4 sec/4 parts). So, T_I = 1 sec.
b. Peak flow cannot be calculated from this information when PCV is in use. Flow depends on the pressure setting, the patient's lung conditions, and any patient effort.
c. If the unit is configured for I:E, then the ratio is constant—even if an inspiratory pause is added. With an I:E of 1:3, T_I stays at 1.0 sec (T_E = 3 sec). An added pause of 0.5 sec shortens delivery time to 0.5 sec. The breath must be delivered in a shorter time so that peak flow has to increase.

Clinical Rounds 12-18

When APV is used during pressure-targeted ventilation (A/C or SIMV), its upper pressure limitation is Pmax – 10 cm H_2O. In this example, Pmax was set at 35 cm H_2O. The ventilator had to deliver 25 cm H_2O to achieve the target volume: 35 cm H_2O – 10 cm H_2O = 25 cm H_2O. The alarm will activate. The therapist might want to increase Pmax to as much as 45 cm H_2O. This would limit pressure to 35 cm H_2O, which is probably the highest pressure advisable to avoid lung injury. (Remember that the ventilator has taken into account changes in patient lung compliance to determine the pressure needed to deliver the target V_T.)

Clinical Rounds 12-19

Problem 1: $\dot{V}_E$ will be 100 mL/min/kg, or 6 L/min (60 kg × 100 mL/kg)
Problem 2: $\dot{V}_E$ will be 200 mL/min/kg IBW × 50%, 5 kg × 200 mL/kg = 1.0 L; 50% of 1 L/min = 0.5 L/min.

Clinical Rounds 12-20

Linear drive pistons normally produce constant (rectangular or square) waveforms (see Chapter 11). However with new technology, even linear drive pistons can be made to produce different waveforms. In the 740 (and the 760) the ventilator will produce square or descending ramp waveforms in volume ventilation.

Clinical Rounds 12-21

Part I: At 1000 mL/sec flow, we can deliver 500 mL in 0.5 seconds. Remember from Chapter 11, T_I = volume/flow.
T_I = 500 mL/1000 mL/sec = 0.5 sec
T_E = TCT – T_I TCT = 60 sec/rate
T_E = 3 sec - 0.5 sec = 2.5 sec
I:E is 0.5:2.5 or 1.5
Part II: Using a descending ramp, the flow begins at the set value of 60 L/min, but progressively decreases. To get the same 500 mL in with the flow descending, the inspiratory time will have to be longer. This will lengthen T_I, shorten T_E, and change the I:E ratio. Fortunately, the 740 and 760 will warn the operator if the ventilator is going into an inverse I:E ratio, in which case the flow may have to be increased. The V_T or respiratory rate could also be changed to alter the ratio, but these two would change the minute ventilation.

Clinical Rounds 12-22

Because the operator is in the process of setting up a mode, the flashing indicator suggests the operator forgot to press the key. The tidal volume key must be pressed, the value adjusted using the control knob (if it is desirable to change V_T), and Accept must be pressed or the operator must press the key and make no changes; this accepts the previous setting. All flashing keys must be pressed before a new mode can be initiated.

Clinical Rounds 12-23

An inspiratory pause would provide compliance and resistance data. This patient has a low V_T compared to the set pressure. An estimated compliance (350 mL/18 cm H_2O) is 19.4 mL/cm H_2O. Also, there is an inspiratory flow at the end of inspiration. It could be that T_I is not long enough for all the pressure to reach the alveolar level since the flow is not zero at this point. So, $P_{plateau}$ might not be equal to set pressure (minus PEEP).

An expiratory pause is indicated to estimate auto-PEEP since there is also flow present at the end of exhalation, suggesting the patient has not had adequate time to completely exhale.

Clinical Rounds 12-24

Part I: A flow of 30 L/min = 30 L/60 sec = 0.5 L/sec.
The tidal volume 365 mL or 0.365 L will now be delivered at a faster rate.
To calculate the new T_I, recall from Chapter 11, Box 11-22.

T_I = volume/flow,
T_I = 0.365 divided by 0.5 L/sec, and T_I = 0.73 seconds.
T_E = TCT − T_I, thus, T_E = 3.75 − 0.73 and T_E = 3.07 seconds.

Part II: T_I will remain constant at 1.00 seconds, and the new TCT will now be 6 seconds (60 sec/rate = TCT, 60 sec/10 = 6 sec). Thus, the new T_E will be TCT – T_I or 6 – 1, T_E = 5 sec.

The operator can change the actual value of a locked parameter and once it is activated it will then become the new constant value. For example, with a rate of 16 breaths/min, T_I = 1.0 sec and T_E = 2.75 sec, if T_I is increased to 2 seconds, T_E will now be 1.75 seconds (TCT – T_I, 3.75 – 2 = 1.75) and TCT will not change since the rate is still 16 breaths/min.

Clinical Rounds 12-25

The graph needs to be rescaled along the y-axis, which displays the flow, so that the entire waveform pattern can be seen.

Clinical Rounds 12-26

For the "DECR RESP RATE FIRST" message to appear, T_I must be > 75% of TCT.

TCT is 60 sec/rate = 60 sec/20 breaths/min = 3 sec
$T_I = V_T$/flow = 1.0 L/(30 L/min)
A flow of 30 L/min is 0.5 L/sec
T_I = 2 sec
75% of 3 sec = 2.25 sec. Because T_I = 2 sec is < 2.25 sec., the error message will not appear.

Clinical Rounds 12-27

Volume added will be 2 mL/cm H_2O × 30 cm H_2O = 60 mL

V_T delivered to the circuit will be 600 mL + 60 mL = 660 mL.

The exhaled V_T will read 600 mL because the computer will subtract the 60 mL of volume that was added.

Clinical Rounds 12-28

The alarm is set incorrectly. The patient was originally in CMV, and the alarm setting was appropriate, but it was not changed when the patient was switched to SIMV. The alarm is being activated because the spontaneous V_T is lower than the alarm setting. The alarm should be set slightly below the average spontaneous V_T.

Clinical Rounds 12-29

If the patient ceases to trigger a breath at a rate of 2 breaths/min, a maximum of 60 seconds could elapse before a machine-triggered mandatory breath would occur. The longest interval that can be set for an apnea period is 60 seconds. Fortunately, a prudent respiratory therapist would have set an apnea interval of no more than 20 seconds so that apnea ventilation would begin long before the 60-second interval had elapsed (see the section on special functions of the 7200 in Chapter 12 for a description of apnea ventilation).

Clinical Rounds 12-30

Problem 1: 10 breaths/min = TCT of 6 sec (60 sec ÷ 10 breaths/min). With an I:E ratio of 1:1, total units in a breath are 1 + 1 =2. Each unit is 6 sec ÷ 2 units = 3 sec. T_I = 3 sec.; T_E = 3 sec. If the rate is changed to 15 breaths/min and T_I is constant, then TCT = 60 sec ÷ 15 breaths/min = 4 sec. With T_I constant at 3 sec, the T_E = TCT – T_I, or 4 sec – 3 sec = 1 sec. The ratio is 3:1.

Problem 2: Old T_I was 3 sec. When rate is increased from 10 to 15 breaths/min and I:E is constant at 1:1, then TCT is 4 sec. With an I:E of 1:1, total units in a breath are 1 + 1 = 2. Each unit is 4 sec ÷ 2 units = 2 sec. T_I = 2 sec.; T_E = 2 sec.

Clinical Rounds 12-31

Problem 1: The therapist should increase the flow on the front panel flow meter until the gauge no longer displays significant negative pressure during inspiration.

Problem 2: The therapist should check the patient's ventilatory pattern to be sure the patient is not coughing. Then check the expiratory limb of the circuit for added resistance from water accumulation or a filter with increased resistance. If the increase in pressure is not being caused by the first two possibilities, then lower the level of SPONT flow set with the flow meter on the face panel.

Clinical Rounds 12-32

The flow is only 30 L/min. With a T_I of only 0.5 seconds and a low flow, there is not enough time for the ventilator to reach the PIP setting for this patient. Of course, this is influenced by patient lung characteristics and patient effort. A flow of 30 L/min may be adequate to achieve the target pressure in a patient with low compliance, but in this case, the therapist should first increase the flow and then reevaluate breath delivery.

Clinical Rounds 12-33

The pressure drop is probably the result of a very small leak in the circuit. The low-pressure alarm activates because the pressure has dropped below the trigger sensitivity level during exhalation and exceeded the time allotted.

Clinical Rounds 12-34

During pressure-targeted ventilation, increasing T_I increases mean airway pressure. During volume-targeted ventilation, however, the therapist might increase PEEP to increase mean airway pressure. If the therapist increases T_I during volume-targeted ventilation, he or she will also increase V_T delivery unless a corresponding decrease in flow is made. Remember that with the Wave during volume ventilation, V_T = flow × T_I.

Clinical Rounds 12-35

Problem 1: The patient is obviously trying, without success, to inhale. The patient's inspiratory effort is demonstrated by the negative inspiratory pressures and the use of accessory muscles. The observed and set breath rates are the same, so no additional breaths are being detected and triggered. This is confirmed by the fact that the Patient Effort indicator is not lighting up. The Sensitivity is most likely set at "- -," or the off position. Even if it was set at 9 L/min, the highest setting, the ventilator would pressure-trigger at –3 cm H_2O during a patient effort if the patient were able to drop the pressure that low. The solution is to set the sensitivity appropriately for the patient. If the physician does not want additional patient breaths, perhaps sedation would be in order. This might be the case if the patient was having seizure activity or was highly agitated.

Problem 2: An appropriate initial setting would be a sensitivity of 2 L/min. Afterward, the respiratory therapist could evaluate how this setting suited the patient's needs and whether auto-triggering was occurring. [*Note*: This would hold true if leak compensation were not available as an option. If leak compensation is on, just set the sensitivity to 2 L/min.]

Clinical Rounds 12-36

This message indicates that both the low minute volume and low peak pressure for spontaneous breath alarms are turned off. The therapist should activate the LMV alarm and note that the LPP alarm is off and consider turning it to "all breaths." It is important, particularly with a spontaneously breathing patient, that a safe minimum minute ventilation is monitored. With CPAP being used, it is also appropriate to have a low peak pressure monitored for spontaneous breaths.

Clinical Rounds 12-37

The flow termination point is 2.5 L/min (10% of 25 L/min). The preset default flow in the LTV is 2 L/min.

Clinical Rounds 12-38

The therapist should change the breath type to Pressure, the mode to SIMV/CPAP, the breath rate to "—," the sensitivity to a level appropriate for the patient, and the pressure support to 15 cm H_2O. Remember that on the LTV the pressure setting for PS is not added to the PEEP value. The PEEP valve/expiratory valve is manually adjusted to a PEEP to 3 cm H_2O. The pressure graph displays the value for the PEEP setting. The exhaled measured tidal volume should also be checked to see if it is appropriate for the patient.

Clinical Rounds 12-39

The "I-Time Too Long" alarm occurs in adults when a pressure support breath is more than 3.5 seconds long (inspiration). The value is 2.5 seconds for pediatric patients.

Most likely a leak has occurred in the circuit. A small leak will result in the ventilator putting more air in the patient circuit during inspiration to maintain the set pressure. A large enough leak can prevent the inspiratory flow from dropping to its termination setting (E-trigger) and flow-cycling inspiration.

Clinical Rounds 12-40

The actual breath rate will be 8 breaths/min. The apnea ventilation rate cannot be set lower than the set mandatory rate in A/C or SIMV ventilation, or it defaults to the set rate for the mode.

Clinical Rounds 12-41

The clinician should check the toggle switch for adult/infant $\dot{V}_E$ ranges because sometimes this is incorrectly positioned. If it is in the infant setting, a $\dot{V}_E$ of 6 L/min will give a high-ventilation alarm.

Clinical Rounds 12-42

Turn the oxygen up to 100%, but remember to turn the oxygen control back to its original setting afterward.

You could press the gas change button briefly to flush the system with 100% oxygen, but this must be done with caution. When the gas change button is pressed, the patient is not being ventilated. Circuit pressure is maintained at 20 cm H_2O, which subjects the patient to high flows and effectively creates 20 cm H_2O of PEEP.

Clinical Rounds 12-43

(1) The tidal volume is determined by the inspiratory pressure level, the characteristics of the patient's lungs, and how much of an inspiratory effort the patient makes. Tidal volume is variable in pressure support.
(2) 19 cm H_2O, or the PEEP level plus the inspiratory pressure level.
(3) Pressure support is designed to stop inspiratory flow if pressure rises above the inspiratory pressure + PEEP + 3 cm H_2O. The upper pressure limit also acts as a safety back-up to release the pressure level.
(4) The inspiratory gas flow will stop when the ventilator measures a T_I equal to 80% of the total cycle time. With a set rate of 15 breaths/min, TCT is 4 seconds. Inspiration will end at 3.2 seconds.

Clinical Rounds 12-44

The ventilator will not permit the T_I to exceed 80% of the TCT. The flashing yellow light next to the PAUSE TIME% control indicates that an attempt has been made to exceed the 80% T_I limit. The ventilator will shorten the pause time so that the T_I is 80%. In this case, because the T_I = 80%, there will be no pause.

Clinical Rounds 12-45

As the patient's rate drops below 12 breaths/min, the ventilator determines that it is not maintaining the set $\dot{V}_E$ even though it is maintaining V_T. To compensate, it will increase the pressure to increase the delivered V_T, thus increasing $\dot{V}_E$.

In this example, the patient's rate dropped to 8 breaths/min. The volume was 500 mL. The machine measures a $\dot{V}_E$ of 4.0 L/min, and the set value is 6.0 L/min. The machine will increase volume delivery (by increasing pressure) to a maximum of 150% of the set value. In this case, the ventilator would go as high as 750 mL of V_T to keep the $\dot{V}_E$ at 6.0 L/min, the set value. Remember that in VS the ventilator cannot alter the rate. $\dot{V}_E$ can be higher than the set value, but not lower.

Clinical Rounds 12-46

SIMV cycle time = 60 sec/SIMV frequency = 60/3 = 20 sec.
SIMV period = 60 sec/CMV frequency = 60/15 = 4 sec.
Spontaneous period = 20 sec − 4 sec = 16 sec.

Clinical Rounds 12-47

The ventilator is time cycling and the plateau feature is enabled. The plateau pressure created at the end of inspiration when flow is zero reflects the alveolar distending pressure. This value can be used in the calculation of static compliance.

Clinical Rounds 12-48

Problem 1: The internal battery charge is almost completely drained. No AC or other DC power source is available. The therapist should reconnect the unit to an AC outlet or an external DC battery to provide sufficient power to continue operation.
Problem 2: This is a high-priority alarm, as shown by the "!!!" message, the 5 tones, and the red LED. The therapist should first try pressing the alarm reset key. If this resolves the alarm, the Savina can be used for ventilation. If pressing alarm reset does not resolve the alarm condition, find an alternative method to ventilate the patient and remove the ventilator from service. Call a Dräger service representative.

Clinical Rounds 12-49

(1) The flow is not constant during volume control ventilation on the Servo^I because the ventilator is designed to provide flow to the patient on demand. When the ventilator senses pressure dropping 2 cm H_2O below current pressure in the circuit, additional flow is delivered to the patient.
(2) The ventilator will cycle out of inspiratory when the flow drops to 30% of 100 L/min or 30 L/min. There is no pause time, so inspiratory time is not extended after this point.
(3) The set tidal volume is delivered and the possibility exists that the patient will receive an additional volume because the patient was actively inspiring. The only circumstance in which volume would not be delivered would be if the upper pressure limit was exceeded. This would end the breath early.

Clinical Rounds 12-50

If the patient's spontaneous V_T is higher than the set V_T during volume support, the ventilator will not provide additional pressure during inspiration. In this case the delivered V_T must be ≥ 450 mL.

Clinical Rounds 12-51

(1) The peak pressure is 25 cm H_2O for mandatory breaths and 20 for PS breaths (the sum of inspiratory pressure and PEEP.)
(2) The flow-cycle is set for 40%; 40% of 50 L/min is 20 L/min. If inspiration ends at 20 L/min, then the breath is most likely flow-cycled. The operator could also check how long inspiration was from the flow-time curve. If T_I is1.5 seconds, then the flow is probably time-cycled.
(3) PS breaths will end when flow drops to 10 L/min. (20% of 50 L/min is 10 L/min)

Clinical Rounds 12-52

The rate will change immediately. The ventilator will change to volume ventilation as soon as the selection is activated.

Clinical Rounds 12-53

The display shows "- -" if the ventilator cannot measure a stable plateau pressure. Remember that an inspiratory pause cannot be accurately obtained if the patient makes any respiratory efforts during this measurement.

Clinical Rounds 12-54

(1) The ventilator will compare the exhaled V_T to the set value and determine that the exhaled V_T is low. It will respond by increasing the pressure in the next breath to achieve the target V_T, but not by more than 6 cm H_2O at a time.
(2) The highest pressure the ventilator will reach is 35 cm H_2O, the set pressure limit.

Bear 1000 Review Questions

1. d
2. c
3. d
4. b
5. This is both true and false. It is true that the Bear 1000 normally operates with air/O_2 high-pressure sources and electrical power. If an air compressor has been added to it, however, it can use the air compressor as a high pressure gas source. If the compressor is the only high-pressure gas source, it cannot deliver a high oxygen percentage.
6. True
7. The lock control may be active. If the LED near the lock control is illuminated, the control needs to be pressed to unlock the panel and allow the tidal volume to be adjusted.
8. Unless the LED next to the V_T control is illuminated, it cannot be adjusted. One likely problem is that the ventilator is in a ventilatory mode in which the V_T control is not active, such as PSV or PCV.
9. No. The sharp rise in pressure that then falls to a plateau indicates that the flow is too rapid at the beginning of inspiration and the pressure sloping feature should be used to adjust it.

10. Volume output = volume added + set volume
Volume output = (25 × 3 mL/cm H_2O) + 0.7 = 0.775 L
11. Because the breath flow cycles and volume delivery are higher than the set value, the patient must be actively breathing.

Bird 8400STi Review Questions

1. c
2. c
3. a
4. b
5. a
6. d
7. d
8. True
9. False; only units that have had the PCV option added will provide this mode.
10. The patient triggers the breath, as suggested by the dip in pressure before inspiration begins. The ventilator reaches the set pressure and sustains it. The patient must have received at least the set $\dot{V}_I$ because there was no rise in pressure at the end of inspiration, which would have occurred if flow had been sustained. Expiration occurs normally. The breath is flow-cycled.

Bird T-Bird AVS Review Questions

1. a
2. a
3. a
4. a
5. a
6. d
7. False; the T-Bird does not require a high-pressure gas source to function.
8. True
9. True
10. Both ventilators flow-cycle out of inspiration when V_T delivery is achieved. The Bear 1000 flow-cycles at 30% of the measured peak flow delivered during inspiration. The T-Bird AVS III flow-cycles when the actual flow value equals the set peak flow.

Dräger Evita Review Questions

1. a
2. b
3. c
4. c
5. c
6. d
7. d
8. True
9. True
10. APRV provides two levels of CPAP (P_{high} and P_{low}) and is intended for use with spontaneously breathing patients. The operator can adjust both pressure levels and the amount of time each level of pressure is applied (see the section on APRV in this chapter).

Dräger E-4 Review Questions

1. d
2. a
3. a
4. d
5. True
6. False; Pmax is a function that limits the amount of pressure that can be provided, particularly with mandatory breath delivery during volume ventilation.
7. False; Neoflow is a feature available for the upgraded version (2.n) of the Evita 4 that allows the unit to be used in neonatal ventilation.
8. The unit's front panel contains touch pads, a dial (rotary) knob, and a computer screen. On the computer screen are images or icons. Some are shaped like knobs and are called "soft" or "cyber" knobs, and some are shaped like touch pads and are called "soft" or "cyber" pads. All these dials and knobs are used to control the unit.
9. Touch the soft pad for V_T on the computer screen to select it (the icon changes from green to yellow). Use the rotary knob to choose the desired value for V_T. Press the rotary knob when the desired value is visible to activate that value. The icon changes back to its original color.
10. This is a top priority warning, indicating that the set high-frequency respiratory rate limit has been exceeded.

Dräger E-2 Dura Review Questions

1. d
2. c
3. b
4. c
5. b
6. True; the purpose of this special function is to measure end-expiratory pressure (auto-PEEP level).
7. False; the Evita 2 Dura is not equipped for neonatal ventilation. Otherwise, both ventilators require you to select the type of patient you are going to ventilate during the initial set-up.
8. True; after a parameter touch pad is pressed, it flashes to indicate that it is activated and can be changed.
9. When an alarm event occurs, either exclamation points or a red or yellow light flashes at the upper right corner of the unit. The number of exclamation points (one, two, or three) or the color that appears designates the level of alarm priority. In addition, an alarm message is displayed at the upper right corner of the computer screen to provide information on the type of alarm limit that has been exceeded. If a low or medium priority alarm occurs and the problem is corrected, the alarm (lights, message, and audible)

switches off. Warning messages, however, must be acknowledged by pressing the alarm reset touch pad.

10. Although the setting of the parameter is slightly different because of the difference in the control panels, the function of Pmax in the Evita 2 Dura is the same as in the E-4. Pmax operates in CMV, SIMV, and MMV modes. When Pmax is operational, the unit will guarantee the set V_T, but limits the pressure delivered during the breath. The pressure in the circuit rapidly reaches the maximum pressure setting (Pmax,), inspiration continues for the set inspiratory time (time-cycled), but the amount of pressure in the circuit does not go above this setting. Flow rises rapidly during inspiration, plateaus, and then becomes a descending flow waveform. The V_T will remain constant at the set value as long as flow drops to zero before the end of inspiration. If flow does not drop to zero for the pressure being provided by the unit, then the volume cannot be guaranteed and a VOLUME NOT CONSTANT alarm is activated.

Hamilton VEOLAR^{FT} Review Questions

1. b
2. b
3. a
4. d
5. c
6. True
7. False; the flush control flushes the circuit at 60 L/min with the oxygen percentage set on the O_2 % control.
8. True, the nebulizer may increase V_T slightly.
9. E% = 75% (100% – 25%); TCT = 60 sec ÷ (15 breaths/min) = 4 sec; T_I = 1 sec; T_E = 3 sec; I:E = 1:3. These are set values; however, if a breath is patient-triggered, it can actually shorten T_E.
10. When HOLD is pressed during exhalation, it stops the delivery of the next breath (valve closes when inspiratory flow is detected) and keeps the exhalation valve closed to measure end-expiratory pressure or auto-PEEP. To read this value, select the PEEP touch pad in the monitoring section.

Hamilton GALILEO Review Questions

1. d
2. c
3. a
4. c
5. False; the highest pressure would be the high-pressure alarm, which is normally set above the pressure level for breath delivery.
6. True
7. The commonly adjusted parameters for any mode appear on the screen. The operator selects the desired parameter, such as tidal volume, by scrolling through the choices using knob C. When the desired parameter is highlighted, the operator pushes knob C to select the parameter. The icon for the parameter then changes from yellow to red. By rotating knob C, the operator changes the numeric value of the parameter. For example, if V_T is highlighted (yellow) and selected (red), the value for V_T can be increased or decreased by rotating knob C. The operator confirms the changes by pressing knob C; the changes will not become active until they are confirmed by pressing knob C.
8. The actual values for any of the alarm parameters are represented by a green horizontal line on the bar graph for the parameter.
9. $\dot{V}_E$ delivery in the adult is 0.1 L/min/kg IBW when the $\dot{V}_E$ support is set at 100%. For a 50 kg adult, the $\dot{V}_E$ will equal 5 L/min.
10. They are very similar except for the way in which the pressures are set. On the VEOLAR^{FT}, the PS level plus CPAP equals the peak pressure. For example, if P_{peak} is 20 cm H_2O and CPAP is set at 5 cm H_2O, the PS level is 15 cm H_2O (P_{peak} – CPAP). In the GALILEO, if you want 15 cm H_2O of PS and the patient is receiving 5 of CPAP, set PS at 15 cm H_2O. P_{peak} will be 20 cm H_2O (PS + CPAP).

Puritan Bennett 740 Review Questions

1. d
2. b
3. c
4. d
5. c
6. c
7. False; when not in use, the ventilator should be in the standby mode to allow the battery to charge. This requires that it be plugged into an AC power source, turned on, and placed into standby using the menu function.
8. False; apnea ventilation works in the spontaneous mode or when the mandatory rate for A/C or SIMV is set at less than 6 breaths/min
9. True
10. Apnea ventilation will not begin, because it is available only in the spontaneous mode. Because the minimum respiratory rate of 3 breaths/min is the lowest possible setting for both A/C and SIMV, a mandatory breath will occur before the apnea time would have elapsed (it actually elapses at 20.2 seconds). However, you would expect a low $\dot{V}_E$ alarm to occur as long as you had set the low $\dot{V}_E$ alarm correctly.
11. a
12. c

Puritan Bennett 760 Review Questions

1. b
2. c
3. d
4. b
5. a

Puritan Bennett 840 Review Questions

1. c
2. d
3. d
4. a
5. True; these settings are always visible as long as the ventilator is operating.
6. d
7. c
8. c
9. a
10. b
11. a
12. True
13. True
14. True
15. d

Puritan Bennett 7200 Review Questions

1. b
2. a
3. d
4. d
5. a
6. b
7. No correct choice is provided. I and IV are not available in Option 30/40.
8. c
9. c
10. Set trigger flow at 2 L/min for this size patient. The base flow must be about twice this value (4 L/min), but the lowest available setting is 5 L/min (maximum is 20 L/min).

Newport Breeze E150 Review Questions

1. c
2. a
3. c
4. d
5. c
6. b
7. b
8. True
9. False; the E150 does not have a tidal volume control.
10. First, the therapist should check the sensitivity setting to be sure it is adjusted to the baseline and fine-tuned to be as sensitive as possible to patient effort. Then the set spontaneous flow setting should be checked because it may be too high for patient need and may be interfering with the ventilator sensing patient effort. In addition, there might be a leak in the circuit.

Newport Wave E200 Review Questions

1. a
2. a
3. Either "a" or "b" is correct, although it is probably better to add an external gas source for nebulization than to change the mode of ventilation to the patient. You would have to monitor the effects of the extra flow on pressures, flows, and volumes. The E200 nebulizer does not work during pressure-control ventilation.
4. d
5. b
6. b
7. True
8. True
9. A 10% discrepancy from delivered V_T is not alarming. It may be the result of a knob setting being slightly off. Another possibility is that the pressure-relief valve setting is being reached during the volume-targeted breath.
10. T_I is constant on the Wave and is based on what is set on the front panel. When you use an inspiratory pause, this actually shortens the time during which inspiratory flow can occur. To achieve the target V_T (based on set flow and T_I), the actual flow increases over the set value. The increase in flow results in a small increase in pressure.

Pulmonetics LTV Series Review Questions

1. c
2. d
3. a
4. b
5. a
6. d
7. b
8. True. There is a "- -" setting for sensitivity which makes the unit unresponsive to patient effort.
9. a
10. c
11. The message LMV LPPS OFF means that both the low minute volume and low peak pressure alarms are turned off.

Respironics Esprit Review Questions

1. d
2. d
3. c
4. a
5. a
6. c
7. d
8. True
9. a
10. c
11. c
12. d
13. b

Siemens Servo 900C Review Questions

1. c
2. c
3. b
4. d
5. c
6. b
7. True
8. True; the set apnea time is 15 seconds.
9. V_T = (12 L/min) ÷ 12 breaths/min = 1.0 L; TCT = 60 sec ÷ (12 breaths/min) = 5 sec. T_I = 0.2 × 5 sec = 1 sec. Flow = (12 L/min) × (100%/20%) = 60 L/min.
10. During PC, the inspiratory pressure control determines the target pressure, and this value is added to the set baseline (PEEP) level.

Siemens Servo 300 Review Questions

1. c
2. d
3. a
4. a
5. d
6. a
7. True
8. False
9. The Servo 300 gives four test breaths when PRVC is initiated. It measures pressures and volumes to calculate the system compliance and uses this information to determine the pressure required to deliver the desired volume.
10. The ventilator will sound an alarm, and the message "LIMITED PRESSURE" appears in the window. The ventilator will not let the pressure rise higher than the upper pressure limit setting minus 5 cm H_2O.

    For this patient, this indicates that more pressure is required to deliver the same volume. The patient's lung characteristics may have changed. For example, the airway resistance may have increased because of secretions in the airway, or the lung compliance may have decreased from a lung problem such as a pneumothorax or developing pulmonary edema. The patient should be carefully evaluated to determine the cause and then treated appropriately.

Dräger Savina Review Questions

1. d
2. a
3. b
4. d
5. d
6. b
7. d

Siemens Servo^i Review Questions

1. b
2. a
3. c
4. a
5. d
6. c
7. d

Viasys Avea Review Questions

1. c
2. d
3. a
4. d
5. a
6. c
7. b
8. b
9. d

Newport e500 Review Questions

1. b
2. a
3. c
4. b
5. c
6. e
7. c
8. b
9. a
10. c

Chapter 13

Clinical Rounds Exercises

Clinical Rounds 13-1

This indicates alarm limits are manually set and the pressure alarms are violated. The respiratory therapist should allow the microprocessor to automatically set them by pressing the button for 3 seconds.

Clinical Rounds 13-2

A "Pressure Setting Incompatible" alarm will occur when the PEEP/CPAP level is set higher than the Inspiratory Pressure control. The therapist needs to evaluate the appropriate setting for both of these controls based on the patient's condition.

Clinical Rounds 13-3

Problem I: The total flow will be the auxiliary gas flow plus the higher setting, either inspiratory or base flow. In this case the total flow is 5 L/min plus 10 L/min = 15 L/min
Problem II: There is more than one possible answer to this question. There could be a leak in the system. Also, the Over Pressure Release Valve may be set at 10 cm H_2O.

Clinical Rounds 13-4

I. The cause of the problem is insufficient internal battery power to run the ventilator.
II. The infant can receive room air because the expiratory valve and the internal safety valve both open.
III. The respiratory therapist should immediately provide another means of ventilation for the patient and then connect the Infant Star to an AC outlet.

Clinical Rounds 13-5

In this situation, the flow is inadequate for the ventilator to deliver the set PIP within the selected inspiratory time. Therefore, the "Low Inspiratory Pressure" alarm will be activated. Increasing the flow should resolve this problem.

Clinical Rounds 13-6

The ventilator rate of 78 breaths/min would permit a total cycle time (the amount of time for one inspiration and one expiration) of 0.77 seconds. If inspiratory time is set at 0.5 seconds, an expiratory time of only 0.27 seconds is possible (0.77 seconds minus 0.5 seconds = 0.27 seconds). Therefore the "Insufficient Expiratory Time" alarm will be activated. For rates below 100 bpm, an expiratory time of less than 0.3 seconds will trigger this alarm.

Clinical Rounds 13-7

This is an example where the patient is probably actively inspiring since the set V_T is less than the delivered V_T. The breath is not volume-cycled. Since flow drops to zero before the end of inspiration, the breath is not flow-cycled.

Clinical Rounds 13-8

The therapist should check to see if the leak compensation is turned on. If it is turned on, the sensitivity control may need to be readjusted. In some cases efforts to remove leaks are preferable to using the leak compensation feature. The therapist should also check to be sure no Auto-PEEP is present, which can make triggering the ventilator difficult.

Clinical Rounds 13-9

With improvement in blood gases and breath sounds, the increase in servo pressure may indicate an improvement in compliance.

Review Questions

1. c
2. b
3. b
4. a
5. a
6. d
7. d
8. a
9. b
10. d
11. c
12. c
13. d
14. a
15. d
16. b
17. d
18. b
19. c
20. a
21. c
22. d
23. b
24. a
25. d
26. b
27. d
28. c.

Chapter 14

Clinical Rounds Exercises

Clinical Rounds 14-1

A change in altitude can affect the ventilator's oxygen blender. The therapist should use the Menu/ESC button to readjust the altitude setting.

Clinical Rounds 14-2

The high peak pressure alarm is about 35 cm H_2O, and the pressure-relief control is at 25 cm H_2O to allow the therapist to start at approximately the same V_T as was set in the volume control mode.

Clinical Rounds 14-3

Yes. The E cylinder can provide approximately 45 minutes of ventilation.

Rate = 15 breaths/min. V_T = 500 mL. Cylinder pressure = 1500 psi.
Tank factor (E cylinder) = 0.28.
Estimated duration = (cylinder pressure × tank factor)/minute ventilation
(Cylinder pressure × tank factor) = (1500 psi) × (0.28) = 336 L
Minute ventilation = (rate) (V_T) = (15 breaths/min) (0.5 L) = 7.5 L/min
Estimated duration = 336 L/7.5 L/min = 44.8 min

Clinical Rounds 14-4

The sensitivity is set by the manufacturer at –2 cm H_2O. The patient must create a drop in the circuit pressure to –2 cm H_2O to trigger a volume-targeted breath. The peak pressure is the sum of the pressures associated with delivery of the set volume plus the baseline pressure. During exhalation, the pressure drops to the value set on the PEEP valve. To overcome this problem, the operator can increase the breath rate to reduce the work of breathing required by the spontaneously triggered breaths.

Clinical Rounds 14-5

10 cm H_2O of the pressure support. The pressure support delivered to the patient is the difference between pressure support and PEEP: 15 – 5 = 10 cm H_2O.

Clinical Rounds 14-6

Problem 1: The tidal volume is equal to the flow (L/sec) times the inspiratory time (seconds.)
60 L/min = 60 sec/60 L/min = 1 L/sec
1 L/sec × 1 second = 1.0 L tidal volume
Problem 2: Total cycle time is 60 sec/20 breaths/min = 3 seconds. T_E = TCT – T_I = 3 sec – 2.5 sec.
T_E = 0.5 sec, estimated V_T is 0.1 L/sec × 2.5 sec = 0.25 L
I:E = (2.5/0.5)/(0.5/0.5) = 5:1)

Since the E100M will limit the ratio to 4:1, if the t_I and rate settings result in an inverse I: E ratio of greater than 4:1, the I: E ratio display adjacent to the t_I control flashes. t_I is then shortened by the ventilator to provide an I:E ratio of no more than 4:1. This results in a reduced tidal volume delivery. To reestablish the desired V_T, the operator can either increase the mandatory flow or reduce the set t_I.

In this case it limits T_I to 2.0 seconds (ratio of 4:1). At a flow of 0.1 L/sec the new V_T will be 0.2 L.

Clinical Rounds 14-7

The sensitivity has to be adjusted. Before the patient took spontaneous breaths, the sensitivity did not need to be set.

Clinical Rounds 14-8

The Bear 33 does not compensate for PEEP on spontaneous breaths. The trigger sensitivity allows for adjustments to mandatory, not spontaneous, breaths. When the patient triggers a spontaneous breath, the demand valve must be opened at –0.2 cm H_2O below atmospheric pressure, regardless of what the baseline pressure is.

Clinical Rounds 14-9

There are several possible answers. There could be a small leak in the circuit, or the measuring device (respirometer) could be inaccurate. The V_T setting on the ventilator may be out of calibration, but most likely, the PEEP attachment is in the wrong position. It should be placed proximal to the exhalation valve when a disposable circuit is used.

Clinical Rounds 14-10

No. The total cycle time is 4 seconds with an inspiratory time of 2.5 seconds. The inverse I:E ratio alarm will sound and limit the I:E ratio to 1:1, thereby limiting the inspiratory time.

Clinical Rounds 14-11

The machine will not cycle from inspiration to expiration when the EPAP setting is equal to or greater than the IPAP setting. Until the IPAP setting is increased or the EPAP setting is decreased, the pressure will remain constant in the circuit (CPAP = 8 cm H_2O) at the IPAP setting.

Clinical Rounds 14-12

None. If the rate setting is 6, the total respiratory cycle is 10 seconds. Because the patient is breathing 20 times a minute, or once every 3 seconds, the time interval for a time-triggered breath is never exceeded, and no time-triggered mandatory breath is delivered.

Clinical Rounds 14-13

The Respironics Vision will not allow EPAP to be set higher than IPAP. The unit will stop the pressure from rising higher than the IPAP setting. This is not unlike the BiPAP S/T, which will treat this as a CPAP setup and keep both the IPAP and EPAP at the same level when EPAP is set higher than IPAP.

Clinical Rounds 14-14

The rise time setting is greater than the % I time. Because this has occurred, the % I time will remain the same, but the rise time setting will be decreased to the maximum setting below the % I time.

Review Questions

1. c
2. d
3. d
4. b
5. a
6. c
7. b
8. d
9. d
10. c
11. c
12. c
13. a
14. c
15. d
16. a
17. c
18. c
19. True
20. False
21. True
22. True
23. False
24. True

Chapter 15

Clinical Rounds Exercises

Clinical Rounds 15-1

Several important facts suggest that Mr. H may have a sleep-related disorder: he has been referred to the laboratory after an automobile accident when he "fell asleep at the wheel." He also reports excessive daytime sleepiness, and his wife says that he snores and that his sleeping pattern has become increasingly restless during the last 6 months. It is also mentioned that he has a long history of smoking cigarettes (possibly indicating the presence of some chronic respiratory problem, such as small airway disease) and that alcohol seems to exacerbate his snoring episodes. All of these findings suggest that Mr. H might have obstructive sleep apnea.

An effective strategy here would be to schedule this patient for an overnight sleep study involving polysomnography. This information, coupled with a complete history and physical examination, should allow for a diagnosis of sleep apnea if that is the case. Furthermore, the results of these studies will provide valuable information on the severity of the disorder, thus helping you to devise an appropriate treatment plan.

Clinical Rounds 15-2

This is a typical polysomnographic recording of a patient with mixed sleep apnea. Notice that an initial central apnea is followed by an obstructive apnea that usually produces significant oxygen desaturation.

Review Questions

1. c
2. Neonates do not follow the pattern of sleep that is typically found in adult sleepers. For example, adults enter sleep through NREM and progress over a period of 90 minutes through NREM Stages 1-4 to REM sleep. Neonates enter sleep through an active sleep state, which is comparable to REM sleep in the adult. Furthermore, as any parent can attest, neonates awaken on a more regular basis, such as every 2-3 hours.
3. As the sleeper passes through the various stages of non-REM sleep, there is a progressive reduction in chemosensitivity and respiratory drive. The reduction in respiratory drive that occurs during the early stages of non-REM sleep (Stages 1 and 2) predisposes the person to periods of apnea (i.e., Cheyne-Stokes respiration) as he or she fluctuates between being awake and being asleep. With the establishment of non-REM slow-wave sleep (Stages 3 and 4), non-respiratory inputs become minimized, and minute ventilation is regulated by metabolic control. Minute ventilation decreases by 1 to 2 L/min when compared with wakefulness. As a consequence, $PaCO_2$ rises by 2 to 8 mm Hg, and PaO_2 decreases by 5 to 10 mm Hg.

   As the sleeper enters REM sleep, breathing becomes irregular as the ventilatory response to chemical and mechanical respiratory stimuli are further reduced and even transiently abolished. There is decreased skeletal muscle activity, including inhibition of the upper airway muscles and the intercostal and accessory muscles of respiration. Inhibition of the upper airway muscles leads to an increase in upper airway resistance, and inhibition of the intercostal and accessory muscles is associated with diminished thoracoabdominal coupling and short periods of central apnea (10 to 20 seconds in duration). $PaCO_2$ and PaO_2 levels are variable but are generally similar to those during the latter stages of non-REM sleep.
4. b
5. True
6. b
7. (1) Oxygen saturation; (2) nasal-oral airflow; (3) respiratory effort.
8. d
9. See Figure 15-7 for the answer to this question.
10. c
11. d
12. c
13. c
14. The AI is the number of apneic periods observed divided by the total number of hours of sleep; the AHI includes both apneic and hypopneic episodes for the total number of hours of sleep. Normative data of asymptomatic individuals from Guilleminault and Dement suggest that males average about seven apneic episodes per 8 hours of sleep, and females average about two episodes per 8 hours of sleep.
15. c

Glossary

A

100% O_2 suction A control on the Puritan Bennett 7200 ventilator that causes the ventilator to deliver 100% O_2 for 2 minutes. Intended for use prior to patient suctioning.
absolute humidity The actual mass or content of water in a measured volume of air. It is usually expressed in grams per cubic meter, or pounds.
absolute zero The temperature at which no molecular motion occurs: –273° C, or 0K.
absorbance sensor An apparatus designed to react to physical stimuli from light or other radiant energy.
accelerating waveform A pressure- or flow-time tracing that indicates upward or increasing movement (acceleration) of the pressure or flow value over time.
accumulator A device that allows a volume of gas to be held for a period and then releases the gas at a preset rate. Used as a timing or limiting mechanism.
accuracy The state or quality of being precise or exact.
acid-fast bacteria Of, or pertaining to, certain bacteria (especially Mycobacteria spp.) that retain red dyes after an acid wash.
acoustics The science of sounds.
action potential An electrical impulse consisting of a self-propagating series of polarizations and depolarizations transmitted across the plasma membrane of nerve and muscles cells.
actual bicarbonate The concentration of HCO_3^- that is present in the plasma of anaerobically drawn blood. It is derived from measurements of pH and $PaCO_2$ using the Henderson-Hasselbalch equation.
adaptive pressure ventilation (APV) A closed-loop (servo-controlled) mode of ventilation available on the Hamilton GALILEO ventilator that provides pressure-targeted ventilation with a volume guarantee.
adaptive support ventilation (ASV) A closed loop mode of ventilation available on the Hamilton GALILEO that uses pressure-targeted ventilation to ensure a certain minute volume. The ventilator predicts tidal volume and respiratory rate based on the patient information entered by the operator, constantly monitors patient and ventilator parameters, and adjusts breath delivery to establish the least amount of work possible for the patient.
adhesion The physical property by which unlike substances are attracted and hold together; also refers to the abnormal formation of fibrous tissues (resulting from inflammation or injury) that bind together body structures that are normally separate.
adjustable reducing valve See adjustable regulator.
adjustable regulator A valve that allows the user to determine (adjust) pressure limits.
adjustable restrictor A mechanism that governs flow or pressure with a series of variable-sized orifices.
aerobe A microorganism that lives and grows in the presence of free oxygen.
aerosol A suspension of solid or liquid particles in a gas.
aerosol mask A device covering both the nose and mouth that is used to deliver aerosols in respiratory care.
airborne Carried in the air via aerosol droplets, droplet nuclei, or dust particles.
airborne precautions Safeguards designed to reduce the risk of airborne transmission of infectious agents.
air-dilution Adding air to a primary gas to reduce the oxygen concentration of the primary gas.
air-dilution control A mechanism that allows the user to set the amount of air dilution in a device.
air-entrainment mask An oxygen mask that uses a Venturi or Pitot type of device to provide precise concentrations of high-flow oxygen to a patient.
air foil A device that acts like an airplane wing to generate pressure differences by creating areas of high and low resistance in an airstream.
air inlet regulator A regulator that determines the inlet pressure on a gas system or ventilator.
air-mix control Another name for an air-dilution control. Used in the Bird Mark and Bennett TV and PR series respirators.
airway pressure Pressure achieved in the patient airway.
airway pressure release ventilation (APRV) A mode of ventilation during which the patient breathes spontaneously at an elevated baseline that is periodically "released" to allow expiration.
airway resistance (Raw) A measure of the impedance to ventilation caused by gas movement through the airways. It is computed as the change in pressure along a tube divided by the gas flow through the tube.
alarm A signal that is a warning of danger, such as a high-pressure or apnea alarm.
alarm silence A control button that silences audible alarms for approximately 60 seconds or until it is pressed a second time.
Allen test A test for the patency of the radial artery. The patient's hand is formed into a fist while the therapist compresses the ulnar and radial arteries. Compression continues while the fist is opened. If blood perfusion through the ulnar artery is adequate, the hand should flush and resume normal (pink) coloration when the ulnar artery compression is released.
alpha wave One of the four types of brain waves, characterized by a relatively high voltage or amplitude and a frequency of 8 to 13 cycles per second. Alpha waves are the "relaxed waves" of the brain and are the majority of the waves recorded by electro-encephalograms. Compare beta wave, delta wave, and theta wave.
alternating current (AC) An electric current that reverses direction according to a consistent sinusoidal pattern. Compare direct current.
alternating supply system A gas supply system that has two supplies of compressed gas (primary and secondary). The secondary system is used when the primary system fails.
alveolar ventilation (VA) The volume of air that ventilates all the perfused alveoli, measured as minute volume in liters per minute. This figure is also the difference between total ventilation and dead space ventilation. The normal average is from 4 to 5 liters/min.
ambient compartment In the Bird Mark ventilator series, the portion of the ventilator casing that is open to the environment and hence to ambient pressures.
ambient inlet filter A portion of an air entrainment device that removes dust particles and other debris from the entrained air before it enters the gas circuit.

AMBU (air-mask-bag-unit) A type of manual resuscitator consisting of a pliable bag, a one-way valve system, and either a mask or an artificial airway connector.
American Standard Indexing A type of safety system for high-pressure gas connections. American Standard connections are noninterchangeable to prevent the interchange of regulator equipment between gases. American Standard Indexing includes separate systems for large and small cylinders.
ammeter An instrument for measuring the strength of an electric current in terms of amperes.
amorphous solids A solid, such as glass or margarine, in which the constituent atoms and molecules are arranged in a fashion that is not rigid. In contrast, the constituent particles of crystalline solids are more rigidly arranged.
amperometric Refers to measuring an electric current at a single applied potential.
amplitude The height of a waveform; usually indicative of intensity.
anaerobe A microorganism that grows and lives in the absence of oxygen.
analog pressure manometer A back-up method of verifying digitally displayed pressure values (peak, mean, and plateau pressure).
analyte Any substance that is measured; usually applied to a component of blood or other body fluid.
AND/NAND gate A monostable fluidic element with two control ports and two outlet ports.
anemometer A gauge for determining the force or speed and sometimes the direction of the wind or air.
aneroid barometer See aneroid manometer.
aneroid manometer A pressure-measuring device that compares a reference pressure to an observed pressure (using one of several methods).
aneroid manometer assist indicator (cycle indicator) A light that signals a pressure change in an aneroid manometer indicating that the patient has generated a negative pressure (assist effort).
anti-suffocation valve An internal, subambient relief valve on a ventilator that opens if the ventilator cannot provide a breath to the patient. The patient can then inhale, open the valve, and receive room air.
AP series A Bennett ventilator series used for IPPB administration. AP stands for air-compressor powered.
apnea alarm A system that warns that the patient is not breathing or being ventilated.
apneic period A reference to a setting that is adjustable from 2 to 60 seconds to warn that a patient is not breathing.
apneic ventilation Emergency back-up ventilation triggered when no patient breath is detected for a certain period of time.
apneustic flow time A reference to a control on the old Bird Mark series ventilators that limited the length of apnea or no flow allowed by the ventilator.
Archimedes's principle States that when an object is submerged in a fluid, it will be buoyed up by a force equal to the weight of the fluid that is displaced by the object.
arousal response A response to sensory stimulation to induce active wakefulness.
artificial nose See heat and moisture exchanger.
automaticity The property of the heart to initiate an action potential in absence of external stimuli.
assist A mode of ventilation in which every breath is patient-triggered.
assist and sensitivity mechanism A device that sets the maximum effort a patient must make (sensitivity) before the ventilator triggers (assists).
assist/control (A/C or ACV) mode Continuous mandatory ventilation (CMV) in which the minimum breathing rate is predetermined, but the patient can initiate ventilation at an increased rate with a set tidal volume or pressure.
assist/control pressure-targeted A mode of ventilation in which the operator selects a pressure for inspiration. Breaths can be patient- or time-triggered.
assisted breaths Breaths in which the patient begins inspiration, but the ventilator controls the inspiratory phase and ends inspiration.
assistor A ventilator that lets the patient initiate inspiration.
assistor/controller A ventilator that can function as an assistor or as a controller.
atmospheric barometric pressure The force exerted by the air column extending from the measuring site to the edge of space (i.e., 760 mm Hg at sea level). Sometimes called ambient pressure.
atmospheric-to-subatmospheric pressure gradient The difference in the force exerted by the ambient pressure and that exerted in a negative-pressure system. May be called driving pressure.
atom The smallest division of an element that exhibits all the properties and characteristics of that element, including neutrons, electrons, and protons. The number of protons in the nucleus of every atom of a given element is the same and is called its atomic number.
atomic theory The concept that all matter is composed of submicroscopic atoms that are in turn composed of protons, electrons, and neutrons. A chemical element is identified by the number of protons in its atoms.
atrial diastole A period of rest of the atria of the heart.
atrial fibrillation A cardiac rhythm characterized by disorganized electrical activity in the atria accompanied by an irregular ventricular response that is usually rapid.
atrial flutter A type of atrial tachycardia with rates greater than 230 beats per minute. The atria lose their ability to contract normally and typically appear to quiver.
atrial premature depolarizations An atrial beat that occurs earlier than expected. Also known as premature atrial beat.
atrial systole The contraction of the atria of the heart which precedes ventricular contraction by a fraction of a second.
autoclave An apparatus that uses steam under pressure to sterilize articles and equipment.
autoflow A dual mode of ventilation that provides pressure-targeted breaths with volume guarantee whenever volume ventilation (CMV, SIMV, MMV) is simultaneously selected in the Dräger E-4 ventilator. It also alters the function of the inspiratory and expiratory valves, allowing patients to receive whatever inspiratory flow they demand—up to 180 L/min in any volume mode—regardless of the volume settings.
automode A ventilator feature (available on the Servo 300A) designed to switch from a control to a support mode of ventilation if the patient triggers two consecutive breaths. The ventilator remains in the support mode as long as the patient keeps triggering breaths.
auto-PEEP Abnormal and usually undetected residual pressure above atmospheric remaining in the alveoli at end-

exhalation due to dynamic air trapping. Also called intrinsic PEEP.

B

Babington/hydrosphere nebulizer A type of nebulizer in which a thin film of water flowed over a hollow glass sphere with a slit in it, through which a high-flow gas stream was passed, creating a high-density aerosol.
bacilli Aerobic or facultatively aerobic, spore-bearing, rod-shaped microorganisms of Bacillaceae spp.
back pressure A reduction in the pressure gradient secondary to downflow resistance.
back-pressure compensation Any method that allows accurate pressures and flows to be read.
back-pressure switch A fluidic element with one control port that has a loop with a built-in restriction and two outlet ports.
back-up rate A control rate set on a ventilator to take over if a patient's assisted ventilation falls below the desired rate.
back-up ventilation (BUV) A mode of volume ventilation (available on the Puritan Bennett 7200 ventilators) with a minimum breath rate that goes into effect if the patient becomes apneic.
bacteria filter A device designed to remove particles and bacteria from the system. Usually rated in pore size or in microns.
bactericide Any drug or other agent that kills bacteria.
baffle Any obstruction in an aerosol's path that breaks the aerosol into smaller particles.
base excess/deficit The number of millimoles of strong acid or base required to titrate a blood sample to a pH of 7.4, a PCO_2 of 40 mm Hg, and a temperature of 37° C.
base flow The flow added to the circuit during exhalation to provide flow triggering; see also bias flow.
baseline pressure The pressure level at which inspiration begins and ends.
beam deflection The change in the direction of a beam or jet of gas when it is hit with another jet of gas moving through a fluid device.
bell factor In a water-sealed spirometer, the number of milliliters of gas that must be displaced to cause a kymograph pen to move 1 millimeter.
bellows accumulator A device used to store a volume of gas that will be pressurized for delivery to the patient. Usually a bag or bellows.
bellows chamber The inside of a bellows containing a volume of gas.
bellows potentiometer A mechanism that senses the volume displacement of a bellows and releases the contents at a preset value, usually through an electrical signal.
Bennett Cascade A specialized, heated passover humidifier employing a water-air froth as a humidifying technique.
Bennett circuit The patient gas delivery tubing that includes all of the tubing and ancillary devices from the machine to the patient and back.
Bennett MA-1 ventilator A mechanical volume ventilator (Mechanical Assistor-1) previously manufactured by the Puritan-Bennett Corporation.
Bennett PR ventilators Bennett Pressure Respirator series (1 and 2) pneumatically powered assistor/controllers. No longer produced.
Bennett valve A drumlike device with pressure/flow sensitive vanes that controls gas pressure and flow in the Bennett PR and AP series respirators.
Berman airway An upper airway device (oropharyngeal airway) used to provide air passage distal to the tongue by keeping the base of the tongue away from the back of the throat.
beta wave One of the four types of brain waves, characterized by relatively low voltage and a frequency of more than 13 cycles per second. Beta waves are the "busy waves" of the brain. Compare alpha wave; delta wave; and theta wave.
bias alert A message provided on the T-Bird AVS ventilator that informs the operator of the bias flow setting after self-testing at start-up.
bias flow Flow in the circuit during the expiratory phase of mechanical ventilation that makes fresh gas immediately available when the patient inhales. Bias flow also reduces the ventilator's response time for triggering a breath.
bilevel continuous positive airway pressure (BiPAP) A variant of continuous positive airway pressure in which both inspiratory and expiratory pressures are set by the operator.
bilevel positive airway pressure (BiPAP) A spontaneous breath mode of ventilatory support that allows separate regulation of the inspiratory and expiratory pressures. Also called bilevel pressure assist or bilevel pressure support.
BiPAP Abbreviation for bilevel continuous positive airway pressure.
bistable A special type of fluidic control unit that acts as a switch mechanism.
bleed hole A small hole in the center body of the Bird Mark series respirators that allows pressure equalization across the center body, or a small hole in an accumulator device that allows the measured escape of gas to "dump" the accumulator contents.
bleed regulator An adjustable bleed hole.
blower A mechanical device sometimes used to control volume delivery in a mechanical ventilator (e.g., a rotating vane that produces a flow of gas).
body humidity The absolute humidity in a volume of gas saturated at a body temperature of 37° C; equivalent to 43.8 mg/L.
body plethysmography A method of studying alveolar pressures, lung volumes, and airway resistance. The patient sits or reclines in an airtight compartment and breathes normally. The pressure changes in the alveoli are reciprocated in the compartment and recorded automatically by the body plethysmograph.
body tank respirator Iron lung; a type of negative-pressure ventilator.
boiling point The temperature at which a liquid begins to turn to a gas. For water at 1 atm: 100° C, 212° F, or 373° Absolute.
Boothby-Lovelace-Bulbulian (BLB) mask An apparatus for administering oxygen; consists of a mask fitted with an inspiratory-expiratory valve and a rebreathing bag.
Bourdon flowmeter A flowmeter that incorporates a Bourdon gauge.
Bourdon gauge A device that indicates pressure measurements from the use of a hollow, coiled tube that attempts to straighten in response to increased pressure.
Bourdon regulator A regulator that incorporates a Bourdon gauge.
BPM (breaths per minute) respiratory rate Usually a digital or analog indicator on the ventilator control panel.
Brownian movement The random movement of molecules/particles caused by the molecules being struck by other molecules/particles.
BTPS Abbreviation for body temperature, ambient pressure, saturated (with water vapor).

bubble humidifier A device that increases the water content of a gas by passing it through a volume of water.
buffer base The total blood buffer capable of binding hydrogen ions. Normal buffer base (NBB) ranges from 48 to 52 mEq/L.

C

calorimetry A method of determining energy expenditure by using the measurements of the amount of heat radiated and absorbed by an organism.
capillary blood gases (CBGs) Gases dissolved in the blood that are obtained from a capillary sample. Results include pH, PCO_2, and PO_2 values, which may differ from arterial blood gas values.
capillary mesh A netlike web with small openings that are used to measure flow and resistance in monitoring devices.
capillary system Microscopic tubes that connect arteries and veins and provide perfusion to tissues and cells.
capnogram A tracing that shows the proportion of carbon dioxide in exhaled air.
capnograph A device that measures and provides a graphic representation of the amount of carbon dioxide in a gas sample. A mainstream capnograph analyzes gas at the airway. With a side-stream capnograph, however, the gas to be analyzed is aspirated from the airway through a narrow-bore polyethylene tube and transferred to a sample chamber.
cardiac cycle The pressure, volume, and flow events that occur in the heart and great vessels during a typical heart beat
cardiac work The product of pressure and volume measurements that accompany ventricular contraction.
cardiopulmonary resuscitation (CPR) A basic emergency procedure for life support involving artificial respiration and manual external cardiac massage.
cascade humidifier A bubble humidifier in which gases travel down a tower and pass through a grid into a chamber of heated water. The displaced water rises above the grid, forming a liquid film that is converted to froth as the gas also rises from the chamber through the grid. The process results in an airflow that can have a relative humidity of up to 100% (see Bennett Cascade).
caudad Toward the tail or end of the body; away from the head.
Celsius (C) Temperature scale in which 0° is the freezing point of water and 100° is the boiling point of water at sea level.
center body The metallic divider in the midportion of the Bird Mark series that was a site for gas channels and control devices.
central processing unit (CPU) The component of a computer that controls the encoding and execution of instructions. Mainly consists of an arithmetic unit, which performs arithmetic functions, and an internal memory, which controls the sequencing of operations. Also called processor.
centrifugal nebulizer A humidification device in which a spinning disk with vanes on it breaks water into particles.
central sleep apnea Absence of breathing as the result of medullary depression, which inhibits respiratory movement; becomes more pronounced during sleep. Compare mixed sleep apnea and obstructive sleep apnea.
cephalad Toward the head.
ceramic switch Part of the Bird Mark series ventilators that controls flow through the gas channels. Consists of a ceramic tube with offset grooves and holes that selectively match up with gas channel inlets in the center body.
chamber An accessory to enhance aerosol deposition from a metered dose inhaler.
check valve A device usually consisting of a one-way valve that prevents back or retrograde gas flow.
chemical analyzer A device that measures the amount of a specific gas in a system by measuring the results of chemical reactions.
chemical potential energy Potential energy stored in a chemical bond, such as petroleum reserves of coal, gas, or oil.
chemical sterilant Any chemical agent that destroys all living organisms, including viruses, in a material.
chemiluminescence monitoring A type of nitrogen oxide monitoring system routinely used during nitric oxide administration. It involves the quantification of gas-specific photoemission. See also electrochemical monitoring.
chest cuirass The shell-like part of a negative-pressure ventilator.
chest shell piece The rigid portion of a cuirass type of negative-pressure ventilator that covers the thorax.
Cheyne-Stokes respiration An abnormal, repeating pattern of breathing characterized by progressive hypopnea alternating with hyperpnea and ending in a brief apnea.
child adult mist (CAM) tent An environmental enclosure that controls oxygen concentration, humidity, and temperature.
circadian rhythm A pattern based on a 24-hour cycle, especially the repetition of certain physiologic phenomena, such as sleeping and eating.
CIRC alarm circuit integrity warning Denotes a leak or disconnection in the patient circuit.
Clark electrode The electrode most commonly used to measure the partial pressure of oxygen.
cleaning The removal of all foreign material, especially organic matter (e.g., blood, serum, pus, and fecal matter) from objects with hot water, soaps, detergents, and enzymatic products.
closed-circuit calorimeter See indirect calorimeter.
closed-loop system A hardware/software combination that controls a mechanical or electronic process without user input.
clutch plate In the Bird Mark series, the steel plates that are connected by a wire shaft and suspended between two magnets. The clutch plates act as on/off switches for gas flow.
Coanda effect A term in fluidics that refers to the sidewall attachment phenomenon of gas streams.
cocci Bacteria that are round, spherical, or oval, such as gonococci, pneumococci, staphylococci, and streptococci.
cohesion The attractive force between like molecules.
collodion A clear or slightly opaque, highly inflammable liquid composed of pyroxylin, ether, and alcohol. It dries to a strong, transparent film that is used as a surgical dressing.
combined power ventilator A ventilator that requires both pneumatic and electric sources for operation. The electric source often powers a microprocessor.
combined pressure device A ventilator that employs both positive and negative pressure during breath delivery. For example, a high-frequency oscillator delivers positive pressure on inspiration and negative pressure on expiration.
combined pressure gradient The additive pressure difference in a multipart system, such as the combined air-to-arterial-to-cell pressure difference.
Combitube A double-lumen device designed to provide a patent upper airway when inserted blindly after failed intubation or in a comatose patient with airway difficulties.

compensated leak alarm A warning that activates when the leak compensation mechanism is engaged.
compensator valve A system designed to provide additional flow or volume to overcome the effects of leaks in a pressurized system.
compound A substance composed of two or more elements, chemically combined in definite proportions, that cannot be separated by physical means.
compressibility factor A mathematical expression of the reduction of volume delivery in a ventilator setting in response to increased pressure in the system.
compressor A machine that uses electrical power to move a piston, fan, or bellows, which in turn reduces the volume of air and increases its pressure.
compressor-driven unit A mechanical ventilator that is powered by an air compressor.
concentration gradient In open or communicating systems, the difference between the amount of a substance in part of the system and the amount of the same substance in another part of the system.
condensation Change of state from gas to liquid, such as with water vapor condensation.
conductivity The property of cardiac muscle to propagate and impulse throughout the heart.
constant positive airway pressure See continuous positive airway pressure (CPAP).
constant positive-pressure breathing (CPPB) A mode of ventilation in which the ventilating pressures are always elevated above zero.
contact precautions Safeguards designed to reduce the risk of transmission of epidemiologically important microorganisms by direct or indirect contact.
continuous flow CPAP system A continuous positive airway pressure (CPAP) system incorporating a constant flow of gas.
continuous flow IMV system A volume ventilator with the addition of an intermittent mandatory ventilation circuit that incorporates a constant flow of gas. The one-way valve going toward the patient circuit is kept open by the continuous flow and does not have to be opened by the patient. Also called a closed-circuit IMV system.
continuous flow ventilation (CFV) A mode of ventilation in which a gas stream constantly passes through the airway and is hence available.
continuous mandatory ventilation (CMV) A mode of ventilation that provides control or assist/control ventilation. Breaths are time- or patient-triggered, volume- or pressure-targeted, and volume- or time-cycled.
continuous nebulizer A nebulizer that runs during the entire ventilatory cycle.
continuous positive airway pressure (CPAP) A method of providing positive pressure for spontaneously breathing patients without mechanical assistance (i.e., mandatory breath delivery). A technique for increasing functional residual capacity and arterial oxygenation.
continuous supply system A mechanism that delivers a gas or an aerosol throughout the ventilatory cycle.
control mode Continuous mandatory ventilation (CMV) in which the breathing frequency is determined by the ventilator without patient initiation according to a preset cycling pattern (time-triggered ventilatory support).
control panel The user interface, with the controls for the operator to set desired parameters.
control pneumatic logic circuit A fluidic circuit that controls the operation of other circuits.
control pressure manometer A gauge that indicates the maximum or control pressure in a ventilator system.
control variables Four elements of breath delivery including flow, volume, pressure, and time. The elements are controlled and/or limited by the ventilator. Numerical values for each element are set on the front panel of the ventilator by the operator.
controlled expiratory time A system that controls rate or end-expiration by limiting expiratory time.
controller A type of ventilator that will not allow spontaneous breathing.
convoluted tube A tube that has many bends and turns.
counterweight A weight used to offset the effects of pressure on a system.
coupling chamber In an ultrasonic nebulizer, the water-filled space between the ultrasonic source and the solution to be nebulized. It transmits the ultrasonic waves from the transducer to the medication chamber.
CPAP Abbreviation for continuous positive airway pressure. A method of pressurized gas delivery whereby the patient breathes spontaneously without mechanical assistance at pressures above ambient.
critical pressure The pressure above which a material cannot exist as a gas.
critical temperature The temperature below which a material cannot exist as a gas.
cryogenic Producing extremely low temperatures.
cuirass The shell-like part of a negative-pressure ventilator.
cupped-disk valve A type of valve that looks like a shallow bowl. The convex side of the disk fits into an orifice, sealing it to end inspiration and inspiratory flow delivery, and begin the expiratory phase during mechanical ventilation.
cyber knob The term given by Drager for the icons on the monitor screen of the Dräger E-4 ventilator that are shaped like knobs and used to control the unit.
cyber pad The term given by Dräger for the icons on the monitor screen of the Dräger E-4 ventilator that are shaped like touch pads and used to control the unit.
cycle rate control The part of the ventilator that determines the length of the ventilatory cycle.
cycle variable The phase variable that is measured and used to end inspiration; the element of breath delivery that determines the end of inspiration. See also control variables.

D

dead space ventilation Ventilation characterized by respired gas volume that does not participate in gas exchange. Alveolar dead space is characterized by alveoli that are ventilated but are not perfused.
dead space volume (VD) The amount of volume during ventilation that is not involved in gas exchange because of lack of pulmonary perfusion to the area.
decelerating taper (ramp) A flow curve in which the flow gradually decreases over time.
decelerating waveform See decelerating taper.
decompression port A gas channel that relieves pressure in part of the gas circuit.

decontamination The process whereby contaminants are removed from objects, usually by simple physical means (e.g., washing).
default Failure to do something when it is required or expected.
delay time control A device that controls the back-up rate on a ventilator by setting a maximum time between cycles.
delta wave The slowest of the four types of brain waves, characterized by a frequency of less than 3.5 cycles per second and a relatively high voltage. Delta waves are "deep-sleep waves" associated with a dreamless state from which an individual is not easily aroused. Compare alpha wave; beta wave; and theta wave.
demand-flow accelerator servo An automatic device that increases patient gas flow in response to patient effort.
demand-flow CPAP system A continuous positive airway pressure (CPAP) system in which the patient must open a one-way valve to receive gas flow from a warmed and humidified blended gas source.
demand-flow IMV system An intermittent mandatory ventilation system in which the patient is required to perform the work of opening a one-way valve. Also called a parallel flow IMV or open-circuit IMV.
demand sensitivity system A subsystem that sets the level of inspiratory effort needed to trigger a ventilator into the inspiratory phase.
demand valve A mechanism that provides pressurized gas when the patient makes an inspiratory effort.
density An expression of the amount of mass per unit of volume a substance possesses.
Diameter Index Safety System (DISS) A safety system for compressed gas fittings. The DISS is used in respiratory care when equipment is connected to a low-pressure gas source (less than or equal to 200 psi).
diameter restrictor A device that controls or reduces flow by reducing the diameter of the flow path.
diaphragm compressor A gas delivery system that operates to reduce gas volume by increasing pressure via movement of a flexible diaphragm.
diaphragm/leaf valves Comparatively thin, flat valves that have many applications in respiratory care. They may separate high- and low-pressure areas as one-way valves or as backflow prevention devices.
diaphragm valve See diaphragm/leaf valves.
diastasis A longer period of reduced filling that typically follows the rapid filling period during the first third of ventricular filling.
diastolic depolarization A phenomenon in which cardiac nodal tissue (i.e., nodal tissue) gradually becomes depolarized during phase 4 of its action potential.
differential area gas blending valve A gas-mixing device that changes the proportions of a gas mixture by varying the size of each gas inlet port.
differential output The difference between the output of O_1 and O_2 in a fluidic element.
diffuser A device used to mix or dissipate gases. Also a device to muffle the sound of a loud turbine or compressor.
diffuser humidifier A device that forces gas flow through a porous material submerged in water, causing the gas to form many bubbles that rise to the surface of the gas.
diffusion The physical process whereby atoms or molecules tend to move from an area of higher concentration or pressure to an area of lower concentration or pressure.
Digital Communications Interface (DCI) A function on the Puritan Bennett 7200 ventilator that provides data reports including data logs, chart summary reports, ventilator status reports, and host reports.
digital flowmeter A flowmeter on the panel of the Newport Breeze E150 that displays and controls the flow during spontaneous breaths and is used to stabilize baseline pressure between mandatory breaths in assist/control.
diluter regulator A mechanism that controls the entrained air in an oxygen diluter system.
diode A high-vacuum type of electron tube with a cold anode and a heated cathode that is used as a rectifier of alternating current.
diplobacilli Bacilli that occur in pairs.
diplococcus A member of the Coccaceae family that occur in pairs because of incomplete cell division. Diplococci are often found as parasites of saprophytes. Also used to describe bacteria of the Coccaceae family that occur as pairs of cocci.
dipole-dipole interaction The interaction of equal and opposite electrical charges.
direct-acting valve A device that provides volume or flow by direct action from a control knob or device, such as the valve connected to a water faucet. As the faucet is turned, the valve opens or closes.
direct contact Mutual touching of two individuals or organisms. Many communicable diseases may be spread by direct contact between infected and healthy persons.
direct current (DC) Current flowing in one direction. Compare alternating current.
direct drive piston A piston whose movement is governed by linear (straight line) movement of a shaft that is connected to the piston head. Also called a linear drive piston. Compare with rotary drive piston.
direct-drive piston ventilator A ventilator that incorporates a linear drive piston.
disconnect ventilation An emergency mode of ventilation available on the Puritan Bennett 7200 ventilator that activates when the microprocessor detects inconsistencies in airway pressures, PEEP, and the gas delivery pressure in the pneumatic system, which can occur in conditions such as tubing disconnects or plugged tubing.
disinfection The process of destroying at least the vegetative phase of pathogenic microorganisms by physical or chemical means.
display window A monitoring screen on the front panel of a ventilator that displays ventilator parameters.
DISS See Diameter Indexed Safety System.
Doppler effect The apparent change in frequency of sound or light waves emitted by a source as it moves away from or toward an observer. The frequency increases as the source moves toward the observer and decreases as it moves away (e.g., the rising pitch of an approaching train and the falling pitch of a departing train). The Doppler effect is also observed in electromagnetic radiation (e.g., light and radio waves).
double circuit A type of ventilator with two distinct gas flows, one of which provides power to deliver a breath, and the other is the actual flow delivered to the patient's airway.
double-lumen endotracheal tube (DLET) A specialized endotracheal tube that allows the right and left lungs to be ventilated separately (i.e., independent lung ventilation).
double-stage reducing valve A pressure-control device that lowers line pressure to working pressure in two steps. Generally from 2200 psig to 750 psig to 50 psig.

drag turbine The name of the flow control device in the T-Bird AVS ventilator.
drive mechanism Refers to the method by which gas flow to the patient is achieved with a mechanical ventilator.
droplet precautions Safeguards designed to reduce the risk of transmitting infectious agents by droplet.
drum vane The air foils on the Bennett valve in the PR, TV, and AP series respirators, which act as sensitivity and flow-cycling mechanisms.
dry powder inhaler A type of metered dose inhaler that delivers a drug as a powder rather than as a liquid aerosol.
dry-rolling seal spirometer A type of device measuring volume changes in the airway opening. Consists of a canister containing a piston sealed to it with a rolling diaphragmlike seal.
dual modes of ventilation A phrase used to describe pressure-targeted ventilation that also guarantees delivery of a set volume.
dual OR/NOR gate See OR/NOR fluidic switch.
duckbill/diaphragm/fishmouth valves Valves made of elastic materials that have a slit in the middle, which opens when pressurized to allow gas flow.
dump port A mechanism that allows expired gas to exit the ventilator. May be part of the expiration valve.

E

effective refractory period A period after firing of an impulse during which cardiac tissue is unable to propagate the impulse.
EGTA See esophageal gastric tube airway.
elastic potential energy The potential energy stored in a compressed spring that will be converted into kinetic energy when the spring is allowed to uncoil.
electrical analyzer A type of gas analyzer that detects changes in electrical current in response to varying gas concentrations.
electrical impedance The total opposition offered by an electric circuit to the flow of an alternating current of electrons. Impedance is a combination of the effects of electrical resistance and reactance.
electrically powered Energy supplied by the activity of electrons or other subatomic particles in motion. Also a mechanical device or ventilator requiring electricity to operate.
electricity A form of energy expressed by the activity of electrons and other subatomic particles in motion, as in dynamic electricity, or at rest, as in static electricity. Electricity can be produced by heat; generated by a voltaic cell; or produced by induction, rubbing on nonconductors with dry materials, or chemical activity.
electrochemical Pertains to the electrical effects that accompany chemical action and the chemical activity produced by electrical influence.
electrochemical monitoring A type of monitoring system routinely used when oxygen or nitric oxide is administered. Gases diffusing across a semipermeable membrane react with an electrolyte solution, generating a current flow between two polarized electrodes as electrons are liberated or consumed. See also chemiluminescence monitoring.
electrochemical sensor An apparatus designed to react to physical stimuli that accompany chemical activity produced by electrical influence.
electrode A contact for the induction or detection of electrical activity. Also a medium for conducting an electrical current from the body to physiologic monitoring equipment.
electromagnetic frequency interference (EFI) The disruption of the operation of a device due to electromagnetic waves in the vicinity.
electromechanical transducer A mechanical device that is activated by electricity and capable of converting one form of energy into another. Commonly used to measure physical events.
electromechanical valve A mechanical valve system that responds to an electrical signal; also called an electrically powered mechanical valve.
electromotive force (EMF) The electrical potential, or the ability of electric energy to perform work. Usually measured in joules per coulomb, or volts. Any device, such as a storage battery, that converts some form of energy into electricity is a source of EMF.
electronic capacitance transducer An electronic component that changes one form of energy to another based on the strength of the electrical charge stored in the unit.
electronic logic In the Bear 3 ventilator, the term applied to the control mechanism that governs ventilator operation.
electronically controlled PEEP valve A PEEP valve whose pressure limits are maintained by electrically operated valves.
element One of more than 100 primary, simple substances that cannot be broken down into any other substance by chemical means. Each atom of any element contains a specific number of protons in the nucleus and an equal number of electrons outside the nucleus. The nucleus contains a variable number of neutrons. An element with a disproportionate number of neutrons may be unstable, in which case the nucleus undergoes radioactive decay into a more stable elemental form.
endotracheal tube A type of artificial airway inserted through the mouth or nose and the larynx into the trachea.
energy expenditure The metabolic cost (in calories or kilojoules) of various forms of physical activity.
entrainment device A device designed to add ambient gas into a primary gas stream. Usually a jet/Venturi device.
entrainment nebulizer A nebulizer designed to entrain gas or liquids into the primary gas stream. See also entrainment device.
entrainment reservoir The part of an entrainment nebulizer that contains the substance to be entrained and nebulized.
EOA See esophageal obturator airway.
esophageal gastric tube airway (EGTA) A type of artificial airway that consists of a double lumen tube that passes through a tight-fitting face mask and extends through the mouth into the esophagus (this portion has an inflatable cuff above the distal opening). The oral portion of the airway has a ventilation tube with holes through which gas from a resuscitation device ventilates the lungs.
esophageal obturator airway (EOA) A type of artificial airway used in emergency situations. Consists of a blind tube that passes through a tight-fitting face mask and extends through the mouth into the esophagus (this portion has an inflatable cuff). The oral portion of the airway has holes through which gas from a resuscitation device is forced into the lungs.
EST See extended self-test.
eukaryotic Of or pertaining to cells with true nuclei bounded by a nuclear membrane and capable of mitosis.
evaporation The process by which liquids change into the vapor state. This occurs because of changes in temperature, pressure, and vapor pressure gradients.

excitability The ability of the heart to respond to a stimulus by producing an action potential.
exhalation timer A control that determines the length of the expiratory portion of the respiratory cycle.
exhalation valve A one-way valve system through which exhaled gases exit the ventilator and its circuit.
exhalation valve leak alarm A device that warns that the integrity of the exhalation valve has failed.
exhausted fuel cell alarm A warning that the sensing mechanism in a fuel cell gas analyzer is not functional.
expiratory flow cartridge In the Bird Mark series, an accumulator cartridge that used an adjustable and controlled leak to vary expiratory time.
expiratory flow gradient control A device that allows for adjustment of expiration by manipulation of back pressure and expiratory pressure gradients.
expiratory hold A mechanical ventilator control that delays mandatory breath delivery when it is pressed during the end of exhalation, used for measuring auto-PEEP.
expiratory hold (end-expiratory pause) The time at the end of exhalation after a mandatory breath during which the ventilator delays delivery of another mandatory breath for the purpose of measuring end-expiratory pressure. Usually performed to check for auto-PEEP.
expiratory pause See expiratory hold.
expiratory positive airway pressure (EPAP) The pressure measured in a patient circuit during exhalation. A parameter that can be set during bilevel positive airway pressure (BiPAP) ventilation that governs pressure delivery during exhalation.
expiratory resistance control An adjustable device that allows back pressure to increase forces opposing expiratory flow.
expiratory retard A device or control designed to increase the resistance to exhaled gas flow, which increases the pressure maintained in the circuit during exhalation and can increase expiratory time.
expiratory servo valve The device that controls the expiratory scissors valve in the Siemens 900 series ventilators.
expiratory tidal volume The volume from a normal inspiration to a normal expiration measured from a patient's exhaled air.
expiratory time The length of time of the expiratory portion of a breath. From the end of inspiration to the beginning of the next inspiration.
expiratory time accumulator See expiratory flow cartridge.
expiratory time control See expiratory flow cartridge.
expiratory timer See expiratory flow cartridge.
expiratory trigger sensitivity (ETS) The adjustable control available on the Hamilton GALILEO ventilator used to establish the percent of peak flow at which pressure support or spontaneous breaths will cycle out of inspiration.
extended self-test (EST) A series of tests that are part of the normal maintenance procedure for the Puritan Bennett 7200 ventilator and that trained personnel perform between patient uses.
external battery A direct current power source sometimes used by ventilators as an alternative power supply when the normal electrical power source is not available.
external circuit The portion of the pneumatic circuit consisting of tubing from a ventilator to a patient. Also called patient circuit or ventilator circuit.
external IMV reservoir A reservoir bag or tubing that provides a volume of gas at a predetermined Fio2 in a sufficient amount to accommodate the patient's volume.
external IMV system A reservoir, tubing, gas source, and valve system attached to the outside of a ventilator. Sometimes referred to as an H-valve assembly because of its design.
external PEEP valve A threshold or flow resistor added to the exhalation valve assembly of a ventilator or breathing device (e.g., resuscitation valve) to provide positive pressure during exhalation.
extreme extension See sniffer's position.

F

facultative Not obligatory; having the ability to adapt to more than one condition (e.g., a facultative anaerobe that can live with or without oxygen).
Fahrenheit (F) A temperature scale in which the boiling point of water is 212° and the freezing point of water is 32° at sea level.
fail-safe baseline metering orifice A variable metering device whose orifice opens during failure of power or pressure.
fail-safe valve A safety measure designed to provide a way for the patient to breathe if the gas delivery devices fail.
feedback channel In pneumatic or fluid devices, a mechanism that provides a signal or flow to a control device.
feedback line See feedback channel.
fenestrated tracheotomy tube A tracheotomy tube with a hole or "window" (fenestra in Latin) on the posterior wall of the outer cannula above the cuff. This allows the patient to speak when the inner cannula is removed, the cuff is deflated, and the tracheostomy tube is occluded at the connector. Fenestrated tubes aid in weaning patients from the artificial airway.
fetal hemoglobin (HbF) A hemoglobin variant that has a greater affinity for oxygen than adult hemoglobin. HbF is gradually replaced over the first year of life by HbA (adult hemoglobin).
F_IO_2 (fraction of inspired oxygen) The ratio (amount) of oxygen to the total volume of a gas mixture; expressed as a decimal.
fishmouth valve See duckbill/diaphragm/fishmouth valves.
fixed orifice A hole in a device that has a specific, unchanging size.
fixed-performance oxygen-delivery system Oxygen therapy equipment that supplies inspired gases at a consistent preset oxygen concentration. Also called a high-flow system.
fixed restrictor A device that is designed to produce a set back pressure (resistance) that inhibits forward flow.
flapper A type of valve system that employs a lightweight diaphragm to occlude an orifice.
flap vane In the Puritan Bennett PR, AP, and TV series ventilators, the winglike protrusions extending from the Bennett valve's internal cylinder that react to the force of airflow to cycle the device.
Fleisch pneumotachometer A device that operates on the principle that the flow of gas through the device is proportional to the pressure drop that occurs as the gas flows across a known resistance (a bundle of brass capillary tubes arranged in parallel.)
flip-flop device See flip-flop unit.
flip-flop unit A fluidic element that contains two outlets and two control ports. The main flow switches flow from one outlet to the other when a signal gas pulse acts on the main flow.
floating electrode ECG electrodes, which consist of a silver-silver chloride electrode that is encased within a plastic

housing. The surface of the electrode is covered with a conductive gel or paste. The entire electrode assembly can be attached to the skin with a double-sided ring, which adheres to the patient's skin and to the plastic housing of the electrode. These electrodes are referred to as "floating" electrodes because the only conductive path between the electrode and the patient's skin is the electrolyte gel or paste.

floating-island nebulizer A type of aerosol production device in which the jet assembly floats underneath a pontoon assembly in a reservoir of water. Also called a Win-Liz nebulizer after the wives of the inventors.

flow acceleration cartridge In the Bird Mark series, a pneumatic device designed to increase inspiratory flow.

flow-and-volume augmented breaths in the Bear 1000 A function that provides additional flow or volume when the patient's inspiratory effort drops pressure below the set baseline pressure.

flow-by option A feature available on the Puritan Bennett 7200 ventilator that provides continuous flow during the expiratory phase to provide fresh gas at the beginning of inspiration and reduce the ventilator response time to patient inspiratory effort (also see bias flow and base flow).

flow control See flow control valve.

flow control valve A device that controls and adjusts inspiratory flow on a ventilator, thus affecting respiratory rate and/or volume.

flow-dependent incentive spirometer A device that encourages a patient to take slow, deep breaths. The patient is encouraged to achieve a specific air flow during inspiration by using a visual cue that indicates air flow.

flow-dependent valve A device that responds to low flow by halting inspiration, the operating principle of the Bennett valve in the AP, PR, and TV series Puritan Bennett respirators. A flow dependent valve measures and displays the inspiratory flow that the patient achieves during a maximum sustained inspiratory effort.

flowmeter A device that controls and measures a flow of gas or liquid. Usually stated in volume per unit of time.

flow rate control See flow control.

flow resistor See flow restrictor.

flow restrictor A device that reduces the flow of a fluid/gas out of a system by providing an in-stream obstruction, usually in the form of a orifice of reduced size, thus causes back pressure in the system. Increases or decrease in gas flow result in increases or decreases in the back pressure created by the restrictor.

flow restrictor/regulator See flow restrictor.

flow sensor A mechanism that detects the movement of a volume of gas.

flow transducer An electronic device that changes one type of signal to another type proportionate to the flow that passes through it.

flow trigger The amount the flow must drop from the base flow value to trigger a breath during mechanical ventilation.

flow triggering When the ventilator detects a drop in gas flow then inspiration is set to occur.

flow waveforms The graphic pattern produced when flow is plotted against time.

fluidic Referring to hydrodynamic principles used to direct gas flow through circuits, resulting in switching of flow directions and signal amplification. Also used in pressure and flow sensing.

fluidic-breathing assistor A device that uses the principles of fluidics to augment the patient's ventilatory efforts.

fluidic drive A type of pneumatically powered ventilator or device that uses fluidic principles (elements). A mechanism to provide the primary power source for gas delivery using fluidics.

fluid logic A method for delivering gas flow that uses fluidic elements that do not require moving parts (see fluidic).

fluorescent sensor An optical blood gas sensor that uses dyes that fluoresce when struck by light in the ultraviolet or near-ultraviolet visible range. The pH, PCO_2, or PO_2 of arterial blood can be determined by using these devices.

flutter valve A mucus clearance device that consists of a pipe-shaped apparatus with a steel ball in a bowl covered with a perforated cap. The flutter valve utilizes the principles associated with positive expiratory pressure and high-frequency airway oscillations.

fomite Nonliving material, such as bed linens or equipment, that may transmit pathogenic organisms.

fractional distillation of liquid air A method of reducing air to its component gases using pressure and temperature changes. See also Joule-Kelvin-Thompson method.

fractional hemoglobin saturation The amount of oxyhemoglobin measured divided by the amount of all four types of hemoglobin present, written as follows: Fractional O_2Hb = $O_2Hb/(HHb + O_2Hb + COHb + MetHb)$.

FRC See functional residual capacity.

freezing point The temperature at which a liquid becomes a solid.

French scale A measurement scale commonly used to delineate the external diameter of catheters; 1 French unit equals approximately 0.33 mm.

French sizes See French scale.

froth A mixture of liquid and gas that forms a dense layer of bubbles, increasing the gas/liquid surface area.

functional hemoglobin saturation The oxyhemoglobin concentration divided by the concentration of hemoglobin capable of carrying oxygen, written as follows: Functional O_2Hb = $O_2Hb/(HHb + O_2Hb)$.

functional residual capacity (FRC) The total amount of gas left in the lungs after a normal, quiet exhalation.

fungicide An agent destructive to fungi.

fusible plug A type of pressure-relief mechanism made of a metal alloy that melts when the temperature of the gas in the tank exceeds a predetermined temperature. Fusible plugs operate on the principle that as the pressure in a tank increases, the temperature of the gas increases, which causes the plug to melt. The melting of the plug releases excess pressure.

G

galvanic analyzer An electric analyzer that measures gas concentrations by measuring the change in resistance of electric current in both reference and sampling circuits.

gas A fluid state of matter with the least organization and definition.

gas-collector exhalation valve A device that allows expired gases to be collected through a one-directional port.

gas streaming Asymmetric velocity profiles that occur when gas flows in both directions through a conductive airway (tube) at the same time as exhaled gas travels on the outside of the tube and inspired gas moves down the center.

geometric standard deviation (GSD) A measure of the variability of particle diameters within an aerosol. The higher the GSD, the more (larger and smaller) particles are present.

germicide A drug that kills pathogenic microorganisms.
Geudel airway An upper airway device (oropharyngeal airway) used to provide air passage distal to an obstructing tongue.
glucose oxidase An enzyme used to coat electrodes when measuring glucose.
gmw See gram molecular weight.
gram molecular weight (gmw) A chemical measurement for the mass of a chemical equal to the atomic weight of its chemical components (expressed in grams); sometimes called the combining weight.
Gram negative Having the pink color of the counterstain used in Gram's method of staining microorganisms. This property is a primary method of characterizing organisms in microbiology.
Gram positive Retaining the violet color of the stain used in Gram's method of staining microorganisms. This property is a primary method of characterizing organisms in microbiology.
Gram stain The method of staining microorganisms using a violet stain and an iodine solution; decolorizing with an alcohol or acetone solution; and counterstaining with safranin. The retention of either the violet color of the stain or the pink color of the counterstain is a primary means of identifying and classifying bacteria. Also called Gram's method.
graphics A visual representation of monitored parameters, such as pressure, volume, and flow per unit time. See also scalars.
gravitational potential energy The potential energy an object can gain by falling, as a result of gravity.

H

Haldane effect The influence of hemoglobin saturation and oxygen on carbon dioxide dissociation.
hardware The mechanical, magnetic, and electronic design, structure, and devices of a computer. Compare software.
heart blocks A group of arrhythmias in which impulses fail to propagate in a normal manner due to an increased refractoriness of one or more conductive paths in the heart. (e.g., AV blocks).
heart sounds A normal series of sounds produced within the heart during the cardiac cycle that can be heard over the precordium.
heat and moisture exchanger (HME) A passive, disposable device that humidifies and warms incoming gases in patients receiving mechanical ventilation using the principles of condensation and evaporation. Also called an artificial nose.
heated blow-by humidifier A type of pass-over humidifier that exposes gas flow to a heated water reservoir, where heat and moisture are transferred into the gas stream.
heated wire See heated wire circuit.
heated wire circuit A type of ventilator circuit in which the inspiratory tubing is heated to reduce water vapor "rain-out" (condensation).
heliox A low-density therapeutic mixture of helium with at least 20% oxygen; used in some institutions as part of large airway obstruction treatment.
Henderson-Hasselbalch equation The chemical formula relating pH, pKa, and the ratio of the conjugate base (bicarbonate) to the weak acid (carbonic acid).
HFFI See high-frequency flow interrupter.
HFJV See high-frequency jet ventilation.
HFO See high-frequency oscillation.
HFV See high-frequency ventilation.
high breathing rate alarm A ventilator warning system that indicates rapid respirations exceeding the desired rate.
high-frequency flow interrupter (HFFI or HIFI) A type of high-frequency ventilator that provides rapid gas pulses to the airway (up to 30 Hz) by periodically interrupting a high-flow gas stream.
high-frequency flow interruption See high-frequency flow interrupter.
high-frequency jet ventilation (HFJV) A type of high-frequency ventilator that provides a jet gas pulse to the airway via a small-lumen catheter within the endotracheal tube at rates of about 100 to 200 pulses/min.
high-frequency oscillation (HFO) A type of high-frequency ventilator that cycles at rates of 60 to 3000 times per minute.
high-frequency oscillatory ventilation (HFOV) See high-frequency oscillation.
high-frequency percussive ventilation (HFPV) Ventilation that incorporates the beneficial characteristics of a conventional positive-pressure ventilator and a jet ventilator. Can be compared with time-cycled, pressure-limited ventilation in which high-frequency pulsations (up to 100 to 225 cycles/min, or 1.7 to 4 Hz) are injected into the airway through a Venturi during the inspiratory phase.
high-frequency positive pressure ventilation (HFPPV) A mode of ventilatory support with rates from 60 to 100/minute and small tidal volumes (often approaching anatomic dead space) using a low-compliance patient circuit.
high-frequency ventilation (HFV) A method of ventilation at rates >80 times per minute. See also high- frequency jet ventilation and high-frequency oscillation.
high-level disinfection Using chemical sterilants at reduced exposure times (less than 45 minutes) to kill bacteria, fungi, and viruses. High-level disinfection does not kill a high level of bacterial spores. Compare intermediate-level disinfection and low-level disinfection.
Holter monitoring Making prolonged (usually 24 hours) electrocardiograph recordings on a portable tape recorder while the patient, wearing appropriate monitoring leads, conducts normal daily activities.
hood An environmental control device that covers the head and regulates the humidity, gas concentration, and temperature of inspired gases.
hot film anemometer A flow-sensing device used in some ventilators that works by measuring the temperature of the gas flow. Similar to hot-wire flow transducers.
humidity The amount of water vapor in a system expressed as weight/volume (e.g., grams/liter). Also water in the molecular form.
humidity deficit A condition in which the available humidity is less than the potential humidity; that is, the percentage relative humidity is less than 100 (e.g., the humidity deficit at a body temperature of 37° C is compared with its capacity of 44 mg/L).
hydrogen bonding The attractive force of compounds in which a hydrogen atom covalently linked to an electronegative element (e.g., oxygen, nitrogen, or fluorine) has a large degree of positive character relative to the electronegative atom, thereby causing the compound to have a large dipole.
hydrometer A device that determines the specific gravity or density of a liquid by comparing its weight with that of an equal volume of water. A calibrated hollow glass device is placed in the liquid being examined, and the depth to which the device settles in the liquid is noted.

hydrophobic The property of repelling water molecules.
hygroscopic The property of attracting and binding water molecules.
hyperbilirubinemia Above-average amounts of the bile pigment bilirubin in the blood; often characterized by jaundice, anorexia, and malaise.
hypertonic A solution of water and chemicals in which the solute to solvent ratio exceeds that of normal body fluids. For salt water, this is greater than 0.9% NaCl.

I

ideal gas A gas acting as if it exactly follows all of the gas laws.
I:E ratio control A ventilator control that regulates the proportions of inspiratory and expiratory time during a respiratory cycle.
I:E ratio limit control A mechanism that prevents high inspiratory to expiratory (I:E) ratios; usually above 1:1.
IMV (pressurized breaths) See intermittent mandatory ventilation.
impedance cardiography A noninvasive technique for measuring cardiac output based on the principle of impedance plethsmography. In this technique two sets of electrodes are placed on the thorax to measure electrical impedance.
impedance plethysmography A technique for detecting blood vessel occlusion that determines volumetric changes in an area of the body (i.e., limb blood flow) by measuring changes in its girth as indicated in the electrical impedance of mercury-containing polymeric silicone (Silastic) tubes in a pressure cuff.
incisura A notch or indentation that appears on the aortic pressure tracing. It is thought to be associated with retrograde flow of blood from the aorta back towards the left ventricle at the end of ventricular systole.
indirect calorimeter A device used for measuring energy expenditure. With a closed-circuit calorimeter, the patient breathes into and out of a container prefilled with oxygen. Oxygen consumption is determined by measuring the volume of oxygen the patient uses. With an open-circuit calorimeter, the volume of oxygen is determined by measuring the volumes of inspired and expired gases along with the fractional concentrations of oxygen in the inspired and expired gases. The volume of oxygen is then determined by calculating the difference between the amount of oxygen in the inspired gas and the amount in the expired gas.
indirect contact Contacting a susceptible host with a contaminated intermediate object (usually inanimate) in the patient's environment.
indirect-drive piston A ventilator power mechanism in which the power gas is driven by a piston but does not go to the patient. For example, the power gas may compress a bellows that contains the patient gas volume.
inertia The tendency of objects to resist changes in position unless acted upon by an outside force (from Newton's laws).
inertial impaction The deposition of particles by collision with a surface; the primary mechanism for pulmonary deposition of larger particles (usually over 5 m in diameter). Large particles tend to travel in a straight line and collide with surfaces in their pathway (e.g., airway branches, baffles).
infection surveillance The procedures of a hospital or other health facility to minimize the risk of spreading of nosocomial or community-acquired infections to patients or staff members.
inflating port An orifice through which ventilating gas flows.
injector A device that adds a quantity of liquid or gas to a main flow source. See also jet.
isovolumetric contraction The period of ventricular systole that occurs during the period between closure of the AV valves and opening of the semilunar valves.
isovolumetric relaxation The period of ventricular diastole that occurs during the period between closure of the semilunar valves and opening of the AV valves.
isothermic saturation boundary (ISB) The point at which gases reach body temperature and full saturation.
inspiratory controls Mechanisms that determine the length and timing of inspiratory gas flow.
inspiratory flow rate control A ventilatory mechanism that sets the gas volume delivered per unit of time during inspiration.
inspiratory hold (plateau) A ventilatory maneuver in which delivered volume is held in the lungs before exhalation. Inspiratory gas flow stops, and the expiratory valve is maintained briefly in the closed position, thus keeping the delivered volume (and pressure) in the lungs. Commonly used to measure plateau pressure for the calculation of static compliance.
inspiratory interrupter switch A control device that terminates inspiration.
inspiratory pause See inspiratory hold.
inspiratory positive airway pressure (IPAP) The pressure measured in a patient circuit during inspiration. A parameter that can be set during bilevel positive airway pressure (BiPAP) ventilation and governs pressure delivery during inspiration.
inspiratory pressure calibration control Allows the inspiratory pressure limit to be set.
inspiratory pressure level The maximum amount of pressure allowed during mechanical ventilation.
inspiratory pressure-relief control A device that sets the "pop-off" pressure on a mechanical ventilator.
inspiratory pressure-time product (PTP) The integration of the area within the curve during inspiration on a pressure/time graph.
inspiratory time (TI) See inspiratory time control.
inspiratory time control Sets the length of inspiration either directly or as a fraction of the I:E ratio.
inspiratory time percent The proportion of the respiratory cycle time devoted to inspiration.
inspiratory timer A control that determines the time allowed for inspiration.
insulator A nonconducting substance that is a barrier to heat or electricity passage.
intensive care unit (ICU) A hospital unit in which patients requiring close monitoring and care are housed for as long as necessary.
intermediate level disinfection Removing vegetative bacteria, tubercle bacteria, viruses, and fungi, but not necessarily killing spores. Compare high-level disinfection and low-level disinfection.
intermittent mandatory ventilation (IMV) (pressurized breaths) A time-triggered ventilatory mode that permits spontaneous ventilation and intersperses required pressurized breaths at predetermined intervals. See also synchronized intermittent mandatory ventilation.
intermittent (inspiratory) positive-pressure breathing (IPPB) A treatment modality in which the inspiratory pressure is elevated above atmospheric but is allowed to return to

atmospheric during exhalation. Another term applied to mechanical ventilation.

intermittent positive-pressure ventilation (IPPV) Intermittent positive-pressure breathing done continuously as a form of mechanical ventilation.

internal battery A direct current power source sometimes used by ventilators as an alternative power supply when an alternating current source is not available.

internal demand valve A device that is triggered to provide gas flow when patient effort decreases pressure or flow below a certain baseline.

internal mechanism A device inside a ventilator or piece of equipment that functions in the operation of the equipment.

internal regulator A device inside a ventilator for adjusting pressure delivery.

International 10-20 EEG system The standard pattern for electrode placement on the scalp to record EEGs during sleep studies.

intrinsic positive end expiratory pressure (PEEPi) The level of pressure in the airway as a result of pressure trapped in the lung at the end of exhalation. Also called auto-PEEP.

invasive Characterized by a tendency to spread or infiltrate. Also refers to the use of diagnostic or therapeutic methods that require access to the inside of the body.

inverse ratio ventilation (IRV) Ventilation in which inspiratory time exceeds expiratory time. See also pressure-controlled inverse ratio ventilation and volume controlled-inverse ratio ventilation.

in vitro Occurring in a laboratory apparatus (of a biological reaction).

in vivo Occurring in a living organism (of a biological reaction).

IPPB flow Gas flow during IPPB breaths.

iron lung A negative-pressure ventilator. Also called a tank ventilator, artificial lung, or Drinker respirator.

isolation procedures Infection control measures that combine barrier-type precautions (e.g., hand washing and the use of gloves, masks, and/or gowns) with the physical separation of infected patients in specific disease categories to disrupt transmission of pathogenic microorganisms.

isolation techniques See isolation procedures.

isotonic A solution of water and chemicals in which the solute concentration equals that of plasma.

J

jet A device using a gas-entrainment mechanism to mix gases or add aerosols to a mainstream gas flow.

jet humidifier A humidifier that uses the jet principle to add water vapor to the main gas flow.

jet nebulizer A nebulizer that uses the jet principle to add water droplets to the main gas flow; contains a baffle.

jet Venturi A jet used to produce a pressure drop for entraining gas or fluid.

joule A unit of energy or work in the meter-kilogram-second system. It is equivalent to 107 ergs, or 1 watt second.

Joule-Kelvin effect A physical phenomenon in which the rapid expansion of a gas without the application of external work causes a cooling of the gas. Used in the liquefication of air to produce oxygen and nitrogen. Also called the Joule-Thompson effect.

Joule-Kelvin-Thompson method See fractional distillation of gases.

Joule-Thompson effect See Joule-Kelvin effect.

junctional escape rhythm Rhythm that is characterized by the AV node becoming the pacemaker of the heart (i.e., intrinsic rate of 40–60 beats/min). This type of rhythm typically occurs in cases of sinus block or sinus arrest.

K

K complexes Large vertical slow waves with amplitudes of at least 75 microvolts with an initial negative deflection.

Kelvin (K) An absolute temperature scale calculated in centigrade units from the point at which molecular activity apparently ceases (–273.15° C). To convert Celsius degrees to Kelvin, add 273.15.

kilowatt Unit of measure of electrical power (1000 watts).

kinetic activity Molecular motion uses energy and produces heat as a by-product.

kinetic energy The energy a body possesses by virtue of its motion.

kinetic flowmeter A flow-regulation device that incorporates a spindle or plunger in place of a floating ball as a flow indicator.

Korotkoff sounds Sounds heard during the taking of blood pressure using a sphygmomanometer and stethoscope.

kymograph A device for graphically recording lung volume changes during spirometry. See also water-sealed spirometers.

L

laryngeal mask airway (LMA) A custom-formed, soft mask with a hollow tube fitting into the pyriform sinuses directly above the larynx. Used to establish and maintain a patent upper airway.

Laryngoscope An endoscope for examining the larynx.

latent heat The amount of heat needed for a substance to change its state of matter.

leaf-type valve See leaf valve.

leaf valve A thin membrane that overlays an orifice and that when closed prevents fluid (gas or liquid) transmission through the opening.

Levy-Jennings charts The most common method of recording quality control data. These charts allow the operator to detect trends and shifts in performance and thus can help avoid problems associated with reporting inaccurate data due to analyzer malfunction.

light-emitting diode (LED) An electronic component that emits light when exposed to current flow. Used in instruments to display digital data.

limiting variable An element of breath delivery including flow, volume, pressure, or time given a set maximum value by the operator that cannot be exceeded during the breath.

linear-drive piston A piston with movement is governed by linear (straight line) movement of a shaft that is connected to the piston head. See also direct drive piston.

Liquefaction The conversion of a substance into its liquid form.

liquid crystal A type of data display surface that indicates data by turning parts of the display on (dark) or off (light).

liquid crystal display See liquid crystal.

lock-out cartridge A control that inhibits (locks out) the functions of other controls or systems.

loop A circlelike graphic display of two variables plotted on the x (horizontal) and y (vertical) axis. Pressure/volume and flow/volume loops are most commonly used.

low battery alarm A warning that the power (charge) remaining in a battery is below acceptable limits.
low inlet gas alarm A warning that system pressure is below optimal pressure standards.
low-level disinfection Killing most vegetative bacteria, some fungi, and some bacteria. Compare high-level disinfection and intermediate-level disinfection.
low-pressure reducing valve A pressure-regulating system designed to operate below 50 psig.
low-pressure regulator A low-pressure–reducing valve combined with a flowmeter.
low-residual-volume, high-pressure cuff A type of endotracheal or tracheostomy tube seal that uses low volumes at high pressures to achieve an airtight seal.
low-resistance/high-compliance system A system in which the forces resisting flow are low and the volume change per unit of pressure exerted is high.
Luer-Loc A glass or plastic syringe with a simple screw-lock mechanism that securely holds the needle in place. Also called Luer syringe.

M

Macintosh blade A curved laryngoscope blade, as opposed to a straight Miller type of blade.
macroshock A shock from an electric current of 1 mA or greater that is applied externally to the skin.
magnetic valve resistors A type of threshold resistor containing a bar magnet that attracts a ferromagnetic disc seated on the expiratory port of a pressurized circuit.
magnetic PEEP valve A valve that maintains a positive end-expiratory pressure by means of a magnetically activated component.
magnetism The branch of physics dealing with magnets and magnetic phenomena; also called magnetics.
main solenoid The master control device governing flow in a gas-delivery system.
mainstream capnograph See capnograph.
mainstream nebulizer A nebulizer that introduces the jet stream into the main gas flow.
mandatory breath A breath initiated and ended by the mechanical ventilator. Mandatory breath delivery is completely determined by the ventilator.
mandatory minute ventilation (MMV) A closed-loop (servo-controlled) mode of ventilation that guarantees delivery of a set minute volume by monitoring patient spontaneous minute volume and supplementing breaths as necessary to achieve the set minute volume.
mandatory minute volume See mandatory minute ventilation.
manifold A system of interconnected devices (e.g., a gas manifold). Two or more cylinders connected to regulators and a metering device or a breathing manifold. The externally mounted exhalation valve, tubing, and nebulizer, which make up a portion of the ventilator circuit.
manometer ports Orifices from which pressure readings are obtained by connecting pressure manometers.
manual trigger A device in which the function is activated by hand.
mass median aerodynamic diameter (MMAD) Regarding aerosol particles, the diameter at which the mass is equally divided. That is, 50% of the particles are lighter than the MMAD and 50% are heavier.
mass spectrometry A sophisticated analysis technique used to analyze the composition of substances by examining a stream of charged particles to separate elements on the basis of atomic mass.
maximum expiratory flow A pulmonary function measurement of the patient's ability to exhale quickly and forcefully (in liters/second).
maximum inspiratory time control The mechanism that determines the length of inspiration allowed.
maximum motor current The highest electrical current the motor will tolerate.
maximum pressure control Sets the highest allowable ventilator pressure. Also called pressure-limit control.
maximum pressure limit (Pmax) The upper pressure value that can be delivered during inspiration. In the Hamilton GALILEO, the Pmax setting also establishes a reference point for pressure delivered during servo-controlled modes of ventilation.
maximum voluntary ventilation (MVV) The maximum volume of air that a person can breathe over a one-minute period.
mean airway pressure (MAP) The average pressure occurring in the airway during a complete respiratory cycle. Mathematically, the area below the pressure/time curve for one breathing cycle divided by the breath cycle time.
measured variables One or more of the four elements of a breath (pressure, flow, volume, and time) monitored during ventilation.
mechanics The branch of physics dealing with the motion of material bodies and the phenomena of the action of forces on them.
melting point The temperature at which solids begin to turn into liquids.
membrane concentrator An oxygen concentrator that separates oxygen from air by means of a selectively permeable membrane.
mercury barometer A device for measuring atmospheric pressure by the change in the height of a mercury column.
message window A monitoring screen on the front panel of a ventilator used to display messages.
metered dose inhaler (MDI) A small pressurized cartridge that contains a propellant and a medication. When the cartridge is activated, a precise amount of aerosolized medication is delivered.
microcuvette A small transparent tube or container with specific optical properties. The chemical composition of the container determines the vessel's use (e.g., Pyrex glass for examining materials in the visible spectrum, or silica for those in the ultraviolet range).
Microprocessor A small, compact computer designed to monitor and control specific functions.
microprocessor-controlled Regulated by a small, compact computer.
microshock A shock from a usually imperceptible electrical current (<1 milliampere) that is allowed to bypass the skin and follow a direct, low-resistance pathway into the body.
microswitche Small control device that institutes or halts processes.
Miller blade A straight laryngoscope blade, as opposed to a curved Macintosh blade.
mini-fluid amp A device that increases the strength of a fluidic signal.

minimal occluding volume (MOV) The least amount of air needed to achieve a seal in a cuffed endotracheal or tracheostomy tube.
minimum minute volume See mandatory minute volume.
minute ventilation The total ventilation per minute. The product of tidal volume and respiratory rate, as measured by expired gas collection for 1 to 3 minutes. The normal value is 5 to 10 liters per minute. Also called minute volume.
minute volume control The mechanism that sets the minute volume delivered by a ventilator.
mixed sleep apnea Repeated episodes of complete airflow cessation for more than 10 seconds during sleep, with characteristics of both obstructive sleep apnea and central sleep apnea. In mixed sleep apnea, the central event usually precedes the obstructive event.
mixer A device that blends or mixes two gases to provide a precise mixture (concentration) of the gases.
mixture A substance composed of ingredients that are not chemically combined and do not necessarily occur in a fixed proportion.
molecular sieve A term used to describe components of a type of oxygen concentrator that filters air and chemically removes nitrogen and some trace gases from the air.
molecule The smallest unit that exhibits the properties of an element or compound. A molecule is composed of two or more covalently bonded atoms.
monitor To observe and evaluate a body function closely and constantly. Also, a mechanical device that provides a visual or audio signal or a graphic record of a particular function (e.g., a cardiac or fetal monitor).
monoplace hyperbaric chamber A hyperbaric unit rated for single occupancy.
monostable A fluidic device or element that can direct gas flow to only one outlet unless the gas flow is acted upon by a separate gas pulse.
multiplace hyperbaric chamber A walk-in hyperbaric unit that provides enough space to treat two or more patients simultaneously.
multistage reducing valve See multistage regulator.
multistage regulator A pressure-reducing valve that has more than one level of pressure reduction between system pressure and working pressure.
murmur A gentle blowing, fluttering, or humming sound, such as a heart murmur.
mustache cannula A type of reservoir nasal cannula that can reduce oxygen supply use from that of a continuous-flow nasal cannula.
myocyte A muscle cell.

N

nasal cannula An oxygen delivery device characterized by small, hollow prongs that are inserted into the external nares.
nasal catheter An oxygen delivery device consisting of a narrow, hollow tubing that is inserted through the nose into the nasopharynx.
nasal trumpet A type of artificial airway. Also called a nasal, or nasopharyngeal, airway.
nasopharyngeal airway A type of artificial airway inserted through the nose with the distal tip in the posterior part of the oropharynx. Also called nasal trumpet or nasal airway.
nasotracheal intubation Using the nose as the entry point for placement of tubes or catheters in the trachea.
nebulization controls Devices on ventilators that regulate the time and/or intensity of the flow output from a connector used to power a nebulizer.
nebulizer A type of aerosol production device that consists of an "atomizer," or jet, and a baffle or baffles.
nebulizer controls See nebulization controls.
nebulizer solenoid A switch mechanism that turns the nebulizer on or off.
nebulizer system The parts of a device that produce, control, and deliver aerosols to the patient.
negative end-expiratory pressure (NEEP) See negative expiratory pressure.
negative expiratory pressure A mode of ventilation in which a small suction is exerted during expiration to assist expiratory flow, reduce mean airway pressure, and decrease expiratory time.
negative extrathoracic pressure A subatmospheric pressure applied to the external chest wall. Used in negative-pressure ventilators.
negative-pressure capability The ability of a device to generate subambient pressures.
negative-pressure control The mechanism that regulates the application of negative pressures in a device.
negative-pressure jet A Venturi or Pitot device that reduces pressure by air entrainment.
negative-pressure Venturi See negative-pressure jet.
negative-pressure ventilator A machine that provides ventilation by generating less pressure than ambient (atmospheric) around the thorax while maintaining the upper airway at ambient. The iron lung and chest cuirass are examples.
Nernst equation An expression of the relationship between the electrical potential across a membrane and the concentration ratio between permeable ions on either side of the membrane.
newton An SI unit of force that would impart an acceleration to 1 kg of mass of 1 meter per second.
nonconstant flow generator A ventilator that reacts to back pressure and resistance by varying the inspiratory flow pattern.
nonforced vital capacity The maximum amount of air that can be slowly exhaled after a maximum inspiration. Also called slow vital capacity.
noninvasive Pertains to a diagnostic or therapeutic technique that does not require the skin to be broken or a cavity or organ of the body to be entered (e.g., obtaining a blood pressure reading by auscultation with a stethoscope and sphygmomanometer).
nonlinear drive piston See rotary drive piston.
non-rapid eye movement sleep See non-REM sleep.
nonrebreathing valve A valve that opens, allowing gas to flow to the patient, then closes, allowing exhaled air to exit by another route. Examples are spring-loaded and diaphragm valves. Diaphragm valves are further subdivided into duckbill (or fishmouth) valves and leaf type valves.
non-REM sleep Non-rapid eye movement sleep. Four observable, progressive stages of sleep that represent three fourths of a typical sleep period and are collectively called non-REM sleep. The remaining sleep time is usually occupied with REM sleep, during which dreaming occurs.
normal body humidity At BTSP, 47 mm Hg vapor pressure or 43.8 gm H_2O/L of air.

normal flora Microorganisms that live on or within a body to compete with disease-producing microorganisms and provide a natural immunity against certain infections.
normal rate control The system that sets the normal breathing frequency on a ventilator.
normal sinus rhythm A cardiac rhythm characterized by the presence of P waves and an effective ventricular rate of 60 to 100 beats per minute.
nosocomial Pertaining to or originating in a hospital (e.g., a nosocomial infection).

O

obstructive sleep apnea (OSA) A condition in which five or more apneic periods (≥10 seconds each) occur per hour of sleep and that is characterized by occlusion of the oropharyngeal airway with continued efforts to breathe. Compare central sleep apnea and mixed sleep apnea.
occlusion pressure (P 0.1) or airway occlusion pressure See P0.1.
ohm A unit of measurement of electrical resistance. One ohm is the resistance of a conductor in which an electrical potential of 1 volt produces a current of 1 ampere.
one-point calibration Adjusting the electronic output of an instrument to a single known standard to help ensure quality assurance. It should be performed before analyzing an unknown sample, unless the analyzer is programmed to automatically perform a one-point calibration at regular intervals (e.g., every 20 to 30 minutes).
open-circuit calorimeter See calorimeter.
open-loop system A microprocessor-controlled system that provides clinical data or advice but defers to the user to take the appropriate action.
open-top tent An environmental control enclosure used for small children; features an open top to facilitate CO_2 washout.
optical encoder The name of the device on the T-Bird ventilator that sends information about the turbine speed to the microprocessor in order to control the precise flow delivered to the patient.
optical plethysmography A technique for measuring blood volume changes in a specific body part (e.g., a digit or earlobe). These blood volume changes are then used to define systolic and diastolic time periods during the cardiac cycle.
optics A field of study that deals with the electromagnetic radiation of wavelengths that are shorter than radio waves but longer than x-rays.
O_2 relay An electronic or mechanical device that controls oxygen flow into a delivery system.
OR/NOR gate A monostable, fluidic element with one control port and two outlet ports.
oropharangeal airway An artificial airway that is inserted into the mouth until the distal tip is behind the base of the tongue, providing an open channel to the laryngopharynx.
outflow valve A control device that regulates the gas exiting a system.
outlet manifold Part of the exhalation valve on a ventilator.
outlet valve A safety valve on a piped-gas system that prevents the high-pressure gas from free flowing.
over-pressure alarm A warning that the pressures in a system have exceeded predetermined levels.
over-pressure relief A device that allows pressure to be released from a system that has exceeded desired pressure limits.
over-pressure–relief valve See over-pressure relief.
oximeter A device that monitors the amount of oxygen in a (physiologic) system. See also pulse oximeter.
oxygen analyzer A device used to determine the concentration of oxygen in a gas mixture.
oxygen blender A device that mixes oxygen with air or other gases to provide precise oxygen concentrations.
oxygen concentrator A device that increases the oxygen content of inspired gas by enriching or concentrating the oxygen in air.
oxygen control A device in a ventilator that regulates the oxygen concentration delivered to the patient.
oxygen controller/blender See oxygen blender.
oxygen exhaust port An opening through which oxygen-enriched gas is expelled to the atmosphere.
oxygen inlet regulator A pressure-control device that governs the pressure of the oxygen entering a system.
oxygen percentage control See oxygen control.
oxygen percentage valve A metering device that regulates the proportion of oxygen in the delivered gas.
oxygen sensor The monitoring probe of an oxygen analyzer.
oxygen system The equipment and devices that distribute, control, and monitor oxygen from the bulk storage unit to the site of patient use.

P

P0.1 The mouth pressure 100 msec after the start of a patient's inspiratory effort that is measured in a closed (occluded) system; a measure of the output of the respiratory center.
$PaCO_2$ Partial pressure of arterial carbon dioxide.
P_ACO_2 Partial pressure of alveolar carbon dioxide.
PaO_2 Partial pressure of arterial oxygen.
P_AO_2 Partial pressure of alveolar oxygen.
paramagnetic Of or pertaining to a characteristic that causes a substance to be attracted to magnetic fields.
parameter A value or constant used to describe or measure a set of data representing a physiologic function or system (e.g., the use of blood acid-base relationships as parameters for evaluating the function of a patient's respiratory system).
paroxysmal atrial tachycardia A rapid atrial rate that begins and ends abruptly.
partial pressure The absolute pressure exerted by one gas in a mixture of gases.
partial-rebreathing mask A kind of oxygen mask that allows patients to reinhale the first third of their exhaled breath.
particle filter A device that removes particulate matter from an area or gas stream.
particle inertia The tendency of a particle to maintain a direction and speed of motion unless acted on by another force.
pass-over humidifier A humidification system in which the patient gas supply flows over a water supply. See also blow-by humidifier.
pasteurization The process of applying moist heat, usually to a liquid such as milk for a specific time to kill or retard the development of pathogenic bacteria.
pathogenic Capable of producing disease.
patient circuit The portion of the pneumatic circuit consisting of tubing from a ventilator to a patient. Also called external, or ventilator, circuit.
patient disconnect alarm A system warning that the patient is not connected to the ventilator; a low-pressure alarm.

patient triggering When pressure, flow, or volume begin the breath; that is, the patient controls the beginning of inspiration.
peak flow A measurement of the maximum amount of gas that can be forcefully exhaled after a maximum inspiration; expressed in liters per minute.
peak flow control A control on the front panel of a ventilator used to set the maximum flow delivered during a mandatory inspiration.
peak flow meter A device that regulates the maximum flow a ventilator delivers.
peak flow setting See peak flow control.
peak inspiratory pressure (PIP) A measurement of the maximum pressure in the patient circuit that occurs during delivery of a mandatory breath from a ventilator. Also called peak pressure (Ppeak).
peak pressure See peak inspiratory pressure.
pedestal ventilator A term used in reference to a Puritan Bennett PR series respirator.
PEEP See positive end-expiratory pressure.
PEEP/CPAP pressure-control valve A mechanism that regulates the pressure limits of the PEEP/CPAP devices in a ventilator system.
PEEP exhalation valve An exhalation valve fitted with a PEEP device.
pendant cannula A type of reservoir nasal cannula that can reduce oxygen supply use (compared with a continuous-flow nasal cannula). The reservoir is attached as connecting tubing that is a conduit to a pendant, which hangs below the chin.
Pendelluft Movement of gas, from "fast" to "slow," filling spaces during breathing. Alternatively, the ineffective movement of gas back and forth (accompanied by mediastinal shifting) from a healthy lung to one with a flail segment; caused by a crushing chest injury.
percent pause time A ventilator control that uses a percentage of the inspiratory time to provide a pause at the end of inspiration, usually lengthening inspiratory time and allowing for an inspiratory hold.
PH Abbreviation for potential hydrogen, a scale representing the relative acidity (or alkalinity) of a solution, in which a value of 7.0 is neutral, below 7.0 is acid, and above 7.0 is alkaline.
pH electrode See Sanz electrode.
PH_2O Partial pressure of water vapor; 47 mm Hg at BTSP.
phase variables During breath delivery, the variables controlled by the ventilator that are responsible for each of the four parts of a breath, including triggering (begins inspiratory flow), cycling (ends inspiratory flow), and limiting (places a maximum on a control variable: pressure, volume, flow, and/or time).
Phonocardiography The recording of heart sounds and murmurs using an electromechanical apparatus.
Photoplethysmography The use of light waves to detect changes in the volume of an organ or tissue. Pulse oximeters use this principle to measure the arterial pulse.
physical analyzer A gas analyzer that uses the principles of physics (heat, electrical flow, etc.) to measure gas concentration.
piezoelectric quality The ability of a substance to change shape in response to and at the frequency of an electrical current, thus changing electrical energy into mechanical energy.
Pin Index Safety System (PISS) A standardized scheme to prevent accidental mismatching of reducing valves and pressurized gases in small capacity cylinders (E or smaller).
PISS See Pin Index Safety System.
piston bag A baglike reservoir that contains a volume of gas to be delivered to the patient when compressed by a piston.
piston compressor A gas source in which a volume of gas is reduced in volume and pressurized by a piston.
plateau pressure (Pplateau) The pressure measured in the patient circuit of a ventilator during an inspiratory hold maneuver. Also the pressure needed to overcome the elastic component of the lungs (static compliance) during breath delivery.
Pneumatic Pertaining to air or gas.
pneumatically powered Supplied energy by high-pressure gas or air.
pneumatic circuit A series of tubing that directs the gas flow in a ventilator and from a ventilator to a patient.
pneumatic drive mechanism A method of operating a ventilator using pressurized gas as a power source.
pneumatic expiratory timing device A gas-powered device that controls expiratory time (e.g., using a controlled leak to deflate a diaphragm and open an inspiratory valve).
pneumatic nebulizer A device that produces an aerosol cloud using a pressurized gas source as the propellant.
pneumatic system An air or gas system.
pneumatic timing mechanisms See pneumatic expiratory timing device.
pneumobelt A corset with an inflatable bladder that fits over the abdominal area. The bladder is connected by a hose to a ventilator that delivers positive pressure at an adjustable rate and pressure. Used to alleviate strain to assist in the respiratory rehabilitation of patients with high cervical injuries.
pneumotachometer A device that measures the flow of respiratory gases. The pressure gradient is directly related to flow, thus allowing a computer to derive a flow curve measured in liters per minute.
pneumotachygraph An instrument that incorporates a pneumotachometer to record variations in respiratory gas flow.
polarographic electrode A device that employs the flow of electric current between the negative (cathode) and positive (anode) electrodes to measure a physical phenomenon such as the partial pressure of oxygen in the blood. See also arterial blood gas analysis.
polysomnography The measurement and recording of variations in airflow, EEG, EOG, and arterial blood gases during sleep. Used in the diagnosis of sleep apnea.
poppet assembly A spool-shaped device used to open or close an orifice in response to pressure differences.
poppet valve See poppet assembly.
positive end-expiratory pressure (PEEP) A form of therapy applied during mechanical ventilation that elevates the baseline pressure from which inspiration is delivered. PEEP increases functional residual volume and mean airway pressure to improve oxygenation.
positive intrapulmonary pressure A condition in which the pressure in the lungs is maintained at levels above physiologic.
positive-pressure ventilator A device that applies positive pressure to the lungs to improve gas exchange.
POST See power-on self-test.
potential energy The energy a body possesses by virtue of its position.
potentiometer An electronic device in which the output signal varies in strength with the strength of the input signal.
potentiometric Refers to measuring voltage.

power A source of physical or mechanical force or energy. Force or energy that can be put to work (e.g., electric power).

power failure alarm A warning device that indicates that the main power source of a piece of equipment has failed. Also known as a power disconnect alarm.

power indicators Monitoring lights or diodes that illuminate to give information about a device's power source.

power-on self-test (POST) An essential test started by the microprocessor as soon as the ventilator is turned on that lasts about 5 seconds. The unit must complete this test before it is functional.

power source The origin of physical or mechanical force or energy. Force or energy that can be put to work (e.g., electric power).

power transmission system Gas or electrically powered mechanical devices that generate a pressure gradient to provide all or part of the work of breathing for a patient. Also called a drive mechanism.

precision/imprecision In measurement, precision is freedom from random errors; imprecision is inaccuracy due to random error.

precision metering device See proportional metering device.

premature ventricular beats A ventricular depolarization occurring earlier than expected.

premature ventricular depolarizations See premature ventricular beats.

preset minute volume The set volume of gas to be delivered in a minute through a ventilator.

preset reducing valve See preset regulator.

preset regulator A device that decreases the pressure from a gas supply system to a predetermined lower pressure.

preset working pressure A predetermined pressure at which pneumatically powered devices function efficiently and safely. Usually below 60 psig.

Pressure The amount of force exerted per unit of area.

pressure augmentation (PAug) A servo-control (closed-loop) mode of pressure-targeted ventilation that guarantees volume delivery on a breath-by-breath basis.

pressure and sensitivity adjustments Mechanisms that let the operator select the pressure and sensitivity values on a mechanical ventilator.

pressure capacitance chamber A device that increases or decreases pressure against a pressure-relief valve in the Bio-Med MVP-10 ventilator.

pressure compartment In the Bird Mark series, the right side of the respirator in which superambient pressures could develop and be transmitted to the patient.

pressure control The mechanism that determines the pressure level generated by the ventilator.

pressure-control ventilation (PCV) A mode of ventilation in which the maximum preset pressure is delivered, regardless of the volume achieved.

pressure-controlled inverse ratio ventilation (PCIRV) Pressure-targeted, time-cycled ventilation in which the inspiratory time exceeds the expiratory time.

pressure differential devices Mechanisms that operate by attempting to balance pressures within the device.

pressure differential transducer A device whose output signal strength depends on the difference between two or more input pressures.

pressure-equalization passage In the Bird Mark series, a hole in the center body that allows for equalization of pressure between the pressure and ambient sides of the respirator.

pressure limit control A dial or button that allows the operator to determine the preset maximum pressure a ventilator will deliver.

pressure-limited A descriptive term indicating that a maximum pressure has been set that cannot be exceeded. Also see pressure-targeted ventilation and pressure ventilation.

pressure-limited resuscitators Emergency ventilation devices that have a preset maximum inspiratory pressure.

pressure-limited ventilation A mode of ventilation in which inspiration is stopped when a selected pressure value is reached.

pressure ramp (Pramp) A ventilator control that determines how rapidly the set pressure is achieved during inspiration. Also called pressure sloping.

pressure-regulated volume control (PRVC) The name given to a mode of ventilation on the Siemens Servo 300 ventilator that provides pressure-targeted, time-cycled ventilation that is volume guaranteed.

pressure release Baseline ventilation in which elevated baseline pressures are periodically allowed to fall to baseline or a pressure-relief safety valve is activated.

pressure-relief valve A safety device that vents pressure in excess of a preset value to atmosphere.

pressure sensor A device that detects pressure or pressure changes.

pressure slope A ventilator control that adjusts the rate at which the set pressure is reached during inspiration. Also called pressure sloping. See also pressure ramp.

pressure support See pressure-support ventilation.

pressure-support ventilation (PSV) A mode of ventilatory support designed to augment spontaneous breathing. Patient-triggered, pressure-targeted, flow-cycled ventilation.

pressure swing absorption (PSA) A technique used in some oxygen sieve concentrators to produce enriched oxygen mixture. In this technique room air is drawn through one or more filters by a compressor and eventually compressed to a pressure of 15–25 psig and then passed through an air-cooled heat exchanger before entering two or more sieve beds containing a porous material such as Zeolite. The PSA method attempts to minimize the problems associated with accumulation of moisture and other contaminants building up on the sieve bed and allows for the pressurization of one sieve bed while the other bed is purged at a rate of 1 to 5 times per minute.

pressure switch A device that responds to changes in or the presence of a pressure signal by instituting an action within the ventilator system.

pressure-targeted ventilation A form of ventilation in which the operator selects a specific pressure for delivery of inspiration.

pressure transducer A mechanism that converts a pressure signal to another form of energy, usually electric.

pressure triggering Inspiration begins when the ventilator senses a drop in circuit pressure.

pressure ventilation Setting a desired pressure. Also called pressure-limited ventilation, pressure-controlled ventilation, and pressure-targeted ventilation.

pressurized metered dose inhaler (pMDI) See metered dose inhaler.

prokaryotic Of or pertaining to an organism that does not contain a true nucleus surrounded by a nuclear membrane. Characteristic of lower life forms, such as bacteria, viruses, and blue-green algae. Division of the organism occurs through simple fission.

proportional amplifier A fluidic control device that boosts or reduces output signal strength in proportion to the strength of the input signal.

proportional assist ventilation (PAV) A method of assisting spontaneous ventilation in which the practitioner adjusts the amount of work the ventilator will perform.

proportional manifold A mechanism that directs blended gas through a series of solenoids to control flow in the Infrasonics Infant Star ventilator.

proportional metering device A mechanism used to provide precise mixtures of gases. As the amount of one gas increases at a given total flow, the amount of the second gas decreases proportionately.

proportional solenoid A valve designed to modify gas flow. Typically, an electrical current flows through an electromagnet, creating a magnetic field that controls a plunger. The plunger governs the valve opening and gas delivery.

proportioning valve A system in which two or more valves vary the amounts of the gases they control entering the gas delivery system. This determines the final composition of the gas mixture.

proximal airway pressure gauge A gauge that indicates the proximal airway pressure.

proximal pressure line A line in the patient circuit to monitor airway pressures at the Y connector.

PSV See pressure-support ventilation.

PSVmax The amount of pressure-support ventilation delivered to achieve a desired volume.

pulmonary vascular resistance The impedance to right ventricular blood flow offered by the pulmonary circulation.

pulse demand oxygen delivery system A system that delivers oxygen to the patient only during inspiration (on demand).

Q

quality assurance Any evaluation of services provided and the results achieved as compared with accepted standards.

quality control A planned, systematic approach to designing, measuring, assessing, and improving performance.

quenching A process of removing or reducing an energy source, such as heat or light. Also, stopping or diminishing a chemical or enzymatic reaction.

quick-connect adapter A device that allows rapid connection and disconnection of compressed gas appliances to high-pressure gas delivery systems.

quick-connect outlet See quick-connect adapter.

R

radio frequency interference (RFI) The disruption of the operation of a device due to specific types of radio waves in the vicinity.

rapid eye movement sleep See REM sleep.

rapid shallow breathing (RSB) index A weaning parameter mathematically defined as the spontaneous respiratory rate divided by the spontaneous tidal volume.

rate The frequency of occurrence stated in incidents per unit of time (e.g., 16 per minute).

rate control A device that allows the number of breaths per minute to be selected.

ratio light A visual warning indicating that the I:E ratio is not within predetermined limits.

real gas A gas that does not fit all of the kinetic theories, as compared with an ideal gas.

rebreathing mask A gas-delivery system in which expired gases are oxygen-enriched and inhaled again by the patient. Characterized by a reservoir bag and a series of one-way valves.

reducing valve A mechanism that decreases the delivery pressure of a gas to a lower "working" pressure.

reference electric potential A constant electrical voltage against which electrical flow in a sampling chamber is compared during gas analysis.

reference potentiometer A device that compares a predetermined, preset signal to other signals within an electrical or fluidic system.

reference pressure A preset pressure level to which other pressures are compared within a control system.

reference pressure-support bias pressure A condition in the Bear-3 ventilator in which spring tension in the adjustable pressure-support regulator equals the PEEP pilot pressure plus the pressure-support setting. This increases the machine-side pressure in the regulator, maintaining pressure support.

relative humidity The ratio of actual to potential water vapor in a volume of gas (i.e., how much is present as opposed to how much could be present).

relative refractory period The time period during phase 3 of a ventricular action potential in which a depressed response is possible to a strong stimulus.

REM sleep (Rapid Eye Movement sleep) Sleep periods, lasting from a few minutes to half an hour, during which dreaming occurs. REM sleep periods alternate with non-REM sleep periods.

reservoir bag A pliable container that holds a volume of premixed gas for use in succeeding ventilations or as a back-up.

reservoir system A collection of bags or tubes that form a device to contain a supply of gas or liquid for later use.

residual volume (RV) The volume of gas remaining in the lungs after a complete exhalation.

respiration rate control The mechanism that controls the number of respirations per minute in a ventilator.

respiratory mechanics Measurable values used to evaluate the capacity for spontaneous breathing, which includes parameters such as maximum inspiratory pressure (MIP, also called negative inspiratory force [NIF]), vital capacity (VC), tidal volume (V_T), respiratory rate (f), compliance (C), and airway resistance (Raw).

respiratory system compliance The distensibility of the lungs and chest wall, which is determined by dividing the tidal volume by the pressure. Normal compliance averages 0.1 L/cm H_2O.

rheostat An electronic device that allows for variable control of the amount of electrical current flowing from the device.

rhythmicity See automaticity.

rocker arm assembly The mechanism that determines piston stroke length to control tidal volume in the Bennett M25A and M25B portable ventilators.

rocking bed A device that rocks a patient from 15 to 30 degrees. Rocking moves the abdominal contents, and the resulting diaphragmatic movement assists lung ventilation.

rotary blower A kind of fan or compressor in which a fanlike device spins at high speeds to produce a pressurized gas flow.

rotary compressor See rotary blower.

rotary drive piston A piston that is connected to a wheel-like device, the movement and speed of which governs it. Also called nonlinear drive piston. Compare direct- or linear-drive piston.

rotary vane respirometer A volume recording device that measures the movement of a drum-like cylinder with blade- or wing-shaped extensions (air foils).

S

safety valve A device that protects a patient-breathing system from complete closure, leading to suffocation, by allowing access to air. Also, a device that prevents excessive pressure in a patient-breathing system.
sample chamber In gas analyzers, the reservoir in which the observed gas (that to be analyzed) is held and compared with the reference gas.
Sanz electrode The standard electrode that measures pH. Composed of two half-cells that are connected by a potassium chloride bridge.
Scalars Graphic displays of pressure, volume, and flow over time.
Schmitt trigger An integrated circuit made up of several proportional devices (three proportional amplifiers and two flip-flop valves) connected in a series. Often used in pressure-cycled fluidic ventilators.
secondary equipment Oxygen delivery equipment extending from the wall outlet or reducing valve to the patient apparatus.
Sedimentation The deposition of insoluble materials at the bottom of a liquid or out of suspension in an aerosol.
semipermeable membrane A biologic or synthetic membrane that only permits the passage of certain molecules (e.g., based on size or electrical charge).
sensing port A connection or opening through which gas pressure, flow, or concentrations are sampled or measured.
sensing/servoing Venturi A Venturi device with known pressure gradients, allowing comparisons with unknown pressures.
sensitivity See sensitivity setting.
sensitivity control See sensitivity setting.
sensitivity setting A setting on a ventilator that determines the amount of patient inspiratory effort necessary to start inspiration. Also called trigger sensitivity and sensitivity control.
separation bubble A low-pressure vortex.
sequencing switch Used in the Bird Mark 7A and 8A respirators to regulate flow through control ports. See also ceramic switch.
service verification test (SVT) A test procedure used on the T-Bird ventilator to evaluate unit function.
servo-controlled A closed-loop system in which a microprocessor compares a set parameter with a measured parameter and alerts the operator and/or makes specific changes to the set value based on its findings.
servo-controlled flow valve A servo valve that varies and controls gas flow in response to feedback from a flow transducer.
servo valve A scissor-like device that controls flow through the patient circuit in the Siemens Servo 900 ventilators.
set tidal volume The preset or desired volume of a ventilator, usually calculated based on the patient's physical characteristics.
Sidestream A gas analyzer that extracts a small sample of gas from the main gas flow for analysis. A nebulizer in which the aerosol cloud is formed outside of the main gas flow.
sidestream capnograph See capnograph.
sidestream nebulizer See sidestream.
Siggaard-Anderson nomogram A graph for calculating actual and standard bicarbonate, buffer base, and base excess concentrations.
sigh rate The frequency, in sigh breaths per hour, that will be delivered by a ventilator.
sigh system The portion of a ventilator dedicated to the production and timing of sigh breaths.
silica gel A crystalline chemical compound that is reversibly hydrophilic. It absorbs water and water vapor; a drying agent.
simple humidifier A device that uses unsophisticated methods of adding water vapor to inhaled gases (e.g., bubble or pass-over type of humidifiers).
simple mask A device consisting of a gas supply line and a cone-like appliance that fits over the mouth and nose of the patient.
SIMV See synchronized intermittent mandatory ventilation.
SIMV breaths/min The number of synchronized mandatory respirations delivered per minute.
SIMV cycle time The length of time between mandatory synchronized inspirations.
SIMV system The part of a ventilator mechanism devoted to producing and monitoring SIMV breaths.
SIMV volume ventilator A ventilator that can deliver volume targeted breaths in the SIMV mode.
sine waveform A graphic representation of the relationship between amplitude and time in which amplitude demonstrates repetitive peaks and valleys.
sine-wavelike curve See sine waveform.
single circuit A ventilator whose source gas powers the machine and is also the gas delivered to the patient's airway.
single-circuit ventilator See single circuit.
single-stage reducing valve See single-stage regulator.
single-stage regulator A pressure-reducing system that lowers primary equipment pressure to working pressure (approximately 50 psig) in one step.
sinus arrhythmia Cardiac rhythm characterized by a waxing and waning of the heart rate. The rhythm appears to be related to the breathing cycle with heart rate increasing during inspiration and decreasing during expiration.
sinus bradycardia Cardiac rhythm characterized by the presence of P waves preceding each QRS complex with an effective ventricular rate of less than 60 beats per minute.
sinusoidal Of or pertaining to the shape of a sine wave.
sinus tachycardia Cardiac rhythm characterized by the presence of P waves preceding each QRS complex with an effective ventricular rate greater than 100 beats per minute.
sleep spindles Waveforms with waxing and waning amplitude that occur at a frequency of 9 to 13 cycles per second.
slip/stream nebulizer See sidestream nebulizer.
slope Any inclined line, surface, position; a slant.
sloping To have an upward or downward inclination. To take an oblique direction, incline, or slant. Also see pressure slope and pressure ramp.
slow vital capacity See nonforced vital capacity.
small-volume nebulizer (SVN) A pneumatic aerosol generator. It may be used with a gas-flow circuit used for IPPB therapy or mechanical ventilation, or as a hand-held nebulizer powered by low-flow oxygen or compressed air.
SmartTrigger The name given to the trigger function on the Bear 1000 ventilator in which the ventilator selects the signal that is most sensitive to the patient's effort with the quickest response.
smart window The name given to part of the display screen on the Dräger E-4 ventilator that gives information about ventilating parameters.

sniffer's position Extension of the occiput with flexion of the lower cervical spine; the optimal position to establish and maintain a patent upper airway, as well as for oral intubation. Also called extreme extension.

software The programs, data, routines, etc. for a digital computer. Compare hardware.

solenoid A magnetically operated, electrically powered switching device in which an electrically charged coil moves in a cylinder.

solenoid valve A valve which has its position controlled by a solenoid.

solubility coefficient An expression of the ability of a liquid to hold dissolved solids or gases.

spacer An accessory to enhance aerosol from a metered dose inhaler.

specific gravity The ratio of the weight of one volume of a substance to the weight of the same volume of water. Usually expressed in grams per liter or grams per cubic meter.

sphygmomanometer An instrument for indirect measurements of arterial blood pressure. It consists of an inflatable cuff that fits around the arm, a bulb for controlling air pressure within the cuff, and a mercury or aneroid manometer.

spinning disk A kind of nebulizer in which a volume of water is broken into particles by the action of a rapidly revolving, toothed disk. Also called a centrifugal humidifier.

spirochete Any bacterium of the genus Spirochaeta that is motile and spiral-shaped with flexible filaments. Spirochete organisms include those responsible for leptospirosis, relapsing fever, and syphilis.

spirogram A graphic representation of lung volumes and ventilatory flow rates.

spirometer A device that measures lung volumes and flow rates.

spirometer alarm A low-volume or patient disconnect warning device.

splitter configuration Part of a fluidic element consisting of an intersection point, toward which the main gas flow is directed. The gas flow hits the splitter, causing the gas stream to split and follow two separate pathways.

spontaneous bag A reservoir device that holds gas to be inhaled during patient-initiated, unassisted respirations.

spontaneous breaths Breaths initiated and ended by the patient with no ventilatory support provided. The ventilatory muscles must assume all responsibility for breathing.

spontaneous indicator (demand indicator) A visual or audio signal denoting patient-initiated breathing.

spring and disk release valve A valve that is opened by a pressure greater than that caused by a spring's pressure on a movable, disk-shaped valve cover.

spring disk A spring of a predetermined tension attached to a flat disk. Used to occlude orifices until the spring tension is exceeded by another pressure source.

spring-loaded bellows A power transmission system for a ventilator that uses a spring to apply force and increase the pressure delivered to the patient.

spring-loaded device A device that functions based on its ability to overcome the tension imposed by a spring.

spring-loaded disk PEEP valve A positive end-expiratory pressure valve that allows for pressure relief when the expiratory pressure exceeds the spring disk's spring tension.

spring-loaded resistors A type of threshold resistor that relies on a spring to hold a disc or diaphragm down over the expiratory port of a pressurized circuit.

spring-loaded valve A valve that functions based on its ability to overcome the tension imposed by a spring.

square-wave flow curve A flow-time diagram that takes the form of a box, indicating a constant flow delivered during inspiration.

square waveform A graphic representation of two variables that form a boxlike shape. Also called a constant, or rectangular, waveform.

standard bicarbonate The plasma concentration of HCO_3 in mEq/liter that would exist if the PCO_2 were normal (40 torr).

standard precautions Guidelines recommended by the Centers for Disease Control and Prevention to reduce the risk of transmission of blood borne and other pathogens in hospitals. Standard precautions apply to blood and all body fluids, secretions, and excretions (excluding sweat) regardless of whether they contain blood, nonintact skin, or mucous membranes.

Staphylococcus spp. A genus of nonmotile, spherical Gram-positive bacteria. Some species are normally found on the skin. Certain species cause severe purulent infections or produce an enterotoxin, which may cause nausea, vomiting, and diarrhea. Life-threatening staphylococcal infections may arise in hospitals.

static compliance A lung characteristic associated with the elastic properties of the lungs such that a delivered volume is associated with a specific delivered pressure under conditions of no gas flow. Mathematically expressed as the change in volume divided by the change in pressure.

Stead-Wells spirometer A type of water-sealed device that uses a plastic instead of a metal bell to measure volume changes in the airway opening.

stepper motor A microprocessor-controlled motor with multiple possible positions. Used to open valves or gas flow channels for quick response to microprocessor signals.

sterilization The complete destruction of all microorganisms, usually by heat or chemical means.

Stoke's law The physical law governing the rainout of aerosol particles in the lung through sedimentation.

streptobacilli Chains of bacilli.

Streptococcus spp. A genus of nonmotile, Gram-positive cocci classified by serologic type (Lancefield groups A through T), hemolytic action (alpha, beta, gamma), reaction to bacterial viruses (phage types 1 to 86), and grown on blood agar. The various species occur in pairs, short chains, and chains. Some are facultative aerobes; some are anaerobic. Some species are also hemolytic, but others are nonhemolytic. Many species cause disease in humans.

subambient overpressure pressure-relief valve (SOPR) See subambient pressure-relief valve.

subambient pressure-relief valve In the Bear 5 and Bear 1000 ventilators, a safety bypass system that lets the patient breathe ambient air if ventilator power fails or inspiratory circuit pressure exceeds 120 cm H_2O.

subambient-pressure valve See subambient pressure-relief valve.

subambient relief valve An internal anti-suffocation valve. If the ventilator cannot provide a breath, the patient can inhale, open the valve, and receive room air.

sublimation The direct transition of a substance from solid to the gas or vapor state.

sulfhemoglobin A form of hemoglobin containing an irreversibly bound sulfur molecule that prevents normal oxygen binding.
supercooled liquid An amorphous solid (e.g., margarine).
supply pressure The driving or operating pressure of a gas-powered device.
sustained maximum inspiration (SMI) A therapeutic breathing maneuver in which patients are coached to inspire from the resting expiratory level up to their inspiratory capacity (IC), with an end-inspiratory pause.
synchronized intermittent mandatory ventilation (SIMV) A mode of ventilation in which the patient breathes spontaneously with mandatory breaths periodically imposed after an inspiratory effort.
synchronous period The period during which a mandatory breath may be imposed.
system failure alarm A warning device that signals that the mechanism being monitored has ceased functioning.
Système International (SI) An internationally accepted scientific system of expressing length, mass, and time in base units (IU) of meters, kilograms, and second, replacing the old centimeter-gram-second system (CGS). The SI system includes the ampere, Kelvin, candela, and mole as standard measurements.
systemic vascular resistance The resistance to left ventricular blood flow offered by the systemic circulation.

T

tank ventilator Another name for the iron lung.
Taylor dispersion The enhanced mixing of gases associated with the turbulent flow of high-velocity gases moving through small airways and their bifurcations.
temperature A measure of molecular activity or motion. Also a reference to the reactive hotness or coldness of a material.
temperature correction Attaining body temperature within a normal range.
terminal flow control A control on the Bennett PR-2 that lets the operator provide a minimum flow to compensate for leaks during inspiration.
thermal conductivity The physical ability of a substance to conduct heat. This principle is used in oxygen analyzers and flow sensors.
thermal flowmeter A device that measures gas flow using a temperature-sensitive, temperature-resistive element.
thermodynamics The science of the interconversion of heat and work.
thermometer An instrument for measuring temperature. Usually consists of a sealed glass tube that is marked in degrees of Celsius or Fahrenheit and contains liquid such as mercury or alcohol. The liquid rises or falls as it expands or contracts according to changes in temperature.
theta wave One of the four types of brain waves, characterized by a relatively low frequency of 4 to 7 cycles per second and a low amplitude of 10 mU. Theta waves are the "drowsy waves" that appear in electroencephalograms when the individual is awake but relaxed and sleepy. Compare alpha wave, beta wave, and delta wave.
Thorpe tube See Thorpe-tube flowmeter.
Thorpe-tube flowmeter A type of flowmeter in which the gas stream suspends a steel ball in a tapered tube. As the ball obstructs a greater proportion of the cross-section of the tapered tube, flow is reduced.
Thorpe-tube/reducing-valve regulator A combination of a pressure-reducing valve and a Thorpe-tube type of flowmeter that can regulate both pressure and flow.
three-point calibration Adjusting the electronic output of an instrument to two known standards, as in a two-point calibration, and then adding a third standard intermediate to the other two to ensure linearity of the response. It should be performed every 6 months or whenever an electrode is replaced.
three-way exhalation valve solenoid An electronic device that determines the direction of flow in an expiratory valve.
threshold resistance Usually the amount of pressure needed to overcome resistance to flow.
threshold resistor In positive airway therapy, a device against which a patient exhales. The pressure generated by a threshold resistor can be set to provide specific expiratory pressures independent of flow.
timing flip-flop A fluidic control device that is an on/off switch.
tonicity An expression of the amount of solute in a solution.
total cycle time (TCT) The time required for both inspiration (T_I) and expiration (T_E). Also called total respiratory cycle and ventilatory cycle time.
total lung capacity (TLC) The total amount of gas in the lungs after a maximum inspiration.
total volume output In ventilators, the sum of nebulizer gas volume and ventilatory gas volume.
tracheal button A device used to provide a temporary seal in a tracheostomy; used to keep the stoma patent.
tracheostomy tube An artificial airway surgically inserted into the trachea through the neck.
transcutaneous electrode A monitoring electrode that measures or indicates changes in physiologic conditions across the skin.
transmission-based precautions In hospitals, safeguards designed for patients documented or suspected to be infected with highly transmissible or epidemiologically important pathogens for which additional precautions (beyond standard precautions) are needed to interrupt transmission. There are three types of transmission-based precautions: airborne precautions, droplet precautions, and contact precautions, which may be combined for diseases with multiple transmission routes. Whether these types are used singularly or in combination, they are to be used in addition to standard precautions.
transport ventilator A mechanical ventilator used to provide ventilatory support while moving a patient from one location to another.
trigger The manner in which a ventilator determines when to begin inspiration (e.g., time-triggering or patient-triggering).
trigger sensitivity The amount of patient effort needed to begin inspiratory gas flow from a ventilator. Usually determined by measured pressure or flow changes.
trigger variable That which begins inspiration. A ventilator may be time-, pressure-, flow-, or volume-triggered.
triple-stage reducing valve A pressure-reducing system that reduces pressure from 2200 to 750 psig, then to 50 psig.
turbine An engine or motor driven by the pressure of steam, water, air, etc. against the curved vanes of a wheel or set of wheels fastened to a driving shaft.
two-point calibration Adjusting the electronic output of an instrument to two known standards to ensure quality assurance. Usually performed at least three times daily, usually every 8 hours.

U

ultrasonic nebulizer (USN) A device that uses high-intensity sound waves to break water into very fine particles.
ultrasonic transducer A mechanism that converts electrical energy into sound waves by means of a piezoelectric crystal.
underwater jet humidifier A device that adds water vapor to a carrier gas by injecting a high-velocity gas stream below the surface of a water reservoir, causing a large amount of small bubbles to form and rise to the water surface.
underwater seal resistor A type of threshold resistor in which tubing attached to the expiratory port of a pressurized circuit is submerged beneath a column of water.
universal precautions An approach to infection control designed to prevent transmission of blood-borne diseases, such as human immunodeficiency virus and hepatitis B, in health-care settings. Universal precautions were initially developed in 1987 by the Centers for Disease Control and Prevention in the United States and in 1989 by the Bureau of Communicable Disease Epidemiology in Canada. The guidelines for universal precautions include specific recommendations for use of gloves, masks, and protective eyewear when contact with blood or body secretions containing blood is anticipated.
upper pressure limit The maximum amount of pressure allowed to be delivered by a ventilator. See also maximum pressure limit and pressure limit.
user interface The control panel; where the operator sets the controls. Also called the front panel.
user verification test (UVT) A ventilator test on the T-Bird AVS that allows the operator to review several ventilator functions, such as a lamp test, a filter test, and a leak test.

V

van der Waals forces Physical intermolecular forces that cause molecules to be attracted to each other.
vapor A transition state between a liquid and a gas during which, through application of pressure/temperature changes, the transition may be reversed.
vaporization The process whereby matter in its liquid form is changed into its vapor or gaseous form.
vapor pressure The force exerted by vapors on a gas or a mixture of gases.
variable performance oxygen-delivery system Oxygen therapy equipment that delivers oxygen at a flow that only provides part of the patient's inspired gas needs. Also called a low-flow system.
variable pressure control A closed-loop mode of ventilation available on the Cardiopulmonary Corp.
variable pressure support A closed-loop mode of ventilation available on the Cardiopulmonary Corp. Venturi ventilator that is patient-triggered, pressure-targeted, flow-cycled, and volume-guaranteed.
variable restrictor A device that reduces flow by incorporating an adjustable orifice.
vector An animal carrier, especially an insect, of infectious organisms.
vehicle Any substance, such as food or water, that can be a mode of transmission for infectious agents.
ventilator A mechanical device that moves gases into and out of the lungs.
ventilator circuit The portion of the pneumatic circuit consisting of tubing from a ventilator to a patient. Also called external circuit or patient circuit.
ventilator inoperative alarm See ventilator inoperative system.
ventilator inoperative system A system that warns of the nonfunctional status of a ventilator.
ventilatory cycle time The time it takes from the beginning of one inspiration to the beginning of the next inspiration. Also called the total cycle time and the total respiratory cycle.
ventilatory pattern The rate, volume, flow, and pressure characteristics of breathing over a period.
ventricular asystole The cessation of ventricular contractions.
ventricular diastole The period of the cardiac cycle that encompasses the filling period for cardiac ventricular muscle.
ventricular systole The contraction period for cardiac ventricular muscle.
ventricular tachycardia Cardiac rhythm that is characterized by at least 3 consecutive ventricular complexes with a rate of more than 100 beats/min. It usually originates in a focus distal to the branching part of the bundle of His.
venturi A device that incorporates a jet device to create pressure flow and admixture changes in a gas stream. Also called an air-entrainment device.
Venturi Ventilator that is pressure-targeted, time-cycled, and volume guaranteed.
Venturi gate Part of a mechanism in the Bird Mark series ventilators that balanced spring tension on a valve cover with driving pressure to adjust flow through a Venturi device.
Venturi PEEP valve A Venturi in which the output pressure opposes gas flow through a one-way valve to increase end-expiratory pressure.
vernier A control that can initiate small changes in a system—usually a dial that can be adjusted in small increments.
vibrio A bacterium that is curved and mobile. Cholera and several other epidemic forms of gastroenteritis are caused by members of this genus.
virucide Any agent that destroys or inactivates viruses.
viscosity The thickness of a fluid; its ability to flow.
vital capacity (VC) The total amount of air that can be exhaled after a maximum inspiration. The sum of the inspiratory reserve volume, the tidal volume, and the expiratory reserve volume.
volt (V) The unit of electrical potential. In an electric circuit, a volt is the force required to send 1 ampere of current through 1 ohm of resistance, or the difference in potential between two points on a conductor carrying a charge of 1 ampere when there is a dissipation of 1 watt between them.
voltmeter An instrument, such as a galvanometer, that measures (in volts) the differences in potential between different points of an electric circuit.
volume-assured pressure support (VAPS) A pressure-targeted mode of ventilation that guarantees volume delivery with each breath. It is a servo-control (closed-loop) mode that is similar in function to pressure augmentation.
volume conductor The heart is surrounded by tissues that contain ions that can conduct electrical impulses generated in the heart to the body surface where these electrical signals can be detected by electrodes placed on the skin.
volume control A dial or setting that determines the volume to be delivered by a mechanical ventilator.

volume-controlled inverse ratio ventilation (VCIRV) A volume-targeted, volume- or time-cycled mode of ventilation in which inspiratory time exceeds expiratory time.

volume-displacement device The mechanism by which some ventilators deliver a positive-pressure breath. The device may be a piston, bellow, concertina bag, or similar "bag-in-chamber" mechanism.

volume-displacement incentive spirometer A device that encourages a patient to take slow, deep breaths (as in sighing or yawning) to inspire a preset volume of air. The device measures and visually displays the volume of air that the patient inspires during a sustained maximum inspiration.

volume hold A ventilator control or a maneuver where a volume of gas is held in the patient's lungs for a period of time so static pressure can be read or gas distribution improved.

volume limit A setting that sets the maximum deliverable volume on a ventilator.

volume support A closed-loop mode of ventilation available on the Siemens Servo 300 ventilator that is patient-triggered, pressure-targeted, flow-cycled, and volume guaranteed.

volume targeted ventilation A form of ventilation in which the operator selects a specific volume for delivery of inspiration.

volume ventilation Setting a desired tidal volume in breath delivery. Also called volume-limited ventilation, volume-controlled ventilation, and volume-targeted ventilation.

vortex shedding A characteristic of flow systems in which changes in flows that contact air foils are proportionate to the velocity of the gas, thus allowing for pressure, flow, and volume to be determined.

W

water-weighted diaphragm A PEEP device in which a water column placed in contact with the diaphragm of an expiration valve creates a PEEP pressure equal to the height of the water column.

watt A unit of power, equivalent to work done at the rate of 1 joule per second.

weighted ball resistors A type of resistor in which a steel ball is placed over a calibrated orifice that is attached directly above the expiratory port of a pressurized circuit.

Wheatstone bridge A particular arrangement of multiple resistors in an electrical circuit.

wick humidifier A type of humidification system in which the flow is exposed to a water-saturated cloth, paper, or polyethylene membrane.

Wolff-Parkinson-White syndrome Cardiac rhythm that is characterized as a pre-excitation syndrome. In this arrhythmia, ventricular depolarizations are initiated when impulses initiated in the atria bypass the AV node and traveling through an ancillary bundle of Kent resulting in the presence of characteristic delta waves.

Wood's metal A metal alloy commonly used in fusible plugs.

work of breathing The amount of force needed to move a given volume into the lung with a relaxed chest wall. It can be reduced when applied properly with mechanical ventilation.

Y

Y connector An adapter shaped like the letter Y that connects the endotracheal tube adapter to the main inspiratory and expiratory lines of a patient circuit used for mechanical ventilation.

Z

zone valve A valve that controls gas flow to specific areas served by a bulk gas system.

Index

A

D

I

J

K

L

M

N

O

P

Q

R

S

U

V

W

X

Y

Z

Frequently Used Formulae and Values

Gas Laws

Definitions of Standard Conditions

Temperature (°C)	Pressure (mm Hg)	Water Vapor
STPD	760	Zero
ATPD	Atmospheric	Zero
ATPS	Atmospheric	Saturated
BTPS	Atmospheric	47 mm Hg

Gas Cylinders

Oxygen cylinder factors for common cylinder sizes

D Cylinder	0.16
E Cylinder	0.28
G Cylinder	2.41
H Cylinder	3.14
K Cylinder	3.14

Flow Rates, and Mixing Air and Oxygen

Air to Oxygen Ratios and Total Flows of Several Common Venturi Devices*

%	Oxygen Flow Rate (L/min)	Air/Oxygen Ratio	Total Flow (L/min)
24%	4	25.3:1	105
28%	4	10.3:1	45
31%	6	6.9:1	47
35%	8	4.3:1	42
40%	8	3:1	32
50%	12	1.7:1	32
60%	24	1:1	48
70%	24	0.6:1	38

Formulas Used with Gas Laws

Boyle's law (solving for pressure): $P_2 = \frac{P_1 \times V_1}{V_2}$

Boyle's law (solving for volume): $V_2 = \frac{P_1 \times V_1}{P_2}$

Charles's law (solving for volume): $V_2 = \frac{V_1 \times T_2}{T_1}$

Gay-Lussac's law (solving for pressure): $P_2 = \frac{P_1 \times T_2}{T_1}$

Combined gas law:

$$V_2 = \frac{V_1 \times P_1 \times T_2}{P_2 \times T_1} \text{ (solving for volume)}$$

Combined gas law:

$$P_2 = \frac{V_1 \times P_1 \times T_1}{V_2 \times T_1} \text{ (solving for pressure)}$$

Combined gas law:

$$T_2 = \frac{P_2 \times V_2 \times T_1}{P_1 \times V_1} \text{ (solving for temperature)}$$

Combined gas law:

$$V_2 = \frac{V_1 \times [P_1 - (PH_2O \text{ @ } T_1)] \times T_2}{[P_2 - PH_2O \text{ @ } T_2] \times T_1}$$

$$\text{Density} = \frac{\text{GMW}}{22.4 \text{ L}}$$

$$\text{Density} = \frac{[(\text{GMW of gas \#1} \times \%) + (\text{GMW of gas \#2} \times \%)}{22.4 \text{ L}}$$

Formulas Used with Cylinders and Liquid Oxygen

$$\text{Cylinder factor} = \frac{\text{cubic feet in full cylinder} \times 28.3}{\text{pressure of full cylinder}}$$

$$\text{Duration (minutes)} = \frac{\text{gauge pressure (psig)} \times \text{cylinder factor}}{\text{oxygen flow rate (liters/minute)}}$$

Duration of liquid oxygen cylinder (min)

$$= \frac{\text{liquid } O_2 \text{ capacity (L)} \times 860 \times \text{gauge reading (\%)}}{\text{oxygen flow rate (L/min)}}$$

$$\text{Duration (min)} = \frac{\text{weight of liquid } O_2 \text{ remaining (pounds)} \times 344}{\text{oxygen flow rate (L/min)}}$$

Formula Used When Mixing Air and Oxygen

$$O_2\ (\%) = \frac{(\text{air flow} \times 21\%) + (O_2 \text{ flow} \times 100\%)}{\text{total gas flow}} \times 100$$

Formulas Used When Calculating Humidity

$$\text{RH (\%)} = \frac{\text{content}}{\text{capacity}} \times 100$$

$$\text{BH (\%)} = \frac{\text{content}}{\text{capacity @ } 37^{\circ}\text{ C}}$$